LONGMAN DICTIONARY

OF

PSYCHOLOGY AND PSYCHIATRY

LONGMAN DICTIONARY

OF

PSYCHOLOGY AND PSYCHIATRY

ROBERT M. GOLDENSON, Ph.D.

Editor in Chief

A WALTER D. GLANZE BOOK

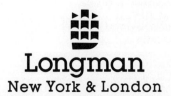

Longman
New York & London

Longman Dictionary of Psychology and Psychiatry

Longman Inc., 1560 Broadway, New York, N.Y. 10036
Associated companies, branches, and representatives
throughout the world.

Developmental Editor: Gordon T. R. Anderson
Production Supervisor: Ferne Y. Kawahara
Manufacturing Supervisor: Marion Hess

Library of Congress Cataloging in Publication Data
Main entry under title:
Longman dictionary of psychology and psychiatry.
    "A Walter D. Glanze book."
    1. Psychology—Dictionaries.   2. Psychiatry—
Dictionaries.   3. Psychology, Pathological—Dictionaries.
4. Psychology, Physiological—Dictionaries. I. Glanze,
Walter D. II. Goldenson, Robert M. [DNLM: 1. Psychology—
Dictionaries.   2. Psychiatry—Dictionaries. WM 13 L856]
BF31.L66 1983   150'.3'21   83-13591
ISBN 0-582-28257-8

Manufactured in the United States of America
Printing: 9 8 7 6 5 4 3 2 1   Year: 91 90 89 88 87 86 85 84 83

CONTENTS

PREFACE

"Nothing that is human is alien to me." This statement might well be the motto of the two great disciplines from which the contents of this work have been drawn: psychology and psychiatry. It means that these two fields, even their technical aspects, touch every phase of our lives—our feelings and emotions, our mentality, our development from womb to tomb, and our relationships to other human beings, individually and collectively. But it also means that a dictionary encompassing both these fields must be broad in scope, and must overflow traditional boundaries to include theories, concepts, and terms from other fields with which they interface.

In conceiving the *Longman Dictionary of Psychology and Psychiatry*, the editors had three objectives in mind. First, to present a comprehensive lexicon on all phases of these two vast areas. Second, to place heavy emphasis on current terms the reader is likely to encounter in the professional literature and professional practice of today, without overlooking older terms that have special historical value. Third, to avoid the limitations of a one-dimensional glossary by giving a maximum amount of information in a minimum number of words, and by including thousands of examples, elaborations, and important details that make the definitions more meaningful and useful to the reader—giving the volume an encyclopedic flavor by adhering to Robert Browning's celebrated lines, "Oh, the little more, and how much it is! And the little less, and what worlds away!"

The rationale for compiling and writing this Dictionary, and its unusual editorial features, are explained in the METHODOLOGICAL NOTES.

Every effort has been made to consult the most authoritative sources and to do full justice to every facet of these fluid, expanding fields. Even a casual glance at the entries will reveal term after term not only from the core of the two basic areas, but from their ramifications and from the interdisciplinary borderland where they interact with other important fields. Among the core areas are psychoanalytic theory and practice, physiological psychology, neuropsychology, psychopharmacology, cognitive psychology, psychotherapy, the categories of mental disorder (DSM-III), genetics, the etiology of mental retardation, psychological statistics, personality theories, psychometrics, cross-cultural psychiatry, hypnosis, educational psychology, and rehabilitation psychology. Among the interface areas are neurology, biofeedback, anthropology, sociology, market research, environmental psychology, treatment and service facilities, evaluation research, semantics, and sexology. In all, there are hundreds of interfacing areas, which in itself indicates the richness of the broad field covered by this Dictionary.

Though numbers might appear cold in the context of a very human book, a few "vital statistics" may be in order: This Dictionary has 21,164 entries, or headwords—twice to five times the number of other dictionaries in these fields. Included are, e.g., entries for 488 kinds of tests; over 300 entries for therapies; 70 entries treating Piaget's work and ideas, 100 treating Jung's; entries for 93 kinds of manias, 61 kinds of neuroses, 72 kinds of psychoses, 36 kinds of complexes; about 500 entries for phobias; 550 entries denoting syndromes and diseases; thousands of entries for individual symptoms and signs; about 300 entries on drugs, with formulae; 150 biographies of historical figures from Aristotle to the present day, plus about 900 brief biographical entries on other investigators, especially those who have lent their names to theories and disorders. In keeping with current tendencies, this Dictionary contains far more neurological, physiological, and medical terms than any comparable work. Also see the INVENTORY OF ARTICLE ENTRIES (page xvi).

The principal contributors are Dr. Robert M. Goldenson (editor in chief) and Kenneth N. Anderson; together with Nancy H. Cohen, they wrote the bulk of the entries (Kenneth N. Anderson's main contribution consisting in entries of a physiological, medical, and pharmacological nature). Walter D. Glanze, who conceived of, produced, and edited this Dictionary, also wrote a large number of entries (including 120 entries in linguistics) and provided the etymologies, pronunciation, combining forms, and most of the 10,750 cross references—the latter providing an encyclopedic context and adding immeasurably to the usefulness of this Dictionary.

The language of the definitions is kept as simple and concrete as an often highly complex and abstract subject permits, and the entry headwords are given in their natural, noninverted word order—as an invitation not only to consult but also to browse in this Dictionary.

ROBERT M. GOLDENSON, Ph.D.

STAFF AND CONSULTANTS

EDITOR IN CHIEF:
Robert M. Goldenson, Ph.D.—see below

THE PRINCIPAL WRITERS:
Robert M. Goldenson, Ph.D.; Adjunct Professor, School of Psychology, Florida
   Institute of Technology; on the faculty of New York Medical College; author of
   many books in the psychosciences, including *The Encyclopedia of Human Behavior*
   (2 volumes, 1970), *All About the Human Mind* (1963), *Mysteries of the Mind*
   (1973); editor in chief of the *Disability and Rehabilitation Handbook* (1978)
Kenneth N. Anderson, B.S.; author and coauthor of over 20 medical books,
   including the *Newsweek Encyclopedia of Family Health and Fitness* (1980); former
   editor of *Today's Health* (American Medical Association)
Nancy H. Cohen, writer and researcher, New York and Boston

PRODUCER AND MANAGING EDITOR:
Walter D. Glanze, of Walter Glanze Word Books Associates; lexicographer;
   author and editor of language and subject dictionaries (managing editor of *The
   Scribner-Bantam English Dictionary*, 1977)

CONTRIBUTORS AND REVIEWERS:
See the METHODOLOGICAL NOTES, paragraph 1.4, for the role of staff writers in
relation to consultants in many fields—too numerous to list. The editors are grateful
to all, but are particularly indebted to the following specialists, who, by writing or
reviewing entries, have contributed greatly to the completeness and authority of this
Dictionary.

Timothy C. Brock, Ph.D.; Professor of Psychology; in collaboration with **Mary Ann
   Brickner**, Ph.D., and **Vernon Padgett**, Ph.D.; all of Ohio State University
   (*evaluation research*)
Peter B. Field, Ph.D.; Adjunct Professor, School of Psychology, Florida Institute of
   Technology; Veterans Administration Medical Center, Baltimore, MD (*statistics,
   experimental psychology*)
Steven Kanor, Ph.D.; Medical Engineer; Consultant, United Cerebral Palsy
   Association of Westchester County, NY (*behavioral engineering*)
Tamara Nieburgs, M.S., CCC-SP; Adjunct Professor, School of Psychology, Florida
   Institute of Technology; Consultant, Institute of Child Development, Hackensack
   Hospital, Hackensack, NJ (*speech and language pathology, audiology, learning
   disabilities*)
Humphry Osmond, M.D., Fellow of the Royal College of Physicians;
   Founder-Member of the Royal College of Psychiatrists; Professor of Clinical
   Psychiatry, University of Alabama—see the entry OSMOND, HUMPHRY
   (*schizophrenia, psychoactive drugs*)
Michael Weintraub, M.D.; Diplomate in Neurology, Phelps Memorial Hospital,
   Tarrytown, NY (*neurology, neurological disorders*)

The editors also are grateful to the American Psychiatric Association for permission
to include the terms and the Classification of the *DSM-III* (see APPENDIX A and the
METHODOLOGICAL NOTES, paragraph 7.1), and to **Barbara Whitney**, M.A., Executive
Director of SIECUS (Sex Information and Education Council of the United States)

ILLUSTRATIONS:
Trudy Oppenheimer, Amherst, MA

RESEARCH AND CLERICAL STAFF:
Lois Anderson, Agnes Glanze, Irene Goldenson, Donna Williams

DEVELOPMENTAL EDITOR:
Gordon T. R. Anderson, Longman Inc.

METHODOLOGICAL NOTES

Walter D. Glanze

1. GENERAL

1.1. The *Longman Dictionary of Psychology and Psychiatry* was created from primary sources of the past two decades to reflect the living vocabulary of the behavioral and cognitive sciences. These primary sources include research papers, journal articles, treatises, and the major textbooks in psychology- and psychiatry-related fields. Only after a headword list from the primary sources was prepared and the bulk of the definitions was written, were terms of historical interest added and were dictionaries and other reference works scanned for additional headwords; such reference sources include, e.g., data bases like the *Thesaurus of Psychological Index Terms*. The American Psychiatric Association gave the editors permission to list in this Dictionary all official terms of the *Diagnostic and Statistical Manual of Mental Disorders* (DSM-III) and to condense the descriptions for this purpose (see 7.1 below), as well as to include the DSM-III Classification (see APPENDIX A).

1.2. The result is the first dictionary of its kind, both in size (over 21,000 entries, over three-quarter million words) and in scope—encompassing the vocabulary of all the psychosciences as well as terms from hundreds of fields with which the psychosciences interact. (See INVENTORY OF ARTICLE ENTRIES, and APPENDIX D.) Moreover, "in keeping with current tendencies, this Dictionary contains far more neurological, physiological, and medical terms than any comparable work," as stated in the PREFACE.

1.3. This Dictionary is also unprecedented in such features as

- considerations of (a) the accessibility of compound entry headwords, together with (b) the consultation value in including or not including a reference entry—which also made it possible to give compound headwords in noninverted, natural word order for greater ease not only in consulting but also in browsing in this Dictionary (see 3.2, 3.3, 2.4);

- the extent of cross-referencing between defined entries (about 10,750 cross references), to provide encyclopedic context, as well as

- the index function of many of the long sequences of cross references (e.g., 93 references to other manias from the entry **mania**, or 39 references to other epilepsy entries from the entry **epilepsy**—see 6.5.1, 3.3);

- the large number of biographical entries (over 1,000), which may be (a) primarily narrative, (b) primarily explaining the origin of the many eponymic terms, or (c) primarily of index nature (the entry **Jung, Carl Gustav**, e.g., providing reference to 99 entries that mention Jung, or the entry **Parkinson, James**, providing reference to 47 parkinsonism-related entries—see 7.2.1);

- a three-level relationship among hundreds of entries on drugs, with formulae (see 7.3);

- choice and styling of hundreds of combining forms for additional access to the meaning and origin of (a) entry headwords, (b) terms used in the definitions, and (c) many terms occurring in other literature (see 7.4);

- editorial consistency (of which the main principles are explained in these Methodological Notes).

1.4. For maximum coherence and readability, about 97 percent of all entries were written by a staff of three principal writers (see STAFF AND CONSULTANTS). All work was done in close consultation with specialists in many fields, who also reviewed the entries before final staff editing.

1.5. One of the marks of a good dictionary is that it is easy to use. We should not be expected to study the editorial rules that underlie the overall structure of a dictionary or the elements of an entry. These Methodological Notes, therefore, are addressed to the reader who loves reference works, and wants to use them to the greatest effectiveness. And while the main purpose of these Notes is to render account of the editors' methods, they may contribute to throwing light on the richness of the subject.

2. ALPHABETICAL ORDER

2.1. Letter by Letter. All entries are in strict alphabetical order. The order is letter by letter, that is, dictionary style (not word by word, which is telephone-book style, though still found in some dictionaries). Example: **Rh factor / -rhin- / Rhine / rhinencephalon /** (then nine more "rh-" entries; only then:) **Rh reaction.** (Note: **MacKenzie** follows **Mach scale; McArdle** follows **MBO**.)

2.2. Alphanumeric. The alphabetization is alphanumeric, that is, words and numbers form a single sequence, numbers being positioned as though they were spelled-out numerals. Example: **chromosome 5 .../ chromosome 4 .../ chromosome number / chromosome 13 ...**

2.3. Subscripts and Superscripts. Small lowered or raised numbers or letters are disregarded. E.g., G_{M1} **gangliosidosis** is positioned as though it were GGANGL ...

2.4. Inversion Comma. Text that follows an inversion comma is disregarded for the purpose of primary alphabetization. Example: **Devic, M. Eugène / device for automated desensitization / Devic's disease**

As the headwords of this Dictionary are given in natural word order (see 3.2), inversions occur only in biographical entries (example: **Devic, M. Eugène**) and in some of the DSM-III terms (example: **conduct disorder, undersocialized, nonaggressive**), as well as in a small number of other headwords with fixed styling, such as certain terms in genetics (example: **chromosome 13, deletion of long arm**).

2.4.1 Secondary Alphabetization. When secondary alphabetization after an inversion comma is needed, the same rules apply. Example: **schizophrenia / schizophrenic disorder, catatonic type / ... / schizophrenic disorder, undifferentiated type /** (only then:) **schizophrenic disorders**

2.4.2. Enumeration Comma. Alphabetization disregards commas that occur in enumerations, and that do not indicate inversions. Example: **existence needs/ Existence, Relatedness, and Growth theory / existential analysis**

2.5. Near-Homographs. In near-homographs, lower-case letters precede capital letters. Examples: **being cognition / Being cognition; Cs / CS**. However, combining forms follow the other headword. Examples: **SCAT / -scat-; sem. / -sem-**

2.6. Homographs. In this Dictionary, **homographs** (see that entry) are not differentiated (as, e.g., through superscript numbers) because they occur rarely, and when they do occur, it is nearly always in the juxtaposition of abbreviations. These abbreviations are two reference entries or a reference entry and a brief article entry. Examples: "**BB** = BLUE BLOATER" and "**BB**: See CREATINE PHOSPHOKINASE"; "**BAL** an abbreviation of *blood-alcohol level*" and "**BAL** = BRITISH ANTI-LEWISITE."

2.6.1. Identical terms that have totally different meanings and are defined, are not listed as separate entries, as homographs, but are given in separate paragraphs of an entry. For examples, see 4.5.5 (a) and (e).

2.7. For combined headwords of adjacent reference entries, see 5.5. (For headword variants of combining-form entries, see 7.4.1.)

2.8. For terms that are not listed with separate headwords as reference entries because they are immediately adjacent to their respective article entry, see 5.6.

2.9. If an entry term is not exactly what the reader may have had in mind, common-sense variations will in many cases lead to the right entry, including (a) singular for plural, and vice versa, e.g., **hallucinogens**, removed by six entries from where "hallucinogen" would appear; (b) spelling variants, e.g., "aetiology" versus **etiology** (and *c* versus *k* in many words of Greek origin); (c) suffixes, e.g., in "alcohol ..." versus "alcoholic ..."; (d) variations such as "color ..." and "chrom- ...," or "social ..." and "socio- ..."

3. THE ENTRY HEADWORD

3.1. Each entry begins with a headword in boldface type. The styling of the headword is the same for article entries (see section 4) and reference entries (see section 5).

(For the sake of simplicity, the term headword applies to any alphabetical definiendum—or dictionary item consulted—be it a single-word or a compound term.)

3.2. Headword Style. Compound headwords are seen as one concept and are therefore given in natural word order. Examples: (a) **delusional mania**, not "mania, delusional"; (b) **genetic map**, not "map, genetic"; (c) **sensory deprivation**, not "deprivation, sensory"; (d) **Klinefelter's syndrome**, not "syndrome, Klinefelter's." (See 3.3.)

3.2.1. For necessary exceptions to this rule, see 2.4.

3.3. Access to Compound Headwords. Many of the last elements of compound headwords of article entries are listed as headwords with their own definition, with a cross reference to the compound headword, and many of the last elements are listed as (or indicated in) a reference entry—depending on the need for additional access to the article headword. E.g., the four entries mentioned in 3.2. represent four different situations:

(a) The entry **mania**, after the general definition of mania, gives cross references to 93 specific manias, including **delusional mania** (See 6.5.1).

(b) A reference entry, "**mapping of genes:** See GENETIC MAP," provides additional access to the article entry **genetic map**.

(c) There is no reference entry referring to **sensory deprivation** because the consultation value of such an entry (perhaps, "deprivation, see sensory deprivation") would be negligible. (And this Dictionary does not include an article entry for "deprivation" alone.) But note that **sensory deprivation** is referred to from other article entries, including **stimulus hunger**.

(d) The article entry **syndrome** does not give cross references to the compound headwords ending in "syndrome." There are various reasons for not doing so: (i) The first element of the compound term is already known when a syndrome is being looked up in the Dictionary, so that there is no need to start at the entry **syndrome**. (ii) "Syndrome" and "disease" are often used interchangeably, so that a listing of syndromes would be meaningful only if all compound headwords ending in "disease" would be included (or if all "syndrome" entries along with "disease" entries would be listed after the entry **disease**.) (iii) The number of "syndrome" entries in this Dictionary is very large—about 385 (to which should be added the approximately 165 "disease" entries of this Dictionary). Also (iv), adding to the arbitrariness of such a listing: many "syndromes" or "diseases" are called neither one nor the other, e.g., **trichorrhexis nodosa with mental retardation**.

3.3.1. Variants of 3.3 (b) are certain reference entries with multiple references such as **family**, which refers to seven compounds ending in "family"; **marriage**, with ten references; **nurse**, with seven; or **leader**, with nine. (A different type of reference entry is, e.g., **Native Americans**, which refers, not to compounds formed with this headword, but to 16 entries dealing with Native Americans, from **berdache** to **yopo**.)

3.4. Headword Abbreviation. The headword is abbreviated—by its first letter, or the first letters of its compound elements—when it recurs in the same entry, provided (a) it shows no inflectional change (**instinct**—instincts, **instincts**

—instinct); (b) it does not assume a possessive form (**Freud** —Freud's, **Weiss**—Weiss') (but see 3.4.1); (c) it is not an element of a solid compound (**cathexis**—countercathexis) (but it may be an element of a hyphenated compound—see 3.4.2.); (d) it consists of more than three letters (but see 3.4.3.); (e) it is not part of a quotation or title of a work (e.g., in the entry **suicide**).

The headword abbreviation occurs by itself in the definition, or as part of a spaced or hyphenated compound term in the definition or in any other element of an article entry. In reference entries in the headwords referred to, as part of a compound term. Examples: "**absolute threshold** ... the a.t. is relative ..."; "**anthropology** ... **cultural a.; social a.**) ..."; "**adaptation syndrome** = GENERAL A.S."

3.4.1. The possessive form of a headword is abbreviated as though it were the basic word. Example: **Heschl's gyrus** —H.g. But see 3.4 (b).

3.4.2. The headword is abbreviated when it is an element of a hyphenated compound (or when it has a modifier). But see 3.4 (c).

3.4.3. According to 3.4 (d), a headword of two or three letters is not abbreviated. However, a two- or three-letter word is abbreviated if it is an element of a spaced or hyphenated compound. Examples: **at risk**—a.r.; **good-me** —g.-m.; **bowing of bones**—b.o.b.

Exceptions to this rule are "No." and "Rh": **Red Dye No. 3**—R.D. No. 3; **Rh factor**—Rh f.

3.4.4. Abbreviations in capital letters that are part of a headword are not further abbreviated. Examples: **GABA** —GABA; **transfer RNA**—t. RNA

3.4.5. When a nonhyphenated compound headword recurs as modifier of another term, no hyphen is inserted in the abbreviation (that is, the rules for hyphenation of compounds—see 9.1—are suspended for the abbreviated headword). Examples: "**leaderless group** ... The l.g. technique may be used ..." instead of "The l.-g. technique ..."

3.4.6. The abbreviation of the headword is understood to represent the headword phonetically, especially when preceded by an indefinite article; the letters do not have their own pronunciation. Example: "**local sign** ... A l.s. helps ..." rather than "An l.s. ..." /an′el′es′/.

3.4.7. In biographical entries the last name is abbreviated in the definition if the rules of 3.4 are satisfied (7.2.2). The name is not abbreviated when it recurs among the cross references.

3.5. For the rules for alphabetical order, see section 2.

3.6. For alphabetically adjacent reference headwords that are combined into one reference entry (and separated by semicolons), see 5.5.

3.7. For the separation of variants of combining forms (and use of semicolons) in combining-form entries, see 7.4.1.

3.8. For reference terms that are not entered as separate headwords because they are alphabetically adjacent to their article entries, see 5.6.

3.9. For the selection of headwords for this Dictionary, see 1.1. Also see 4.5.4.

3.10. For count and classification of entries, see section 10, and INVENTORY OF ARTICLE ENTRIES.

4. ARTICLE ENTRIES

4.1. An article entry defines its headword (and often contains additional information).

4.2. Entry Elements. The principal elements of an entry (in their usual order) are
the headword—see section 3;
pronunciation—see section 8, and PRONUNCIATION KEY;
the main definition—see 4.5.1, 4.5;
a definition expansion—see 4.5.2., 4.5.;
etymology—see 4.6.;
subentries in boldface or lightface type—see 5.2.2 (a), 5.2.2 (b);
abbreviations of the headword as alternative terms—see 4.8., 5.2.2 (a);
alternative terms (including trademarks)—see 4.9, 5.2.1;
inflected forms and parts of speech—see 4.10, 5.2.2 (a);
cross references—see section 6;
identification of DSM-III entries—see 7.1.

4.3. Headword. See section 3.

4.4. Pronunciation. See section 8, and PRONUNCIATION KEY.

4.5. Definition. All entries have a main definition (4.5.1), and most entries have a definition expansion (4.5.2). Different meanings of a headword may be discriminated in the main definition as well as in the definition expansion (4.5.3). With few exceptions (4.5.5), entries consist of one paragraph.

4.5.1. The main definition is written in dictionary style, that is, the definition is always in the same part of speech as the headword; thus it is never a sentence. (Most noun definitions begin with the definite or the indefinite article; many adjective definitions begin with expressions such as "denoting," "consisting of," "suitable for," or "situated . . ."; all verb definitions begin with the particle "to.")

4.5.2. The definition expansion consists of one or several complete sentences.

4.5.3. Meaning Discrimination. Multiple meanings are not numbered. In the main definition they are separated by semicolons. Field labels are added where needed. Examples: "**behavioral variability** the diversity of behavior; the fact that . . . ; also, the fact that . . ."; "**parameter** in psychoanalysis, a technique that . . . ; in statistics, a value of . . . ; in mathematics, a quantity that . . . ; in general, a standard or determining factor; in colloquial usage, a limit."

(Also single-meaning definitions make frequent use of field labels. Example: "**sport** in genetics, an organism that has undergone mutation and . . .")

In the definition expansion, meanings are separated narratively, often with field labels. Example: "**orientation** . . . In industrial psychology, o. is the process of . . . In environmental psychology, the term refers to . . . Other meanings include . . ."

4.5.4. Words Used in Definitions. Words occurring in definitions include (a) as many plain English words as the nature of the entry permits; (b) terms that are, in turn, headwords of article or reference entries; (c) many technical terms that are defined where they are used (10.1.2); (d) technical terms whose meaning may be understood through the combining-form entries (7.4); (e) relatively few technical (mainly medical and chemical) terms that are not directly explained in this Dictionary—occurring primarily in entries that are likely to be consulted by the reader to whom they are not unfamiliar.

4.5.4.1. Because of the wide coverage of this Dictionary, almost all terms germane to its subjects are of the foregoing types (b), (c), and (d), but mainly of type (b). Therefore, if a technical term is not defined at the point of use, the reader may assume, generally, that it is entered as a headword. And there was, thus, no need to impair the readability of a definition by burdening the syntax with references to other entries, through a change of typeface, "q.v.," or other distracting devices—notwithstanding the abundance of cross references (10,750) that follow the entries.

4.5.4.2. Access Entries. This Dictionary includes brief article entries that might not be expected to be found in a work of this nature, but which were added to give *access* to the meaning of certain terms used in the definitions though not explained there because of their repeated occurrence. Examples are **acrosome, cation**, and **macrophage**.

4.5.5. Paragraphs. A small number of entries have more than one paragraph. These exceptions are made
(a) to separate totally dissimilar meanings of the headword—of the same or different origin (examples: the entries **humor**, as fluid and as a state of mind, and **soma**, the body and an alternative term for "fly agaric") (also see 2.6.1);
(b) to set off an afterthought to the definition (examples: the entries **IQ, origin-of-language theories, suicide**, and **trademark**);
(c) to continue the definition after a sequence of cross references (example: the entry **disfigurement**);
(d) to set off long sequences of cross references, as a concession to the eye (examples: the entries **neurosis** and **Jung**);
(e) to add a cross reference that is unrelated to the meaning of the headword—a cross reference actually standing for a reference entry whose headword coincides here with the headword of an article entry (thus, a reference entry that appears in the guise of a cross reference); example:

> **possession** in the two-word stage of language development, an expression of ownership, as in "Mommy dress."
> Also see DEMONIC P.

4.6. Etymology. Etymological information is given when the editors thought it contributes to the understanding of a term or is intriguing for other reasons.

4.6.1. Etymology may be indicated
(a) in parentheses, usually in or at the end of the main definition (with the etymon set in italics); examples: "**epistemic** . . . (from Greek *episteme*, "knowledge")"; "**foreunpleasure** a term employed by Anna Freud (from German *Vor-Unlust*) to denote . . ."; "**locus** the place or position (Latin, "place") of an . . ."
(b) as an integral part of the wording of the main definition or the definition expansion; for examples, see the last paragraph of 4.6.2.

4.6.1.1. Etymologies may include inflected forms of the etymon (example: the entry **Gestalt**) or pronunciation of the etymon (for an example, see 8.3).

4.6.2. An example of entries in which etymology is essential is **phonomania**, which is derived from Greek *phonos*, "murder," yet appears in a long sequence of entries that all begin with "phono-," derived from Greek *phone*, meaning "sound" or "voice."

An example of entries in which the etymology may simply add to the understanding of the headword is **sex**—derived from Latin *sexus*, with the original meaning of "division, *section*," and related to *secare*, "to cut."

For examples in which an explanation of the headword's origin is not really needed but is of historical interest, see the entries **psychedelics, syphilis, peeping Tom, Tadoma**, and **storm-and-stress period**.

4.6.3. In addition to etymology provided within entries, there are two kinds of entries that serve etymological purposes: (a) the combining forms (see 7.4); (b) all biographical entries that are eponymous, that is, that have cross references to headwords that are derived from the respective name (see 7.2). Example: **Gilles de la Tourette**, for whom **Tourette's disorder** was named.

4.7. Subentries. Many definitions include terms that are not defined in separate article entries but are explained here directly or implicitly, and which are listed as reference entries in their alphabetical place.

4.7.1. Most of these subentries are set in boldface, others in lightface type (the choice depending not only on their importance but on juxtaposition with other terms occurring in the definition). For examples, see 5.2.2 (a), 5.2.2 (b). Also see 4.5.4.

Also see 5.6, for boldface terms that would immediately precede or follow the article headword in alphabetical order.

4.7.1.1. Note that a boldface subentry indicates that this term need not be looked up under that headword; it is not defined there.

4.7.2. Nearly all special terms employed in a definition are explained within that definition or are defined in another article entry. See 4.5.4.

4.8. Abbreviations. Abbreviations that may be used as alternative terms for the headword are preceded by "Abbrev.:" They are set in boldface and listed as reference entries in their alphabetical places. For an example, see 5.2.1.

4.8.1. If the abbreviation rather than the full term is the generally used version, the abbreviation is the headword. An example is the article entry **IQ**, to which **intelligence quotient** refers as a reference entry.

4.9. Alternative Terms. Alternative terms for the headword are preceded by "Also called" or, if pronounced alike, "Also spelled." They are set in boldface type here and listed as reference entries in their alphabetical places. For examples, see 5.2.1.

4.9.1. If the alternative expression is a proprietary term,

it is preceded by "Trademark:" See 7.3.1. (But there are entries in which the trademark itself is the headword.)

4.10. Inflected Forms and Parts of Speech. Inflected forms of the headword and headword-derived parts of speech are set in boldface type here and listed as reference entries in their alphabetical places; see 5.2.2 (a). Such forms are preceded by the respective designation and a colon. Examples: "**locus** ... Plural: **loci**"; "**taxes** ... Singular: **taxis**. Adjectives: **tactic; taxic**."

4.11. Cross References. See section 6. Cross references are the last element of an entry with the exceptions mentioned in 4.5.5 (c) and with the exception of 4.12.

4.12. DSM-III. The entries corresponding to the 238 terms that are listed in the DSM-III Classification (Appendix A) and an additional 22 entries are identified at the end of each such entry by the designation "(DSM-III)." See 7.1.2.

5. REFERENCE ENTRIES

5.1. While an article entry defines its headword, a reference entry refers to a definition in one or more article entries. The entries referred to are set in small capital letters. (For headword style, see section 3.)

5.2. Reference entries are of two types—synonymous references (5.2.1) and nonsynonymous references (5.2.2).

5.2.1. Synonymous References. If the headword is followed by an equal sign, this headword is an alternative term for the headword referred to. It is given there in boldface type and preceded by "Also called," "Also spelled," or "Abbrev.:" (and, occasionally, by designations such as "Trademark:"). (See 4.9, 4.8.) Examples: "**myotonic pupillary reaction** = ADIE'S SYNDROME"; "**aboulia** = ABULIA"; "**AChE** = ACETYLCHOLINESTERASE."

5.2.1.1. In many instances the reader will be satisfied with this information and may choose not to consult the definition. However, pronunciation, etymology, or inflected forms of the alternative term—whenever they are provided—would be found in the article entry only.

5.2.2. Nonsynonymous References. If the headword is followed by a colon plus "See," a direct or indirect explanation of that term is included under the headword or headwords referred to:

(a) The term may appear in the article entry in boldface type, either as a subentry in the definition (4.7.1) or added to the definition (4.10). Examples: "**viscerotonic temperament**: See ENDOMORPH" and "**endomorph** ... with a **viscerotonic temperament** (tendency toward love of ...) ..."; "**run amok**: See AMOK" and "**amok** ... a culture-specific syndrome ... Verb: **to run a.**"

(b) The term may appear in the definition of the article entry, set as a subentry in lightface type (4.7.1). Example: "**feeling-talk**: See CONDITIONED-REFLEX THERAPY" and "**conditioned-reflex therapy** ... to say what they feel ("feeling talk") ..."

(c) The term may be implied in the article entry. Exam-

ple: "**compulsive gambling**: See PATHOLOGICAL GAMBLING" and "**pathological gambling** ... failure to resist ..."

(d) The term may be derived from the headword. Example: "**mapping of genes**: See GENETIC MAP." (3.2)

5.3. A reference entry may be a combination of the two types of 5.2.1 and 5.2.2. Example: "**dependence** = DEPENDENCY. Also see PSYCHOLOGICAL D."

5.4. A small number of reference headwords are followed by a parenthetic explanation. Example: "**combination** (in genetics) = MIXOVARIATION."

5.5. Combined Reference Headwords. If two or more reference headwords are immediately adjacent to each other and refer to the same article entry, the reference entries are combined, with a semicolon separating the headwords. (Such combined headwords count as separate entries—see 10.1.1.) Example: "**echomatism; echomimia** = ECHOPRAXIA."

5.6. Hidden Reference Headwords. Reference entries that would be derived from a boldface term in an immediately adjacent article entry are not listed as separate headwords (also see 10.1). Examples: "**agglutination** ... Adjective: **agglutinative**." / "**aggregation problems** ..." ("agglutinative" would immediately follow the entry); "**acute shock psychosis** ..." / "**acute stress reaction** ... Also called **acute situational reaction**." ("acute situational reaction" would immediately precede the entry)

Therefore, if an entry is not found in its expected place, it may be among the boldface terms of an immediately adjacent entry.

5.6.1. This rule thus does not apply to reference entries that do not have a corresponding boldface term in the adjacent article entry, that is, subtypes 5.2.2 (b), (c), and (d). Example: "**vicious circle** ..."/ "**victim psychology**: See VICTIM RECIDIVISM." / "**victim recidivism** ..."

5.7. For reference entries with index function, see 6.5.2.

6. CROSS REFERENCES

6.1. A cross reference always refers to an article entry, never to an undefined headword.

6.2. Style. Cross references are set in small capital letters. Multiple cross references are separated by semicolons —and occasionally by commas, depending on syntax.

6.3. Position. Cross references are usually given

(a) at the end of an entry, preceded by "See," "Also see," or "Compare"; examples: "**UFOs** ... See MYTHOLOGICAL THEMES; MANDALA"; "**abience** ... Also see AVOIDANCE. Compare ADIENCE."

(b) at the end of a definition (or very close to the end), followed by "See this entry" or "See these entries"; example: "**acrosome** a hoodlike formation on the front end of a SPERMATOZOON. See this entry."

For certain drug entries (7.3) and a small number of other entries, cross references are given

(c) in the body of the definition, immediately followed by "(see this entry)" or "(see these entries)"; example:

"**psychedelics** ... Miscellaneous p. include AMYL NITRITE, BENACTYZINE (see these entries), **benzene**—C_6H_6, **carbon tetrachloride**—CCl_4, ..."

Also see 4.5.5 (c).

6.4. Directions. "See" and "Also see" refer to entries with related information, "See" referring primarily to essential information that expands or supplements the preceding definition; the reference may be one-directional or reciprocal. "Compare" refers to a contrasting term; this reference is usually reciprocal.

6.4.1. Occasionally, the use of "See" is modified, as in "For the individual types, see ..."

6.5. Adjacent Entries. Adjacent entries are usually not referred to. (Among the exceptions are entries that are of immediate relevance; e.g., the ten cross references at the end of **herpes infection** include the subsequent entry **herpes simplex encephalitis**.)

Therefore, the reader is advised to glance at the entries that precede and follow the consulted entry.

6.5.1. This advice applies especially where multiple cross references are given to compound headwords that contain the headword of the entry—that is, where a cross reference has *index function*. (More on index function in 3.3.) E.g., the entry **superego** shows these seven references: "Also see DOUBLE S.; GROUP S.; HETERONYMOUS S.; PARASITIC S.; PRESUPEREGO; PRIMITIVE S.; REWARD BY THE S." But no reference is made to the four entries that follow the entry **superego**, namely, **superego anxiety, superego lacunae, superego resistance**, and **superego sadism**.

Other representative examples: While **epilepsy** has 39 cross references, they do not include the 12 subsequent entries beginning with "epileptic," "epilepti-," and "epilepto-," from **epileptic absence** to **epileptogenic lesion**. While **self** has 13 cross references, they do not include the 84 subsequent entries beginning with "self-." While **dreams** has 16

cross references, they do not include the seven subsequent entries or the six *preceding* entries beginning with "dream."

6.5.2. The same advice applies to certain reference entries; e.g., **family** refers to seven compounds ending in "family" but does not list the 12 subsequent entries beginning with "family" (or the nine preceding entries beginning with "familial").

6.6. For the index function of cross references from the biographical entries, see 7.2.1, 7.2.2 (f).

6.7. The entries **DSM-III, test, psychological test, therapy**, and **psychotherapy** are cross-referenced to the respective Appendixes (A, B, and C) of this Dictionary. Summary references are made at the entries **Freud** (over 200 entries), **phobia** (250 article entries and 250 reference entries), **psychiatry** (42 headwords), **psychoanalysis** (47 headwords), **psychology** (82 headwords), **reflex** (about 80 headwords), and **syndrome**—see 3.3 (d).

6.8. For implied cross references, see 4.5.4.1.

7. ENTRIES WITH SPECIAL STYLE

7.1. DSM-III Entries. This Dictionary includes, with the permission of the American Psychiatric Association, the official terms of the *Diagnostic and Statistical Manual of Mental Disorders* (Third Edition, 1980). See the entry **DSM-III** and APPENDIX A.

7.1.1. The definitions were condensed for this Dictionary, and a few editorial changes were made in coordinating the Classification with the dictionary entries. The hyphenation of compound terms was made consistent and adapted to the style of this Dictionary. (Alternative terms and cross references that precede the designation "(DSM-III)" at the end of an entry were not necessarily suggested by the *DSM-III*.)

7.1.2. DSM-III entries differ from the regular style of this Dictionary in several details: (a) headword inversion—see 2.4, 3.2; (b) "(DSM-III)" as the last element of an entry—see 4.11, 4.12. Also, (c) when a DSM-III, DSM-II, or DSM-I term is used as part of a definition and is not set in boldface type (a subentry) or in small capital letters (a cross reference), the term is put in quotation marks.

7.1.3. Passages from the *DSM-III* are quoted in several entries that do not have DSM-III headwords and the designation "(DSM-III)." Example: the entry **psychosis**.

7.2. Biographical Entries. This Dictionary includes more than 1,000 biographical entries, of which about 150 are in narrative form. These entries—with few exceptions—are (a) names that correspond to eponymic headwords (see 4.6.3), and (b) names that are mentioned under other headwords.

7.2.1. Many biographical entries have index function; e.g., the entry **Jung** lists 99 cross references to headwords in or under which Jung is mentioned, and **Piaget** has 69 such cross references (30 of the names have more than 15 such cross references each).

7.2.2. Entry style: (a) Alternative names are added to the headword, e.g., **Descartes, René (Renatus Cartesius)**. (b) Pronunciation is given for most of the foreign last names (and a few first names such as **Jean** /zhän/—see 8.7). (c) The basic added data are nationality, occupation, and years of birth and death. (d) For headword abbreviation in biographical entries, see 3.4.7. (e) Headword-derived parts of speech are given occasionally to show usage, spelling, or pronunciation; e.g., **Rogers—Rogerian; Descartes—Cartesian;** Piaget /pē·äzhe′/—**Piagetian** /pē·äzhā′tē·ən/; **Mesmer—to mesmerize** and **mesmeric** /-mer′-/.

(f) Cross references from biographical entries include, in this order: (i) headwords that are or contain eponyms of the name, e.g., "**Feil** ... See KLIPPEL-FEIL SYNDROME"; (ii) headwords under which an eponymic term appears as an alternative term, with the eponymic term (and "also called") added in parentheses in boldface, e.g., "**Berger** ... See BRAIN WAVES (also called **Berger rhythms**)"; (iii) headwords under which an eponymic term appears as a boldface or lightface subentry, with the eponymic term (and "there:") added in parentheses in boldface if it is not mentioned in a preceding cross reference, e.g., "**Kugelberg** ... See PROGRESSIVE SPINAL-MUSCULAR ATROPHY (there:

Wohlfart-Kugelberg-Welander disease)," but "**Balo** ... See BALO'S DISEASE; PROGRESSIVE DEGENERATIVE SUBCORTICAL ENCEPHALOPATHY"—where Balo's disease also appears in the definition: (iv) headwords under which the name is mentioned in other ways, e.g., "**Maslow** ... See HIERARCHY OF NEEDS ..."; "**Casanova** ... See DON JUAN"; (v) general cross references.

7.2.3. Eponymic compounds ending in "syndrome" or "disease" have an apostrophe for one person, e.g., **Kraepelin's disease** or **Treacher Collins' syndrome**, but have no apostrophe for more than one person, e.g., **Dollinger-Bielschowsky syndrome**. (Among the few exceptions is **Munchausen syndrome**.)

7.2.4. For the pronunciation of eponyms and proper names, see 8.7.

7.2.5. Not all names have separate biographical entries. The exceptions include (a) units of physics (e.g., **angstrom, bel**) and several other eponymic headwords (e.g., **Barnum effect, Munchausen syndrome**)—for which the biographical information appears in the definition; (b) entries such as **Siamese twins** (about Eng and Chang, 1811–74); (c) names for which data were unavailable. (For revised editions of this Dictionary, the editors welcome any information on missing or incomplete biographical data.)

7.3. Drug Entries. This Dictionary includes about 300 pharmacological entries, of which most are drugs with their formulae.

Nearly all are given in a three-level relationship: The level-one entries represent 14 general categories, namely **analgesics, anorexics, antidepressants, antiepileptics, antimanics, antiparkinson drugs, anxiolytics, migraine-neuralgia analgesics, narcotic analgesics, narcotic antagonists, neuroleptics, psychedelics, sedative-hypnotics**, and **stimulants**. Each of these 14 level-one entries mentions its subgrouped level-two entries; e.g., **antimanics** lists, among others, PHENOTHIAZINES. A level-two entry, in turn, (a) describes an individual drug, with its formula, as a boldface level-three subentry, or (b) refers to a separately defined individual drug, as a level-three article entry; e.g., **phenothiazines** describes, among others, "... **thioproperazine** —$C_{22}H_{30}N_4O_2S_2$," but also refers to THIORIDAZINE (6.3). The definition of a level-three article entry begins with the formula, and includes a reference or is followed by a reference to the level-two entry for the larger context; e.g., "**thioridazine** $C_{21}H_{26}N_2S_2$—a ... See PHENOTHIAZINES."

7.3.1. Trademarks. See the entry **trademark** for a definition of this term. Trademarks appear as (a) article headwords (followed by "a trademark for") or (b) alternative terms to a headword or a subentry (see 4.9.1). When a trademark is the headword of a reference entry, it is not labeled "trademark" there, only in the article entry referred to. Nearly all trademarks in this Dictionary are drugs (an example of the exceptions is **Optacon**).

NOTICE: Any term that to the best knowledge of the editors of this Dictionary is a trademark is identified as such; but neither the editors nor the publishers of this Dictionary are expressing an opinion on the legal status of any term by designating or not designating it as "trademark" or, in general, by entering or not entering any term in this Dictionary.

7.4. Combining Forms. The combining-form entries—about 300—are an important feature of this Dictionary. They serve two purposes:

(a) They provide additional information on many entries, including an indication of etymology (see 4.6.3). E.g., while **hysterectomy** is defined as a headword, its components are better understood by consulting the two combining-form entries **-hyster-; -hystero-** and **-ectomy**.

(b) They give access to many terms that are not listed in this Dictionary but occur in its definitions or may be encountered in other literature. E.g., the definition of **de Lange's syndrome** mentions "microbrachycephaly"; the approximate meaning of this term will be understood by consulting the three combining-form entries **-micr-; -micro-, -brachy-,** and **-cephal-; -cephalo-**.

7.4.1. A combining-form entry may have a headword that consists of variants of the combining form, which are separated by semicolons. Such multiple combining forms count as one entry (10.1.1). In alphabetizing, all variants after the first semicolon are disregarded (2.7), as in the entries **-hum-; -hom-** and **-scler-; -sclero-** (which is followed by **sclera**). While combining-form entries themselves have an etymological purpose, most of them, in turn, are given with etymology (4.6.3).

7.4.2. Especially helpful may be the many combining-form entries that interpret two or more meanings. Example: "**-ped-** a combining form relating (a) to children (from Greek *pais*, "child"), (b) to the feet (from Latin *pes*, "foot")." Also see, as examples, the entry **-rad-** (which includes the adjectives **radical** and **radial**, of different origin), the cross-referenced entries **-troph- . . .** and **-tropic- . . .**, and the juxtaposed entries **-brom-; -broma-** (relating to food) and **-brom-; -bromo-** (relating to bromine).

8. PRONUNCIATION

8.1. Generally, pronunciation is given whenever inquiry patterns have shown it is likely to be needed.

8.2. System. See the PRONUNCIATION KEY. All symbols for English sounds are ordinary letters of the alphabet with few adaptations, and with the exception of the schwa, /ə/ (the neutral vowel). For the three symbols used for foreign sounds, see 8.5.

The accent mark follows the stressed syllable; only primary stresses are shown. A raised dot shows that two vowels or two consonants are pronounced separately (as in "**maieusiophobia** /mä·oosē·ō-/" and "**principle of Prägnanz** /preg·nänts′/." Pronunciation is often given in truncated form.

Examples: "**ptosis** /tō′sis/"; "**rachischisis** /rakis′kəsis/"; "**epididymis** /-did′-/"; "**satyriasis** /-rī′ə-/"; "**allophasis** /-lof′-/" "**alloplasty** /al′-/"; "**amblyopia** /-i·ō′-/," "**amblyo-scope** /am′-/," and "**amblystomas** /-blis′-/"; "**-pnea-; -pneo-** /-nē·ə-; -nē·ō-/"; "**cerebrum** /ser′-/ or /sərēb′-/"

8.3. Position. Pronunciation may be given for any part of an article entry. Examples: "**real anxiety** . . . the *Realangst* /rä·äl′ängst/ of Freud . . ."; "**primiparous** /-mip′-/ . . . as a **primipara** /-mip′-/ . . . **primigravida** /-grav′-/ . . . Also called **uniparous** /-nip′-/."

8.4. Letterword versus Acronym. If the pronunciation of an abbreviation is not mentioned, the abbreviation is usually a letterword (read letter by letter), e.g., "**ABO** . . ." (read /ā′bē′ō′/). If the abbreviation is an acronym (read as a word), this is indicated by pronunciation, e.g., "**ECHO virus** /ek′ō/," or in the wording of the definition, e.g., "**CAGE** an acronym derived from . . ." Some abbreviations are used as letterword *or* acronym, e.g., "**UFOs** /yoo′ef′ōs′/ or /yoo′fōs/" and "**ESL** /es′əl/ or /ē′es′el′/."

8.5. Foreign Sounds. The only special symbols used are /œ/ for the *eu* in French *deux* and for the *ö* in German *schön*, /kh/ for the *ch* in Scottish *loch* and the second *ch* in German *Rorschach*, and /N/, which does not represent a sound but indicates that the preceding vowel is a nasal as in French *bon* /bôN/ or *fin* /feN/. Because this Dictionary is not a language dictionary, other foreign sounds are merely approximated by the closest equivalents among the English

symbols of the PRONUNCIATION KEY. (These native sounds have to be heard to be learned; no amount of printed explanation could render them. The reader who is familiar with the native sounds will make the appropriate substitutions.) Thus, this Dictionary generally shows /sh/ for the *ch* in German *Reich* /rīsh/ or *nichts* /nishts/; /i/ for the short *ü* in German *Müller* /mil′ər/; /ē/ for the long *ü* in German *für* /fēr/ or *Gemüt* /gemēt′/ and for the *u* in French *une* /ēn/ or *rue* /rē/. (The latter, e.g., is a closer and much more realistic improvisation than the customary but more misleading /ōon/ and /rōo/.)

French compound terms are usually transcribed as though they were one word, e.g., "**arc de cercle** /ärk′dəser′kl/"; "**folie à trois** /fōlē′ätrō·ä′/."

8.6. Latin Terms. Most of the numerous Latin terms in this Dictionary appear without pronunciation, mainly because there are different ways (all of them understood) in which Latin is pronounced by the English speaker and may be pronounced in general. However, guidance is given in many cases, often to reflect common usage. Examples: "**potency** . . . Also called **potentia coeundi** /kō·ä·ōon′dē/"; "**b.i.d.** . . . (Latin *bis in die* /dē′ä/"; "**focus** . . . Plurals: **focuses; foci** /fō′sī/ or /fō′kē/"; "**spina bifida** /spī′nə bi′fədə/ or /spē′nä bif′idä/"

8.7 Eponyms and Proper Names. The pronunciation for eponymic entries, if included, is given in the corresponding biographical entries.

English proper names and names of immigrants to English-speaking countries are usually not shown with pronunciation. (Examples of exceptions: **Yerkes, Selye, Szasz.**) Pronunciation is given for most foreign last names in the biographical entries (and occasionally for first names —see 7.2.2). While these pronunciations apply also to the corresponding eponymic terms, the latter are often used without awareness of their origin, and the reader should not hesitate to follow whatever is usage in his or her working or social environment. Examples: "**Froin, Georges** /frô·eN′/," but one may hear /froinz/ in **Froin's syndrome**; "**Morvan, A. M.** /môr·väN′/," but one may hear /môr′vanz/ in **Morvan's disease.**

9. ASSORTED STYLE NOTES

9.1. Spelling preferences and hyphenation compatible with *The Scribner-Bantam English Dictionary*, followed by *The Random House Dictionary*. End-of-line hyphenation also according to *The Medical & Health Sciences Word Book* and *The Word Book* (both Houghton Mifflin).

Common prefixes form solid compounds (including, e.g., "antiintraception" and "posttraumatic"). Restrictive clauses use the specific "that" rather than the ambiguous "which." Both U.S. and metric measurements; one added to the other in parentheses. Nine, ten, 11, 12; but "grades 2 to 11."

Modifying subcompounds are hyphenated according to their function—important for clarity in a work that has

many long compounds. (Even the DSM-III terms—see 7.1.1—were adapted to this principle.)

Because of the frequency of its occurrence, "central nervous system" becomes "CNS" when it is part of a headword or when it modifies a noun or adjective.

Straightforward syntax; simple, concrete words—helpful in a work in which the specialized vocabulary is complex and abstract. Whenever the common term fits, the rarer term is avoided. Examples: aggravate, not exacerbate; behind, not dorsal to; clefts, not invaginations; positions, not loci; that do not respond to, not that are refractory to. Also see 4.5.4 (a)

No special abbreviations, except "Abbrev." itself.

"Native American" and "nation" (not "American Indian" and "tribe").

9.2. Basic typeface is 8-point Times Roman (8/9); com-

puter-set. (Length of Dictionary proper—pages 1 to 807 —corresponds to approximately 5 million characters.)

10. ENTRY COUNT AND TAXONOMY

10.1. Entry Count. This Dictionary has a total of 21,164 entry headwords. Counted as entries are (a) the large boldface headwords set flush left, whether article entries or reference entries (for multiple headwords, see 10.1.1), and (b) certain reference headwords that occur in what would be an immediately adjacent article entry and are therefore not set flush left as separate headwords (see 5.6). The total of article entries (section 4) is 15,909; the total of reference entries (section 5) is 5,255.

Of the 5,255 reference entries, 2,572, or 49%, are alternative terms (5.2.1); 2,683, or 51%, are other, nonsynonymous referred terms (5.2.2).

10.1.1. For reference entries that refer to the same article entry and are immediately adjacent to each other, the headwords are combined (and separated by semicolons). As they are really separate entries, they are counted separately (5.5). (However, variants of a combining form—also separated by semicolons—are part of the same headword and thus are counted as one article entry.)

10.1.2. Not included in the entry count are thus (a) any other types of terms that are loosely referred to as "entries" in these Methodological Notes, such as the "subentries" in 4.7; (b) terms that in some dictionaries are called "hidden entries" (hidden, usually, in a definition), including formulae, symbols, names of genus and species, but primarily the vast number of terms that are defined where they are used —see 4.5.4 (c)—but which are not accessible in their alphabetical place through reference entries.

10.2. Inventory of Article Entries. See page xvi. This list is meant to be merely an overview; it is not without arbitrariness: (a) The categories could be grouped differently. (b) More—or fewer—"interface areas" could be singled out; in particular, see the headwords listed in APPENDIX D, many of which could categorize additional "interface areas." (c) Most categories overlap (especially with the large category "psychiatry"), and the assignment of a

number of entries to a category is approximate in most cases.

10.2.1. For statistical data not singled out in this inventory, see also (a) the numbers mentioned or referred to below (10.2.2); (b) the numbers mentioned at the end of the dictionary entries **psychology, psychiatry, psychoanalysis, reflex**, and **Freud** (6.7); (c) the numbers mentioned as examples in the PREFACE.

10.2.2. The following are footnotes to the small superscript numbers in the INVENTORY OF ARTICLE ENTRIES.

(1) For an approximate distinction between "core areas" and "interface areas," see also the PREFACE.

(2) Included are (i) 385 "syndrome" and 165 "disease" entries—see 3.3 (page x); (ii) about 250 "phobia" (and "fear") entries—not counting here another 250 "phobia" reference entries.

(3) See APPENDIX C for a list of most of the therapy entries.

(4) Included are the 488 test entries listed in APPENDIX B.

(5) For drug entries, see 7.3 (page xiii).

(6) For the Classification of DSM-III entries, see APPENDIX A, and 7.1 (page xiii).

(7) For biographical entries, see 7.2 (page xiii).

(8) Included are (i) about 300 combining forms—see 7.4 (page xiv); (ii) the 24 letters of the Greek alphabet; (iii) abbreviations such as **TPR** ("*t*emperature, *p*ulse, and *r*espiration"); (iv)—at the request of paraprofessional personnel—abbreviations used in prescriptions, such as **p.r.n.** (*pro re nata*, "as needed").

(9) See 10.2 (b), above.

10.3. Cross References. The large number of cross references—10,750—between article entries is meant to establish encyclopedic coherence within categories of entries or from entries in one category to entries in another category (section 6, especially 6.5.1).

INVENTORY OF ARTICLE ENTRIES

For general comments and for explanations of the small superscript numbers,
see METHODOLOGICAL NOTES, 10.2 (page xv)

CORE AREAS[1]:
General Psychology: 720
Abnormal Psychology; Clinical Psychology: 440
Psychiatry[2]—specific entries: 3,310
Cross-Cultural Psychiatry: 90
Psychoanalysis: 1,180
Physiological Psychology; Neuropsychology;
    Genetics: 1,550
Cognitive Psychology: 140
Personality Psychology: 90
Educational Psychology: School Psychology;
    Learning Disabilities: 470
Child Psychology; Developmental Psychology;
    Mental Retardation: 1,260
Speech Pathology; Audiology: 320
Rehabilitation Psychology: 520
Social Psychology; Social Work: 340
Applied Psychology (including Operations
    Research, Human Engineering, and Industrial,
    Consumer, and Advertising Psychology): 220
Psychotherapy; Counseling[3]: 480
Hypnosis: 100
Psychometrics (Tests and Testing)[4]: 590
Psychological Statistics; Experimental Psychology:
    520
Psychopharmacology; Neuropharmacology;
    Drugs[5]: 310
DSM-III entries[6]: 260

Biographical entries (including 150 narrative
    Biographies)[7]: 1,039
Combining Forms and miscellaneous entries[8]: 400

INTERFACE AREAS[9]:
Anthropology: 50
Behavioral Medicine: 70
Biofeedback: 60
Community Psychology: 100
Comparative Psychology: 150
Environmental Psychology: 150
Evaluation Research: 60
Facilities and Services: 70
Forensic Psychology and Psychiatry: 70
Humanistic Psychology: 90
Linguistics: 130
Philosophical Psychology: 40
Proxemics: 40
Psychological Esthetics: 120
Semantics: 40
Sexology: 320

Total of article entries above: 15,909
Reference entries, not included in this inventory:
    5,255
Total dictionary entries: 21,164

PRONUNCIATION KEY

For further details, see METHODOLOGICAL NOTES, section 8 (page xiv).

SYMBOLS	KEY WORDS	SYMBOLS	KEY WORDS	SYMBOLS	KEY WORDS
/a/	hat	/oi/	boy	/ng/	sing, drink
/ä/	father	/o͝o/	book	/ngg/	finger
/ā/	fate	/o͞o/	move	/s/	sell
/e/	flesh	/ou/	sound	/sh/	shoe, lotion
/ē/	he	/u/	cup	/th/	thin
/er/	air	/ur/	fur	/th/	than
/i/	sit	/ə/	ago, focus	/v/	very
/ī/	eye	/ər/	murder	/w/	work
/o/	proper	/ch/	much	/y/	yes
/ô/	saw	/g/	good	/z/	zeal
/ō/	nose	/j/	gem	/zh/	azure, vision

No key words are needed for /b/, /d/, /f/, /h/,
/k/, /l/, /m/, /n/, /p/, /r/, and /t/.

/œ/, /kh/, and /N/ are symbols for foreign sounds; see 8.5, page xiv.

A

A; Å = ANGSTROM.

āā an abbreviation used in prescriptions, meaning "of each" (Latin *ana*)

AA = ACHIEVEMENT AGE.

AA = ALCOHOLICS ANONYMOUS.

ab- a combining form meaning (a) away from, (b) on the opposite side.

A/B/A design an experimental design in which a baseline or other initial condition (A) is followed by a changed condition (B), and then is returned to the initial condition (A).

Abadie, Charles /äbädē'/ French ophthalmologist, 1842–1932. See ABADIE'S SIGN.

Abadie's sign insensitivity of the Achilles tendon to pressure in cases of early tabes dorsalis.

abalienation an obsolete term for mental illness. Adjective: **abalienated**.

abandonment reaction a feeling of emotional deprivation, loss of support, and loneliness experienced by children who have been deserted or neglected by one or both parents. A.r. is also experienced by adults who have lost a loved one on whom they have depended.

abandonment threat a threat to abandon a child or send him to a "bad boy's home," used deliberately as a disciplinary measure, or expressed impulsively in a fit of anger. Such threats usually arouse acute anxiety and a tendency to cling to the parents.

abasement a desire or compulsion to submit to aggressive or punishing acts, or to humble or degrade oneself. See MASOCHISM.

abasia: See ASTASIA-ABASIA.

abclution the rejection of acculturation or of the established behavior patterns of the culture.

abderite /ab'dərīt/ an obsolete term for simpleton (from the ancient Greek town of Abdera, whose inhabitants were considered stupid).

abdominal bloating = BLOATING.

abdominal epilepsy a pathologic condition in which an abnormal discharge of nerve cells from the brain results in spasms of pain in the abdomen.

abdominal ganglion aplasia the total or partial failure of an abdominal ganglion to develop normally.

abdominal melancholia a term sometimes used to identify a type of depression accompanied by delusional fixation involving the gastrointestinal tract and complaints of constipation, flatulence, belching, and dyspepsia.

abdominal nephrectomy: See NEPHRECTOMY.

abdominal reflex a contraction of muscles of the abdominal wall in response to tactile stimulation of the area.

abducens nerve the sixth cranial nerve of the human body, carrying somatic fibers for control of the lateral rectus muscle of the eye. The a.n. is referred to as "cranial nerve VI." Also called **abducent nerve**.

abducens nucleus a collection of nerve cells in the fourth ventricle of the brain, from which the abducens nerve originates. See ABDUCENS NERVE.

abducent nerve = ABDUCENS NERVE.

abductor any muscle that draws away from the median plane of the body or the axial line of a limb or digit of the body. The **a. hallucis** flexes the large toe.

Aberdeen system a 19th-century industrial-social movement which established a series of schools emphasizing the rights of children, family ties, day care rather than residential placement, and meeting the needs of the whole child and his or her family.

aberration any deviation from the normal or typical. In vision, a. is failure of light rays to converge on the same point. See MENTAL A.

abience /āb'-/ the type of response or behavior that results in movement away from a stimulus either by physical withdrawal or by activity designed to sever contact with the stimulus; avoidance. Adjective: **abient**. Also see AVOIDANCE. Compare ADIENCE.

ability competence, or capacity, to perform a physical or mental act. A. may be either innate or acquired by education and practice.

ability grouping the assignment of pupils to school classes on the basis of their learning ability. A.g. may also be the process of dividing a class into sections based on the students' ability in one area, e.g., the practice of assigning elementary-school children to reading groups for fast or slow readers.

ability test any standardized test designed to

measure aptitude or intelligence. The term is also applied to tests measuring achievement.

abiotrophic atrophic dementia = ATROPHIC DEMENTIA.

abiotrophy /-ot′-/ the loss of resistance to a disease through degeneration or failure of a body system, e.g., the decline of an individual's immune system with aging, resulting in an increased risk of cancer growth as the antibodies lose ability to reject the tumor cells. A. also may be accelerated by a genetic defect, as in Huntington's chorea which usually does not produce symptoms until middle age. Adjective: **abiotrophic** /-trof′-/.

ablation the surgical excision of all or part of an organ, usually to study its function. Also called **extirpation**. See BIOPSY.

ablatio penis the surgical excision of the penis or a portion of the penis. It is an operation performed in the treatment of diseases, e.g., cancer or gangrene, of the organ, or in a sex-change procedure.

-ablemo- a combining form meaning feeble.

ablutomania a morbid preoccupation with washing or bathing. It is a symptom of obsessive-compulsive disorder. Also see DIRT PHOBIA.

Abney, Sir William de Wiveleslie English chemist and physicist, 1843–1920. See ABNEY'S LAW.

Abney's law the principle that the luminance (strength) of a given monochromatic light is proportional to the luminosity (brightness) of the light and the radiance (radiant energy).

abnormal in psychiatry and psychology, pertaining to any deviation from what is considered normal; pathological; maladjustive. In statistics, the term denotes scores that are outside the normal or expected range. Noun: **abnormality**.

abnormal behavior behavior that is regarded as evidence of a mental or emotional disturbance ranging from minor adjustment problems to severe mental disorder; a neurosis, psychosis, or personality disorder.

abnormality: See ABNORMAL.

abnormal psychology the branch of psychology concerned with the study of mental and emotional disorders, including neuroses, psychoses, personality disorders, organic mental syndromes, psychophysiologic disorders, and mental retardation.

ABO blood-group incompatibility an immune reaction that can occur when blood of one genetic type is transfused into the body of a patient whose own blood is of another genetic type. The original major grouping of blood types as A, B, and O was introduced in 1900 by Karl Landsteiner. A fourth, the AB type, was added in 1920. Incompatibility is characterized by an agglutination, or clumping, that occurs when a substance in the red blood cells of a donor contacts an antibody in the blood serum of the recipient. The recipient's blood reacts in a manner similar to the introduction of any foreign substance into the bloodstream, such as insect venom or an infectious bacterium.

aboiement /äbô·ämäN′/ a speech disturbance in which animalistic sounds, such as barking, are involuntarily and uncontrollably produced (French, "barking"). It is a symptom occurring in chronic advanced schizophrenia and Tourette's disorder.

aboriginal therapies psychotherapy practiced in primitive societies, including folk healing, sorcery, and the incantations of a shaman or witch doctor. See DEMONOLOGY; WITCHCRAFT.

abortifacient any agent, such as ergot, that is used to produce an abortion. A type of seaweed, laminaria, sometimes is used to induce an abortion by dilating the cervix; a small stem of laminaria is inserted into the cervix where it absorbs moisture and expands, forcing the cervical canal to enlarge. Also called **abortient; abortigen**.

abortion the expulsion of an embryo or fetus before it has reached the stage of viability (ability to live outside the uterus), that is, before about 20 weeks of gestation. A. may be either spontaneous or induced. See SPONTANEOUS A.; INDUCED A.; THERAPEUTIC A.

aboulia = ABULIA.

Abraham, Karl German psychoanalyst, 1877–1925. One of Freud's earliest disciples, A. became the first German analyst and made significant contributions to the study of manic-depressive states, schizophrenia, the relation between dream symbolism and myths, and the formation of the oral and anal characters through pregenital fixation.

abreaction a therapeutic technique, originated by Josef Breuer, in which the patient discharges repressed emotions by reviving and reliving painful experiences that have been buried in the unconscious. A. refers to the process; catharsis to the end-result, the discharge of tension. Also see RETENTION HYSTERIA.

abscissa the horizontal coordinate in a graph or data plot; the X axis. Also see ORDINATE.

absence a brief loss of consciousness during a hysterical or epileptic attack, with suspended or automatic activity followed by amnesia.

absenteeism in industrial psychology, a record of the number, duration, and cause of absences from work. This record is frequently used as one criterion of job performance and job satisfaction.

absent-mindedness a form of habitual inattention, marked by a tendency to be occupied by one's own thoughts, but less severe than withdrawal or autism.

absent state a vacant, dreamlike state of detachment that frequently occurs in temporal-lobe epilepsy.

absinthe the dried leaves and flowering tops of wormwood, Artemisia absinthium, which grows wild or under cultivation in North America,

Europe, Africa, and Asia. The principal ingredient, absinthin—$C_{30}H_{40}O_6$—produces gastrointestinal and CNS effects. A. is classed as a convulsant that can induce cerebral convulsions of an epilepsy type while involving limited muscle groups. It is used as a flavoring in certain alcoholic beverages and is alleged to be an aphrodisiac. See WORMWOOD.

absolute accommodation the visual accommodation of either of the eyes when tested separately.

absolute bliss: See TRANSCENDENTAL MEDITATION.

absolute impression a judgment based on implied or vague standards, such as "It was a bright day."

absolute inversion a Freudian term for a kind of homosexuality that is so well entrenched that interest in the opposite sex is implausible and even the thought of the opposite sex may evoke repugnance. Also see AMPHIGENOUS INVERSION.

absolute limen = ABSOLUTE THRESHOLD.

absolute luminosity the measure of luminosity in standard units of light reflectance, e.g., lumens per watt.

absolute measurement a measurement made directly, and independently of comparison with other variables.

absolute pitch the frequency of a tone as measured in cycles per second, e.g., A at 440 vibrations per second; also, the ability to identify an isolated tone.

absolute rating scale a type of rating instrument in which the given dimensions are evaluated according to absolute values, that is, the dimensions or subjects to be rated are not compared with other dimensions or subjects but are judged according to independent criteria.

absolute refractory period a brief period after the firing of a neuron when it cannot be discharged again.

absolute scale a scale that is measured in equal intervals from a base point of absolute zero.

absolute scotoma: See SCOTOMA.

absolute sensitivity the minimum stimulus needed to produce a sensation. See ABSOLUTE THRESHOLD.

absolute threshold the minimum amount of nervous stimulation required to trigger a reaction or produce a sensation. It is the lowest or weakest level of stimulation that can be detected on 50 percent of trials, e.g., the slightest, most indistinct sound the ear can detect. Although the name suggests a fixed level at which stimuli effectively elicit sensations, the a.t. is relative and fluctuates according to alterations in receptors and environmental conditions. Also called **detection threshold; absolute limen (AL).**

absorbed mania a mental state in which the patient has concentrated his attention on inner thoughts so intensely that he has excluded himself from reality.

absorption an extreme involvement or preoccupation with one object, idea, or pursuit with inattention to other aspects of the environment.

abstinence the act of refraining from the use of alcohol, drugs, or certain foods, or from sexual intercourse. See RULE OF ABSTINENCE. Also see WITHDRAWAL.

abstinence delirium a type of delirium that is a part of the withdrawal symptoms of alcoholism or drug dependence. See ALCOHOL-WITHDRAWAL DELIRIUM; DELIRIUM.

abstinence rule = RULE OF ABSTINENCE.

abstinence syndrome: See WITHDRAWAL

abstract attitude a term coined by Goldstein for a set of cognitive abilities that comprise the capacity to use general concepts, as opposed to thinking concretely and in terms only of immediate experience. This capacity is usually impaired in patients with organic brain syndromes. Also called **categorical attitude.** Also see ABSTRACT THINKING. Compare CONCRETE ATTITUDE.

abstract conceptualization the process of forming abstract concepts such as liberty and integrity. See ABSTRACT ATTITUDE; ABSTRACT THINKING.

abstract expressionism the practice of depicting subjective generalizations which interpret the observations or experiences of the artist.

abstract idea a generalized concept considered apart from concrete examples, e.g., time flow.

abstract intelligence the intellectual ability to think in terms of abstract concepts. See ABSTRACT THINKING. Compare CONCRETE INTELLIGENCE.

abstraction the formation of general concepts derived from particular instances; also, the concepts themselves, such as goodness and beauty. In schizophrenia and mental retardation the ability to abstract is usually impaired.

abstract modeling an extension of the original social-learning theory, proposing that we learn and acquire behavior patterns by extracting from a series of observations common elements and principles or common structural features that are incorporated into later patterns of behavior. Earlier social-learning theory assumed that children imitate precisely what they observe. A.m. modifies this early belief by proposing that children discern general patterns in the behavior they observe; based on these observational patterns, they develop their own guiding principles that may generate behavior quite different from specific behaviors observed.

abstract perceptions uncanny and unlocalized experiences in and around the body, such as floating through space, awareness of hazy rotating objects, and sensations of crescendo and decrescendo. A.p. occur most often in dreams, while falling asleep, or in stress situations, and may be echos of infantile subjective experiences. See ISAKOWER PHENOMENON.

abstract thinking thinking characterized by the

ability to use abstractions and generalizations. A.t. is specifically the ability to grasp essentials and common properties, to keep different aspects of a situation in mind and shift from one to another, to predict and plan ahead, and to think symbolically and draw conclusions. Also see ABSTRACT ATTITUDE.

abstract-versus-representational dimension a system of evaluating the psychological reaction to a work of art based on the amount and pattern of detail referred to or denoted in the art. At the representational end of the dimension, a work of art will be characterized by a great amount of detail. At the abstract end of the scale, detail and pattern of detail will be highly selective and some detail will be excluded.

absurdities test the type of test in which subjects must identify absurdities, inconsistencies, or incongruities in a picture, story, or other written paragraph. The Binet test incorporates absurdity tasks.

absurdity an idea or expression that is obviously nonsensical, incoherent, or meaningless.

abulia an extreme loss of initiative and will power; inability to make decisions or perform voluntary actions. A. is a rare symptom found in schizophrenia and occasionally in profound depression. Also spelled **aboulia**. See HYPOBULIA.

abundancy motive the tendency to want and strive for a greater degree of gratification than that required to fill a particular physical need, e.g., eating more food than the amount actually needed to reduce tension associated with hunger. Compare DEFICIENCY MOTIVE.

abused child: See BATTERED-CHILD SYNDROME.

abuse liability the measure of the ability of a drug to reinforce drug-taking behavior. Factors may include tolerance and dependence effects that may or may not be subjective. Amphetamines have a high degree of a.l. because of their CNS effects. Nicotine also has a.l. because of its use in tobacco, which is socially acceptable.

a.c. an abbreviation used in prescriptions, meaning "before meals" (Latin *ante cibum*).

academic pertaining to any line of inquiry or research that is theoretical in purpose, thus intended to expand existing knowledge but not intended for direct application to a practical problem; also, pertaining to formal education.

academic inhibition: See ADJUSTMENT DISORDER WITH WORK OR A.I.

academic-underachievement disorder an "academic problem" (DSM-III category) characterized by a pattern of failing grades or significant underachievement in spite of adequate intellectual capacity, stimulation, and teaching, but without evidence of a specific developmental disorder or other mental disorder to account for the problem. Also see UNDERACHIEVER.

acalculia an inability to perform arithmetic operations. It is a form of aphasia, usually due to damage to the parietal lobe. In some cases the individual may also be unable to read or write numbers. Also called **anarithmia; dyscalculia**.

acanthesthesia a form of skin sensation in which the individual experiences the feeling of pin pricks in the absence of an external stimulus. Such sensations may result from disease or abuse of certain drugs. e.g., alcohol or methaqualone.

-acaro- a combining form meaning (a) short, (b) momentary (from Greek *acari*, "mite").

acarophobia a morbid fear of skin parasites (mites), ants, worms, and, by extension, small objects such as pins and needles. The condition is believed to be related to the sensation of insects crawling on or under the skin, which occurs in alcoholism, cocaine use, narcotic addiction, and delirium resulting from meningitis, encephalitis, rheumatic fever, or diphtheria. See FORMICATION; LILLIPUTIAN HALLUCINATION. Also see PARASITOPHOBIA; ENTOMOPHOBIA.

acatalepsia an inability to comprehend or reason. The term was formerly used as an alternative for dementia.

acatamathesia the absence or loss of the ability to comprehend perceptions of objects or situations; also, inability to comprehend speech.

acataphasia the use of inappropriate or grammatically incorrect words and expressions. A. is a speech disturbance frequently found in schizophrenic and aphasic patients. Also spelled **akataphasia**. See SYNTACTICAL APHASIA; AGRAMMATISM.

acathexis in psychoanalysis, the absence of feeling ordinarily associated with emotionally charged ideas. The patient is detached or indifferent when significant unconscious material is brought to the surface, or when he or she is told about an event that usually arouses a happy or angry response.

acathizia = AKATHISIA.

ACCD: See SELF-HELP GROUPS.

Acceleranstoff an epinephrinelike substance secreted by sympathetic nerve fibers that innervate the heart muscle of the frog. When the substance released by the accelerans nerve of one frog is applied to the heart of a second frog, the rate of contractions of the second heart accelerates. A. may be produced by heart nerves of mammals, including humans, but evidence of its presence has not been verified.

accelerated interaction the heightened level of emotional interaction reached, e.g., by members of a marathon group, due to continuous proximity for an extended period of time. See MARATHON GROUP; TIME-EXTENDED THERAPY.

acceptance the receptive, approachable, caring quality of psychotherapists and teachers who convey an implicit respect and regard for their patients and students as individuals. A. is objective in nature, ideally excluding value judgments and emotional involvement. In general, a. is a favorable attitude toward an idea or person.

accessible receptive or responsive to external stimuli. In psychiatry, a patient is a. if he responds to the therapist in a way that facilitates the development of rapport.

accessory nerve a name sometimes applied to the eleventh cranial nerve because one of its functions is that of serving as an accessory to the tenth, or vagus, nerve. The a.n. is referred to as "cranial nerve XI."

accessory symptoms a term used by Bleuler for secondary symptoms that are not fundamental in schizophrenia, such as hallucinations, delusions, memory disturbances, verbigeration, neologisms, and asyndesis.

accidental crisis in community psychology, one of two major types of crisis, characterized by a period of acute disorganization of behavior or affect precipitated by a stressful and somewhat unpredictable life experience such as the death of a family member, illness, accident, surgery, loss or change of job, or marital disruption. Also called **situational crisis; unanticipated crisis**. See MATURATIONAL CRISIS.

accidental error any error in measurement due to unpredictable, unknown, or uncontrollable factors.

accidental homosexuality homosexuality in which a male or female chooses another male or female as a sexual object when no individuals of the other sex are available. See SITUATIONAL HOMOSEXUALITY; FAUTE DE MIEUX.

accidental hypothermia: See HYPOTHERMIA.

accidental stimuli dream stimuli that are of an external sensory nature, such as the sound of a telephone ringing or a cramped muscle pain.

accident behavior unsafe behavior that might result in injury to the individual or other persons, or in physical damage to equipment or the environment. Accidents are associated with such situational factors as a risky job, atmospheric conditions, a fatiguing work schedule, and equipment failure; or such personal factors as inattention, perception errors, risk-taking, and decision errors.

accident neurosis = COMPENSATION NEUROSIS.

accident prevention application of scientifically tested methods for preventing as many accidents as possible. Major methods include a psychological study of accident repeaters and accident proneness; redesign of equipment such as cars and industrial machines; improved signs and warnings; study of circumstances in which accidents occur (icy roads, crowded workplace); reduction of personal stress and tension through counseling and psychotherapy; and such educational techniques as group discussion of safety problems in schools, role-playing, goal-setting by the student safety council and the school safety court, and driver-training programs.

accident-prone personality a hypothetical personality type marked by such characteristics as impulsiveness, risk-taking, and a fatalistic outlook, which are believed to lead to multiple accidents under different circumstances. Also called **accident repeater**. See ACCIDENT PRONENESS; VICTIM RECIDIVISM.

accident proneness a chronic susceptibility to accidents; the tendency to be an "accident repeater" in different situations. This tendency has been ascribed to a set of personality traits such as impulsiveness, intolerance of authority, emotional instability, and an inclination to trust to luck. Recent studies, however, question the existence of a fixed accident-prone profile. Many people are temporarily accident-prone due to inattention, boredome, "highway hypnosis," and the like, and a few individuals may unconsciously invite accidents as a means of "paying the piper" for guilty behavior. See PURPOSIVE ACCIDENT.

accident reduction reduction in the number and severity of accidents through such measures as safety-education programs, alcohol-detection tests, penalties for drunk or reckless driving, use of safety helmets, warnings of poor road conditions, and administration of psychological tests, such as the Siebrecht and Hannaford scales, that elicit attitudes associated with accidents.

accident repeater: See ACCIDENT-PRONE PERSONALITY.

acclimatization the alterations in physiological adaptation mechanisms involved in moving to a different climate. The term may also be used to refer to any emotional or mental adjustment to new circumstances or environmental conditions. Also called **acclimation**.

accommodation contraction or relaxation of the ciliary muscles of the eyes to adjust the lens to far or near vision. A. also involves changes in convergence and pupil size. Absolute a. refers to each eye separately; binocular a. is the simultaneous a. of both eyes. Also called **visual a**.

accommodation reflex the reflexive action involved in adjusting vision for various distances by the convergence of the eyes, constriction of the pupils, and changing the shape of the lens through contracting or relaxing of the ciliary muscles.

accomplishment quotient an obsolescent term for achievement quotient.

accountability in psychiatry, the responsibility of a hospital, clinic, or other facility to outside agencies such as the state mental-health department, its board of trustees, citizen organizations, professional societies, universities assisting in training and research, Medicare and Medicaid authorities, the public-health department, and the Joint Commission on Accreditation of Hospitals.

accreditation the process by which an institution or program is evaluated to determine if it complies with standards established by an appropriate professional group. A. is a voluntary process conducted by a nongovernmental body. Examples include the Accreditation Council for Psychiatric Facilities and Accreditation Council for Facilities for the Mentally Retarded.

accretion in environmental psychology, the accumulation of objects or material in the environment, e.g., littering, which may be taken as a measure of the degree of individual responsibility of persons who use a particular area. The term may also be applied to a form of learning resulting from the cumulative effect of repeated associations and reinforcements. Compare EROSION.

acculturation the processes by which social and broader cultural values, ideas, beliefs, and behavioral patterns are instilled. A. may also refer to an adult's attitudinal and behavioral adjustment to conform to a new culture, e.g., a new country. In social anthropology, a. is the adoption by a distinct people or group of alien cultural patterns as in Japan's adoption of Western customs beginning in the 19th century.

accumulation objects amassed without meaning or purpose, unlike a collection. See SOTERIA.

accuracy test a test scored for correctness and not for other criteria such as speed.

acedia /asē′-/ an obsolete term for apathy (from Greek *a-*, "not," and *kedos*, "care").

acenesthesia a loss of the sensation of physical existence; a lack of awareness of one's own body. See DEPERSONALIZATION.

-aceous /-āsh′əs/ a combining form referring to the characteristics of something.

acerophobia a morbid fear of sourness (from Latin *acer*, "sharp, sour").

acetaminophen: See ANILIDES.

acetanilide: See ANILIDES.

acetazolamide: See CARBONIC ANHYDRASE INHIBITORS.

ACE test the American Council on Education test of intelligence for upper high-school students and college students, yielding a language score (L) a quantitative score (Q), and a total score.

acetone /as′-/ a colorless volatile liquid with a sweet, fruity odor that occurs in excessive amounts in the blood and in the urine of diabetics and persons affected by other metabolic disorders. A. also is a normal metabolite of ethyl alcohol and a sign of alcoholism. Also called **dimethyl ketone**.

acetophenetidin: See ANILIDES; ASPIRIN COMBINATIONS.

acetoxycycloheximide an oral diabetic agent of the sulfonylurea group used in control of blood glucose in cases of maturity-onset diabetes.

acetylcholine /-kō′lēn/ a substance occurring in many body tissues where it is involved in various physiological functions, mainly as a neurotransmitter that facilitates the transfer of a nerve impulse across the synaptic gap between nerve cells. An excess or deficiency of a.

may result in a neuromuscular block. Abbrev.: **ACh**.

acetylcholine receptors receptors that are stimulated by acetylcholine or acetylcholinelike substances. They include (a) effector cells of the postganglionic parasympathetic fibers, (b) preganglionic autonomic fibers connecting to sympathetic and parasympathetic ganglion cells and to the adrenal medulla, (c) somatic motor nerve fibers connecting to the skeletal muscles, and (d) some CNS fibers.

acetylcholinesterase /-es′-/ an enzyme that splits acetylcholine into chlorine and acetic acid after the neurotransmitter has been utilized by a nerve impulse. Abbrev.: **AChE**.

acetylphosphate a high-energy molecule that is involved in the contraction of muscle fibers. The a. energy is released through the action of an enzyme, acetylphosphatase, which splits the a.

acetylsalicylic acid: See ASPIRIN EFFECTS; ASPIRIN POISONING; SALICYLATES.

acetylureas drugs that are chemical analogs of hydantoins and are used in the management of psychomotor epilepsy. The a. include **phenacemide**—$C_9H_{10}N_2O_2$—and **ethylphenacemide**—$C_{11}H_{14}N_2O_2$. Because of adverse side effects the a. are administered mainly in cases that do not respond to other antiepileptics.

ACh = ACETYLCHOLINE.

achalasia a gastrointestinal disorder caused by failure of the smooth muscles of the digestive tract to relax. The specific cause of the disorder is unknown, but it is associated with degeneration of nerve cells at one of the junctions of the tract, particularly in the region where the esophagus joins the stomach. The attacks are precipitated or aggravated by anxiety or emotional distress. Because of proximity to the heart, attacks are sometimes called **cardiospasms**. A. is derived from Greek *a-*, "not," and *chalasis*, "relaxation."

AChE = ACETYLCHOLINESTERASE.

achievement in general psychology, personal accomplishment, or attainment, of goals set by the individual or by society. In educuational psychology, the term applies to a specified level of proficiency in academic work in general or in a specific skill such as reading or arithmetic. Also see NEED FOR A.

achievement age the achievement rating of an individual as measured in terms of the norm or standard for a particular chronological age. Abbrev.: **AA**.

achievement battery any group of achievement tests designed to provide an index of a person's knowledge or specific skills across a range of related topics. See ACHIEVEMENT TESTS.

achievement drive a strong impulse to exert one's best efforts to achieve a high goal and, usually, to be recognized and approved for attaining it. Students with a strong a.d. have been found to make better grades than equally gifted students with a weaker a.d. Also, studies of the literature of different societies (McClelland, 1958, 1961) indicate that achievement themes predominate during periods of rapid economic growth. Also see ACHIEVEMENT MOTIVATION.

achievement ethic a cultural standard or ideal embodying a high level of accomplishment. Also see WORK ETHIC.

achievement motivation as used by H. Murray, the need to overcome obstacles and strive to master difficult challenges. High scorers in a.m. are likely to set higher standards and work with greater perseverance than equally gifted low scorers. McClelland found a significant relationship between high a.m. and a history of early independence in childhood; in addition, high a.m. positively correlates with actual achievement in later life. See NEED FOR ACHIEVEMENT; ACHIEVEMENT DRIVE.

achievement quotient the ratio of actual performance, usually on a standardized test, to expected performance or age norm. Abbrev.: **AQ**.

achievement tests standardized tests intended to measure an individual's present level of skill or knowledge in a given subject. Often the distinction is made that a.t. emphasize ability acquired through formal learning or training whereas aptitude tests emphasize innate potential. In addition to use in academic areas, a.t. are employed for a variety of vocational, professional, and diagnostic purposes.

Achilles reflex a reflex action of the ankle when the Achilles tendon is lightly tapped. Also called **ankle jerk**.

achluophobia a morbid fear of night or darkness. Also called **nictophobia; nyctophobia; noctiphobia; scotophobia; night phobia**. Also see FEAR OF DARKNESS.

-achondr-; -achondrio-; -achondro- a combining form relating to insufficient or defective cartilage.

achondroplasia a form of autosomal-dominant dwarfism in which the bones derived from cartilage develop at a slower rate than the bones derived from connective tissue. This results in an enlarged cranial vault and abnormally high forehead. Motor development of infants with this disorder may be slow and the individual may or may not be mentally retarded. About one-third of one group studied had subnormal intelligence. Also called **achondroplastic dwarfism**. Also see DWARFISM.

ACh receptors nerve receptors that react to acetylcholine or substances that have the same physiological effects as the parasympathomimetic agent.

achromatic-chromatic scale a scale of color values ranging through the chromatic spectrum of hues and including the achromatic shades of black through gray to white.

achromatic colors colors without saturation and hue, that is, black, white, and gray. Compare CHROMATIC COLORS.

achromatic response the reaction of a subject to a visual test in which color is not a factor, as in responses to the Rorschach inkblots that involve variations in shading or texture but not color, or giving noncolor responses to inkblots that do involve color.

achromatism a rare condition marked by the inability to distinguish any colors. Everything is seen in different shades of gray. The major cause of the disorder is a congenital lack of retinal cone cells, often associated with albinism, although it may also result from injury or from optic neuritis, lead poisoning, or carbon disulfide poisoning. Also called **achromatopsia; monochromatism; total color blindness**. Also see DICHROMATISM; TRICHROMATISM.

acid a slang term for LSD. See PSYCHEDELICS.

-acid- a combining form relating to (a) acid, literally something that is sour or sharp to the taste (introduced into English by Francis Bacon in 1626, from Latin *acidus*, "sour"), (b) a pointed object or needle (from Greek *ake*, "point").

acidity: See HYDROGEN-ION CONCENTRATION.

-acidno- a combining form meaning feeble, weak.

acidosis a disorder caused by a loss of the normal acid-base balance of body chemistry resulting in an increase in the level of acidity in the blood and tissues or a depletion of alkaline reserves. The condition results in neurologic abnormalities such as muscle twitching, disorientation, and coma. Heart arrythmias also may be an effect. Compare ALKALOSIS.

Ackerman, Nathan W. Russian-born American psychoanalyst, 1908–71. His work was concerned with the position of the child in the family and family problems. See FAMILY THERAPY.

acme /ak′mē/ a summit; the highest point of sexual pleasure (Greek, "point"). Also called **summa libido**.

acmesthesia a form of paresthesia in which a cutaneous stimulus normally sensed as pain is perceived instead as touch or pressure. Also called **acuesthesia**.

acoasm = ACOUSMA.

aconite: See SORCERY DRUGS.

aconuresis = ENURESIS.

acoria /-kō′-/ an excessive appetite, marked by gluttony or greediness rather than persistent hunger. See BULIMIA.

Acosta, José de Spanish Jesuit missionary and geographer, 1539–1600. See ACOSTA'S SYNDROME.

Acosta's syndrome a form of altitude sickness resulting from lack of oxygen at high altitudes. Symptoms include dizziness, blue skin, weakness, and impaired mental processes. Also called **mountain-climber's syndrome; Acosta's disease; D'Acosta's syndrome**.

-acou- a combining form relating to hearing.

acousma an auditory sensation that is perceived in the absence of a stimulus. The a. often is heard as a buzzing, ringing, or roaring sound. In the absence of an organic cause, it may be considered an elementary auditory hallucination. Also called **acoasm; akoasm.**

acoustical resonance an effect of extension and intensification of sound frequencies received as vibrations by the middle- and inner-ear structures. The resonant frequencies are a step in the conversion of external sound waves to the sounds perceived in the brain and determine the range of hearing. A.r. also may refer to the resonant effect of one's own vocal sounds contributed by sinuses and other cavities in the skull.

acoustic irritability hypersensitivity to auditory stimulation, a characteristic of traumatic neurosis.

acoustic-mnestic aphasia a form of aphasia due to lesions in the central portions of the left temporal area or deep portions of the temporal cortex. It is marked by difficulty in recalling word lists, comprehension and reproduction of long sentences, comprehension of words, and inability to name objects. Also called **acoustico-amnestic aphasia.**

acoustic nerve = STATOACOUSTIC NERVE.

acoustic neurinoma a tumorous growth either benign or malignant in the region of the eighth cranial nerve between the cochlea and the brainstem, which may cause a sensorineural hearing loss through pressure exerted on the nerve trunk.

acousticoamnestic aphasia = ACOUSTIC-MNESTIC APHASIA.

acousticophobia a morbid fear of noise. Also spelled **akousticophobia.** Also see PHONOPHOBIA.

acoustic papilla = ORGAN OF CORTI.

acoustic pressure the waves of air pressure that are of sufficient intensity and frequency to be perceived as sounds. The pressure variations of the air required to produce acoustic effects are very small compared with atmospheric pressure, which is equivalent to one million dynes per square centimeter. A very loud undesirable sound may represent an a.p. change of one thousand dynes per square centimeter. A.p. of a sound that is just below the normal human threshold of audibility would be measured at about 1/1,000 of a dyne per square centimeter. The human range of perceivable a.p., therefore, is approximately one million to one.

acoustic radiation a band of fibers that function as a relay in the auditory pathway from the thalamus to the cerebral cortex.

acoustic reflex an automatic reaction to the intensity of a sound. The a.r. frequently is employed in routine hearing tests involving sounds of different frequencies. Kinds of acoustic reflexes include blink, condition-oriented, Moro, stretch, and sucking reflexes. An infant's blinking may be considered a positive response to a low-decibel hearing-test sound.

acoustics the science of sound including the production, transmission, and effects of mechanical vibrations and waves in any medium, whether audible or not.

acoustic spectrum = SOUND SPECTRUM.

acoustic trauma a form of sensorineural hearing impairment resulting from exposure to intense noise. Even brief periods of exposure to jet-aircraft engine noise, gunfire, and heavy drills may cause permanent damage to the nerve fibers in the cochlea.

acquiescent-response set the tendency on the part of subjects in an experiment to agree with statements of attitude regardless of their content. Acquiescence or yea-saying can distort the results of personality inventories and attitude scales.

acquired agraphia: See AGRAPHIA.

acquired drive any drive that is learned, as opposed to an inborn drive such as hunger.

acquired folie morale /fōlē'mōräl'/ a form of schizophrenia marked by antisocial behavior, the psychotic manifestations appearing as delusions, auditory hallucinations, stupor, or agitation.

acquisition any new type of response, idea, or information that is added to the individual's repertoire.

acquisitiveness the tendency, impulse, or desire to acquire and accumulate objects or possessions. The term should be distinguished from hoarding. Also called **acquisitive instinct.**

acquisitive spirit the drive to possess and accumulate money, property, or objects of personal or social value, as in collecting coins or figurines. See ANAL CHARACTER; COLLECTING MANIA; HOARDING CHARACTER.

acrai an Arabian term that is synonymous with nymphomania and satyriasis.

acrasia a pathological absence of self-control; extreme intemperance. Also called **acrasy.**

-acro- a combining form relating to (a) the extremities, (b) intensity, (c) height.

acroanesthesia an absence of sensitivity in the extremities as a result of disease or an aftereffect of anesthesia. Also see ACROPARESTHESIA. Compare ACROESTHESIA.

acrocentric chromosome a chromosome in which the centromere is near one end, making one arm of the replicating chromosome shorter than the other. An a.c. may be much smaller than others and may occur as additional genetic material in disorders such as cat's-eye syndrome.

acrocephalopolysyndactyly = CARPENTER'S SYNDROME.

acrocephalosyndactyly = APERT'S SYNDROME.

acrocephalosyndactyly, Type VI = PFEIFFER'S SYNDROME.

acrocephalosyndactyly, Type III = CHOTZEN'S SYNDROME.

acrocephaly a high, pointed condition of the skull. Also called **oxycephaly**.

acrocinesia the excessive motion or movement that is sometimes observed in hysteria or the manic phase of bipolar disorder. Also called **acrocinesis**.

acrocyanosis a bluish coloration of the skin of the extremities sometimes observed in schizophrenia patients, particularly asthenic types, due to inadequate blood circulation.

acrodynia /-din'-/ or /-dīn'-/ a pinkish coloration of the skin that occurs in infants and small children suffering from mercury poisoning. A. also is associated with peripheral neuropathy and cerebral damage. Also called **pink disease; erythredema; erythromelalgia**.

acroesthesia an abnormal sensitivity to stimuli applied to the extremities. Compare ACROANESTHESIA; ACROPARESTHESIA.

acrohypothermia an abnormal coolness of the skin of the extremities found in certain schizophrenia patients, particularly those with acrocyanosis.

acromania an obsolete term for violent incurable insanity.

acromegaloid-hypertelorism-pectus carinatum syndrome a congenital condition, believed to be hereditary, marked by short stature, mental retardation, hypertelorism, and skeletal anomalies including an enlarged head and a deformed sternum. Only males are known to be affected. All show slow psychomotor development and IQs estimated in the 20s.

acromegaloid personality a personality pattern observed in a large proportion of patients with acromegaly. The chief features are frequent changes in mood, impulsiveness, temper outbursts, impatience, and, in advanced cases, loss of initiative, egocentricity, and somnolence.

acromegaly an abnormal enlargement of the skeletal extremities, such as the arms, legs, and parts of the skull. The condition is rare and usually occurs in adults whose normal bone growth has already stopped. The cause is a pituitary-gland abnormality that results in hypersecretion of the growth hormone. In growing children, whose bones are still developing, the effect is known as GIGANTISM. See this entry.

acromicria a type of underdevelopment marked by abnormally small fingers, toes, or facial features. The term is sometimes applied to Down's syndrome.

acroparesthesia a feeling of numbness, tingling, or other abnormal sensation in the extremities. Kinds of a. include Nothnagel's a., which is accompanied by circulatory disorders, and Schultze's a., marked by peripheral-nerve irritability but without circulatory abnormalities. Also see ACROANESTHESIA. Compare ACROESTHESIA.

acrophobia a morbid fear of high places. In psychoanalysis, the fear of falling from heights may represent fear of punishment for forbidden wishes or impulses. Also called **hyposophobia; height phobia**.

acrosome a hoodlike formation on the front end of a SPERMATOZOON. See this entry.

ACT = ATROPINE-COMA THERAPY.

ACT Assessment a college admission program developed by E.F. Lindquist, comprising four *a*cademic *c*ollege *t*ests: English Usage, Mathematics Usage, Social Studies Reading, and Natural Science Reading, each of which provides a set of work samples of college work that focuses on the basic intellectual skills required for satisfactory performance in college. Also called **American College Testing Program**.

act ending the termination of an act that was performed to relieve tension. Normally, a.e. follows tension release or satiation, but in cases of mental disorder, such as childhood schizophrenia, the a.e. function is impaired so that the action, e.g., eating, continues beyond satiation.

ACTH = ADRENOCORTICOTROPHIC HORMONE.

act-habit a habit or personality trait rooted in cultural or environmental influences, e.g., overprotectiveness, or a scientific attitude.

actin one of two muscle-fiber proteins that function together to produce contractions and relaxations of muscle groups. The second protein is **myosin**. The protein team sometimes is identified as **actomyosin**. Also see MUSCLE CONTRACTION.

acting in a form of resistance in which the patient discharges repressed wishes during the analytic hour through actions instead of words, e.g., by getting up and walking around the room (Eidelberg).

acting out the uncontrolled release of impulses, usually sexual or aggressive, to gain relief from tension or anxiety. The term is also applied to the psychotherapeutic release of repressed feelings, as in movement therapy or psychodrama. In addition, a.o. is frequently applied to antisocial or delinquent behavior in general.

actinic keratosis: See KERATOSIS.

actinomycin-D a member of the actinomycin family of antibiotics, several of which also are used in the treatment of cancer as well as in the control of bacterial infections.

action current = ACTION POTENTIAL.

action group a task-oriented group engaged in accomplishing a specific goal or goals that are intended to produce an effect on a group, organization, business, institution, or social unit. An a.g. may be contrasted to a therapy group, personal-growth group, or study group. Whereas a therapy group attempts to change individuals in their interpersonal relations, an a.g. seeks, in some manner, to have a direct impact on and achieve a modification of the environment.

action-group process activities undertaken by an organized group to solve specific problems or attain specific objectives, such as improving interpersonal relations in an industrial plant or campaigning for a nonpolluted environment.

action-instrument in the two-word stage of language development, a verbal expression indicating knowledge of the use of instruments, as in "eat-fork."

action interpretation the nonverbal reaction of a therapist to acts or remarks by a patient.

action-location in the two-word stage of language development, an expression indicating location of an action, as in "sleep-bed."

action painting = TACHISME.

action potential the change in electric potential caused by physiological activity, such as the contraction of a muscle or the transmission of a nerve impulse. Also called **action current**.

action-recipient in the two-word stage of language development, an indication of the recipient of an action, as in "cookie-me."

action research a form of scientific study or research directed toward a practical goal, usually an improvement in a particular process or system in contrast to purely experimental research. In industry, a.r. is a group technique or T-group that seeks to develop leadership skills, communication skills, and greater self-awareness and cooperation among executives.

action stream: See STREAM OF ACTION.

action system a term used to identify the body's mechanism for fulfilling a need or desire. The term was introduced by Kardiner to explain the cause of traumatic neuroses, which he believed were due to damage of an a.s.

activated sleep an alternative term for REM sleep, characterized by rapid conjugate eye movements during D-state sleep.

activation the process of alerting an organ or body system for action, particularly arousal of one organ or system by another. See RETICULAR ACTIVATING SYSTEM.

activation pattern in EEG interpretation, a suppression of alpha waves and shift to low-voltage rapid activity when the subject opens his eyes to view a displayed object. The alpha desynchronization may be localized or general as measured in various cerebral areas, and transient or sustained.

activation theory of emotion the concept that any emotion may be located over a spectrum that ranges from no activity, as in sleep, to a maximum, as observed in violent action.

activator a substance that stimulates the activity of a second substance, particularly a chemical that stimulates an inactive enzyme to become functional.

active analysis = ACTIVE ANALYTIC PSYCHOTHERAPY.

active analytic psychotherapy the therapeutic approach of Wilhelm Stekel in which the analyst gives more attention to the intrapsychic conflicts in the patient's present life than to exploring early childhood experiences. In dealing with these conflicts, the therapist, Stekel believed, should play an active role by (a) intervening in the process of free association to discuss important issues, (b) attacking the patient's resistances directly, (c) offering advice and exhortation at appropriate times, and (d) helping the patient interpret his dreams intuitively in the light of current attitudes and problems. Through these methods, and by avoiding many of the Freudian steps such as analysis of the transference, he sought to shorten the therapeutic process to six months or less. Also called **active analysis**. See STEKEL.

active castration complex the ideas and emotions associated with the fear of losing the penis, as distinguished from the **passive castration complex** in which the individual has a castration wish or believes castration has already occurred.

active concretization the process of transforming anxieties into concrete form, as in the paranoid schizophrenic's tendency to express his feeling that the whole world is hostile to him in the form of a hallucination that bad odors are emanating from his body, or that derogatory voices are emanating from the air conditioner.

active-daydream technique a form of imagery therapy advocated by Jung. The patient is encouraged to allow autonomous images to appear, and then react to them as if they were real, e.g., by hiding from a threatening figure, or by talking to it. Interacting with unconscious material would, Jung believed, have a more beneficial effect than passively accepting and watching it.

active fantasying a therapy technique in which the patient spontaneously describes his imagery which the analyst studies for clues to sources of inner conflicts.

active immunity: See IMMUNITY.

active introversion a type of introversion, or inward-directed libido, that is willed by the subject.

actively aggressive reaction type a personality-trait disturbance characterized by a pattern of overt hostility and resentment, irritability, low frustration tolerance, rebellion against authority, argumentativeness, and in some cases violent behavior. This DSM-I category corresponds closely to the DSM-III categories of "conduct disorder, undersocialized, aggressive," "conduct disorder, socialized, aggressive among children and adolescents," and "antisocial personality disorder among adolescents and adults."

active mode of consciousness: See CONSCIOUS PROCESSES.

active negativism active resistance to demands or suggestions. E.g., a catatonic patient may remain mute when asked a simple question, or continue to stand up when he is invited to sit down to lunch.

active recreation a form of recreational therapy, e.g., dancing, in which the patient is an active participant, as opposed to passive recreation.

active therapist a psychotherapist who does not remain neutral or anonymous, as in orthodox psychoanalysis, and does not hesitate to express opinions and interpretations, make suggestions and recommendations, and even, on occasion, issue injunctions and prohibitions. See ACTIVE ANALYTIC PSYCHOTHERAPY; PASSIVE THERAPIST.

active therapy a brief form of psychotherapy in which the therapist actively intervenes in the patient's mental and actual life by giving his own interpretations or by urging the patient to master anxiety by facing dreaded situations directly. See FERENCZI.

active transport the movement of ions across a cell membrane by a mechanism other than simple osmosis. E.g., the movement may depend upon a special affinity between ions, a metabolic reaction, or some other energy-consuming process. A.t. is presumed to be involved in the movement of sodium and potassium ions across a membrane of a nerve cell. Compare PASSIVE TRANSPORT.

active vocabulary the working vocabulary, or actual number of words used by an individual. Compare PASSIVE VOCABULARY.

activism the theory or practice of direct, positive, vigorous action or involvement to achieve an end, in particular a political goal. In philosophy, a. is the doctrine that any relationship between thought and reality is characterized by continuous activity on the part of the mind rather than passive receptivity.

activities of daily living the normal functional actions of people, such as getting out of bed in the morning, dressing, eating, using the toilet and bath, performing other personal grooming tasks, getting into bed, and using chairs and other household or working objects. While taken for granted by normal persons, disabled individuals may be required to relearn such activities with new techniques, e.g., with a wheelchair, walker, or special utensils. Abbrev.: ADL.

activity deprivation lack of opportunity for physical activity, e.g., during incarceration in a small cell or extended confinement in a cardiac unit. A.d. generates an intense need to move about, and a high degree of frustration. For this reason it has been used as a form of torture. See ACTIVITY DRIVE.

activity drive the general urge for bodily activity as expressed in a spontaneous need to move about or to engage in some other activity. Many psychologists believe this drive is basic and unlearned, since animals such as rats that have been conditioned to press a bar for a food reward will continue to press it when their only reward is an opportunity to run; and humans become pent-up when deprived of the opportunity to move about freely. The satisfaction of the activity drive may therefore be pleasurable in itself. See ACTIVITY DEPRIVATION.

activity-group therapy a form of group therapy developed by S.R. Slavson for children and young adolescents. The emphasis is on revising faulty attitudes and reactions, such as aggressiveness or timidity, through active participation in hobby groups conducted in a permissive, nonthreatening atmosphere. The children are given an opportunity to release tensions and feelings of hostility, test out new ways of relating to others, and gradually experience the satisfactions of creative effort and normal give and take.

activity-interview group psychotherapy an analytic technique applied by S.R. Slavson to children in the latency period. Hobbies and recreational activities are used to stimulate communication and the expression of conflicts and fantasies. During the process, the therapist asks questions which encourage the children to understand how their immediate problems such as fears are affecting their behavior and attitudes; e.g., a child may learn that though his hostile feelings may be directed at his parents, they are really meant for a younger brother or sister.

Activity, Interest, Opinion: See PSYCHOGRAPHICS.

activity level the amount of movement occurring at a given time. Among humans, the a.l. tends to be low during a depressive state (except for the agitated type) and high during a manic episode or in the hyperkinetic syndrome. Among animals, it rises when they get hungry or thirsty or are denied activity for short periods, and decreases when these needs are satisfied.

activity log a diary kept by an experiment director or the experimental subject of hourly activities in various environmental settings. A typical a.l. includes data regarding the location of the subject by time period, e.g., at home, at work, or traveling, and whether the time is spent alone or with family, friends, or work associates. An a.l. as a method of obtaining data is superior to interviews based on a subject's memory. Also see ACTIVITY RECORD.

activity-play therapy a controlled play technique developed by J.C. Solomon (1948) in which the child is given a set of dolls and encouraged to express and explore his feelings about them, including sadness, guilt, and hostility, on the theory that he will then become less afraid of these emotions and will no longer repress them.

activity pleasure the satisfaction derived from activity in and of itself. The term is frequently used to denote the pleasure that infants and children experience in sheer physical movement and manipulation. By extension, a.p. includes intellectual activities that satisfy the child's curiosity.

activity quotient a measure of a subject's emotionality as determined by the ratio of verbs to adjectives used in his communications.

activity record the written or recorded data detailing a student's extracurricular involvement in school activities, clubs, or special projects. Also see ACTIVITY LOG.

activity system = BEHAVIOR SYSTEM.

activity therapy in psychiatry, a form of adjunctive therapy in which patients are encouraged to engage in various activities such as arts and crafts, exercises, music, and dramatics groups. Activity programs are designed to keep interest alive, increase self-esteem, and prevent patients from lapsing into a state of apathy and passivity. See SOCIAL-BREAKDOWN SYNDROME; TOTAL-PUSH THERAPY.

activity wheel a revolving drum that turns by the weight of an animal running inside. The a.w. may be used to exercise the animal or in various energy-related experiments such as endurance tests while the animal is deprived of a nutrient.

actomyosin: See ACTIN.

act psychology a philosophical concept of the psychology of consciousness proposed by Franz Brentano, who held that act and content of psychological processes were separate functions, e.g., the act of seeing color leads to a perception of the visual content, or image. However, acts, not contents, are the proper subject of psychology, in contrast to Wundt's emphasis on introspection and conscious contents.

actualization the process of mobilizing one's potentialities and expressing them in concrete form. See INDIVIDUATION; SELF-ACTUALIZATION.

actual neurosis a neurosis which, according to Freud, stems from current sexual frustrations, such as coitus interruptus, forced abstinence, or incomplete gratification, as contrasted with psychoneurosis, which stems from experiences in infancy or childhood. The term was applied primarily to anxiety neurosis, hypochondriasis, and neurasthenia, but is rarely used today.

actuarial statistical, as opposed to clinical. This term suggests the counting up, as by a clerk or actuary, of prior instances in order to estimate likelihood or risk of a particular outcome.

acuesthesia = ACMESTHESIA.

acuity grating a device used to measure the visual acuity of a subject. The a.g. consists of alternating black and white lines spaced very closely together, testing the ability of the subject to determine the boundaries. Also see VISUAL ACUITY.

aculalia nonsensical speech associated with the lack of comprehension of written or spoken language. A. is a form of aphasia resulting from lesions in the left temporal lobe. It is similar to jargon aphasia. See WERNICKE'S APHASIA.

acupuncture a technique of relieving disorders and/or producing anesthesia in certain body areas or organs by piercing specific places on the skin with fine needles (from Latin *acus*, "needle"). A has been practiced in China for several thousand years to relieve pain, to induce anesthesia for surgical procedures, and as a form of therapy. It is based on an Oriental concept that "meridians" or pathways of energy flow between places on the skin (and perhaps peripheral nerves) and the body's organ systems.

-acusia a combining form relating to hearing.

acute denoting a state of being sharp, keen, or very sensitive, e.g., an a. pain, or a. sense of hearing; also, denoting a sudden, short, intense attack of illness.

acute affective reflex a term introduced by Kretschmer to describe the initial involuntary emotional reaction (usually tremors) to a severe stress.

acute alcoholic myopathy a condition of severe pain, tenderness, and swelling of the muscles accompanied by cramps and muscular weakness, that develops after a period of heavy drinking. The effects may be general or focused on one body area. In some cases, muscle fibers may undergo necrosis. Recovery may require several weeks to several months.

acute anxiety a sudden feeling of dread and apprehension precipitated by a threatening situation such as an examination or court hearing. The feeling usually subsides as soon as the situation is over. See PERFORMANCE ANXIETY.

acute anxiety attack = ANXIETY ATTACK.

acute ascending paralysis: See LANDRY'S PARALYSIS.

acute brain disorder an organic brain syndrome resulting from temporary, reversible impairment of brain-tissue functioning, ranging from mild changes in mood to acute delirium, and involving more or less serious personality and behavior disturbances. In DSM-I, this category included syndromes associated with intracranial infection, systemic infection, drug or poison intoxication, alcohol intoxication, brain trauma, circulatory disturbance, convulsive disorder, metabolic disturbance, intracranial neoplasm, and diseases of unknown cause such as multiple sclerosis. See ORGANIC BRAIN SYNDROMES; ORGANIC MENTAL DISORDERS.

acute cerebellar ataxia; acute cerebral tremor = ZAPPERT'S SYNDROME.

acute confusional state a severe stress reaction typically experienced by adolescents who are required to face an unfamiliar situation such as going away to college. The disorder is usually precipitated by a minor frustration, and consists of intense anger followed by inability to concentrate, feelings of alienation and loneliness, depersonalization, and despondency—all of which subside as the individual adapts to the situation.

acute delusional psychosis a reactive psychosis, particularly a schizophrenic episode which has no strong evidence of a genetic link, and which has a favorable prognosis, in contrast to nuclear or process schizophrenia. Disorders of this kind are also known as **bouffées délirantes** /bŏŏfā′dālēräNt′/ (French, "delirious outbursts"), **schizophrenic states, pseudoschizophrenias, cycloid psychoses**, and **acute schizophrenic reactions**. Also see ACUTE SCHIZOPHRENIC EPISODE; CYCLIC ILLNESS.

acute depression a state of depression characterized by marked retardation in thought, speech, and general activity along with extreme feelings of guilt, isolation, futility, and unreality as well as delusions, loss of interest in the outside world, utter pessimism, and suicide attempts. See MANIC-DEPRESSIVE REACTION.

acute dystonia an acute form of dystonia, a lack of normal muscle tone.

acute gout: See GOUT.

acute hallucinosis sudden onset of hallucinations resulting from alcohol or drug intoxication or a traumatic event. The condition usually subsides within weeks.

acute head trauma: See HEAD TRAUMA.

acute lymphoblastic leukemia: See LEUKEMIA.

acute mania a mood disorder seen in the manic phase of manic-depressive reaction and characterized by an extremely unstable euphoric mood of grandiose optimism with hyperactivity, excessively rapid thought and speech, completely uninhibited and un-self-conscious behavior, and flight of ideas. Hypomania and hypermania are the less and more intense expressions of the manic phase. See MANIC-DEPRESSIVE REACTION.

acute myeloblastic leukemia: See LEUKEMIA.

acute otitis media: See OTITIS MEDIA.

acute paranoid disorder a paranoid disorder of less than six months duration, which usually develops suddenly in individuals who have experienced drastic environmental changes, e.g., immigrants, refugees, POWs, inductees, or people leaving home for the first time. See PARANOID DISORDERS. (DSM-III)

acute peritonitis: See PERITONITIS.

acute polyneuritis the severe inflammation of a number of spinal nerves at the same time, accompanied by pain, paralysis, and muscle atrophy. Causes may include drug reactions, viral or other infections, and metabolic disorders, e.g., vitamin-B deficiencies. A form of infectious polyneuritis is the Guillain-Barré syndrome that follows a viral infection. Also see POLYNEURITIS.

acute posttraumatic stress disorder: See POSTTRAUMATIC STRESS DISORDER.

acute preparation an experimental animal that must be destroyed at the end of a study for humane reasons.

acute psychotic break a sudden loss of contact with reality accompanied by florid symptoms of severe mental disorder, such as hallucinations, delusions, incoherence, and disorganized, violent, or catatonic behavior.

acute schizophrenic episode a schizophrenic episode of sudden onset and usually short duration. Episodes of this kind may occur in the form of an acute psychotic break among men and women with no previous history of overt mental disorder. The episode, however, usually follows an emotional upheaval precipitated by a loss or separation. The patient isolates himself or herself and experiences a rapid flight of ideas and insights of extraordinary intensity, and within hours or days may become confused, disoriented, delusional, and hallucinatory.

acute schizophrenic reactions: See ACUTE DELUSIONAL PSYCHOSIS.

acute shock psychosis a wartime psychiatric disorder in which the patient becomes unconscious and lacks sensitivity to pain and external stimuli. The eyeballs are rolled upward and outward and the eyelids flutter. The condition, which is temporary, usually occurs in combat situations.

acute stress reaction a severe emotional reaction to extreme environmental stress, such as a natural catastrophe, bankruptcy, divorce, or combat experience. In DSM I (1952) stress disorders were categorized as "transient situational personality disorder"; in DSM II (1968) they were termed "transient situational disturbances"; and in DSM III, the less severe conditions were categorized as ADJUSTMENT DISORDER, and the more severe, as POSTTRAUMATIC STRESS DISORDER. See these entries. Also called **acute situational reaction**.

acute tolerance a type of tolerance that can develop rapidly and in response to a small dose of a particular drug. Barbiturates may produce a.t., as indicated by blood levels of the drug that may be higher hours after administration than immediately following administration.

acute traumatic disorder a temporary impairment of brain functions associated with a severe blow to the head. If a concussion with loss of consciousness occurs, the symptoms are usually confusion, headache and disorientation, as well as a partial or total amnésia for the event. In cases involving contusion (displacement and bruising of the brain), unconsciousness may last for hours or days followed by clouding of consciousness, restlessness, and often delirium. If an actual rupture of brain tissue, or laceration, occurs, the symptoms are similar but more severe and may be followed by permanent intellectual and motor defects.

acute undifferentiated schizophrenia: See UNDIFFERENTIATED SCHIZOPHRENIA.

acute viral hepatitis: See HEPATITIS.

-ad- a combining form meaning to, on the outside,

or toward the middle. (The **-al** of adjectives is replaced by **-ad** to form adverbs.)

Adamantiades, B. French physician, fl. 1931. See BEHCET'S DISEASE (also called **Adamantiades-Behcet syndrome**).

adaptability capacity to make appropriate responses to changed or changing situations; ability to modify or adjust one's behavior in meeting different circumstances or different people.

adaptation in general, the modification of an organism in structure or function to accommodate its ability to survive in a new or different environment. More specifically, a sense organ may undergo transient a. to changing conditions, as when the pupil of the eye adjusts to dim or bright light. For psychological a., see SENSORY A.; SOCIAL A.; A.-LEVEL THEORY.

adaptational approach a psychodynamic approach developed by S. Rado, which avoids the orthodox analytic emphasis on childhood experience and the role of the therapist as a substitute parent, and focuses instead on the nature and development of the patient's maladaptive behavior, and the steps he should take in the direction of new, more effective patterns. Also called **adaptational psychodynamics**.

adaptation-level theory Helson's theory that the conditions to which one is presently adapted form a standard against which new stimuli are evaluated. E.g., the traffic in a small town may seem heavy to the farmer and light to the city dweller; and Beethoven's music sounded cacophonous to audiences of his time, but seems melodious to nearly all of us. A common abbreviation of adaptation level is **AL**.

adaptation mechanisms according to Piaget, biological adaptation through the interplay between the assimilation of data of experience and modification of the organism to accommodate new data into its mental framework. See ADJUSTMENT PROCESSES.

adaptation period a period of time during which a subject becomes accustomed to instrumentation or experimental apparatus.

adaptation syndrome = GENERAL A.S.

adaptation time the period of time from the start of a stimulus through the end of the effect in the sense organ stimulated.

adaptive act the process whereby an organism makes appropriate responses to stimuli needed for an adjustment to the environment.

adaptive approach a psychological approach built around the concept that psychological reactions must be viewed in their relationship to external reality, and emphasizing the principle that man and society must constantly adapt and readapt to each other in the interest of survival. Horney and Erikson are prime exponents of this approach.

adaptive behavior any behavior that enables the individual to adjust to the environment appropriately and effectively. See ORIENTATION.

Adaptive Behavior Scale a test developed by the American Association on Mental Deficiency for assessing the effectiveness of mental retardates in coping with the demands of the environment. Observers provide information on ten behavior domains, such as independent functioning, language development, physical development, and socialization; and also on maladaptive behavior such as withdrawal, hyperactivity, and destructive behavior.

adaptive delinquency: See DYSSOCIAL REACTION.

adaptive hypothesis in H. Hartmann's version of ego psychology, the view that the functioning of the primary autonomous ego is to cope with an "average expectable environment" through perception, memory, and motility.

adaptive processes = ADJUSTMENT PROCESSES.

adaptive skills activities that require self-management, such as controlling impulses, willingness to accept criticism and direction, and an ability to adjust to a new environment and to learn new things.

adaptive testing a testing technique designed to adjust to the response characteristics of individual examinees (usually applied with the aid of a computer). E.g., all examinations may start with an item of intermediate difficulty, and if the subject's response is correct, he or she will be routed upward to the next more difficult item, and if the response is wrong, will be moved downward to the next easier item.

addiction psychological and in some cases physiological dependence on the use of alcohol, narcotic drugs, tobacco, or other substances. The criteria for addiction are a compulsive craving leading to persistent use, a need to increase the dose due to increasing tolerance, and acute withdrawal, or abstinence, symptoms if the substance is sharply reduced or withdrawn. In psychiatry, the term a. is being replaced by the term SUBSTANCE DEPENDENCE. See this entry. Also see PHYSIOLOGICAL DEPENDENCE.

addictive alcoholism = GAMMA ALCOHOLISM.

addictive personality a hypothetical personality pattern characterized by a strong tendency to become psychologically and physically dependent on one or more substances, such as alcohol, heroin, amphetamines, tobacco, or barbiturates. Such individuals develop a craving for the substance involved, as well as a tendency to use it in increased amounts. See SUBSTANCE-USE DISORDERS.

Addison, Thomas English physician, 1793–1860. See ADDISON'S DISEASE; ADDISON-BIERMER ANEMIA; ADRENOCORTICAL INSUFFICIENCY; ANEMIA; ATYPICAL OR MIXED ORGANIC BRAIN SYNDROME.

Addison-Biermer anemia a form of chronic megaloblastic anemia involving vitamin-B_{12} deficiency and associated with gastric mucosa atrophy in stomach diseases. The condition often is a cause of neurologic disorders, including loss of the senses of taste and smell, ataxia, incoordination, apathy, irritability, and psychoses. Also called **Biermer's anemia; Biermer-Ehrlich anemia; pernicious anemia; Addison's anemia**.

Addison's disease a disorder caused by a malfunction of the adrenal glands resulting in a deficiency of adrenal hormones. A major symptom is muscle fatigue with trembling, due in part to an inability to maintain a stable level of blood sugar for energy. Mental effects include depression, anxiety, and mood changes. The disease is named for Thomas Addison, the 19th-century English physician who first described the disease.

additive mixture the process and effect of combining colored lights, as manifested in new, composite colors; e.g., in stage lighting, red and green spotlights are blended to form yellow. The color in television is another example of a.m. See COLOR MIXTURE.

additive scale a scale with all points distributed equally so that a result can be obtained by addition, e.g., a metric ruler.

adducted aphonia a loss of voice as a result of contractions of the adductor muscles that move the vocal cords.

adductor a muscle that draws toward the median plane of the body or the axial line of a limb or digit. The **a. pollicis muscle** draws the thumb toward the palm of the hand.

ademonia = AGITATED DEPRESSION.

ademosyne /-mos'inē/ an obsolete term for nostalgia.

-aden-; -adeno- a combining form relating to glands.

adenine molecule /ad'ənēn/ a purine compound that is present in the nuclei of plant and animal cells. Adenine and guanine are the essential components of the nucleic acids, DNA and RNA. When adenine is metabolized, the end product is uric acid.

adenohypophysis /-pof'-/ the anterior lobe of the hypophysis, or pituitary gland. The a. secretes adrenocorticotropin, follicle-stimulating hormone, growth hormone, luteinizing hormone, prolactin, and thyrotropin. Compare NEUROHYPOPHYSIS.

adenoid type an individual whose pharyngeal tonsil or adenoid is pathologically enlarged and associated with constitutional anomalies such as cretinism, deaf-mutism, or oxycephaly.

adenoma sebaceum a type of skin lesion that develops as a benign tumor of the sebaceous glands, often appearing in a pattern of multiple yellowish papules on the face. A.s. often occurs as a butterfly rash on the bridge of the nose in cases of TUBEROUS SCLEROSIS. See this entry.

adenosine /əden'-/ $C_{10}H_{13}N_5O_4$—a naturally occurring chemical of most living cells, consisting of the adenine molecule of the RNA base and a sugar molecule. It functions as an energy source in metabolic activities at the cellular level. In combination with three phosphate units, a. forms a high-energy bond that is easily split when a cell requires quick energy and is associated with nerve-impulse transmissions.

adenosine 3′, 5′ -monophosphate = CYCLIC AMP.

adenosine triphosphate a nucleotide compound present in all living cells and the source of chemical energy for muscle contractions. Abbrev.: **ATP**.

adenyl cyclase /ad'-/ a form of adenylic acid that functions as an enzyme acting on adenosine triphosphate to form cyclic AMP, which in turn functions as a "second messenger" in hormone functions. Also called **adenylate cyclase**.

adenylic acid /-nil'-/ a ribonucleic-acid derivative of the purine base adenine. A.a. is a precursor of adenosine triphosphate and plays an important role in such functions as muscle contraction, carbohydrate metabolism, and fermentation. Also see ADENOSINE TRIPHOSPHATE.

adephagia an obsolete term for bulimia.

adequate stimulus a stimulus of sufficient potential to trigger an impulse that excites a receptor. See SPIKE POTENTIAL; ALL-OR-NONE LAW; GRADED POTENTIALS.

ADH = ANTIDIURETIC HORMONE.

adhesive otitis media a condition resulting from prolonged presence of fluid in the middle ear despite elimination of infection with antibiotics. The remaining fluid thickens, becomes gluelike and interferes with the movement of the ossicles.

adiadochokinesis the loss of ability to perform rapid alternating movements, as in fanning oneself, due to cerebellar disorder (from Greek *a-* and *diadochos*, "successive," and *kinesis*, "movement"). Also called **adiadokokinesis; adiadokokinesia**.

Adie, William John English neurologist, 1886–1935. See ADIE'S SYNDROME; TONIC PUPIL OF ADIE.

Adie-Holmes syndrome = ADIE'S SYNDROME.

adience /ād'-/ movement or action toward a stimulus. **Adient behavior** is approaching behavior or behavior designed to sustain or prolong contact with a particular stimulus. Compare ABIENCE.

Adie's syndrome a neurologic disorder involving both ocular and tendon reflexes. The ocular effects include very slow changes between near and far vision, slow or absent response of dilated pupils to light, and accommodation difficulties. Ankle and knee-jerk reflexes, and various other tendon reflexes, usually are absent. Also called **Adie–Holmes syndrome; Weill's syndrome; myotonic pupillary reaction**.

-adip-; -adipo- a combining form relating to fat, or meaning fatty (from Modern Latin *adiposus*, "fatty").

adipocytes /ad'-/ the special cells that store body fat. A far larger number of a. are present in the bodies of obese persons than in those of normal weight. The level of fat cells is determined by genetic factors and nutritional patterns in infancy and childhood; a high level is considered a predisposing factor to obesity since this level remains constant in adulthood. Dieting reduces the size but not the number of a.

adipose /ad'-/ the fat in the cells of a. tissue.

adiposogenital dystrophy = FRÖHLICH'S SYNDROME.

adipsia an abnormal avoidance of water or beverages, usually because of an absence of thirst A. is associated with lesions in the ventrolateral hypothalamus.

adjective check list a psychological testing technique in which a list of adjectives is constructed and subjects are required to check those that apply to the person or object being investigated. The methodology is used, e.g., in the assessment of a product image, or "personality," in advertising research, and in determining an individual's self-concept as in the Adjective Check List by Gough (1952).

adjunctive therapist a member of a treatment or rehabilitation team whose functions are ancillary to the core of a therapeutic program, e.g., a hospital recreation director.

adjustment the modification of attitudes or behavior to meet the demands of life effectively, such as carrying on constructive interpersonal relations, dealing with stressful or problematic situations, handling responsibilities, or fulfilling personal needs and aims.

adjustment disorder a maladaptive reaction occurring within three months after the individual is subjected to specific, identifiable stress, such as divorce, business crises, family discord, a natural disaster, persecution, going to school, becoming a parent, or retirement. The maladaptive character of the reaction is not merely a single instance of overreaction, but involves impairment in social or occupational functioning and unexpectedly severe symptoms which generally subside when the stress ceases or when a new level of adaptation is reached. (DSM-III)

adjustment disorder with anxious mood an adjustment disorder characterized by nervousness, worry, and jitteriness, but distinguishable from anxiety disorders. (DSM-III)

adjustment disorder with atypical features a residual adjustment-disorder category involving symptoms that cannot be attributed to specific categories. (DSM-III)

adjustment disorder with depressed mood an adjustment disorder characterized by depressed mood, tearfulness, and hopelessness, but distinguishable from both major depression and uncomplicated bereavement. (DSM-III)

adjustment disorder with disturbance of conduct an adjustment disorder characterized by conduct that violates the rights of others or major norms and rules of society appropriate to the individual's age, as differentiated from conduct disorder and antisocial disorder. Examples are vandalism, truancy, reckless driving, fighting, and defaulting on legal responsibilities. (DSM-III)

adjustment disorder with mixed disturbance of emotions and conduct an adjustment disorder predominantly involving impaired ability to work or perform academically (e.g., to study or write papers and reports) in an individual whose performance has been adequate in these areas. Though anxiety and depression are frequently involved, the disturbance is differentiated from anxiety disorders and depressive disorders. (DSM-III)

adjustment disorder with mixed emotional features an adjustment disorder involving various combinations of depression, anxiety, or other emotions, but distinguishable from depressive and anxiety disorders. An example would be reactions of ambivalence, depression, anger, and increased dependency in an adolescent who moves away from home. (DSM-III)

adjustment disorder with withdrawal an adjustment disorder characterized by social withdrawal without significant depressed or anxious mood, and differentiated from depressive disorders. (DSM-III)

adjustment disorder with work or academic inhibition anxiety focused on school or occupational performance, including inability to write reports, examination anxiety, and difficulty in concentrating despite satisfactory intellectual or performance ability. (DSM-III)

adjustment inventory a survey form used to evaluate a subject's emotional and social adjustment as compared with a large and representative sample of individuals. See BELL ADJUSTMENT INVENTORY.

adjustment mechanism a habitual behavior pattern that enables the individual to meet the demands of life.

adjustment method a psychophysical technique in which a subject adjusts a variable stimulus to match a constant or standard. E.g., the subject may be asked to draw a figure as nearly identical as possible to a standard figure.

adjustment of observations the reinterpretation of observed data or weighting of data to correct for atypical information; also, use of the least-squares method to determine the best probable value of a measurement series.

adjustment processes a general term for any functions or activities through which we attempt to adjust to environmental demands. Examples are defense mechanisms through which we protect our ego while adapting to reality; language, which enables us to solve problems by gathering information and communicating with others; perception, which enables us to recognize and interpret experiences and events; memory, which stores knowledge to be called upon when needed; and imagination, which enables us to envisage new ideas and solutions. Also called **adaptive processes**.

adjustment reaction a type of disorder subsumed under the heading of "transient situational personality disorders" in DSM-I, comprising adjustment reactions of infancy, childhood, adolescence, and later life, defined in general terms as "reactions which are more or less transient in character and which appear to be an acute symptom response to a situation without underlying personality disturbance." In DSM-III this description most nearly applies to adjustment disorders. See A.R. OF INFANCY; A.R. OF CHILDHOOD; A.R. OF ADOLESCENCE; ADJUSTMENT DISORDER.

adjustment reaction of adolescence a situational stress disorder (DSM-I) associated with emancipatory strivings and inability to control impulses and emotions (including truancy, vandalism, sexual acting out, running away, stealing, defiance of school rules).

adjustment reaction of childhood a situational stress disorders (DSM-I) classified into habit disturbance (including nail-biting, thumb-sucking, enuresis, masturbation, temper tantrums, feeding problems), conduct disturbances (including truancy, stealing, destructiveness, sexual offenses, fire-setting, vandalism, cruelty, use of alcohol, running away), and neurotic traits (such as tics, somnambulism, stuttering, overactivity, phobias).

adjustment reaction of infancy a situational stress disorder (DSM-I) associated most frequently with the birth experience, feeding problems, sleeping difficulties, and maternal rejection or overprotection.

adjustment reaction of later life a situational stress disorder (DSM-I) stemming from involutional physiological changes, retirement from work, loss of family members and friends, illness, decline in attractiveness, financial insecurity, dependency on relatives, or the prospect of death.

adjuvant therapy secondary or subsidiary methods of treating mental disorders as an addition to psychotherapeutic techniques (from Latin *adjuvans*, "aiding"). A.t. may include the use of drugs and hypnosis.

ADL = ACTIVITIES OF DAILY LIVING.

Adler, Alfred /äd′lər/ Austrian psychiatrist, 1870–1937. A. was the first disciple of Freud to break away and form his own school, individual psychology, which was based on the theory that human beings are governed by a conscious drive to express and fulfill themselves, as opposed to Freud's theory of dominance by early sexual trauma and blind unconscious instincts. The school revolved around such concepts as the striving for superiority, feelings of inferiority, the inferiority complex, compensation and overcompensation, social interests, and the creative development of an individual style of life that incorporates both personal and social goals. Adjective: **Adlerian** /ädlär′ē·ən/. See ANALYST; BASIC MISTAKE; BIRTH ORDER; COM-PENSATION; COMPLEX; CONFRONTATION; CREATIVE SELF; DEPTH PSYCHOLOGY; DIRECTIVE FICTION; EFFECTIVE MOTIVE; EGO PSYCHOLOGY; FEMININE IDENTIFICATION; FICTION; FICTIONAL FINALISM; FINAL TENDENCY; GUIDING FICTIONS; INDIVIDUAL PSYCHOLOGY; INFERIORITY COMPLEX; KEY QUESTION; LIFE GOAL; LIFE LIE; LIFE PLAN; LONG-TERM PSYCHOTHERAPY; MASCULINE ATTITUDE; MASCULINE PROTEST; MORPHOLOGICAL INFERIORITY; NEO-FREUDIANS; NEUROTIC FICTION; NEUROTIC HUNGER STRIKE; NUCLEAR COMPLEX; ORGAN INFERIORITY; ORGAN JARGON; OVERCOMPENSATION; PARAPATHETIC PROVISO; PERSUASIVE THERAPY; RECONSTRUCTIVE PSYCHOTHERAPY; SEGMENTAL INSUFFICIENCY; SELF; SOCIAL INSTINCT; SOCIAL INTEREST; TELEOLOGY; WILL TO POWER.

ad lib. an abbreviation used in prescriptions, meaning "freely" (Latin *ad libitum*).

administration the application of a drug or other agent in the diagnosis or treatment of a disorder. Routes of a. include topical application, in which the agent is applied to the body surface, **oral a.**, **rectal a.**, **vaginal a.**, and **injection a.**, the latter may be through a vein (intravenous injection), into a muscle (intramuscular injection), or under the skin (subcutaneous injection). A. may also be done by enema, or through the digestive tract. Drugs used for disorders of the nervous system usually follow **systemic routes of a.**, that is, oral, rectal, or injection routes. Also see TOPICAL APPLICATION; INTRAVENOUS INJECTION; INTRAMUSCULAR INJECTION; SUBCUTANEOUS INJECTION.

administrative psychiatry an area of psychiatry concerned with the organization and management of mental-health facilities such as public and private mental hospitals, psychiatric units of general hospitals, and mental-health clinics and centers. Administration of these institutions involves policy formation, a cost-effective approach, development of a system of accountability, and the exercise of leadership that will enable the staff to make its maximum contribution. More specific areas of responsibility are supervision over business administration, labor relations, legal rules and regulations, public relations, and citizen involvement.

admission: See FIRST A.; RATE OF ADMISSIONS; READMISSION; VOLUNTARY A.

admission certification in psychiatry, review of a patient's case record to determine the necessity for admission to the institution and for the particular services it provides.

admission procedures in hospital psychiatry, the process of admitting patients to the institution, which includes such steps as putting them at ease; obtaining necessary information from them, from their family, or from the referral agency; conducting a preliminary psychiatric interview; and giving them a brief, reassuring account of the type of help they will be offered.

adolescence the period of transition from childhood dependence and immaturity to the greater maturity and independence of adulthood. The period starts with puberty and roughly spans ages 12 to 21 in girls and 13 to 22 in boys. During this period, major, and often disturbing, changes occur at varying rates in sexual characteristics, body image, sexual interest, social roles, intellectual development, and self-concept. See DEVELOPMENTAL TASKS. Also see AUTISTIC-PRESYMBIOTIC ADOLESCENT.

adolescent counseling the provision of professional guidance to adolescents through personal interviews, analyzing case-history data, and use of psychological tests. Because adolescents expect tolerance of their activities, counselors may need to take an open and nondefensive position about such matters as sexual behavior outside marriage.

adolescent crisis the emotional changes of adolescence that accompany the normal drive by the ego to achieve independence by casting off old emotional ties and developing new relationships as well as adapting to a changed body.

adolescent homosexuality homosexual contacts of an erotic nature during the pubertal period. It has been estimated that at least 20 percent of boys and three percent of girls have experienced homosexual contacts resulting in orgasm before the end of adolescence, and about twice that number have had casual or relatively uninvolved homosexual experiences during adolescence.

adolescent pregnancy pregnancy that occurs during the period of adolescence. Girls who begin to menstruate at age 12 can become pregnant at that age, but pregnancies at ages younger than 12 are rare in Western societies.

adolescent psychiatry diagnosis and treatment of adolescent mental disorders, which according to E.J. Anthony (in *American Handbook of Psychiatry*, 1975) fall roughly into four categories: (a) those beginning in childhood and terminating in adolescence (many cases of enuresis, asthma, and epilepsy), (b) those beginning in childhood and continuing through adolescence into adult life (various personality disorders), (c) phase-specific disorders beginning and ending in adolescence (situational maladjustment, identity confusion, and some cases of obesity and anorexia nervosa), (d) those beginning in adolescence and continuing into adult life (schizophrenia and some manic-depressive psychoses). The classical neuroses may fall into any of the four categories; and most of the syndromes involve mood swings, acting out, identity problems, episodic changes of behavior, sexual conflicts, and egocentrism.

adolescent psychotherapy according to P. Blos and S.M. Finch (in *American Handbook of Psychiatry*, 1975), psychotherapy that begins after evaluation of the young person and his family, and encompasses three phases, each of which must be "interesting" to the patient: (a) the "opening moves" devoted to getting ac-

quainted with the patient and creating a non-threatening, nonjudgmental atmosphere, (b) a middle phase in which the patient gradually overcomes his resistances, works through his problem, and reaches a new plateau of insight, and (c) a terminal phase in which the therapist and patient review what they have talked about and compare the patient with what he was before treatment began.

adolescent sex changes the physical and physiological changes that occur in males and females during puberty. They include accelerated development of sex organs and secondary sexual characteristics, such as appearance of pubic hair, and occurrence of first seminal ejaculation by boys and first menstruation by girls.

adoption studies estimation of the degree of heritability of a given trait or disorder by such methods as comparing the incidence of schizophrenia in adoptive and biologic parents when an adoptee has been diagnosed schizophrenic; and comparing the incidence of schizophrenia among adoptees whose biologic parents were schizophrenic with the incidence among adoptees whose parents were not schizophrenic.

Adorno, Theodor Wiesengrund /vē′zəngrōōnt/ German philosopher and musicologist, 1903–69. See ANTIINTRACEPTION; AUTHORITARIAN AGGRESSION; AUTHORITARIAN SUBMISSION; F SCALE; PROJECTIVITY.

-adren- a combining form meaning near or relating to the kidneys.

adrenal cortex /ədrēn′əl/ the outer layer of the adrenal gland and the source of a number of hormones, including the androgens, glucocorticoids, and mineralcorticoids. A.c. functions are controlled by the ACTH hormone of the pituitary gland. Loss of 80 percent or more of the a.c. can result in death within two weeks.

adrenal-cortical hyperfunction the excessive production of one or more of the hormones of the adrenal cortex. The manifestations vary with the hormone; e.g., adrenal virilism is a characteristic of androgen hypersecretion; excessive production of glucocorticoids results in Cushing's syndrome; and hypersecretion of aldosterone causes hypertension, sodium retention, and, in Conn's syndrome, paresthesia, weakness, and transient paralysis. Because more than one hormone may be hypersecreted, the symptoms can overlap. Causes may include a benign or malignant tumor or adrenal hyperplasia, which may be congenital or acquired.

adrenalectomy the surgical removal of one or both of the adrenal glands. A. may be performed in the treatment of cancer, hypertension, or excessive production of adrenal hormones. Also called **suprarenalectomy**.

adrenal gland a small yellowish body lying atop the kidney on both sides of the body and supplied with blood from the renal and phrenic arteries and innervated by branches of the splanchnic nerves. Two separate parts, the medulla and cortex, secrete several important hormones. Also called **suprarenal gland**. See ADRENAL CORTEX; ADRENAL MEDULLA.

adrenal hyperplasia a usually congenital disorder marked by increased adrenal production of cortisol precursors and androgens. Increased secretion of androgens during intrauterine life causes masculinization of female genitalia and an enlarged penis in boys. The children grow rapidly at first, but skeletal maturation is premature so that they are below average in height as adults.

adrenaline = EPINEPHRINE.

adrenaline-Mecholyl test a test employed to determine the probability that a mental patient will benefit from electroconvulsive-shock treatment. The test is conducted by injecting the patient intravenously with epinephrine hydrochloride, a form of adrenaline, one day and intramuscularly the next day with Mecholyl, a trademark for methacholine. If Mecholyl increases the blood pressure significantly, the patient is regarded as a poor candidate for electroshock. Also called **Funkenstein test**.

adrenal medulla the central portion of the adrenal gland. The a.m. secretes two hormones, epinephrine (or adrenaline) and norepinephrine (or noradrenaline). Both hormones are similar to those of the sympathetic nervous system. Unlike the adrenal cortex, the a.m. and its hormones are not essential to survival.

adrenal virilism : See ADRENAL-CORTICAL HYPERFUNCTION.

adrenergic /-nur'jik/ pertaining to the activity or effects of epinephrine or similar substances released by the adrenal medulla or nerve fibers, or introduced into the system as a drug. The term means literally adrenalinelike.

adrenergic blocking agents substances that inhibit certain responses to adrenergic nerve activity which key the organism up. The term also is applied particularly to drugs that block the action of epinephrine and norepinephrine. Ergot alkaloids were first discovered to alter responses to sympathetic nerve stimulation. A.b.a. are selective in action and are classed as **alpha a.b.a.** (or **alpha blockers** or **alpha-receptor blocking agents**) and **beta a.b.a.** (or **beta blockers** or **beta-receptor blocking agents**), depending upon which types of adrenergic receptors are affected by them. Also see ADRENERGIC DRUGS.

adrenergic drugs substances that stimulate the activity of epinephrine or mimic the functions of epinephrine. A.d. are part of a group of sympathomimetic amines that includes ephedrine, amphetamines, and isoproterenol. A.d. may be produced naturally in plants and animals or developed synthetically. They include **benzphetamine hydrochloride**—$C_{17}H_{22}ClN$, **chlorphentermine hydrochloride**—$C_{10}H_{15}Cl_2N$, **diethylpropion**—$C_{13}H_{19}NO$, **phendimetrazine**

—$C_{12}H_{17}NO$, **phenmetrazine**—$C_{11}H_{15}NO$, **phentermine hydrochloride**—$C_{10}H_{16}ClN$. See ADRENERGIC BLOCKING AGENTS. Also see ANALEPTICS.

adrenergic neurons = CATECHOLAMINERGIC NEURONS.

adrenergic reaction the response of autonomic-nervous-system fibers to stimulation by norepinephrine or epinephrine, the adrenergic hormones. Kinds of a.r. include increased blood-pumping by the heart and constriction of blood vessels. The a.r. generally occurs at a synapse where norepinephrine is released An a.r. can occur at a CNS site, but the activity is mainly in the autonomic system.

adrenergic-response state a physiological reaction pattern of increased pulse, heart rate, and blood-sugar levels.

adrenergic system the part of the autonomic nervous system, including receptor sites, that is influenced by adrenergic drugs. The nerves included in the a.s. vary somewhat with species but generally include all postganglionic sympathetic fibers. Also see CHOLINERGIC SYSTEM.

adrenochrome /ədren'-/ a chemical produced by the oxidation of adrenaline, or epinephrine. It is used to control capillary or other localized bleeding and as a psychotomimetic drug. An association has been observed between high levels of a. and schizophrenia.

adrenocortical atrophy with diffuse cerebral sclerosis a neurologic syndrome marked by adrenal-cortex atrophy and widespread loss of myelin in the cerebral hemispheres and brainstem. A dusty brown pigmentation covers all or most of the body. Neurologic signs usually begin between the ages of five and 15, with visual problems, arm or leg weakness, indistinct speech, and mental deterioration.

adrenocortical insufficiency a condition caused by failure of the adrenal cortex to produce adequate levels of hormones required for normal metabolic functions. Symptoms may include muscle weakness and fatigue, dizziness, and depression. See ADDISON'S DISEASE.

adrenocorticotrophic hormone a substance secreted by the pituitary gland to control the release of steroid hormones from the adrenal cortex. Also called **corticotropin**. Abbrev.: **ACTH**.

adrenoleukodystrophy /-dis'-/ a disease involving the white matter of the brain, either because of faulty myelin formation or myelin degeneration. A. is characterized by adrenal insufficiency, blindness, deafness, and mental retrogression and affects mainly children between the ages of five and ten years. Also called **sudanophilic leukoencephalopathy; Schilder's disease**.

adult-ego state the component of the personality that represents a mature capacity to deal with current reality, characterized by Eric Berne as **neopsychic**, since it represents the individual's own views, as contrasted with **exteropsychic**

tendencies, borrowed from the parents, and **archaeopsychic** relics of childhood. See TRANS-ACTIONAL ANALYSIS.

adult foster home = BOARDING HOME.

adult home: See REST HOME.

adult Huntington's chorea: See HUNTINGTON'S CHOREA.

adult motivation: See PROPRIATE STRIVING.

adultomorphism = ENELICOMORPHISM.

adult polycystic disease: See INFANTILE POLYCYS-TIC DISEASE.

adult sensorineural lesions organic damage to structures of the auditory system that develop from the inner ear to the brain areas in which sound is perceived. The lesion generally will be located in the cochlea or the eighth cranial nerve. A sensory lesion in the cochlea may be due to Ménière's disease, prolonged exposure to loud noises, a viral infection, or drug effects. A lesion of the eighth cranial nerve frequently is caused by a tumor.

adult situational reaction a transient personality disorder (DSM-I) in which such symptoms as anxiety attacks and insomnia occur as a result of overwhelming stress associated with such situations as marital discord, pregnancy, premature birth, spontaneous abortion, job difficulties, financial insecurity, menopause, acute illness, or surgery. See TRANSIENT SITUATIONAL PERSONALITY DISORDER.

adult spinal-muscular atrophy: See PROGRESSIVE SPINAL-MUSCULAR ATROPHY.

advanced placement examinations achievement tests which give high-school students an opportunity to gain admission to college with advanced standing in one or more subjects (the **College Entrance Examination Board Advanced Placement Program**), or to evaluate college-level education acquired through independent study and other nontraditional procedures (the **CEEB College Level Examination Program**).

advantage by illness a method of gaining social approval and sympathy by the exploitation of neurotic symptoms. Once a.b.i. is gained, the patient may resist therapy that would threaten the gain. The term is sometimes used as an alternative for EPINOSIC GAIN. See this entry.

advantage law: See LAW OF ADVANTAGE.

adventitia cells connective-tissue cells that form a loose outer covering over an organ or body part.

adventitious deafness a loss of hearing that results from injury or illness following a period of normal hearing ability. Compare CONGENITAL DEAFNESS.

adventurousness the tendency of children to engage in activities that involve exploration and risk, as well as to run, climb, wrestle, and wander.

adversary model the method of assigning the approach to truth to two opposing parties, as in the legal profession or in sanctification proce-dures of the Roman Catholic Church (with an *advocatus diaboli*, "devil's advocate"). "The hope is that through their adversary positions, one presenting the evidence as negatively as possible and the other as positively as possible, truth will emerge" (S. Anderson, S. Ball, and T. Murphy, *Encyclopedia of Educational Evaluation*, 1975). There are few examples of the use of this model in the practice of program evaluation.

adverse drug reactions any physical or mental disorders associated with the use of a drug administered for therapeutic purposes or self-administered. Reactions may be highly individual and related to genetic susceptibility, interactions with other drugs or dietary items, or chronic or acute health problems. Monoamine oxidase inhibitors, e.g., may react with wines, cheese, or other foods that contain tyramines, to produce a hypertensive crisis.

advertising psychology the psychological study of the techniques and effectiveness of all types of advertising, including the motives that prompt consumers to buy, the use and value of slogans, and the physical characteristics of ads in terms of such factors as color, size, and position in print media and different elements of commercials such as jingles, animated figures, and repetition. See ADVERTISING RESEARCH.

advertising research the study of (a) the selection of effective appeals for specific products or commodities, (b) the creation of product images including trade names and package designs, and (c) the development of methods of measuring the effectiveness of advertising campaigns in different media. A.r. also may be applied to generic advertising, e.g., advertising of an industry or product category such as cigars or coffee, rather than specific brands. Also see ADVERTISING PSYCHOLOGY.

advocacy research the form of research in social psychology that analyzes the impact of specific social institutions on the poor or powerless. A.r. is explicitly activist, often combining direct social action with research that seeks to identify social ills and develop concrete programs for change. See ADVOCATE; ACTIVISM.

advocate in the field of mental health, mental retardation, and rehabilitation, an individual who represents the "consumer," especially when he is disadvantaged, to protect his rights to effective care and treatment, training, housing, and public assistance. There are two general types of advocates: **case a.**, in which a single individual is represented, and **class a.**, in which a whole group is represented. Advocates other than lawyers are frequently termed linkage workers, mental-health counselors, or mental-health workers. Also see OMBUDSMAN; EXPEDITER; MENTAL-HEALTH WORKER.

adynamia = ASTHENIA.

aedoeomania /ēdē·omā′-/ an obsolete term for nymphomania.

aelurophobia = AILUROPHOBIA.

-aemia; -emia a combining form relating to blood.

AEP an abbreviation of *average evoked potential.*

AEq = AGE EQUIVALENT.

-aer-; -aero- a combining form relating to air or gas.

AER: See AVERAGE-EVOKED-RESPONSE TECHNIQUE.

aerial perspective a monocular cue to depth perception consisting of the relative clearness of objects under varying atmospheric conditions. Nearer objects are usually clearer in detail and color whereas farther objects are less distinct.

aeroacrophobia /erō·ak-/ a morbid fear of open and high spaces, especially when flying in a plane.

aeroneurosis neurotic behavior observed in some airplane pilots who exhibit anxiety, restlessness, headache, and other physical symptoms. Also called **aeroasthenia.**

aerophagia swallowing of air as a neurotic symptom (Greek, "air-eating"). Gulping air may accompany a rapid-breathing attack during anxiety or panic, and in some cases may be due to an unconscious desire for pregnancy, since the abdomen becomes distended. Also called **aerophagy; air-drinking.** See HYPERVENTILATION.

aerophobia a morbid fear of air, drafts, gases, or airborne noxious influences. Also called **air phobia.**

aerumna /ērōŏm'nə/ an obsolete term for depression caused by physical suffering.

aeschromythesis /eskrōmithē'sis/ an obsolete term for obscene speech.

affect the psychiatric term for any experience of feeling or emotion, ranging from the utmost pain to the utmost pleasure, from the simplest to the most complex sensations, and from the most normal to the most pathological emotional reactions. Affect, or "feeling tone," colors our entire psychic life and is experienced on both a conscious and an unconscious level. Adjective: **affective.** See AFFECTIVE DISORDERS.

affectability an obsolete term for emotional susceptibility.

affectate an obsolete term meaning to arouse emotions.

affectation an artificial manner or behavior assumed to impress others. It is a symptom of certain cases of hysteria or the manic phase of bipolar disorder.

affect-block a condition marked by inability to show strong emotions because of a fear of emotional ties. It is characteristically seen in schizophrenics and obsessive-compulsives.

affect-energy the energy generated by the excitement of a stimulus that affects the entire human organism.

affect-fantasy a term employed by Jung to denote a fantasy or imagined experience laden with strong emotion.

affect fixation: See FIXATION OF AFFECT.

affect hunger a craving for affection and loving care, especially among small children who have been emotionally deprived.

affect inversion: See REVERSAL.

affectio hypochondriaca an obsolete term for hypochondriasis.

affection a general term for feelings of tenderness and attachment, especially when such feelings are nonsexual.

affectional attachments affectionate relationships toward a primary love object (often but not always the mother), as well as other members of the family including pets. Expressions of affection begin toward the end of the first year of life and are generated by cuddling, kissing, words and acts of endearment, and attitudes of kindness and consideration, as well as demonstrations of affection between the parents.

affectional bonds feelings of affection and emotional attachment between human beings, between animals, and between human beings and animals. A.b. are manifested by such activities as clinging, cuddling, stroking, and embracing. Evidence of a.b. also lies in the sense of loss, grief, and anxiety experienced if separation occurs. See SEPARATION ANXIETY.

affectional drive the urge to give and to receive affection, both of which are believed by most psychologists to be innate, since the infant responds to cuddling and being held from the very start of life and expresses love as soon as he is capable of patting and stroking others. Moreover, children who are treated coldly and mechanically usually show signs of unhappiness and even suffering. Freudians, however, claim that the child becomes attached to the mother or mother surrogate only because of the role they play in gratifying his basic needs. See EMOTIONAL DEPRIVATION; MATERNAL DEPRIVATION.

affective: See AFFECT.

affective ambivalence a manifestation of an ambivalence in which the same person, object or event simultaneously arouses pleasant and unpleasant feelings, or friendly and hostile feelings. A schizophrenic patient, e.g., may express great love for his mother but almost in the same breath ask how to kill her.

affective amnesia a form of amnesia that is not related to organic cerebral conditions and which is not characterized by patterns of behavior-associated dementia or cortical amnesia. The term may be applied in cases of memory defects associated with functional psychological disorders, e.g., the Ganser syndrome.

affective-arousal theory the theory of D.C. McClelland that motives derive from changes in affective states.

affective discharge = CATHECTIC DISCHARGE.

affective disharmony a characteristic of schizophrenia in which there is an absence of conformity between emotional reaction and ideational content.

affective disorders a group of disorders in which there is a prolonged, pervasive disturbance of mood (either depression or elation) accompanied by a full or partial manic or depressive syndrome not due to any other physical or mental disorder. In DSM-III these disorders include major affective disorders (manic episode, major depressive episode, bipolar disorders), other specific affective disorders (cyclothymic disorder, dysthymic disorder), and atypical affective disorder. (DSM-III)

affective eudemonia the use of mental illness as a means of escaping from the fears or frustrations of reality. The Ganser syndrome is an example of a.e., as well as faxen psychosis and hypochondriasis. See FLIGHT INTO ILLNESS.

affective experience any experience of emotion or feeling including any degree of pleasure or pain, whether normal, pathological, conscious, or unconscious. See AFFECT.

affective feeble-mindedness an apparent loss of intellectual ability that is secondary to depression or another emotional state.

affective hallucination a hallucination associated with feelings of depression or elation, and involving grandiose ideas or self-depreciation, or such depressive content as poverty, disease, or guilt.

affective interaction interpersonal relationships carried out on an emotionally-charged level, as in group psychotherapy or family therapy.

affective monomania a now-obsolete term used by Esquirol, which appears to correspond to the manic phase of manic-depressive (bipolar) disorder. See ESQUIROL. Also see MONOMANIA.

affective psychosis a psychotic reaction characterized by a severe disturbance of mood. Major types are manic depressive disorder (now termed "bipolar disorders"), psychotic depressive reaction (now termed "major depression"), and involutional psychotic reaction (now categorized as "major depression" or "paranoid disorder," according to the symptomatology.) Extreme elation or depression are the basic characteristics of affective psychoses, although they may also involve thought disorder (such as delusions or hallucinations), or behavior disorder (such as psychomotor agitation, or suicidal tendencies). For details, see MAJOR DEPRESSIVE EPISODE; MANIC EPISODE; BIPOLAR DISORDER, MANIC; BIPOLAR DISORDER, DEPRESSED; BIPOLAR DISORDER, MIXED.

affective ratio the ratio of the total number of responses to the colored cards in a Rorschach test to the total number of responses to the achromatic cards. The significance of the a.r. is in the effect of color on the degree of responsiveness, and is therefore an index of affectivity.

affective rigidity a condition in which emotions or feelings remain unchanged through varying situations in which affect changes normally would occur. A.r. is common in obsessive-compulsive neuroses and schizophrenia.

affective separation a situation among infants in which the mother figure is physically present but not adequately stimulating or responsive. The infants frequently become detached and indifferent and lose hope for good relationships. Also called **masked deprivation**.

affective slumber the middle stage of Alzheimer's disease in which the patient becomes phlegmatic and dull, and it is hard to arouse attention and emotional response—in addition to other symptoms such as disorientation, perplexity, alexia, and echolalia.

affective state any emotional, subjective, or psychological state associated with any feeling of any degree of intensity. The feelings in questions may be pleasurable, painful, normal, pathological, conscious, or unconscious. Affective states influence and are influenced by perception, cognition, memory, and somatic factors. See AFFECT.

affective suggestion an emotional relationship that is established between a hypnotist and his subject while in a hypnotic setting. Also called **hypotaxia**.

affective tone the mood or feeling associated with a particular experience or stimulus.

affectivity the degree of response to pleasure, pain and other emotional stimuli. Evaluation of a. is an important component of the psychiatric examination; the diagnostician may look for evidence of such reactions as BLUNTED AFFECT, INAPPROPRIATE AFFECT, LOSS OF AFFECT, AMBIVALENCE, DEPERSONALIZATION, ELATION, DEPRESSION, or ANXIETY. See these entries.

affectomotor patterns a combination of overactivity and emotional excitement, as seen in such conditions as INTERMITTENT EXPLOSIVE DISORDER and BIPOLAR DISORDER, MANIC. See these entries. (DSM-III)

affectualization a term coined by Bibring and colleagues (1961) for a defense mechanism in which the emotional repercussions of unwelcome issues confronting the patient are overemphasized by the patient in order to avoid a rational understanding of them.

affectus animi /än'imē/ an obsolete term for mental disposition in general.

Affenliebe = MONKEY LOVE.

afferent /af'-/ conducting or conveying toward a point, as when a. nerves conduct impulses toward the brain or spinal cord. Noun: **afference**. Compare EFFERENT.

afferent motor aphasia a type of motor aphasia caused by a lesion in an afferent part of the nervous system.

afferent stimulus interactions the theory that all afferent impulses interact and modify each other.

affiliation the need to associate; a fundamental social drive to be involved with other people in close interdependent relationships, friendships, and various kinds of social groups and organizations. Many theorists believe that the early relationship between mother and child sets the pattern for the individual's a. need. Also see AFFILIATIVE DRIVE.

affiliative bonding = BONDING.

affiliative drive the urge to associate, form friendships and attachments, and depend on others; the tendency to join organizations and enjoy social gatherings. Affiliation appears to be a basic source of emotional security; without it, most individuals have been found to feel lost, anxious, and frustrated, for among normal persons there is probably no more intensely unpleasant feeling than loneliness. Also see GREGARIOUSNESS; AFFILIATION.

affiliative need a term used by H.A. Murray to denote a fundamental **determinant need** to seek cooperative, friendly association with other individuals.

affinal /afī'-/ related by marriage.

affinity the relationship by marriage between a man or woman and his or her spouse's blood relatives. The term also applies to attraction, as between two persons or between chemicals that form compounds.

affirmative action in industrial psychology, a government policy designed to reach the goal of equal opportunity for all, by requiring firms with federal contracts or subcontracts to develop and submit plans for hiring, training, and promoting minorities, including the handicapped, and to keep extensive records of their progress toward these goals.

affirming the consequent a term sometimes used to identify an error in logic in which it is assumed that a particular effect is always due to the same cause.

affordance the functional property of any object encountered by an organism in its own environment. The term is applied broadly to include food, shelter, and other items that afford some benefit to the individual, e.g., an object that can be used as a seat affords sittability. The a. of an object varies with the organism, e.g., a tree may afford food, shelter, or fuel to different organisms.

affricate /af'-/ a speech sound consisting of a plosive, e.g., /t/, followed by a fricative, e.g., /sh/, as the /ch/ in "chair" or the /dj/ in "jam." Also called **semiplosive**. Also see PLOSIVE; FRICATIVE.

A fiber a myelinated fiber of the somatic nervous system. A fibers generally have a diameter between one and 22 microns and transmit impulses at a velocity of five to 120 meters per second. Also see SOMATIC NERVOUS SYSTEM.

African sleeping sickness = ECONOMO'S DISEASE.

afterbirth the placenta, fetal membranes, and the remainder of the umbilical cord expelled from the uterus after childbirth.

aftercare a continuing program of outpatient treatment and rehabilitation services provided to patients who have been discharged from the hospital. The program is directed to mainte-

nance of improvement, prevention of relapse, and adjustment to the community.

aftercurrent = AFTERPOTENTIAL.

afterdischarge a nerve impulse that continues to discharge after the stimulus producing the muscle contraction or other activity has been removed.

aftereffect the aftersensation or continuation of a sensation after the stimulus has ended.

afterexpulsion the prevention of the return of the repressed idea or impulse. Also called **secondary repression; repression proper**. See REPRESSION.

afterimage the image that remains after a stimulus ceases or is removed. A **positive a.** occurs rarely, lasts a few seconds, and is caused by a continuation of receptor and neural processes following cessation of the stimulus; it is approximately the color and brightness of the original stimulus. A **negative a.** is more common, often more intense, and lasts longer; it is usually complementary to the original stimulus in color and brightness; e.g., if the stimulus was bright yellow, the negative a. will be dark blue. See AFTERSENSATION.

afterpotential the action potential that remains after the electrical charge involved has reached its peak, or spike. Also called **aftercurrent**.

aftersensation the sensation that remains or continues after a stimulus ceases or is removed. The term is essentially synonymous with afterimage, although afterimage nearly always refers to visual experience whereas a. may sometimes refer to experience in the other sense modalities, such as taste or pressure.

aftertest: See BEFORE-AFTER DESIGN.

agape /ägä'pā/ a Greek-derived term for a complex form of love. A. involves the practice of erotic, or sensual, love of the body and also feelings of tenderness, protectiveness, self-denial, and esthetic preference for the features, gestures, speech, and other traits of a person. A. sometimes is used to describe an unselfish love as taught by such religious figures as Jesus and the Buddha. Also called **agapism**.

agastroneuria a deficiency of nervous control of the stomach.

AGCT = ARMY GENERAL CLASSIFICATION TEST.

age: See ACHIEVEMENT AGE; ANATOMICAL AGE; BASAL MENTAL AGE; CEILING AGE; CHRONOLOGICAL AGE; CYBERNETIC THEORY OF AGING; DENTAL AGE; DEVELOPMENTAL AGE; EDUCATIONAL AGE; EVERSION THEORY OF AGING; GESTATIONAL AGE; MENSTRUAL AGE; MENTAL AGE; OVERAGE; PHYSIOLOGICAL AGE; SECONDARY AGING; SIZE-AGE CONFUSION; VINELAND SOCIAL MATURITY SCALE.

age-appropriate maturity psychological maturity, or the ability to deal effectively and resiliently with experience, and to perform developmental tasks (biological, social, cognitive) characteristic of one's age level.

âge critique /äzh'krētēk'/ the menopausal years (French, "critical age").

âge de retour /äzh'dərəto͞or'/ the years of senility (French, "age of return," namely, to childhood).

age effects the social and other results of being identified according to a chronological age. An example of a.e. is the attitude that a person over the age of 65 is senile or that an individual under the age of 21 is not competent or responsible, or that "you can't trust anyone over 30." Also see AGEISM.

age equivalent any score or measure of development expressed in chronological age. Abbrev.: **AEq.**

age-equivalent scale a system of expressing test scores in terms of age norms or averages.

age-grade scaling a method of standardizing a test by establishing norms based on a sample of children who are at the normal age for their grade in school.

ageism the tendency to stereotype the aged or aging as debilitated, inadequate, or unable to fend for themselves, and therefore to overlook their potential for making positive contributions to society and to the solution of their own problems. The term is also applied to discrimination against the middle-aged, especially in employment.

agency-centered consultation: See PSYCHIATRIC CONSULTATION.

agenesis /əjen'-/ the failure of a body part, such as an organ, to develop normally. An example is a. of the corpus callosum which may be manifested by lack of motor-coordination or epilepsy. However, in many cases the condition is not detected until a postmortem examination is conducted for other reasons.

agenetic /-net'-/ defective in development; also, nongenetic. See AGENESIS.

age norm the chronological age associated with an average or expected level of achievement as indicated by statistics based on test scores. Age norms are derived from the results of standardized tests administered to large numbers of children.

agent, action, and object in the two-word stage of language development, an expression indicating an agent's action on an object, in which only two components of the thought are used, as in "John ball" for "John throw ball."

agent provocateur /äzhäN'prōvōkätœr'/ the precipitating factor of factors, usually of a psychological character, that bring about symptoms, defensive reactions, dreams, or disorders.

agerasia literally, eternal youth (Greek); the quality of not appearing aged.

age ratio a rough indication of the predictive power of an aptitude test, obtained by dividing the subject's chronological age at one administration by his age at a later administration.

age regression a hypnotic technique in which the therapist helps the subject recapture a crucial experience by inducing amnesia for the current date, then suggesting that he return, year by year, to the earlier age when the experience took place.

ager naturae /ä'gər näto͞o'rī/ the uterus (Latin, "nature's field").

age scale: See AGE-EQUIVALENT SCALE.

age score a test score expressed in terms of the norm or average for the age of the subject.

ageusia /əgo͞o'-/ absence or impairment of the sense of taste (from Greek *a*- and *geusis*, "taste"). Some cases are organic, as in defective taste buds due to injury, disease, or senility; others are psychiatric, occurring primarily as a conversion symptom, or in depression and schizophrenia. Also called **ageusis; ageustia**.

agglutination the formation of words by adding forms that remain independent words or elements, e.g., "mankind," "peaceful," or "don't." Adjective: **agglutinative** /əglo͞ot'-/.

aggregation problems in evaluation research, the difficulty of separating individual effects from contextual effects when established groups or institutions are used as the unit of analysis in an evaluation. E.g., investigators are likely to attribute characteristics of the institution to the individual.

aggression behavior motivated by anger, hostility, or overcompetitiveness, and directed toward harming, destroying, or defeating other people or, in some cases, the self. In the Freudian theory, the aggressive impulse is innate and instinctive; in anthropological studies, it is a response to cultural factors, since some societies are highly aggressive and others nonaggressive; and in the psychological research of Dollard and Miller, a. is interpreted as a common reaction to frustration. Also see DIRECT A.; ANIMAL A.

aggressive behavior: See AGGRESSION.

aggressive instinct: See DEATH INSTINCT.

aggressiveness a behavioral trait consisting of self-assertiveness, social dominance, and a tendency toward hostility.

aggressive-predatory type: See AGGRESSIVE TYPES.

aggressive socialized reaction : See CONDUCT DISORDER, SOCIALIZED, AGGRESSIVE.

aggressive types subgroups of the antisocial personality, according to their characteristic aggressive behavior, e.g., B. Karpman's **aggressive-predatory type**, S. Arieti's **simple type**, who acts on pure impulse, and Arieti's **complex type**, who plans his activities in the manner of a professional bankrobber or swindler. There is little agreement on such classifications.

aggressive undersocialized reaction; See CONDUCT DISORDER, UNDERSOCIALIZED, AGGRESSIVE.

aging theory: See CYBERNETIC THEORY OF AGING; EVERSION THEORY OF AGING.

agitated depression a type of depression in which the patient wears an anguished look, wrings his hands, and paces restlessly about, bemoaning his lot. Also called **ademonia**.

agitation a state of extreme tension, restlessness, and anxiety. The individual is overwrought, anguished, and may pace up and down and bemoan his fate. Also see AGITATED DEPRESSION.

agitographia very rapid writing with unconscious omission and distortion of letters, words, or parts of words.

agitophasia very rapid and cluttered speech in which sounds, words, or parts of words are unconsciously omitted or distorted. Also called **agitolalia**.

aglossia a peripheral expressive speech disorder resulting from loss of the tongue.

agnosia loss or impairment of the ability to recognize objects, grasp the meaning of words and other symbols, or interpret sensory stimuli (from Greek *a-* and *gnosis*, "knowledge"). The condition may be due to organic brain damage or, in some cases, to emotional factors, as in schizophrenia, hysteria, or depression. See ANOSOGNOSIA; ASTEREOGNOSIS; AUTOTOPAGNOSIA; FINGER A.; LITERAL ALEXIA; APRACTAGNOSIA; VERBAL ALEXIA; VISUAL A.; VISUOSPATIAL A.; AUDITORY APHASIA; TIME A.; SIMULTANAGNOSIA; TOPOGRAPHAGNOSIA.

agnosic alexia a form of word blindness that may occur in the absence of speech or writing disorders. The patient usually is able to write spontaneously or to take written dictation but is unable to copy printed material or read sentences that have just been read to him and discussed. The condition often is associated with agenesis or lesions of the corpus callosum fibers in the occipital lobe.

agonist /ag'-/ a drug that affects a nerve receptor by binding to the surface and producing a physiological change. The change could involve stimulation of a neuron, thereby causing a nerve impulse to be fired, or it could provide the mediation needed to inhibit a nerve-cell discharge. Also, an a. is a contracting muscle whose action is opposed by another muscle.

agonistic behavior competitive interactions among individuals of a group in vying for food, shelter, or a mate. The interactions usually are marked by expressive movements such as heavy breathing, baring of teeth, hissing, barking, or crouching posture.

agoraphobia an anxiety disorder characterized by marked fear of being alone or in public places (crowds, tunnels, bridges, elevators, public transportation) from which escape might be difficult or help unavailable in case of need. The disorder (a) occurs without panic attacks (**a. without panic attacks**) or (b) begins with a panic attack (**a. with panic attacks**) and develops to a point where normal activities are increasingly restrictive, until the fear and avoidance behavior dominate the individual's life. Compare CLAUSTROPHOBIA. (DSM-III)

agrammatism a form of aphasia characterized by extremely ungrammatical speech to the point of incoherence. It is frequently seen in Pick's disease and Alzheimer's disease, and occasionally in schizophrenia. Some authors apply the term a. to syntactical aphasia. Also called **agrammata; agrammataphasia; agrammaphasia; agrammatologia; agrammalogia**.

agranular cortex a type of cerebral cortical tissue found in the posterior portions of the frontal lobes. This type of tissue, composed of cells without granules, is found in Brodmann areas 4 and 6 and parts of areas 8 and 44. A.c. cells often are associated with motor functions.

agranulocytosis a pathological condition marked by a reduction in the number of white cells circulating in the bloodstream, resulting in increased susceptibility to bacterial infections and ulcers of the mucous membranes. A. can be caused by chemotherapeutic drugs, e.g., phenothiazine derivatives, used in treatment of psychiatric disorders.

agraphia the total inability to write, or the ability to write letters but not syllables, words, or phrases. The defect is most frequently due to stroke, head injury, encephalitis, or other conditions resulting in brain damage (**acquired a.**), but is occasionally due to a localized congenital defect that may not result in other impairment. Some authorities also apply the term to cases of emotional inhibition, parallel to cases of psychogenic mutism. See APHASIA; VISUAL A.

agriothymia /-thim'-/ an obsolete term for homicidal insanity.

agriothymia ambitiosa an obsolete term denoting an obsession to destroy nations. Also called **Alexanderism**.

agriothymia hydrophobica a compelling urge to bite.

agriothymia religiosa an obsolete term denoting an obsession to destroy other religions and their followers.

agromania a morbid desire to live alone, especially in rural seclusion. A. is an occasional symptom of schizophrenia.

agrypnia = INSOMNIA.

agrypnocoma = COMA-VIGIL.

agrypnotic /-not'-/ inducing wakefulness; also, any substance acting in this manner, such as caffeine.

agyiophobia /ajē·ō-/ a morbid fear of streets. Also see TOPOPHOBIA; DROMOPHOBIA.

agyria /əjī'-/ absence of convolutions in the cerebral cortex due to development defect (from *a-* and *gyrus*). The condition results in severe to profound mental retardation. Also called **lissencephaly** ("smooth brain"). Also see LISSENCEPHALY SYNDROME.

aha experience a descriptive term for the emotional reaction that typically occurs at a moment of sudden insight following a long process of learning, problem-solving, or psychotherapy. It is the moment when the separate elements of a problem seem to come together and make sense; in psychotherapy, a.e. usually refers to sudden insight into unconscious motives.

ahistorical denoting the perspective of behavior in terms of contemporary causative factors; denoting emphasis on the here-and-now.

ahypnia; ahypnosia = INSOMNIA.

aichmophobia a morbid fear of pointed objects such as nails, forks, or knives (from Greek *aichme*, "spear, point"). The patient avoids these objects because they arouse threatening impulses to use them against others.

aide a nonprofessional staff member with limited training, such as a nurse's aide, social-work aide, or psychiatric aide, who assists in the care and rehabilitation and in some cases treatment of patients with physical disabilities, mental retardation, or mental disorders. See PSYCHIATRIC AIDE.

aidoiomania = EROTOMANIA.

ailurophobia /īlo͞oro͞o-/ a morbid fear of cats (from Greek *ailouros*, "cat"). It is often interpreted as a dread of being scratched or bitten in the genital area. Also called **aelurophobia; galeophobia; gatophobia; cat phobia**.

aim in psychoanalytic theory, the activity through which an instinct or impulse is gratified or "discharged"; e.g., kissing may satisfy the oral-erotic impulse.

aiming test a test of visuomotor coordination, precision, and speed. The subject (a) thrusts a stylus into a series of progressively smaller holes momentarily uncovered by a rotating shutter, or (b) places dots in small circles as rapidly as possible.

aim inhibition a Freudian term for suspending or altering the original activity that gratified an instinctual drive, in favor of another form of gratification; e.g., "biting sarcasm" may be an expression of an aim-inhibited wish to bite.

aim-transference the transfer of a patient's objectives from one life situation to another where they will be easier to achieve or will be more satisfactory as a goal.

AIO: See PSYCHOGRAPHICS.

air blade the narrow stream of air passing through the slit formed by placing the inner surface of the lower lip lightly against the tips of the upper teeth, in producing a fricative such as /f/.

air-bone gap the difference between the air-conduction and bone-conduction hearing levels at specific frequencies. This indicates the amount of conductive impairment in the ear tested.

air conduction the normal process of conducting sound waves through the ear canal to the eardrum which is set into vibration by the compression and rarefaction of air adjacent to it.

air-conduction testing an audiological procedure for the purpose of measuring a person's threshold for pure tones in each ear at individual frequencies.

air-drinking = AEROPHAGIA.

air encephalography /-log'-/ a diagnostic technique utilized to examine brain areas by injecting air into the cerebrospinal fluid. The air outlines the ventricles of the brain and the meningeal membranes that follow surface contours of the cortex. Because of the difference in opacity between the air and brain tissues, the air appears as a dark shadow on X-rays. The location of· the air in the brain can be manipulated by changing the patient's posture. The development of the CAT scan has reduced the need for this test.

air hunger the need for air in the lungs, which is physiological since oxygen is constantly required not only to burn the body's fuel and supply energy but to flush out carbon dioxide. The need increases as exertion and therefore metabolism increases and oxygen debt or oxygen deprivation (as in mountaineering or near-drowning) produces severe physiological and psychological effects. For details, see ANOXEMIA; ASPHYXIA; HYPOXIA; CARBON-MONOXIDE POISONING.

air phobia = AEROPHOBIA.

air-pollution adaptation the acceptance by a local population of levels of air pollution through gradual loss of sensitivity to the health and esthetic effects. In industrial communities, a high level of air pollution may be regarded as a sign of prosperity as large amounts of fossil fuels are consumed by factories, while some tourists find the smog of large American cities to be a visual attraction. See AIR-POLLUTION SYNDROME.

air-pollution syndrome a set of signs and symptoms associated with exposure to high levels of air pollutants. The a.-p.s. is characterized by headache, fatigue, insomnia, eye irritation, impaired judgment, depression, and irritability. One of the common air pollutants, carbon monoxide, can be a contributing factor to such disorders as visual and hearing impairment, parkinsonism, epileptic seizures, memory disturbances, psychoses, and retardation. Abbrev.: **APS**.

air-pressure effects any abnormal mental or physical condition caused by a significant variation from normal atmospheric pressure of 14.7 pounds per square inch, or one atmosphere. A.-p.e. at high pressures—e.g., more than two atmospheres as experienced in diving more than 33 feet (10 meters) beneath the surface of the sea—may include breathing difficulty, nitrogen poisoning marked by light-headedness and mental instability, and oxygen poisoning caused by breathing oxygen under extreme pressure. A.-p.e. at lower pressures—e.g., those experienced in high mountain-climbing or during airplane flights without oxygen or air-pressure modification—are characterized by oxygen starvation, with impaired performance and eventual loss of consciousness and death. Also see DECOMPRESSION SICKNESS.

akataphasia = ACATAPHASIA.

akathisia an anxiety reaction characterized by inability to sit down (Greek, "not sitting"); also, inability to sit still, accompanied by extreme restlessness and jitteriness due to heavy doses of phenothiazines, a major tranquilizer. In addition, patients with brain diseases affecting the striopallidal area may be unable to sit at all, and continually pace the floor or move their limbs in bicycle fashion. Also called **akatizia; acathizia**.

Akerfeldt test a physiological test for schizophrenia in which ceruloplasmin in the blood of the patient tends to be increased in acute but not chronic cases. The test involves the oxidation of N-N-dimethylparaphenyline diamine by a sample of blood from a schizophrenia patient.

-akine- a combining form relating to absence of motion or impaired motion.

akinesia the absence or lack of control of the voluntary muscles. The term is applied to a wide range of voluntary-muscle-control deficiencies, including (a) the catatonic state of schizophrenia, (b) a. algera, marked by paralysis due to the intense pain of muscle movement, (c) a severe muscle weakness caused by heavy metals, e.g., lead toxicity, (d) a neurosis accompanied by paretic symptoms, (e) the tremors and rigidity of parkinsonism, (f) **a. amnestica**, characterized by loss of muscle power due to disuse, (g) akinetic epilepsy, marked by sudden collapse of the patient, and (h) a condition caused by certain drugs that affect the nervous system, e.g., phenothiazines. Also called **akinesis**.

akinesia algera /al'-/ a condition in which pain is experienced with any body movement, a disorder often associated with cases of hysteria.

akinesthesia the absence, loss, or impairment of the kinesthetic sense.

akinetic-abulic syndrome a group of symptoms frequently resulting from treatment with tranquilizers, including slowing of movement (bradykinesia), tremors, hypertonia, reduced mental drive, and loss of interest.

akinetic apraxia loss of the ability to perform spontaneous movements.

akinetic epilepsy = AKINETIC SEIZURE.

akinetic mania a form of mania that is accompanied by a lack of movement and may actually be a symptom of schizophrenia.

akinetic mutism an absence or gross reduction in voluntary movements and speech. The patient lies inertly in bed, and has to be fed and toileted, but shows some slight signs of alertness, such as following eye movements. The condition is often associated with a tumor of the third ventricle, which is believed to interfere with the reticular activating system. Also see COMA-VIGIL.

akinetic psychosis a state of extreme catatonia in which the patient exhibits stupor, waxy flexibility, and little if any perceptible movement.

akinetic seizure a form of petit mal seizure involving a sudden muscular collapse accompanied by head nodding or falling. Also called **akinetic epilepsy**.

akinetic stupor = CAIRNS'S STUPOR.

akoasm = ACOUSMA.

akousticophobia = ACOUSTICOPHOBIA.

-al a combining form meaning of, or having to do with.

AL: See ABSOLUTE THRESHOLD.

AL: See ADAPTATION-LEVEL THEORY.

Alajouanine, Theophile French neurologist, 1890—. See ALAJOUANINE'S SYNDROME.

Alajouanine's syndrome a congenital neurological disorder involving lesions of the sixth and seventh cranial nerves, double facial paralysis, and convergent strabismus. Double clubfoot also is associated with the condition.

alalia the inability to speak due to the absence or impairment of muscles and sense organs involved in speech.

Al-Anon an organization composed of the families of alcoholics who belong to Alcoholics Anonymous. It was formed to deal with problems generated by living with an alcoholic.

alarm reaction a response to sudden stress, marked by hyperactivity, increase in heart rate, and, if prolonged, adrenocortical enlargement, ulcers, or other damage to the gastrointestinal tract. The a.r. usually is associated with the GENERAL ADAPTATION SYNDROME. See this entry.

Al-a-Teen an organization composed of the children of alcoholics, aimed at helping them gain increased understanding of their parent's problem, at enlisting their cooperation in the parent's efforts to find a solution, and at enabling them to face the social and emotional difficulties that they themselves are experiencing as a result of this problem.

-alb-; -albin-; -albino- a combining form meaning white (Latin *album*).

albedo a measure of the ratio of light reflected from the surface of an object to the amount of light falling upon it.

albinism a genetic disorder marked by a failure of melanocytes to produce normal melanin pigments in the skin, hair, and eyes. A. often is due to a metabolic defect marked by a lack of the enzyme tyrosinase. **Tyrosinase-negative a.** is the classic form of the disorder, affecting about three persons per 100,000, both blacks and whites, and characterized by skin and hair that appear unpigmented and an ocular fundus that is bright red. A form of a. that affects blacks more frequently than whites is **tyrosinase-positive a.**, which is marked by a lack of melanin at birth, but pigmentation increases with age. Other forms include **ocular a.**, in which only the eyes are affected, and **cutaneous a.**, a dominant genetic trait marked by a triangular white forelock and other a. effects limited to skin and hair. Photophobia, nystagmus, and strabismus may accompany a.

Albright, Fuller American physician, 1900–69.

See ALBRIGHT'S DISEASE; PSEUDOHYPOPARATHY-ROIDISM (also called **Albright's hereditary osteodystrophy**).

Albright's disease a disorder caused by a pituitary-hypothalamic dysfunction, characterized by pigment abnormalities, skeletal pseudocysts, and precocious puberty in females.

Albright's hereditary osteodystrophy = PSEUDO-HYPOPARATHYROIDISM.

alchemy a medieval philosophy that combined some knowledge of chemistry with various superstitions, including the belief that gold could be produced from common elements and that a proper mixture of elements would yield an elixir that would cure any disease and prolong life indefinitely.

alcohol a class of chemical compounds characterized by a hydroxyl group (-OH) attached to a nonbenzenoid carbon atom. The group includes ethyl alcohol—C_2H_5OH, commonly consumed in alcoholic beverages, methyl (or wood) alcohol—CH_3OH, glycerol—$C_3H_5(OH)_3$, sorbitol—$C_2H_4(OH_2)$ $(CHOH)_4$, and cholesterol—$C_{27}H_{45}OH$. Nearly 60 different alcohols are known. The primary effect of ethyl alcohol on the central nervous system is depression of the ascending reticular activating system, releasing the cerebral cortex from control of inhibition, release of the spinal reflexes from CNS control, disturbances of the cerebellar and vestibular functions, resulting in staggers, anesthesia, and prolonged secretion of cerebrospinal fluid which increases the intracranial pressure that produces adverse aftereffects. Changes in brain-wave rhythms can be monitored by EEG as a. effects progress through the central nervous system. Also see CHOLESTEROL; ETHANOL.

alcohol abuse the pathological use of alcohol for at least a month, characterized by (a) a daily need for alcohol in order to function, (b) repeated unsuccessful efforts to control drinking, (c) periodic binges, blackouts, and occasional consumption of a fifth or the equivalent, (d) impaired functioning, as indicated by violence or traffic accidents while intoxicated, and (e) absence from work, loss of job, arrests, and arguments with family or friends over excessive use of alcohol. (DSM-III)

alcohol-amnestic disorder a rare amnesia syndrome involving both long- and short-term memory, resulting from vitamin deficiency associated with prolonged heavy use of alcohol. The memory impairment often follows an acute episode of Wernicke's disease, and usually persists indefinitely. Also called **Korsakoff's disease**. (DSM-III)

alcohol dependence a disorder characterized by either a pattern of alcohol use or impaired functioning (as described under alcohol abuse), with either tolerance (need to increase consumption markedly for the desired effect, or diminished effect if the regular amount is consumed) or withdrawal (e.g., morning shakes, nausea,

malaise) after cessation or reduction of drinking. Also see ALCOHOLISM. (DSM-III).

alcohol derivatives drugs that utilize the sedative and hypnotic effects of alcohols for therapeutic purposes. In the 1890s, it was found that compounds derived from methyl alcohol had CNS-depressant effects. In the 1950s, a new generation of alcohol-based compounds with greater hypnotic activity was introduced. They include **ethchlorvynol**—C_7H_9ClO, a short-acting drug with the effects of certain barbiturates, and ETHINAMATE (see this entry), which also has a barbituratelike effect but is a more potent sleep inducer than ethchlorvynol. The a.d. are prescribed mainly for treatment of mild insomnia.

alcohol hallucinosis an organic hallucinosis following cessation or reduction in heavy drinking by an alcohol-dependent individual. The condition usually lasts a few hours or days, and the hallucinations are typically of the auditory type, consisting of derogatory, threatening voices to which the individual may respond by calling the police or arming against invaders. (DSM-III)

alcoholic addiction = ALCOHOLISM.

alcoholic blackout amnesia experienced by an alcoholic for his or her behavior during a drinking bout. Even though the individual may not be fully intoxicated, a blackout indicates that brain damage is starting to occur, though the damage is still reversible.

alcoholic brain syndrome any one of several brain syndromes produced by prolonged heavy use of alcohol, such as alcohol-amnestic disorder and dementia associated with alcoholism.

alcoholic dementia a syndrome associated with progression of Korsakoff's psychosis in which there is intellectual and memory impairment, emotional instability, carelessness in dress and personal cleanliness, and, in some cases, delusions of marital infidelity. See DEMENTIA ASSOCIATED WITH ALCOHOLISM.

alcoholic deterioration : See DEMENTIA ASSOCIATED WITH ALCOHOLISM.

alcoholic epilepsy = RUM FITS.

alcoholic jealousy persistent delusions of jealousy experienced by chronic alcoholics. It is not considered an independent syndrome in DSM-III but is diagnosed instead as "alcohol dependence with an additional diagnosis of paranoid disorder." Also see ALCOHOLIC PARANOIA.

alcoholic myopathy : See MYOPATHIES.

alcoholic neuropathies a collection of neurologic disorders including numbness, tingling, and tenderness of the extremities, foot drop, and loss of reflexes. In severe cases, vision and hearing may be affected. The symptoms also are those of beriberi, especially lassitude, suggesting a B-vitamin deficiency factor. The term is used because the condition is rarely observed in the Western world except in persons diagnosed as alcoholics.

alcoholic organic mental disorders organic

mental disorders attributed to the ingestion of alcohol. (DSM-III)

alcoholic paranoia in DSM-II, a paranoid state characterized by the alcoholic spouse's or lover's pathological jealousy and delusions of infidelity. Also called **alcoholic psychosis, paranoid type**.

alcoholic pseudoparesis a form of periodic paralysis associated with alcoholism and characterized by muscular weakness, particularly in the lower limbs, accompanied by numbness, loss of reflexes, and other symptoms of polyneuritis and myopathy. The condition usually can be corrected by diet and medical treatment.

alcoholic psychoses organic mental disorders resulting from excessive use of alcohol. The common denominator of these disorders is an acute or chronic inflammation of the brain which produces psychotic symptoms such as hallucinations, delusions, delirium, clouding of consciousness, memory impairment, confabulation, severely impaired judgment, and, in advanced cases, general mental deterioration. In DSM-II, these disorders comprise "alcoholic deterioration," "alcoholic hallucinosis," "alcoholic paranoia" (or "alcoholic psychosis, paranoid type"), "delirium tremens," and "Korsakoff's psychosis." In DSM-III, the corresponding categories are DEMENTIA ASSOCIATED WITH ALCOHOLISM, ALCOHOL HALLUCINOSIS, ALCOHOL-WITHDRAWAL DELIRIUM, and ALCOHOL-AMNESTIC DISORDER. See these entries.

Alcoholics Anonymous a voluntary organization of alcoholics and ex-alcoholics which seeks to control the compulsive urge to drink, through understanding, fellowship, and emotional support. The program is based on (a) the individual's admission that he cannot control his drinking, (b) recognition of a supreme spiritual power which can give him strength, (c) a searching examination of past errors, carried out with another member who serves as "sponsor," (d) making amends for these errors, (e) development of a new code and style of life, (f) sharing of experiences and problems at meetings, and (g) helping other alcoholics who are in need of support. Abbrev.: **AA**.

alcoholic twilight-state a condition associated with pathological drunkenness in which twilight states are released, often involving illusions, hallucinations, and excessive emotions of rage and anxiety.

alcohol idiosyncratic intoxication a rare disorder characterized by a marked behavioral change associated with drinking an amount of alcohol that is insufficient to intoxicate most people. The behavior is not typical of the individual when not drinking; e.g., a shy, retiring, mild person may become belligerent and assaultive, followed by amnesia for the episode. (DSM-III)

alcohol intoxication a disorder associated with overuse of alcohol, and marked by (a) maladaptive behavior, as in fighting, impaired judgment, and defective social and occupational functioning, (b) one or more physiological signs, such as flushed face, slurred speech, unsteady gait, incoordination, and nystagmus, and (c) one or more psychological signs, such as loquacity, impaired attention, irritability, euphoria, and emotional lability. Other frequent features are blackouts and behavioral change (e.g., from suspicious to paranoid, and from withdrawal to conviviality). (DSM-III)

alcoholism chronic dependence on alcoholic beverages, characterized by compulsive drinking and consumption of alcohol to such a degree that it produces mental disturbance and interferes with social and economic functioning. Major signs of addiction are increasing consumption; sneaking and gulping drinks; morning drinking; excessive drinking when alone; confusion and tremors; prolonged "benders"; uncontrolled behavior; blackouts; and severe withdrawal symptoms. Also called **alcohol addiction**. Also see ALCOHOL DEPENDENCE; FETAL ALCOHOL SYNDROME; STATISTICS.

alcoholophilia a morbid craving for alcohol. Also called **alcoholomania**.

alcohol-paranoid state an atypical paranoid disorder in alcoholics, characterized by excessive jealousy, suspiciousness, and delusions of the spouse's infidelity.

alcohol psychosis, paranoid type = ALCOHOLIC PARANOIA.

alcohol withdrawal a condition developing several days after cessation or reduction of heavy, prolonged alcohol consumption, involving such symptoms as coarse tremors, nausea and vomiting, malaise or weakness, rapid heartbeat, sweating, elevated blood pressure, anxiety, depressed mood, or irritability, but without delirium. (DSM-III)

alcohol-withdrawal delirium a condition developing within a week after cessation or reduction of heavy drinking, and characterized by (a) clouding of consciousness, perceptual disturbance, incoherent speech, and disorientation, (b) autonomic hyperactivity (rapid heartbeat, sweating, elevated blood pressure), and, in most cases, (c) delusions, hallucinations (usually visual), agitation, and coarse, irregular tremors. Also called **delirium tremens (DT)**. (DSM-III)

alcoolisation: See BETA ALCOHOLISM.

aldehydes /al′dəhīdz/ a group of chemical compounds formed by the oxidation of primary alcohols. The a. correspond to the alcohols used. Further oxidation of a. produces corresponding acids; e.g., ethyl alcohol—C_2H_5OH—is oxidized to acetaldehyde—CH_3CHO—which is oxidized to acetic acid—CH_3COOH. Kinds of a. include **benzaldehyde, formaldehyde**, and **fufuraldehyde**. A. may produce CNS depression or other toxic effects, e.g., pulmonary edema, when oxidized from alcohols in body tissues.

aldolase /al'-/ an enzyme normally found in muscle tissue where it serves to split a complex sugar molecule. Excessive levels of a. in the blood may be an early indication of muscle-function abnormality and a clue in the diagnosis of muscular dystrophy.

aldosterone /al'-/ a mineralcorticoid hormone secreted by the adrenal cortex. A. acts on mineral and water metabolism and often is involved in salt retention by the body tissues. Excessive secretion of a. may be associated with hypertension, muscle weakness, and polydipsia.

aldosteronism a pathological condition caused by excess secretion of the adrenal-cortex hormone aldosterone. A. is marked by headaches, urinary disturbances, fatigue, and hypertension. It may be primary, due to an adrenocortical disorder, or secondary, as a result of a liver, heart, or kidney disease affecting the adrenal glands. Also called **Conn's syndrome**.

alector a person afflicted with insomnia.

alert inactivity an infant state marked by facial relaxation, calm and even breathing, open, luminous eyes, and considerable visual exploration.

alerting mechanisms systems within the central nervous system that trigger a response or direct the attention of higher brain centers to possible threats. Most important is the arousal reaction mechanism of the reticular activating system in the brainstem that awakens an animal or human from deep sleep in response to unexpected stimuli. See RETICULAR ACTIVATING SYSTEM.

alertness the quality of being awake, aware, attentive, and ready to act or react; the opposite state of being dull and drowsy. In neurological terms, a. is a high degree of cortical activity resulting from stimulation of the reticular formation, or alerting system. Also see AROUSAL.

Alexander, Franz Hungarian-American psychoanalyst, 1891–1964. A. was professor of psychoanalysis at the University of Chicago, and a contributor to psychosomatic medicine and brief analytic therapy. See COMMON COLD; CORRECTIVE EMOTIONAL EXPERIENCE; DYNAMIC REASONING; PRINCIPLE OF INERTIA; SPECIFIC-DYNAMIC PATTERN; ULCER PERSONALITY.

Alexander, W. Stewart English pathologist, fl. 1949. See ALEXANDER'S DISEASE.

Alexanderism = AGRIOTHYMIA AMBITIOSA.

Alexander's disease a type of megalencephaly associated with hyaline pan-neuropathy (generalized nervous disorder). The patients show a severe deficiency of myelin and an accumulation of eosinophilic bodies in the white matter. Most show severe psychomotor retardation early in infancy; some also have generalized seizures, and a few are unable to raise their heads. Most of those afflicted die before the age of three years, but one has lived to age 15.

alexia the inability to understand written language. A. is a form of aphasia due to brain lesions in the parietal or occipital-parietal lobe. The condition may be congenital, due to prenatal toxicity, injury, or anoxia; or it may be acquired, due to encephalitis, head injury, stroke, or brain disease (Alzheimer's, Pick's, or cerebral arteriosclerosis). The term may be applied to persons who merely have difficulty in reading words. Also called **word blindness; visual aphasia**. Also see AGNOSIC A.; LITERAL A.; VERBAL A.; CONGENITAL A.

alexithymia a condition of limited fantasy and emotional life. According to P. Sifneos, patients with this condition have trouble recognizing and describing their emotions and "give the impression that they do not understand the meaning of the word 'feeling'" (*Short-Term Psychotherapy and Emotional Crisis*, 1972).

-alg-; -algia-; -algy; -algesia a combining form denoting pain (Greek *algos*).

ALG = ANTILYMPHOCYTE GLOBULIN.

algedonic pertaining to pain associated with pleasure. **Algedonics** is the study of the mixture of pleasure and pain.

algesia the ability to experience the sensation of pain. Compare ANALGESIA.

algesimeter /-sim'-/ an instrument used to measure the sensitivity of an individual to pain. The a. contains a calibrated needle that is pressed against a body surface in order to determine the subject's pain threshold. Also called **algometer**.

algesthesia the sensitivity to pain.

algolagnia a psychosexual disorder in which sexual excitement is achieved by experiencing or inflicting pain. See SEXUAL MASOCHISM; SEXUAL SADISM.

algometer = ALGESIMETER.

algophily /-gof'-/ a seldom used term for masochism.

algophobia a morbid fear of pain. Also called **odynophobia; pain phobia**.

algopsychalia a symptom of pain recognized by the patient as of mental rather than physical origin, an effect observed in certain cases of hypochondriasis and schizophrenia. Also see PSYCHIC PAIN.

algorithm /al'-/ a rote or mechanical procedure for solving a problem, e.g., opening a combination lock by trying all the possible numbers in order. Computer programs often make use of a. (The word is derived from the name of the ninth-century Arab mathematician *al-Khuwarizmi*.) Also called **algorism**.

Alice in Wonderland effect: See METAMORPHOPSIA.

alienatio mentis a legal term for insanity (Latin, "alienation of the mind").

alienation the breakdown of any sociological, interpersonal, or experimental relationship. In psychiatry, a. denotes estrangement from oneself and others, including estrangement from one's own feelings which are excluded from awareness through defensive maneuvers. A. is characteristic of obsessive-compulsive states; it is seen in a more drastic form in schizophrenia. Also, a. is a general term for mental illness, occasionally used in court cases but no longer in psychiatry. Also see SELF-A.

alienation coefficient: See COEFFICIENT OF ALIENATION.

alienist a physician (usually but not always a psychiatrist) who serves as an expert witness on mental competence and mental health or illness. The term is seldom used today.

alienus /alē·ā′-/ an obsolete term meaning delirious.

alimentary orgasm a term used by S. Rado for the intense pleasure experienced by the infant during satiation of hunger, which he considered the prototype of adult sexual orgasm. The desire to experience a.o. again has been suggested as a basis for adult drug abuse and overeating.

-aliphat- a combining form relating to oil or fat (from Greek *aleiphar*, "oil, fat").

aliphatic chains /-fat′-/ compounds of fatty acids that form chains of carbon atoms with other atoms attached. The chains may be open or branched. The alcohols and their corresponding compounds occur in a.c. Fatty acids are released into the bloodstream as an automatic response to a variety of stimuli and provide a quick source of energy for flight-or-fight reactions.

aliphatic phenothiazines a group of phenothiazine tranquilizers with an aliphatic (fatty-acid) side chain in the molecular structure. The a.p. include chlorpromazine, promazine, and triflupromazine. The a.p. are the least potent of the phenothiazine drugs.

alkalinity: See HYDROGEN-ION CONCENTRATION.

alkalosis a pathologic condition caused by an abnormally high level of alkalinity in the blood and tissues of the body. It also may result from a depletion of acids, thereby upsetting the body's acid-base balance. The condition often is marked by slow, shallow breathing but also may include such symptoms as muscle weakness, muscle twitching, confusion, irritability, and, in severe cases, convulsive seizures. Compare ACIDOSIS.

alkylating agent a synthetic chemical compound which acts on the DNA in the nuclei of cells when used in cancer chemotherapy. However, an a.a. damages normal as well as malignant cells because it is not selective. Also called **nitrogen mustard**.

-all-; -allo- a combining form meaning other.

-allach- /-alak-/ a combining form meaning elsewhere.

allachesthesia the sensation of touch experienced in a place other than the point of stimulation. Also called **allesthesia; alloesthesia**. Also see VISUAL A.

Allan Dent disease a disorder characterized by the presence in the urine and cerebrospinal fluid of argininosuccinic acid, resulting from an inborn error of metabolism and accompanied by epilepsy and mental retardation. The term is often used interchangeably with ARGININOSUCCINIC ACIDURIA. See this entry.

allele /al′ēl/ or /əlēl′/ alternative forms of a gene (from Greek *allelon*, "of one another"). Each person normally has two alleles for each gene, one inherited from each parent. The alleles normally are located at precisely the same position, or locus, on each of the pairs of matching chromosomes inherited from the mother and father.

Allen, F.H. American psychologist, 1890—. See NONDIRECTIVE PLAY THERAPY; RELATIONSHIP THERAPY.

allergens /al′-/ substances that are capable of producing a sensitivity reaction in an individual. An allergen, which may be a food item, house dust, animal dander (scales from hair or feathers), plant pollen, or tissues of another organism, does not produce an allergic reaction directly, but initiates the immune-response system that produces the antibodies to resist the invading allergen.

allergic potential scale a scale for evaluating a predisposition to allergic reaction, based on family history of allergy, eosinophilic count, skin-test reactions, and the relation between certain allergens and clinical symptoms.

allergy a hypersensitivity of body tissues to an antigen of foreign substance, producing irritation in various degrees.

allesthesia = ALLACHESTHESIA.

allied health professional a trained nonmedical specialist who contributes to the prevention, treatment, and rehabilitation process. The following allied health professions and professionals are particularly involved in the fields of psychiatry and clinical psychology: OCCUPATIONAL THERAPY; PHYSICAL THERAPY; PSYCHIATRIC SOCIAL WORK; SPEECH PATHOLOGY; DANCE THERAPY; MUSIC THERAPY; ART THERAPY; INDUSTRIAL THERAPY; SOCIAL WORKER; PSYCHIATRIC NURSE; REHABILITATION NURSE; EDUCATIONAL THERAPIST; REHABILITATION COUNSELOR. See these entries.

allied reflexes two or more simultaneous or closely successive reflexes that appear as a single reaction.

allobarbital a barbiturate drug of the intermediate-acting class. It usually is administered in combination with a mild analgesic in the treatment of migraine, neuralgia, and similar disorders.

allochiria /-kī′-/ the transfer of pain or touch sensations to a point on the opposite side of the body corresponding to the place actually stimulated. Also spelled **allocheiria**. See HYSTEROGENIC ZONES.

allocortex /-kôr′-/ the archipallium or rhinencephalon regions of the cerebral cortex associated with olfactory and related functions.

alloeroticism the outward extension of erotic

feelings toward others, as opposed to autoerotism.

alloesthesia = ALLACHESTHESIA.

allolalia any speech defect, especially when associated with disease affecting the speech center.

allopathy /əlop'-/ a method of treating disease through the use of agents that produce effects different from those caused by the disease. A psychological example might be the use of relaxation in desensitizing a patient to phobic situations. See DESENSITIZATION. Compare HOMEOPATHY.

allopatric species: See SYMPATRIC SPECIES.

allophasis /-lof'-/ an obsolete term for disorganized speech.

allophone: See PHONEME.

alloplasty /al'-/ a psychoanalytic term for a form of adaptation in which the libido is directed to altering the external environment in accordance with the reality principle rather than the pleasure principle. See AUTOPLASTY.

allopsyche /-sī'-/ the psyche or mind of another person.

allopsychic referring to the assignment or projection of one's own thoughts or ideas to people or events in the outside world. Also see ALLO-PSYCHOSIS.

allopsychic delusion: See AUTOPSYCHIC DELUSION.

allopsychosis a delusional or hallucinatory syndrome in which the patient's own feelings or impulses are projected into others. E.g., if the patient feels hostile, he may become convinced that other people are conspiring to harm him.

allopurinol /-pyōō'-/ a drug administered in the treatment of gout, or gouty arthritis, by preventing the formation of uric acid. The disabling symptoms of gout result from the accumulation of uric-acid salts in the joints. A. blocks the action of the enzyme xanthine oxidase which normally produces uric acid from other substances in the bloodstream.

all-or-none law the principle that if a stimulus is strong enough to produce a nerve impulse, the entire impulse is discharged (a weak stimulus never triggers a weak impulse). However, some nerve fibers require a greater minimal stimulus to fire than others. Also called **all-or-none principle**. Also see ACTION POTENTIAL.

-allotrio- a combining form meaning perverted, offensive, strange (from Greek *allotrios*, "strange, perverted").

allotriogeusia /-gōō'-/ a perverted sense of taste, or an abnormal appetite. Also called **allotriogeustia**. See ALLOTRIOPHAGY.

allotriophagy /-trē·of'-/ a desire to eat offensive food. Also called **allotriophagia** /-fāj'-/.

allotriorhexia the compulsion to pluck and usually to swallow threads from clothing.

alloxan /al'oksan/ or /əlok'sən/ a substance produced by the oxidation of uric acid. It is capable of producing a condition of hypoglycemia by stimulating insulin secretion by the pancreas,

followed by hyperglycemia and destruction of the insulin-secreting cells, an effect called **a. diabetes**.

Allport, Gordon Willard American psychologist, 1897–1967. A. is widely recognized as the originator of a theory of personality based on common and unique traits and as coauthor of two personality inventories, the ALLPORT-VERNON-LINDZEY STUDY OF VALUES and the ALLPORT A–S REACTION STUDY. See these entries. Also see ALLPORT'S PERSONALITY-TRAIT THEORY; ASSIMILATION; CARDINAL TRAIT; CENTRAL TRAIT; COMMON TRAITS; DIRECTEDNESS; FUNCTIONAL AUTONOMY OF MOTIVES; GROUP-RELATIONS THEORY; HUMANISTIC PERSPECTIVE; PERSONAL-DOCUMENT ANALYSIS; PERSONALISTIC PSYCHOLOGY; PROPRIATE STRIVING; PROPRIUM; SELF; SELF-EXTENSION; SELF-OBJECTIFICATION. Also see PERSONALITY STRUCTURE; INDEX OF ADJUSTMENT AND VALUES.

Allport A-S Reaction Study a personality test designed to measure the relative strength of two traits, *a*scendance and *s*ubmission, by presenting standardized life situations and asking the subject to choose his own way of meeting such situations.

Allport's personality-trait theory the theory that the individual's personality traits are the key to the uniqueness and consistency of his behavior. Traits are conceived as dynamic forces that interact with each other and determine the characteristic actions or reactions that define our self, or " proprium." Our traits develop largely from experience, learning, and imitation, and fall into three main categories: cardinal traits or master qualities like overweening ambition; central traits, or clusters of distinctive attitudes and characteristics; and secondary traits, which are more limited and not essential to personality description.

Allport-Vernon-Lindzey Study of Values a personality test designed to show the relative importance of six basic values in the subject's life: theoretical, economic, athletic, social, political, religious. The categories are based on Edward Spranger's Types of Men, 1928, and are presented in the form of statements and questions to which the subject responds.

allusive thinking a type of thinking marked by inference and suggestion rather than direct communication, with concepts that may seem diffuse and indistinct.

alogia the inability to speak due to lesions in the central nervous system or mental impairment.

alogous /al'-/ an obsolete term meaning irrational.

Alpers, Bernard Jacob American neurologist, 1900—. See ALPERS' DISEASE.

Alpers' disease a condition characterized by progressive degeneration of the cerebral cortex in infancy. After an apparently normal early infancy, psychomotor development slows and first symptoms of spasticity occur. The head may become microcephalic, accompanied by cerebral atrophy and a brain weight loss of as much as

20 percent. The child becomes inattentive or unresponsive and dies before the age of five years. Also called **progressive infantile cerebral poliodystrophy**.

alpha /al'fə/ first letter of the Greek alphabet (A, α).

alpha adrenergic blocking agents: See AD-RENERGIC BLOCKING AGENTS.

alpha alcoholism one of the classifications of E.M. Jellinek, characterized by undisciplined drinking and psychological dependence on the effects of alcohol for the relief of physical or psychological pain, but without losing control or being unable to abstain. A.a. is also described as **problem drinking, escape drinking, dyssocial drinking, thymogenic drinking, reactive alcoholism**, or **symptomatic alcoholism**.

alpha apparent = ALPHA MOVEMENT.

alpha-arc the simple sequence of a basic neural impulse routing from stimulus to motor response. Also see BETA-ARC.

Alpha, Beta, Gamma hypotheses three divergent theories: Alpha—repetition frequency enhances learning; Beta—repetition frequency has no effect; Gamma—repetition frequency hinders learning.

alpha block the suppression of alpha waves by a factor such as a visual stimulus that produces beta waves on EEG tracings. See ACTIVATION PATTERN.

alpha blockers: See ADRENERGIC BLOCKING AGENTS.

alpha cells: See ISLANDS OF LANGERHANS.

alpha-endorphin: See ENDORPHIN.

Alpha examination a World War I military-personnel test of verbal ability.

alpha-ketoglutarate: See GABA SHUNT.

alpha level the probability set for rejecting the null hypothesis, usually .01 or .05; also, the probability of making a Type I error, that is, rejecting the null hypothesis when it is true.

alpha movement a visual illusion in which an object appears to change in size as parts are presented successively. Also called **alpha apparent**.

alphaprodine: See SYNTHETIC NARCOTICS.

alpha receptor an adrenergic nerve receptor that is stimulated by norepinephrine and blocked by dibenamine. Alpha receptors represent a part of the autonomic nervous system that is distinguished from the beta-receptor category. Compare BETA RECEPTOR.

alpha-receptor blocking agents: See ADRENERGIC BLOCKING AGENTS.

alpha state a state of relaxed wakefulness achieved by subjects who produce alpha brain waves (7.5 to 13.5 cycles per second) as a result of biofeedback training. See ALPHA-WAVE TRAINING.

alpha-2-globulin: See BERGEN'S FRACTION.

Alpha verbal test: See ARMY TESTS.

alpha waves a pattern of brain waves as recorded by encephalograph that indicates the human mind is in a wakeful but relaxed state. The waves occur at a frequency of between 7.5 and 13.5 cycles per second. A.w. are utilized in biofeedback training to reduce blood pressure or other manifestations of anxiety and tension. Also called **alpha rhythms**.

alpha-wave training a type of biofeedback training in which the subject learns to achieve a state of peaceful wakefulness and relaxation by controlling his alpha waves. The technique usually involves a tone that changes pitch or disappears when the alpha state of mind has been reached.

alpinism a general term applied to mental disorders such as the asthenia syndrome associated with living at high altitudes or other low-atmospheric-pressure environments.

Alport, Arthur Cecil English physician, 1879–1959. See ALPORT'S SYNDROME.

Alport's syndrome a familial condition characterized by hematuria (bloody urine), nephropathy, and deafness. The hematuria may first appear in infancy while the deafness is likely to develop around the age of puberty. The condition also may be accompanied by cataracts and mental retardation.

ALS = AMYOTROPHIC LATERAL SCLEROSIS.

als ob: See AS-IF PERSONALITY.

Aström, Carl Henry Swedish physician, 1907—. See ALSTRÖM-HALLGREN SYNDROME.

Alström-Hallgren syndrome a familial disorder characterized by obesity, deafness and visual disorders, and diabetes. The syndrome occasionally is associated with mental disorders.

-alt-; -alter- a combining form meaning other, another, second (Latin *alter*).

alter an individual's concept of another person; also, the other person in a social interaction.

altered state of consciousness a modification of the state of awareness, especially with regard to the quality and intensity of perception, cognition, and affectivity. Intoxication by drugs and infections may produce delirious states involving clouding of consciousness and disorientation, but when psychedelic or hallucinogenic drugs are ingested, the change in perception and other mental functions usually occurs in a clear sensorium. Many other phenomena are also associated with alterations in consciousness: epilepsy (twilight sleep), catatonic stupor, coma, dreaming, hypnagogic states, dissociative states (fugue, somnambulism), as well as religious and mystical experiences. Abbrev.: **ASC**.

alter ego an intimate, supportive friend with whom the individual can share all types of problems and experiences, as if he or she were "another self."

alter-egoism an altruistic concern or a feeling of empathy for another person in the same situation as oneself.

alternate binaural loudness-balance test a test for recruitment, or abnormal sensitivity to loud sounds. The patient hears two tones of the same frequency played alternately into the two ears, but the intensity of the sound at one ear is set at a level 20 decibels higher than the other. If the patient perceives the two sounds as having the same loudness, it indicates that one ear is more sensitive to loudness.

alternate form a scale of items so closely similar to another scale that each is considered a different version of the same test.

alternate hemiplegia: See HEMIPLEGIA.

alternate-response test a test requiring the subject to choose the correct response of two alternatives.

alternate-uses test a test of divergent thinking which requires the subject to cite possible uses for a specified object, other than its common use. E.g., a newspaper can be used for starting a fire or packing objects in a box.

alternating personality a dual personality with components that alternately appear. See DUAL PERSONALITY.

alternating perspective: See AMBIGUOUS FIGURE; NECKER CUBE; RUBIN'S FIGURE.

alternating psychosis the circular form of manic-depressive psychosis (bipolar disorder), in which there is an alternation between elation and depression.

alternating role periodic shifting from one pattern of behavior to another, e.g., from an authoritarian to a democratic role and back to an authoritarian role.

alternating vision the alternate use of only the right or left eye for seeing, one eye usually being dominant.

alternation the replacement of an emotional problem with a physical condition. The term applies also to A. METHOD. See this entry.

alternation method a technique used in the study of thinking, language, and problem-solving among animals and human beings, in which the subject is required to follow an increasingly complex sequence of activities in order to reach a goal or receive a reward. An example is RRR LLL, or triple alternation: turning right three times, then left three times.

alternation-of-response theory a concept based on experimental evidence that proper division and parsing of a stream of stimuli is an important control mechanism in short-term memory tasks. E.g., extending the time interval between right-left alternation-task couplets reduces the rate of errors. Also see VOLLEY THEORY.

alternative group session a meeting of a therapy group that is held at scheduled intervals without the presence of the therapist.

alternative hypothesis a prediction that experimental effects or relationships will be found. The a.h. is accepted when the null hypothesis is rejected at a predetermined level of significance. Symbol: H_1. Also see NULL HYPOTHESIS.

alternative reinforcement a response-maintenance technique in which reinforcement occurs according to either a fixed-ratio or fixed-interval schedule, whichever is satisfied first.

altitude sickness: See ACOSTA'S SYNDROME.

altitude test a type of test intended to calculate the student's or subject's ability in a particular area as indicated by the level of difficulty he can reach.

altricial an ornithological term meaning helpless at hatching and requiring parental care for a period of time (from Latin *altrix*, "nourisher, foster mother").

altrigenderism a socially approved, nonsexual attraction and association between individuals of the opposite sex.

altruism unselfish concern for the interests of others—a term coined by Auguste Comte in 1830 from French *vivre pour autrui*, "to live for the sake of others" (from Latin *alter*, "another"). In Freudian theory, the infant is completely egoistic and narcissistic, but under the impact of sibling rivalry and the need to share the mother's love, gradually learns that a. can satisfy the ego as well as the demands of society.

altruistic behavior acting in the interest of others; putting concern for others above concern for oneself. Examples of a.b. cover a wide range, including expressions of interest, support, and sympathy; doing special favors for others; active defense of the rights of the deprived; engagement in volunteer activities for the mentally or physically handicapped; and martyrdom.

altruistic suicide a term used by Durkheim for what he described as suicide associated with excessive integration with a group (as contrasted with egoistic, asocial motives), as exemplified by the suicide of kamikaze pilots, or of older people who believe they are a burden to their families.

alucinatio an obsolete term for hallucination.

alusia an obsolete term for mental derangement.

alusia hypochondriaca an obsolete term for hypochondriasis.

alveolar /əlvē′ələr/ a speech sound made with the tongue touching or near the gum ridge above the upper teeth (called the **a. ridge**), e.g., /d/, /t/, /n/, or /s/. Accurate placement of the tongue tip or tongue blade in this area is necessary for precise articulation. Also called **gingival**. Also see FRICATIVE; PLOSIVE.

alveolus /-vē′-/ any small, hollow chamber of a body organ or tissue, such as a tooth socket or follicle of a gland. The term is commonly applied to the myriad thin-walled chambers of the lungs where blood vessels are able to release carbon dioxide and admit oxygen during respiration cycles. Plural: **alveoli**. Also see ALVEOLAR.

alysm an obsolete term denoting a patient's restlessness or anguish. Also called **alysmus**.

alysosis extreme boredom usually associated with the simple form of schizophrenia. Also called **otiumosis**.

Alzheimer, Alois /älts′hīmər/ German neurolo-

gist, 1864–1915. See ALZHEIMER'S DISEASE;
AFFECTIVE SLUMBER; AGRAMMATISM; ALEXIA;
ARGENTOPHILIC PLAQUES; ATROPHIC DEMENTIA;
BIOLOGICAL VIEWPOINT; BRAIN ATROPHY; BRAIN
DISEASES; CONGOPHILIC MATERIAL; DEMENTIA; DE-
SCRIPTIVE PSYCHIATRY; ECHOLALIA; LOGOCLONIA;
LONG-TERM CARE; MIRROR SIGN; MYOCLONIC DE-
MENTIA; NEUROFIBRILLARY DEGENERATION; NEURO-
LOGICAL IMPAIRMENT; NURSING HOME; PALILALIA;
SENIUM PRAECOX; SENILE PLAQUES.

alzheimerization of brain tissue: See NEUROFI-
BRILLARY DEGENERATION.

Alzheimer's disease presenile dementia due to
widespread degeneration of brain cells into
tangled, threadlike structures, first described by
the German neurologist Alois Alzheimer in
1907. Cortical atrophy begins around 50 years
of age and progresses rapidly through three
stages: (a) a gradual loss of memory, poor
perception and reasoning, inefficiency in everyday tasks, (b) intellectual and emotional impairment with confabulation, depression, irritability, restless wandering, slurred speech, inability to read or write, and (c) increasing disorientation, incoherence, misidentification of
relatives, and emaciation, usually followed by
death in four or five years.

amacrine cells /am'-/ nerve cells in the retina
that have short branching dendrites but appear
to lack axons. The a.c. are located in the inner
nuclear layer, about halfway through the ten
cellular layers of the retina.

Amalric's syndrome a condition in which deafness is associated with central vision defects.

amantadine: See ANTIVIRAL DRUGS.

Amat: See MARIN A.

amathophobia a morbid fear of dust or sand.

amaurosis the partial or complete loss of sight
without evidence of organic abnormality of the
affected eye or eyes (Greek "dimming"). The
condition may be hereditary, as in Leber's congenital a., a transient condition, or a part of a
syndrome such as amaurotic familial idiocy. The
cause often is a lesion of the brain or the optic
nerve. The term is also occasionally used for
psychogenic, or hysterical, blindness.

amaurotic familial idiocy: See TAY-SACHS DIS-
EASE.

amaurotic idiocy a neurological disease marked
by progressive degeneration of the cortical
neurons. Signs and symptoms include loss of vision, increasing muscular weakness and paralysis, and mental retardation. Death often occurs
before the age of five. See TAY-SACHS DISEASE.

amaxophobia a morbid fear of being in or meeting in a moving or stationary vehicle.

ambenomium: See MYELASE.

-ambi- a combining form meaning both (from
Latin ambo, "both, two").

ambidextrous the ability to use either hand with
equal skill.

ambient conditions the physical variables in a
particular environment, such as temperature,

humidity, air quality, noise level, and intensity
of light that, taken as a whole, create an **ambi-
ence** or atmosphere that may evoke a distinct
feeling or mood.

ambient temperature the surrounding temperature conditions; the atmospheric temperature
conditions.

ambiguity in psychoanalysis, the side-by-side existence of contrasting affects without affecting
each other, as in dreams that reveal a wish to
both love and destroy a parent; also, a slip of
the tongue that expresses our underlying
thoughts in disguise, as in describing an individual as "erotic" instead of "erratic."

ambiguity tolerance the ability to cope with conflicting situations without undue distress.

ambiguous figure a figure that can be interpreted
in different ways, or in which the perspective
appears to change. See NECKER CUBE; RUBIN'S
FIGURE.

ambiguous genitalia sex organs that are not fully
differentiated, as in cases of girls born with a
clitoris that could be mistaken for a penis. The
clitoris, labia, and other genitalia develop from
primordial structures which, if exposed to
androgen stimulation during the embryo stage,
develop into male genitalia. Also see HER-
MAPHRODITE.

ambilevous /-lē'-/ denoting a person who lacks
normal manual "dexterity" in both hands (from
Latin ambi- and laevus, "left").

ambisexuality sexual behavior that accommodates erotic interest in both males and females;
also, the possession of sexual characteristics
that are identified with both male and female
sexes. An example of an ambisexual or bisexual
trait is pubic hair, which is common to both
sexes. The term was introduced by Ferenczi to
identify the psychological aspects of BISEXUAL-
ITY. See this entry. Also see HERMAPHRODITE;
TRANSSEXUALISM.

ambivalence /-biv'-/ the simultaneous existence
of contradictory feelings and attitudes, such as
love and hate, toward the same person, activity, or goal. Conflicting feelings are particularly
strong toward parents, since they are agents of
both discipline and affection. Indecisiveness
about getting married or taking a certain job is
frequently due to ambivalent feelings stemming
at least partly from sources beyond awareness.
Bleuler, who originated the term, viewed extreme a. as a major symptom of schizophrenia.
See AFFECTIVE A.

ambivalence of the intellect a condition in which
ideas and counterideas are held at the same
time. E.g., a schizophrenic patient may vehe-
mently deny he hears voices, yet describe what
they are saying.

ambivalence of the will a condition observed in
its most extreme form in schizophrenia. The patient may at the same time desire and not desire
to perform an action, e.g., demand food or
work but adamantly refuse it when it is offered.

ambiversion a personality with approximately

equal amounts of introversion and extraversion traits.

amblyopia /-i·ō′-/ the functional loss of vision in the absence of organic or refractive defect (from Greek *amblys*, "blunt," and *ops*, "eye"). It is frequently due to alcoholism, drugs, albinism, or color blindness.

amblyoscope /am′-/ an instrument used to find the point where two separate visual stimuli fuse.

amblystomas /-blis′-/ salamanders of the Amblystoma genus that are used for experimental purposes because they have larval and adult stages that tend to overlap. They may, e.g., be able to breed in the larval stage but retain their larval gills in the adult stage. The axolotl is the larva of the tiger salamander and typical of the genus.

ambulation the act of walking. A. training often is necessary in the rehabilitation of patients who have suffered a spinal injury, stroke, or other disorder affecting the neuromuscular system, and in the physical therapy of individuals affected by certain genetic or congenital defects, e.g., achondroplastic dwarfism.

ambulatory care medical or psychological treatment provided to patients who are not bedridden or otherwise confined. Generally, the term is applied to care that is rendered patients who are able to travel to a doctor's office, hospital out-patient department, or health center, but sometimes a.c. is offered as an emergency home-care service. Most drug rehabilitation programs, e.g., methadone-maintenance centers, are operated as a.c. facilities.

ambulatory insulin treatment = SUBCOMA INSULIN TREATMENT.

ambulatory psychotherapy psychological treatment on an out-patient basis.

ambulatory schizophrenia a schizophrenic condition in which the patient manages to stay out of the hospital, but is marginally adjusted and eccentric in behavior. In many cases these individuals wander aimlessly about, make peculiar grimaces, talk to themselves, and put an extreme burden on their families.

ambulatory services in psychiatry, services such as psychotherapy and counseling provided on an out-patient basis. See WALK-IN CLINIC.

ambulatory treatment any therapy that can be administered to a person on an out-patient basis, such as in a doctor's office, as distinguished from treatment that would be given a patient confined to a hospital.

amelectic a seldom used term meaning emotionally indifferent.

ameleia morbid apathy or indifference.

amenomania a term applied by Benjamin Rush to a morbidly elevated affective state, equivalent to the manic phase of bipolar disorder today.

amenorrhea the absence of the menses, or failure to menstruate, during the period from puberty to menopause. When menstruation fails to be-

gin after puberty, the condition is called **primary a**. If menstrual periods stop, in the absence of pregnancy or menopause, after starting, the condition is known as **secondary a**. Changes in physical or mental health can be a causal factor.

amentia an obsolete term (Latin, "lack of mind") for profound, congenital mental retardation, or "primary mental deficiency." The term has had other applications, e.g., the Viennese school of psychiatry used it to denote the acute hallucinatory confusion that frequently occurs in delirium. See STURGE-WEBER SYNDROME. Also see ISOLATION A.; DEVELOPMENTAL A.; ECLAMPSIC A.

American Coalition of Citizens with Disabilities: See SELF-HELP GROUPS.

American College Testing Program = ACT ASSESSMENT.

American Home Scale one of several indices of the home environment (another is the **Home Index**) which contain questions on parental status (occupational and educational level) and such data as size and nature of the home, telephones, refrigerators, vacuum cleaners, books and magazines, and the esthetic and civic involvement of the family.

American Law Institute Guidelines a set of rules adopted in 1962 that combine the M'Naghten rules and irresistible-impulse concepts in determining criminal responsibility by a person suspected of a mental disease or defect.

American Psychiatric Association code; American Psychological Association code: See CODE OF ETHICS.

Ames, Adelbert, Jr. American educator, 1880–1955. See AMES DEMONSTRATIONS; DISTORTED ROOM (also called **Ames distortion room**); HONI PHENOMENON.

Ames demonstrations a series of illusions, designed by A. Ames, Jr., e.g. distorted rooms used to test depth perception. See DISTORTED ROOM.

amethopterin: See AMINOPTERIN.

amethystic a theoretical drug that would have the effect of countering the intoxicating effects of alcohol. Also called **antiintoxicant**.

ametrophia a dioptric defect of the eye resulting in refractive errors of acuity or accommodation (from Greek *ametros*, "irregular").

amimia the inability to convey meaning through appropriate gestures (**motor a**. or **expressive a**.) and, in some cases, to interpret the gestures of others (**sensory a**. or **receptive a**.). A. is a language, or communication, disorder. See APHASIA.

amine group /əmēn′/ or /am′in/ a family of chemicals derived from ammonia through the replacement of one or more of the hydrogen atoms by a hydrocarbon or other radical. Kinds of amines include epinephrine, norepinephrine, and dopamine, the catecholamines that are involved in stimulation of the adrenergic nerves.

aminoacetic acid = GLYCINE.

amino-acid imbalance a disorder, genetic or acquired, characterized by a deficiency in the body's ability to normally transport or utilize certain amino acids. The cause usually is an absence or lack of an enzyme needed to carry an amino acid or its components through a step of a metabolic cycle. More than 80 kinds of a.-a.i. have been identified and many, e.g., phenylketonuria and hyperglycemia, affect the central nervous system.

amino acids organic compounds that contain an amino, or NH_2, and carboxyl, or COOH, group. They occur naturally in plant and animal tissues and are the building blocks of protein molecules. Eight of the more than 20 a.a. in the human diet are essential and must be obtained from foods. The human body normally is able to synthesize the other a.a. from various food sources in the diet.

aminopterin /-nop'-/ a folic-acid antagonist sometimes used to induce abortions. Surviving infants show teratogenic effects such as hydrocephalus, craniosynostosis with skull defects, and mild-to-moderate retardation. A related drug, **amethopterin**, has similar teratogenic effects.

aminopyrine: See PYRAZOLONES.

amitriptyline; amitriptyline hydrochloride: See TRICYCLIC ANTIDEPRESSANTS.

amixia a custom of requiring that husband and wife be of the same ethnic or cultural group, religion, caste, or color.

ammonium-sulfate test = ROSS-JONES TEST.

-amnes- a combining form relating to loss or impairment of memory (from Greek *amnesia*, "forgetfulness").

amnesia a partial or complete, temporary or permanent, loss of memory due to (a) organic factors, as in head injury, alcoholic intoxication, epileptic seizure, stroke, general paresis, senile dementia, or (b) psychogenic factors, as in unconscious repression of painful or traumatic experiences. In the latter case, the a. is usually more circumscribed than in the organic cases since it serves as a defense against anxiety and distress, or as a way of escaping from specific situations. See FUGUE; AFFECTIVE A.; ALCOHOL AMNESTIC DISORDER; ANTEROGRADE A.; AUDIOVERBAL A.; AUDITORY A.; AUTOHYPNOTIC A.; CATATHYMIC A.; CIRCUMSCRIBED A.; CONTINUOUS A.; CORTICAL A.; DISSOCIATIVE A.; EPISODIC A.; EPOCHAL A.; GLOBAL A.; HYSTERICAL A.; INFANTILE A.; LOCALIZED A.; NEUROLOGIC A.; ORGANIC A.; POLYGLOT A.; POSTENCEPHALITIC A.; POSTHYPNOTIC A.; POSTTRAUMATIC A.; PSYCHOGENIC A.; RETROGRADE A.; TACILE A.; VERBAL A.; VISUAL A.; BARBITURATE OR SIMILARLY ACTING SEDATIVE OR HYPNOTIC AMNESTIC DISORDER.

amnesic aphasia = AMNESTIC APHASIA.

amnesic confabulation fanciful tales and experiences unconsciously fabricated to fill gaps in memory. It occurs in Korsakoff's and other organic psychoses. See CONFABULATION.

amnesic-confabulatory syndrome an alternative name for Korsakoff's psychosis, based on the two most striking symptoms of this syndrome: memory defect and confabulation. See CONFABULATION; KORSAKOFF'S PSYCHOSIS.

amnesic misidentification: See MISIDENTIFICATION.

amnesic syndrome a syndrome in which the most prominent behavioral symptom is a difficulty to retain new information. A second symptom is polyneuritis. The a.s. originally was believed to be due to alcoholism associated with thiamine deficiency. However, in recent years it has been reported to follow a viral encephalitis infection, unilateral anterior-temporal lobectomy in the language-dominant hemisphere, and lesions near the central axis of the brain. Also called **axial amnesia; Korsakoff amnesia**. Also see AMNESTIC SYNDROME.

amnestic pertaining to loss or impairment of memory, as in A. APHASIA, A. SYNDROME, or ALCOHOL-A. DISORDER. See these entries.

amnestic aphasia impaired ability to recognize the meaning of words and to find the right name for objects. Mild forms may be due to anxiety, fatigue, intoxication, and senility; severe forms are indicative of a focal lesion between the angular gyrus and the first temporal gyrus on the left side. Also called **amnesic aphasia; nominal aphasia**.

amnestic apraxia an inability to remember and therefore carry out a command although there is no loss of ability to perform the task.

amnestic syndrome an impairment in both short- and long-term memory (learning new material and recalling past information), without clouding of consciousness as in delirium or intoxication, and without general loss of intellectual abilities, as in dementia. Onset is often rapid and may be associated with organic factors such as head injury, surgery, thiamine deficiency, alcohol abuse, or insufficient oxygen supply to the brain. The patient is usually disoriented, and may deny his problem or fill memory gaps with fictitious events. See ALCOHOL-AMNESTIC DISORDER; KORSAKOFF'S PSYCHOSIS. Also see AMNESIC SYNDROME. (DSM-III)

amniocentesis /-sentē'-/ a method of examining the chromosomes of fetal cells obtained from amniotic fluid during the period of gestation (from Greek *amnion*, and *kentein*, "to puncture"). A sample of fluid can be extracted after the 12th week of pregnancy for direct examination to determine the sex of the fetus and certain other information, such as the F body, a part of the Y chromosome that fluoresces when stained with quinacrine. A more detailed examination requires the culturing of the fetal cells so that they can be observed during cell division when the chromosomes replicate. A. often is recommended when there is a pregnancy in which the risk of a chromosomally abnormal fetus appears to be more important than the risk of damage to the fetus through the a.

procedure itself, which is relatively safe when performed by experienced personnel in a well-equipped medical center. A. may be ued to detect dozens of different inherited disorders in embryos and fetuses, such as Down's syndrome, PKU, and sickle-cell anemia.

amnion /am'ni·ən/ the innermost of the fetal membranes containing the developing offspring and the amniotic fluid.

amniotic fluid an albumin-rich fluid in which the fetus floats within a membranous sac in the uterus. The a.f. helps protect the fetus against injury and provides a constant temperature environment. It is normally clear and present in amounts between 500 and 1,500 milliliters. Excessively large or small amounts of a.f. or discoloration of the fluid usually is a sign of a fetal abnormality.

amobarbital $C_{11}H_{18}N_2O_3$—a barbiturate that is used both as a sedative and hypnotic. It is short-acting, that is, its effects develop rapidly and it is metabolized and excreted more quickly than other barbiturates. However, a. abuse can result in addiction, narcosis, and death. See BARBITURATES.

amoebic dysentery /əmē'bik dis'-/ an infection of the digestive tract by a protozoal parasite, Entamoeba histolytica. The disease is acquired by ingesting the organism in contaminated food or water, usually through asymptomatic food handlers in hotels and restaurants. The incidence ranges from less than five percent in the United States to more than 50 percent in countries with poor sanitation. Cases that do not respond to drugs may require treatment by ileosotomy.

amok /əmok'/ a culture-specific syndrome observed among schizoid males in Malay, the Phillipines, and parts of Africa (Malay *amoq*, "in a frenzy"). The individual experiences a period of brooding and depression, then begins a wild, unprovoked, and indiscriminate attack on any person or animal nearby, usually killing or maiming a dozen individuals before being overpowered or collapsing from exhaustion or killing himself. The patient has complete amnesia for the event and may commit suicide. The causes suggested include alcoholic intoxication, social factors such as rejection by the family of a prospective bride, a side effect of malaria, a type of epileptic attack, or a psychosis. Before the advent of Western culture, a . was accepted as a way of reacting to a frustration. Also **amuck**. Verb: **to run a**. See FUROR; PSEUDOAMOK SYNDROME; PUERTO RICAN SYNDROME.

amoralia an obsolete term for moral imbecility.

amor Lesbicus an obsolete term for Lesbianism.

amorous paranoia an obsolete term used to identify a type of jealousy or infidelity delusion which, in some cases, represents a denial of unconscious homosexuality. See DELUSIONAL JEALOUSY.

amorphosynthesis /-sin'-/ an inability to perceive a specific form based on tactile sensations.

The failure of the brain to synthesize an image from neural impressions received by touching an object is a type of a. known as astereognosis. The cause may be a parietal-lobe lesion, although a. also reportedly may be experienced by subjects under the influence of psychedelic drugs. See ASTEREOGNOSIS.

amotivational syndrome a personality pattern (rather than a recognized clinical entity) consisting of apathy, passivity, loss of drive for achievement, a tendency to drift, low frustration tolerance, and difficulty in concentrating and following routines. This pattern has been attributed by some investigators to the deteriorating effects of marijuana and LSD, though others suggest that it is primarily a function of the hippie life-style. Still others believe the pattern is due to a combination of both factors, or that it can be ascribed to preexisting personality tendencies.

amour fou /ämo͞orfo͞o'/ a seldom used term for obsessive love or infatuation (French).

amphetamine $C_9H_{13}N$—a CNS stimulant closely related in structure and activity to ephedrine. It is used in the treatment of narcolepsy, certain forms of parkinsonism, and hyperkinesis. A. is a catecholamine-releasing drug, causing sympathetic-nervous-system fibers to release stored norepinephrine. Also see AMPHETAMINES; DEXTROAMPHETAMINE.

amphetamine dependence: See AMPHETAMINE OR SIMILARLY ACTING SYMPATHOMIMETIC DEPENDENCE.

amphetamine or similarly acting sympathomimetic abuse a disorder of at least a month's duration characterized by (a) pathological use, that is, inability to curtail use, (b) intoxication throughout the day, (c) use of the substance nearly every day for at least a month, (d) episodes of delusional disorder or delirium, and (e) impaired functioning, as manifested in fights, loss of friends, absence from work, loss of jobs, and repeated legal difficulties. (DSM-III)

amphetamine or similarly acting sympathomimetic delirium a disorder whose essential feature is a delirium occurring within 24 hours and usually lasting over six hours, during which the user may experience a delirious state associated with such reactions as tactile and olfactory hallucinations, and violent or aggressive behavior. (DSM-III)

amphetamine or similarly acting sympathomimetic delusional disorder a syndrome that occurs in chronic users who take a large dose of amphetamine or an amphetaminelike substance. The symptoms develop rapidly, last for a week or more, and include delusions of persecution with at least three of the following: ideas of reference, aggressiveness and hostility against misperceived "enemies," anxiety, and agitation. Also common is the hallucination that bugs are crawling on or under the skin (formication). (DSM-III)

amphetamine or similarly acting sympatho-mimetic dependence a condition characterized by tolerance (need for increased amounts to achieve the desired effect, or decreased effect from regular use of the same amount) or development of withdrawal syndrome (depressed mood with fatigue, disturbed sleep, or increased dreaming) when use of the substance is suspended or reduced. (DSM-III)

amphetamine or similarly acting sympatho-mimetic intoxication a disorder with the following DSM-III criteria: at least two psychological symptoms developing within one hour of use (agitation, elation, grandiosity, loquacity, and hypervigilance, or excessive wakefulness); at least two physical symptoms (tachycardia, pupillary dilation, elevated blood pressure, perspiration or chills, nausea or vomiting; and such behavioral effects as fighting, impaired judgment, and interference with social or occupational functions. (DSM-III)

amphetamine or similarly acting sympatho-mimetic withdrawal a syndrome that develops among long-term, heavy users of these substances when the dose is terminated or substantially reduced. The essential characteristics are depressed mood plus fatigue, disturbed sleep, or increased dreaming. (DSM-III)

amphetamine psychosis: See AMPHETAMINE OR SIMILARLY ACTING SYMPATHOMIMETIC DEPENDENCE; AMPHETAMINE OR SIMILARLY ACTING SYMPATHOMIMETIC INTOXICATION; AMPHETAMINE OR SIMILARLY ACTING SYMPATHOMIMETIC DELIRIUM; AMPHETAMINE OR SIMILARLY ACTING SYMPATHOMIMETIC DELUSIONAL DISORDER.

amphetamines a group of phenylethylamine-derived drugs that stimulate the reticular activating system and cause a release of stored norepinephrine. The effect is a prolonged state of arousal and relief from feelings of fatigue. A. were introduced in 1932 and have been used in the treatment of narcolepsy, certain forms of parkinsonism, hyperkinesis, and obesity. During World War II, millions of a. were dispensed to combat soldiers to enable them to remain alert for periods of up to 60 hours. Tolerance develops progressively with continued use until the patient reaches a point of exhaustion and sleeps continously for several days. The prototype of a. is AMPHETAMINE (see this entry) which closely resembles ephedrine in molecular structure and activity. Other forms include **dextroamphetamine sulfate**—$C_{18}H_{28}N_2O_4S$, used in the treatment of mental depression, alcoholism, encephalitis, narcolepsy, and obesity; **methamphetamine**—$C_{10}H_{15}N$, sometimes used to combat hypotension; and **amphetamine sulfate**—$C_{18}H_{28}N_2O_4S$. In addition to a. developed for therapeutic purposes, some forms of the drug have been manufactured as psychedelics, e.g. **methyldimethoxyamphetamine (DOM, STP)**—$C_{12}H_{19}NO_2$. See PSYCHEDELICS.

amphierotism /-i·er'-/ a condition in which a

person is able to conceive of himself in erotic terms as a male or a female or both.

amphigenesis a form of sexuality in which a person who is primarily homosexual is able to have normal sexual relations with a member of the opposite sex.

amphigenous inversion /-fij'-/ a term for psychosexual hermaphroditism in which a homosexual may engage in sexual intercourse with members of either sex. Also see ABSOLUTE INVERSION.

amphimixis /-mik'sis/ a psychoanalytic term (Greek, "mingling of two components") for the integration of anal and genital erotism in the development of heterosexuality. A. denotes also the merging of the germ plasm of two organisms in sexual reproduction, so that both parents are responsible for inheritance.

amplitude in acoustics, a measure of loudness or intensity of sound; the distance through space a vibrating body moves.

amplitude distortion a hearing disorder in which loud sounds are distorted or misjudged.

amplitude of response: See RESPONSE AMPLITUDE.

ampulla any saccular dilation of a duct or passageway through body tissues or organs. **Ampullae** located at each end of the semicircular canals of the inner ear contain hair cells that help maintain the normal sense of balance.

amputation the surgical removal of a limb or other appendage from the body (from Latin *amputare*, "to shorten, prune"). A. generally is performed as a life-saving measure following an injury or disease, e.g., diabetes, to prevent the spread of a pathogenic condition, such as gangrene or cancer, toward the body core. Because of the resulting handicap, the patient may require psychological as well as physical rehabilitation.

amputation doll a play-therapy doll that can be taken apart, to encourage expression of feeling. The basic a.d. is a mother doll, but in appropriate situations the therapist can increase the family with brother and sister dolls.

Amsterdam dwarf disease; Amsterdam type of retardation: See de LANGE'S SYNDROME.

amuck = AMOK.

amurakh a culture-specific syndrome occurring among Siberian women. The term means "copying mania," since the principal symptom consists of mimicking other people's words or behavior. Also see COPYING MANIA.

amusia a type of auditory agnosia in which the subject is unable to recognize melodies. The condition usually is associated with a lesion in the left parietal lobe of right-handed persons. A. also may be applied to a loss of musical expression, or **expressive a.** Also see MOTOR A.; SENSORY A.

amychophobia /amikō-/ a morbid fear of being scratched.

amygdala /əmig'-/ an almond-shaped mass of nerve tissue located immediately below the cerebral cortex. In most animals, the a. functions mainly as an olfactory organ, but in humans it is associated with a wide range of behavior patterns involving sexual activity, digestion and excretion, heart rate, arterial blood pressure, and muscle tone. Also called **amygdaloid body; amygdaloid complex**.

amygdaloidectomy the removal of a portion of the amygdala as a therapeutic effort to reduce hallucinations or other abnormal reactions. Ablation of various areas of the amygdala can produce a sense of fear, aggressiveness, hypersexuality, and compulsive oral responses, depending upon the area affected. Also called **amygdalectomy**.

amygdaloid stimulation an experimental procedure in which mild stimulation of the basolateral portion of the amygdaloid nucleus of animals produces a searching response and more intense stimulation initiates defensive-aggressive reactions. Nerve pathways run directly to the hippocampus and hypothalamus from the amygdala, making a.s. an important behavioral-research tool.

amyl nitrate $C_5H_{11}NO_2$—a member of a family of drugs that act primarily on the cardiovascular system. They produce a relaxation of the smooth muscles of the arteries. The effect on the heart is one of dilating the coronary arteries, accelerating heart action, and reducing blood pressure. Most of the pharmacologic properties of a.n. are equivalent to those of amyl nitrite, and the substances often are used interchangeably. Also see PSYCHEDELICS.

amyloidosis a disorder marked by the accumulation of an **amyloid**, a complex starchlike protein substance, in the tissues. The cause is believed to be an immune-deficiency disease. A. eventually is destructive because it interferes with normal function of tissues, forming tumors in the respiratory tract, liver, kidney, and other organs. Major kinds of a. are **primary a.**, in the absence of other diseases, and **secondary a.**, when associated with a chronic disease.

amyostasia a type of muscle tremor frequently observed in locomotor ataxia.

amyosthenia = APHORIA.

amyotony = APHORIA.

amyotrophic lateral sclerosis a motor-neuron disease marked by progressive degeneration of the corticospinal nerve tracts. Muscular atrophy and weakness begin spontaneously in the hands and spread to the arms and legs, the symptoms usually starting after age 40. Spasticity and increased reflexes may be observed before other signs of the disease such as respiratory distress. The sensory nerves are not affected. The victims usually are male. Also called **progressive muscular atrophy; anterior-horn-cell disease**. A popular alternative term for a.l.s. is **Lou Gehrig's disease**, named for New York Yankees baseball player Henry (Lou) Gehrig (1903–41), who died of a.l.s. after establishing a reputation as the "iron man" of baseball; Gehrig's illness did much to promote interest in the cause and treat-

ment of a.l.s. A more general term that is often specifically applied to a.l.s. is MOTOR-NEURON DISEASE. See this entry. Also see PROGRESSIVE BULBAR PALSY. A.l.s. is often abbreviated as **ALS**.

Amytal ablation a presurgical and diagnostic technique for determining hemispheric functions by injecting a small dose of the anesthetic sodium Amytal into the internal carotid artery on one side of the brain. The anesthetic effect clears in a few minutes, but dysphasia effects may continue for 30 minutes if the hemisphere injected is dominant for language.

Amytal interview = SODIUM-A.I.

-an-; -a- a combining form meaning (a) not or without, (b) in, at, (c) to, toward.

-ana- a combining form meaning up, back, against.

anabolic phase the building-up phase of a metabolic process, as in the example of the formation of rhodopsin molecules in the retinal receptors to replace the visual purple consumed during exposure to illumination.

anabolic system a constitutional body type in which the abdomen is more prominent than the chest due to the presence of large visceral organs.

anabolism /ənab'-/ a constructive stage of metabolism in which dietary nutrients are used to build or restore tissues or are stored for future use. Adjective: **anabolic** /-bol'-/. See METABOLISM.

anaclisis /ənak'-/ an extreme dependence on another person for emotional and in some cases physical support, just as an infant is dependent on the mother for the satisfaction of its basic needs. Freud introduced the term to describe the attachment of the sex drive to the satisfaction of another instinct, such as hunger or defecation. Adjective: **anaclitic** /-klit'-/; **anaclinic**.

anaclitic depression an acute reaction of lethargy and apparent despondency in infants abruptly separated from their mother or deprived of mothering care, as in impersonal institutions or foster homes.

anaclitic object choice in psychoanalysis, the selection of a mate or other love object who will provide the same type of assistance, comfort, and support that the individual has received from the mother during infancy and early childhood.

anaclitic therapy a form of psychotherapy in which the patient is encouraged to regress to an infantile state of dependence on the therapist. The object is to have him revive and relive early experiences which have produced the feelings and fixations that are blocking normal adjustment. In some cases the patient is kept in isolation and fed and "mothered" by the therapist.

anacusis total deafness. Also called **anacusia; anacousia**. Adjective: **anacusic**.

Anadenanthera genus name for a group of plants indigenous to Latin America and used by local populations as a source of a mind-altering snuff. The plant materials contain bufotenine and dimethyltryptamine, both known hallucinogens.

anaesthesia = ANESTHESIA.

anaglyptoscope a shadow-perspective study instrument that reverses light and dark patterns.

anagogic interpretation Jung's view that dreams and other unconscious material are expressions of ideals and spiritual forces, as contrasted with the sexual interpretations of psychoanalysis (from Greek *anagoge*, "leading upward").

anagogic symbolism the indirect representation of objects associated with moral, spiritual, or idealistic concepts.

anagogic tendency: See KATAGOGIC TENDENCY.

anal-aggressive character in psychoanalysis, a personality type characterized by obstinacy, obstructionism, defiance, and passive resistance. Such traits are believed to stem from the anal stage in which the child asserted himself by withholding his feces. See ANAL CHARACTER.

anal birth a symbolic desire to be reborn through the anus as expressed in dreams or fantasies with anal erotic content.

anal castration anxiety a displacement of the fear of castration by a regressive anal manifestation, e.g., various toilet phobias.

anal character in psychoanalysis, a pattern of personality traits believed to stem from the anal phase of psychosexual development, when defecation was a primary source of pleasure. According to this theory, a child who derives special satisfaction from retention of the feces tends to develop a personality marked by the **anal triad** of frugality, obstinacy, and orderliness; and, as an adult, such a person will probably be compulsive, meticulous, rigid, and overconscientious. Also called **anal personality**.

analeptics stimulants other than amphetamines that produce subjective effects similar to those caused by amphetamine use. The effects may include alertness, elevated mood, increased feeling of energy, decreased appetite, irritability, and insomnia. The group includes **diethylpropion**—$C_{13}H_{19}NO$, **methylphenidate**—$C_{14}H_{19}NO_2$, and **pipradrol**—$C_{18}H_{21}NO$. The a. also may include certain psychostimulants, such as COCAINE. See this entry. Also see ANOREXICS.

anal eroticism = ANAL EROTISM.

anal-erotic traits in psychoanalysis, personality traits characteristic of obsessive individuals: overcautiousness, overmeticulousness, stubbornness, miserliness, overconcern with detail. See ANAL EROTISM; ANAL CHARACTER.

anal erotism in psychoanalysis, pleasurable sensations associated with expulsion, retention, or observation of the feces. These sensations first arise in the anal phase of psychosexual development, between the ages of one and three. Individuals who are fixated at this stage may later derive special gratification from elimination, manipulation of the anal region, or anal intercourse. Also called **anal eroticism**. See ANAL CHARACTER; ANAL PHASE; COPROPHILIA.

anal-expulsive stage a phase of the anal stage in which pleasure is obtained by expelling feces.

anal fantasies fantasies of anal intercourse or anal

pregnancy and birth, not uncommon in children. If retained on an unconscious level, these fantasies may give rise to gastrointestinal conversion symptoms years later.

analgesia an insensitivity to pain due either to organic disorder or to psychological factors. Loss of pain sensation occurs most frequently in conversion, or hysterical, disorder, and schizophrenia. Also called **analgia**. Compare ALGESIA.

analgesics drugs or other agents that alleviate pain. Analgesic drugs usually are classed as narcotic or nonnarcotic, depending upon their potential for physical dependence. Narcotic a. are generally more effective in relieving pain symptoms. The milder nonnarcotic a. include the ANILIDES, SALICYLATES, INDOLE DERIVATIVES, and PYRAZOLONES. See these entries.

analgia = ANALGESIA.

anal humor jokes that involve the anal zone. According to psychoanalytic theory, the tendency to appreciate such humor harks back to the anal stage when the child derived pleasure from the stimulation of this zone by retention or elimination of feces. A preoccupation with a.h. may be indicative of a fixation at this stage.

anal impotence an inability to defecate except under certain conditions, e.g., absolute privacy.

anal intercourse a form of sexual activity in which pleasure is achieved through anal intromission of the penis. According to some psychiatrists, a craving for anal-erotic satisfaction is the basis for homosexuality. Also called **coitus analis; coitus in ano**. Also see SODOMY.

anal itching irritation of the skin and surrounding tissues of the perianal region. Causes include allergies to soap or clothing, systemic diseases such as diabetes mellitus, hemorrhoids, or parasitic agents such as pinworms. A yeast infection, moniliasis, often is a cause of a.i. as a result of anal intercourse involving a male partner with moniliasis of the glans penis. Also see MONILIASIS.

anality erotic pleasure associated with the anal region.

anal masturbation a form of anal erotism in which sexual excitement is achieved through manual or mechanical stimulation (usually self-stimulation) of the anus.

analog denoting a continuous or graded representation of information, in contrast to digital or binary representation. Also spelled **analogue**.

analogies test a test of the subject's ability to comprehend the relationship between two items and then extend that relationship to a different situation; e.g., paintbrush is to paint as pen is to _____.

analogue = ANALOG.

analogue experiment an experiment in which a phenomenon related to the study objective is produced in order to obtain an improved perspective toward the situation. Examples of an a.e. include the use of hypnosis, mind-altering drugs, and sensory deprivation to produce brief periods of abnormal behavior which simulates that of psychopathological conditions.

analogue study a research method in which a type of treatment is evaluated under well-controlled conditions analogous to those in a clinic.

analogy-principle response: See RESPONSE-BY-ANALOGY PRINCIPLE.

anal personality = ANAL CHARACTER.

anal phase in psychoanalysis, the second stage of psychosexual development, occurring during the second year of life, in which the child's interest and sexual pleasure are focused on the expulsion and retention of the feces. Also called **anal stage**.

anal-rape fantasy a fear or concept of sexual attack via the anus, a fantasy that may occur in either men or women.

anal retention: See ANAL CHARACTER.

anal-retentive stage a phase of the anal stage marked by pleasure in retaining feces and thereby defying the parent.

anal sadism in psychoanalysis, the expression of destructive and aggressive impulses in the anal stage of psychosexual development, as well as their expression in later life.

anal-sadistic stage in psychoanalysis, the second part of the anal stage, when the child manifests aggressive, destructive, and negativistic tendencies. One expression of these tendencies is withholding the feces in defiance of parental urging.

anal stage = ANAL PHASE.

anal triad: See ANAL CHARACTER.

analysand in psychoanalysis, the patient who is under analysis.

analysis in general, the division of any complex entity, such as a chemical compound or a personality type, into its component parts. In psychiatry, a. is an abbreviated term for psychoanalysis, but is also used for other approaches in which the deeper levels of the psyche are probed.

analysis-by-synthesis the theory of perception stating that the perceiver first breaks down (analyzes) a stimulus object into its constituent elements and then assembles (synthesizes) the significant components to form a percept in accordance with the object's context and the perceiver's previous experience.

analysis in depth in psychiatry, any therapeutic approach based on exploration of unconscious processes, especially psychoanalysis and Jung's analytic psychology. See DEPTH PSYCHOLOGY.

analysis of covariance an extension of analysis of variance which adjusts means for the influence of a correlated variable or covariate. A.o.c. is appropriate when experimental groups are known to differ on a background-correlated variable, in addition to the differences attributed to the experimental treatment.

analysis of the resistance a basic procedure in psychoanalysis, in which the patient's tendency to maintain the repression of unconscious impulses and experiences is subjected to analytic scrutiny. The process of explaining resistances is believed to be a major contribution to self-understanding and self-change. See RESISTANCE.

analysis of transference in psychoanalysis, the interpretation of a patient's early relationships and experiences as they are reflected and expressed in his present relationship to the analyst. See TRANSFERENCE; TRANSFERENCE RESISTANCE.

analysis of variance a statistical procedure, developed by R. A. Fisher, that isolates the joint and separate effects of independent variables upon a dependent variable, and tests them for statistical significance. Abbrev.: **ANOVA**.

analysis unit: See ELEMENT.

analyst a term most frequently applied to followers of Freud, or psychoanalysts, but also used for followers of Jung, or analytic psychologists, followers of Adler, or individual psychologists, and followers of Meyer, or psychobiologists. See PSYCHOANALYST.

analytic couch = COUCH.

analytic group psychotherapy a form of group psychotherapy developed by S. R. Slavson, based on the application of psychoanalytic concepts and techniques to three principal age groups. In play-group psychotherapy—for preschool children—internal conflicts, fantasies, and interpersonal communication are elicited by play activities and materials, and the children are encouraged to understand how their problems, such as fears or sibling rivalries, are affecting their behavior and feelings. In activity-interview group psychotherapy—for children in the latency period—hobby and recreational activities open the way to interpretation of the child's attitudes and feelings, not only by the therapist but by members of the group; e.g., the child gains analytic insight into hostile reactions by recognizing that he is taking out his frustrations or anger on others (displacement). In interview group psychotherapy—for adolescents and adults—the groups are selected on the basis of therapeutic balance, and six analytic principles are applied: transference, catharsis, achievement of insight, development of ego strength, reality testing, and sublimation through discussions, drawing, and other activities.

analytic insight in psychoanalysis, an awareness of the unconscious origin and meaning of behavior and symptoms, especially as a result of working through resistances which, as Freud (1914) claimed, "effects the greatest changes in the patient and which distinguishes analytic treatment from any kind of treatment by suggestion." See RESISTANCE.

analytic interpretation in psychoanalysis, the therapist's formulation of the patient's early experiences, dreams, character defenses, resistances, and other productions in terms that are meaningful to the patient.

analytic neurosis a type of neurosis that may result from overextended psychoanalysis, characterized by a neurotic attitude based on emotional dependency on analysis and analysts.

analytic patient a person receiving analytic treatment. According to Freud, psychoanalysis is most effective between the ages of 15 and 50, since children do not have sufficient reasoning power and older people do not have enough elasticity to profit by the process. In general, the patient must be self-motivated, willing to cooperate with the therapist, able to reason, not in an acute or dangerous state, and willing to remain in therapy for a lengthy period. Freud found that classical analysis is most effective with relatively young, educated, and intelligent patients afflicted with conversion hysteria and, with only slight changes in method, with patients suffering from phobias and obsessive-compulsive reactions.

analytic psychology Carl Gustav Jung's system in which the psyche is interpreted primarily in terms of philosophic values, racial images and symbols, and a drive for self-fulfillment. His basic concepts are (a) the ego, which maintains a balance between conscious and unconscious activities, and gradually develops a unique self (individuation), (b) the personal unconscious, made up of memories, thoughts, and feelings based on personal experience, (c) the collective unconscious, or residual of racial ideas (archetypes) which exert a basic influence on consciousness, (d) dynamic polarities, or tension systems, which derive their psychic energy from the libido, and influence the development and expression of the ego: conscious versus unconscious values, introversion versus extraversion, sublimation versus repression, rational versus irrational. The object of life, and of Jungian therapy, is to achieve a creative balance among all these forces.

analytic rules the three rules laid down by Freud for conducting psychoanalytic therapy: the "fundamental rule" of free association, which gives free reign to the unconscious to bring repressed impulses and experiences to the surface; the rule of abstinence, which discourages gratifications that might drain off energy that could be utilized in the therapeutic process; and the rule against acting out feelings and events instead of talking them out. See ACTING OUT; BASIC RULE; RULE OF ABSTINENCE.

analytic stalemate: See ID RESISTANCE.

analyzer a theoretical part or function of a sensory nerve system responsible for making sensitivity evaluations. The concept was introduced by Pavlov.

anamnesis in psychiatry and clinical psychology, the patient's personal account of his developmental, family, and medical history prior to the onset of his illness (Greek, "recollection"). A. is an integral part of the psychiatric examination, first suggested by Adolph Meyer as an aid to diagnosis and exploration of possible causes of the patient's disorder. Also see PSYCHIATRIC HISTORY.

anamnestic analysis a Jungian term for analysis that emphasizes the patient's historical account of his problem with added material from family and friends.

anancasm repetitious, stereotyped behavior which the individual feels impelled to carry out in order to relieve tension and anxiety. Also spelled **anankasm**. See COMPULSION.

anancastic personality a personality disorder characterized by excessive perfectionism, overconscientiousness, lack of warmth, preoccupation with form and details, and inability to "loosen up" and enjoy leisure-time activities. Also called **anancastia**. See COMPULSIVE-PERSONALITY DISORDER. Also see COMPULSIVE CHARACTER.

anandria the absence of masculinity.

anankasm = ANANCASM.

ananke /ənang′kē/ the Greek term for external necessity, or fate, conceived to be the counterpart of inner necessity arising from Eros, the life instinct, and Thanatos, the death instinct. These two forces, internal and external, were viewed as the parents of human culture.

anaphase a stage of mitotic cell division in which the chromosomes migrate to the poles of the spindle to form daughter chromosomes.

anaphia the absence or loss of ability to perceive tactile sensations or stimuli (from Greek *an-* and *haphe*, "touch").

anaphrodisia an obsolete term for lack of sexual feelings.

anaphrodisiac any drug or other agent that functions as a sexual sedative to reduce or repress sexual desire. Among substances claimed to have an a. effect are potassium bromide, heroin, and camphor. Members of religious orders reportedly have cultivated the bitter herb rue (Ruta graveolens) in their cloister gardens for its a. effect. Anaphrodisiacs also may be a cause of sexual anesthesia or frigidity.

anaphylaxis hypersensitivity to the introduction of an allergen into body tissues, resulting from previous exposure to it. The reaction may be sudden and violent, marked by convulsions, coma, breathing difficulty, shock, and death, depending upon individual sensitivities. Anaphylactic reactions may occur after a wasp sting or after an injection of penicillin. In psychiatry, the term **psychiatric a.** is applied more broadly to reactivation of earlier symptoms, such as hives, by an activating event which is emotionally similar to the one that produced the original sensitivity. E.g., the sensitizing agent might have been social embarrassment in the teen years, and the presently activating event might be anxiety produced by rejection by a social organization.

anaplasia cellular tissue that lacks structural differentiation. The term also may be applied to a cell or tissue that has reverted to a more primitive or embryonic stage. Cancer tissue often develops as a.

anaplastic astrocytoma a form of brain tumor that contains astrocytelike glioma cells that are poorly differentiated. It may be composed of young, immature tumor cells.

anarchic behavior lawless, antisocial behavior; also, rebellion of children against rules and regulations in an effort to achieve independence, or to get attention.

anarithmia = ACALCULIA.

anarthria /ənär′thrē·ə/ the inability to speak due to brain lesions or damage to peripheral nerves that affect the articulatory muscles.

anastomoses alternate pathways formed by branches of main circuits. A. may be found in nerves or blood or lymphatic vessels. The brain is served by **arterial a**. which help insure a continuing blood flow to as many areas of brain tissue as possible in the event one pathway is blocked by a blood clot or rupture of a blood vessel.

anatomical age a measure of the state of physical development of an individual, based on the condition of certain skeletal features as compared with the normal state of the bones for a specified chronological age. Also see CHRONOLOGICAL AGE; MENTAL AGE.

anchor a reference point used by subjects when making series of judgments. E.g., in an experiment in which subjects gauge distances between objects, the experimenter introduces an a. when he or she informs subjects that the distance between two of the stimulus objects is a given value. That value then functions as a reference for subjects in their subsequent judgments.

anchoring point a reference point for subjective judgments, e.g., rating sunsets on a scale of one to ten. See ANCHOR.

anchor test a test used in establishing comparable norms for tests in the same field, e.g., the use of the reading comprehension and vocabulary subtests of the Metropolitan Achievement Test as a basis for comparing various reading achievement tests and developing a single score scale (the National Reference Scale).

Andersen, Dorothy Hansine American pediatrician, 1901–63. See ANDERSEN'S DISEASE; ANDERSEN'S SYNDROME.

Andersen's disease a familial disorder marked by cirrhosis of the liver with involvement of the heart, kidneys, muscles, and nervous system. The disease is due to a deficit of an enzyme needed to convert glucose carried from the digestive tract into glycogen for storage by the liver.

Andersen's syndrome a disorder consisting of three pathologic conditions, which are cystic fibrosis of the pancreas, celiac disease, and vitamin-A deficiency. The condition may be marked by symptoms of depression, muscle wasting, and hypotonia. Children may show difficulty in walking or standing. Also called **Andersen's triad**.

Anderson, Rose Gustava American psychologist, 1893—. See KUHLMANN-ANDERSON TESTS.

-andr-; -andro- a combining form meaning male.

Andrade, Corino M. de English physician, fl. 1952. See ANDRADE'S SYNDROME.

Andrade's syndrome a form of amyloidosis. The major effects of the amyloid are flaccid paralysis, sensory disorders, impotence, and premature menopause. Also called **familial Portuguese polyneuritic amyloidosis; Corino de Andrade's paramyloidosis; Wohlwill-Corino Andrade syndrome**.

androgen hypersecretion: See ADRENAL-CORTICAL HYPERFUNCTION.

androgenic: See ANDROGYNY.

androgens any substances that produce male sexual characteristics. The main a. are androsterone and testosterone, which are manufactured mainly by the testes and circulate in the bloodstream as **androgenic hormones**. They contribute to the development of facial hair, a deep masculine voice, and the growth of bones and muscle that account for the normally greater size and strength of men as compared with women. A. may also be produced synthetically, and in small quantities by the adrenal cortex. An adrenal tumor can result in excessive production of a., causing serious masculinization effects in women as well as men.

androgynous sex role a mixture of sex roles in which there is a confusion or uncertainty about gender identity and behavior that may be labeled both masculine and feminine. A male may play an effeminate role and prefer a partner of his own sex, or a female may play a masculine role and prefer a partner of her own sex.

androgyny /-droj′-/ a combination of male and female characteristics in one individual. The term is usually applied to a male with feminine traits. Also called **androgyneity; androgynism**. Adjectives: **androgynous; androgenic**. See BISEXUALITY; GYNANDROMORPH; HERMAPHRODITE.

andromania = NYMPHOMANIA.

androphobia a morbid fear of men.

androphonomania an obsolete term for homicidal insanity.

androsterone /-dros′-/ a steroid hormone metabolite with weak androgenic effects. A. is a substance commonly found in the urine of males.

anechoic chamber an enclosure scientifically designed to eliminate sound reverberations and echoes. It is an environment typically used in audiological testing centers.

anecdotal evidence evidence based on uncontrolled personal observations, e.g., behavior of one patient.

anecdotal method a technique of presenting data based on personal observation rather than scientific experimentation with controlled variables. The a.m., like epidemiology findings, may not reveal causal relationships but can offer clues as to areas of investigation that warrant scientific studies.

anecdotal record in education, a factual, written record containing spontaneous, succinct, cumulative descriptions of a student's behavior. Such observations are usually considered significant because they highlight a given aspect of the student's personality and may prove useful in future evaluations.

-anem-; -anemo- a combining form meaning wind, air current.

anemia a blood disorder marked by a lower-than-normal number of red blood cells or a deficiency of hemoglobin in the red blood cells. The condition is a sign of several possible diseases or abnormalities that can include loss of blood through hemorrhage, bone-marrow disease, exposure to toxic substances in the environment, or an inadequate diet. One form of a., sickle-cell a., is hereditary. (A. comes from the Greek word *anaimia*, "lack of blood.") Also see ADDISON-BIERMER A.; COOLEY'S A.; SICKLE-CELL A.; CEREBRAL A.

anemophobia a morbid fear of wind or strong drafts.

anemotaxis: See JOHNSTON'S ORGAN.

anemotropism an orientation response of the body to air currents.

anencephaly /-sef'-/ the congenital absence of a brain. The condition may range from complete lack of cerebral hemispheres to the presence of only small masses of cerebral tissue. Also called **anencephalia** /-fãl'-/.

anergasia a term applied by A. Meyer to a psychosis or loss of functional activity due to a structural brain disorder.

anergia absence of energy; extreme passivity. Also called **anergy**. Adjective: **anergic**. Also see BURNED-OUT.

anergic schizophrenia any form of schizophrenia that is marked by passivity or lack of energy. See BURNED-OUT.

anergic schizophrenic = BURNED-OUT.

anergy = ANERGIA.

anesthesia a loss or impairment of sensitivity to stimuli due to nerve damage or destruction, narcotic drugs, hypnotic suggestion, or conversion (hysterical) disorder. The latter condition involves loss of sensation in specific areas that do not correspond to the distribution of nerve fibers, such as glove, stocking, girdle, wrist, or trunk anesthesia. Also spelled **anaesthesia**.

anesthetic leprosy = DANIELSSEN-BOECK DISEASE.

anesthetics agents that produce anesthesia as characterized by loss of sensation, unconsciousness, relaxation of skeletal muscles, reduction of motor activity and reflexes, amnesia, or a combination of such effects. Kinds of a. include **general a.**, which may be administered by inhalation, intravenous injection, or retention enema, **regional a.**, administered by injection or topical application, and other a. techniques, e.g., acupuncture and hypothermia.

anethopathy behavior marked by an absence of ethics or moral inhibitions, accompanied by narcissistic sexual behavior and egocentrism. A. patients are usually "disease-fast," or unresponsive to psychotherapy. See ANTISOCIAL-PERSONALITY DISORDER.

aneuploidy an irregular number of chromosomes such as 45 or 49, instead of the normal 46. A. is frequently associated with neurologic defects or mental retardation, or both. The condition often can be detected through amniocentesis, which may reveal the addition or loss of one or more chromosomes, or parts of normal chromosomes.

aneurysm /an'yərizəm/ a permanent dilation at some point in an artery caused by the pressure of blood on weakened tissues (from Greek *aneurysmos*, "dilation"). Also spelled **aneurism**.

angel dust a street name for phencyclidine and related substances of abuse which produce acute organic mental disorders. See PHENCYCLIDINE; PSYCHEDELICS.

Angell, James Rowland American psychologist and educator, 1869–1949. A. was a founder, with John Dewey, of the functionalist approach which stresses the practical utility of thinking, emotions, and other mental processes in enabling the organism to adjust to the environment. See FUNCTIONALISM.

Angelman syndrome = HAPPY-PUPPET SYNDROME. Also see LAUGHTER.

anger a reaction of tension and hostility aroused by frustration, physical restraint, threats, derogatory remarks, unfairness, injustice, or discrimination. Feelings of a. involve such autonomic responses as increase in blood pressure, respiration, and heart rate; perspiration; and release of blood sugar, all of which serve to put the organism on a "war footing." Expressions of a. vary from person to person and from age to age, ranging from temper tantrums, hitting, kicking, biting, and obstinacy in the early years, to teasing, surliness, fighting, and name-calling during the school years, to scapegoating, nursing of grievances, caustic remarks, swearing, irritability, and righteous indignation at later ages.

anger-in hostility turned inward, particularly as a source of depression. Freud held that depression can be distinguished, e.g., from normal mourning by the anger and guilt one feels toward the self due to feelings of aggression toward the lost love object (*Mourning and Melancholia*, 1917). See SELF-ACCUSATION.

-angi-; -angio- a combining form relating to blood vessels or lymph vessels.

anginophobia = PNIGOPHOBIA.

angiography the visualization of blood vessels, usually through X-rays or similar radiological techniques. A. is a diagnostic aid in conditions such as heart attacks and cerebrovascular accidents. In a., a substance that is opaque to X-rays is injected into one of the blood vessels to follow the path of blood blow. Any obstruction, aneurysm, or rupture in the blood vessel will be revealed as a white contrasting pattern on black film (**angiogram, arteriogram**). Also called **arteriography**. Also see CEREBRAL A.; DIGITAL A.

angiokeratoma corporis diffusum = FABRY'S DISEASE.

angioneurotic edema a disorder marked by recurrent episodes of noninflammatory swelling of certain body tissues, particularly the skin, mucous membranes, viscera, and central nervous system. The disorder may begin suddenly and last for hours or days, sometimes causing death. Attacks may be triggered by food or drug allergies, insect stings or bites, or viral infection. A hereditary form may be associated with emotional stress. Also called **Quincke's disease**.

angioscotoma a type of visual-field disorder caused by blood-vessel shadows on the retina.

angiotensin a polypeptide substance in the blood that functions as a vasopressor to stimulate contractions of the walls of arteries and capillaries. A. is formed by the action of the enzyme renin on a globulin molecule in the blood. A. also is a stimulator of aldosterone secretion by the adrenal cortex.

angry-woman syndrome a personality disorder marked by obsessive neatness, perfectionism, punctuality, outbursts of unprovoked anger, marital troubles, critical attitude toward others, and a tendency to drug and alcohol abuse. The patient also may make serious attempts at suicide.

Angst /ängst/ a key concept (German, "fear, anxiety, anguish") of the existentialist approach which seeks to understand the fundamental structure of human existence. Rollo May has described A. in these terms: "anxiety is the inward state of my becoming aware that my existence can become lost, that I can lose myself and my world, that I can become 'nothing.' Anxiety strikes at the center of the person's experience of himself as a being. Fear, in contrast, is a threat to the periphery of his existence" (in *American Handbook of Psychiatry*, 1959).

angstrom a unit used in expressing extremely small dimensions, such as wavelengths of light or X-rays. An a. is equivalent to 0.1 millimicron. It was named for the Swedish physicist **A. J. Ångström** (1814–74). Abbrev.: **A; Å**.

angular gyrus a folded convolution in the inferior parietal lobe formed by a junction of the superior and middle temporal gyri. The a.g. arches over the end of the superior temporal sulcus and becomes continuous with the middle temporal gyrus.

anhedonia the inability to derive pleasure from experiences that are normally pleasurable. A. is a symptom of schizophrenia, especially the pseudoneurotic type, as well as depressive disorder. Also called **dystychia**.

anhidrosis an abnormal deficiency of sweat. Also spelled **anhydrosis**.

aniconia an absence of mental imagery.

anilerdine: See SYNTHETIC NARCOTICS.

aniliction = ANILINGUS.

anilides nonnarcotic analgesics that are aniline derivatives. The first in the series of a. was **acetanilide**—C_8H_9NO—which was discovered in 1852 but was not employed therapeutically until 1886, when German physicians found as a result of a prescription error that acetanilide can reduce symptoms of fever. Other a. include **acetaminophen**—$C_8H_9NO_2$—and **acetophenetidin (phenacetin)**—$C_{10}H_{13}NO_2$.

anilingus the practice of applying the mouth to the anus as a form of sexual activity. According to some investigators, the identification of the anus as a source of sexual pleasure probably is due to the common ancestry of the anus and reproductive tract as represented by the cloaca in lower animals. Also called **aniliction**.

anima a Jungian term with two meanings: (a) the individual's inner self, which represents feelings and attitudes that stem from unconscious sources, as contrasted with the outer self, or persona, which the individual presents to the world, and (b) an archetype which represents feminine characteristics, in contrast to the animus, which represents masculine characteristics. See ARCHETYPE; PERSONA; ANIMUS.

animal aggression various types of aggression among animals, including, among others, (a) **maternal aggression**, when the female's young are threatened, (b) **predatory aggression**, when prey are sighted, (c) **dominance aggression**, to maintain status or rank, (d) **sexual aggression** in the male, for purposes of mating, (e) **antipredatory aggression**, for defense of territory, (f) **fear-induced aggression**, incited by confinement or threat, (g) **intermale aggression**, elicited by a male competitor.

animal-cry theory: See ORIGIN-OF-LANGUAGE THEORIES.

animal magnetism a hypothetical magnetic fluid which, according to Mesmer, emanates from the heavenly bodies and pervades the atmosphere. This fluid, he held, could be focused on ailing parts of the body with curative effect through the use of a magnetized wand, magnetized rods, and magnetized baths. See BAQUET; MESMER.

animal phobia a morbid fear of animals in general (zoophobia) or of a particular animal such as snakes (ophidiophobia), cats (ailurophobia), dogs (cynophobia), insects (acarophobia), mice (musophobia), or spiders (arachneophobia). Phobias of this kind frequently arise from the warnings of others, from traumatic experiences, or from unconscious symbolism. See LITTLE HANS.

animal psychology: See COMPARATIVE PSYCHOLOGY.

animal spirits a vaguely defined substance which Galen in the second century and Descartes in the 16th pictured as flowing through hollow tubes from the brain to all parts of the body—a precursor of the modern concept of the nerve impulse. Descartes, however, also anticipated the modern concept of the peripheral nervous system by maintaining that nerves conduct in either direction between the muscles and sense organs.

animal starch = GLYCOGEN.

animatism the tendency to assign psychological qualities to inanimate objects; personification. It is a common symptom in schizophrenia.

animism the belief that natural phenomena, such as rivers and clouds, possess souls or spirits. Freud held that primitive man modeled this picture of the world after his own mind, and held that the creation of spirits was man's first theoretical achievement. Also see SOCIAL A.

animistic thinking a stage in the development of the child's cognitive processes in which he attributes friendly or hostile intentions to inanimate objects such as sticks or stones (Piaget). The term also applies to irrational or superstitious thought processes based on the effects of nonliving objects on our lives, as in carrying or stroking a charm to bring luck.

animus in Jungian analytic psychology, the masculine component of the female personality, an archetype representing the racial experiences of women with men, which are stored in the collective unconscious.

anions /anī′əns/ ions that carry a negative charge.

aniridia-oligophrenia-cerebellar ataxia syndrome a rare form of mental retardation in which the patient also suffers from lack of normal muscle control and has speech difficulty. Lenses and corneas may be normal, but the eyes lack irises and visual acuity is in a range between 20/100 and 20/200.

aniseikonia a difficulty in binocular vision in which the two eyes perceive images of unequal size or shape.

ankle clonus a series of rapid calf-muscle contractions and relaxations causing foot tremors.

ankle jerk = ACHILLES REFLEX.

-ankyl-; -ankylo-; -ancylo- a combining form meaning bent, crooked.

ankyloglossia the restricted movement of the tongue due to abnormal shortness of the lingual frenum. Normal speech production may be affected. Also called **tongue tie**.

ankylosing spondylitis an inflammation of the vertebrae that results in a permanent stiffening of the vertebral column in a kyphosis, or hunchback, position. The vertebrae and intervertebral disks usually are eroded or destroyed, causing a collapse of the spine. A.s. may be associated with Pott's disease, a form of tuberculosis, or other infectious diseases, e.g., brucellosis. A chronic rheumatoid form of a.s. is called **Marie-Strümpell disease**.

ankylosis an immobility and consolidation of a joint, usually due to the destruction of membranes lining the joint or to a bone-structure defect. A. may occur naturally, as in rheumatoid arthritis, or by surgical fusion (arthrodesis).

Anlage /än′läge/ a genetic factor that predisposes the individual to a particular trait; also, the individual's hereditary disposition as a whole (German, "aptitude").

Anna O.: See TALKING CURE.

annihilation anxiety the fear of destroying oneself or of being destroyed. A.a. is frequently felt by drug users just before or just after taking a heavy dose of a psychedelic drug. It may also be a form of death anxiety experienced by depressive patients.

anniversary excitement a term introduced by Bleuler to identify episodes of agitation or other mental disturbances that tend to occur on the anniversary of a significant date in the life of the patient. The event usually is related to the cause of the patient's conflict. Also see ANNIVERSARY REACTION.

anniversary hypothesis a generalization that the first admission for a mental patient who lost a parent in childhood is likely to occur within a year of the time when his or her eldest child reaches the age of the patient when the parent died.

anniversary reaction the unconscious revival of symptoms, or the aggravation of a psychophysiologic illness (e.g., arthritis), on the anniversary of a disturbing event such as the death of a loved one or a severe disappointment. Also see ANNIVERSARY EXCITEMENT.

annoyer an irritating or unpleasant stimulus which the subject seeks to terminate.

annulment in psychiatry, a mental phenomenon in which disagreeable ideas or events are erased from the mind instead of being relegated to the unconscious, as in repression.

annulospiral receptor a sensory end organ of a muscle spindle cell. Its function is to detect changes in the stretch reflex.

anodal polarization a condition in which the flow of electrical current is toward the positive pole. In a typical nerve cell, the positive pole would be in extracellular fluid and the current flow would be from the inside toward the outside of the cell membrane.

anodontia a congenital absence of normal dentition resulting in faulty articulation if uncorrected.

anodyne /an′ōdīn/ any agent or procedure that relieves pain, including aspirin, opium, anesthetics, or acupuncture.

anoesia an obsolete term for mental deficiency.

anoesis a form of noncognitive consciousness or mere feeling, in which the individual lacks knowledge of or reference to objects.

anogenital relating to the anatomical region in which the anus and genitalia are located.

anoia an obsolete term for insanity, or for a psychosis that is functional or lacking in somatic origin.

anomalopia = ANOMALOUS TRICHROMATISM.

anomaloscope a spectral device employed in determining color weakness through the use of the Rayleigh equation, which states the proportion of red and green stimuli required to match a given yellow. Anomalous trichromats, who are either red-weak or green-weak, require either more red or more green for a match.

anomalous dichromatism partial color blindness in which only two colors (usually blue and yellow) are seen.

anomalous trichromatism a form of color blindness or color weakness marked by a diminished capacity to respond to the red-green color system. The ability to distinguish these colors increases in proportion to their intensity, that is, less brilliant shades are less easily identified. Also called **anomalopia**.

anomaly in psychiatry, a personality that is on the outer fringes of what is considered normal, e.g., character neuroses or schizoidism. In general, an a. is anything that is irregular or abnormal, or any deviation from the natural order. Also see CONGENITAL ANOMALIES.

anomia a form of aphasia characterized by an impaired ability to recall the names of objects. The term was also used by Benjamin Rush for a defective moral sense. Also called **anomic aphasia; dysnomia**.

anomic suicide a term introduced by Durkheim to identify a type of suicide caused by the disorientation of the individual after an unfavorable change in financial or social situations. The subject believes his expected life-style is no longer possible.

anomie /anˈəmē/ a sense of alienation and despair arising from a disorganization of personal and social values during a period of catastrophe, such as a war or depression. Also see ANOMIC SUICIDE.

anomie scale in consumer psychology, a system of evaluating the deviance of an individual from accepted social behavior. The scale is based on the responses to questions that reveal the subject's attitudes toward sexual chastity, cheating on tax returns, smuggling, bribing police, cheating on examinations, and similar issues. Studies indicate that a.s. responses on consumer surveys reveal attitudes toward the credibility of advertising appeals.

anophthalmia: See X-LINKED A.

anopia blindness, usually the result of a defect in the eyes.

anorexia the absence or loss of appetite for food, usually as a chronic or continuing condition as opposed to a temporary lack of appetite. Because appetite is regarded as a primarily psychologic function, it is assumed that a. also is psychologic. However, a. also may be associated with a physiologic disorder, e.g., hypopituitarism. Adjectives, nouns: **anorectic; anorexic**. See A. NERVOSA. Also see ELECTIVE A.; SOCIAL A.; BULMOREXIA; APPETITIVE BEHAVIOR.

anorexia nervosa a persistent lack of appetite and refusal of food, often accompanied by amenorrhea, vomiting, severe weight loss, and wasting (cachexia). The condition occurs most frequently in adolescent girls, and is often explained as an urge to remain "as thin as a boy" and thereby escape the burdens of growing up and assuming a female sexual and marital role. Characteristically, they "feel fat" even when dangerously thin, deny their illness, and in some cases develop an active disgust for food. Also see PHAGOPHOBIA; NEUROTIC HUNGER STRIKE.

anorexiant: See APPETITE SUPPRESSANT.

anorexic: See ANOREXIA.

anorexics drugs that suppress the appetite and are used in the treatment of obesity. Most a. are adrenergic drugs that also produce insomnia, a factor that limits their effectiveness in reducing the appetite in the evening when many obese patients consume most of their daily intake of calories. The efficacy of a. in controlling obesity has been challenged because the benefits tend to be short-term, calorie intake must be restricted during administration of the a., and the a. often produce adverse effects involving the central nervous system. See ADRENERGIC DRUGS. Also see ANALEPTICS.

anorgasmia the inability to achieve orgasm. Also called **anorgasmy**. Adjective: **anorgasmic**.

anorthopia a type of visual distortion, sometimes associated with strabismus.

anosmia the absence of a sense of smell, which may be general or limited to certain odors. Also called **anosphresia**.

anosognosia the failure or refusal to recognize the existence of a defect or disease, such as deafness, poor vision, aphasia, disfigurement, or even loss of a limb. A. is a form of denial, or of denial of reality. See DENIAL.

anosphresia = ANOSMIA.

ANOVA = ANALYSIS OF VARIANCE.

anovulatory menstrual cycle a menstrual cycle that occurs without ovulation. It results from an imbalance between hormone production of the pituitary gland and the ovaries and is marked by irregular menstruation. An a.m.c. is most likely to be associated with menarche or menopause.

anoxemia the absence or deficiency of oxygen in the blood, a condition that frequently results in loss of consciousness and brain damage.

anoxia: See CARBON-MONOXIDE POISONING.

ANS = AUTONOMIC NERVOUS SYSTEM.

-ant-; -ante-; -antero- a combining form meaning before, in front of, coming before.

-ant-; -anti- a combining form meaning opposed to, counteracting, relieving.

Antabuse a trademark for a drug used in the control of alcoholism because it interferes with the metabolism of alcohol by the liver enzymes. By inhibiting oxidation of the aldehyde metabolite of alcohol, A. causes an accumulation of aldehyde in the blood that results in disagreeable symptoms. The symptoms include nausea, vomiting, heart arrhythmias, difficult breathing, flushing, and sweating.

antagonist a substance that inhibits another agent by blocking or reducing its functional pathways. An a. may occupy the receptor site of the other agent without activating the receptor. Or an a. may compete with other substances at a receptor site. Also see AGONIST.

antagonistic cooperation a phrase used by W. G. Sumner for the normally expected conflict that occurs in a competitive society in which groups such as unions cooperate but at the same time use their power to derive greater benefits from that cooperation.

antagonistic muscles muscle groups that oppose each other in function. E.g., the biceps flexes the arm at the elbow while the opposing triceps straightens the arm.

antecedent an event or factor that precedes a situation or outcome and that may be investigated for its influence or effect on that outcome.

antedating response a response that occurs earlier than anticipated or scheduled.

anterior = FRONTAL.

anterior cerebral artery a branch of the internal carotid artery that begins near the lateral cerebral sulcus and passes above the optic nerve to the beginning of the longitudinal fissure. After joining the opposite a.c.a., the two arteries run parallel in the longitudinal fissure, then curve back along the upper surface of the corpus callosum and finally end by joining the posterior cerebral arteries.

anterior choroidal artery a relatively narrow artery that is a posterior branch of the middle cerebral artery, which also is a continuation of the internal carotid artery. It passes across the optic tract toward the temporal horn of the lateral ventricle and into the choroid plexus, hippocampus, thalamus, amygdaloid complex, and related deep structures.

anterior commissure a bundle of white fibers in the brain connecting parts of the two cerebral hemispheres. It also contains fibers of the olfactory tract and is involved in certain disorders, e.g., tumors and syphilis, that are marked by loss of the sense of smell.

anterior communicating artery an artery that forms a link between the left and right anterior cerebral arteries at about the beginning of the longitudinal fissure. It is a very short blood vessel that sometimes is absent, the two anterior cerebral arteries in such cases forming a single trunk that soon divides again.

anterior forceps fibers of the corpus callosum that bend around the cleft between the frontal lobes of the right and left hemispheres. The fibers form a forceps-shaped pattern in that region of the brain. Also called **forceps minor**.

anterior fossa: See FOSSA.

anterior-horn-cell disease = AMYOTROPHIC LATERAL SCLEROSIS.

anterior horns the ventral gray matter of the spinal cord and site of the large motor neurons.

anterior nephrectomy: See NEPHRECTOMY.

anterior orbital gyrus: See ORBITAL GYRI.

anterior pituitary the larger of the two lobes of the pituitary gland, sometimes identified as the adenohypophysis. It secretes hormones affecting body growth, ovaries, mammary glands, and the pancreas, adrenal cortex, and thyroid glands.

anterior pituitary gonadotropin: See GONADOTROPIN.

anterior-posterior development gradient rapid growth of the head region as contrasted with lower areas of the body during fetal development. In the early embryonic stages, the head and brain make up 50 percent of the entire body mass, and at birth represent one quarter of the infant's total height. See CEPHALOCAUDAL DEVELOPMENT.

anterior rhizotomy: See RHIZOTOMY.

anterior-spinal-artery syndrome = BECK'S SYNDROME.

anterior thalamic nuclei a small bundle of gray matter in the optic thalamus portion of the brain. The nuclei contain relay fibers that extend to other areas in the interior of the cerebrum.

anterograde amnesia the loss of memory for events subsequent to the psychological or physical trauma that produce the amnesia. E.g., a boxer who receives a heavy blow to the head may not remember finishing the fight. Also see AMNESIA. Compare RETROGRADE AMNESIA.

Anthony, Saint Egyptian monk, 251–356. See SAINT ANTHONY'S FIRE; CHOREA (there: **Saint Anthony's dance**); ERGOTISM.

-anthr-; -anthra- a combining form relating to coal, dust, carbon.

anthracosis = BLACK-LUNG DISEASE.

-anthrop-; -anthropo- a combining form relating to the human race (from Greek *anthropos*, "man, human").

anthropocentrism literally, human-centered; the explicit or implicit assumption that human experience is the central reality and, by extension, the idea that all phenomena can be evaluated in light of their relationship to man.

anthropoid manlike; pertaining to or resembling a human being. The term is usually applied to the tail-less apes, specifically, gorillas, orangutans, chimpanzees, and gibbons.

anthropology the study of human beings (a) from the viewpoint of their origin, evolution, and adaptation to a changing environment (**physical a.**), and (b) from the viewpoint of the development of their customs, beliefs, and institutions (**cultural a., social a.**). In *Totem and Taboo* (1913) and subsequent works, Freud applied basic psychoanalytic concepts, such as the Oedipus complex, incest prohibitions, and the death instinct, to the study of folklore.

anthropometry the science of body measurements, with emphasis on ethnic, sexual, cultural, and other variables.

anthropomorphism /-môr′-/ the attribution of human characteristics to nonhuman entities such as God or gods, animals, plants, or inanimate objects. In comparative psychology, a. is the tendency to interpret the behavior and mental processes of lower forms of life in terms of human abilities. In the 19th century, those who used this approach were frequently called **anthropomorphs**. Adjective: **anthropomorphic**. Also see LLOYD MORGAN'S CANON.

anthropophobia the fear of people or the fear of human qualities or humankind.

anthropos the Jungian archetype of primal man.

anthroposcopy the practice of judging the body build of an individual by mere inspection, as distinguished from the use of anthropometric techniques of body measurement.

anthrotype the human phenotype or biological type. Also see BIOTYPOLOGY.

anti. an abbreviation of "antidote."

antianalytic procedures a term applied by psychoanalysts to measures that reduce or block the capacity for insight and understanding by interfering with thinking, remembering, and judging, e.g., administration of certain drugs, facile reassurance, and the assumption by the analyst of the role of a past figure such as a loving parent who might make the patient feel better ("transference cure").

antiandrogenic agent a substance that reduces the physiological effects of androgenic hormones on tissues normally responsive to the hormones. An a.a may function by producing antagonistic effects or by inhibiting the androgenic reaction. Kinds of antiandrogenic agents include the female sex hormone estrogen and the synthetic steroid drug cyproterone.

antiandrogen therapy medical treatment directed toward correction of the effects of excessive levels of male sex hormones. A.t. agents may include female sex hormones or more potent substances, e.g., cyproterone acetate. A.t. may control cancer of the prostate and precocious puberty in the male and masculine traits such as facial hair in the female.

antianxiety medications: See ANXIOLYTICS.

antibiotics drugs that are used to destroy pathogenic or noxious organisms. A. may be produced by or obtained from living cells, e.g., molds, yeasts, or bacteria, or manufactured as synthetic chemicals with effects similar to natural a. Some a. act by interfering with the ability of a bacterium to reproduce, others may disrupt normal life functions of a pathogen. A. generally are not effective in treating viral diseases.

antibody a modified protein molecule produced by the body's immune system having the ability to interact with an antigen, or molecule of foreign tissue. Each a. is designed to interact with a specific antigen that is identical with an antigen that has invaded the body tissues previously. Each new antigen is identified in an a. template that is used by the immune system to produce countless copies of the defensive a. in any future contact with the same antigen. See ANTIGEN; TRANSPLANTATION REACTIONS.

antibrain antibody an antibody, termed taraxein, which Heath and colleagues (1957) claim to have found in the blood of schizophrenics. The investigators believed this substance is created to work against a "unique antigen" contained in the septal-basal caudate region of the brain. The antigen resembles histamine and may be produced either by stress or by constitutional defect. Accordingly, they hypothesized that schizophrenia is basically an immunologic disease. Also see TARAXEIN.

anticathexis = COUNTERCATHEXIS.

anticholinergics drugs that block or otherwise interfere with cholinergic activity, e.g., acetylcholine transmission of impulses along parasympathetic routes. In large doses, a. may interfere also with actions of histamine, serotonin, and norepinephrine. Natural a. include ATROPINE and SCOPOLAMINE (see these entries). Scores of synthetic a. are used in treatment of nervous-system disorders, many as antiparkinson drugs. They include **benztropine mesylate**—$C_{22}H_{29}NO_4S$, **cycrimine hydrochloride**—$C_{19}H_{30}ClNO$, **procyclidine**—$C_{19}H_{29}NO$, and **trihexyphenidyl hydrochloride**—$C_{20}H_{32}ClNO$, which are administered primarily to relieve the symptoms of muscular rigidity. The a. often are used in combinations to control specific patient symptoms. See ANTIHISTAMINES; ANTIPARKINSON DRUGS.

anticholinergic syndrome a disorder produced by cholinergic blocker substances, marked by ataxia, drowsiness, slurred speech, confusion and disorientation, hallucinations, and memory deficits, particularly short-term memory impairment. Scopolamine, curare, and hexamethonium are drugs that can cause a.s.

anticholinesterase a substance that inhibits or deactivates acetylcholinesterase. So-called nerve gases and organophosphate insecticides cause muscle paralysis by blocking normal acetylcholinesterase activity since further nerve impulses cannot be transmitted in the affected area.

anticipation looking forward to the future; basing expectation on past and present experience. In psychoanalysis, a. of the future in imagination is a major function of the ego. However, when a. takes the form of anxious expectation of danger, it becomes a neurotic symptom. Also see EXPECTATION.

anticipation method a verbal-learning method in which the subject is prompted to give the correct answer if he hesitates or makes an error. Success may be measured by the number of prompts needed to master the material. Also called **prompting method**.

anticipatory autocastration in psychoanalysis, an explanation for feminine behavior in males as an unconscious symbolic self-castration intended to reduce the fear of actual castration.

anticipatory error an error made by responding prematurely in a serial-learning situation.

anticipatory guidance counseling and educational services provided to individuals or families before they reach a turning point, or normative crisis, in their lives. Examples are parental guidance before a child enters school, consultation provided to attorneys dealing with clients petitioning for divorce, or counseling of workers soon to reach retirement age.

anticipatory-maturation principle: See PRINCI-
PLE OF ANTICIPATORY MATURATION.

anticipatory mourning a term applied by Futter-
man and colleagues to a series of adaptive processes experienced by parents and other relatives during the fatal illness of a child, including
acknowledgment of the inevitability of death,
grief and grieving, reconciliation to the expected
death while preserving the values of the child's
life, detachment in the sense of withdrawal of
emotional investment from the child as a growing being, and memorialization through investment in the image and memory of the child, replacing investment in the real child. These
steps take place before death occurs. See GRIEF.

anticipatory response a response that occurs before the stimulus, that is, "jumping the gun."

anticonformity in social psychology, behavior that
contradicts group standards, specifically behavior motivated by a rebellious need to challenge the power of the group. Compare
CONFORMITY.

anticonvulsants: See ANTIEPILEPTICS.

antidepressants drugs administered in the treatment of psychotic and psychoneurotic depression. A. are believed to elevate depressed mood
by increasing the availability of catecholamines
at CNS receptor sites. The primary kinds of
a. are the tricyclic antidepressants and the
monoamine oxidase inhibitors, or MAOI. Some
stimulants also may function as a. See TRICYCLIC
ANTIDEPRESSANTS; MONOAMINE OXIDASE INHIBI-
TORS.

antidiuretic hormone a hormone normally secreted by the neurohypophysis of the pituitary
gland but also produced synthetically. Its main
action is to contract smooth muscles, particularly of blood vessels. It suppresses the secretion of
urine and is used in the treatment of diabetes insipidus. Also called **vasopressin.** Abbrev.: **ADH.**

antidromic phenomenon the passage of a nerve
impulse in a reversed direction (from axon to
dendrite) produced for experimental purposes.

antiepileptics drugs used to reduce the frequency
or severity of epileptic seizures, or to terminate
a seizure already underway. Until the advent of
hydantoin drugs in the 1930s, a. consisted mainly of bromides and barbiturates. The barbiturates and barbituratelike drugs and the hydantoins are prescribed for grand mal epilepsy and
focal cortical seizures. Petit mal seizures usually
are treated with oxazolidinediones and succinimides. Psychomotor epilepsy may be treated
with one of the hydantoins or an acetylurea
medication. One of the tricyclic antidepressant
drugs, **carbamazepine,** also is used in some
countries in the control of psychomotor
epilepsy. Also called **anticonvulsants.** See
HYDANTOINS; BARBITURATES; OXAZOLIDINE-
DIONES; SUCCINIMIDES; CARBONIC ANHYDRASE
INHIBITORS; BENZODIAZEPINES; TRICYCLIC ANTI-
DEPRESSANTS; ACETYLUREAS; PRIMIDONE.

antiestrogenic: See PROGESTOGENS.

antifetishism a characteristic tendency of latent
homosexuals to find aversions to the physical
features of members of the opposite sex, as a
protection against recognition of their true sexual interests.

antigen any agent that is capable of inducing the
production of antibodies in an organism and of
reacting with the antibodies. The agent may be a
virus, a bacterium, or a toxin (such as bee
venom) of the tissues such as blood or skin cells
of another individual with different genetic characteristics. Also see ANTIBODY.

antigen-antibody reactions a part of a natural defense mechanism of the body tissues of an animal against the introduction of a foreign substance, which may be a bacterium or virus, into
the host tissues. The antibody is a protein molecule produced by white cells in the bloodstream
with the specific role of neutralizing the foreign
substance, which becomes the antigen. Once the
individual's immune system has developed antibodies to fight a certain type of antigen, the antibodies can be mobilized quickly to destroy any
repeated invasion by the antigen; the first antigen attack thus having induced an immunity to
future attacks. The ability of an individual to
produce antibodies is influenced in part by age
and heredity. Older people lose some immunity,
and some individuals fail to inherit the genetic
mechanism needed to manufacture the protein
molecules that resist certain kinds of antigens.
As a result, some people are more susceptible to
a particular type of disorder, such as respiratory
disease or infections by pus-forming bacteria.

antigonadal action the blocking of gonadal function by an agent or process, such as a lesion in
the pituitary gland or amygdala.

antihistamines drugs that inhibit the effects of histamine, a substance produced by the breakdown
of the amino acid histidine, which occurs naturally throughout the body. Histamine dilates
blood vessels, constricts bronchial smooth-
muscle tissue, and produces headaches. A. may
have sedative or hypnotic effects and are used
for that purpose. Some a., such as SCOPOLAMINE
(see this entry), an anticholinergic drug, are
sedatives in moderate doses but produce agitation rather than sleep in large doses. Certain
tricyclic antidepressant drugs have antihistamine
and anticholinergic effects. A few a., e.g.,
chlorphenoxamine—$C_{18}H_{22}ClNO$—and **diphen-
hydramine hydrochloride**—$C_{17}H_{22}ClNO$—
function as antiparkinson drugs. Other a. include CYPROHEPTADINE (see this entry), **methapyrilene**—$C_{14}H_{19}N_3S$, and **dimenhydrinate**—
$C_{24}H_{28}ClN_5O_3$, a commonly prescribed remedy
for motion-sickness. See ANTICHOLINERGICS;
ANTIPARKINSON DRUGS; MIGRAINE-NEURALGIA
ANALGESICS.

antiintoxicant = AMETHYSTIC.

antiintraception a personality trait marked by
rejection and denial of the subjective element
in life, including the rejection of imaginative,

artistic, emotional, and intellectual experiences. A. was identified by Adorno and Frenkel-Brunswik as one of the traits associated with the authoritarian personality. Also see AUTHORITARIANISM.

antilibidinal ego the portion of the ego structure that is similar to Freud's superego in W. R. D. Fairbairn's object-relations theory. The a.e. develops out of the unitary ego present at birth when the infantile libidinal ego (similar to the id) experiences deprivation and frustration at the hands of the parent, and the infant suppresses the needs that are not met. But the parents also do meet some of the infant's needs; and out of this positive experience of good relations and understanding, the infant develops the central ego (similar to Freud's ego) which is the conscious self of everyday living.

antilymphocyte globulin a substance used in organ transplants as an adjunct to drugs that suppress the immune response. It is the gamma-globulin portion of antilymphocyte serum. Abbrev.: **ALG**. Also called **antithymocyte globulin**.

antimanics a group of drugs that reduce symptoms of mania, or manic episodes of manic-depressive disorders (or may be used as neuroleptics). The main kinds of a. are butyrophenones, lithium, and phenothiazines. The general effects of a. include psychomotor inhibition, although each of the various types of a. may produce somewhat different pharmacologic actions. See BUTYROPHENONES; LITHIUM; PHENOTHIAZINES. Also see NEUROLEPTICS.

antimetabolite a substance that has a molecular structure so similar to that of another substance required for a normal physiological function that it may be accepted as the required molecule, thereby disrupting a normal metabolic process. The anticoagulant drug bishydroxy-coumarin functions as an a. by interfering with the vitamin-K role in producing the blood-clotting agent prothrombin.

antimicrobial agents substances produced by chemical synthesis or derived from bacteria or molds that are effective as antibacterial, anti-rickettsial, or antifungal agents. A.a. generally function by interfering with the microbe's cell-wall building, the permeability of the cell wall, or its processes of reproduction or protein synthesis.

antimotivational syndrome a behavior pattern associated with chronic use of cannabis. The concept that use of marijuana or its chemical agent is a cause of personality changes, e.g., loss of drive and initiative, is mainly conjectural and based on observations of the life-styles of chronic cannabis users in various cultures around the world.

antinodal behavior the period of quietude that follows nodal peaks of aggressive, disorderly, or excessively active behavior.

antiparkinson drugs drugs that reduce the severity of signs and symptoms of parkinsonism,

e.g., tremors of voluntary muscles, movement and gait abnormalities, and muscle rigidity. With a few exceptions, a.d. generally are of two types, (a) natural or synthetic anticholinergic drugs, e.g., atropine and scopolamine, and (b) dopamine-related substances that are administered with antihistamines. The exceptions include drugs that are primarily antivirals or neuroleptics such as phenothiazines with anti-parkinson effects. Also called **antiparkinsonian agents**. See ANTICHOLINERGICS; ANTIHISTAMINES; ANTIVIRAL DRUGS; PHENOTHIAZINES; DOPAMINERGICS.

antipredatory aggression: See ANIMAL AGGRESSION.

antipsychiatry opposition to psychiatry based on the idea that mental illness does not exist, that psychiatry is only a form of social repression, that treatment is a disguised form of punishment, and that mental hospitals should be closed because they make the patients worse (Szasz).

antipsychotics drugs that are classed as major tranquilizers, or neuroleptics, and used mainly to treat schizophrenia and certain manic states. For details, see NEUROLEPTICS.

antipyretics drugs that help control fever or other forms of hyperthermia by action on the thermo-regulatory center in the hypothalamus. A. generally act by resetting the center to maintain a lower body temperature. A. also may help the body to dissipate heat faster by dilating peripheral arteries. Aspirin and other non-narcotic analgesics often function as a. Also see PYRAZOLONES.

antipyrine: See PYRAZOLONES.

antirabic serum-induced demyelinating encephalopathy a rare complication of immunization against rabies, marked by the destruction of white matter in the brain. The disorder is believed to be caused by antigens present in the vaccine; in some cases live rabies virus was found in the vaccine. Young children are seldom affected, but about one percent of young adults immunized with antirabies vaccine have been afflicted.

antireward system a performance-effect process in which an unsatisfactory stimulus is given for an unsuccessful task effort. An a.s. may develop as a rebound effect when a reward that induces a reinforcing activity is no longer offered.

anti-Semitic scale = A-S SCALE.

anti-Semitism prejudice against the Jews as a group, frequently expressed in terms of (a) a distorted, unflattering picture of so-called Jewish traits, (b) acts of discrimination and persecution, and (c) use of this minority group as a scapegoat for personal frustrations and aggressive drives and the ills of society.

antisocial aggression any act of aggression that has socially destructive and undesirable consequences. See AGGRESSION. Compare PROSOCIAL AGGRESSION.

antisocial behavior aggressive, impulsive, and sometimes violent actions that flout social and ethical codes such as laws and regulations relating to personal and property rights. Compare PROSOCIAL BEHAVIOR.

antisocial compulsion an irresistible impulse to commit antisocial acts such as stealing. See ANTISOCIAL BEHAVIOR. Also see CONCEALED ANTISOCIAL ACTIVITY.

antisocial-personality disorder a personality disorder characterized by chronic and continuous antisocial behavior when this is not due to severe mental retardation, schizophrenia, or manic episodes. This behavior pattern, which is more common in males than females, starts before age 15 with such infractions as lying, stealing, fighting, truancy, vandalism, theft, drunkenness, or substance abuse. It then continues after age 18 with at least four of the following manifestations: inability to work consistently; inability to function as a responsible parent; repeated violations of the law; inability to maintain an enduring sexual relationship; frequent fights and beatings inside and outside the home; failure to repay debts and provide child support; travel from place to place without planning; repeated lying and conning; and extreme recklessness in driving and other activities. (DSM-III)

antisocial reaction a character disorder marked by impulsive, egocentric, unethical behavior, rejection of authority and discipline, extreme irresponsibility, absence of anxiety, lack of foresight, and absence of genuine loyalty to individuals or groups. The category includes a varied assortment of confidence men, quacks and shysters, unscrupulous businessmen, prostitutes, and crooked politicians. The disorder was once termed constitutional psychopath and constitutional psychopathic inferior, which then became psychopathic personality, and has been renamed ANTISOCIAL-PERSONALITY DISORDER in DSM-III. See this entry.

antithymocyte globulin = ANTILYMPHOCYTE GLOBULIN.

antitussives drugs that suppress coughing. A. work by their effect on a cough-control center in the medulla oblongata. Because the cough center is one of the brain areas sensitive to narcotics, opium derivatives are effective in suppressing cough. Morphine, codeine, and similar narcotic components of a. have been replaced in recent years by synthetic substances, e.g., dextromethorphan, which lack addictive properties.

antiviral drugs substances that interfere with normal functions of viruses. A.d. may act by blocking host-cell enzyme systems required for viral reproduction; blocking signals carried in messenger RNA; and uncoating the nucleic-acid molecule of the virus. A.d. are difficult to manage in clinical practice because chemicals that block viral life processes also may interfere with the patient's normal cell functions. Anti-

virals occasionally interact with substances in human tissues to yield unexpected benefits, as with **amantadine**—$C_{10}H_{18}ClN$, which can be used as an antiparkinson drug because it helps control brain-dopamine levels by delaying normal metabolic destruction of the neural substance.

antivitamins substances that interfere with the functions of vitamins. Most a. are chemicals that are similar in structure to the vitamins they render ineffective. A. are employed mainly in studies and tests of vitamin deficiencies.

antlophobia a morbid fear of floods.

Anton, Gabriel German neuropsychiatrist, 1858–1933. See ANTON'S SYNDROME; BABINSKI'S SYNDROME.

Anton's syndrome a disorder marked by a patient's denial of blindness despite clinical evidence of the loss of vision. A.s. may occur in cases of either complete or incomplete blindness. The patient usually confabulates an explanation for his inability to see; e.g., he may claim it is night or there are no lights in the room where he is being examined. Also called **Anton-Babinski syndrome; denial visual hallucination syndrome; hemiasomatognosia.** Also see HYSTERICAL BLINDNESS; BABINSKI'S SYNDROME.

antonym test the type of test in which the subject must identify the opposite of each word in a given series.

anulospiral ending a type of nerve-fiber ending in muscle tissue in which the nerve is wrapped around one or more muscle fibers near the center of the spindle. Compare FLOWER-SPRAY ENDING.

anus: See LIBIDINAL PHASES.

anvil = INCUS.

anxietas tibiarum a form of nervous agitation marked by a need to change the position of the legs.

anxiety a pervasive feeling of dread, apprehension, and impending disaster. A. should be distinguished from fear. Fear is a response to a clear and present danger; a. is a response to an undefined or unknown threat which in many cases stems from unconscious conflicts, feelings of insecurity, or forbidden impulses within ourselves. In both, however, the body mobilizes itself to meet the threat, and muscles become tense, breathing is faster, and the heart beats more rapidly. See ACUTE A.; ANAL CASTRATION A.; ANNIHILATION A.; BASIC A.; CATASTROPHIC A.; CHRONIC A.; DEATH A.; EGO A.; EROTIZED A.; EXAMINATION A.; EXISTENTIAL a.; FREE-FLOATING A.; GENERALIZED A. DISORDER; HETEROSEXUAL A.; ID A.; INSTINCTUAL A.; MANIFEST A.; MORAL A.; NEUROTIC A.; ORAL A.; ORGANIC A.; PAN-A.; PERFORMANCE A.; PHOBIC A.; PRE-RELEASE A. STATE; PRIMAL A.; REAL A.; SEPARATION A.; SIGNAL A.; SOCIAL A.; STRANGER A.; SUPEREGO A.; TRAUMATIC A.; URETHRAL A.; VIRGINAL A.

anxiety attack a sudden eruption of acute anxiety, which starts with pounding of the heart, difficulty in breathing, excessive perspiration, and dizziness, and in many cases mounts to a full-scale panic in which the patient experiences unbearable tension, fear of suffocation, and a feeling that he is going to die or that some unnamable disaster is going to befall him. Also called **acute a.a.**

anxiety discharge any anxiety-reducing activity associated with normal daily functions, e.g., sexual intercourse, as an alternative to suppression of anxiety.

anxiety disorders a group of disorders in which anxiety is either the predominant disturbance or is experienced in confronting a dreaded object or situation, or in resisting obsessions or compulsions. The disorders include agoraphobia, social phobia, simple phobia, panic disorder, generalized-anxiety disorder, obsessive-compulsive disorder, posttraumatic-stress disorder, and atypical anxiety disorder. Not included are disorders in which the anxiety is due to another disorder, such as schizophrenic or affective syndromes. See the specific a.d. (DSM-III).

anxiety disorders of childhood or adolescence a DSM-III subclass in which anxiety is the predominant feature. The category includes SEPARATION-ANXIETY DISORDER; AVOIDANT DISORDER OF CHILDHOOD OR ADOLESCENCE, in which anxiety is focused on specific situations; and OVERANXIOUS DISORDER, in which the anxiety is generalized to a variety of situations. See these entries. (DSM-III)

anxiety disturbance a condition marked by a high level of anxiety, with extreme sensitivity, self-consciousness, and morbid fears.

anxiety fixation the continuation of an anxiety reaction from one developmental stage to another.

anxiety hierarchy the ordering of stimuli that produce anxiety in a specific individual, starting with the object or situation causing the least fear. An a.h. may be constructed for use in desensitization of phobic patients. Desensitization proceeds from the least threatening situation and progresses along the hierarchy. See COUNTERCONDITIONING; DESENSITIZATION.

anxiety hysteria a neurosis in which the anxiety generated by unconscious sexual conflicts is expressed in phobic symptoms, such as an irrational fear of dirt or open spaces, and in physical disturbances known as conversion symptoms. The term was originated by Freud; it is seldom used today, since it combines disorders that are now classified separately. See ANXIETY STATE; PHOBIC DISORDERS; CONVERSION DISORDER.

anxiety neurosis a psychoneurotic disorder characterized by persistent apprehensiveness, feelings of impending disaster, and "free-floating fear" accompanied by such symptoms as difficulty in making decisions, insomnia, loss of appetite, and heart palpitations. Chronic anxiety of this kind may occasionally erupt into an acute anxiety or panic attack. The source of the anxiety is believed to be unresolved conflicts, forbidden impulses, or disturbing memories that threaten the individual. In his original theory, Freud attributed a.n. to a buildup of sexual tension resulting from frustrated discharge. In DSM-III, anxiety neuroses are called **anxiety states.** See GENERALIZED-ANXIETY DISORDER; PANIC DISORDER; OBSESSIVE-COMPULSIVE DISORDER; ACTUAL NEUROSIS. (DSM-III)

anxiety object an object that represents the original source of anxiety; e.g., a nonhuman object is feared because it represents the father who caused the original anxiety. See LITTLE HANS.

anxiety preparedness the increased state of alertness and motor tension that normally accompany fear or anxiety.

anxiety-relief responses in behavior therapy, the repetition of reassuring or tranquilizing words (e.g., "calm") in anxiety-provoking situations.

anxiety resolution the resolution of anxiety by therapeutic processes that uncover the unconscious roots of the problem so that they can be understood and mastered.

anxiety scales tests designed to measure manifest anxiety as opposed to assessing hidden sources or effects. Among these tests are the children's and adult forms of the Manifest Anxiety Scale ("I get nervous when someone watches me work," "I blush easily," etc.), the General Anxiety Scale for Children (fear of snakes, being along, etc.), and the Sarason Test Anxiety Scale. See PERFORMANCE ANXIETY.

anxiety state an obsolete term applied by Freud to a traumatic neurosis precipitated by a wartime experience in which the ego-ideals of war conflict with customary ideals. See ACTUAL NEUROSIS.

anxiety states: See ANXIETY NEUROSIS.

anxiety tolerance the ability to cope with a high level of anxiety without psychological harm.

anxiolytics a group of drugs that are minor tranquilizers or antianxiety medications. A. resemble barbiturates in their actions and side effects and are often prescribed for patients who experience severe anxiety or tension. A. also may be employed in the treatment of petit mal epilepsy. Kinds of anxiolytics include BENZODIAZEPINES, CHLORMEZANONE, TYBAMATE, DIPHENYLMETHANES, and PROPANEDIOLS. See these entries.

anxious depression a depression involving a high anxiety level but without agitation.

anxious expectation a sense of apprehension that is experienced in situations that are novel, unexpected, or unusual.

anxious intropunitiveness a frequently observed symptom pattern found by Lorr (1962) and included in an Inpatient Multidimensional

Psychiatric Scale, consisting of self-blame, apprehensiveness, self-depreciation, guilt and remorse, suicidal threats, morbid fears, and ideas of sinfulness.

aortic-arch syndrome a disorder caused by progressive obliteration of the main branches of the aortic arch because of arteriosclerosis, aneurysm, or a related problem. Usually only one or two of the branches are involved, affecting blood flow to a local area. If the carotid or vertebral arteries are involved, the brain will be affected. The patient may experience fainting spells, epilepsylike seizures, temporary blindness, paralysis on one side of the body, aphasia, or memory disturbances, or a combination of symptoms. A typical effect is the **carotid-sinus syndrome** in which the patient faints after turning the head. Collateral circulation may develop to compensate for some degree of interrupted blood flow but progressive loss of vision may occur in the meantime.

aortic stenosis: See STENOSIS.

APA an abbreviation meaning (a) American Psychological Association, (b) American Psychiatric Association, (c) American Psychoanalytic Association, or (d) American Psychopathological Association.

Apalache tea: See CASSINA LEAVES.

apallic syndrome a long period of disturbed consciousness that may follow a head injury. Symptoms include mutism, akinesia, disorders of reflexes, and muscle contractions.

apandria a feeling of aversion toward the male sex.

apareunia the inability to perform sexual intercourse; also, abstinence from coitus.

apastia a psychiatric symptom manifested by an abstinence from food.

apathetic hyperthyroidism an acquired myopathy associated with thyrotoxicosis. In contrast to other types of hyperthyroid conditions, a.h. usually is characterized by lethargy or otherwise unexplained congestive heart failure.

apathetic withdrawal a retreat from society with loss of interest and initiative.

apathy the absence of emotional response, or affect, and indifference to one's surroundings. It is a common symptom in severe depression and schizophrenia.

apathy syndrome an expression sometimes used to describe the pattern of emotional insulation (indifference, detachment) adopted by many prisoners-of-war and other victims of catastrophes in an effort to maintain their stability.

APC: See ASPIRIN COMBINATIONS.

apeirophobia a morbid fear of infinity or of the thought of endlessness.

aperiodic reinforcement a type of reinforcement that is irregular or intermittent.

Apert, Eugène /äper'/ French pediatrician, 1868–1940. See APERT'S SYNDROME; DISFIGUREMENT.

Apert's syndrome a form of craniosynostosis accompanied by mental retardation and syndactyly. The syndactyly usually involves both hands and feet and may result in fusion of the skin alone or of the skin and bones. Partial fusion is designated Type II while Type I is marked by "mitten hands" and "sock feet" in which the digits are fused. Also called **acrocephalosyndactyly.**

apertural hypothesis the hypothesis that the psychological representations of the primary instinctual functions center on the apertures of organs that serve primary instincts (mouth, anus, urethra, vagina). According to this view, the phase of a woman's hormonal cycle can be predicted from the analysis of her dreams and fantasies.

aperture color a film color seen in holes or spaces in neutral screens.

Apgar, Virginia American anesthesiologist, 1909—. See APGAR SCORES.

Apgar scores ratings of the neonate on five factors: color, respiration, heartbeat, reflexes, and muscle tone. Tests are administered at one and again at five minutes after birth to assess the degree of physical normality and the ability to survive independently. Each factor is scored 0, 1, or 2, with a maximum total of ten points. Infants with low scores at five minutes usually have neurologic damage if they survive.

aphagia a lack of appetite. See ANOREXIA.

aphakia the absence of the lens from the eye, a condition that may be congenital or the result of disease, injury, or surgery. Adjective: **aphakic.**

aphalgesia = HAPHALGESIA.

aphanisis /əfan'isis/ a term used by Ernest Jones for total extinction of the capacity for sexual enjoyment, which he believed to be at the root of all neuroses (from Greek *aphanes*, "invisible, unnoticed").

aphasia the loss or impairment of the ability to understand or express language due to brain injury or disease. Impaired ability to understand words, signs, or gestures is termed sensory, impressive, or receptive a.; impaired ability to speak, write, or make meaningful gestures is termed motor or expressive a. Major causes of the cerebral damage are stroke, brain tumor, encephalitis, and head trauma. For specific types of a., see ALEXIA; AGRAPHIA; ANOMIA; AUDITORY A.; CENTRAL A.; BROCA'S A.; EXPRESSIVE A.; ACALCULIA; AMIMIA; ECHOLALIA; AMUSIA; SYNTACTICAL A.; SEMANTIC A.; AMNESTIC A.; CONGENITAL A.; ACOUSTIC-MNESTIC A.; AFFERENT MOTOR A.; CONDUCTION A.; DEVELOPMENTAL DYSPHASIA; EFFERENT MOTOR A.; SENSORIMOTOR A.; WORD SALAD; ACATAPHASIA; COMBINED TRANSCORTICAL A.; TRANSCORTICAL A.; EXPRESSIVE A.; RECEPTIVE A.; WERNICKE'S A.; MOTOR A. Also see DYSPHASIA; EXAMINING FOR APHASIA.

aphemia the loss of speech ability, usually due to a CNS lesion or an emotional disorder.

aphemia pathematica an obsolete term for a loss of speech due to fright.

aphemia plastica an obsolete term for voluntary mutism.

aphephobia = HAPHEPHOBIA.

aphonia the loss of voice due to organic defect or emotional disorder. Also called **aphony**. See HYSTERICAL A.; MUTISM; FUNCTIONAL A.; WHISPER A.; ADDUCTED A.

aphoria a condition of weakness that cannot be improved through exercise, especially as manifested by neurotics (Janet). Also called **amyosthenia; amyotony**.

aphraenous an obsolete term for insane.

aphrasia the inability to utter or understand words arranged in phrases, even though individual words may be used or understood.

aphrenia an obsolete term for dementia, also for apoplexy.

aphrodisia a state of sexual excitement.

aphrodisiacs substances that stimulate sexual activity in humans or animals. The agent may be an odor, e.g., perfumes, a food, or a drug. Alcohol, various alkaloids, e.g., yohimbine, cantharidin from the Spanish fly, vitamin E, amyl nitrite, raw oysters, and chestnuts are among a. accepted by humans as sexual stimulants although evidence of their efficacy is lacking.

aphrodisiomania a state of extreme sexual excitement.

aphronesia an obsolete term for dementia.

aphthongia a rare form of spasmodic vocal neurosis which affects verbal communication (especially public speaking). A. may be a variety of occupational neurosis analogous to writer's cramp.

apiphobia = MELISSOPHOBIA.

aplasia the arrested development or failure of body tissue to grow. See AGENESIS.

aplestia extreme greediness.

Aplysia a genus of gastropods used in laboratory studies of neurons. An abdominal ganglion of Aplysia depilans contains neurons that have been utilized in single-cell-conditioning experiments.

apnea /ap'nē·ə/ temporary suspension of respiration, as in catching one's breath, or in **sleep a**. The latter, which usually terminates in a loud snore, body jerk, arm flailing, or standing without awakening, is frequently caused by obstruction of the airway by mucus or by excessive tissue (e.g., pharyngeal fat deposits) which may in some cases require surgery. If the **apneic period** is a long one, the heart may be slowed (bradycardia), and EEG changes may occur. The condition is also found in many disorders such as major epilepsy and concussion.

-apo- a combining form meaning away from, without, separated.

apocarteresis self-destruction by deliberate starvation.

apoclesis absence of a desire for food.

apoenzyme /apō·en'zīm/ the protein component of an enzyme. A second component, a coenzyme, is required to make the enzyme functional.

Apollonian attitude a state of mind that is well-ordered, rational, clearly defined, and harmonious (from *Apollo*, Graeco-Roman god of male beauty and wisdom). This modern use of the term Apollonian was proposed by Friedrich Nietzsche, who contrasted it with Dionysian. Compare DIONYSIAN ATTITUDE.

apomathema an obsolete term for loss of memory.

apomorphine $C_{17}H_{17}NO_2$—a morphine derivative used as an expectorant and to induce vomiting.

aponeurosis a flat fibrous sheet of connective tissue that attaches muscle to bone. In the pharynx it lies under the mucosa.

apopathetic behavior behavior influenced by the presence of others although not directed toward them, as in boasting about one's exploits.

apoplectic type a term used by Hippocrates for a body type characterized by a heavyset, rotund physique which roughly corresponds to Kretschmer's pyknic type and Sheldon's endomorphic type. Also called **habitus apoplecticus**. See PYKNIC TYPE; ENDOMORPH.

apoplexy: See STROKE.

apparent movement an illusion of motion or change of size, as in television animation. Also called **illusory movement**. See ALPHA MOVEMENT; BETA MOVEMENT; DELTA MOVEMENT; EPSILON MOVEMENT.

apparition a visual illusion or hallucination that results from distortion of a perceived object, often interpreted as threatening, and usually associated with an organic or toxic disorder such as alcoholic delirium.

apparitions: See GHOST IMAGES.

appeals efforts to arouse a sympathetic response from an individual or group, particularly from consumers who are the targets of advertising a. A. may be based on psychological studies of consumer desires or needs, which may be as overt as a practical package design or as subtle as an implied suggestion that the product might enhance the purchaser's sexual attractiveness. Advertising a. also may be directed toward the purchaser's competitive drives.

appeasers a descriptive term for parents who avoid exercising authority and who fear confrontation and conflict with their children. Their behavior is conciliatory, and they attempt to circumvent problems rather than face them directly. (Lafore, 1945) Also see COOPERATORS; DICTATORS; TEMPORIZERS.

apperception the awareness of the meaning and significance of an object, idea, or perception by relating it to an already-existing body of knowledge and experience; also, the simpler process of clear perception or recognition.

appersonation a delusion, most often observed in schizophrenia, in which the individual identifies with another person and assumes his or her characteristics. Also called **appersonification**.

appetite an urge, desire, or bodily need, especially for food, water, sex, and air. Our appetites are affected by experience and learning as well as physiological factors; e.g., when we are hungry, we may have a desire for one type of food and not another due to cultural conditioning or individual preferences and aversions.

appetite control a mechanism or method of increasing or decreasing the rate of food intake by an organism. A.c. is both psychologic and physiologic, and may be stimulated by the sight, smell, and memory or mental associations of food, as well as by anger, anxiety, or fear. Physiologic factors may include metabolic disorders and use of drugs, e.g., amphetamines. See ANOREXIA; APPETITE SUPPRESSANT; SELF-SELECTION OF DIET.

appetitive behavior feeding activity that may be excessive, adequate, or deficient, as influenced by nuclei of the hypothalamus. Lesions of the ventromedial nucleus result in voracious eating while lesions of the lateral hypothalamic nuclei cause anorexia. The ventromedial nucleus is regarded as the satiety center.

appetite suppressant any anorexiant, such as drugs, used in the treatment of obesity. An a.s. may be an amphetamine, a sympathomimetic amine such as phentermine hydrochloride, or a phenylpropanolamine salt, all of which stimulate metabolism. Some a.s. drugs contain a mild anesthetic that dulls the taste buds so that normally appetizing foods seem to lack flavor and aroma. See APPETITE CONTROL.

applied psychoanalysis the application of psychoanalytic principles to areas beyond clinical practice, e.g., to the study of art, religion, anthropology, biography, history, philology, and philosophy. Freud's own interpretation of Leonardo da Vinci, Moses, and Hamlet, as well as his studies of folklore and mythology, are prime examples.

applied research research aimed at answering a practical question rather than developing a theory; also, engineering as opposed to science. Compare PURE RESEARCH.

applied psychology the application of the theories, principles, and techniques of psychology to practical problems, e.g., political campaigns, consumer affairs, industry, human engineering, education, advertising, vocational guidance, and environmental issues.

apport the alleged supernatural transport of an object by poltergeists or during a seance.

apprehension = APPREHENSIVENESS.

apprehension span a measure of the number of items a subject can perceive in a fixed time.

apprehensive expectation: See GENERALIZED-ANXIETY DISORDER.

apprehensiveness a relatively mild form of anxiety and uneasiness, especially about what might happen in the future. Also called **apprehension**.

apprentice complex a behavior pattern in which the boy expresses a desire to be like his father and is willing to serve as his apprentice.

approach-approach conflict a conflict situation involving a choice between two almost equally desirable but incompatible goals, e.g., when a child is torn between separated parents, both of whom he loves. Also called **double-approach conflict**. Also see APPROACH-AVOIDANCE CONFLICT; AVOIDANCE-AVOIDANCE CONFLICT.

approach-avoidance conflict a conflict situation involving strong attraction and strong repulsion toward the same goal, e.g., when a highly desirable job requires long separation from one's family. Also see APPROACH-APPROACH CONFLICT; AVOIDANCE-AVOIDANCE CONFLICT; DOUBLE APPROACH-AVOIDANCE CONFLICT.

approach gradient the graduated variation in the strength of a positive drive as we approach the goal to which it is directed. E.g., eagerness to get married usually increases, and hesitations are gradually put aside, as the wedding date approaches. See GRADIENT.

appropriate affect feeling-tone in harmony with the accompanying thought, reaction, or verbal expression.

approval need: See NEED FOR APPROVAL.

approximation in speech and language disorders, the bringing together of the vocal cords. An abnormal a., caused by a tumor, paralysis, or structural defect in the throat tissues, can be the cause of a voice pitch that is not appropriate for the age and sex of the person, or cause the voice to be inaudible to others. According to Travis, most clinical voice problems involve faulty vocal-fold a. For a different use of the term a., see WORD A.

approximation conditioning = SHAPING.

approximation method = METHOD OF SUCCESSIVE APPROXIMATIONS.

appurtenance a Gestalt term for interaction or mutual influence between parts of a perceptual field.

apractagnosia an impaired ability to organize movements in space, to remember such movements, or to analyze spatial relationships. The condition is due to lesions in the lower part of the occipital and parietal lobes. Also called **spatial a**.

apraxia the loss of ability to perform purposeful movements such as dressing or driving a car. The condition is believed to be due to damage to the parietal lobe of the brain, which affects the memory for a series of acts or skills without producing paralysis or loss of sensation. For various types, see DRESSING A.; A. OF GAIT; CONSTRUCTIONAL A.; IDEATIONAL A.; IDIOKINETIC A.; MOTOR A.; AKINETIC A.; AMNESTIC A.; LEFT-SIDED A.; DYNAMIC A.

apraxia of gait impairment or loss of ability to walk due to lesions in the motor cortex but not involving sensory impairment or paralysis. Also called **a. for gait**.

apraxic dysarthria inability to articulate clearly due to spasticity, paralysis, or lack of coordination of the muscles used in speaking. Also see APRAXIA.

aprobarbital $C_{10}H_{14}N_2O_3$—an intermediate-acting barbiturate drug. It has been used mainly as a hypnotic, to induce sleep, but also may be administered in a lighter dosage for its sedative effect. Also see BARBITURATES.

aprosexia the loss of the ability to maintain attention, due to a brain lesion or psychiatric disorder, e.g., productive mania or marked depression (from Greek *a-* and *prosechein*, "to heed"). However, a. may be selective for certain subject areas.

APS = AIR-POLLUTION SYNDROME.

apsychia an obsolete term for loss of consciousness.

apsychognosia a lack of consciousness of one's own personality or behavior, e.g., an alcoholic's absence of awareness of other people's attitude toward his behavior.

aptitude the capacity to acquire competence or skill through training. Individuals who can learn to play the piano or perform arithmetical calculations with relative ease are frequently said to have a **natural a.** for these activities. **Specific a.** is potential in a particular area, e.g., artistic or mathematical aptitude; **general a.** is potential in several fields.

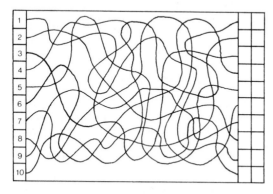

APTITUDE TESTS. Visual pursuit: Follow each numbered line with the eyes only, and number the box where the line terminates.

aptitude tests tests designed to measure (a) individual concrete abilities such as dexterity, visual acuity, and clerical performance, (b) selection of candidates for professional training, such as in medicine, law, or nursing, and (c) a wide range of basic abilities required for academic or vocational success, such as verbal comprehension, numerical ability, mechanical knowledge, and reasoning.

AQ = ACHIEVEMENT QUOTIENT.

aq. dest. an abbreviation used in prescriptions, meaning "distilled water" (Latin *aqua destillata*).

-aqua- a combining form relating to water or a waterlike fluid.

aquaphobia a morbid fear of water or bathing and swimming. Also see WATER PHOBIA.

aqueduct of Sylvius a cerebral canal or passage that extends vertically through the mesencephalon to link the third and fourth ventricles of the brain.

aqueous humor the clear fluid that occupies the anterior chamber of the eye between the cornea and the lens. See HUMOR; EYE STRUCTURE.

Aquinas: See THOMAS A.

ara-A an antiviral drug used to treat herpes simplex eye ulcers, a major cause of corneal blindness. The name is derived from the components, *a*denine *ara*binoside. Also called **vidarabine**. Trademark: **Vira-A**.

-arachn-; -arachno- a combining form relating to a spider or to something cobweblike (from Greek *arachne*, "spider"). Adjective: **arachnoid**.

arachneophobia a morbid fear of spiders. Also called **arachnophobia; spider phobia**.

arachnoid: See -ARCHN-.

arachnoid granulations a series of extensions of the arachnoid layer of the meningeal membranes through the dura mater layer that permits circulating cerebrospinal fluid to drain into the bloodstream.

arachnoid layer the weblike membrane between the pia mater and dura mater meninges covering the brain and spinal cord.

arachnoid mater the middle layer of the meningeal membranes covering the surface of the brain and spinal cord. It is identified by strands of tissue that resemble spider webs. The meningeal membranes follow closely all of the various contours of the brain and spinal cord.

arachnoid tissues: See MENINGES.

arachnophobia = ARACHNEOPHOBIA.

Aran, François Amilcar /äräN'/ French physician, 1817–61. See ARAN-DUCHENNE DISEASE; PROGRESSIVE SPINAL-MUSCULAR ATROPHY.

Aran-Duchenne disease a progressive form of muscular atrophy that affects the spine. It is a motor-neuron-system disease that involves the anterior horn cells of the spinal cord and produces marked weakness in the hands at onset. Muscle wasting spreads to the arms, shoulders, and legs, eventually reaching even the tongue muscles. A.-D.d. progresses very slowly, and the patient may suffer from the ailment for as long as 25 years. A.-D.d. is a variation of AMYOTROPHIC LATERAL SCLEROSIS. See this entry.

arbitrary symbols a term used in the study of language for the arbitrary relation between a word's meaning and the sound or written symbol used to express it. E.g., diverse languages use different-sounding words to convey the same idea or refer to the same object.

arbor virus: See EQUINE ENCEPHALITIS.

arc de cercle /ärk'dəser'kl/ a rigid arching of the body concavely, convexly, or, rarely, laterally (French, "arc of a circle"). In psychiatry, the condition may be interpreted as a conversion symptom; according to Freud, the concave and convex types represent an unconscious "invitation to sexual relations." Also see OPISTHOTONOS; EMPROSTHOTONOS.

archaeopsychic: See ADULT-EGO STATE.

archaic brain the brain structures included in the paleocortex, e.g., the olfactory functions, which represent the furthest stage of cortical development by lower animals. The paleocortex is retained in the human brain but is subverted by development of the neocortex, or higher brain areas.

archaic inheritance a term applied to presumed phylogenetic influences in the development of the individual's mental processes, including the racial unconscious and archetypes of Jung.

archaic residue in Jung's analytic psychology, the remnants of inherited primitive mentality in the form of symbolic function-engrams imprinted on the racial unconscious.

archaic thought a type of thinking observed in schizophrenia that is dominated by concreteness, perception, and feeling, and lacks abstractness and reasoning.

archaism the unconscious memories that Jung believed to be inherited from the prehistoric past as influences on the modern psyche.

archetype as used by C. G. Jung, a structural component of the mind which derives from the accumulated experience of humankind. These inherited components, which Jung also refers to as primordial images, imagos, and mythological images, are stored in the collective unconscious and serve as a frame of reference with which we view the world, and also serve as one of the major foundations on which the structure of the personality is built. Examples are anima, animus, persona, the shadow, energy, supreme being, earth mother, hero, unity, magic, power, death, rebirth, the demon, the elder wise man, the creation myth, the Virgin Birth, the Sphinx, Hercules, and the philosoper king. Also called **archetypal image.** See IMAGO; PRIMORDIAL IMAGE.

archicerebellum the primitive part of the brain that during embryonic life develops into the cerebellum. The a. first appears around the fourth or fifth week of intrauterine life as a vesicle of the hindbrain. Thick plates of tissue form a roof over the a., and during the third month, fissures begin to form in the surface and the structure becomes easily identifiable as the future cerebellum.

archicortex the primitive areas of the cortex, including the hippocampus and olfactory system. Also called ARCHIPALLIUM.

architectonic structure = CYTOARCHITECTONICS.

architectural barriers building designs that hamper the mobility and functioning of persons who are blind, paraplegic, or otherwise handicapped. The term also is applied to hampering persons who lack normal mobility because of pregnancy, childhood, physical size, or old-age frailty. Local laws in some areas require barrier-free construction of public buildings as well as curb cuts and convenient parking places. See BARRIER-FREE ENVIRONMENT.

archival research the use of books, documents, manuscripts, and other records or cultural artifacts in scientific research. As in other research methods, experimenter bias and sampling procedures must be controlled.

Arctic hysteria a culture-specific syndrome occurring among the natives of Northern Siberia, characterized by a high degree of suggestibility and a tendency to imitate the movements and actions of other people.

arcuate fasciculus a bundle of nerve fibers that connects the superior and middle frontal gyri with parts of the temporal lobe. The a.f. fibers are associated with conduction aphasia; patients manifest normal comprehension but poor reception.

arcuate nuclei small groups of gray matter on the surface of the medulla oblongata that are believed to be components of the neighboring pons portion of the brainstem. They are associated with the somesthetic senses of the face.

arcuate zone of the brain the bow-shaped portion of the reticular formation extending from the spinal cord to the cerebellum that includes the internal and external arcuate fibers and arcuate nuclei. The arcuate fibers are concentrated in the olive portion of the medulla.

areal brain stimulation: See BRAIN STIMULATION.

area sampling a method of selecting persons for interview in public-opinion research, in which a specific neighborhood, street, or house is designated in advance as the source of respondents.

arecoline $C_8H_{13}NO_2$—a parasympathomimetic drug obtained from the seeds of the Areca catechu plant and used to produce temporary remissions in certain cases of schizophrenia. Also see BETEL NUT.

areflexia an absence of reflexes. The condition may occur when a person is unconscious as after administration of a general anesthetic. Individual reflexes involve motoneuron synapses associated with specific peripheral-nerve tracts. Absence of a particular reflex indicates a lesion or disease affecting the associated neural pathway. The condition may be general or involve one or more specific tendons, as in the absence of the normal knee-jerk reflex.

Aretaeus (of Cappadocia) Greek physician, 2nd century A.D. A. was an acute observer of mental disorders, who accurately described and differentiated mania, melancholia, senile conditions, and mental deterioration; and attributed mental illness to both physical and psychological determinants rather than divine inspiration.

-argent-; -argento- a combining form meaning silver (Latin *argentum*).

argentophilic plaques structures found in the brain tissues of older persons and identified as argentophilic because they absorb tissue stains containing silver. The a.p. appear under a microscope as wispy fibers in the frontal cortex and hippocampus. The a.p. are associated with Alzheimer's disease in humans and also have been found in the brains of aging animals. Also called **argyrophilic plaques**.

argininosuccinic aciduria a form of moderate-to-severe mental retardation, often accompanied by grand mal seizures in childhood. Clinical signs include sparse, dull, friable hair on the scalp and body. Large quantities of argininosuccinic acid are present in the urine. Treatment is based on control of protein intake to prevent hyperammonemia. The trait is transmitted by an autosomal-recessive gene.

argumentativeness contentiousness; a persistent urge to dispute and argue. In extreme form, a. may be a core symptom in manic episodes.

Argyll-Robertson, Douglas Moray Cooper Lamb Scottish ophthalmologist, 1837–1909. See ARGYLL-ROBERTSON PUPIL; GENERAL PARESIS; WERNICKE'S ENCEPHALOPATHY.

Argyll-Robertson pupil a myotic pupil that does not respond to light, reacts slowly to mydriatic drugs, and responds to accommodation. The A.-R.p. is a diagnostic sign of several CNS conditions, such as neurosyphilis, brain tumor, and multiple sclerosis. Also called ARGYLL-ROBERTSON SIGN; ARGYLL-ROBERTSON SYNDROME.

argyrophilic plaques = ARGENTOPHILIC PLAQUES.

arhinencephalia = ARRHINENCEPHALY.

Arieti, Silvano Italian-born American psychiatrist, 1914–82. See AGGRESSIVE TYPES; BASIC TRUST; CLAIMING TYPE OF DEPRESSION; CLASSICAL DEPRESSION; DEFORMATION OF THE SELF; DESUBJECTIVIZATION OF THE SELF; LISTENING ATTENTION; PROGRESSIVE TELEOLOGIC REGRESSION; TERTIARY-PROCESS THINKING; STORMY PERSONALITY.

aristogenic an obsolete term referring to persons presumed to be best suited eugenically for parenthood.

Aristotelian relying on historical explanations rather than contemporary causation or dynamic interaction, and therefore prescientific. A. approaches seek to account for frequently occurring cases but leave exceptional or individual cases unexplained. This meaning of the term—used, e.g., in statistics—was originated by Kurt Lewin. Compare GALILEAN.

Aristotle Greek philosopher, 384–322 B.C. A. was an early student of Plato and founded his own Peripatetic School in Athens. He was the author of the first treatise on psychology, *De Anima*, which viewed the soul, or psyche, as part of the natural rather than supernatural world. "The soul is to the body as cutting is to the

ax." A. investigated such psychological activities as sensation, perception, learning, memory, emotion, imagination, and reasoning, as well as a "common sense" that integrates material from the individual senses to form such concepts as unity, time, and motion. See ARISTOTELIAN; ARISTOTLE'S ILLUSION; ASSOCIATIONISM; GALILEAN; PHYSIOGNOMY; SENSUS COMMUNIS; SOCIAL INSTINCT; SOUL; VITALISM.

Aristotle's illusion the tactile perception that a single object is two objects when held in the crossed index and middle fingers.

arithmal mania = ARITHMOMANIA.

arithmetic disability a disturbance in calculation and reasoning associated with neurological impairment.

arithmetic disorder: See DEVELOPMENTAL A.D.

arithmomania a persistent, uncontrollable impulse to count, such as counting the pickets in fences or the steps in stairways. A. is an obsessive-compulsive symptom. Also called **arithmal mania**.

Army General Classification Test a group intelligence test developed in World War II to classify inductees according to their ability to learn military duties. Three subtests (vocabulary, arithmetic, block-counting) were used to measure verbal comprehension, quantitative reasoning, and spatial perception. Abbrev.: AGCT.

Army tests group intelligence tests for classifying inductees, developed by L. M. Terman and others during World War I. The **Alpha verbal test** measured information, reasoning, and ability to follow directions; the **Beta test** presented nonverbal problems to illiterate subjects and foreigners who were not proficient in English.

Arnold, Julius German pathologist, 1835–1915. See ARNOLD-CHIARI MALFORMATION.

Arnold, Matthew English poet and critic, 1822–88. See ZEITGEIST.

Arnold-Chiari malformation a deformity caused by premature closing of the cranial sutures. A result is an extension of the medulla and cerebellum through the foramen magnum, the large opening at the base of the skull, so that the cerebellum overlaps the top of the spinal cord. There are several variations of the A.-C.m., but hydrocephalus and meningomyelocele are commonly associated with the different types of the deformity. Also called **Arnold-Chiari syndrome; Arnold-Chiari deformity**.

aromatic hydrocarbons a category of chemical compounds containing carbon and hydrogen atoms arranged in closed rings and characterized by a fragrant odor. Benzene is an example of a.h. The a.h. molecules provide important olfactory stimuli that help an individual evaluate differences between edible and inedible substances.

arousal a state of alertness and readiness for action; a pervasive state of cortical response believed to be associated with sensory stimulation and activation of corticofugal (afferent) nerve fibers from the reticular formation. Also called **a. function; a. state**. See ALERTNESS. Also see SEXUAL A.

arousal boost the measurable increase in the arousal level of a subject as a result of a stimulus. The stimulus may affect arousal through either the extrinsic or intrinsic cortex.

arousal boost-jag in psychological esthetics, the feeling of pleasure and reward that may accompany activation of both arousal-boost and arousal-reduction mechanisms in succession. The individual experiences a moderate rise in arousal followed by a drop in arousal. See AROUSAL-BOOST MECHANISM; AROUSAL-REDUCTION MECHANISM.

arousal-boost mechanism any stimulus pattern produced by visual or other contact with a work of art that produces a measurable hedonic or pleasure effect. The arousal is measured by various psychological tests as a subject views a selection of paintings by various masters. The term was introduced in 1967 by D. E. Berlyne as part of his theory of positive hedonic value as a psychological effect of art. See AROUSAL BOOST; AROUSAL-REDUCTION MECHANISM.

arousal detection detection of increased arousal by measuring such physiological signs as brainwave activity, skin-temperature changes, increased heart rate or blood pressure, or GSR. Arousal signs are associated with environmental factors, such as heat, humidity, crowding, and noise, that may heighten performance or induce aggressive behavior. See AROUSAL; AROUSAL THEORY.

arousal function = AROUSAL.

arousal jag the excitation provided by gambling, sports activities, or adventurous challenges, whether real or imagined. It has been speculated that many individuals have a need or desire for an a.j., which may be satisfied either by active participation in great challenges or by viewing films or television programs that portray such activities.

arousal-reduction mechanism any stimulus or inhibitory reaction that decreases the degree of arousal of an individual after arousal has reached an uncomfortably high level. According to D. E. Berlyne, a sharp increase in arousal can have unpleasant or aversive effects, but an a.-r.m. can produce positive hedonic value by lowering the arousal curve. An a.-r.m. may have a natural inhibitory effect on CNS circuits to strong stimulation, or a stimulus that conveys a sense of harmony or concinnity. See AROUSAL-BOOST MECHANISM; CONCINNITY.

arousal state = AROUSAL.

arousal theory in environmental psychology, the concept that arousal increases when personal space is diminished, and that when personal space becomes inadequate for an individual, his level of arousal may become excessive. At that point, arousal may be expressed as aggressive behavior. See AROUSAL; AROUSAL DETECTION.

ARP tests tests of divergent thinking conceived by Guilford and his associates in the Southern California Aptitude Research Project. Test items include writing a series of words containing a specified letter (word fluency), writing titles for short-story plots (ideational fluency, originality), writing words similar in meaning to a given word (associational fluency), writing sentences containing words beginning with given letters (expressional fluency), and listing different consequences of a hypothetical situation, such as people no longer needing sleep. See CREATIVITY TEST; DIVERGENT THINKING; TORRANCE TESTS OF CREATIVE THINKING.

arreptio an obsolete term for insanity.

arrested testis a testis that lies within the inguinal canal but is unable to descend into the scrotum because the normal passage is obstructed. Also called **undescended testicle**. See CRYPTORCHID.

arrest reaction the response to stimulation of an inhibitory nerve circuit in an anesthetized animal. The animal may freeze in its tracks as it might when surprised or frightened.

arrhinencephaly a congenital defect characterized by a failure of the rhinencephalon, the part of the brain associated with the sense of smell, to develop normally. In various forms, the olfactory lobe of the brain and external olfactory organ may be absent or imperfectly developed on one or both sides of the body. Also called **arrhinencephalia; arhinencephalia**.

arrhythmia any variation from the normal rhythm of the heart beat, which is between 72 and 78 beats per minute in human adults. Changes in the heart rhythm are relatively important in terms of diagnosis and therapy. Normal rhythm for an infant may be as high as 150 beats per minute which would be considered tachycardia (any rate above 100 per minute) and a sign of a cardiac emergency for an adult. A rate of less than 60 per minute, bradycardia, also may be a sign of heart disease. Other kinds of arrhythmias include premature beats, atrial flutter in which one of the upper chambers contracts at a rate of as much as 400 times per minute, and heart block, marked by failure of the heart to contract because of the interruption or delay of an electrical stimulus needed to trigger the contraction.

arrhythmokinesis a lack of ability to perform voluntary movement in a rhythmic pattern, or to maintain a rhythmic sequence of movements.

arsenic poisoning a state of acute toxicity characterized in the early stages by vomiting and watery, bloody diarrhea, and in the terminal stages by seizures and coma. Major symptoms in chronic cases are burning sensations, optic neuritis, and gastrointestinal disorders.

Artemidorus (Daldianus) Greek author of books on dreams and ancient rites, fl. 170 A.D. See INSOMNIUM DREAM.

-arter-; -arteri-; -arterio- a combining form relating to arteries.

arterial anastomoses: See ANASTOMOSES.

arterial circle a ring of blood vessels in the brain,

formed by links between the major arteries feeding blood to the brain, the internal carotid, and the vertebrobasilar arteries. The arrangement provides alternate pathways of blood flow in the event of a cerebral hemorrhage or another disorder that could interrupt circulation in one part of the brain. Also called **circle of Willis**.

arterial stenosis a narrowing of an artery so that the normal flow of blood through it is reduced. Atherosclerosis, or a filling in of the lumen of the vessel by plaque, is a common cause of a.s. The reduced blood flow results in turn in malfunction of the neurons or other cells nourished by the blood.

arteriogram; arteriography: See ANGIOGRAPHY.

arteriole reaction an autonomic-nervous-system response marked by a change in the diameter of the arterioles, which control the flow of blood from the arteries to the capillaries. Smooth-muscle walls of the arterioles are particularly sensitive to sympathetic nerve impulses and may react to anger, fear, or other affects by producing dramatic blood-pressure changes.

arteriopathia hypertonica a form of arterial degeneration associated with hypertension. The muscle and elastic tissue of the walls of the arterial system increases and forms layers that are eventually replaced by connective-tissue fibers. The condition can be both a cause and an effect of hypertension, leading to cerebrovascular accidents if not controlled by medication.

arteriosclerotic brain disorder an organic disorder caused by constriction or blocking of the cerebral arteries, which reduces the blood flow to the brain, resulting in damage to neural tissue and loss of mental functions. If small blood vessels are ruptured, a small stroke occurs with temporary physical and mental symptoms such as dizziness, drowsiness, and irritability. If a major or apoplectic stroke (cerebrovascular accident) occurs, or if there is a series of strokes (termed multiinfarct), the patient usually becomes confused and comatose, and suffers permanent loss of brain functions with such symptoms as paralysis, disorientation, delirium, incoherence, and convulsions, with increasing mental deterioration. See MULTIINFARCT DEMENTIA.

arteriosclerotic dementia a disorder marked by progressive and irreversible cerebral dysfunction caused by arteriosclerosis of the arteries supplying blood to the brain. The condition often begins with restricted blood flow in arteries in the neck feeding into the brain tissues. A.d. most commonly occurs in men in their 60s and may be associated with hypertension. The disorder usually progresses through stages of aggravation of neurologic symptoms of depression, suicidal impulses, spontaneous crying or laughing, partial paralysis, and signs of parkinsonism.

arteritis an inflammation of an artery or more than one artery. A common form of a. is **cranial a.**, or **temporal a.**, marked by the appearance of giant multinucleated cells in the arteries of the temporal lobe, or retinal or intracerebral blood vessels. The symptoms include severe temporal-area headaches on both sides and visual disturbances, including loss of sight in one eye. Also called **giant-cell a.** Also see PANARTERITIS.

-arthr-; -arthro- a combining form relating to joints.

arthritic diathesis a predisposition to arthritis which, according to some researchers, occurs especially in the heavy "megalosplanchnic hypervegetative" constitution. Others, however, attribute a.d. to a tendency to sclerosis, or hardening of tissue due to primary hyperplasia (overgrowth), and irritability of connective tissue. Also called **arthritism**.

arthritis any inflammation of a joint. A. may be accompanied by stiffness of the muscles and bones surrounding the joint, a condition that is often painful. It is estimated that more than 16,000,000 persons in the United States alone are afflicted by one of the several forms of a. Kinds of a. include **gonococcal a.**, caused by infection of the joint by gonococcal bacteria; **gouty a.**, or gout, due to the accumulation of uric-acid salts in the joint; **psoriatic a.**, a form of the disease associated with severe psoriasis mainly affecting the ends of the toes and fingers; **rheumatoid a.**, a chronic systemic form of the disease that is associated with inflammatory changes throughout the body's connective tissues and which may be an autoimmune disorder; and **osteoarthritis**, a degenerative joint disease affecting mainly the weight-bearing joints and caused by normal-aging wear and tear on the joint tissues. Also see GOUT.

arthritism = ARTHRITIC DIATHESIS.

arthrodesis: See ANKYLOSIS.

arthrogryposis multiplex congenita a congenital disorder, possibly hereditary, marked by distorted joints in different body areas, clubfoot, and a greater-than-average incidence of mental retardation. In some cases, arms are rotated inward, the hips are dislocated, and the muscles are small, weak, and hypotonic. The term itself means "crooked-joint disorder." A postmortem examination of one child who died at the age of six years found a brain that weighed less than half the normal for a six-year-old. Four separate types of the disease are known. Also called, for short, **arthrogryposis**. Also see FLEXION CONTRACTURES.

arthropathy any inflammatory, neuropathic, or other disease involving a body joint. See NEUROPATHIC A.

arthropod-borne: See EQUINE ENCEPHALITIS.

Arthur, Mary Grace American psychologist, 1883— . See ARTHUR POINT SCALE OF PERFORMANCE TESTS.

Arthur Point Scale of Performance Tests performance tests of intelligence that are particularly applicable to the physically handicapped and foreign-born. The nonverbal materials include such items as form boards, block designs, mazes, and picture completions.

articulate speech oral language that is meaningful and intelligible.

articulation disorder: See DEVELOPMENTAL A.D.

articulation index the relative frequency with which the different sounds of speech occur in speech and the various positions in which they occur within words.

articulation test the phonetic analysis and recording of the speech of an individual with faulty sound production according to such criteria as developmental sequence, correct placement of the articulators, and intelligibility.

articulators: See MOTOKINESTHETIC METHOD.

artifact any man-made object but particularly a product of primitive art or craftsmanship. In psychological research, an a. is a misleading signal or an erroneous observation. A. may refer to static, to noise, to electrical interference.

artificial abortion = INDUCED ABORTION.

artificial body parts prosthetic devices that may be attached or implanted as replacements or aids for missing or defective natural body organs or tissues. A.b.p. may include heart pacemakers, plastic arteries and heart valves, electronic hearing aids, artificial kidneys, skull plates, and artificial hip joints. The category also may be extended to include such equipment as electronic reading machines for the blind.

artificial disorders: See FACTITIOUS DISORDERS.

artificial dream a dream that appears to be initiated by sensory stimulation. According to Freud's viewpoint, a dream may be induced by sensory stimuli but the content has other sources.

artificial insemination the use of medical or surgical techniques to achieve conception by implanting male spermatozoa in the reproductive tract of a female. Human a.i. involves placing semen from a male donor in the vagina below the cervix and injecting additional semen into the cervix. More than one a.i. may be needed to achieve fertilization but the rate of success is approximately 75 percent. Also called **euptelegenesis**. Also see INSEMINATION.

artificial intelligence a term denoting the solution of intellectual problems by computer; "computer thought."

artificialism precausal thinking in which either God or man is regarded as the maker of all natural things.

artificial-kidney dialysis: See DIALYSIS.

artificial neurosis = EXPERIMENTAL NEUROSIS.

artificial penis = DILDO.

artificial selection the selection of plants or animals for breeding, as opposed to natural selection.

arts and crafts creative activities directed by recreational or occupational therapists in rehabilitation programs. The activities may include painting, weaving, woodworking, or leatherworking. For the physically disabled, a.a.c. may be directed toward retraining of muscles, coordination of eyes and limbs, or similar functions. For psychiatric patients, as well as the physically disabled, the purpose may be to help establish confidence, self-esteem, or other behavioral qualities.

art tests tests designed to identify special abilities required for painting, architecture, and other arts, or to assess creativity in the arts, or to evaluate art productions. Varied techniques are utilized for these different purposes such as comparing the subject's judgment of pictures with that of experts, reproducing an object from memory, and identifying errors in a drawing.

art therapy the use of artistic activities such as painting and clay-modeling in psychotherapy and rehabilitation. These activities offer patients a nonthreatening emotional release, a means of restoring confidence and self-esteem, an opportunity for nonverbal communication and expression, and a means of reestablishing social relationships. They also provide the therapist with an avenue to unconscious impulses and hidden sources of emotional problems. Also see DANCE THERAPY; MUSIC THERAPY.

arugamama: See MORITA THERAPY.

aryepiglotticus the anatomical area relating to the arytenoid cartilage and to the epiglottis. It is part of the mechanism involved in speech production.

arylcyclohexylamine compounds substances that have an action similar to phencyclidine such as ketamine (Ketalar) and the thiophene analogue of phencyclidine (PCP).

arytenoids /-ten'-/ the pitcher-shaped pair of cartilages that are mounted on the cricoid cartilage and attached to the vocal bands. The movements of the a. approximate the vocal bands in vocalization.

asapholalia a type of speech that is mumbling or indistinct.

ASC = ALTERED STATE OF CONSCIOUSNESS.

A scale a questionnaire used in evaluating tolerance or intolerance for vagueness, ambiguity, and indefiniteness.

ascendance; ascendancy: See DOMINANCE.

ascendance-submission a behavior continuum ranging from extreme dominance to extreme subordination. Also called **dominance-submission**.

ascending hemiplegia: See HEMIPLEGIA.

ascending reticular system the pathways of nervous impulses from the reticular tissues of the mesencephalon, or midbrain, upward through the thalamus to all parts of the cerebral cortex.

asceticism /əset'isizəm/ a character trait or lifestyle characterized by renunciation of physical pleasures, withdrawal from society, and in many cases dedication to unworldly ideals. Self-denial of this kind is often interpreted in terms of anxiety or guilt generated by sexual impulses, and may be a source of masochistic pleasure. Adjective: **ascetic** /əset′ik/.

Asch, Solomon E. American psychologist, 1907—. See ASCH SITUATION.

Ascher, Karl Wolfgang Czech-born American ophthalmologist, 1887—. See ASCHER'S SYNDROME.

Ascher's syndrome a pathologic condition that is characterized by three types of abnormalities, including a goiter, a double upper lip, and eyelids that are hypertrophied with a loss of elasticity. Also called **Laffer-Ascher syndrome**.

Aschner, Bernhardt /äsh′nər/ Austrian physician, 1883–1960. See ASCHNER TREATMENT.

Aschner treatment an obsolete term for a type of treatment for schizophrenics promoted by Bernhardt Aschner. It consisted of emetics, cold baths, purgatives, and blood-letting.

Asch situation an experimental situation designed by S. E. Asch (1951) to test the degree of a subject's conformity to group opinion. In the A.s. the subject is asked to state his opinion after having been led to believe that it differs from that of all the other members of the group.

Asclepiades (of Bithynia) /asklēpī′adēz/ Greek physician, ca. 100 B.C. A. was one of the first to attribute mental illness to emotional disturbances and to advocate humane treatment in the form of harmonious music, baths, massage, a gently swaying bed, fresh air, and congenial activities.

ascorbic acid the chemical name for vitamin C, the antiscurvy nutrient found in many fruits and vegetables, particularly citrus fruits. A deficiency can result in scurvy, marked by bleeding gums and delayed wound healing. Neurological disorders associated with a.a. deficiency include femoral neuropathy and Sjögren's syndrome.

ASCP: See BLOOD-BANK TECHNOLOGIST.

ascriptive responsibility a term introduced by Szasz to describe a social judgment that society should inflict punishment on somebody who has been found guilty of committing an illegal act. The term is applied in forensic psychiatry in cases in which a criminally responsible person is ascribed legal responsibility. Also see DESCRIPTIVE RESPONSIBILITY.

-ase a combining form relating to an enzyme.

asemia a loss of the ability to understand or utilize language; a general communication disorder that includes such conditions as alexia, agraphia, and amimia, which involve the comprehension and use of communicative signs, symbols, or gestures (from Greek *a-* and *sema*, "sign"). A. is sometimes used interchangeably with asymbolia. Also called **asemasia**.

aseptic a term used to identify an object or substance that is free of infectious or septic material, hence sterile in a hygienic sense (from Greek *a-* and *sepsis*, "decay").

aseptic meningitis: See MENINGITIS.

asexual lacking sexual characteristics or drive; also, being capable of reproduction without the process of impregnation. A. reproduction is common among lower animal species which reproduce by budding or are capable of regenerating an entire animal from separate parts when cut into pieces. An example of a. reproduction can be observed in Hydra species.

Asher, Richard British physician, fl. 1951. See MUNCHAUSEN SYNDROME.

Asian influenza the common name applied to an H2N2 strain of influenza virus that first appeared in north China in 1957. The mortality rate was not high, but the infection was complicated by severe staphylococcal pneumonia in many cases. Some cases also were complicated by postinfluenzal asthenia with psychogenic factors.

as-if hypothesis a term used by Hans Vaihinger for the necessity of guiding our thoughts and actions by unproven or contradictory assumptions which we must treat as if they were true. Also see AS-IF PERSONALITY.

as-if performances a term used by H. S. Sullivan for the process of adopting various roles in order to avoid punishment or to obtain sympathy from other persons.

as-if personality a type of schizophrenic personality in which the individual behaves as if well-adjusted, by doing only what is expected (from German *als ob*, "as if"), and is unable to behave in a warm, genuine, spontaneous manner. According to Helene Deutsch this condition is frequently found in schizophrenics before they reach the psychotic stage. (The term was borrowed from *Die Philosophie des Als Ob*, the main work of the German philosopher Hans Vaihinger, 1911.) Also see AS-IF HYPOTHESIS.

-asis; -osis a combining form relating to a disease condition.

asocial behavior that lacks social sensibility; absence of social customs or values.

asociality a lack of involvement with other people, withdrawal from society, or indifference to social values and customs. Hermits, recluses, and many regressed schizophrenics are characterized as asocial.

asonia a form of sensory amusia characterized by inability to distinguish differences of pitch. Also called **tone deafness**.

asoticamania a self-destructive squandering of money, frequently manifested in manic episodes.

Asperger, Hans /äs′pergər/ Austrian physician, ca. 1844–1954. See AUTISTIC PSYCHOPATHY (also called **Asperger's syndrome**).

aspergillus flavus: See MOLDY-CORN POISONING.

aspermia failure of the male reproductive organs to produce or emit semen. Also called **aspermatism**. Also see PSYCHOGENIC A.

asphyxia a condition in which the level of oxygen in the blood falls below normal levels while the proportion of carbon dioxide increases. A. may be associated with dyspnea or labored or difficult breathing, and marked by signs of pallor or cyanosis. Choking, drowning, electric shock, inhaled smoke or toxic fumes, or disease or injury involving the respiratory system can be causes. Also see NEONATAL A.

aspirational group a group of persons that an individual wishes or aspires to join. An a.g. may have a formal structure, e.g., a professional association, or be an informal collection of other individuals with similar interests, economic status, and proximity. Compare DISSOCIATIVE GROUP.

aspiration level the standard used by the individual in setting his significant goals; the level of performance to which he aspires. The a.l. is an important component of the person's self-image and may reflect a reasonable evaluation of himself, or be unrealistically high or low. As pointed out by Lewin and others (1944), success tends to raise the a.l. and failure to lower or at least restrict it, especially when the judgment of failure reflects group rather than individual standards. Also called **level of aspiration**.

aspirin: See SALICYLATES.

aspirin combinations drug mixtures that include aspirin (acetylsalicylic acid) with various analgesics or stimulants. A common formulation includes *a*spirin, *p*henacetin (acetophenetidin), and *c*affeine, marketed as an **APC** mixture—$C_9H_8O_4/C_{10}H_{13}NO_2/C_8H_{10}N_4O_2$, the term being derived from initials of the ingredients. A.c. also may include antacid medications, codeine, meperidine, or other drugs. Certain individuals with emotional problems or personality disorders often consume large amounts of a.c., particularly those medications that can be obtained without a doctor's prescription, causing gastrointestinal symptoms such as peptic ulcer, and other toxic effects. See CAFFEINE EFFECTS; ASPIRIN EFFECTS; ASPIRIN POISONING.

aspirin effects therapeutic effects of aspirin, or acetylsalicylic acid, which are primarily antipyretic, antiinflammatory, and analgesic. Aspirin alleviates pain mainly by peripheral mechanisms with little risk of CNS side effects. In controlling fever, aspirin helps reset the body's temperature-control mechanism. Adverse effects include occasional allergic reactions, gastric irritation and hemorrhage, and altering effects of other drugs by displacing them in target areas.

aspirin poisoning an effect of overdoses of acetylsalicylic acid. Acute a.p. is more likely to occur in small children because of their low body weight, and the risk is greatest for children who have been taking aspirin for therapeutic reasons. Salicylate effects include CNS stimulation, vomiting, hyperactivity, and abnormally heavy breathing. The breathing activity causes depletion of carbon dioxide in the body and, in turn, an increase in blood alkalinity, or respiratory alkalosis. The kidneys react to the alkalosis

by excreting bicarbonates, sodium, potassium, and organic acids. If not corrected, the condition can progress to dehydration, respiratory failure, and collapse. As adult aspirin tablets usually contain five grains, compared with 1.25 grains for children's tablets, a.p. is more likely with overdoses of adult tablets. (Even more toxic is **oil of wintergreen**, which contains methyl salicylate. The methyl form can provide a fatal dose to a child in an amount as small as one teaspoonful. The effects are similar to those of a.p.) Also called **salicylism**.

assaultive behavior in psychiatry, violent attacks on individuals (child-beating, wife-beating, rape, unprovoked fights) associated with such conditions as alcoholic intoxication, temporal-lobe seizures, Huntington's chorea (occasionally), dyscontrol syndrome, and isolated or intermittent explosive disorder.

A-S scale a scale for measuring anti-Semitism in psychological surveys.

assertion-structured therapy a systematic approach to psychotherapy developed by E. Lakin Phillips, based on the theory that neurotic tendencies can be traced to faulty assumptions and expectations about people and relationships. Neurotic individuals tend to repeat these erroneous assumptions in a self-defeating manner even when they are "disconfirmed" by reality, and the therapist's objective is to help the patient become aware of them and to replace them with more realistic patterns of behavior.

assertiveness training a behavior-therapy technique that seeks to bring about change in emotional and other behavioral patterns by teaching the patient to assert himself. E.g., a timid patient will become less anxious if he is first made to realize that giving voice to his feelings is appropriate, and if he is shown how to behave more assertively in different situations, such as complaining about poor service, chastising a subordinate, or expressing appreciation. Role-playing, or **behavioral rehearsal**, is often used to prepare the patient for real-life situations. Also called **assertive training**. See DESENSITIZATION.

assessment center an office or department where individuals are evaluated with regard to their future growth and development within an organization. The a.c. may be operated only for currently employed personnel or for job applicants, or both.

assets-liabilities technique a counseling method in which the patient lists all his assets and liabilities for study.

assimilation in psychology, (a) the tendency to fit an account or a rumor into one's own attitudes or expectations (Allport and Postman, 1947), (b) an alteration in the reproduction of a geometrical figure to make it resemble a real object (Wulf, 1922), (c) the adoption of attitudes of other people with whom we are closely identified, (d) altering an object or situation to fit the needs of the self (Jung), (e) modifying new material to make it part of existing knowledge.

assimilation effect a shift in judgment toward an anchor when it is introduced in an experiment. Judgments of relative distance or weight will usually be evenly distributed along a scale before the experimenter provides an anchor. If, once the anchor is introduced, judgments cluster around the anchor, assimilation effects are said to have occurred. Also see CONTRAST EFFECT.

assimilation law: See LAW OF ASSIMILATION.

associated movement movement involving the skeletal muscles of one part of the body in association with muscle activity of another body area, as in kicking or biting an opponent who is restraining the subject's arms.

association in psychology and psychiatry, a connection (bond, relationship) between ideas or feelings on a conscious or unconscious level. Associations are established by learning or experience, and may be expressed spontaneously, as in the free-association method, or may be deliberately elicited, as in word-association tests. Also see FREE A.

association area = INTRINSIC CORTEX.

association by contiguity: See CONTIGUITY OF ASSOCIATIONS.

association coefficient a relationship index between discontinuous variables, e.g., big-little.

association cortex a region of the cerebral cortex composed of layers of short-axon neurons whose function is to integrate incoming stimuli impulses into the necessary patterns of response. The a.c. has been identified with pyramidal cells in the second and third layers of the cortex.

association-deficit pathology one of the terms applied to MINIMAL BRAIN DYSFUNCTION. See this entry.

association fibers nerve fibers that transmit impulses between different parts of a hemisphere. A.f. may be long or short, joining distant or nearby brain areas, but they do not extend beyond the hemisphere in which they originate. See COMMISSURAL FIBERS.

associationism the theory that attributes complex mental processes such as thinking, learning, and memory to associative links formed between ideas according to specific laws and principles. Aristotle was the first to cite some of these laws (similarity, difference, contiguity in time or space, etc.), but the theory did not come to fruition until the 17th and 18th centuries with the contributions of Thomas Hobbes (1588–1679), who held that all knowledge is compounded from relatively simple sense impressions, John Locke (1632–1704), and other members of the empirical school who developed the laws and applications of association: Bishop Berkeley (1685–1753), David Hume (1711–76), David Hartley (1705–57), James Mill (1773–1836), John Stuart Mill (1806–

73), Alexander Bain (1818–1903), and Thomas Brown (1778–1820). The approach was relatively static and nonexperimental, but there are echoes of a. in Freud (free association), Jung (word association), and Pavlov (the conditioning process). Also see CONTINUITY HYPOTHESIS.

associationists = S-R PSYCHOLOGISTS.

association nuclei nerve cells that are a part of the association pathways of the cerebral cortex.

association of ideas the process of combining perceptions and ideas into totalities of varying degrees of complexity and abstractness, e.g., connecting the relatively simple ideas of four legs, furry coat, a certain shape and size, etc., into the compound concept of cat. Much of the behavioral tradition (learning theory) rests on the philosophical underpinnings provided by Thomas Hobbes, John Locke, and the British empiricists. See ASSOCIATIONISM. Also see EMPIRICISM.

association-reaction time in a word-association test, the elapsed time between stimulus and response.

associations disturbances: See DISTURBANCES OF ASSOCIATIONS.

association-sensation ratio a learning-ability index based on the ratio of the association areas to the sensory cortex.

association test a method of determining reactions to specific stimuli such as colors or words. The subject is required either to say whatever comes to mind or to respond in a specified manner.

associative anamnesis an interview technique developed by Felix Deutsch, in which the patient gives an autobiographical account of his history and difficulties, while the therapist listens for key words and expressions which he then uses to establish **associative linkages** that will bring the patient closer to the unconscious roots of his disturbance. See SECTOR THERAPY.

associative fluency the ability to generate many answers, responses, or potential solutions; particularly, the ability to generate many original responses. High a.f. has been identified as an aspect of creativity that in many individuals is not positively correlated with high intelligence. Also see DIVERGENT THINKING.

associative inhibition the weakening of an established association when a new one is formed, or interference of a former association with a new one.

associative learning a type of learning in which bonds are formed between stimulus-response units.

associative linkage: See ASSOCIATIVE ANAMNESIS.

associative memory revival of the memory of a past event or place by recalling something associated with it.

associative shifting the principle that responses to one set of stimuli can be evoked by other stimuli in a similar situation (E. L. Thorndike).

associative strength the strength of a stimulus-response link as measured by memory persistence.

associative thinking a relatively uncontrolled cognitive activity that takes place during reverie, daydreaming, and free association. Such thinking may express the individual's inner needs and desires, and since it is free and untrammeled, may be a source of deeper understanding and creative ideas.

assonance a similarity in the vowel sounds of words, e.g., through and flute, sane and stay.

assortive mating the mating of individuals with similar physical or mental characteristics, or of individuals who are genetically similar but not related. Also called **assortative mating**.

assumed mean = WORKING MEAN.

assumed similarity the degree of correlation between one's own traits and one's perceptions of another individual. A.s. is essentially equivalent to the defense mechanism of projection. In social psychology, it may represent a response set in certain tests. See PROJECTION.

astasia-abasia an inability to stand (astasia) or walk (abasia); ability to walk only with a wobbly, staggering gait, though control is normal while lying down. A.-a. is a hysterical symptom possibly motivated by a desire for secondary gains of sympathy and support. Also called **hysterical ataxia**.

astereognosis the loss or marked impairment of the ability to identify familiar objects or geometrical forms by touch. A. is believed to be due to a lesion in the parietal lobe caused by disease or injury. Also called **tactile agnosia; astereognosia**. See APHASIA; ASYMBOLIA. Also see AMORPHOSYNTHESIS.

asterixis transient loss of a fixed position of the hands or arms followed by a jerking recovery movement, usually occurring in association with tremulousness caused by metabolic disorders. Also called **flapping tremor**.

-asthen- a combining form relating to weakness (from Greek *asthenes*, "weak"). Adjective: **asthenic**.

asthenia a condition of severe weakness or loss of strength. A. may be marked by general fatigue and muscular pain or by breathlessness, giddiness, and heart palpitations. One form of a. caused by pituitary-gland dysfunction is characterized by loss of appetite, constipation, hypoglycemia, hypothermia, loss of muscle tone, and, in women, amenorrhea. A. is a common symptom in depressive and neurasthenic disorders. Also called **adynamia**. See DYSTHYMIC DISORDER; ASTHENIC PERSONALITY; NEURASTHENIA. Also see HEAT-INDUCED A.; DA COSTA'S SYNDROME; MENTAL A.

asthenic: See -ASTHEN-.

asthenic personality in DSM II, a personality disorder characterized by persistent mental and physical lassitude, aches and pains, low tolerance for stress, diffuse "nervousness," and lack of enthusiasm. Asthenic individuals are chronic complainers, "wet blankets," and hypochondriacs who magnify minor problems to major proportions. See NEURASTHENIA.

asthenic type the frail, long limbed, narrow-chested type of individual who, according to E. Kretschmer, tends to be shy, sensitive, and introversive in temperament. Also called **leptosome type**. See CONSTITUTIONAL TYPE.

asthenology the study of structural or functional disorders characterized by weakness or debility.

asthenophobia a morbid fear of weakness (of being weak, of showing weakness, or of dealing with weakness).

asthenopia a descriptive term for weakness or fatigue involving the eyes and eye muscles, usually due to strain.

atherosclerosis: See ARTERIAL STENOSIS.

asthma a disorder in which blocking of the bronchial passages by spasmodic contractions and mucus produce wheezing and gasping. Though the precipitating cause is usually an allergen (dust or pollen) or hypersensitivity to bacterias, psychological factors, such as anxiety and stress, may aggravate or even precipitate an attack. Some analysts, including Freud, interpret these attacks as a dependent person's cry for help when the relation to the mother is threatened. (A. is a Greek word meaning "hard-drawn breath.") Also called **bronchial a**. Also see EXTRINSIC A.

astigmatism a visual disorder caused by a cornea that is not evenly curved. The effect is an aberration or distortion of the visual image not unlike the reflection seen in an amusement-park mirror. The cause may be injury or inflammation and, according to some ophthalmologists, pressure produced by frequent rubbing of closed eyes. A. symptoms often overlap with those of other ocular disorders, e.g., nearsightedness.

-astr-; -astro- a combining form relating to stars or anything star-shaped (from Greek *aster*, "star").

astral projection a hypothetical psychic phenomenon in which influences from the stars are believed to control the actions, health, personality, and destiny of human beings. Also see ASTROLOGY.

astraphobia a morbid fear of thunder and lightning. Also called **astrapophobia**. These terms are also loosely used (a) for a morbid fear of thunder specifically, which is more properly called **brontophobia** or **tonitophobia**, and (b) for a morbid fear of lightning specifically, which is more properly called **keraunophobia**.

astroblastoma a type of astrocytoma, or tumor composed of neuroglia cells. An a. usually forms about a small blood vessel as a young cancer cell with multiple nuclei. It attaches itself to the blood-vessel wall by means of short fibrils. An a. develops most frequently in the cerebrum, but also may be found in the cerebellum. Also called **grade II astrocytoma**.

astrocyte: See ASTROCYTOSIS.

astrocytoma: See ASTROBLASTOMA.

astrocytosis a pathologic condition marked by a proliferation of **astrocytes**, or neuroglial cells with fibrous processes. The astrocytes spread into CNS tissues in which normal neurons have undergone necrosis as a result of lack of oxygen or glucose, as during episodes of hypoxia or hypoglycemia.

astroglia a group of astrocyte cells organized as a body tissue.

astrology a pseudoscience based on the belief that the movements of the planets and stars influence the lives of individuals and determine the course of events. As one example, Paracelsus applied medications derived from minerals which were supposed to capture the beneficial magnetic forces emanating from the heavenly bodies. Even today many individuals believe that their horoscope, or map of the heavens at the time of their birth, can be used in determining their personal characteristics, tendencies to particular diseases of mind or body, and liability to good fortune or calamity.

astyphia an obsolete term for sexual impotence.

astysia an obsolete term for sexual impotence.

asyllabia a type of aphasia marked by an inability to form syllables from letters of the alphabet.

asylum a term applied to a refuge for criminals in the classical era (from Greek *asylon*, "sanctuary"), later used to designate an institution for the protection of the mentally ill—an **insane a**. A. and insane a. are obsolete terms, discarded because of their association with criminal behavior and their emphasis on refuge rather than treatment. See MENTAL INSTITUTION.

asylum lunacy an obsolete term for social-breakdown syndrome.

asymbolia an inability to understand or use symbols of any kind, including words, gestures, signals, musical notes, chemical formulae, or signs. A. is a communication, or language, disorder diagnosed as a form of aphasia due to a cortical lesion. Also see ASEMIA.

asymmetrical distribution an irregular or unbalanced statistical distribution in which the frequency of scores above the mean does not match that below the mean.

asymptomatic not showing any symptoms. A disease may be present or not.

asymptomatic neurosyphilis a form of neurosyphilis in which physical signs and laboratory findings show involvement of the nervous system although the patient does not show symptoms of the disease.

asymptote /as'-/ the straight line which a regular curve approaches but never reaches. The term is used in psychology for the approach to a full level of response after many learning trials.

asymptotic curve a curve that approaches an axis more and more closely, but never quite touches it. An example is the normal curve, which has two tails that approach but never touch the abscissa.

asynchrony /əsin'-/ lack of coincidence in time between different processes, e.g., the development of different components of the body (arms, legs, etc.) at different times during puberty, resulting in asymmetry and, frequently, self-consciousness and transient maladjustment.

asyndesis /-sin'-/ disjointed speech in which disconnected ideas are thrown together. A. is a communication disorder most frequently observed in schizophrenia, and occasionally in organic brain syndromes.

asyndetic thinking thought processes in which ideas and images have no intrinsic connection with each other; fragmented thinking resulting from loosening of associations, particularly in schizophrenia.

asynergia a faulty coordination of muscle groups, which may result in difficulty in standing or walking (**major a. of Babinski**), or in kneeling or sitting up from a recumbent position (**minor a. of Babinski**).

asynergic speech = CEREBELLAR SPEECH.

asynesia an obsolete term for severe mental retardation.

ataque a culture-specific disorder observed mainly among Puerto Ricans and manifested as a convulsive seizure believed to be a conversion defense against aggressive urges.

ataractic: See ATARAXY.

ataractics agents that have a calming or quieting effect, producing a state of ataraxy. The term was introduced as an alternative to the general term tranquilizer. Also called **ataraxics; tranquilosedatives**. See ATARAXY; TRANQUILIZER.

Atarax: See DIPHENYLMETHANES.

ataraxia; ataraxic: See ATARAXY.

ataraxics = ATARACTICS.

ataraxy /at'-/ a state of mind that is characterized by perfect peace or detached serenity without loss of mental abilities or clouding of consciousness. Also called **ataraxia**. Adjectives: **ataraxic; ataractic**.

atavism /at'-/ a genetic trait that is inherited from a remote ancestor but did not appear in nearer ancestors; a throwback, a reversion to an earlier type (from Latin *atavus*, "ancestor").

ataxia a neuromuscular disorder marked by failure of the muscles to perform coordinated movements, such as walking or reaching for an object. A. may be due to injury, drugs such as phenytoin, or disorders affecting muscular coordination, such as cerebral palsy or multiple sclerosis. See BIEMOND'S A.; BRIQUET'S A.; CEREBELLAR A.; FRIEDREICH'S A.; INTRAPSYCHIC A.; LOCOMOTOR A.; MARIE'S A.; VOLUNTARY A.; ANIRIDIA-OLIGO-PHRENIA-CEREBELLAR A. SYNDROME; BEHR'S SYNDROME; WESTPHAL-LEYDEN SYNDROME; ZAPPERT'S SYNDROME.

ataxia muscularis = THOMSON'S DISEASE.

ataxia-telangiectasia = LOUIS BAR'S SYNDROME.

ataxic diplegia a neurologic disorder marked by loss of motor coordination on both sides of the body. A.d. may result from separate successive strokes, each affecting an area such as the internal capsule, in opposite hemispheres.

ataxic dysarthria a speech disorder characterized by slurring, uncontrolled volume and sudden spastic irregularities of vocal-cord function. It is usually associated with cerebral diseases, e.g., cerebral palsy.

ataxic feeling: See INTRAPSYCHIC ATAXIA.

ataxic gait a gait in which the patient watches his legs and slaps his feet on the ground when walking, depending upon sound and sight to tell where his feet are. A.g. is due to effects of damage to the posterior-column nerves.

ataxic speech = CEREBELLAR SPEECH.

ataxic writing uncoordinated or irregular writing caused by lack of skill or CNS damage.

ataxophemia an incoherent, disordered coordination of words in forming sentences.

-ate a combining form describing a characteristic feature of a structure.

-atel-; -atelo- a combining form relating to defective development.

atelesis a term applied to schizophrenic dysjunctions, e.g., dysjunction of the psyche and the environment as manifested in autism; also, disintegration, or splitting, of the contents of consciousness.

ateliosis a general term for incomplete development, applied to either physical or mental growth: infantilism, dwarfism, mental retardation.

atephobia a morbid fear of ruin or being ruined (from Greek *ate*, "infatuation, blind impulse").

atheromatosis a pathologic condition caused by the accumulation of **atheromas**, or atherosclerotic plaques, in the smooth-muscle tissue of the walls of arteries. The condition begins in childhood as a series of fatty streaks which develop into plaques over a period of time. If a. develops in a cerebral artery or an artery in the neck that supplies the brain, the plaques may cause occlusion of an artery, depriving the brain tissues of oxygenated blood.

atherosclerosis a common form of arteriosclerosis in which the primary sign is the accumulation of **atheromas**, or yellowish lipid plaques, on the inner walls of large and medium-size arteries.

atherosclerotic plaque: See PLAQUE.

athetoid dysarthria a speech disorder characterized by noisy irregular breathing, hoarseness, and articulatory problems which may result in extreme unintelligibility, or slight distortions. It is usually associated with cerebral palsy.

athetosis a disorder characterized by slow, involuntary, recurrent movements of the fingers, toes, arms, or legs, due to extrapyramidal lesions. It is a common symptom of cerebral palsy.

athetotic dysarthria the loss of articulation associated with slow, writhing involuntary movements of the extremities, as in cerebral palsy.

athletic type the muscular, well-proportioned, broad-shouldered type of individual who, according to Kretschmer, tends to be energetic, aggressive, and schizothymic in temperament. See CONSTITUTIONAL TYPE.

athymia a Hippocratic term for melancholia.

athyreosis a form of hypothyroidism found in children with anatomic dysgenesis of the thyroid gland. The patient is a cretin with no thyroid gland or a gland that is abnormally small and whose essential elements are replaced by fibrous tissue. Also called **athyreotic cretinism**.

atmosphere effect behavioral habits that may be stimulated by the environment, even when inappropriate, such as automatically applauding a poor speech. The term applies also to errors in thinking resulting from an impression made in the statement of the problem.

atmospheric conditions various aspects of the atmosphere (temperature, humidity, air flow, barometric pressure, composition, toxic conditions) as they affect worker comfort and performance or the general public in their homes or in their institutional environment, such as theaters, schools, and hospitals.

atmospheric perspective one of the cues that aid in perception of depth and distance. A.p. is the acquired ability to differentiate near and distant objects on the basis of their clear or indistinct appearance, taking into account dust, smoke, and smog. Also see DEPTH PERCEPTION.

atomism in psychology, the view that psychological phenomena can best be understood by analyzing them into elementary units such as sensations, associations, or conditioned reflexes, and by showing how these units combine to form thoughts, images, and perceptions. Also called **atomistic psychology; elementarism; molecularism**. Also see REDUCTIONISM; STRUCTURALISM.

atonement in the psychiatric sense, acts of atonement, such as apologies, repentance, and restitution, by which we attempt to relieve anxiety generated by guilty impulses or behavior. For pathological forms of a., see UNDOING.

atonia a deficiency or absence of normal muscle tone. The condition may occur with a number of diseases characterized by flaccidity or lack of muscle tension, particularly in the extremities. A. of smooth-muscle tissue can be serious if the loss of tone is in the circulatory, digestive, or other systems which would not be able to maintain arterial blood flow, peristalsis of the gut, or similar functions. By extension, a. is sometimes used in psychiatry to describe patients whose **psychic tone** is lowered due to depression, that is, patients who show a marked reduction in emotional and intellectual responsiveness, energy, and initiative. Also called **atony; atonicity**. Adjective: **atonic**.

ATP = ADENOSINE TRIPHOSPHATE.

atrabilious an obsolete term denoting depression.

atresia in general, closure of a normal opening; a

congenital malformation of the outer ear and occluded external canals, resulting in a conductive hearing loss.

-atri-; -atrio- a combining form relating to an atrium, especially to one of the upper heart chambers. Adjective: **atrial**.

atrial flutter: See ARRHYTHMIA.

at risk vulnerable to disorder, physical or mental. Children of schizophrenics are often considered a.r. for schizophrenia; a fetus carried by a mother who contracts rubella is a.r. for cerebral palsy; and heavy cigarette smokers are a.r. for emphysema and cancer.

atrophic dementia a general term sometimes used to refer to presenile organic brain disorders, e.g., Alzheimer's disease. Also called **abiotrophic atrophic dementia**.

atrophy /at′rəfē/ a wasting away of the body or a part it, as from lack of nourishment; also, a degeneration from disuse (from Greek *atrophos*, "not fed"). Adjective: **atrophic** /ətrof′-/. Verb: **to atrophy** /at′-/.

atropine $C_{17}H_{23}NO_3$—an anticholinergic alkaloid derived from belladonna, hyoscyamus, or stramonium. A. also can be produced synthetically. Its effects include increased heart rate and rate of respiration, relaxation of smooth muscles, and decreased rate of secretions. It can be used as a cerebral stimulant and is most commonly employed in eye examinations to dilate the pupil. A. is closely related in chemical structure and actions to SCOPOLAMINE. See this entry. Also see ANTICHOLINERGICS.

atropine-coma therapy a method of treating tense, agitated, and anxious psychotics by administering atropine sulfate to induce coma. Abbrev.: **ACT**.

atropinics drugs that inhibit the action of acetylcholine in tissues innervated by postganglionic parasympathetic nerves. The affected tissues include the eyes, salivary glands, heart, lungs, urinary bladder, intestine, and other structures. A. therefore can inhibit gastric secretion, urination, and accommodation of the pupil of the eye, and increase the heart rate. Atropine is one of the a.

attachment the tendency of young animals to become physically identified with certain older individuals. Human infants seek a. to their mother as a step in establishing a feeling of security. See A. BEHAVIOR.

attachment behavior in humans, a type of behavior toward the mother-figure that develops from six months onward and is conceived, in general, "as any form of behavior that results in a person obtaining or retaining proximity to some other differentiated and preferred individual, usually conceived as stronger and/or wiser . . . Such behavior includes following, clinging, crying, calling, greeting, smiling, and other more sophisticated forms" (John Bowlby, in *American Handbook of Psychiatry*, 1975).

attachment bond the primary, enduring, and special relationship that gradually develops between an infant and its real or surrogate mother. In the latter half of the first year of life, the baby clearly knows and recognizes its mother.

attachment disorder the failure of an infant to thrive because of emotional neglect or social isolation. A.d. is characterized by apathy and unresponsiveness. Also see the DSM-III term REACTIVE-A.D. OF INFANCY.

attachment theory according to John Bowlby (in *American Handbook of Psychiatry*, 1975), a theory that is "a way of conceptualizing the propensity of human beings to make strong affectional bonds to particular others and the many forms of distress and disturbance which include anxieties, anger, and depression to which unwilling separation and loss give rise." See AFFECTIONAL BONDS; ATTACHMENT BEHAVIOR.

attack behavior an aggressive use of force or violence against an adversary, usually with intent to harm. Animals, and some humans, may use attack as a form of defense. Compare DEFENSE BEHAVIOR.

attendant care a service for severely handicapped individuals who are able to live independently except that help is required for part of the day in dressing, undressing, and feeding. A.c. service is provided by students, housewives, religious missionaries, or mildly retarded or mildly handicapped persons; in many cases two or more attendants work together as a team. A.c. usually is financed by Medicaid or a similar government-funding source.

attending behaviors in counseling, all the verbal, nonverbal, observable, and unobservable behavior engaged in by the counselor while listening and giving attention to the client. Full involvement in listening and observing is felt to be a cornerstone of the counselor's general ability.

attensity the sensory clearness or attention-producing effect of a sensation. The term was applied by E. B. Titchener.

attention a state of conscious awareness, accompanied by sensory clearness and CNS readiness for response to stimuli; the act of focusing on specific stimuli or specific aspects of the environment. The process is a selective one in which the focus is determined by such internal factors as (a) past experience (we notice things that have a meaning for us), (b) the activity in progress (e.g., reading, or waiting for the starting gun of a race) and our physiological condition (a hungry person is especially aware of restaurants), and (c) such external determinants as intensity, movement, repetition, contrast, and novelty of stimuli.

attention-deficit disorder, residual type a disorder affecting individuals who have experienced attention-deficit disorder with hyperactivity. The symptoms of inattention and impulsivity persist, and interfere with social and occupational behavior, but the hyperactivity is no longer present. (DSM-III)

attention-deficit disorder with hyperactivity a childhood disorder with onset before age seven, and involving (a) inattention (failure to finish things, not listening, distractibility, and difficulty in concentrating in school, work, or play activities), (b) impulsivity (acting before thinking, shifting from activity to activity, difficulty in organizing work and taking turns in games, calling out in class, needing extra supervision), and (c) hyperactivity (as in excessive running about or climbing on things, inability to stand still, excessive movement during sleep, and being always on the go as if driven). (DSM-III)

attention-deficit disorder without hyperactivity a childhood disorder with onset before age seven and involving inattention and impulsivity but not hyperactivity. See ATTENTION-DEFICIT DISORDER WITH HYPERACTIVITY. (DSM-III)

attention disorder a learning disability and one of the terms used interchangeably with MINIMAL BRAIN DYSFUNCTION. See this entry. Also see LEARNING DISABILITIES.

attention fluctuation: See FLUCTUATION OF ATTENTION.

attention-getting denoting a type of behavior, usually inappropriate, that is used to gain attention, e.g., childhood tantrums; also, such behavior itself.

attention overload a psychological condition that results from excessive demands for attention to intense, unpredictable, or uncontrollable stimuli. The effect is temporary depletion of available attention and an inability to cope with tasks that demand attention. A.o. can occur in students preparing for an examination or in work tasks, such as supervising commercial-aircraft activity in an airport control tower. See INFORMATION OVERLOAD.

attention reflex a change in the size of the pupil when attention is suddenly fixed.

attention span the number of objects that can be distinctly perceived in one brief presentation. The term may be used, in addition, for the length of time an individual can concentrate on one subject. Also called **span of apprehension; span of attention**. See TACHISTOSCOPE.

attentiveness the state of being alert and actively paying attention; also, the quality of actively attending to the needs of others.

attenuation in statistics, a reduction in size of a true effect because of errors of measurement.

attenuators the calibrated devices that accurately control the decrease in the intensity of tones, or light, on electronic instruments such as audiometers, stereophonic sound systems, or video equipment.

atticomastoidectomy surgical removal of the upper portion of the tympanum and part of the mastoid bone.

attitude a relatively stable predisposition or readiness to react in a specific way to a person, group, idea, or situation. Attitudes are complex prod-
ucts of learning, experience, and emotional processes and include, e.g., our enduring preferences, prejudices, superstitions, scientific or religious views, and political predilections and aversions.

attitude scale a scale used in attitude surveys to measure the strength of opinions. See LIKERT SCALE; THURSTONE ATTITUDE SCALES.

Attitude Scale Toward Disabled Persons a scale devised by H. D. Yuker, J. R. Bloch, and W. J. Campbell to reveal attitudes toward disability.

attitude survey a questionnaire-type study used to measure the attitudes or opinions of a group.

attitude theory a concept of psychosomatic medicine that there is a specific disease condition or set of symptoms associated with each attitude of a patient toward a disturbing situation. The a.t. is demonstrated by hypnotizing the patient and asking him to assume an attitude the patient held at the time he experienced hives or some other disorder. Physiological changes associated with the disorder develop during the hypnotic state.

attitude therapy a form of reeducative treatment that emphasizes current attitudes of the patient in terms of their origins, present purpose, and distortions.

attitude tic a postural attitude due to tonic rigidity in the limbs, head, or upper body area, e.g., torticollis.

attitudinal group any personal growth or therapy group in which members are given the chance to express and exchange feelings and thoughts in an accepting environment. The purpose of an a.g. is greater insight leading to improved interpersonal functioning.

attitudinal reflexes reflexes that help put the organism in a position or condition to make a complex response, as in an animal preparing to attack an adversary.

attitudinal type a Jungian term for either an introvert or extrovert who expresses attitudes of his appropriate type toward the world and himself.

attonity a clinical state of stupor similar to that observed in catatonia but also occurring in cases of severe depression.

attraction in environmental psychology, the act of adjusting proximity relationships between individuals, depending upon such factors as their liking for each other. Male-female couples and female-female pairs who like each other position themselves closer to each other than do pairs who feel no personal a. toward each other; male-male pairs generally do not display a. as a sign of liking each other. Environmental influences, e.g., noise, heat, and humidity, decrease a. between pairs of individuals.

attribute the essential quality or character of a person, sensation, or object, e.g., the tonal a. of a note.

attribution in the two-word stage of language development, a noun qualified by an attribute, as in "blue car."

For a different use of the term, see A. THEORY.

attribution error in the process of explaining behavior, the tendency to underestimate environmental or circumstantial influences while overestimating personal or psychological factors. Attributing behavior to psychological factors is termed dispositional attribution; attributing behavior to environmental factors is termed situational attribution.

attribution theory the study of the processes by which people ascribe motives to their own and others' behavior (F. Heider), e.g., interpreting others' behavior in internal, psychological terms while interpreting one's own behavior in external circumstantial terms.

attrition dropout or loss of subjects during an experiment; or withdrawal of patients during a clinical trial. Also called **mortality**.

atypical affective disorders disorders that include (a) **atypical bipolar disorder**, in which an individual has experienced a major depression episode and now undergoes an episode of relatively mild manic symptoms, and (b) **atypical depression**, a residual category for individuals with depressive symptoms that do not meet the criteria for a major affective or adjustment disorder. (DSM-III)

atypical anxiety disorder a diagnostic category used when the individual appears to have an anxiety disorder that does not meet the criteria for other anxiety conditions. (DSM-III)

atypical bipolar disorder: See ATYPICAL AFFECTIVE DISORDERS.

atypical child a child who deviates markedly from the norm in some basic characteristic, e.g., a boy or girl who is brain-damaged, learning-disabled, mentally retarded, exceptionally intelligent, or emotionally disturbed. See EXCEPTIONAL CHILD; SPECIAL CHILD.

atypical childhood psychosis: See CHILDHOOD-ONSET PERVASIVE DEVELOPMENTAL DISORDER.

atypical conduct disorder a pattern involving violation of either the basic rights of others or social norms and rules, but without conforming to the criteria of other conduct disorders. These are CONDUCT DISORDER, SOCIALIZED, AGGRESSIVE; CONDUCT DISORDER, SOCIALIZED, NON-AGGRESSIVE; CONDUCT DISORDER, UNDER-SOCIALIZED, AGGRESSIVE; CONDUCT DISORDER, UNDERSOCIALIZED, NONAGGRESSIVE. See these entries. (DSM-III)

atypical depression: See ATYPICAL AFFECTIVE DISORDERS.

atypical development a term sometimes used to identify childhood schizophrenia or early infantile autism.

atypical disorder in psychiatry (especially the DSM-III classification), a residual category which includes unusual or uncharacteristic variations of standard mental disorders, such as "atypical paranoid disorder" and "atypical dissociative disorder."

atypical dissociative disorder a residual category applying to individuals who do not have specific dissociative disorders, but who experience trancelike states, a persistent feeling that the external world is unreal (derealization), or dissociative states resulting from prolonged brainwashing, thought reform, or indoctrination during captivity by terrorists or cultists. (DSM-III)

atypical eating disorder a residual diagnostic category for eating disorders that cannot be adequately classified among other eating disorders. (DSM-III)

atypical factitious disorder with physical symptoms a residual category for factitious disorders that do not require hospitalization, such as dermatitis artifacta (induced by excoriation or chemicals) and voluntary dislocation of the shoulder. (DSM-III)

atypical gender-identity disorder a residual category for disorders of gender identity that are not classifiable as any specific gender-identity disorder. (DSM-III)

atypical impulse-control disorder a category comprising disorders of impulse control other than pathological gambling, kleptomania, pyromania, or explosive disorders. (DSM-III)

atypical, mixed, or other personality disorder a category that includes cases of personality disorder in which there is insufficient evidence for a more specific designation. The term "mixed" applies to cases that involve features of several personality disorders without meeting the criteria for any one type; and the term "other" is applied to unclassified cases, such as masochistic, impulsive, or immature personality disorder. (DSM-III)

atypical or mixed organic brain syndrome a residual category of organic syndromes, such as Addison's disease, in which the clinical picture does not meet the·criteria of other organic brain syndromes. (DSM-III)

atypical paranoid disorder a residual category for paranoid conditions not classified under paranoid disorders. (DSM-III)

atypical paraphilia a residual category comprising such paraphilias as coprophilia (feces), frotteurism (rubbing), klismaphilia (enema), mysophilia (filth), necrophilia (corpses), telephone scatologia (lewdness), and urophilia (urine). (DSM-III)

atypical pervasive developmental disorder a category that includes children with multiple disturbances in the development of language and social skill, but not classifiable as infantile autism or childhood-onset pervasive developmental disorder. (DSM-III)

atypical psychosexual dysfunction a category that includes psychosexual dysfunctions outside the standard specific categories, such as absence of erotic sensations despite physiologically normal sexual excitement and orgasm, or the female equivalent of premature ejaculation. (DSM-III)

atypical psychosis a residual category for cases involving psychotic symptoms that do not meet the criteria for any specific mental disorder. It includes such conditions as (a) persistent auditory hallucinations as the only disturbance, (b) postpartum psychoses that do not meet the criteria for other mental disorders, and (c) very brief psychoses for which there is no precipitating stress. (DSM-III)

The term has also been applied to an episodic and sometimes intermittent psychotic state characterized by clouding of sensorium and symptoms of schizophrenia. This condition is called oneirophrenia by Meduna, and may be related etiologically to epilepsy.

atypical somatoform disorder a residual category for conditions such as an imagined defect in physical appearance (dysmorphophobia) that cannot be explained organically, but for which there appear to be psychological factors. (DSM-III)

atypical specific developmental disorder a residual category comprising developmental disorders other than reading, arithmetic, language, or articulation deficits. (DSM-III)

atypical stereotyped-movement disorder a childhood condition involving repetitive head-banging, rocking, and rhythmic finger or hand movements which, unlike tics, are voluntary, do not cause distress, and are often associated with mental retardation, pervasive developmental disorder, or inadequate social stimulation. (DSM-III)

atypical tic disorder a diagnostic category for tics that cannot be adequately classified among stereotyped-movement disorders. (DSM-III)

Aubert, Hermann /ou'bert/ German physiologist and psychologist, 1826–1892. See AUBERT PHENOMENON; AUBERT-FÖRSTER PHENOMENON.

Aubert-Förster phenomenon the principle that small near objects are easier to distinguish than larger distant objects even though the latter subtend the same visual angle.

Aubert phenomenon the illusion that a vertical line tilts in the opposite direction from where the head is tilted when viewing the line.

-audi-; -audio- a combining form relating to sound or hearing.

audibility range: See RANGE OF AUDIBILITY.

audible thought a type of hallucination in which the patient hears his own thoughts as if they were projected into him by an inner voice. Although a.t. appears to be a hallucination of perception, it actually is one of conception.

audience: See CROWD BEHAVIOR.

audile pertaining to a person who is ear-minded, or who learns more easily from spoken as opposed to written language.

auding a level of auditory reception that involves hearing, listening, and comprehension of the information.

audio brain stimulation: See BRAIN STIMULATION.

audiogenic seizure an epilepsylike seizure induced by high-frequency sound waves.

audiogram a recording of a subject's range of hearing. The a. is made with an audiometer which is usually designed to measure the ability of the subject to hear frequencies ranging from 500 to 6,000 cycles per second and at intensities of from 0 to 80 decibels.

audiology the study of hearing including the anatomy and function of the ear, impairment of hearing, and habilitation or rehabilitation of persons with hearing loss. The **audiologist**, who is usually also a speech pathologist, conducts individual and group examinations for hearing loss, contributes to the diagnosis of hearing disorders and the selection of an appropriate hearing aid, and directs or participates in the retraining and rehabilitation of individuals with hearing defects.

audiometric zero the level of sound intensity that is regarded as the normal threshold for human hearing. Commercial **audiometers** are calibrated so that threshold readings will always be at the zero level for any sound frequency that would be perceived by the person with normal hearing. Also see ELECTROENCEPHALIC AUDIOMETRY; BEKESY AUDIOMETER.

audiometry the measurement of hearing acuity with electronic audiometers to determine the nature and extent of hearing impairment as a guide to the use of hearing aids, aural habilitation, and possible surgical intervention. Also see PSYCHOGALVANIC SKIN-RESISTANCE A.; PURE-TONE A.; SCREENING A.; SPEECH A.

audiotape instruction: See COMPUTERIZED THERAPY.

audioverbal amnesia a type of auditory aphasia in which the patient may be able to retain and repeat certain single words presented acoustically but is unable to retain and repeat series of words. The condition often is associated with a lesion in the middle temporal gyrus.

audiovisual training the use of audio and/or visual aids such as films, slides, filmstrips, videotapes, audiotapes, and television, in academic education as well as personnel training. Also called **audiovisual method**.

audit an evaluation or review, such as a patient-care a. or medical a.

audition = HEARING.

auditory acuity hearing sensitivity in which a minimum stimulus is detected half of the time.

auditory agnosia = AUDITORY APHASIA.

auditory amnesia the loss of ability to comprehend sounds or speech. See WERNICKE'S APHASIA.

auditory aphasia a defect or loss in the ability to comprehend spoken language due to disease, injury, or maldevelopment in the left hemisphere of the brain. It is a form of receptive aphasia. Also called **auditory agnosia; word deafness**.

Auditory Apperception Test a projective test designed primarily for blind subjects, who respond to a variety of recorded sounds by telling stories with a beginning, a middle, and an ending based on their interpretation of what is heard.

auditory blending the ability to synthesize the individual sounds, or phonemes, of a word so that the whole word can be recognized.

auditory canal the short tubelike structure that extends between the external ear and the tympanic membrane of the middle ear.

auditory closure the ability to fill in missing parts that were omitted in auditory presentation, and to produce a complete word. It is an automatic process in a normal functioning individual.

auditory cortex the sensory area for hearing, located in the temporal lobe of the cerebral cortex.

auditory discrimination the ability to discriminate between sounds of different frequency, intensity, and pressure-pattern components; the ability to distinguish one speech sound from another; also, the ability to identify other auditory qualities, such as timbre, from a spectrum of sound waves.

auditory disorder any dysfunction in the processes related to hearing, such as total or partial deafness, frequency gaps, hypersensitivity to sound, or auditory aphasia.

auditory distance cues: See DISTANCE CUES.

auditory fatigue = EXPOSURE DEAFNESS.

auditory feedback the act of hearing our own speech, which enables us to adjust its intensity or clarity. Experiments show that delaying the feedback by using an electronic device (**delayed a.f.**) will cause stuttering, slurring, increased intensity, pitch distortion, and emotional disturbances in normal subjects but not in schizophrenic children, possibly because they do not use a.f. in monitoring their speech.

auditory hallucination a false auditory perception; hearing sounds without external stimulation. Examples are accusatory or laudatory voices, strange noises, muffled or disconnected words or commands which in some cases appear to emanate from the patient's own body, or from a light fixture or imaginary telephone. Hallucinations of this type frequently occur in acute alcoholic hallucinosis, paranoid disorder, senile dementia, and occasionally in psychotic depression.

auditory imagery: See IMAGERY.

auditory memory the memory for information obtained by hearing processes. Individuals who are ear-minded tend to have greater ability to grasp ideas that are presented through sound than persons who are more dependent upon visual stimuli in learning. A.m. is particularly important in tonal discrimination.

auditory memory span the ability to immediately recall sequences of related or unrelated orally presented material. Also see MEMORY SPAN.

auditory nerve = ACOUSTIC NERVE.

auditory pathways nerve fibers that transmit impulses translated from sound waves by the inner ear. A.p. include the cochlear nerve, the dorsal and ventral cochlear nuclei, the trapezoid body, superior olivary nucleus, inferior colliculus, and medial geniculate body, leading to the auditory cortex.

auditory perception the ability to interpret and organize sensory information received through the ear.

auditory perceptual disorders a series of language-cognition difficulties associated with lesions in various brain areas. A right-hemisphere lesion may result in acoustic agnosia marked by an inability to discriminate among nonverbal sounds. A lesion in the superior temporal gyrus may cause difficulty in phoneme discrimination so that "bitch" and "pitch" sound the same.

auditory processing the ability to recognize, remember, organize, and interpret what is heard.

auditory projection area the temporal-lobe brain region where sound impulses are received and perceived.

auditory radiations the acoustic impulses that spread from the medial geniculate bodies to the cortex of the cerebrum, and specifically to Heschl's gyrus in the temporal lobe.

auditory sequencing the ability to recall the order of items presented orally, e.g., days of the week, sequences of numbers, or the alphabet. It is a skill associated with reading.

auditory skills the skills related to normal hearing, including auditory acuity, auditory memory, comprehension of speech and music, and auditory-feedback control.

auditory space perception perception of the direction and distance of the source of sound. Perception of direction is dependent on three types of auditory cues: (a) time difference, that is, the fact that sounds often reach our two ears at different times, (b) loudness, that is, a sound appears to be more intense to the nearer ear, and (c) phase difference, that is, when one ear faces the source of sound more directly than the other, the maximum positive pressure of the sound wave reaches this ear first. In contrast, perception of distance depends on the monaural cues of intensity, frequency, and complexity.

auditory span the number of simple items, such as words or numbers, that can be repeated by a person after hearing the series one time. The a.s. of a person indicates the capacity of his immediate memory.

auditory stimulus any sound waves that are within the normal range of the subject's hearing ability. For an adult human, the a.s. range is between 16 and 20,000 cycles per second. Newborn infants and some animals respond to sound waves of higher frequencies. The a.s. normally is received through the tympanic membrane but also can be transmitted through bones of the skull, a route frequently used when deafness is due to middle-ear disease or injury.

auditory system the general organization of the external, middle, and inner ears, including the auditory canal, tympanic membrane, ossicular bones composed of the malleus, incus, and stapes, and the cochlea. The cochlea converts the sound vibrations to nerve impulses carried by the auditory nerve to the brain.

auditory threshold the minimum level of sound that can be detected by a subject. The average normal a.t. varies with the frequency of the sound wave, the human ear being most sensitive to sounds of about 1,000 cycles per second at 6.5 decibels. The threshold for sounds of 125 cycles per second may require an intensity level of 45.5 decibels.

auditory training the instruction and training of the hearing-impaired individual as to the most effective use of his remaining hearing. This may or may not include use of a hearing prosthesis.

Aufgabe /ouf′gäbə/ a German word for task or homework used by the Würzburg School in their introspective experiments on mental processes. An A.—renamed "determining tendency" by Narziss Ach and "mental set" by later psychologists—is a preparation or predisposition which unconsciously determines the way we handle a situation; e.g., if the problem is $\frac{6}{4}$ and the A. is adding, we get 10, but if the A. is subtracting, we get 2. The concept therefore helps to explain the relation between attitude and meaning.

augmentation an increase in the amplitude of average evoked responses (AER). Experiments with bipolar patients, e.g., have shown a greater rate of a. with increasing intensity than was shown in unipolar patients, an effect which diminished somewhat during lithium-carbonate treatment. Also see AVERAGE-EVOKED-RESPONSE TECHNIQUE.

aulophobia a morbid fear of any wind instrument shaped like a flute. It may be the fear of a phallic symbol.

-aur-; -auri- a combining form relating to (a) the ear (from Latin *auris*, "ear"), (b) gold or anything golden (from Latin *aurum*, "gold").

aura in psychiatry, subjective sensations that warn the individual of an impending epileptic seizure or migraine attack: strange tastes or odors, colored lights, numbness, weird sounds, feelings of unreality, stomach distress, or déjà vu. Individual patients experience their own typical auras, which may or may not give them time to prepare for or abort a seizure. The term is also used in parapsychology to denote halos and emanations which some individuals claim to see. (A. is a Greek word meaning "breeze.") Also see EPILEPTIC A.; MIGRAINE A.; VISUAL A.

aura cursoria a condition marked by aimless running immediately preceding an epileptic seizure.

aural microphonics = WEVER-BRAY EFFECT.

auricle: See EXTERNAL AUDITORY MEATUS.

auroraphobia a morbid fear of northern lights (or aurora borealis).

aurothioglucose an organic compound containing gold, used as a medication for the treatment of certain cases of lupus erythematosus and rheumatoid arthritis.

auscultation a diagnostic method in which the examiner listens for sounds occurring inside the body through the use of a stethoscope or by applying the ear to the surface of the body.

Aussage test /ou′sägə/ a test devised by the early forensic psychologist Wilhelm Stern to "illustrate the limitations of witnesses" (German *Aussage*, "declaration"). In one version, a class is suddenly interrupted by an intruder who berates the instructor. After the incident, the students are asked detailed questions about the scene, which usually reveals that their accuracy in observing the event is less than 30 percent.

-aut-; -auto-; -auth- a combining form meaning (a) self, (b) caused by or from itself (from Greek *autos*, "self").

autarchy a period of infancy when the child exerts autocratic power over others, including the parents who satisfy all his instinctual demands.

autemesia a form of idiopathic vomiting usually due to psychogenic causes.

authenticity in psychiatry, the quality of being genuine and real, as applied to an individual's conscious thoughts, feelings, and perceptions.

authoritarian aggression a personality trait marked by hostile, punitive attitudes and behavior usually toward weaker persons or groups who appear to be outside conventional standards. A.a. was identified by Adorno and Frenkel-Brunswick as one of the traits associated with the authoritarian personality. See AUTHORITARIANISM. Compare AUTHORITARIAN SUBMISSION.

authoritarian character; authoritarian character structure = AUTHORITARIAN PERSONALITY.

authoritarian conscience the term used by E. Fromm for the tendency to be guided by fear of an external authority, e.g., parents or a representative of the state. Fromm contrasts a.c. with HUMANISTIC CONSCIENCE. See this entry.

authoritarianism the belief that human beings should be controlled by a superior power, whether in the form of a person, state, group, or idea, and that the individual should have no rights of his own apart from such a power.

authoritarian leader the type of leader who imposes his own goals and methods on group members, making all decisions, rejecting suggestions, and dominating interactions through frequent criticism and threats of punishment. In studies by Lewin, Lippitt, and White, groups with an a.l. showed more fear, anxiety, apathy, and aggression in addition to less independence and originality, and lower group morale than groups with a democratic leader. Productivity (defined as number of tasks completed) was, however, somewhat higher. Compare DEMOCRATIC LEADER; LAISSEZ-FAIRE LEADER.

authoritarian parent a parent who tries to control the child's activity according to relatively rigid standards of behavior. An a.p. stresses obedience, deemphasizes collaboration and dialogue, and employs strong forms of punishment to deter unwanted behavior. Baumrind distinguishes between the not-rejecting a.p. and the rejecting-neglecting a.p. Also see AUTHORITATIVE PARENT; PERMISSIVE PARENT; REJECTING-NEGLECTING PARENT.

authoritarian personality a personality pattern characterized by preoccupation with power and status, strict adherence to conventional values, identification with authority figures, a demand for subservience or obedience on the part of others, and hostility toward minority or other out-groups. Also called **authoritarian character; authoritarian character structure**.

authoritarian rejecting-neglecting parent: See REJECTING-NEGLECTING PARENT.

authoritarian submission a personality trait marked by the need for unquestioning blind submission to a dominant leader or authority. A.s. was identified by Adorno and Frenkel-Brunswik as one of the traits associated with the authoritarian personality. Also see AUTHORITARIANISM. Compare AUTHORITARIAN AGGRESSION.

authoritative parent according to Baumrind, a parent who directs the child's activities in a rational, relatively flexible way, encouraging collaboration and dialogue, yet exercising authority when necessary. Obedience is not valued for its own sake, but firm control is used to handle conflicts if a reasoned approach fails. Also see AUTHORITARIAN PARENT; PERMISSIVE PARENT; REJECTING-NEGLECTING PARENT.

authority complex a pattern of emotionally invested concepts of authority that are partially or completely repressed. Unconsciously motivated reactions to authority, either in the form of rebellion or submission, are common in neuroses.

authority figure in psychoanalysis, an individual who represents power, influence, and standards of right and wrong, such as a parent, teacher, or therapist.

authority principle the concept that each member of a social hierarchy is expected to comply with the wishes of those above him.

autia a personality trait characterized by nonconformity, impracticality, dissociative behavior, and an autistic intellectual life (Cattell).

autism retreat from reality into a private world of fantasies, thoughts, and, in extreme cases, delusions and hallucinations. A. was once thought to be the prime characteristic of schizophrenia, but is now recognized in other disorders, such as senile psychosis, Kanner's syndrome (early infantile autism), and some cases of depression. The autistic person is turned inward, a "shut-in" personality, completely preoccupied with his or her own needs and wishes, which are gratified largely or wholly in imagination. Also see EARLY INFANTILE A.; INFANTILE A.; INFANTILE A., RESIDUAL STAGE.

autisme pauvre /ō'tism pōv'(r)/ a term used to describe the withdrawal and detachment from reality observed in schizophrenia patients (French, "impoverished autism").

autistic child a child who has lost or never achieved contact with other people and is totally withdrawn and preoccupied with his own fantasies, thoughts, and stereotyped behavior such as twirling objects or rocking. Other characteristics are indifference to parents or other people, inability to tolerate change, and defective speech or mutism. The condition is interpreted by some as organically based, and by others as a form of schizophrenia. See INFANTILE AUTISM.

autistic phase according to M. S. Mahler, the first phase of development of the sense of self, during which self and object are not differentiated. During this stage, which occurs in the first few weeks of life, instinctual responses to stimuli are on a reflex and thalamic level and the ego is not integrated. Also called **normal autism.**

autistic-presymbiotic adolescent according to D. B. Rinsley (in *American Handbook of Psychiatry*, 1974), one of two types of adolescent candidates for residential treatment, characterized by nuclear schizophrenia, severe disorganization, perceptual, affective, and cognitive defects, and lack of meaningful relations with others. The condition apparently stems from failure to achieve a satisfying relationship with a mothering figure during infancy. The other type, designated symbiotic or borderline, has experienced this relationship but failed to separate from it, and became either floridly psychotic or highly neurotic, though sometimes gifted.

autistic psychopathy a personality disorder characterized by a lack of sensitivity and understanding, and one-sided communications in which only the patient's views are expressed, usually at the expense of the feelings of others. The patient builds a world of his own within the real world. He not only shows a lack of understanding and sensitivity, but speaks in proclamations rather than in a manner that permits communication with others. Also called **Asperger's syndrome.**

autistic psychosis a form of infantile psychosis in which the child has a constitutionally defective ego structure and cannot maintain a symbiotic mother-child relationship. Characteristically, the child adopts autism as a defense against both external and internal stimuli (M. S. Mahler).

autistic thinking narcissistic, egocentric thought processes, such as flights of fancy and daydreaming, which have little or no relation to reality. See AUTISM; DEREISM.

However, a.t. often is a source of arousal and motivation. E.g., a person may decide to buy a cheeseburger merely as a result of thinking about the food item, even though he may not be hungry. Advertising appeals frequently utilize a.t. mechanisms.

autoaggressive activities behavior in which the individual hurts or mutilates himself, as in some cases of chronic schizophrenia or Lesch-Nyhan syndrome. L. Kanner found that in infantile autism, in which the child has failed to develop a feeling for his own body, he may attempt to arrive at self-awareness by biting himself or knocking his head.

autoallergy = AUTOIMMUNITY.

autobiography in counseling, a technique designed to elicit information regarding a client's behavioral patterns and feelings by means of a life history written by the client from his own point of view. A **structured a**. is based on explicit questions or topic guidelines supplied by the counselor. An **unstructured a**. contains no guidelines and may uncover more latent content, especially if the client is highly verbal.

autocatharsis a form of therapy in which a patient releases disturbing emotions by writing down experiences or feelings that are upsetting.

autochiria an obsolete term for suicide.

autochthonous /ôtok'thənəs/ native, indigenous, original (from Greek *autochthon*, "from the land itself, from the soil").

autochthonous delusion a delusion that appears suddenly and without an apparent cause or explanation. An a.d. usually involves a disturbance of symbolic meaning (e.g., the idea that the universe will be twisted out of shape) as opposed to disturbances of perception or intellect.

autochthonous Gestalt a perceptual pattern induced by internal factors rather than an external stimulus.

autochthonous idea a thought that originates within the mind, usually from an unconscious source, yet appears to arise independently of the individual's stream of consciousness. Examples are fantasies, dreams, delusions, and the repetitious thoughts of obsessive-compulsive individuals.

autochthonous variable any change that develops from internal, as opposed to external, factors.

autocorrelation in statistics, the correlation of a time series with itself, separated by one or more steps or lags. A. is computed in order to estimate the amount of serial dependency.

The term also applies to the theory that groups of individual nerve fibers collaborate to transmit auditory nerve impulses representing frequencies higher than 1,000 cycles per second. This concept is based on evidence that a single fiber is unable to transmit impulses faster than 1,000 per second, thus fibers must function as a team with one firing at one cycle, another at the next cycle, and so on.

autodysosmophobia a morbid fear or a delusion of having an offensive odor. Also see BROMODROSIPHOBIA; AUTOMYSOPHOBIA.

autoecholalia a type of stereotyped behavior observed in catatonic schizophenia in which the patient continuously repeats the same word or phrase. See CATAPHASIA.

autoechopraxia a form of stereotyped behavior in which the patient, usually schizophrenic, repeats an action he has previously experienced, e.g., kneeling for hours or days in the same spot.

autoerotism a term applied by Havelock Ellis to "those spontaneous solitary sexual phenomena of which genital excitement during sleep may be said to be the type." In its broadest sense, a. denotes any self-induced sexual excitement, not only through masturbation, but through self-stimulation of the lips or anus, and fantasies involving self-gratification. Psychoanalysts believe autoerotic satisfactions first appear in the earliest phase of psychosexual development, the oral sucking stage. Also called **autoeroticism**. Adjective: **autoerotic**. Also see SECONDARY A.

autogenic training a relaxation technique developed by the German neurologist J. H. Schultz (1970) in which a quasihypnotic state is self-induced and relaxation is achieved through breathing exercises, muscular decontraction, and head, heart, and abdominal exercises. The method, usually accompanied by a meditative technique, is used to correct functional irregularities of organs and for general intellectual and physical invigoration.

autogenital stimulation any form of stimulation by a human or an animal of its own genitalia. Such a.s. may take the form of pelvic thrusts, masturbation, or self-stimulation preceding sexual intercourse. A.s. may occur in the presence of members of the same or opposite sex or in the absence of other individuals.

autohypnosis self-induced hypnosis. This type of hypnosis may occur spontaneously, as in looking fixedly at bright lights or listening to monotonously repeated sounds; or it may be achieved through training in autosuggestion. Also see SELF-HYPNOSIS.

autohypnotic amnesia a Jungian term for repression.

autoimmunity a condition in which the body's immune system fails to recognize its own tissues as "self" and attempts to reject its own cells as if they were bits of foreign protein. A. increases with age when the immune system deteriorates and is a primary factor in the development of such diseases as rheumatoid arthritis. Also called **autoallergy**.

autointoxication a form of poisoning caused by toxins generated within the patient's own body. The self-poisoning could occur through absorption of products of dead tissue cells, such as tissue destroyed by gangrene, or by absorption or accumulation of products of metabolism that are potentially toxic.

autokinesis any movement that is voluntary.

autokinetic effect the tendency to see movement in a static spot of light in a dark room. The a.e. has been utilized in certain psychological experiments, as in investigating suggestibility or the establishment of group norms. Also called **autokinetic illusion; Charpentier's illusion**.

autolysis /ôtol'-/ the destruction of cells or tissues by enzymes that are produced in other cells within the same organism. A., a form of self-digestion, may be a beneficial activity as it provides a means for the disposal of cells that have died or degenerated. Another form of a. may occur during periods of starvation or malnutrition when protein tissues may be digested in order to obtain glucose molecules to be burned for cellular energy.

automated assessment a system of evaluating psychological information about an individual by the use of computer devices which can utilize data banks of previously acquired information for making comparisons, diagnoses, and prognoses.

automated clinical records a standardized record-keeping system suitable for computerized retrieval of information for such purposes as monitoring patient care, providing data for administrative decisions, and assisting the clinician in understanding and treating patients.

automated desensitization: See DEVICE FOR A.D.

automatic action an act that is performed without conscious awareness.

automatic decisions: See ROLE SPECIALIZATION.

automatic drawing the act of drawing images or objects while in a hypnotic trance or in a situation in which attention is distracted. The drawings are produced without volition and usually represent unconscious fantasies or impulses. A.d. is sometimes used as a technique in hypnoanalysis.

automatic memory a rarely used term for a reactivated feeling or emotional complex (e.g., déjà vu). It is experienced although the person is not aware of the association to an earlier situation.

automatic obedience pathological behavior in which the individual blindly and uncritically or mechanically repeats the speech or actions of others. It is a symptom most frequently found in catatonic schizophrenia. See ECHOLALIA; ECHOPRAXIA; COMMAND AUTOMATISM; OBEDIENCE.

autonomatic reactivity an individual reaction tendency that begins in infancy and continues into adult life as manifestations of sensitivity differences to aversive stimuli. Examples of a.r. may include individuals who are pulse reactors, stomach reactors, and hypertensive reactors to emotional situations.

automatic seizures a form of psychomotor epilepsy in which actions may be carried out automatically, such as continuing to work, with later amnesia.

automatic speech the mechanical repetition of consecutive words such as days of week, numbers, and various kinds of accessory expressions; also, speech that erupts involuntarily, or without conscious control, as in senility or highly emotional states.

automatic writing the act of writing without conscious awareness, as during a hypnotic trance. A.w. sometimes provides a therapist with access to unconscious material.

automatism an activity performed mechanically, without intention, and frequently without awareness. Examples range from reflex responses and habitual acts, such as repeatedly using the same phrase (like "as it were"), to complex activities, such as sleepwalking, automatic writing, and behavior in a fugue state. Automatic behavior is characteristic of various disorders: Patients with psychomotor epilepsy may continue to perform a job during a seizure; vic-

tims of Pick's disease may move the pieces of a jig-saw puzzle around mechanically; catatonic schizophrenics may automatically repeat what others say or do (echolalia, echopraxia); and individuals with senile brain disease may perform the same activity, such as making, unmaking, and remaking a bed, all day long. Kinds of a. include **confusional a.**, in which the patient seems to continue the action in which he was involved at the start of the attack, **verbal a.**, and **gestural a.**

automatization the development of a skill or habit to a point where it becomes routine and requires little if any conscious effort or direction. The term is also applied by some writers to neurotics or psychotics who obey their infantile or compulsive impulses so automatically that they may be described as automata.

automaton a machine that simulates human functions, such as a robot spot-welder, or the "machina docilis" which was capable of conditioning, motility, problem-solving, avoiding obstacles, and obeying a whistle (Walter, 1953), and automatic machines that run mazes, take shortcuts, and even "choose" between goals. See CYBERNETICS; FEEDBACK.

automaton conformity a type of behavior in which the individual follows submissively the dictates of the group that establishes the culture pattern of his environment. A.c. is one way of dealing with the sense of separateness and isolation that pervades today's world.

automorphic perception the perception of others in terms of oneself while ignoring differences.

automysophobia a morbid fear of smelling bad or being unclean. Also see BROMIDROSIPHOBIA; AUTODYSOSMOPHOBIA.

autonomasia a type of amnesic aphasia in which the person is unable to recall nouns or names.

autonomic apparatus the total vital organs, including the ductless glands and viscera, that are controlled by the autonomic nervous system.

autonomic balance the complementary interfacing of sympathetic and parasympathetic nerve actions.

autonomic conditioning gaining conscious control over autonomic processes (such as heart rate) through conditioning.

autonomic disorganization overmobilization of the autonomic nervous system occurring during a situation of extreme stress and resulting in confusion, with weakness, fright, and behavioral disorganization.

autonomic epilepsy a type of seizure that may affect otherwise normal individuals by a sudden diffuse discharge of autonomic-nerve impulses. The person may experience fever, chills, tearing, flushing, salivation, hiccoughs, or blood-pressure changes. The condition may involve either the sympathetic or the parasympathetic system, or both.

autonomic hyperactivity: See GENERALIZED-ANXIETY DISORDER.

autonomic motor pools the cell bodies and dendrites of the motor neurons in the ventral horns of the spinal cord before they exit through the ventral motor roots.

autonomic nerve any nerve that is a part of the autonomic nervous system, such as the nerve involved in regulating activity of the heart muscle or the various glands of the body.

autonomic nervous system the portion of the central nervous system and peripheral nervous system involved primarily in internal, involuntary bodily functions such as those of the circulatory, digestive, and respiratory organs. It is divided into sympathetic and parasympathetic systems. Abbrev.: **ANS**.

autonomic responses any smooth-muscle or glandular activity that occurs as a result of stimuli received through the autonomic nervous system. In certain instances, a.r. can include contractions of skeletal muscles.

autonomic seizure a recurrent epileptic attack involving the autonomic nervous system, and characterized by heart palpitations, vomiting, sweating, temperature changes, tearing of the eyes, and abdominal distress.

autonomic side effect a visceral reaction such as increased blood pressure or heart rate and decreased stomach secretions, associated with a situation of stress or with ingestion of certain psychotropic drugs.

autonomic-sympathomimetic drugs agents that can mimic the actions of natural substances in controlling functions of the sympathetic nervous system. Amphetamine is an example of a.-s.d. as it has the ability to release stored epinephrine from terminals of sympathetic-system nerves, resulting in stimulation of organs and glands innervated by sympathetic nerves.

autonomous activity a term used in general-systems theory for the fact that the organism is not passive and inert, and that it is not wholly dependent on responses to external stimuli, the reduction of tension, or the reestablishment of equilibrium. Rather, it is intrinsically active; and spontaneous, autonomous processes are a primitive form of behavior taking many forms, such as play, exploration, and intellectual and esthetic pursuits for their own sake and not merely as a means of reducing tension or satisfying biological drives.

autonomous depression according to R. D. Gillespie's classification, a type of depression characterized by restlessness, self-accusation, and more activity than in reactive depression, as well as less hypochondriasis than in involutional depression.

autonomous morality = AUTONOMOUS STAGE.

autonomous respiratory center = PNEUMOTAXIC CENTER.

autonomous stage Piaget's second stage of moral development wherein the older child gradually comes to rely less on parental authority and more on individual and independent morality. In the a.s., the child disciplines himself; in the earlier heteronomous stage, discipline is im-

posed by parents. Also called **autonomous morality**. Compare HETERONOMOUS STAGE.

autonomous word = CONTENT WORD.

autonomy a state of independence and self-determination, either in a society or in an individual. According to E. Erikson, the a. drive first appears between the ages of two and four. Compare HETERONOMY.

autonomy-heteronomy the balance between the biological individual and the environment in a world where there are no sharp boundaries but only degrees of ego proximity and ego distance.

autonomy of motives = FUNCTIONAL A. O. M.

autonomy versus doubt stage two of the eight stages of man in Erikson's system of human development. During the second and third years, the child develops a degree of independence if allowed to be active at his own pace, but may begin to doubt his ability to control himself and his world if his parents are overcritical, overprotective, or inconsistent. See ERIKSON'S EIGHT STAGES OF MAN.

autophagy /ôtof'-/ the chewing or eating of one's own flesh.

autophobia a morbid fear of being alone or the fear of oneself. The terms **eremiophobia** and **eremophobia** are similar and refer to fear of solitude and desolate, uninhabited places. A. is also called **monophobia**.

autophonic response the echolike reproduction and vibration of one's own voice, commonly referred to as "hearing one's own voice." A.r. is usually due to middle-ear or auditory-canal disease in which the Eustachian tube remains open. Also called **autophonia; autophony** /ôtof'-/.

autoplasty a psychoanalytic term for the process of adapting to reality by modifying one's own behavioral patterns, particularly those manifested in neurotic behavior.

autopsy a procedure in which the body of a person is examined after death in an effort to determine the exact cause and time of death. Because of legal, religious, and cultural reasons, an a. generally cannot be performed without permission of the next of kin or an order of the public authorities. The procedure usually requires a detailed dissection of body tissues, laboratory tests, and other techniques when the death occurs under suspicious circumstances. Also called **necropsy; post-mortem examination**. Also see BIOPSY; PSYCHOLOGICAL A.

autopsychic characterizing ideas and impulses that originate in the self or relate to the subject's own personality.

autopsychic delusion a delusion that refers to the patient's own personality. The a.d. is one of the Wernicke categories, which also include **allopsychic delusions**, which refer to the outside world, and somatic delusions, which refer to the patient's body. See SOMATIC DELUSIONS.

autopsychic orientation the perception of one's own personality or psychic self, particularly the awareness of changes in one's personality.

autopsychosis a form of paranoid disorder in

which the patient maintains distorted ideas about himself, such as the delusion that he is the world's savior, the devil incarnate, or an unrecognized genius. Such ideas are autopsychic in the double sense of pertaining to the self and arising from within the psyche.

autopsy-negative death a death that cannot be explained by autopsy. The term is sometimes applied to cases of lethal catatonia among mental patients who suddenly develop fever, hyperactivity, delusions, and hallucinations, then die without other warning. See BELL'S MANIA.

autoradiography a technique for producing an image of an object containing radioactive chemicals by placing the object on a sheet of photographic film. A. may be used to study distribution of a psychomimetic drug in a laboratory animal's tissues by tagging the drug with a radioactive atom. Also called RADIOAUTOGRAPHY.

autoscope any device or instrument that magnifies small muscular movements.

autoscopic syndrome a rare delusional disorder in which the patient sees a "double" who looks, talks, acts, and dresses like himself. The image, which may occur only once or repeatedly, is generally hazy, filmy, and colorless. In some cases (**symptomatic autoscopy**) there is evidence of an organic basis, since the condition appears to be associated with epilepsy and migraine; in others (**idiopathic autoscopy**), the basis is probably psychogenic, since it may occur in schizophrenics and depressives, or may follow a disturbing experience. Also called **autoscopic phenomenon; autoscopy** /ôtos'-/.

autosexuality any form of sexual arousal or stimulation that occurs without participation of another person or animal, e.g., masturbation, sexual dreams, and sexual fantasies.

autosomal /-sō'-/ denoting a genetic characteristic located on or transmitted by an autosome.

autosomal aberrations any alterations in the structure of one of the pairs of chromosomes that are not sex chromosomes. A.a. may appear as **translocations** of genetic material from a normal location in a particular chromosome to another, deletion of genetic material from a chromosome, or rearrangement of genetic material to form a ring. An example of an autosomal aberration effect is Down's syndrome. The abnormality may be autosomal-dominant as in Huntington's chorea or autosomal-recessive as in amaurotic familial idiocy, or Tay-Sachs disease. Also called **autosomal abnormalities; autosomal anomalies**.

autosomal-dominant pertaining to a gene or inherited trait that determines a physical or other feature of the offspring even if it is located on only one of the two autosomes, or chromosomes that are not sex chromosomes. See AUTOSOMAL-RECESSIVE.

autosomal-dominant inheritance: See DOMINANT INHERITANCE.

autosomal-recessive pertaining to a gene or hereditary trait that can determine a physical or other feature of an offspring only if it is present on homologous chromosomes that are not sex chromosomes, the homologous chromosomes being identical in both visible structure and the location of the gene segments on the chromosomes. See AUTOSOMAL-DOMINANT.

autosomal trisomy of Group G = DOWN'S SYNDROME.

autosome a chromosome that is not an X or Y sex chromosome. A human normally has 22 pairs, or a total of 44 autosomes, although irregular numbers may occur through the loss or addition of one or more autosomes. The occurrence of three rather than paired autosomes is identified as a trisomy condition.

autosuggestibility susceptibility to being influenced by one's own ideas, attitudes, or by internal commands, as in autohypnosis.

autosuggestion self-suggestion, the process of giving suggestions to oneself to improve morale, induce relaxation, or promote recovery from illness. A. has evolved from the crude techniques of Emile Coué ("Day by Day, in Every Way, I Am Getting Better and Better," 1922), and the early "pep talk" approach, to today's use of autohypnosis as an adjunct to hypnotherapy and relaxation techniques. See AUTOGENIC TRAINING; AUTOHYPNOSIS.

autosymbolism "the direct transformation of abstract dream-content into concrete pictures which can be observed in the dream itself" (Eidelberg, *Encyclopedia of Psychoanalysis*, 1968).

autotomia a term that literally means the casting off of a body part, as when a lizard sheds its tail to escape from a predator. In psychiatry, a. may be applied to the acts of some mental patients who perform self-mutilation of body parts that may offend them.

autotopagnosia an inability to recognize, identify, and locate parts of one's own body. A. is a type of agnosia due to lesions in the thalamoparietal pathways of the cortex. Also called **somatotopagnosia**. See AGNOSIA; APHASIA.

-aux-; -auxo- a combining form relating to growth, enlargement, increase.

auxiliary a word that has no complete meaning and function in itself and is used in combination with other words that do have independent meaning and function. Examples of auxiliaries are prepositions, conjunctions, and some a. verbs such as "may."

auxiliary ego in psychodrama, a trained person who helps to advance the therapeutic process by playing the role of a significant figure in the protagonist's life, and in some cases by acting out the protagonist's hallucinations, delusions, and fantasies, or by exchanging roles with the patient.

auxiliary organ: See EXECUTIVE ORGAN.

auxiliary solution a Horney term for a partial or

temporary solution to an intrapsychic conflict, as in the examples of compartmentalization and externalization.

auxiliary therapist a cotherapist in psychotherapy that is conducted simultaneously by two or more therapists. See MULTIPLE THERAPY.

ava = KAVA.

avalanche conduction: See LAW OF AVALANCHE.

Avellis, Georg German laryngologist, 1864–1916. See AVELLIS' SYNDROME.

Avellis' syndrome a complex of neurologic abnormalities resulting from lesions of the nucleus ambiguus and pyramidal tract. The condition involves unilateral paralysis of the larynx and soft palate with loss of pain and temperature sensations on the opposite side of the body through the trunk and extremities. Vagus and cranial nerves may become involved. The disorder becomes complicated by dysphagia.

average deviation a measure of the dispersion or spread of scores, obtained by finding the average absolute difference between each score and the mean. This measure, also called the **mean deviation**, has now been supplanted by the STANDARD DEVIATION. See this entry.

average-evoked-response technique a method of differentiating between different electrical responses in the cortex despite background "noise," by averaging evoked responses (**AER**), usually with the aid of a digital computer. E.g., if the same stimulus is repeated over and over, we can expect that the subject will respond each time in more or less the same way. Also see AUGMENTATION.

averse conditioning = AVERSIVE CONDITIONING.

aversion a feeling that an individual, object, or situation should be avoided, usually accompanied by a desire to withdraw or turn away from it.

aversion reaction a response expressed by avoiding a distasteful or threatening stimulus.

aversion response turning away from a distasteful stimulus or situation, such as unpalatable food or the use of alcohol if it induces nausea. See AVERSIVE THERAPY; AVOIDANCE CONDITIONING.

aversion therapy = AVERSIVE THERAPY.

aversive conditioning a form of counterconditioning that functions as a type of punishment and is used therapeutically in the treatment of alcoholism and sex deviations. Also called **averse conditioning**. See AVERSIVE THERAPY.

aversive racism a form of racism marked by a dichotomy between conscious attitudes and behavior; specifically, racist behavior coupled with nonracist attitudes, indicating unconscious denial. Studies in this area ascertain subjects' attitudes and then observe their behavior in experimental interracial interactions.

aversive stimulus any object or occurrence that tends to produce an avoidance reaction.

aversive therapy a form of behavior therapy in which the patient is conditioned to avoid unde-

sirable behavior or symptoms by associating them with painful or unpleasant experiences, such as a bitter taste (for nail-biting), nausea (for alcoholism or homosexuality), or an electrical shock (for enuresis). Also called **aversion therapy**. Also see SHAME-AVERSION THERAPY.

Aveyron boy: See WILD BOY OF AVEYRON.

aviator's neurasthenia a syndrome of gastrointestinal disorders, irritability, insomnia, emotional stress, and mental fatigue that occurs in aviators, particularly in pilots of military aircraft.

aviophobia = FEAR OF FLYING.

avoidance a defense mechanism in which situations, activities, or objects that recall or represent painful events are avoided. In Freudian theory, these events are always related to unconscious sexual or aggressive impulses, especially when they involve a fear of punishment. An example is a phobia for pointed objects, called AICHMOPHOBIA. See this entry.

avoidance-avoidance conflict a conflict situation involving a choice between two equally objectionable alternatives, e.g., when a pacifist must choose between going to jail or leaving the country in time of war. Also called **double-avoidance conflict**. Also see APPROACH-APPROACH CONFLICT; APPROACH-AVOIDANCE CONFLICT.

avoidance behavior any act that enables the individual to avoid or escape from unpleasant or painful situations, stimuli, or events, including conditioned aversive stimuli. See AVOIDANCE CONDITIONING.

avoidance conditioning the training of an organism to withdraw from, or to remove, a stimulus associated with punishment. E.g., the subject becomes conditioned to avoid an unpleasant or painful stimulus, such as an electric shock, a hot radiator, or the sight of a mouse that inspires fear. In a typical conditioning experiment a buzzer is sounded, then a shock is applied to the subject—a dog—until he jumps over a fence. After several trials, the dog jumps as soon as the buzzer begins sounding in order to avoid the shock. Also called **avoidance learning**.

avoidance gradient the graduated variation in the strength of a negative drive as we approach the goal to which it is directed; e.g., fear and desire to avoid an examination usually increase step by step as the day of the examination approaches. See GRADIENT.

avoidance learning = AVOIDANCE CONDITIONING.

avoidance response a response in which the organism moves away from a stimulus, usually because it is threatening or noxious. A.r. is a form of abient behavior. Also called **avoidance reaction**.

avoidant disorder of childhood or adolescence a disorder lasting at least six months between the ages of two and a half and 18 years, and involving persistent, excessive shrinking from strangers. The avoidant behavior (timidity, withdrawal) is severe enough to interfere with peer relationships, although warm and satisfying relationships with family members and other familiar figures are generally maintained. (DSM-III)

avoidant personality disorder a personality disorder characterized by (a) hypersensitivity to rejection and criticism, (b) a demand for uncritical acceptance, (c) social withdrawal in spite of a desire for affection and acceptance, and (d) low self-esteem. This pattern is long-standing and severe enough to cause objective distress and seriously impair the ability to work and maintain relationships. (DSM-III)

awareness a consciousness of internal or external events or experiences. Also see CONSCIOUSNESS; SENSORY A.

awareness defect impaired consciousness or perception; lack of alertness, or inability to be cognizant of internal or external events.

awareness-training model an approach in psychology and education that stresses self-awareness, self-realization, exploration, and interpersonal sensitivity. The a.-t.m. is associated with such writers as Fritz Perls and William Schutz.

a wave a portion of a tracing of the venous pulse caused by the contraction of the right atrium of the heart.

Awl, William M. American psychiatrist, 1799–1876. With twelve others A. organized the Association of Medical Superintendents of American Institutions for the Insane, which later evolved into the American Psychiatric Association.

axial amnesia = AMNESIC SYNDROME.

axial gradient the difference in development or metabolic rate of tissues along the body axis.

axial hyperkinesia thrusting pelvic movements occasionally occurring in tardive dyskinesia and other extrapyramidal disorders, as well as in barbiturate and other drug intoxications. A.h. is also a rare conversion symptom.

axiodrama: See PSYCHODRAMA FORMS.

axiology the philosophical study of values, such as those of ethics, religion, and esthetics. See ALLPORT-VERNON-LINDZEY STUDY OF VALUES.

axiom self-evident truth; a universally accepted principle that is not capable of proof or disproof (Greek *axioma*, "worthy thing").

axis a reference line for measuring or defining relationships, such as a body's head-to-tail (cephalocaudal) a.

axis cylinder the central or conducting core of an axon, consisting of a plasm (**axoplasma**) surrounded by a sheath called the **axolemma**.

axo-axonal synapse a synaptic junction between two nerve cells in which the nerve impulse travels from one axon to the other, rather than between axon and dendrite or axon and cell body. See SYNAPSE.

axodendritic synapses; axodendrosomatic synapses: See SYNAPSE.

axolemma: See AXIS CYLINDER.

axon the cylindrical process of a nerve cell that normally carries an impulse away from its associated cell body and dendrites. An a. may range in thickness from one-fourth to as much as ten microns. Axons extending from the spinal cord to the foot may be nearly a meter in length. Also spelled **axone**. See NEURON.

axon reflex a peripheral-nerve reflex believed to be mediated by collateral afferent neurons.

axoplasma: See AXIS CYLINDER.

axosomatic synapses: See SYNAPSE.

ayahuasca = CAAPI.

aypnia = INSOMNIA.

azathioprine $C_9H_7N_7O_2S$—a drug used to suppress the immune response. It is the most widely used drug in support of organ transplantation and other potentially severe cases of immune reactions. A. may be administered simultaneously with allopurinol when it is necessary to control uric-acid-formation side effects. Trademark: **Imuran**.

-azo-; -azoto- a combining form relating to a nitrogenous compound.

azoospermia an absence of viable sperm in the semen, usually as a failure of spermatogenesis.

azotemia a form of uremia marked by the presence of nitrogen compounds in the blood. A. may be prenal or nonrenal if the cause is not a primary kidney disease, or postrenal when associated with a kidney-tubular dysfunction. In certain diseases, e.g., diabetes, a. may be a diagnostic sign of approaching kidney failure.

B

Baader, Ernst W. German physician, 1892—. See STEVENS-JOHNSON SYNDROME (also called **Baader's dermatostomatitis**).

babbling prespeech sounds such as "dadada" made by infants around six months of age. B. is usually regarded as practice in vocalization, which has the effect of facilitating later speech development. Also called **babble**. See PRESPEECH DEVELOPMENT; BABY TALK.

Babinski, Joseph François Félix French neuropathologist, 1857–1932. See BABINSKI-NAGEOTTE SYNDROME; BABINSKI REFLEX; BABINSKI'S SYNDROME; ANTON'S SYNDROME (also called **Anton-Babinski syndrome**); ASYNERGIA (there: **major asynergia of Babinski, minor asynergia of Babinski**); PITHIATISM.

Babinski-Nageotte syndrome a congenital or acquired condition of nystagmus, cerebellar hemiataxia, contralateral hemiparesis, and disturbances of sensibility associated with lesions of the pontobulbar or medullobulbar transitional region as a complication of the Bernard-Horner syndrome. Also called **hemibulbar syndrome; medullary tegmental paralysis**. See BERNARD-HORNER SYNDROME.

Babinski reflex the reflex in which the healthy infant extends toes upward when the sole is gently stimulated. This response disappears by the time the baby walks, but it may reappear in adults if there is a loss of function of the upper motor neurons. Also called **Babinski's sign**. See REFLEX.

Babinski's syndrome a condition in which a person suffering from hemiplegia denies the existence of the defect in his own body despite clinical evidence to the contrary. The B.s. is regarded as a defense mechanism that enables the patient to explain away the possibility that he might be afflicted by a disorder that also affects other persons. Also see ANTON'S SYNDROME.

baby talk sounds used by the normal-speaking child in the early stages of speech development; also, a speech disorder characterized by the production of such speech sounds. Also called **pedolalia**. See INFANTILE SPEECH; PRESPEECH DEVELOPMENT; BABBLING.

bacillophobia a morbid fear of germs.

back-clipping: See CLIPPING.

backcrossing the process of crossbreeding a hybrid species with a member of the genetic line from which the hybrid was originally derived. B. is applied to both plants and animals. The offspring of the mating is known as a **backcross**.

back-formation the formation of a word through elimination of a prefix or suffix from an existing word; also, the word formed in this manner, e.g., "enthuse" from "enthusiasm." Also called **inverse derivation; retrogressive formation**. Also see CLIPPING.

background noise: See WHITE NOISE.

backward association the forming of an associative link between a present item and an item previously learned or experienced; or the forming of an associative link between one item and an item that precedes it in a sequence. Compare FORWARD ASSOCIATION.

backward conditioning a form of pseudoconditioning in which presentation of the unconditioned stimulus precedes presentation of the conditioned stimulus. Although this procedure may elicit responses that appear conditioned, such responses are not believed to represent genuine learning but rather oversensitization to the conditioned stimulus. Also see PSEUDOCONDITIONING.

backwardness a term used by Tredgold for educational retardation due to extrinsic forces (environmental, social, physical) which are said to account for approximately one-third of cases.

Bacon, Francis English essayist, philosopher, and statesman, 1561–1626. See -ACID-.

bacteremia = BLOOD-POISONING.

bacterial cerebral infection: See CEREBRAL INFECTION.

bacterial endocarditis a systemic disease in which the primary symptom is an inflammatory infection of the heart tissues by a bacterial or fungal agent. B.e. usually involves the heart valves with the formation of colonies of the infectious organism on the valve tissues. B.e. is one of several types of infections associated with "mainlining," or intravenous injections of drugs of abuse, such as amphetamines. Also see ENDOCARDITIS.

bacterial infection any of the pathologic conditions caused by invasion of normal body tissues by one of the minute unicellular microorganisms possessing genetic and cytoplasmic materials necessary for growth and reproduction by utilizing dissolved materials in the cellular and extracellular fluids of the host. Infection effects may result from poisons produced by the bacteria, bacterial enzymes that have adverse effects, e.g., hemolysin which destroys red blood cells, or substances such as hyaluronidase which helps the disease agent spread by dissolving a substance that holds body cells together. Bacteria also may release a poison into the host body when the bacteria are destroyed. The poisons produced by some bacteria are more toxic than any substances derived from plant or mineral sources.

bacterial meningitis an inflammation of the meningeal membranes that form a protective covering for the brain and spinal cord, caused by an infection of a meningococcal or a tuberculous bacterium. **Meningococcal meningitis** is an epidemic type of infection and the commonest form of b.m. It is highly contagious because the bacteria are in the throat as well as the cerebrospinal fluid. The tuberculous form is caused by the same bacterium that is associated with tuberculosis of the lungs. B.m. effects can include paralysis, mental retardation, blindness, and deafness if antibiotic treatment is delayed. See TUBERCULOUS MENINGITIS.

bad breast according to Melanie Klein, that part of the breast which is experienced as a bad object, reflecting the death instinct, during the first year of life. This experience, however, is repressed. Compare GOOD BREAST.

bad-me according to H. S. Sullivan, the child's rudimentary organization of impulses and behavior that are disapproved by his parents and therefore arouse anxiety. See PERSONIFIED SELF.

bad object the negative side of the psychoanalytic dichotomy of good versus bad, in which the b.o. of the moral conscience, or superego, represents something sexual or dirty, and in the unconscious the b.o. represents the devil.

bad-people fear = SCELEROPHOBIA.

bad self a term used in psychoanalysis for the tendency of both the patient and the therapist to project their guilty feelings upon each other, each making the other a whipping boy. If analysis is to be effective, this tendency must be controlled.

bad trip an acute psychotic episode that can be an adverse effect of the use of psychedelic drugs, e.g., LSD (lysergic acid diethylamide). The episodes can lead to chronic psychotic conditions, irreversible behavioral changes, and confinement of the LSD user to a mental institution. The b.t. also may be marked by flashbacks at a later date.

Baertschi-Rochaix: See BÄRTSCHI-ROCHAIX.

Baglivi, Giorgio Italian physician, 1669–1707. See TARANTISM.

Bailey, Percival British (?) neurologist and neuro-surgeon, 1892–1973. See SYNDROME OF OBSTINATE PROGRESSION.

Baillarger, Jules /bāyärzhä'/ French psychiatrist, 1809–90. B. is known for his research in manic-depressive conditions.

Bain, Alexander Scottish philosopher and psychologist, 1818–1903. B. extended the associationist approach to all areas of psychological functioning, including habit and learning; coined the term "trial and error"; wrote the first textbook on psychology in English (1855, 1859); and founded the first psychological journal, *Mind*, in 1876. See ASSOCIATIONISM.

bait shyness the avoidance by animals of food that previously had been associated with gastric distress or other adverse effects. The reaction is observed in rats returned to a magnesium-rich diet after being deprived of the mineral. Because the first magnesium meal causes illness, the rats avoid magnesium-rich foods as they would a known poison.

BAL an abbreviation of *blood-alcohol level*.

BAL = BRITISH ANTI-LEWISITE.

balance a harmonious relationship of opposing forces, as in emotional equilibrium.

balance control a form of recreational or physical therapy employed in the rehabilitation of patients who may experience difficulty in maintaining balance when standing or walking. B.c. training often utilizes trainer bicycles, tricycles with body supports and foot attachments, stilts, pogo sticks, rocker boards, and a trampolinelike rubber bouncing tube.

balanced scale a scale in which half the items have opposing values, e.g., a true-false test.

balance theory in social psychology, the theory that people tend to embrace attitudes and opinions they consider compatible while avoiding or rejecting attitudes they find less acceptable.

balbuties /bälbōo'tē·ās/ stammering or stuttering, sometimes identified by the age of appearance: **b. praecox**, during the first three years of life; **b. tarda**, beginning after the age of seven; and **b. vulgaris**, starting between the ages of three and seven.

Baldwin, James Mark American psychologist, 1861–1934. Founder of the psychological laboratories at Toronto and Princeton Universities, B. was one of the first to recognize the influence of social factors on personality development. He wrote a two-volume *Dictionary of Philosophy and Psychology* (1901–02) and established the *Psychological Review* with Cattell in 1904.

Baldwin, Ruth Workman American pediatrician, 1915—. See BESSMAN-BALDWIN SYNDROME.

Balint, Rezsoe Hungarian physician, 1874–1929. See BALINT'S SYNDROME.

Balint's syndrome a disorder caused by lesions in the parieto-occipital portion of the brain. Optic ataxia, visual-attention disorders, and psychogenic paralysis of visual fixation are the main effects of the condition. Also called **psychic paralysis of visual fixation**.

ball-and-field test a Stanford-Binet test item in which the child demonstrates by drawing how he would search for a ball or other object in a large field.

Ballet, Gilbert /bäle'/ French neurologist, 1853–1916. See BALLET'S DISEASE.

Ballet's disease a disorder marked by the loss of movements of the eye and pupil while autonomic responses remain normal. The condition is associated with hyperthyroidism disorders such as exophthalmic goiter. Also called **Ballet's sign; ophthalmoplegia externa**.

ballet technique a structured form of dance therapy which is particularly appropriate for persons who are unable to handle the emotions aroused by free movement.

ballistophobia a morbid fear of missiles.

Balo, Jozsef Matthias Hungarian neurologist, 1895–. See BALO'S DISEASE; PROGRESSIVE DEGENERATIVE SUBCORTICAL ENCEPHALOPATHY.

Balo's disease a neurologic disorder in which white matter of the brain becomes demyelinated in concentric circles which alternate with normal layers of white matter. Effects of the disorder may include optic atrophy, dementia, and bilateral spasticity. See ADRENOLEUKODYSTROPHY.

Bamatter, Fred /bä'mätər/ Swiss physician, fl. 1950. See BAMATTER'S SYNDROME.

Bamatter's syndrome a hereditary condition of progeria with neurologic complications that include congenital glaucoma, microcornea and microphthalmia, and corneal opacity. See PROGERIA.

Bamberger, Eugen /bäm'bergər/ Austrian physician, 1858–1921. See BAMBERGER'S DISEASE.

Bamberger's disease a neuromuscular disorder characterized by clonic spasms of the leg muscles and involuntary jumping or springing actions.

bandwagon effect the tendency for large numbers of people, in social and sometimes political situations, to align themselves or their stated opinion with the majority opinion as they perceive it.

bangungut a culture-specific syndrome observed mainly among young Filipino and Laotian males in which the individual seems to be frightened to death by nightmares—dreams apparently frightening enough to cause fatal cardiac arrhythmia. (B. is a Filipino word for nightmare.) Also called **nightmare-death syndrome; Oriental nightmare-death syndrome**.

baquet /bäke'/ a term (meaning "tub" in French) that has a special place in the early history of psychiatry, or pseudopsychiatry, when Anton Mesmer constructed a huge tub containing magnetized water, with metal rods protruding from all sides, and had his patients place the rods on ailing parts of their bodies so that they would experience its healing power. See ANIMAL MAGNETISM; MESMER.

-bar-; -baro- a combining form relating to gravity, atmospheric pressure, or weight. See -BARY-.

Bar: See LOUIS-BAR.

baragnosis an inability to judge the weights of objects when held in the hand, a condition attributed to a parietal-lobe lesion.

Bárány, Robert Austrian physician, 1876–1936. See BÁRÁNY'S SYNDROME; BÁRÁNY TEST.

Bárány's syndrome a complex of neurologic difficulties that include headaches that occur on one side of the back of the head, periods of deafness that alternate with periods of normal hearing, vertigo, ringing in the ears, and loss of ability to point a finger accurately. Also called **hemicrania cerebellaris**.

Bárány test a test designed to reveal whether the semicircular canals are functioning properly by rotating a subject in a special chair with his head in each of the planes that bring the three canals vertical to the direction of rotation. The resulting nystagmus indicates whether the canals are functioning properly.

Barbara, Saint virgin martyr, fl. 3rd century. See BARBITURATES.

barbaralalia use of melodic patterns and speech sounds of a speaker's native language when learning to speak a new language. Also called **foreign accent**.

barbed-wire psychosis a type of mental disturbance experienced by prisoners of war, with symptoms of irritability and amnesia for events preceding the war.

barbiturate: See BARBITURATES.

barbiturate addiction physical and psychological dependence on barbiturate drugs. See BARBITURATE OR SIMILARLY ACTING SEDATIVE OR HYPNOTIC DEPENDENCE.

barbiturate intoxication: See BARBITURATE OR SIMILARLY ACTING SEDATIVE OR HYPNOTIC INTOXICATION.

barbiturate or similarly acting sedative or hypnotic abuse a substance-use disorder characterized by a pathological pattern consisting of (a) inability to cut down or curtail use of the drug, (b) intoxication throughout the day, with amnesia, and (c) impaired functioning, as manifested in fights, loss of friends, absence from work, loss of job, and repeated legal difficulties. (DSM-III)

barbiturate or similarly acting sedative or hypnotic amnestic disorder a disorder whose criteria are temporary impairment in long- and short-term memory without clouding of consciousness, following prolonged heavy use of a barbiturate or similarly acting sedative or hypnotic. See AMNESTIC SYNDROME. (DSM-III)

barbiturate or similarly acting sedative or hypnotic dependence a substance-use disorder characterized by either (a) tolerance for the drug, that is, a need for increasing the amount taken to achieve the desired effect or markedly decreased effect when the same amount is taken regularly, or (b) withdrawal, that is, nausea, vomiting, malaise, depressed mood, and other symptoms cited under barbiturate or similarly acting sedative or hypnotic withdrawal. (DSM-III)

barbiturate or similarly acting sedative or hypnotic intoxication a type of intoxication that involves (a) at least one psychological sign (mood shifts, uninhibited impulses, irritability, loquacity), (b) at least one neurological sign (slurred speech, incoordination, unsteady gait, impaired attention or memory), and (c) maladaptive behavior (impaired judgment, defective social or occupational functioning, failure to meet responsibilities). The danger of death due to overdose is far greater than in alcohol intoxication. (DSM-III)

barbiturate or similarly acting sedative or hypnotic withdrawal a condition resulting from cessation or reduction of these substances, producing at least three of the following reactions: nausea and vomiting; malaise or weakness; rapid heartbeat, sweating, elevated blood pressure; anxiety; depressed mood or irritability; orthostatic hypertension (drop in blood pressure when standing); and sometimes coarse tremors. (DSM-III)

barbiturate or similarly acting sedative or hypnotic withdrawal delirium a disorder that occurs within a week of cessation or reduction in the heavy use of these substances. It is characterized by clouding of consciousness, disorientation and other symptoms of delirium, with rapid heartbeat, sweating, and elevated blood pressure. (DSM-III)

barbiturates drugs derived from barbituric acid and used as sedative-hypnotics. B. act by depressing metabolic functions in several body systems, but the central nervous system is more sensitive to their effects than other tissues. B. were introduced in 1903, replacing narcotics, chloral hydrate, and other sleep-inducing drugs used at that time. Until the advent of benzodiazepines, in the 1950s, b. represented the largest and most widely used group of sedatives and hypnotics. B. are named for Saint Barbara because barbituric acid was discovered on the day honoring the saint, in 1864. Excessive doses of b. can result in physical dependence and adverse effects ranging from skin eruptions to circulatory collapse and death; fatal overdoses are taken in suicide attempts, and in use as a sleeping medicine because of a consciousness clouding effect in which the patient ingests repeated doses accidentally. A prototype b. is **pentobarbital sodium**—$C_{11}H_{17}N_2NaO_3$, a commonly employed sedative-hypnotic that is short-to-intermediate-acting and may be administered in psychotherapy to make a subject less inhibited and therefore able to express himself more effectively. **Thiopental sodium**—$C_{11}H_{17}N_2NaO_2S$—is an ultrashort-acting barbiturate used as an intravenous anesthetic that produces almost immediate loss of consciousness; it also is used as an antidote in the treatment of stimulant overdose cases and toxic convulsions. Other b. include AMOBARBITAL, APROBARBITAL (see these entries), **mephobarbital**—$C_{13}H_{14}N_2O_3$, **phenobarbital**—$C_{12}H_{11}N_2NaO_3$, **secobarbital sodium**—$C_{12}H_{17}N_2NaO_3$, and **vinbarbital sodium**—$C_{11}H_{15}N_2NaO_3$. See SEDATIVE-HYPNOTICS; LONG-ACTING BARBITURATES; SHORT-TO-INTERMEDIATE-ACTING BARBITURATES; ULTRASHORT-ACTING BARBITURATES; MALONIC ACID; ANTIEPILEPTICS; PRIMIDONE.

barbiturate withdrawal: See BARBITURATE OR SIMILARLY ACTING SEDATIVE OR HYPNOTIC WITHDRAWAL.

barbituric acid: See MALONIC ACID.

Bard, Philip American psychologist, 1898–1977. See CANNON'S THEORY (also called **Cannon-Bard theory**). Also see CANNON.

Bardet, Georges /bärde'/ French physician, 1885—. See LAURENCE-MOON-BIEDL SYNDROME (also called **Laurence-Moon-Biedl-Bardet syndrome**).

bar diagram a chart showing variable items in the form of bars. See BAR GRAPH.

barefoot doctors medically trained personnel who provide health care in communities or areas not served by modern hospitals or clinics. The personnel may or may not be physicians and the areas served may be remote rural districts or impoverished urban communities. The term is derived from a program established by the People's Republic of China which trained thousands of medical paraprofessionals to provide health services for remote populations.

baresthesia the sensation of weight or pressure.

bar graph a chart that represents data by showing bars of varying heights. The length of each bar represents the frequency, size, or amount of a variable. Also called **histogram**. For an illustration, see STATISTICS.

bar hustlers: See MALE HOMOSEXUAL PROSTITUTION.

barking: See ABOIEMENT.

Barnum effect a term denoting the widespread tendency to believe that general and vague predictions or personality descriptions have specific application to individuals, e.g., the predictions of palmists or astrologers. The term was inspired by the remark, "There's a sucker born every minute," which is attributed to the American showman Phineas T. Barnum (1810–91).

barognosis the ability to detect weight differences of objects held in the hand.

barophobia a morbid fear of gravity, of feeling the pull of gravity.

Barr, Murray Llewellyn Canadian microanatomist, 1908—. See EPSTEIN-BARR VIRUS; SEX CHROMATIN (also called **Barr body**); INFECTIOUS MONONUCLEOSIS.

Barré, Jean Alexandre French neurologist, 1880—. BARRÉ-LIÉOU SYNDROME; GUILLAIN-BARRÉ SYNDROME; ACUTE POLYNEURITIS; INFECTIOUS MONONUCLEOSIS.

bar reflex a pathological phenomenon in which the

movement of one leg of a recumbent patient laterally or vertically is followed by a similar movement of the other leg. The b.r. usually is a diagnostic sign of a prefrontal lesion such as a brain tumor.

Barré-Liéou syndrome a disease condition that includes symptoms of occipital headache, dizziness, ringing in the ears, and other neurologic deficits resulting from irritation of a nerve plexus around the vertebral artery. Also called **Neri-Barré syndrome**.

barrier a "protective envelope" which, according to Freud, surrounds the organism and protects it from overstimulation and traumatic situations. The b., which is both a neural and psychological line of defense, is "a shield against stimuli that seek to paralyze the psychical functions" (Eidelberg). As the ego matures, it develops a capacity to cope with the stimuli that filter through. For barriers in social psychology, see PRIVACY. Also see ARCHITECTURAL BARRIERS.

barrier-free environment an environment that is free of obstacles to individuals whose daily normal movements are uncontrolled or unsteady, or who require the use of prosthetic devices, e.g., artificial limbs, or wheelchairs. Environmental barriers can include street curbs, revolving doors or doors too narrow to admit wheelchairs, inaccessible toilets and washbowls, coin-operated telephones beyond the reach of users, elevator buttons that cannot be "read" by blind persons.

barrier responses: See BODY BOUNDARIES.

Barron-Welsh Art Scale a test in which the subject records whether he or she likes or dislikes each of 86 black and white figures which have been selected because they differentiated between criterion groups of artists and nonartists. Performance has been related to creativity in art and other fields, as well as personality variables; e.g., low scorers tend to yield to social pressure, and high scorers tend to form independent judgments.

Bartholin, Caspar Danish anatomist, 1655–1738. See BARTHOLIN'S GLANDS; BARTHOLINITIS; BULBOURETHRAL GLANDS.

bartholinitis an inflammation of the Bartholin's glands on either side of the vaginal orifice. A common cause is gonorrhea but chronic b. more often is due to a nongonococcal infection, e.g., T-mycoplasma or Chlamydia trachomatis.

Bartholin's glands mucus-secreting glands located on either side of the vaginal orifice. Their function is believed to be the production of mucus during sexual excitement in order to lubricate the vagina. Similar glands, called bulbourethral glands, are found in the urethra of the male.

Bartley v. Kremens a Pennsylvania court decision (1976) that extended due-process protection and provision of legal counsel to children committed to mental facilities by their parents.

Bärtschi-Rochaix, Werner /rôshe'/ Swiss physi-

cian, 1911—. See BÄRTSCHI-ROCHAIX'S SYNDROME.

Bärtschi-Rochaix's syndrome a disorder characterized by headaches, dizziness, stiff neck, depressed vision, and paresthesia due to compression of a cerebral artery. Also called **cervical migraine; cervical vertigo syndrome**.

-bary- a combining form meaning heavy or difficult (from Greek *barys*, "heavy").

barylalia thick, blurred, and indistinct speech. It is frequently noted in cases of general paresis.

baryphony a type of dysphasia characterized by a thick, heavy voice quality.

basal age = BASAL MENTAL AGE.

basal body temperature the average normal body temperature of an individual as recorded immediately after awakening in the morning and before getting out of bed. The b.b.t increases by 0.5° to 1.0°F (0.25° to 0.5°C) for a woman on the day she ovulates, and the information is used to indicate the fertility peak in her reproductive cycle.

basal cell papillomas: See SKIN CANCER.

basal ganglia a collection of gray matter in the telencephalon portion of the brain. The area includes the corpus striatum, amygdaloid body, and claustrum. The b.g. help control posture and coordination. Also see CAUDATE NUCLEUS.

basal mental age the mental age at which all items on a standardized test such as the Stanford-Binet are passed. Also called **basal age**.

basal metabolism minimum energy expenditure, measured in calories, required to maintain the vital functions of the body while at rest.

basal reader approach a method of teaching reading through the use of a series of books. The vocabulary, content, and sequence of skills are determined by the authors. A teacher's manual and children's workbooks accompany the series.

basal-resistance level the normal autonomic-response level of an individual's emotional state as measured by galvanic skin response and other factors. An emotional disturbance causes secretion of sweat and generation of a small electrical current by the smooth muscles, which causes a drop in resistance. The resistance level then returns to its predisturbance point indicated by monitoring devices.

Basedow, Karl Adolph von /bä'zədōv/ German physician, 1799–1854. See GRAVES' DISEASE (also called **Basedow's disease**); EIDETIC IMAGE.

base line a measure of behavior under control conditions or before experimentation begins. Later experimental treatments are expected to modify the b.l.

base rate the incidence of a given phenomenon in a given population; the rate of occurrence.

basic anxiety a feeling of uneasiness, dread and impending disaster which, according to Karen Horney, originates in indifference and coldness or excessively high standards and constant criticism on the part of the individual's parents—attitudes that make the child feel isolated, helpless, and insecure in a hostile world. She held that neurosis arises out of maladaptive "strategies" which the individual adopts in attempting to control this anxiety, strategies such as spiteful or hostile behavior, placating and submissive attitudes, exertion of power over others, or withdrawal from what appears to be a threatening world. See HORNEY.

basic conflict a term introduced by Horney to describe neurotic behavior characterized by conflicts between two opposing psychic forces, e.g., the proud self versus the despised self.

BASIC ID: See MULTIMODAL BEHAVIOR THERAPY.

basic mistake Adler's term for early childhood factors, e.g., attitudes and incidents, that affect a person's life-style in later life and which may need to be corrected in order to resolve conflicts.

basic mistrust the unsuccessful resolution of the first stage in Erikson's eight stages of man in which the baby in the first year of life comes to experience a fundamental distrust of his environment, often due to neglect, lack of love, or inconsistent treatment. The acquisition of basic trust or hope is considered essential for the development of self-esteem and normal relatedness. Compare BASIC TRUST.

basic personality As used by A. Kardiner, the shared behavioral traits of persons raised (as children) in the same culture and subjected to the same type of child-rearing practices.

basic rest-activity cycle cyclic alternations between activity and nonactivity during sleep (now termed REM and NREM sleep) as contrasted with the early concept of sleep as a unitary state. Abbrev.: **BRAC.**

basic rule the fundamental rule of psychoanalysis that the patient must feel free to put all spontaneous thoughts, feelings, and memories into words, and thereby bring unconscious impulses and experiences to the surface, where they can be analyzed. See FREE ASSOCIATION.

basic skills in educational psychology, reading, writing, and arithmetic. Proficiency in the b.s. has traditionally been viewed as essential for scholastic achievement.

basic trust the successful resolution of the first of Erikson's eight stages of man in which the baby in the first year of life comes to feel that his world is trustworthy. B.t. is the first task of the ego, laying the foundation for self-esteem and constructive interpersonal relations. The growth of b.t. is attributed to the mother or "mothering one" who is responsively attuned to the baby's individual needs while herself (or himself) conveying the quality of trustworthiness. Compare BASIC MISTRUST.

As described by S. Arieti, b.t. is a feeling that predisposes a person to expect good things, which leads in turn to the development of self-esteem. An example is the b.t. a mother has that her child will become a mature and healthy person; her expression of that b.t. enhances the child's self-esteem.

basilar artery a single trunk formed by the joining of two vertebral arteries at the base of the skull. The b.a. extends to the pons and divides into the two posterior cerebral arteries. Along its path, the b.a. sends on either side pontine, labyrinthine, anterior inferior cerebellar, superior cerebellar, and posterior cerebral branches.

basilar membrane a band of tissue within the cochlea that supports the organ of Corti. See COCHLEA; ORGAN OF CORTI.

basophile adenoma a tumor of the anterior lobe of the pituitary gland that is associated with the various mental and physical symptoms of CUSHING'S SYNDROME. See this entry.

basiphobia a morbid fear of walking.

basophobia a morbid fear of standing erect.

Bassen, Frank Albert American physician, 1903—. See BASSEN-KORNZWEIG SYNDROME.

Bassen-Kornzweig syndrome an autosomal-recessive-trait disorder marked primarily by degenerative changes in the cerebellum and long tracts of the central nervous system, with demyelination. Symptoms include ataxia, amaurosis, retinitis pigmentosa, areflexia, and acanthocytosis.

Bastian, Henry Charlton English neurologist, 1837–1915. See WERNICKE'S APHASIA (also called **Bastian's aphasia**).

Bateson, Gregory British-American anthropologist and philosopher, 1904—. See DOUBLE BIND.

bathing fear = AQUAPHOBIA.

bathophobia a morbid fear of depth, of looking down from high places (from Greek *bathos*, "depth"). See ACROPHOBIA. Also see CREMNOPHOBIA.

bathyesthesia sensitivity of the deep tissues of the body to pressure, pain, or muscle and joint sensations.

batophobia a morbid fear of being on or passing by high objects such as skyscrapers (from Greek *batos*, "passable").

batrachophobia a morbid fear of frogs.

bat radar: See ECHOLOCATION.

Batten, Frederic Eustace English ophthalmologist, 1865–1918. See BATTEN'S DISEASE; CURSCHMANN-BATTEN-STEINERT SYNDROME; CEREBROMACULAR DEGENERATION; NEURONAL LIPIDOSIS.

Batten's disease a rare hereditary disorder characterized by myotonia of muscles of the mouth and hands, testicular atrophy, cataracts, frontal baldness, "hatchet-face" features, and mental retardation. It usually develops between puberty and early adulthood. Also, B.d. may be a juvenile form of amaurotic familial idiocy, or Tay-Sachs disease. See NEURONAL LIPIDOSIS.

Batten-Steinert syndrome = CURSCHMANN-B.-S.S.

battered-child syndrome the pattern of child abuse by parents or parent surrogates who intentionally and repeatedly injure their children, often to the extent that hospitalization is required. Injuries may include bone fractures, burns, lacerations, hemorrhages, neurological damage, and sexual abuse. A broader definition includes severe physical, emotional, or nutritional neglect. In addition to physical trauma, the child may show signs of intellectual retardation and abnormal behavior, such as excessive hostility or submissiveness. The b.-c. s. often recurs within families, that is, battered children tend to become battering parents. Also see CHILD MOLESTATION.

battered wives women who are physically abused by their husbands. Wife-beating is considered to surpass rape as the most underreported act of violent assault in the United States. Accurate statistics are not available, but wife-beating is believed to be common and to occur in all social classes. Initial studies of b.w. report that subjects tend to come from conservative or repressive families that model traditional sex roles while to some extent encouraging attitudes of dependency and submissiveness in women.

battery of tests = TEST BATTERY.

battle fatigue: See COMBAT FATIGUE.

Bayes, Thomas English clergyman and mathematician, 1702–61. See BAYES' THEOREM; BAYESIAN APPROACH.

Bayesian approach in evaluation research, the use of conditional probabilities as an aid in selection or diagnostic procedures. Given some prior information, such conditional probabilities can often be calculated by Bayes' theorem. Although Bayes' theorem is not controversial, the question of its appropriate use has been of some controversy. Also called **decision-theoretic approach**.

Bayes' theorem a formula for estimating inverse probability, that is, the probability that a particular antecedent was responsible for, or associated with, an observed event. An example might be the probability that atherosclerosis of the cerebral arteries preceded the symptoms of stroke.

Bayle, Antoine Laurent Jesse /bel/ French physician, 1799–1858. See BAYLE'S DISEASE; GENERAL PARESIS.

Bayle's disease a severe form of neurosyphilis, first described in 1822 by the French physician Antoine Bayle, marked by atrophy of the cerebral cortex and thickened and cloudy meninges. Deterioration of the neurons and blood vessels of the meninges results in apathy, emotional in-

stability, disorientation, delusions, and inability to concentrate. The term was replaced by GENERAL PARESIS. See this entry. Also see SYPHILIS.

Bayley, Nancy American psychologist, 1899—. See BAYLEY SCALES OF INFANT DEVELOPMENT.

Bayley Scales of Infant Development a three-part scale for assessing the developmental status of children between two months and two and a half years. A variety of test objects such as form boards, blocks, and utensils are used. The **Mental Scale** samples such functions as perception, memory, and vocalization; the **Motor Scale** measures motor ability such as sitting, stair-climbing, and manual manipulation; and the **Infant Behavior Record** assesses aspects of personality development such as social behavior, attention span, and persistence.

BB = BLUE BLOATER.

BB: See CREATINE PHOSPHOKINASE.

B cognition = BEING COGNITION.

Beard, George Miller American psychiatrist, 1839–83. See BEARD'S DISEASE; NEURASTHENIA.

Beard's disease an alternative term for NEURASTHENIA. See this entry.

beast fetishism a paraphilia involving contact with animal furs or hides which serve as an aphrodisiac.

beat a periodic change in sound intensity produced by two similar tones sounded together.

beat generation the generation, or the part of it termed **beatnik**, which came of age in the late 50s. The b.g. rejected traditional values and adopted unconventional dress and behavior.

beating fantasies in psychoanalysis, a girl's fantasy that her father is beating another child, which means "He loves only me," or her fantasy that he is beating *her*, which is interpreted as a masochistic expression of guilt over incestuous feelings toward him. When a boy fantasizes being beaten by the father, it is also an unconscious expression of love; and when he sees himself beaten by his mother instead, it is interpreted as a defense against homosexual impulses.

beatnik: See BEAT GENERATION.

Beaufort, Sir Francis English naval officer, 1774–1857. See BEAUFORT WIND SCALE.

Beaufort wind scale a system of measuring wind velocities, developed in 1806 by Admiral Sir Francis Beaufort. The scale ranges from 0, for winds of less than one mile per hour, when smoke rises vertically, to 12, when sustained winds of at least 73 miles an hour occur, as during a hurricane. Discomfort generally increases with perceived windiness, as evidenced by increased rates of blinking by subjects, increased time required by subjects to select words from lists, and increased times of from 20 to 30 percent for subjects to put on coats or headscarves. Several studies show increased accident rates and decreased performance immediately before or during the approach of windy weather. In some Middle Eastern countries, persons who commit crimes on days of "disturbing winds" are given lenient treatment.

Bechtereff: See BEHKTEREV.

Beck, Karl Maria Otto Hans German neurologist, 1880—. See BECK'S SYNDROME.

Beck's syndrome a disorder caused by interruption of the blood flow in the anterior spinal artery and marked by an assortment of possible symptoms ranging from paresthesia and pain to weakness, cramps, and loss of hearing. Motor abnormalities usually are related to the level of the occlusion. Some sensory effects may include loss of pain and temperature sensations. Also called **anterior-spinal-artery syndrome**.

Beckwith, John Bruce American physician, 1933—. See BECKWITH-WIDEMANN SYNDROME.

Beckwith-Widemann syndrome a condition marked by neonatal hypoglycemia, macroglossia, large abdominal hernia, and visceromegaly. Microcephaly and mental retardation are associated with the syndrome in some cases, possibly due to severe, prolonged neonatal hypoglycemia. Because the disorder occurs in siblings, it may be an autosomal-recessive genetic defect.

bedlam a term derived from St. Mary's of *Bethlehem*, in London, founded as a monastery in 1247 and officially proclaimed a "lunatic asylum" by Henry VIII in 1547. The term is synonymous with wild confusion, since many of the patients were in a state of frenzy, and turmoil prevailed due to the fact that they were shackled, starved, beaten, and exhibited to the public for a penny a look. The term became a common name for any mental institution, and **bedlamism** was used for psychotic behavior, and **bedlamite** for a psychotic individual.

bedsores ulcerlike lesions that develop in the skin of bedridden patients due to prolonged pressure of the body against the bedding. B. are a common complication of neuromuscular diseases, e.g., multiple sclerosis, or injuries that require periods of immobilization of the patient. Also see DECUBITI.

bed-wetting involuntary discharge of urine, especially during sleep. For persistent b.-w., see FUNCTIONAL ENURESIS.

bee fear = MELISSOPHOBIA.

Beers, Clifford W. American founder of the mental hygiene movement, 1876–1943. B. was secretary of the International Committee for Mental Hygiene, founded in 1909 to disseminate information on the nature and prevention of mental illness. Beers' interest in this field originated when, after attempting suicide, he was hospitalized with manic-depressive disorder. During the manic phase of the illness, he began to direct his unbounded energy to public officials, demanding reform and improvement of conditions in mental institutions. He wrote *A Mind That Found Itself*, which vividly describes the phases of his illness and recovery, and advo-

cated an enlightened approach to prevention and treatment. See MENTAL HYGIENE. Also see MEYER.

before-after design the administration of a **pretest** and an **aftertest** to an experimental group and its control group.

beginning spurt = INITIAL SPURT.

behavior an individual's psychological actions, reactions, and interactions in response to external or internal stimuli, including objectively observable activities, introspectively observable activities, and unconscious processes.

behavioral assessment a technique of studying the behavior of individuals by observation, interviews, and other methods of sampling attitudes and feelings in a situational context, in addition to or instead of relying on the use of psychological tests.

behavioral consistency in industrial psychology, a technique for predicting future job performance on the basis of samples of current and past job behavior.

behavioral contingency the relationship between a specific response and the frequency, regularity, and amount of reinforcement.

behavioral contract = CONTRACT.

behavioral dynamics the motivational patterns, or causes, underlying behavior.

behavioral endocrinology the study of the effects of endocrine-gland functions on behavior. Gonadal and adrenal functions have a direct effect on behavior patterns as expressed through sexually related and general activity. Animal experiments show relationships between the size of endocrine glands and activity states; e.g., wild rats that are more physically active than laboratory rats generally have larger adrenal glands.

behavioral facilitation in environmental design, the construction of a setting to facilitate the work or activity performed there. B.f. includes functional conformance and spatial conformance. **Spatial conformance** is the organization of spatial arrangements, e.g., the optimal proportion of locker space to showers to dressing space in a school gymnasium. Also see FUNCTIONAL CONFORMANCE; CONFORMANCE.

behavioral genetics = BEHAVIOR GENETICS.

behavioral medicine the application of behavior-therapy techniques, such as biofeedback and relaxation, to the prevention and treatment of such medical and psychophysiological disorders as hypertension, cardiovascular problems, chronic pain, migraine headaches, and epileptic seizures. Other areas of application include self-control disorders such as cigarette-smoking, overeating, and alcohol abuse. B.m. is a multidisciplinary field in which physicians, psychologists, psychiatrists, physiatrists, social workers, and others work together to develop prevention strategies and improved health-care delivery.

behavioral metamorphosis a change in behavior patterns, personality, or life-style that is significant and usually abrupt. An example from literature is *The Strange Case of Dr. Jekyll and Mr. Hyde* (1886) by Robert Louis Stevenson.

behavioral model a systematic description or conceptualization of psychological disorders in terms of overt behavior patterns. Compare MEDICAL MODEL.

behavioral modeling a personnel-training technique that provides instruction and rehearsal for supervisory and management-level workers in appropriate methods of dealing with subordinates in such matters as poor work quality, absenteeism, and discrimination problems. For behavior modification, see MODELING.

behavioral neurochemistry the study of the relationships between behavior and biochemical influences such as the effects of drugs on metabolic processes within the brain, or the roles of different neurotransmitters and neuroregulatory substances.

behavioral oscillation variations in a subject's reaction potential while performing a test or task.

behavioral prostheses biofeedback devices employed to assist a patient in learning preferred behavior patterns. Examples include portable devices that produce a mild electric shock when the patient's behavior departs from a prescribed course, or a miniature metronome worn like a hearing aid to help stutterers pace their speaking rate.

behavioral psychiatry psychiatric treatment in which behavior modification and learning-theory techniques are applied.

behavioral psychotherapy = BEHAVIOR THERAPY.

behavioral rehearsal: See ASSERTIVE TRAINING.

behavioral research in industrial psychology, evaluation of job performance that utilizes criterion and predictor factors as dependent and independent variables respectively within a statistical concept.

behavioral sciences scientific disciplines in which the actions and reactions of human beings and animals are studied through observational and experimental methods, especially psychology, psychiatry, sociology, psychopharmacology, and anthropology.

behavioral sink a pen in which many experimental animals are crowded together, resulting in disruption of vital modes of behavior such as nest-building, courting, and care of the young (J. D. Calhoun, 1962).

behavioral toxicity an adverse behavioral change produced by antipsychotic drugs, e.g., insomnia, toxic confusional states, bizarre dreams, and reduced psychomotor activity. Dose-related effects can often be alleviated by changing dosage or drugs.

behavioral variability the diversity of behavior; the fact that the same stimulus or environmental condition evokes dissimilar responses in different persons; also, the fact that the same stimulus situation elicits dissimilar responses in one person at different times.

behavior analysis a method, or model, developed by B. F. Skinner based on the experimental analysis of behavior. One basic concept in this approach is the conviction that the subject matter of psychology is the observable interaction between an individual and environmental events defined in physical and functional terms (that is, stimuli, other organisms, and the functioning individual). Another basic concept is that some responses are conditioned by antecedent stimuli (respondent or Pavlovian conditioning), and some by consequent stimuli (operant conditioning), which can be used in replacing undesirable behavior with desirable behavior (behavior modification). See EXPERIMENTAL ANALYSIS OF BEHAVIOR.

behavior chaining = CHAINING.

behavior check list a system of screening learning-disabled children at the preschool level by evaluating specified categories of perceptual-motor skills. The b.c.l. technique was developed from studies showing that early warning signs of learning disability appear in linguistic traits of three- and four-year-old children, particularly in the area of language delays.

behavior-constraint theory the concept that an individual may acquire "learned helplessness" when repeated efforts fail to gain control over excessive or undesirable environmental stimuli. According to the b.-c.t., the normal pattern of coping with crowding, weather, or other environmental threats is (a) perceived loss of control, (b) reaction by attempting to regain control, and (c) helplessness which may lead either to death or to a change in life-styles. E.g., a person who is threatened by a heat wave usually will try to cope with the stimulus by using air-conditioning, wearing lighter clothing, drinking cold beverages, and swimming. If those measures fail to relieve the symptoms of discomfort, the individual may feel helpless and move to a cooler climate or simply try to tolerate the heat, with possibly fatal consequences. Also see GENERAL ADAPTATION SYNDROME; LEARNED HELPLESSNESS.

behavior control a term primarily applied to the possible misuse of invasive or intrusive treatments to achieve control over the lives of patients (e.g., drugs or aversive conditioning).

behavior determinant any variable factor that produces a behavioral effect.

behavior disorder any form of behavior that is considered inappropriate by members of the social group. Premarital-sex practices may be regarded as a b.d. in one culture but a normal activity in another group. B.d. is also a general term for any functional disorder or abnormality.

behavior field any stimuli or conditions, or accumulation of factors, that produce a behavioral effect.

behavior genetics the study of familial or hereditary behavior patterns. An example is the increase in incidence of schizophrenia in certain families over a range from distant relatives to identical twins. Since the twins have the same genes, they have the highest risk of developing the symptoms.

behaviorism an approach formulated by J. B. Watson in 1913, who held that a genuinely scientific psychology must be based on objective, observable facts rather than subjective, qualitative processes such as feelings, motives, and consciousness. To make psychology a naturalistic science, he proposed to limit it to quantitative events such as stimulus-response, the effects of conditioning, physiological processes, and a study of animal behavior—all of which can best be investigated through laboratory experiments that yield statistically significant results. See WATSON. Also see RADICAL B.; DESCRIPTIVE B.; NEOBEHAVIORISM.

behavior language a term used to identify the body language of a child who has not learned to speak and must express himself through crying, smiling, tenseness, or other means.

behavior-mapping a technique of studying the performance of individuals in different environmental situations, e.g., children in a variety of classroom designs. By observing the children in various activities, it may be determined that some individuals achieve better performance in an open-structured learning area whereas others function better in an old-fashioned classroom setting.

behavior method a behaviorism-derived approach to the study of stimulus-response roles in organisms.

behavior modification the use of operant conditioning, biofeedback, modeling, aversive conditioning, reciprocal inhibition, or other learning techniques as a means of changing human behavior, improving adaptation, and alleviating symptoms. See BEHAVIOR THERAPY.

behavior-rating the recording and ranking or scoring of specific types of behavior such as the number of times a child has a temper tantrum.

behavior record a chronicle of observations intended to provide a complete and accurate account of an organism's behavior in a specified time frame. As a guidance term, b.r. refers to a teacher's written observations regarding a student's behavior and personality, e.g., an ANECDOTAL RECORD. See this entry.

behavior rehearsal a technique for learning or improving fundamental social or work-related skills. The therapist-teacher instructs and models effective interpersonal strategies or work procedures to be practiced and rehearsed by the client or patient.

behavior reversal a behavior-modification method in which the patient practices more desirable responses to interpersonal conflicts under the supervision of the therapist.

behavior-sampling the recorded observation of a subject's behavior in a designated time frame.

B.-s. may be conducted over several periods of observation in natural or laboratory settings with or without the awareness of the subject. The data may then be utilized in appraising personality traits or the consistency or inconsistency of the subject's behavior.

behavior setting a term coined by R. Barker and H. Wright for the geographical and social situation as it affects relationships and behavior. E.g., people in a resettlement community tend to "sort themselves out" according to interests, nationality background, and social attitudes.

behavior-shaping = SHAPING.

behavior-specimen recording a method of studying behavior of a single individual by continuously observing him for a period of one or more days and recording all details, including his conversations, how he interacts with other persons, and the number of rooms he uses during the period of observation. The data may be analyzed in the context of environmental influences of working or living areas on the behavior of the subject.

behavior system different activities that can be undertaken to reach the same goal or carry out the same function; e.g., we can communicate through writing, speaking, or gestures. In addition, the term is used by Whiting and Child (1953) for important motives (e.g., hunger, sex, aggression) which are expressed in different ways in different cultures, and among different individuals who have been subjected to different training and experiences within the same culture. Also called **activity system**.

behavior therapy a form of psychotherapy which focuses on modifying faulty behavior rather than basic changes in the personality. Instead of probing the unconscious or exploring the patient's thoughts and feelings, behavior therapists seek to eliminate symptoms and modify ineffective or maladaptive patterns by applying basic learning techniques, such as PAVLOVIAN CONDITIONING, OPERANT CONDITIONING, AVERSIVE THERAPY, and RECIPROCAL INHIBITION. See these entries. Also called **behavioral psychotherapy**.

behavior types personality classifications based upon distinct patterns of behavior, e.g., Jung's division into extraverts and introverts. See TYPOLOGY.

Behcet, Halushi Turkish dermatologist, 1889–1948. See BEHCET'S DISEASE; REITER'S SYNDROME.

Behcet's disease a disorder that affects mainly men in their 20s with ulcers of the mouth, throat, and nasal mucosa. The ulcers are small and red, except for a central yellowish base. Similar ulcers also develop on the genitalia. The central nervous system eventually becomes involved, with meningoencephalitis, brainstem lesions, cranial-nerve plasies, spinal-cord defects, and psychosis, and followed by death from nervous-system complications. Also called **Behcet's syndrome; Behcet's aphthae; Gilbert-Behcet syndrome; Adamantiades-Behcet syndrome**.

Behn-Eschenburg, H. /bān-/ German psychologist, fl. 1927, 1935. See BEHN-RORSCHACH TEST.

Behn-Rorschach Test a variation on the Rorschach test used for research with subjects who are excessively familiar with the standard ink blots.

Behr, Carl /bār/ German physician, 1876—. See BEHR'S SYNDROME.

Behr's syndrome a disorder of the nervous system that is characterized by temporal-nerve atrophy, optic atrophy, ataxia, loss of coordination, and mental retardation. The disease is hereditary or familial and usually begins in infancy. Also called **optic atrophy-ataxia syndrome**.

being cognition in the existential approach, awareness of the inner core of one's existence, that is, one's self, or identity. This general term should be distinguished from Maslow's Being cognition.

Being cognition according to A. Maslow, the ability to perceive reality objectively, a quality ascribed by Maslow to "self-actualizers." Also called **B cognition**.

being-in-the-world the term applied by existentialists to the unique pattern of each person's experience. By drawing on this pattern, the individual will be himself and actualize himself, and his behavior will stem from his own existence and not from the attitudes and dictates of others (or a deity), or the necessities of circumstance.

Being love according to A. Maslow, a form of love characterized by mutuality, genuine concern for another's welfare, and reduced dependency, selfishness, and jealousy. B.l. is one of the qualities Maslow ascribes to "self-actualizers." Also called **B love**. Compare DEFICIENCY LOVE.

Being motivation = METAMOTIVATION.

Being values = METANEEDS.

Bekesy, Georg von Hungarian-born American biophysicist, 1899—. See BEKESY AUDIOMETER.

Bekesy audiometer the first automatic audiometer with patient-controlled push-button responses and an ink recorder to graph the audiogram throughout the testing process. It yields tracings for continuous and interrupted tones at controlled frequencies for site-of-lesion information.

Bekhterev, Vladimir Mikhailovich Russian neuropathologist, 1857–1927. B. studied conditioning independently of Pavlov and proposed an "objective psychology," later named reflexology, in which all behavior, including thought, was viewed as a compounding of motor reflexes. Also spelled **Bechtereff**. See BEKHTEREV'S NYSTAGMUS; BEKHTEREV-MENDEL REFLEX; REFLEXOLOGY; BEHAVIORISM.

Bekhterev-Mendel reflex the dorsal flexion of the foot accompanied by a flexion of the knee and hip on the same side when the foot is bent in a plantar direction, then released. The reflex is one of several diagnostic tests for pyramidal-tract lesions.

Bekhterev's nystagmus a form of nystagmus that develops after the loss of a second labyrinth.

Nystagmus occurs after the destruction of the first of the two labyrinths, but eventually subsides, only to recur as a compensatory effect after loss of the second labyrinth. Also called **compensatory nystagmus**.

bel a unit of measure of sound intensity based on a logarithmic scale. An increase of one bel indicates a doubling of sound intensity; a decibel represents a ten-fold increase. The unit was named for **Alexander Graham Bell** (1847–1922), one of the inventors of the telephone. See DECIBEL.

belching the sudden ejection of gas or air from the stomach via the oral cavity. Causes of b. may include aerophagia in persons who unconsciously swallow quantities of air, an irritable gastrointestinal tract, and the use of medications such as antibiotics that inhibit bacterial metabolism of hydrogen in the gastrointestinal tract so that hydrogen gas accumulates in the stomach. B. may be a psychophysiologic reaction occurring when the patient inhibits speech while struggling to keep from exploding with a torrent of words. Also called **eructation**.

belief system an individual's more or less organized set of attitudes, opinions, and convictions that implicitly or explicitly affect his behavior, interpersonal relationships, and attitudes toward life. Also see CONCEPTUAL SYSTEM.

belief-value matrix the set of judgments and values a subject uses in interfacing with his environment.

Bell, Charles Scottish anatomist, 1774–1842. See BELL'S PALSY; BELL-MAGENDIE LAW; INFECTIOUS MONONUCLEOSIS.

Bell, Hugh McKee American psychologist, 1902—. See BELL ADJUSTMENT INVENTORY; ADJUSTMENT INVENTORY.

Bell, Luther Vose American physician, 1806–62. See BELL'S MANIA; AUTOPSY-NEGATIVE DEATH; CATATONIC CEREBRAL PARALYSIS.

Bell Adjustment Inventory a personality questionnaire that emphasizes home, health, and social and emotional factors.

belladonna alkaloids substances obtained from the shrub Atropa belladonna, also known by the common name of deadly nightshade. B.a. were known to the ancient Hindus and were used in the Middle Ages as a source of poison. The pharmacology of b.a. was unknown to medical science, however, until the 1860s when they were found to affect heart rate, salivary secretion, and other body functions. Atropine is the best known of the b.a. Also see NIGHTSHADE POISONING; BELLADONNA DELIRIUM.

belladonna delirium an effect on the central nervous system of large doses of belladonna alkaloid drugs, e.g., atropine. Symptoms, in addition to delirium, include hallucinations and overactive coordinated limb movement. The term belladonna is derived from the botanical name of its source, Atropa belladonna, a plant of the genus named in turn for Atropos, the eldest of the mythological Furies who cuts the thread of life. Also see NIGHTSHADE POISONING; BELLADONNA ALKALOIDS.

bell and pad a technique for controlling nocturnal enuresis, or bed-wetting, in children. If the child urinates, an electric circuit is closed via the wetted pad and a bell rings, awakening the child.

belle indifférence: See LA B.I.

Bell-Magendie Law the principle that ventral spinal roots are motor in function, dorsal are sensory.

Bell's mania a form of acute maniacal excitement first described in 1849 by Luther Vose Bell as "resembling some advanced stages of mania and fever", which might lead to unexplained death (autopsy-negative death). Also called **exhaustion death; lethal catatonia; deadly catatonia**. Also see DELIRIOUS MANIA; HYPERMANIA.

Bell's palsy a form of facial-nerve paralysis involving one side of the face and characterized by facial-muscle weakness and a distorted expression. The onset of B.p. usually is sudden, often beginning as a pain behind the ear and progressing to paralysis within a few hours. The condition may result from a viral infection leading to a swollen nerve that becomes compressed in its passage through the temporal bone.

belonephobia /bəlōnē-/ a morbid fear of needles (from Greek *belone*, "needle").

belonging the feeling of being accepted and approved by another individual or group, especially the feeling of having a place in a certain group or in society as a whole. Schizophrenics frequently feel they do not belong anywhere, and are strangers here on earth. The term is often used interchangeably with BELONGINGNESS. See this entry.

belongingness the feeling of being accepted by another person or group. E. Fromm uses the term to mean a sense of certainty, security, and rootedness which he contrasted with the anxiety induced by individuality and freedom.

For a different use of the term, see PRINCIPLE OF B.

belongingness and love needs = LOVE NEEDS.

bemegride a chemical with a structure similar to that of the barbiturates. However, it functions as an analeptic and is used in EEG experiments as a brain stimulant. B. was introduced originally as a specific antagonist that would compete with barbiturates at nerve receptors although evidence of that effect is lacking.

Bem Sex-Role Inventory a masculinity-femininity instrument (1981) in which the items are selected in terms of judges' ratings of desirability for males and females and the degree to which they characterize each sex in our society. Masculinity and femininity are treated as independent variables, and persons high in both types of favorable traits (e.g., assertiveness plus warmth) are classified as androgynous.

benactyzine $C_{20}H_{25}NO_3$—an anxiolytic drug that produces very mild CNS depression. B. is about one-fifth as potent as atropine in cholinergic blocking actions. B. slows mental activity and induces relaxation without sedative or hypnotic effects. However, it can cause dizziness and ataxia. The effects of b. can be observed in EEG recordings. Also see PSYCHEDELICS.

benactyzine hydrochloride: See DIPHENYLMETHANES.

Bence Jones, Henry English physician, 1814–73. See MULTIPLE MYELOMA (there: **Bence Jones proteins**).

Benda, Clemens German-born American neuropathologist, 1899–1975. B. is known for his research on mongolism. See DOWN'S SYNDROME.

Bender, Lauretta American neuropsychiatrist, 1897—. See BENDER GESTALT TEST; CHILDHOOD SCHIZOPHRENIA; FACE-HAND TEST; CEREBRAL-DYSFUNCTION TESTS; DOUBLE-SIMULTANEOUS TACTILE SENSATION (there: **Fink-Green-Bender test**).

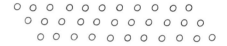

Gestalten to be copied

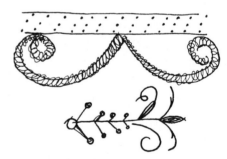

A manic patient's version

BENDER-GESTALT TEST (Portion of Plate 51 of the Bender® Visual Motor Gestalt Test, Monograph, 1938)

Bender-Gestalt test a personality test in which the subject copies nine geometrical figures, such as a circle tangent to a diamond, and a row of dots. Interpretation of these configurations, or Gestalten, and the subject's spontaneous comments, throw light on (a) perceptual ability, (b) visual-motor maturation, (c) personality characteristics such as impulsivity and flattening of affect, and (d) the diagnosis of both functional and organic disorders. The full name is **Bender Visual-Motor Gestalt Test**.

bends a severe form of DECOMPRESSION SICKNESS. See this entry.

beneceptor a nerve receptor whose stimuli are generally beneficial to the organism. Compare NOCICEPTOR.

Benedikt, Moritz Austrian physician, 1835–1920. See BENEDIKT'S SYNDROME.

Benedikt's syndrome a neurologic disorder marked by oculomotor paralysis, ataxia, hyperkinesis, and contralateral tremor.

Benemid a trademark for **probenecid**, a drug employed in the urinary excretion of uric acid, thereby protecting the patient against the risk of gouty-arthritis symptoms. See ALLOPURINOL.

benign /binīn'/ a disease condition that is relatively mild or transient, as opposed to a **malignant** /məlig'nənt/ disease (Latin *benignus* and *malignus*). In psychiatry, a b. disorder usually is one that has a favorable prognosis.

benign hereditary tremor = ESSENTIAL TREMOR.

benign neoplasm: See NEOPLASM.

benign stupor a state of unresponsiveness, immobility, and indifference to surroundings from which the patient is likely to recover or improve. An example is the depressed stupor observed in manic-depressive patients, termed benign because it is associated with a favorable prognosis; some authors, however, contend that this type of b.s. actually is a sign of a form of schizophrenia that progressively deteriorates.

Bennett, George Kettner American psychologist, 1904—. See BENNETT DIFFERENTIAL APTITUDE TEST; BENNETT MECHANICAL COMPREHENSION TEST.

Bennett Differential Aptitude Test a battery of tests designed for grades 8 to 12, measuring verbal, numerical, mechanical, and abstract reasoning, as well as language usage, spatial relations, and clerical speed and accuracy.

Bennett Mechanical Comprehension Test a test for high school students and adults in which a wide variety of mechanical problems are presented in printed form, corresponding to different scientific principles and processes, and different levels of difficulty.

Benommenheit /bənôm'ənhīt/ a term applied by Bleuler to an acute schizophrenic condition in which all mental processes are slowed, and comprehension and ability to deal with complex situations are impaired, although the patient is not dejected or self-deprecatory (German, "benumbing, haze").

Bentley, Arthur Owen physician, 1898–1943. See SYNTHETIC NARCOTICS (there: **Bentley's compound**).

Benton, Arthur Lester American psychologist, 1909—. See BENTON VISUAL RETENTION TEST; CEREBRAL-DYSFUNCTION TESTS.

Benton Visual Retention Test a measure of visual perception, immediate memory, psychomotor reproduction, and possible brain damage. The subject draws ten geometrical designs after each is exposed for ten seconds and removed.

benzaldehyde: See ALDEHYDES.

Benzedrine dependency a form of drug dependency in which Benzedrine, a trademark for amphetamine, is inhaled or taken by mouth, and characterized by inability to abstain, increased tolerance, and such symptoms as restlessness, insomnia, irritability, loss of impulse control, ideas of reference, delusions of persecution, and hallucinosis.

benzene: See PSYCHEDELICS.

benzodiazepines anxiolytic drugs that produce effects of sedation and skeletal-muscle relaxation. B. are used in treatment of alcoholism, petit mal epilepsy, and psychoneuroses. They are a drug of choice for certain patients because of the extreme difficulty of ingesting a fatal overdose of the medication. However, prolonged use of b. can lead to physical dependence. The prototype drug of the b. is **chlordiazepoxide**— $C_{16}H_{14}ClN_3O$. Other b. are **chlordiazepoxide hydrochloride**—$C_{16}H_{15}Cl_2N_3O$, **chlorazepate dipotassium**—$C_{16}H_{11}ClK_2N_2O_4$, **chlorazepate monopotassium**—$C_{16}H_{10}ClKN_2O_3$, **diazepam** (trademark: **Valium**)—$C_{16}H_{13}ClN_2O$, **flurazepam dihydrochloride**—$C_{21}H_{25}Cl_3FN_3O$, **lorazepam**—$C_{15}H_{10}Cl_2N_2O_2$, **oxazepam**—$C_5H_{11}ClN_2O_2$. Diazepam is used as an antiepileptic while **flurazepam**—$C_{21}H_{23}ClFN_3O$— and **nitrazepam**—$C_{15}H_{11}N_3O_3$—are employed as sedative-hypnotics.

benzodiazepines pharmacotherapy the use of benzodiazepines in the treatment of alcoholism and anxiety. B.p. also is employed in disorders that require muscle-relaxant drugs.

benzothiadiazides = THIAZIDES.

benzphetamine hydrochloride: See ADRENERGIC DRUGS.

benztropine mesylate: See ANTICHOLINERGICS.

berdache /bərdash'/ a Native American male who wears female clothing and performs the work traditionally assigned to women.

bereavement a feeling of deprivation and grief, particularly at the loss of a loved one.

Bergen's fraction a plasma fraction (alpha-2-globulin) which J. R. Bergen and his associates claim to be characteristic of schizophrenia, and identical with the protein factor found by C. E. Frohman in the serum of schizophrenics (**Frohman factor**).

Berger, Hans German neurologist, 1873–1941. See BRAIN WAVES (also called **Berger rhythms**); ELECTROENCEPHALOGRAPH.

Bergson, Henri /bergsôN'/ French philosopher, 1859–1941. Though B. wrote in philosophical rather than psychological terms, he contributed heavily to the dynamic point of view. To him, consciousness as well as the whole of reality is in constant flux and contains a creative spirit, or *élan vital*, which can be known by feeling and intuition (empathy, insight) rather than intellect. See VITALISM; COMIC.

beriberi /ber'ēber'ē/ a disease, chiefly of the Orient, caused by vitamin-B_1 deficiency. Also see WERNICKE'S DISEASE.

Berkeley, George English philosopher and bishop, 1685–1753. See ASSOCIATIONISM.

Berlyne, D. E. Canadian psychologist, fl. 1967. See AROUSAL-BOOST MECHANISM; AROUSAL REDUCTION MECHANISM; CIRCULAR-PATTERN RESPONSES; CORTICAL-AROUSAL FACTOR; EXPRESSIONISM FACTOR; HEDONIC-TONE FACTOR; IMPRESSIONISM FACTOR.

Bernard, Claude /bernär′/ French physiologist, 1813–78. See BERNARD-HORNER SYNDROME; BABINSKI-NAGEOTTE SYNDROME; SPINAL-CORD DISEASE; WALLENBERG'S SYNDROME.

Bernard-Horner syndrome a disorder caused by lesions of sympathetic nerve fibers resulting in ocular and cutaneous abnormalities. Ocular manifestations may include ophthalmoplegia, ocular hypotonia, and apparent enophthalmos. Skin signs are facial hyperemia, anhidrosis, and vasodilation. The lesions may occur at any point between the hypothalamus and sympathetic fibers of the sweat glands.

Berne, Eric Canadian-born American psychoanalyst, 1910–70. See ADULT-EGO STATE; EGO STATE; LIFE SCRIPT; PAY-AND-DON'T-GO; SCRIPT ANALYSIS; TRANSACTION; TRANSACTIONAL ANALYSIS.

Bernheim, Hippolyte-Marie French physician, 1837–1919. An early exponent of hypnotherapy, B. held that practically everyone can be hypnotized, since hypnosis is basically an intensification of suggestion, and everyone is suggestible to some degree. Also see LIEBEAULT.

Bernoulli effect a theory relating the velocity of air flow and the pressure exerted on a surrounding surface. This theory has been applied to the effects of air impulses during vocal-cord approximation in speaking.

Bernreuter, Robert Gibbon American psychologist, 1901—. See BERNREUTER PERSONAL ADJUSTMENT INVENTORY.

Bernreuter Personal Adjustment Inventory a six-trait questionnaire on personality and behavior factors yielding measures of neurotic tendency, introversion-extraversion, self-sufficiency, sociability, self-confidence, and dominance-submission.

berserk denoting a behavioral disorder marked by violent rage. The term may come from a Nordic word for bearshirt, the uniform of the Norse warriors who fought with blind, hysterical fury. The **berserkers**, or Norse warriors, also were said to howl like animals and foam at the mouth while attacking their enemies. The berserkers are believed by some to have inspired tales of werewolves. Verb: **to go berserk**.

Bessman, Samuel Paul American biochemist, 1921—. See BESSMAN-BALDWIN SYNDROME.

Bessman-Baldwin syndrome a familial disorder characterized by cerebromacular degeneration and excessive urinary excretion of carnosine, anserine, and histidine. The cerebromacular effects include convulsions, retinitis pigmentosa, blindness, and mental deterioration. The signs and symptoms begin around the age of seven years. Also called **imidazole syndrome**.

best-answer test a test in which the subject examines several possible solutions to a problem or reasons for a situation, and chooses the one he considers most appropriate. Also called **best-reason test**.

bestiality = ZOOERASTY.

best-reason test = BEST-ANSWER TEST.

beta /bēt′ə/ or /bāt′ə/ second letter of the Greek alphabet (Β, β).

beta adrenergic blocking agents: See ADRENERGIC BLOCKING AGENTS.

beta alcoholism a type of alcoholism in which drinking has progressed to the point of physical complications such as effects on the stomach, liver, pancreas, or kidneys, and polyneuropathy, but does not yet involve physical or psychological dependence (E. M. Jellinek, 1952). The patient often exhibits nutritional-deficiency symptoms and diminished job efficiency. B.a. corresponds to the French category **alcoolisation** /älkôlizäsyôN′/. Also called **somatophatic drinking**.

beta-arc the arousal of higher cortical pathways by the functioning of an alpha-arc, leading to a sensation rather than simple awareness. B.-a. is roughly the same as a delayed response or implicit behavior, as contrasted with an immediate response. Also see ALPHA-ARC.

beta blockers: See ADRENERGIC BLOCKING AGENTS.

beta cells: See ISLANDS OF LANGERHANS.

beta-endorphin: See ENDORPHIN.

beta error = TYPE II ERROR.

beta-glucuronidase deficiency /glo͞oʹkəron′-/ one of a group of mucopolysaccharidoses, which are disorders of **glycosaminoglycans (GAG)**. B.-g.d. is characterized by hepatosplenomegaly, dermatan sulphate in the urine, dysostosis multiplex, white-cell inclusions, and mental retardation.

Beta hypothesis: See ALPHA, BETA, GAMMA HYPOTHESES.

beta level the probability of accepting (failing to reject) the null hypothesis when it is in fact false, that is, making a Type II error.

beta movement an illusion in which successive stimuli of different sizes produce apparent motion.

beta receptor one of two basic types of adrenergic-nervous-system receptors, the other type being the alpha receptor. B.r. responses to natural or synthetic biochemical agents are generally inhibitory; an exception is a stimulant effect in heart muscle. B.r. functions include vasodilation, bronchial and intestinal relaxation, and, in some animal species, relaxation of the uterine smooth muscle. Compare ALPHA RECEPTOR.

beta-receptor blocking agents: See ADRENERGIC BLOCKING AGENTS.

beta-stimulant activity the reaction produced by stimulation of the beta portion of the adrenergic nerves. The responses associated with beta-receptor stimulation are primarily inhibitory with the exception of myocardial stimulant effects. Beta activity includes vasodilation, bronchial and intestinal relaxation, and cardioacceleration.

Beta test: See ARMY TESTS.

beta waves an EEG wave pattern that is associated with an alert and activated cerebral cortex. The frequency generally is above 12 cycles per second and may range upwards of 40 cycles per second. Beta activity is recorded during intense mental activity, but it also occurs as a sign of anxiety or apprehension.

beta weight a multiplier coefficient used to quantify the relative predictive power of a variable in a regression analysis.

betel nut the seed of a variety of palm tree, Areca catechu, that is chewed as a stimulant by local populations of India and the islands of the Indian and Pacific Oceans. The b.n. contains a drug, arecoline, which stimulates smooth muscles and glands that respond to postganglionic cholinergic agents. The drug, related to the muscarine agent of certain poisonous mushrooms, is used in veterinary medicine to eliminate internal parasites. See ARECOLINE.

bethanechol chloride $C_7H_{17}ClN_2O_2$—a cholinergic drug used in the control of autonomic-nervous-system complications of diabetes. B.c. is not destroyed by cholinesterase, as are other cholinergics, and is used mainly to treat neuropathy of the urinary and gastrointestinal tracts. See CHOLINERGIC DRUGS.

Bettelheim, Bruno Austrian-born American psychologist and social activist, 1903—. Among his many publications are *Love Is Not Enough—The Treatment of Emotionally Disturbed Children* (1950), *Truants from Life* (1955), and *Freud and Man's Soul* (1983).

betweenbrain = DIENCEPHALON.

between-groups variance a variation in scores attributable to membership in different experimental groups, and therefore reflecting the effect of the experimental variable. Also see WITHIN-GROUPS VARIANCE.

Betz, Vladimir Aleksandrovich Russian anatomist, 1834–94. See BETZ CELLS; CELLULAR LAYERS OF CORTEX.

Betz cells large pyramidal ganglion cells found in the fifth layer of the cerebral cortex. B.c. are associated with muscle movement at a very low threshold of stimulation. Betz-cell lesions result in convulsive seizures, spasticity, and flaccid paralysis. See MOTOR NEURONS.

bewildered a term applied to a patient who appears lost, dazed, and puzzled but apathetic about his confusion. The condition is associated with ambivalence. preoccupation, and autistic thinking.

Bezold-Brücke phenomenon a shift of red and green hues toward yellow and blue hues when illumination increases.

B fibers myelinated preganglionic axons of the autonomic nervous system. They are approximately three microns in diameter and carry nerve impulses at speeds of between three and 15 meters per second. See A FIBER; C FIBER.

bhang one of several preparations of cannabis sativa. B. is a milder form of the active ingredient of marijuana than charas or ganja and, according to studies conducted in India, is associated with a lower incidence of adverse health effects than other cannabis preparations. (B. is a Hindi word meaning "hemp.")

-bi-; -bis- a combining form meaning two, twice, double (from Latin *bis*, "twice").

Bianchi, Leonardo /bē·än′kē/ Italian psychiatrist, 1848–1927. See BIANCHI'S SYNDROME; PROCESSOMANIA.

Bianchi's syndrome a neurologic disorder associated with lesions in the left parietal lobe. It may be caused by injury or disease and is marked by symptoms of hemianesthesia, hemiplegia, agraphia, apraxia, and alexia.

bias an error in a particular direction; a tendency to produce erroneous or misleading conclusions because of the use of data that are incomplete or drawn from a sample that is not representative of the group studied.

biased sampling: See SYSTEMATICALLY B.S.

bibliophobia a morbid fear of books or of having to read books.

bibliotherapy a form of supportive therapy in which carefully chosen readings are recommended for such purposes as (a) helping the patient gain insight into his personality dynamics, (b) facilitating communication with the therapist, (c) bolstering morale, (d) imparting appropriate information on such subjects as sex, vocations, and new interests (e) relieving tensions by stimulating fantasy, and (f) inculcating basic principles of mental health.

Bichat, Marie François Xavier /bēshä′/ French anatomist, 1771–1802. See LAW OF BICHAT.

Bickerstaff, Edwin Robert English physician, fl. 1951. See BICKERSTAFF'S ENCEPHALITIS.

Bickerstaff's encephalitis a complex neurologic disorder believed to be caused by a Herpes simplex virus infection and marked by progressive deterioration of all midbrain functions associated with fibers from the brainstem. Symptoms include headaches, drowsiness, double vision and nystagmus, and loss of hearing. Also called **brainstem encephalitis**.

b.i.d. an abbreviation used in prescriptions, meaning "twice a day" (Latin *bis in die* /dē′ā/).

bidet /bidā′/ or /bide′/ a low, oblong vessel with fixtures of running water, used for washing one's external genital and anal areas (and for urinating) while sitting on it as one would sit on a toilet seat. Though eminently practical, the b. is not widely used outside France. (The term was originally a French word for a small horse.)

Bidwell, Shelford English physicist, 1848–1909, See BIDWELL'S GHOST.

Bidwell's ghost a second visual afterimage that appears in a hue complementary to the stimulus. Also called **Purkinje afterimage**.

Biedl, Arthur /bē′dəl/ Austrian physician, 1869–1933. See LAURENCE-MOON-BIEDL SYNDROME.

Bielschowsky, Alfred /bēlshôfs′ kē/ German ophthalmologist, 1871–1940. See BIELSCHOWSKY'S DISEASE; CEREBROMACULAR DEGENERATION.

Bielschowsky, Max /bēlshôfs′kē/ German neurologist, 1869–1940. See DOLLINGER-BIELSCHOWSKY SYNDROME; NEURONAL LIPIDOSIS (there: **Bielschowsky-Jansky disease**); SPHINGOLIPIDOSES.

Bielchowsky's disease a condition marked by the temporary loss of the ability to move the eyes in a vertical direction, up or down, in a synchronized manner.

Biemond, A. /bēmôN′/ French physician, 1902—. See BIEMOND'S ATAXIA; BIEMOND'S SYNDROME.

Biemond's ataxia a hereditary form of ataxia caused by a loss of Purkinje cells in the cerebellum and degeneration of the dorsal column and large fibers of the dorsal roots. See FRIEDREICH'S ATAXIA.

Biemond's syndrome a disorder that combines mental retardation, hypophyseal infantilism, coloboma of the iris, and polydactyly.

Biermer, Anton /bēr′mər/ German physician, 1827–92. See ADDISON-BIERMER ANEMIA; ANEMIA.

Biermer-Ehrlich anemia; Biermer's anemia = ADDISON-BIERMER ANEMIA.

bifactorial theory of conditioning the theory that attitudes determine probability of conditioning and stimulus properties determine the magnitude of response.

bigamy the state of being married to two persons at the same time. While b. is considered illegal in some cultures, it is accepted in others, e.g., in Muslim communities. Multiple simultaneous marriages constitute polygamy. (B. is derived from Latin *bi-*, "two," and Greek *gamos*, "marriage.")

Big Brother Program: See DEATH NEUROSIS.

bigeminal pregnancy: See PREGNANCY.

big lie a propaganda measure in which a false statement of extreme magnitude is constantly repeated in order to persuade the public, on the theory that it would be more impressive and less likely to be challenged than a lesser falsehood.

Big Sister Program: See DEATH NEUROSIS.

-bil-; -bili- a combining form denoting bile or the bile-producing system. Adjective: **biliary**.

bilabial a speech sound made with both lips which stop or modify the air stream, e.g., /b/, /p/, /m/, or /w/. Also called **labiolabial**. Also see LABIODENTAL.

bilateral lesion a lesion that begins in one hemisphere but produces dysfunction in the other because of a disruption of blood flow, metabolism, tumor spread, edema, or other complications.

bilateral speech speech function that is represented in both the left and right hemispheres of the brain. As a general rule, right-handed subjects have speech representation in the left hemisphere and are more likely to experience speech deficits following a left-hemisphere lesion.

bilateral transfer the transfer of training from one side of the body to the other through the contralateral distribution of nerve fibers between the two hemispheres. Thus, the training of the left hand to perform a task should condition, or at least precondition, the right hand to perform the same task. Studies show b.t. is most feasible in visual-learning activities.

bilharziasis = SCHISTOSOMIASIS.

biliary: See -BIL-.

bilingualism the ability to speak two languages fluently; strictly, the simultaneous learning of two languages in childhood. Some studies indicate possible intellectual advantages for bilingual children.

bilirubin an orange bile pigment produced from breakdown products of the hemoglobin of red blood cells. Normally, the human body produces one-fourth of a gram of b. per day, all of which is excreted in feces and urine. An excess of b. is a sign of a disorder such as abnormal destruction of red blood cells and may be marked by deposits of yellowish pigments in the skin and other tissues, a condition commonly known as JAUNDICE. See this entry. Also see HEPATITIS.

bilirubin encephalopathy a degenerative disease of the brain caused by the deposition of bilirubin in the basal ganglia and brainstem nuclei. The condition results, in turn, from the overproduction or undersecretion of bilirubin, a breakdown product of old or damaged red blood cells. A newborn child may lack the bacteria needed to metabolize bilirubin into other products.

bill of rights in psychiatry, the civil rights of patients, including (a) the right to treatment, (b) the right, or objective, of the least-restrictive alternative (less treatment rather than more), (c) the right not to be subject to unusual or hazardous treatment methods without expressed and informed consent, (d) the right of children committed to mental institutions to due-process protection and provision of legal counsel, (e) the right of a nondangerous person not to be custodially confined if he can survive safely in freedom, (f) the right to refuse treatment that may be invasive, intrusive, or hazardous, and (g) the right to a humane environment and adequate staffing.

bimodal distribution a set of scores having two modes (two peaks), reflecting a tendency for scores to cluster around two separate values. A b.d. of recall would be found if some subjects recalled nothing and others recalled several events.

binasal hemianopia: See HOMONYMOUS HEMIANOPIA.

binaural pertaining to both ears.

binaural beat periodic intensity fluctuations produced when tones of slightly different frequency are perceived separately by the two ears. See BINAURAL SHIFT.

binaural fusion: See FUSION.

binaural shift a periodic shift in the localization or

intensity of the sound which is heard when two tones of slightly different frequency are perceived separately by each ear, the rate of fluctuation corresponding to the frequency difference.

Binet, Alfred /bine'/ French psychologist, 1857–1911. B. was a pioneer investigator of suggestion and the thought processes of the mentally gifted and mentally retarded. Opposing J. M. Cattell's reduction of mental abilities to sensory capacities, as measured by "brass instruments," B. developed a variety of verbal and numerical test items in 1905 (with the assistance of Théodore Simon) that could be used to determine the child's mental age and to differentiate between mentally defective pupils and others who had the ability to succeed. Later revisions, in 1908 and 1911, led ultimately to the development of the Stanford-Binet Intelligence Scale, which is in wide use today. See BINET TEST; STANFORD-BINET INTELLIGENCE SCALE; STANFORD-BINET SCALE; ABSURDITIES TEST; BALL-AND-FIELD TEST; BASAL MENTAL AGE; CATTELL INFANT SCALE; CEILING AGE; DEVIATION IQ; HUNT-MINNESOTA TEST FOR ORGANIC BRAIN DAMAGE; INDIVIDUAL TEST; INTELLIGENCE TEST; IQ; SUPERIOR INTELLIGENCE. Also see GODDARD; TERMAN.

Binet Test the original Binet-Simon verbal test developed to assess the intellectual ability of French children in 1905.

binge drinking = EPSILON ALCOHOLISM.

binge-eating syndrome a recurrent disorder in which the individual eats huge quantities of any food he can lay his hands on. The condition is most apt to occur after a stressful event. See BULIMIA.

Binger, Carl American psychoanalyst, 1890–1976. B. is known for his work in psychosomatic medicine.

Bini, Lucio Italian psychiatrist, 1908–64. See ELECTROCONVULSIVE TREATMENT.

binocular accommodation: See ACCOMMODATION.

binocular cells cortical cells that respond to a stimulus presented to either the left or right eye. The effect has been observed in cells associated with the retinal area centralis of cats. Stimulation of both eyes simultaneously results in a **summation effect**.

binocular cues visual cues that require the use of both eyes functioning in parallax. Depth perception generally requires b.c. Also see MONOCULAR CUES.

binocular disparity = RETINAL DISPARITY.

binocular fusion: See BINOCULAR VISION; FUSION.

binocular parallax the differences in the two retinal images due to separation of the eyes.

binocular perception the interaction of the two eyes resulting in the fusion of the two visual fields in three dimensions.

binocular rivalry = RETINAL RIVALRY.

binocular vision the normal coordinated function of the right and left eyes that permits viewing of the surroundings in three dimensions. The term **binocular fusion** is applied to the merging of the two retinal images such that the perceived object is experienced as a single image.

binomial distribution an approximation to the normal probability curve for data in binary form (0-1, yes-no, etc.).

binomial test a test of the significance of the deviation of binary (two-valued, yes-no, or 0-1) data from their expected or chance frequency.

Binswanger, Otto /bins'vängər/ German psychiatrist, 1852–1929. See BINSWANGER'S DISEASE.

Binswanger's disease a progressive neurologic disorder beginning after middle age and characterized by memory disorders, paranoia, emotional instability, speech disorders, and hallucinations. The changes are associated with demyelination of the white matter, apparently due to arteriosclerosis of the brain. The gray matter is not affected. Also called **Binswanger's dementia; subcortical arteriosclerotic encephalopathy; progressive subcortical encephalopathy; demyelinating encephalopathy**.

-bio- a combining form relating to life or a living organism (from Greek *bios*, "life").

bioanalysis a term coined by M. Solomon (1915) for an analytic approach that focuses on somatic symptoms as well as the psychic phenomena, such as unconscious impulses and conflicts, that are at the core of psychoanalysis.

biochemical approach in psychiatry, the study of behavioral patterns, including mental disorders, from the standpoint of chemical changes, e.g., the view that schizophrenia can be explained in terms of an excess or deficiency of certain substances in the nervous system, such as serotonin. The term also applies to the use of psychotropic drugs in the treatment of mental disorders.

biochemical defects any of a number of chemical imbalances or aberrations in brain tissue that may be associated with neurologic disorders. High calcium levels have been found during periods of catatonia. Other studies have found relationships between schizophrenia and monoamine-oxidase activity, dopamine metabolites, and defective conversion of tryptophan or serotonin into a substance that is chemically related to hallucinogens.

biodata = BIOGRAPHICAL DATA.

bioelectric potential the electric potential of a nerve, muscle, and other living tissue.

bioenergetics according to a leading exponent, Alexander Lowen, "a way of understanding personality in terms of the body and its energetic processes, and a way of relieving the individual's chronic muscular tensions and rigidities resulting from emotional stress and unresolved emotional conflicts," a process which helps him "regain his full aliveness and emotional well-being." Major techniques used for his purpose are respiratory exercises, free expression of feelings, and improvement in the body image, and therefore the self-image, through a form of movement and posture therapy. The approach is based on the work of Wilhelm Reich.

bioengineering the branch of engineering that specializes in the research and design of equipment and environmental features that enhance the performance of human tasks. E.g., a **bioengineer** may be assigned the responsibility of developing electronic devices that enable a quadriplegic individual to dress himself.

biofeedback the organism's internal regulatory systems that are responsible for control of the organic processes. Impulses are received from muscles, visceral organs, and the nervous system, and control over these organs is maintained at a physiologically desirable level. The term also applies to the use of a monitoring device, such as an electromyograph, psychogalvanometer, or electroencephalograph. Also called **sensory feedback**. See B. TRAINING.

biofeedback training the use of a monitoring device, such as an electromyograph, psychogalvanometer, or EEG, to inform the individual about changes occurring in his muscles, brain waves, heart rate, temperature, blood pressure, or other bodily processes over which he ordinarily has no control. This information, conveyed by sight or sound, frequently enables the subject to gain control over these processes and relieve such conditions as high blood pressure, torticollis, uncontrolled head movements, faulty posture, and headache.

biogenesis: See BIOGENETICS.

biogenetic law = RECAPITULATION THEORY.

biogenetics the scientific study of the principles and processes governing the production of living organisms from other living organisms (**biogenesis**), including the mechanisms of heredity.

biogenic amines a group of psychoactive amines, including epinephrine, norepinephrine, and serotonin. Epinephrine and norepinephrine are catecholamines and serotonin is an indoleamine. The b.a. are sometimes identified as neurohormones because they activate the autonomic nervous system during periods of physical or psychic stress.

biogenic psychosis a term applied by Kraepelin and others to schizophrenia, manic-depressive psychosis, paranoia, and involutional states that are due to a single major cause. They are all, in this view, abnormal reactions to experiences that normally should develop the personality and the individual's ability to master life.

biogram a pattern of possible events involved in learning a biofeedback experience. The b. may begin as a conscious memory device but through repeated trials eventually becomes subconscious in a manner similar to other learning experiences acquired through repeated trials.

biographical data information gathered about a client's history and behavioral patterns from those who know him. B.d. serve to either supplement or substitute for an autobiography; the term is often resorted to if the client is, for some reason, unable to write an autobiography. In industrial psychology, the term applies to information on job candidates for use in personnel selection. The data are usually obtained from application forms or special questionnaires and include such items as age, sex, education, work experience, marital status, relevant physical characteristics (height, weight), medical history, interests, and use of leisure time. Also called **biodata**. See AUTOBIOGRAPHY.

biographical method the use of personal data in studying factors affecting a subject's life.

biological aging: See SECONDARY AGING.

biological clock the mechanism within an organism that controls periodic changes or rhythms in various physiological and behavioral functions, such as variations in body temperature or blood pressure that tend to repeat at approximately the same time each day. Also see CIRCADIAN RHYTHMS.

biological determinism the concept that psychological and behavioral characteristics are entirely the result of constitutional and biological factors.

biological drives the unlearned arousal states that result from depletion or deprivation of survival necessities, e.g., water, oxygen, food, and sleep. Whenever physiological equilibrium is disrupted, the organism is impelled to engage in behavior designed to restore physiological balance.

biological factors in psychiatry, organic, or biogenic, conditions associated with mental disorder, e.g., cerebral arteriosclerosis, lead poisoning, hyperthyroidism, syphilitic infection, chromosomal aberrations, or phencyclidine intoxication.

biological intelligence a level of innate mental ability required primarily for cognitive activity. The term was introduced by W. C. Halstead to differentiate forebrain-functioning ability from traditional concepts of intelligence. B.i. is measured with a battery of tests that also indicate evidence of brain injury.

biological measures: See PRIMARY PREVENTION.

biological psychiatry a psychiatric field focused on biochemical, pharmacological, and neurological factors in the study of the causes and in the treatment of mental disorder.

biological rhythm periodic variations in physiological and psychological functions such as energy level, sexual desire, hunger, sleep, elimination, the estrus in animals, and menstruation. These rhythms vary considerably from person to person and from one period of life to another, but tend to be a basic characteristic of each individual. Also called **endogenous rhythm; life rhythm; internal rhythm**. See CIRCADIAN RHYTHMS; INFRADIAN RHYTHM; ULTRADIAN RHYTHM; DIURNAL RHYTHM. Also see BIORHYTHMS.

biological stress a condition that imposes severe demands on the physical and psychological defenses of the organism. Examples include acute or chronic disease, a congenital or acquired disability or defect, exposure to extreme heat or cold, malnutrition or starvation, hallucinogens or other drugs, and the ingestion of toxic substances. Also see STRESS.

biological taxonomy the science of the classification of plants and animals into categories based on their relationships in nature. Also called **systematics**.

biological therapy any method that seeks to treat mental disturbance by altering physiological processes, such as through the use of drugs, electric shock, or psychosurgery. Also called **biomedical therapy**. See CLINICAL PSYCHOPHARMACOLOGY; ELECTROCONVULSIVE TREATMENT; PSYCHOSURGERY; PSYCHOTROPIC DRUG.

biological viewpoint an approach to abnormal psychology based on causative factors that are organic, such as the senile plaques that are an assumed causative factor in Alzheimer's disease.

biomechanics the study of body functions and their relationship to working situations, e.g., problems of work tolerance, human-performance effectiveness, and methods of preventing disabling accidents on the job.

biomedical engineering the branch of engineering that specializes in research and development of equipment for medical treatment, rehabilitation, and special needs, e.g., devices to monitor the physiological condition of astronauts in space. The development of ultrasound devices for outlining (e.g., through a **sonogram**) the position of a fetus in the uterus in order to perform amniocentesis is another example of b.e.

biomedical therapy = BIOLOGICAL THERAPY.

biometry a term meaning literally the measurement of life, including the mathematical calculations associated with the study of exogenous and endogenous factors that may affect the duration of life.

bion a hypothetical microscopic vesicle charged with sexual energy, postulated by Wilhelm Reich (1942) as the ultimate source of the orgasm. See ORGONE; ORGONE THERAPY.

bionomics the study of relationships between organisms and environmental influences.

biophysical system a term used by Masters and Johnson to identify the hormonal and genital functions of the sexual response system.

biophysics the interface of biology and physics; the study of biological structures and processes by means of the methods of physics, e.g., the application of principles of physics in the study of vision or hearing.

biopsy the surgical removal and study of a small amount of tissue from an organ or body part that is believed to be diseased or otherwise abnormal. The b. sample usually is examined under a microscope for signs of malignancy or other clues that would help determine the proper course of therapy. A b. often is performed during exploratory or corrective surgery. Also see AUTOPSY.

biopsychic pertaining to psychological phenomena that play a role in the development and life of the individual.

biopsychology a branch of psychology concerned with the effect of biological factors, such as glands, blood pressure, and nervous-system functioning on adaptation and behavior.

biopsychosocial system in general-systems theory applied to psychiatry, a systematic integration of biological, psychological, and social approaches to the study of mental health and specific mental disorders.

biorhythms a pseudoscience based on the belief that every person is biologically programed by three precise rhythms (physical, emotional, and intellectual), beginning at birth and continuing unaltered until death, and that good and bad days for various activities can be calculated accordingly. As with astrology, the predictions, however, do not differ significantly from chance. Until the term became preempted by this fad, biorhythm was a reputable synonym of BIOLOGICAL RHYTHM. See this entry.

biosocial pertaining to the interplay or mingling of biological and social forces, e.g., human behavior that is influenced simultaneously by complex physiological processes and learned social meanings.

biosocial determinism the viewpoint that individual behavior is the result of interaction between biological and social influences.

biosocial theory a personality theory, such as that of G. Murphy, based on observation of the individual's dynamic relations and interactions with the social or ecological environment, as contrasted with theories that view personality as a self-contained unit.

biosphere the total area of the earth and its atmosphere in which living organisms subsist; the environment in which biological processes take place.

biotaxis the powers of living cells for selecting and arranging themselves with respect to their environment. Also see NETWORK B.; NEUROBIO-TAXIS.

biotechnology the scientific study of the relation between human beings and machines, particularly in the work process. The study involves the design, use, and placement of mechanical equipment with the efficiency and safety of the worker in mind. See ENGINEERING PSYCHOLOGY; HUMAN ENGINEERING.

biotype a group of individuals who are genotypically the same (alike in heredity) although they may vary in phenotypical (visible) features.

biotypology the classification of human beings according to basic, or constitutional, anatomical, physiological, and psychological characteristics. See CONSTITUTIONAL TYPE.

biovular twins = DIZYGOTIC TWINS.

bipedal locomotion walking or running on two feet and in an upright position, as in man, birds, and, for short periods, in simians and bears, especially when the animal is carrying food, traveling over wet ground, or looking for something to eat.

biphasic symptom a symptom of compulsive behavior characterized by two contradictory parts, the second of which is the reverse of the first. An example is a compulsion to open a window, followed by a compulsion to close it again.

bipolar cells nerve cells with two processes, an axon and a dendrite. Cells of this type are found in the eye and ear.

bipolar disorder, depressed an affective disorder in which the individual has experienced one or more manic episodes, but in which a major depressive episode occurs currently or most recently. See MANIC EPISODE; MAJOR DEPRESSIVE EPISODE. (DSM-III)

bipolar disorder, manic an affective disorder in which a manic episode occurs currently or most recently. See MANIC EPISODE. (DSM-III)

bipolar disorder, mixed an affective disorder in which the current or most recent episode involves all features of both manic and depressive episodes, intermixed or rapidly alternating every few days, and in which depressive symptoms are prominent and last at least a full day. See MANIC EPISODE; MAJOR DEPRESSIVE EPISODE. (DSM-III)

bipolar neuron a nerve cell characterized by two long processes, the axon and dendrite, which extend in opposite directions. Other nerve cells, by comparison, such as sensory neurons, usually consist of an axon that appears continuous with a dendrite while the cell body, or nucleus, is offset at an angle to the processes.

bird phobia = ORNITHOPHOBIA.

Birnbaum, Karl /bĕrn′boum/ German psychiatrist, 1878—. B. is known as a pioneer in forensic psychiatry.

birth adjustment the set of major adaptations that must be made by the infant during the interval of 15 to 30 minutes after birth, including adjustment to a temperature of 70°F (21°C) instead of 100°F, obtaining oxygen by inhalation, taking nourishment via the mouth, and eliminating waste products through the rectum and urethra. During this period and for several days thereafter, the baby usually loses weight and shows many signs of behavior disorganization, such as gasping, coughing, sneezing, and difficulties in sucking and swallowing. The extent of this disorganization is dependent on the mother's emotional state during pregnancy and the type of birth experienced by the infant. Also see BIRTH EXPERIENCE.

birth control voluntary regulation of the number and spacing of offspring, including prevention of conception through intrauterine devices, contraceptive pills, spermicides, rhythm method, male contraceptive devices, surgical methods of sterilization (salpingectomy, vasectomy), and termination of pregnancy by artificially induced abortion. Also see STERILIZATION; VASECTOMY; RHYTHM METHOD.

birth cry the initial reflexive sound produced by a newborn infant when respiration begins.

birth defect a malformation, sensory or intellectual defect, or disease process that is present at birth and due to such factors as heredity, prenatal conditions, chromosomal aberration, biochemical defect, or birth injury. Examples of malformation are spina bifida and cleft palate; of prenatal defect: hypothyroidism, and cerebral palsy due to rubella; of sensory defect: deafness and blindness; of neurological disease: Huntington's chorea and phenylketonuria; of chromosomal aberration: Down's syndrome; of biochemical defect: Tay-Sachs disease; of birth injury: cases of brain damage that result in mental retardation.

birth experience the abrupt change from a parasitic existence within the warmth of the womb to a condition of independent survival, accompanied by a flood of internal and external stimulation. According to Freud and, especially, Otto Rank, this sudden adjustment gives rise to the infant's first, basic experience of anxiety. See BIRTH TRAUMA. Also see BIRTH ADJUSTMENT.

birth injury physical damage incurred during the birth process, especially malformation or brain injury. Damage is most likely to occur in transverse or breech births, in instrumental deliveries, in premature infants, and among twins.

birth order the ordinal position of the child—firstborn, second-born, middle, or youngest—particularly in relation to personal adjustment and status in the family. Alfred Adler was the first to maintain that b.o. is an important factor in personality development. He held, e.g., that the youngest child will either expect attention and help later in life, or develop a strong impulse to surpass others. This generalization, and practically all others on the subject of b.o., have been challenged by later studies. It appears that the attitudes of the parents have a far greater influence than b.o. on the development of the child, and that the child's *psychological* position may bear no relation to his ordinal position in the family. Also see CONFLUENCE MODEL.

birth trauma the psychological shock of being born; the sudden transformation from the blissful security of the womb to being bombarded with stimuli from the external world. Freud viewed birth as the child's first anxiety experience; to Otto Rank, it was the crucial fact of life. Rank maintained that if the basic "separation anxiety" is successfully worked through, the individual will make a normal adjustment; if not, there will be a lasting predisposition to neurosis and psychosis.

-bis-: See -BI-.

biserial correlation a measure of relationship between a continuous and dichotomous variable. It is frequently used to determine discriminatory power of a test item.

bisexual behavior a condition in which the individual is attracted sexually to either sex. The subject usually is able to achieve orgasm in contact with members of both sexes.

bisexuality the existence of male and female genitals in the same person, usually accompanied by psychological characteristics of both sexes. The term is also used for equal sexual attraction to both sexes. Freud held that every individual displays a mixture of masculine and feminine character traits. See HERMAPHRODITE; INTERSEX; AMBISEXUALITY.

bit in information theory, the quantity of information that decreases uncertainty or the germane alternatives of a problem by one half; e.g., "Suppose a twenty dollar bill has been placed in one of sixteen identical books standing side by side on a shelf, and our task is to guess which one it is by asking a minimum number of questions that can be answered only by a yes or a no. The best way to proceed would be to begin by asking if the book is to the right or the left of center. The answer to this question would provide one 'bit'..." (R.M. Goldenson, *The Encyclopedia of Human behavior*, 1970). (Bit is a contraction of *bi*nary digi*t*.)

BITCH test = BLACK INTELLIGENCE TEST OF CULTURAL HOMOGENEITY.

bitemporal hemianopia: See HOMONYMOUS HEMIANOPIA.

biting attack a form of aggressive behavior in which the teeth are used as a weapon. Small children and young animals often go through a normal period of biting attacks which may be regarded as a form of fighting or playing, unless or until the behavior undergoes displacement. B.a. was identified by Freud as oral sadism. Also see ORAL-BITING PERIOD.

biting mania a 15th-century epidemic of mass hysteria in which a German nun developed a compulsive urge to bite her associates, who in turn bit others, until the mania spread to convents throughout Germany, Holland, and Italy. See MASS HYSTERIA.

biting stage in psychoanalysis, the second stage of the oral period of psychosexual development, during which the child from the eighth to the 18th month feels increasingly independent of the mother, develops ambivalent attitudes toward her, and expresses hostility by biting her breast or the nipple of the bottle. When she attempts to wean him later on, the urge to bite may take the form of nail-biting, spitting, sticking out the tongue, or chewing on a pencil or gum.

bivariate characterized by two variables.

bizarre behavior one of the specific symptoms of consciousness changes in cases of brain damage and psychosis, especially schizophrenia. B.b. may be related to other symptoms, e.g., misunderstandings, confusion of dreams with reality, states of fear or anxiety, which often develop when consciousness returns after a period of coma or semiconsciousness. The precise form of b.b. may depend upon the part of the brain affected, such as the speech center, visual cortex, or other area.

bizarre delusion a belief that is patently absurd and fantastic, as in a schizophrenic patient's conviction that half of him is on this planet while the other half is in outer space.

black box a euphemism for a device that produces a predictable effect as a result of a specific input although the exact cause-and-effect relationship is not revealed to the observer. In biofeedback training, the subject may be identified as a b.b., reacting in a predictable manner to a given stimulus.

Black Intelligence Test of Cultural Homogeneity a cross-cultural test in which black and white respondents are compared as to their understanding of typical in-group slang used by black Americans. Abbrev.: **BITCH test**.

black-lung disease a form of emphysema that results from the gradual deposit of coal dust throughout the lungs and development of coal macules around the bronchioles. B.-l.d. is caused by more or less continuous exposure to coal dust in mining operations. Severity of the symptoms varies and appears to be independent of the amount of exposure to coal dust. The condition may be aggravated by cigarette-smoking. Also called **anthracosis**.

black-market source: See GRAY MARKET.

blackout total loss of consciousness produced, e.g., by sudden lowering of the blood supply to the brain; by decreased oxygen supply, as in mountain-climbing; or in alcoholic intoxication. Also see ALCOHOLIC BLACKOUT.

blackout threshold the point at which an oxygen-deprived person loses consciousness.

Blacky pictures a set of dog cartoons with human analogies used in analyzing emotional problems of children, such as family conflicts, oedipal situations, and sibling rivalry.

bladder cancer any of several types of malignant tumors that can invade the lining or musculature of the urinary bladder. Common symptoms include blood in the urine, a burning sensation during urination, and frequent urination. B.c. occurs most frequently among cigarette smokers and workers in dye, rubber, and asbestos industries, and about twice as often in men as in women.

bladder control the ability to regulate urination to a sufficient extent to void in the proper place and at the proper time. Generally speaking, b.c. begins during the 15th or 16th month, but daytime control is not achieved until the child is two or two and a half years old, and nighttime control about a year later. See TOILET TRAINING.

bladder training: See BLADDER CONTROL.

blanket group a group that lacks criteria for membership.

blank experiment an experiment that uses irregular or meaningless conditions to prevent the subject from guessing or giving automatic responses.

blank hallucination a type of sensation of equilibrium and space, involving rotating or rhythmically moving objects, usually localized in the mouth, hands, or skin, and also in the space immediately surrounding the body. In psychoanalysis, b.h. is associated with primal-scene material.

blank screen in psychoanalysis, the metaphoric backdrop on which the patient projects his feelings and fantasies during the transference process. The screen is the analyst, and is described as blank because the analyst remains passive and neutral, so that the patient will feel free to give voice to his innermost ideas and attitudes.

-blast-; -blasto- a combining form relating to a germ, a sprout, a formative cell.

blastocele: See BLASTULA.

blastocyst the mammalian embryo at a very early stage of development when it consists of an inner mass of cells and a yolk sac forming a tiny sphere that is enclosed in a thin layer of trophoblast cells that help implant the b. in the uterine lining. The b. stage in human development occurs around the beginning of the second week following conception.

blastomere one of the cells formed by cleavage of the zygote, forming the **blastoderm**.

blastula a somewhat spherical group of cells formed by cleavage of the zygote, consisting of a single layer of cells surrounding a fluid-filled cavity (the **blastocele**).

-blenn-; -blenno- a combining form relating to mucus.

blepharospasm a tonic spasm of the eyelid muscle that is manifested by an involuntary blinking.

Bleuler, Eugen /bloi′lər/ Swiss psychiatrist, 1857–1939. Working with Freud and Jung, B. held the first conclave on psychoanalysis, in 1908, and was instrumental in organizing the International Psychanalytic Association two years later. His major contributions were a recognition of the psychological causes of mental illness, as opposed to the prevailing organic theory of Kraepelin; and an attempt to apply Freud's psychological interpretation of neurosis to psychoses, such as dementia praecox, which he renamed schizophrenia. See ACCESSORY SYMPTOMS; AMBIVALENCE; ANNIVERSARY EXCITEMENT; BENOMMENHEIT; BLUNTED AFFECT; CONDENSATION; CONSTITUTIONAL DEPRESSIVE DISPOSITION; CONSTITUTIONAL MANIC DISPOSITION; DEMENTIA PRAECOX; DETERIORATION OF ATTENTION; DIRECTIVE PROGNOSIS; DISTURBANCES OF ASSOCIATIONS; DOUBLE ORIENTATION; FRAGMENTATION; FUNDAMENTAL SYMPTOMS; MORAL IDIOCY; MORAL IMBECILITY; PARALOGIA; PRELOGICAL THINKING; PSEUDOMOTIVATIONS; SCHIZOID-MANIC STATE; SCHIZOPHRENIC DISORDERS; SECONDARY SYMPTOMS; SIMPLE SCHIZOPHRENIA; THYMOPATHIC; WILL DISTURBANCES. Also see BRILL.

blind alley a type of maze pathway or passage whose only exit is its entrance. Also called **blind; dead end; cul-de-sac** /kēdəsäk′/ or /kul′dəsak′/ (plural: **culs-de-sac**).

blind analysis a diagnosis made by studying test results and data without briefing about the patient or contact with the patient.

blindism the mannerism of blind persons, e.g., rubbing the eyes or fanning the fingers before the eyes, as observed in some otherwise normal children who eventually discontinue the behavior.

blind-matching technique a validation procedure by matching different protocols or sets of diagnostic data.

blindness the inability to see; the total inability to receive visual stimuli. However, b. is legally defined as 20/200 vision in the better eye with correction. Major causes of organic blindness include inoperable cataracts, uncontrolled glaucoma, retinitis pigmentosa, diabetic retinopathy. More infrequent causes include macular degeneration, rubella, and severe head trauma. Functional or psychogenic blindness may be a conversion symptom, and is frequently termed hysterical blindness. Personality studies indicate that people who are born blind have more personality problems than those who have lost their sight later in life; but, as a whole, R. G. Barker and colleagues (1953) found that the total amount of personality disturbance among the blind is relatively small. Also see BLUE-YELLOW B.; COLOR B.; CORTICAL B.; DAY B.; HYSTERICAL B.; NIGHT B.; RED-GREEN B.; SNOW B.; NORRIE'S DISEASE.

blind spot in psychiatry, a persistent lack of insight or awareness which serves as a defense against recognition of one's true motives; in psychoanalysis, a form of resistance to disclosure of repressed impulses or memories that would threaten the patient's ego. Also called **mental b.s.** Also see SCOTOMA; SCOTOMIZATION.

blink response abrupt closing of the eyelids in response to bright light, shifting attention, or irritation of the eye. Also called **blinking reflex**. See BLEPHAROSPASM.

bliss: See TRANSCENDENTAL MEDITATION.

BLM *bucco*l*ingual* *m*asticatory syndrome. This is the most common form of tardive dyskinesia, characterized by repeated involuntary movements of the tongue, lips, and mouth. Also called **oral-lingual dyskinesia**. See TARDIVE DYSKINESIA.

bloating a gastrointestinal symptom which may be physical or psychogenic: The patient usually feels, falsely, that his abdomen is distended, and complains of belching, flatus, and indigestion. The reaction is usually hysterical or hypochondriacal, and may result from an unconscious pregnancy fantasy. B. due to air-swallowing (aerophagia) is a common psychophysiologic disorder. Also called **abdominal b**.

block in experimental design, a group of conditions or measures that are treated as a unit, or pooled.

blockage a term used by the Horney school for defensive techniques employed by patients to ward off awareness of inner conflicts and self-hate, e.g., by minimizing, ignoring, pseudoaccepting, intellectualizing, or attacking interpretations.

block design an experimental design that divides subjects into "blocks" or relatively homogeneous categories. Each block is exposed to experimental conditions and evaluated as a unit.

block-design test an intelligence test in which the subject is asked to use colored blocks to match a specified design. The b.-d.t. also is utilized in the diagnosis of mental disorder and mental deterioration.

blocking an abrupt, involuntary interruption in the flow of thought or speech. The individual suddenly cannot recall what he wanted to say or find words to express himself. Transient blockage occasionally occurs in normal individuals who are overwhelmed by grief, terror, or anger. In psychiatric cases, b. may be an attempt to keep threatening or distasteful ideas out of consciousness. In catatonic schizophrenia all thought and speech may be obstructed for a prolonged period. Also called **thought deprivation; thought obstruction; emotional b.**

block sampling a survey technique for compiling a final sample from each of several larger samples representing different segments of the population.

Blocq, Paul Oscar /blôk/ French physician, 1860–96. See BLOCQ'S SYNDROME.

Blocq's syndrome a fear of standing or walking, or hysterical inability to stand or walk. See ASTASIA-ABASIA.

blood-bank technologist a registered medical technologist who has received an additional 12 months of training in an approved blood-bank school. The school must be approved by the American Association of Blood Banks. The b.-b.t. bears the official designation of M.T. (ASCP) B.B., where ASCP is an abbreviation for American Society for Clinical Pathologists.

blood-brain barrier a semipermeable membrane surrounding blood vessels of the central nervous system and designed to allow certain nutrients and ions to enter areas of vital brain tissues while screening out substances that might prove harmful. Physiological mechanisms of the central nervous system also influence the entry or exclusion of certain amino acids and other molecules.

blood clotting the process by which a fibrous mesh of jellylike material forms on rough or damaged surfaces of blood vessels. B.c. begins when platelets flowing in the bloodstream contact a rough surface and rupture, releasing substances that trigger the 12-stages of the b.c. mechanism. The absence of one or more of the 12 b.c. factors is responsible for such disorders as Christmas disease or hemophilia.

blood disorder any disease or defect, congenital or acquired, that interferes with the normal functions of blood in general or its various components. Kinds of b.d. include Cooley's anemia, in which both lack of hemoglobin and red blood cells limit oxygen distribution to brain and body tissues; hemophilia, characterized by a deficiency of a blood-clotting factor; leukemia, a disease of the blood-forming organs; Hodgkin's disease, a disorder of the lymphatic system that manufactures blood-plasma cells and white blood cells; and sickle-cell anemia, marked by the formation of distorted red blood cells that carry inadequate

amounts of oxygen and tend to form "logjams" in the capillaries. Also see BLOOD GROUP; RH BLOOD-GROUP INCOMPATIBILITY; RH FACTOR.

blood dyscrasia an abnormal condition of the blood, usually the result of an accumulation or imbalance of certain cellular elements. B.d. often is a chronic condition associated with another disorder such as a tumor of the bone-marrow cells. B.d. also may be caused by an adverse reaction to drugs which may produce hemolytic anemias, defects in blood clotting, or other complications.

blood group a category of a broad spectrum of different inherited red-blood-cell traits. The basic categories are A, B, O, and AB. In addition, there are more than 20 other b.g. systems within the ABO categories, such as at least 33 types of Rh factors, 16 types of Kell factors, and so on. An individual red blood cell may possess more than 60 different antigens or factors.

blood-letting removing blood for therapeutic reasons, usually by cutting into a vein. B.-l. may be performed in cases of congestive heart disease or for polycythemia in which the bloodstream contains an abnormally high proportion of red blood cells. Also called **phlebotomy; venesection.**

blood levels the relative amounts of various substances in a measured amount of blood as compared with amounts that may be determined to be normal or average, or toxic. The amount may be expressed in percentage, milligrams or micrograms per 100 milliliters, milliequivalents per liter, or a similar measure. Normal b.l. of iron would be 60 to 280 micrograms per 100 milliliters.

blood phobia = HEMATOPHOBIA.

blood-poisoning a common term for a severe or significant bacterial infection of the bloodstream, usually by microorganisms invading from an infection site elsewhere in the body. B.-p. may be characterized by fever, chills, and skin eruptions. A particularly hazardous complication is spread of the infection to tissues of the nervous system. Also called **bacteremia; septicemia.** Also see SEPSIS.

blood pressure the pressure exerted by contractions of the heart as it pushes blood from the left ventricle into the general body circulation. B.p. also is influenced by the viscosity and amount of blood in the vessels and the elasticity of the artery walls and resistance of the arterioles. B.p. is measured as an extrapolation of the height that it will cause a column of mercury to rise in a glass tube when the blood flow in a major artery is interrupted by air pressure pumped into a rubber cuff placed over the artery. The higher b.p. measurement represents the force of the heart contraction and is called systolic; the lower figure represents blood pressure in the artery during relaxation of the heart and is termed diastolic. The readings usually are recorded as systolic/diastolic, and the upper limit of normal b.p. is approximately 140/90 millimeters of mercury for an adult. Also see DIASTOLIC B.P.; SYSTOLIC B.P.; HIGH B.P.

blood-pressure phobia a morbid fear of high blood pressure, which may produce enough tension to feed back and aggravate existing hypertension.

blood sugar the glucose circulating in the bloodstream as immediately available energy for body cell activities. The normal fasting level of blood sugar is about 80 milligrams per 100 milliliters. Abnormally high levels, hyperglycemia, indicate diabetes mellitus, hyperthyroidism, or hyperpituitarism. Levels below 40 milligrams per 100 milliliters, hypoglycemia, suggest hypopituitarism or hyperinsulinism. See GLUCOSE-TOLERANCE TEST.

blood type: See BLOOD GROUP.

blood volume the amount of blood available to any or all of the body's tissues, as a source of oxygen and nutrients for cellular metabolism. The human nervous system consumes about 20 percent of the entire body's oxygen reserves as carried by the **erythrocytes**, or red blood cells. The b.v. of an individual can be measured by injecting a sample of the person's own red blood cells tagged with a radioactive tracer into his circulation. A second measured sample removed about ten minutes later and analyzed for radioactivity levels will reveal the amount of dilution and by extrapolation the amount of blood in the subject's body. Also called **blood supply.**

B love = BEING LOVE.

blow = COCAINE.

blue bloater a popular term for a patient who is afflicted with **Type B chronic bronchitis**. The individual may appear healthy except for signs of cyanosis in the lips and fingernails. During a period of respiratory infection, such as a cold or influenza, the b.b. shows definite signs of bluish lips and nail beds, due to lack of oxygenated blood, and edema, which may cause the body to swell. Abbrev: **BB.** Also see PINK PUFFER.

blue-collar therapy a therapeutic approach developed by the William Alanson White Institute and worker organizations for low-income patients who do not relate well to middle-class therapists and their techniques. The emphasis is on external or physical causes, present situations rather than early childhood experiences, the alleviation of symptoms, a directive approach, and concrete solutions to problems. Other features are role-playing centered on the patient's problems, the use of nonprofessional auxiliaries, or "indigenous nonprofessionals," as helpers, and involvement in activity groups.

blue-yellow blindness a rare type of partial color blindness marked by blue and yellow confusion.

blunted affect a disturbance of affectivity in which feeling tone is dulled. It was cited by Bleuler as one of the basic symptoms of schizophrenia, but is also observed in presenile and senile brain disease.

blushing an involuntary autonomic rush of blood to the skin (**hyperemia**) as a normal reaction to embarrassment or self-consciousness, or, if persistent, a conversion symptom stemming from unconscious feelings of guilt, sexual reactions, or shame. Also see ERYTHROPHOBIA.

B motivation = METAMOTIVATION.

boarding homes community-living facilities for the mentally retarded or mentally ill who may be able to work in business or industry or sheltered workshops. Also called **adult foster homes**. The terms boarding home and adult foster home are often used interchangeably with HALFWAY HOUSE. See this entry.

boarding-out system a system in which psychotic patients are cared for in private homes. See GHEEL COLONY.

bodily ego feeling the bodily self or the experienced composite representation of the body that is the core of the ego. See BODY EGO.

body awareness the perception of one's body structure as a component of the image of self. The body image is derived from internal sensations, movement, and contact with the external world. In emotionally disturbed children, b.a. may be lacking or distorted.

body boundaries a component of the body image, consisting of the definiteness or indefiniteness of the boundary of the body. Rorschach responses such as turtle with shell and man in armor and other such **barrier responses** indicate a definite body boundary, while responses like person bleeding, a torn coat, and other penetration responses indicate indefinite boundaries. High barrier scores are characteristic of individuals with rheumatic arthritis and conversion symptoms, while low barrier scores correlate with gastric ulcers and colitis.

body buffer zone the physical distance toward a second person which the subject experiences as uncomfortable. The distance is shorter toward the front than toward the rear, and studies show that the greater the b.b.z., the more aggressive the individual.

body build a general measure of the body in terms of trunk, limb length, and girth.

body-build index an index of constitutional types proposed by H. J. Eysenck. Individuals are grouped according to this formula: height times 100 divided by six times the transverse chest diameter. Mesomorphs fall within one standard deviation of the mean; leptomorphs one standard deviation or more above the mean; and eurymorphs one standard deviation or more below the mean.

body cathexis the investment of psychic energy in the subject's own body; the emotional attachment to one's body.

body cell a term sometimes applied to a tissue cell that is not a germ cell. Also called **somatic cell**.

body concept the thoughts, feelings, and perceptions that comprise the way we view our body; the conceptual image of one's body. See BODY PERCEPT.

body-contact-exploration maneuver an encounter-group technique in which the participants touch or stroke each other in order to increase awareness of the sensations and emotions evoked by this type of experience.

body ego the nucleus around which all the perceptions of the self are grouped, that is, our individual memories, sensations, ideas, wishes, strivings, and fantasies.

body-ego concept the mental representations of the body as the nucleus of the self, or ego. The b.-e.c. is derived from sensations, perceptions, fantasies, feelings, and emotions associated with our BODY IMAGE. See this entry.

body ideal the body type considered attractive and age-appropriate by one's culture.

body identity the concept of one's own body, independently and apart from all other objects in space.

body image the mental picture we form of our body as a whole, including both its physical and functional characteristics (body percept), and our attitudes toward these characteristics (body concept). Our b.i. stems from both conscious and unconscious sources and is a basic component of our concept of self. See BODY EGO; BODY SCHEMA.

body-image distortion a term used to refer to the perceptual distortion of the body experienced during altered states of consciousness; e.g., an individual may feel detached from his body, or parts of the body may be experienced differently or appear larger or smaller than usual.

body-image disturbance psychological maladjustments stemming from deformity, disfigurement, or dismemberment (Schilder, 1950). Reactions vary from slight self-consciousness to deep depression and paranoid states, and are relatively mild where the defect is congenital or acquired early in life, since the defect is likely to be incorporated in the body image during the process of development. Also see PHANTOM LIMB; BREAST-PHANTOM PHENOMENON.

body-image hallucinations false perceptions or fantasies of one's body, particularly with respect to size. Examples of b.-i.h. are found in *Gulliver's Travel* and *Alice in Wonderland* stories. Some psychotic patients experience b.-i.h. in which body parts appear to be transplanted to other regions of the body. See LILLIPUTIAN HALLUCINATION.

body language the expression of unconscious feelings, impulses, and conflicts through organs of the body, as in conversion symptoms, or through posture, gesture, facial expression, and other forms of nonverbal communication. One of the major objectives of psychotherapy is to translate and interpret the language of the body. The term is often used interchangeably with organ language.

body-mind dichotomy the division between the somatic and psychic spheres in psychosomatic medicine, which raises theoretical questions about the relation between the two sets of factors in the etiology of disease: Why do they covary? Which takes the lead? Is there feedback between them? Is constitutional predisposition a factor? Where do social and ecological influences enter in?

body-mind problem the question of the relationship between mental and physical processes, between psyche and soma. The major concepts are (a) **interactionism**, or mutual influence, (b) **parallelism**, or separate processes with a point-to-point correspondence, (c) **idealism**: only mind exists, and the soma is a function of the psyche, (d) **double-aspect theory**: body and mind are both functions of a common entity, (e) **epiphenomenalism**: mind is a by-product of bodily processes, (f) **materialism**: body is the only reality and the psyche is non-existent, and (g) **dualism**: mind and body are distinct entities, each functioning according to its own principles.

body-monitoring a term introduced by B. Neugarten for close observation of one's body functions, especially changes in sexual response, vigor, and general health during middle and old age, which leads to various strategies to preserve performance and appearance.

body narcissism an exaggerated concern with the body and its erotic zones. According to psychoanalytic theory, this is particularly evident in the phallic-oedipal years when both boys and girls become preoccupied with body functions, explore their bodies, and have an extreme dread of any body injury.

body odor the odor produced by the action of bacteria on skin secretions, such as perspiration which itself is nearly odorless. Attitudes toward b.o. vary in different cultures; e.g., Americans consider b.o. offensive while in certain Middle Eastern countries it is inoffensive. In environmental-psychology tests, subjects generally agree that b.o. is associated with fat, nervous, unintelligent, unsociable, dirty, unattractive, unhealthy people.

body percept the mental image we form of the physical characteristics of our body, that is, whether we are slim or stocky, strong or weak, attractive or unattractive, tall or short. The b.p. may or may not conform to reality since it is influenced by our body concept. See BODY CONCEPT; BODY IMAGE.

body protest a term introduced by E. L. Richards for physical disorders that serve as an outlet for frustrations and anxieties.

body schema the pattern of the body as viewed by the individual; the body percept formed on the basis of touch, movement, posture, and overall structure. Also called **body scheme**.

body sores: See DECUBITI.

body therapies the relief of psychological tensions and other symptoms through body manipulation, relaxation, massage, breathing exercises, and changes in posture and position of body parts, on the theory that the body and its functioning embodies the individual's basic personality and way of life. See BIOENERGETICS; ROLFING; RELAXATION THERAPY; AUTOGENIC TRAINING.

body type a classification of individuals according to body build or physique. For examples, see CONSTITUTIONAL TYPE; ECTOMORPH; ENDOMORPH; MESOMORPH; ASTHENIC TYPE; ATHLETIC TYPE; DYSPLASTIC TYPE; PYKNIC TYPE.

Boeck, Karl Wilhelm Norwegian dermatologist, 1808–75. See DANIELSSEN-BOECK DISEASE.

Boehm Test of Basic Concepts a test designed to assess knowledge of concepts frequently used but often misunderstood by kindergarten and first-grade children. The concepts are classified under **Space** (location, orientation, dimension), **Quantity** (including numbers), **Time**, and miscellaneous. Examples are: marking pictures that show an equal number of lollipops, and marking a box that is away from a table.

Boerjeson: See BÖRJESON.

Bogardus, Emory Stephen American sociologist, 1882—. BOGARDUS SOCIAL-DISTANCE SCALE; FAD.

Bogardus social-distance scale a measure of the degree of acceptance or rejection between individuals and members of different ethnic, national, and social groups.

Bogen cage /bō'gən/ a maze test in which a ball is moved with a stick toward the exit by the shortest possible route.

Bogorad, F. A. Russian physician, fl. 1928. See BOGORAD'S SYNDROME.

Bogorad's syndrome a disorder apparently caused by an anomaly of cranial-nerve fibers resulting in profuse lacrimation by the patient when eating or drinking. The condition sometimes follows an attack of facial palsy. Also called **crocodile tears; gustolacrimal reflex**.

Bohemian unconcernedness a group of personality traits consisting of a tendency toward unconventionality, eccentricity, and hysterical upsets. R. B. Cattell considered these to be underlying traits, or source traits, of a particular type of personality, parallel to such traits as cyclothymic and schizothymic in personalities of these types.

boiler-makers deafness a high-frequency hearing loss resulting from exposure to high-intensity noise. The condition has been known for many years and is especially relevant today due to the increased noise of highly industrialized society. Acoustic trauma may also be due to the intense sound-level pressures of contemporary music.

bolek-hena: See JUSTITIA PECTORALIS STENOPHYLLA.

Bolgar, Hedda Swiss-born American psychologist, 1909—. See BOLGAR-FISCHER WORLD TEST.

Bolgar-Fischer World Test a projective test in which the subject reveals his attitudes and orientation to reality by constructing a miniature "world" out of toy houses, animals, figurines, cars, trees, and a wide variety of other objects which he selects from a chest containing 200 different items.

BOLT = USES BASIC OCCUPATIONAL LITERACY TEST.

bondage a form of mock enslavement of one person by another to arouse sexual pleasure in one or both partners. The b. scenario, which usually is accompanied by threats or acts of danger and humiliation, may involve heterosexual or homosexual participants. The enslaved person may be immobilized with ropes, straps, chains, or other restraining devices.

bondage and discipline a phase of sexual bondage that is accompanied by acts of sadomasochism such as whipping. B.a.d. sometimes is offered as a service of prostitutes. Because of the potential physical danger, the partners usually agree upon a signal to be used when the erotic activity exceeds the pleasurable limits.

bonding a close attachment, or affiliation, between individuals and groups, which is present in normal behavior but absent in some psychiatric disorders such as in the sociopathic personality. Also called **affiliative b.**

bone bowing: See BOWING OF BONES.

bone conduction the transmission of sound waves to the inner ear through vibrations of bones in the skull.

bone-conduction testing an audiological procedure to determine if the hearing loss detected in air-conduction testing is due to conductive or sensorineural factors. It is performed at controlled frequencies with a small bone-conduction vibrator, attached to a headband, placed on the temporal bone behind the ear.

bone disease any pathologic change in bone tissue that may be congenital or acquired. Kinds of b.d. include osteoporosis, characterized by brittleness and porosity in the bone; osteomyelitis, caused by an infection that spreads to the bone tissue; osteomalacia and rickets, the adult and childhood versions of a softening of the bones due to an imbalance of calcium and phosphorus in the bone tissue; osteoma, a bone tumor that can be either benign or malignant; and osteitis fibrosa cystica, marked by the replacement of bone calcium by fibrous tissue because of a malfunction of the parathyroid glands. Several types of dwarfism are due to hereditary defects in bone development, e.g., pseudoachondroplasia, diastrophic dwarfism, and achondroplasia.

bone marrow a soft spongelike material in the hollow areas of bones, particularly in the long bones. The b.m. actually consists of blood vessels and special connective tissue fibers plus fat and blood-forming tissues. The function of b.m. is the production of red and white blood cells and blood platelets. The b.m. is highly sensitive to diseases and environmental agents, e.g., chemicals and radiation.

bone-marrow diseases diseases in which the bone marrow is underactive or overactive. In Cooley's anemia it is hyperactive in order to compensate for the rapid destruction of red blood cells, sometimes resulting in brittle bones and thickening of the cranial bones, which may produce a protuberant upper jaw and mongoloid facial features. In leukemia there is an underproduction of red blood cells (and overproduction of abnormal white cells) due to dysfunction of the bone marrow as well as the lymph nodes and spleen.

bone-pointing: See VOODOO DEATH.

Bonhoeffer, Karl /bôn′hœfər/ German psychiatrist, 1868–1948. See BONHOEFFER'S SYMPTOM.

Bonhoeffer's symptom the loss of muscle tonus associated with chorea.

Bonnet, Charles /bône′/ Swiss naturalist, 1720–93. See CHARLES BONNET'S SYNDROME.

Bonnet's syndrome = CHARLES BONNET'S SYNDROME.

Bonnevie, Kristine Elisabeth Heuch Norwegian biologist, 1872–1950. See BONNEVIE-ULLRICH SYNDROME; NIELSEN'S DISEASE.

Bonnevie-Ullrich syndrome an apparently congenital disorder involving abnormalities of bones and muscles, associated with disorders of the cranial nerves. The condition sometimes is found as a part of Nielsen's disease with symptoms of the Klippel-Feil syndrome that include deafness and mental retardation. Also see NIELSEN'S DISEASE.

Bonnier, Pierre /bônyā′/ French physician, 1861–1918. See BONNIER'S SYNDROME.

Bonnier's syndrome symptoms of vertigo, locomotor weakness, apprehension, tachycardia, somnolence, and trigeminal neuralgia caused by lesions of Deiters' nucleus, which receives incoming fibers from the vestibular nerve. Also called **Deiters' nucleus syndrome**.

book fear = BIBLIOPHOBIA.

books for the blind: See TALKING BOOKS.

borderline pertaining to any phenomenon difficult to categorize because it straddles two distinct classes, showing characteristics of both. Thus, b. intelligence shows characteristics of the normal and deficient categories. In psychiatry, a **b. state** shows both neurotic and psychotic reactions, as in a person who is likely to become psychotic but who at present retains contact with reality.

borderline disorders a relatively vague term denoting a group of psychological conditions that lie between normality and neurosis, between neurosis and psychosis, or between normal intelligence and mental retardation. Schmideberg (1959) includes such subgroups as "depressives, schizoids, paranoids, querulents, hypochondriacs, antisocials, and mixed cases." DSM-III categories include SCHIZOID-PERSONALITY DISORDER, SCHIZOTYPAL-PERSONALITY DISORDER, BORDERLINE PERSONALITY DISORDER, and BORDERLINE INTELLECTUAL FUNCTIONING. See these entries. Also see BORDERLINE SYNDROME.

borderline intellectual functioning an intelligence level between low normal and mentally retarded. Also called **borderline intelligence**. (DSM-III)

borderline mental retardation a level between clearly normal and clearly subnormal intelligence. Some researchers define it as an IQ between 68 and 83, others as any IQ in the 70s.

borderline personality disorder a personality disorder characterized by a long-standing pattern of instability in mood, interpersonal relationships, and self-image which is severe enough to cause extreme distress or interfere with social and occupational functioning. Among the manifestations of this disorder are self-damaging behavior, in such areas as gambling, sex, spending, overeating, and substance use; intense but unstable relationships; uncontrollable temper outbursts; uncertainty about self-image, gender, goals, and loyalties; shifting moods; self-defeating behavior, such as fights, suicidal gestures, or self-mutilation; and chronic feelings of emptiness and boredom. (DSM-III)

borderline psychosis a condition in which the individual exhibits psychotic tendencies and employs psychotic mechanisms when under stress, but on the whole is still in touch with reality. According to Fenichel, "to this group belong . . . psychopaths, abortive paranoids, and many 'apathic' individuals whom one may call hebephrenoid personalities." For specific types, see AMBULATORY SCHIZOPHRENIA; PRESCHIZOPHRENIC EGO; PSEUDONEUROTIC SCHIZOPHRENIA.

borderline schizophrenia a term sometimes applied to the condition of an individual who is potentially schizophrenic but has not broken with reality, although he may exhibit schizophrenic reactions when faced with frustrations.

borderline state: See BORDERLINE.

borderline syndrome a general, loosely used term applied to patients who exhibit a combination of characteristics and tendencies associated with neurosis, psychosis, or character disorders, yet do not show a specific symptom pattern. Among these characteristics are low tolerance for frustration, poor judgment, inability to establish normal sexual or love relationships, lack of repression, and absence of empathy or feeling for others. Borderline individuals usually give up one job after another and are likely to drift into unemployment, alcoholism, and petty crime. Also see BORDERLINE DISORDERS.

boredom loss of interest in a particular activity accompanied by wandering attention and lack of motivation. Inability to respond to any activity, no matter how meaningful or stimulating it is to others, is considered pathological. B. is a common sociopsychological problem among adolescents, the aged, and workers in monotonous jobs. Also see DIVERSIVE EXPLORATION.

Börjeson, Mats Gunnar Swedish physician, 1922—. See BÖRJESON-FORSSMAN-LEHMANN SYNDROME.

Börjeson-Forssman-Lehmann syndrome a disorder characterized by microcephaly, severe mental retardation, short stature, and hypogonadism. All patients showed IQs estimated at between 20 and 40, and had little or no pubic hair, even as adults. The syndrome may be related to an X-linked recessive mutant gene.

bottle feeding: See FEEDING TECHNIQUES.

botulineal spores the spores of the bacterium Clostridium botulinum that produce the highly active neurotoxin botulin. The term is derived from the Latin word *botulus*, "sausage," referring to the earlier association between botulism and sausage poisoning.

Bouchard, Charles Jacques /bōōshär′/ French physician, 1837–1915. See CHARCOT-BOUCHARD ANEURYSM.

bouffées délirantes: See ACUTE DELUSIONAL PSYCHOSIS.

Bouillaud, Jean B. /bōōyō′/ French physician, 1796–1881. See BOUILLAUD'S DISEASE.

Bouillaud's disease acute rheumatic fever with carditis (inflammation of the heart).

boulimia = BULIMIA.

boundary detectors optic-nerve fibers that respond to a sharp edge in a receptive field, regardlesss of brightness or contrast on either side of the edge. B.d. are part of the specialized visual system of amphibia.

boundary system in general-systems theory, the semipermeable boundaries between living systems, permitting information to proceed in either direction but posing the question of how much interpenetration and interdependence is feasible in a given social system. Also see EGO BOUNDARIES.

bound energy ego energy that is used to deal with reality rather than fantasy or repression.

Bourneville, Désiré-Magloire /bōōrnvēl′/ French neurologist, 1840–1909. See TUBEROUS SCLEROSIS (also called **Bourneville's disease**).

boutons terminaux = SYNAPTIC KNOBS.

bovarism failure to differentiate between fantasy and reality (a theme of the Flaubert novel *Madame Bovary*).

bowel control the ability to regulate defecation so that elimination occurs in the proper place at the proper time. On the average, b.c. begins at about six months of age and is fairly complete by age two. See TOILET TRAINING.

bowel disorders in psychiatry, disorders of the bowels that frequently occur as responses to stress and anxiety. In some cases, transient disturbances such as constipation and diarrhea may occur as side effects of psychotropic drugs. Major b.d., which may be psychologically caused or aggravated, include chronic constipation, irritable-bowel syndrome, mucus colitis, and ulcerative colitis.

bowel training: See BOWEL CONTROL.

bowing of bones deformities of bone structure generally associated with faulty mineralization of the tissues, as in osteomalacia and rickets, resulting in a softening of the long bones, which become bowed rather than straight. The condition occurs most frequently in weight-bearing bones, e.g., the femur and tibia. In true bowlegs, or genu varum, the knees are farther apart than normal and the patient tends to walk with the feet turned inward. In knock-knee, or genu valgum, the knees are abnormally close together when the patient is standing. A third variation of the leg-bone deformity is genu recurvatum, marked by a hyperextension of the knees with little ability to flex them. B.o.b. may be an occupational deformity, e.g., of jockeys or cowboys, and also can result from PAGET'S DISEASE. See this entry.

bowlegs: See BOWING OF BONES.

bow-wow theory: See ORIGIN-OF-LANGUAGE THEORIES.

boxer's dementia a chronic, slowly progressive brain disorder resulting from scattered petechial hemorrhages produced by repeated blows to the head. Common symptoms of being "punchdrunk" are mild mental confusion, uncertain balance, inability to concentrate, and involuntary movements. The term is often applied to the more advanced cases, while **boxer's traumatic encephalopathy** refers to all types of cases. Also called **dementia pugilistica**.

Boyle's disease = GENERAL PARESIS.

BPRS = BRIEF PSYCHIATRIC RATING SCALE.

BRAC = BASIC REST-ACTIVITY CYCLE.

braces devices that give support to a moving part of the body, e.g., the limbs. B. are intended for permanent or long-term use, as opposed to splints, which are used for temporary support. B. may be jointed to permit flexion and often are attached to garments, such as shoes. For patients with neuromuscular damage, b. may be designed to assist in movement of the affected limb or limbs.

-brachi-; -brachio- a combining form relating to the arm.

brachium a part of the interior structure of the cerebellum, forming the lateral wall on either side of the fourth ventricle. Its fibers originate in the dentate nucleus and are a part of the cerebellorubrospinal pathway. The term also is applied to the midbrain structures: the **superior b.**, which carries visual-cortex fibers, and the **inferior b.**, which carries auditory-cortex fibers.

brachium conjunctivum a peduncle or band of fibrous tissue extending upward from each hemisphere of the cerebellum. The b.c. from one side joins the other to form the walls and part of the roof of the fourth ventricle of the brain.

Brachman-de Lange syndrome: See DE LANGE'S SYNDROME.

-brachy- a combining form meaning short.

brachycephaly a condition marked by a skull that is abnormally short and wide. On the cephalic index scale of head proportions, a b. skull is rated between 81 and 85. Also called **brachycephalism**. Adjective: **brachycephalic**.

brachymorph a body type characterized by an abnormally short, broad physique. Also called

brachytype; brevitype. Adjectives: **brachymorphic; brachylineal; brevilineal.**

brachyskeletal a term applied to a person with abnormally short bones, particularly short leg bones.

brachytype = BRACHYMORPH.

-brady- a combining form meaning slow.

bradyarthria = BRADYLALIA.

bradycardia a slow heartbeat due to an organic or psychogenic condition. See ARRHYTHMIA.

bradyglossia slowness of speech that is due to organic causes, e.g., neural lesions or a disease or anomaly involving the mouth or tongue.

bradykinesia abnormal slowness of movements with a decrease in spontaneous motor activity, due to psychogenic or organic factors. **Functional b.** is most commonly found in depression and schizophrenia. Also caled **bradykinesis.**

bradylalia abnormally slow speech. It is common in depression, senile brain disorder, general paresis, and emotionally inhibited individuals. Also called **bradyarthria.**

bradylexia extreme slowness in reading. It is a common symptom of depression, mental retardation, and learning disability.

bradylogia a functional disorder marked by abnormally slow speech.

bradyphrasia = HYPOPHRASIA.

bradyphrenia sluggish mental processes associated with severe anxiety or depression, since intense emotional states tend to interfere with thinking. The term is sometimes used as a synonym for psychomotor retardation, and is occasionally used for mental retardation.

bradypragia slowness of action due to an organic disorder such as myxedema.

Braid, James British medical writer, ca. 1795–1860. B. is chiefly noted for his attacks on animal magnetism and his introduction of the term hypnotism, which he described as a state of sleep induced by psychological rather than physical forces. See BRAID'S STRABISMUS; BRAIDISM.

braid-cutting a sadistic hair fetish in which the victim's hair is cut. In psychoanalysis, b.c. is regarded as a symbol of castration in which knowledge that the hair will grow back is a reassurance that castration need not be final.

Braidism an obsolete term for hypnotism, named for James Braid, who coined the word hypnosis.

Braid's strabismus a form of strabismus in which hypnosis can be induced by causing the eyes to converge and turn upward.

braille /brāl/ a system of letters, numbers, punctuation marks, and scientific and musical symbols adapted as a written language for the blind from combinations of raised dots or points, as on the surface of a sheet of paper. The basic alphabet consists of six dots organized in two parallel vertical columns. A dot in the No. 6 position makes the following letter a capital; dots in the 3,4,5,6 positions advise the reader that the following character is a number rather than a letter. More than 200 contractions, short-form words, or re-

curring letter combinations can be formed by different patterns of the six dots; e.g., the word "and" is represented by dots 1,2,3,4,6, while dot No. 5, placed before a combination of dots 1,4,5 (the code for the letter "d"), becomes a contraction for the word "day." The system was devised by the French teacher Louis Braille.

Braille, Louis /brä′yə/ or /brel/ French teacher, 1809–52. See BRAILLE /brāl/.

Brailsford, James Frederick English radiologist, 1888—. See MORQUIO'S SYNDROME (also called **Brailsford-Morquio syndrome**).

brain the mass of CNS nerve tissues, including the cerebrum and related structures, within the skull. Though the b. weighs only about three pounds, the outer layer (the cortex) alone contains over ten billion nerve cells of two general kinds: association fibers, which connect one part of the brain to another, and projection fibers, which carry messages to and from organs in the rest of the body. The complexity of the b. is indescribable, but in gross anatomy it is divided into two hemispheres bridged by the corpus callosum, and is divided by deep fissures into four lobes, each with special functions. Also called **encephalon.** See FRONTAL LOBE; OCCIPITAL LOBE; PARIETAL LOBE; TEMPORAL LOBE; SPLIT B.; CEREBRUM; ARCHAIC B.; ARCUATE ZONE OF THE B.; FOREBRAIN; EVOLUTION OF B.

brain abscess a circumscribed collection of pus that may occur in any part of the brain. The infection may produce an organic mental disorder, or neurological symptoms such as dysarthria or hemiparesis.

brain atlas a collection of illustrations of details of brain structure.

brain atrophy degeneration of cerebral nerve fibers occurring, e.g., in senile dementia, cerebral arteriosclerosis, epidemic encephalitis, Alzheimer's disease, Pick's disease, Huntington's disease, and Charcot-Marie-Tooth disease.

brain bank a parkinsonism-research program established by the Columbia University Medical School to enable medical scientists to conduct intensive pathological studies into causes and treatments of the disease. The b.b. consists of a registry of parkinsonism patients who have agreed to bequeath their brains for research.

brain control the manipulation of brain functions by electrical, chemical, or other devices, for experimental or therapeutic purposes. An example is psychic surgery.

brain damage injury to the brain caused by such conditions as prenatal infection, Rh incompatibility, birth injury, head trauma, toxic agents, brain tumor, brain inflammation, severe seizures, certain metabolic disorders (e.g., Wilson's disease), vitamin deficiency, intracranial hemorrhage, stroke, and surgical procedures. B.d. usually is identified as a lesion and is reflected in a behavioral or functional abnormality; e.g., persons with lesions of the frontal lobes of the brain tend to perform poorly on tests of abstraction.

brain-damage language disorders any loss of ability to communicate effectively by means of symbolic stimuli. It includes sensory and motor aphasias. See APHASIA; ALEXIA.

brain death the cessation of neurologic signs of life. In 1973, the American Neurological Association adopted a definition of b.d. as that of human death; and a 1974 California law states that a person shall be "pronounced dead if it is determined that the person has suffered total and irreversible cessation of brain function." The concept of b.d. has been accepted by the Roman Catholic Church. There are variations in the interpretation of the b.d. concept, but generally excluded are cases of brain-damaged persons living in a vegetative state, cases involving hypothermia or cases of drug overdose marked by absence of normal brain-wave activity. Medical criteria include absence of reflex response or response to noxious stimuli, absence of blinking, swallowing, or movement of eyeballs when ice water is injected into the ear canals, and absence of EEG activity. However, absence of EEG activity alone is not a final diagnostic sign. But a diagnosis of b.d. cannot be made if there is any sign of EEG activity.

brain-disease fear = MENINGITOPHOBIA.

brain diseases a group of diseases that affect the brain and its functions. Examples include epidemic encephalitis, senile brain disease, presenile brain disease (Pick's; Alzheimer's), Parkinson's disease, cerebral meningitis, meningovascular syphilis, and tuberous sclerosis.

brain disorders a DSM-I term for a group of acute or chronic mental disorders caused by or associated with impairment of brain-tissue function, and characterized by mild-to-severe impairment of orientation, memory, judgment, general intellectual functions, and affect. Also called **brain syndromes**. In DSM-II, the term b.d. was replaced by "organic brain syndromes," and in DSM-III, by ORGANIC MENTAL DISORDERS. See this entry. Also see ACUTE BRAIN DISORDER; CHRONIC B.D.

brain-injured child a child who before, during, or after birth suffered from an infection or injury to the brain. The results of such organic impairment are reflected in communication and learning problems.

brain lesion any damage to an area of brain tissue caused by injury, surgery, tumor, CVA, or infection.

brain nuclei clusters of cells within the cerebrum.

brain pathology the study of any disorder of the brain due to disease or injury.

brain potential the electrical potential of brain cells. See ELECTROENCEPHALOGRAPH.

brain research investigation of the structure and functions of the brain through scientific experimentation and naturalistic observation. Among the specific techniques used are (a) psychological and neurological tests administered after lesions have occurred in various areas, (b) observation or measurement of the effects of stimulation or extirpation of parts of the animal brain, (c) behavioral methods that demonstrate the systematic collaboration of several areas of the brain in complex functions like writing, (d) the study of the electrical properties of the cortex, as well as the nature and functions of chemicals involved in neurotransmission, and (e) the use of such methods as electroencephalography, radioisotopic encephalography, and the CAT scan to assess the extent and location of brain damage associated with such conditions as epilepsy, brain hemorrhage, and brain tumor.

brain scan a diagnostic technique in which radioisotopes are injected into the patient's blood. The brain is then examined with a scanning device that detects the distribution of the radioactivity. Normal brain tissue will show little if any uptake of radioactive material, but the radioactive substance will tend to accumulate in a region of tissue abnormality; this represents alteration of the blood-brain barrier. The CAT scan has reduced the need for and performance of this test. Also see POSITRON EMISSION TOMOGRAPHY; DIGITAL ANGIOGRAPHY; COMPUTERIZED AXIAL TOMOGRAPHY.

brain-splitting surgical separation of the cerebral hemispheres. The procedure may be experimental in laboratory animals but is performed in humans for therapeutic purposes, as in the treatment of infantile hemiplegia, to remove a malignant tumor, or for control of a severe adult form of epilepsy. See HEMIDECORTICATION.

brainstem the nervous tissues of the brain, including the pons, medulla oblongata, and midbrain, that connect the cerebral hemispheres with the spinal cord.

brainstem encephalitis = BICKERSTAFF'S ENCEPHALITIS.

brain stimulation stimulation of all of the brain or activation of specific areas of the brain, such as the amygdala, as a means of determining their effects on behavior. Kinds of b.s. include **areal b.s.**, when an extended portion of a sense organ is stimulated, **audio b.s.**, when the sense of hearing is stimulated, and **cerebral b.s.**, when the cerebrum is stimulated, as in learning situations. See BRAIN RESEARCH.

brainstorming stimulation of innovative ideas by creating a "wild and free" atmosphere where "anything goes." The technique was first used in advertising to stimulate the creation of original solutions to problems. In b. sessions, people working alone or more commonly in groups are encouraged to freely suggest any idea or solution without group criticism or any evaluation until all ideas have been expressed.

brain syndromes = BRAIN DISORDERS.

brain trauma physical injury to the brain produced, e.g., by a blow to the head, a gun wound, or a cerebrovascular accident. See HEAD TRAUMA; ACUTE TRAUMATIC DISORDER; CHRONIC TRAUMATIC DISORDER; INTRACRANIAL HEMORRHAGE.

brain tumor any abnormal tissue growth within the confines of the skull. The skull itself is a limiting factor for the space a tumor can occupy, so any new growth is likely to compress neighboring brain tissue and disrupt normal brain functions. The cause of b.t. is unknown, but it can occur at any age, producing initial symptoms of headache, nausea, or sudden vomiting without apparent cause. As the b.t. progresses, the patient usually experiences disturbances of perception in the visual, auditory, and olfactory senses, loss of coordination, weakness, and paralysis. Convulsions sometimes are caused by a b.t. Personality changes may take the form of memory lapses, absent-mindedness, loss of initiative, or generally slow reactions to mental stimuli. Surgery is the method of b.t. treatment.

brainwashing the combination of coercive propaganda techniques systematically applied to political prisoners or prisoners of war under planned conditions of physical and emotional intimidation. The ultimate goal is to produce attitude changes through subversion of the prisoner's morale and system of values followed by imposition of a new system of beliefs.

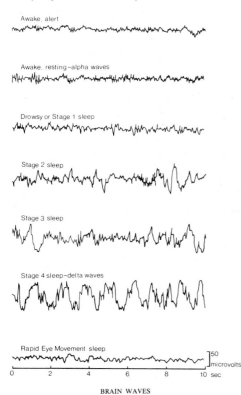

Awake, alert

Awake, resting–alpha waves

Drowsy or Stage 1 sleep

Stage 2 sleep

Stage 3 sleep

Stage 4 sleep–delta waves

Rapid Eye Movement sleep

50 microvolts

0   2   4   6   8   10 sec

BRAIN WAVES

brain waves spontaneous, rhythmic electrical impulses emanating from different areas of the brain as long as it is alive. The first substantial account of these waves was given by the German physiologist Hans Berger in 1929, which arose out of an investigation of the possibility of ex-

trasensory perception and psychic phenomena. Brain-wave patterns appear to be relatively stable for each individual and are currently used in diagnosing brain lesions, tumors, and epilepsy, but not neurotic or psychotic disorders. Also called **Berger rhythms**. See ALPHA WAVES; BETA WAVES; DELTA WAVES; GAMMA WAVES; KAPPA WAVES; THETA WAVES; SPINDLE WAVES; SAW-TOOTH WAVES; SPIKE-WAVE ACTIVITY; ELECTROENCEPHALOGRAPH.

brain weight the weight of a brain, between 1,200 and 1,500 grams for an adult human. B.w. for elephants and whales may exceed 7,000 and 9,000 grams respectively. Human brain sizes usually increase until around the age of 21, then gradually diminish. B.w. apparently is not related to intellectual ability; one of the smallest brains ever examined belonged to French writer and Nobel Prize winner Anatole France.

branching program a form of programed instruction that provides additional steps, or branches, to be followed if the material has not been adequately mastered to the point in question. See PROGRAMED INSTRUCTION.

brand loyalty the tendency of consumers to purchase a particular brand consistently.

brand preference preference for a particular brand of cigarette, beer, margarine, or other products. Two types of tests are frequently used to determine if consumers can recognize their own brands: blindfold testing, and submission of unlabeled packages or bottles to a consumer panel.

brand-use survey a test of advertising psychology in which consumers are interviewed to determine whether they purchased a particular brand of product that was featured in a specific advertising appeal. The b.-u.s. may be accompanied by use of the pantry-check technique to validate results of the survey.

Bray, Charles William American otologist, 1904—. See WEVER-BRAY EFFECT.

breakdown: See NERVOUS B.

breakthrough a major or significant advance in knowledge, research, or treatment; also, a sudden forward step in therapy, especially after a plateau.

breast complex in psychoanalysis, the substitution of the possessed penis for the mother's breast that has been withheld or denied. The b.c. may manifest itself as breast envy or a form of homosexuality in which the penis unconsciously represents the breast. Also see GOOD BREAST; BAD BREAST.

breast envy the psychoanalytic theory that males who have repressed a breast complex as infants may later ignore the female breasts and develop overt homosexual traits, or that they may deny the importance of the female breasts by becoming sexually excited only if the female partner sucks their breasts. See BREAST COMPLEX.

breast feeding: See FEEDING TECHNIQUES.

breast-phantom phenomenon the illusion that an amputated breast is still there. The breast, or breast prosthesis, is still included in the body image, and in many cases the woman feels tingling and, occasionally, painful sensations in the missing organ, and in some instances she denies that it has been removed. Also see PHANTOM LIMB.

breast self-examination a technique for the early detection of breast tumors in women who train themselves to perform the monthly procedure. The procedure includes seven steps of visual examination before a mirror and palpation of each quarter of the breast and armpit on each side. B.s.-e. is performed immediately after menstruation when the breasts are usually soft. If any lump is felt during the examination, it is reported to a physician.

breathing the mechanism of respiration, or the cycles of alternate inhalation and exhalation. The term often is accompanied by an adjective to identify a particular type of b., such as abdominal b. or diaphragmatic b.

breathy voice a voice characterized by an excessive emission of breath. When the voice is both weak and breathy, the condition is sometimes described as **phonasthenia**. B.v. may be due to tension, defense against voicing unacceptable feelings, or debility.

breech birth: See BIRTH INJURY.

Brentano, Franz German philosopher and psychologist, 1838–1917. In opposition to Wundt's emphasis on mental contents, B. described all psychological phenomena in terms of mental processes or "acts" of three kinds: ideating, judging, and feeling. His views paved the way to Gestalt psychology, with its emphasis on perception; and to the psychodynamic approach, which views the mind as an agent rather than a receptor. See ACT PSYCHOLOGY; INTENTIONALITY.

Breuer, Josef /broi'ər/ Austrian physician, 1842–1925. B. was an early collaborator of Freud and introduced the "cathartic method" in which the patient talked out sexual feelings under hypnosis. He published *Studies in Hysteria* with Freud in 1895, recognized as the first book on psychoanalysis. See HERING-BREUER AFFECT; ABREACTION; CATHARSIS; DEFENSE HYSTERIA; HYPERESTHETIC MEMORY; STRANGULATED AFFECT; TALKING CURE.

brevilineal; brevitype: See BRACHYMORPH.

bridge to reality: See REMOTIVATION.

brief group therapy group therapy conducted on a crisis-intervention model, as contrasted with long-term group therapy.

Brief Psychiatric Rating Scale a system of evaluating clinical psychiatric signs on the basis of 18 factors, such as bizarre thinking, hostility, withdrawal, and anxiety. Abbrev.: **BPRS.**

brief psychotherapy = SHORT-TERM THERAPY.

brief reactive psychosis a syndrome involving emotional turmoil and at least one psychotic symptom (incoherence or loosening of associations, delusions, hallucinations, disorganized or catatonic behavior), following a period of stress involving, e.g., loss of a loved one. The condition develops suddenly and lasts from two hours to two weeks. (DSM-III)

brief-stimuli technique electroconvulsive therapy in which stimuli lasting from one-sixth to one-third millisecond are used. Some authorities claim that this technique diminishes the duration of memory impairment.

brief-stimulus therapy a mild form of electroconvulsive therapy.

Briggs, Lloyd Vernon American psychiatrist, 1863–1941. See BRIGGS' LAW.

Briggs' law a Massachusetts law which requires a psychiatric examination for a defendant in a criminal case who has been convicted or indicted previously for an offense. The purpose is to determine if the defendant suffers a mental illness that affects his responsibility.

Briggs-Myers Type Indicator = MYERS-BRIGGS TYPE INDICATOR.

Brigham, Amariah American physician, 1798–1849. Superintendent of the Hartford Retreat and later the New York State Lunatic Society, B. with twelve others organized the Association of Medical Superintendents of American Institutions for the Insane, which later evolved into the American Psychiatric Association. A strong advocate of humane treatment, he opposed blood-letting and physical restraint, and insisted that mental illness can be cured in its early stages.

brightness a dimension of color that correlates with the intensity of the physical stimulus; the dimension of brilliance, ranging from white (the highest value) to black (the lowest value). Bright colors reflect light to a greater extent than dark colors.

brightness adaptation a decrease in the brilliance of stimuli as general illumination increases.

brightness constancy the tendency to perceive a familiar object as having the same brightness under different conditions of illumination. That is, the object is experienced in the same way even though its stimulus properties have altered. B.c. is one of the perceptual constancies. Also see OBJECT CONSTANCY; PERCEPTUAL CONSTANCY.

brightness contrast the apparent brightness increment resulting from prior stimulation or simultaneous stimulation. E.g., a gray disk looks darker on a white background than on a black background.

brightness discrimination the ability to distinguish differences in brightness, which may appear to vary according to the wavelength of light.

brightness threshold the minimum intensity of light of a designated wavelength that can be detected against a surrounding field.

bril a brightness measurement equivalent to 1/100 of a millilambert.

Brill, Abraham Arden Austrian-American psychiatrist, 1874–1948. B. studied under Freud and Bleuler in Europe, and later became one of the first exponents of psychoanalysis in America, devoting himself to the translation of Freud's works, and applying a flexible Freudian approach to psychotic as well as neurotic patients. See SCHIZOID-MANIC STATE.

Briquet, Pierre /brike′/ French physician, 1796–1881. See BRIQUET'S ATAXIA; BRIQUET'S SYNDROME.

Briquet's ataxia a form of hysterical ataxia marked by loss of sensation in the skin and leg muscles.

Briquet's syndrome symptoms of apnea and aphonia due to hysterical paralysis of the diaphragm. As a polysymptomatic form of hysteria, B.s. is characterized by a vague but often dramatic medical history beginning in early adulthood, with numerous visits to many physicians, and a long list of disabling symptoms for which no organic disorder can be found.

Brissaud, Edouard /brisō′/ French neurologist, 1852–1909. See BRISSAUD'S DISEASE; BRISSAUD'S INFANTILISM; VARIABLE CHOREA OF BRISSAUD.

Brissaud-Meige syndrome = BRISSAUD'S INFANTILISM.

Brissaud's disease a neurogenic or psychogenic condition in which spasms or sudden recurrent movements are initiated voluntarily but cannot be stopped by voluntary control. The disorder is most likely to occur during childhood. See HABIT SPASM.

Brissaud's infantilism a developmental anomaly in which infantile mental and physical characteristics continue past puberty. The condition is the result of faulty functioning of the thyroid gland. Also called **infantile myxedema; Brissaud-Meige syndrome**.

British anti-Lewisite a poison antidote developed as an anti-gas-warfare agent, effective against Lewisite. B.a.-L. is used therapeutically to treat cases of poisoning by arsenic, gold, or mercury in humans and by heavy metals in general in animals. **Lewisite** was invented by an American chemist, W. Lee Lewis, as a lethal lung irritant for use in gas warfare. Abbrev.: **BAL**. Also called **dimercaprol**.

Broadbent, Sir William Henry English physician, 1835–1907. BROADBENT'S APOPLEXY; BROADBENT TEST.

Broadbent's apoplexy a type of cerebrovascular accident in which the hemorrhage originates outside the ventricles but continues until it infiltrates the interior of the ventricles by its own pressure. Also called **Broadbent's syndrome**.

Broadbent test a test of temporal-lobe-lesion effects, using a stereophonic tape recorder with headset that feeds different sets of digits into each ear at the same time. The lobe with the lesion is unable to compete effectively with the normal lobe, as measured by the ability of the patient to repeat the digits heard in the ear on the opposite side. Words and music may be substituted for digits.

Broadman; Broadmann: See BRODMANN.

broad-thumb-hallux syndrome = RUBINSTEIN-TAYBI SYNDROME.

Broca, Paul French physiologist and surgeon, 1824–80. B. was an authority on aphasia and the localization of function, including speech, in the cerebral cortex. See BROCA'S AREA; BROCA'S APHASIA; DESCRIPTIVE PSYCHIATRY; EXPRESSIVE APHASIA; LANGUAGE CENTERS; LANGUAGE LOCALIZATION; SPEECH AREAS; SPEECH IMPAIRMENT; SYMPATHETIC DYSPRAXIA; TRANSCORTICAL APHASIA; WORD FLUENCY.

Broca's aphasia primarily an expressive aphasia in which the patient has difficulty in speaking or writing words, but may still be able to use gestures. It is associated with a lesion in the posterior part of the inferior frontal convolution, a region of the brain sometimes identified as area 44. The patient is usually emotionally upset with this type of aphasia.

Broca's area a region of the posterior portion of the inferior frontal convolution of a hemisphere that is associated with the control of speech. It is located on the left hemisphere of right-handed persons and on the right hemisphere of left-handed individuals.

Brodmann, Korbinian /brōt′män/ German neurologist, 1868–1918. (His name is occasionally spelled Broadman or Broadmann.) See BRODMANN'S AREA; AGRANULAR CORTEX; CYTOARCHITECTONICS; ENTORHINAL-CORTEX LESION; INTERMEDIATE PRECENTRAL AREA; LIMBIC LOBE; MOTOR AREA; PRESTRIATE AREA; VISUAL CORTEX.

Brodmann's area one of several areas of the cerebral cortex characterized by six cell layers. They are identified by numbers and are believed to be associated with specific brain functions. Brodmann's original cerebral-cortex map identified 47 different areas; investigators in the past 50 years have expanded the mapping to identify more than 200 distinctive cortical areas. Also called **Brodmann's cytoarchitectonic area**.

Brodmann's area 4 = MOTOR AREA.

Brodmann's areas 18 and 19 = PRESTRIATE AREA.

Brodmann's area 6 = INTERMEDIATE PRECENTRAL AREA.

Brodmann's area 24 = LIMBIC LOBE.

Brodmann's cytoarchitectonic area = BRODMANN'S AREA.

broken home a single-parent home resulting from death, divorce, separation, desertion, or institutionalization.

-brom-; -broma- a combining form relating to food, nourishment (from Greek *broma*, "food").

-brom-; -bromo- a combining form denoting the presence of bromine (from Greek *bromos*, "noisome smell").

bromide an ion of the halogen category of elements that is widely used in medications and has a depressant effect on the central nervous system. The depressant action occurs gradually over a period of several days. B. may be administered to induce prolonged sedation or for its anti-

epileptic effects. Single doses required to produce sedative effects also cause vomiting. High
blood levels of b. cause impaired memory,
ataxia, disorientation, delirium, and coma.
Acute intoxication rarely occurs because overdoses result in vomiting. Chronic intoxication,
a condition called b. intoxication, is not uncommon, and CNS symptoms can mimic a wide variety
of psychiatric conditions. See B. INTOXICATION.

bromide hallucinosis an extended hallucinatory
state accompanied by marked fear reactions
occurring as a result of bromide intoxication.

bromide intoxication a toxic disorder caused by
excessive use of bromides, usually ingested to
relieve tension, induce sleep, or combat the
aftereffects of alcohol. The first signs are weakness, drowsiness, inability to concentrate, memory defect, dulling, tremor, acne, and unsteady
gait. Continued use may lead to **bromide
psychosis**, a schizophreniform psychosis characterized by apprehension, confusion, disorientation, delirium with hallucinations, paralysis, and clouding of consciousness, which may
last for ten days to two months. Also called
brominism.

bromidrosiphobia a morbid fear of offending with
one's body odors. Also see AUTOMYSOPHOBIA;
AUTODYSOSMOPHOBIA.

brominism: See BROMIDE INTOXICATION.

-bronch-; -bronchi-; -broncho-; -bronchio- a
combining form relating to the bronchial system.

bronchi /brong′kı/ the two main branches of the
windpipe (Greek *bronchoi*). Singular: **bronchus**.
Adjective: **bronchial**.

bronchial asthma = ASTHMA.

bronchial spasm: See SPASM.

bronchioles the smaller respiratory channels that
branch off from the bronchi. The b. become successively smaller as they extend into lung tissue,
becoming eventually a part of an alveolar terminus.

bronchodilator medications drugs administered
to patients afflicted with asthma, bronchitis, and
related respiratory disorders. The b.m. may include antibiotics, corticosteroids, and theophylline combinations. Some b.m. may produce
adverse neurologic effects; e.g., a combination
of the antibiotic erythromycin ethylsuccinate can
interfere with normal clearance of theophylline
asthma medications, resulting in severe overstimulation of the central nervous system, with
convulsions.

bronchus: See BRONCHI.

brontophobia: See ASTRAPHOBIA.

brooding compulsion a compelling drive to pon-
der anxiously about trivial details or abstract
concepts as an escape from unacceptable or
threatening impulses. It is a common symptom
of obsessive-compulsive disorder. See INTELLEC-
TUALIZATION; OBSESSIONAL BROODING.

brother complex = CAIN COMPLEX.

brotherliness the term used by Erich Fromm to denote the feeling of human unity or solidarity as

expressed in productive involvement and caring
for the well-being of others and society as a
whole. According to Fromm, b. represents the
positive or ideal resolution of the search for
rootedness. Also see ROOTEDNESS NEED. Compare INCESTUOUS TIES.

Brown, Roger American psychologist and linguist,
1925—. See COGNITIVIST; PRODUCTIVITY; SEMAN-
TICITY.

Brown, Thomas Scottish physician and philosopher, 1778–1820. See ASSOCIATIONISM.

Brown, W. English scientist, fl. 1910. See SPEAR-
MAN-BROWN PROPHECY FORMULA.

Brown-Sequard, Charles Edouard /sekär′/ French
physiologist, 1818–94. See BROWN-SEQUARD'S
SYNDROME; SPINAL-CORD DISEASE.

Brown-Sequard's syndrome a pathologic condition caused by damage to a lateral half of the
spinal cord. It is characterized by a set of symptoms that include contralateral loss of the sense
of pain and temperature, loss of vibratory, joint,
and tendon sensations, and spastic paralysis on
the same side as the lesion.

brucellosis a generalized infection of the body's re-
ticuloendothelial system caused by a strain of
bacteria transmitted from domestic animals,
such as goats, cattle, and pigs. The main symptoms include an undulant fever, malaise,
headache, and anemia. The disease is transmitted by drinking infected milk or by contact with
the carcass of an infected animal. Because of the
fluctuating fever symptom, the disease sometimes is called **undulant fever**.

brucine $C_{23}H_{26}N_2O_4$—a poisonous alkaloid
obtained from the Brucea genus of shrubs. It resembles strychnine but is less poisonous and
often is used as a component of nux vomica.

Bruck, F. /brook/ German physician, fl. 1889. See
DE LANGE'S SYNDROME (there: **Bruck-de Lange
type**).

Brugsch's index a system of measuring the chest
circumference in anthropometric studies. The
procedure involves multiplying the chest circumference by 100 and dividing the result by
height of the individual.

Bruininks-Oseretsky Test of Motor Proficiency
a battery of 46 items grouped into eight subtests,
which yield three scores: **Gross Motor Composite** (performance of large muscles, shoulders,
trunk, legs), **Fine Motor Composite** (performance of small muscles of fingers, hands, and
arms), and a **Total Battery Composite**.

Bruner, Jerome S. American psychologist, 1915
—. See CONCEPT-ATTAINMENT MODEL; COGNITIVIST;
DISCOVERY METHOD; ENACTIVE MODE; ENACTIVE
PERIOD; ICONIC CONTENT; ICONIC MODE; ICONIC
STAGE; SYMBOLIC MODE.

Brunhes, S. French physician, fl. 1938. See CHA-
VANY-BRUNHES SYNDROME.

Brunhilde (I) virus: See LEON (III) VIRUS.

Bruns, Ludwig /broons/ German neurologist,
1858–1916. See BRUNS' SYNDROME.

Bruns' syndrome a series of effects caused by

postural changes in the position of the head when the normal flow of cerebrospinal fluid is blocked. The symptoms include vertigo, vomiting, headaches, and visual difficulties. Tumors, cysts, or other obstacles in the third or fourth ventricles are usually a cause of the disorder. Also called **Bruns' sign.**

Brunswik, Egon American psychologist, 1903—. BRUNSWIK RATIO; CAUSAL TEXTURE; ECOLOGICAL VALIDITY.

Brunswik ratio a mathematical expression of perceptual constancy as environmental factors vary.

Brushfield, Thomas English physician, fl. 1924, 1927. See BRUSHFIELD-WYATT SYNDROME.

Brushfield-Wyatt syndrome a form of mental retardation associated with several other anomalies including an extensive port-wine birthmark, paralysis on the side opposite to the causal lesion, contralateral hemiplegia, and cérebral tumor.

brute pride: See PRIDE.

bruxism persistent grinding or gnashing of teeth, usually during sleep. It is generally regarded as a tension symptom or interpreted as an unconscious expression of repressed anger or resentment. Also called **stridor dentium; bruxomania**.

Bryngelson, Bryng American speech pathologist, 1892—. See BRYNGELSON-GLASPEY TEST.

Bryngelson-Glaspey test a test that evaluates proficiency in articulation of speech sounds by presenting stimulus pictures that elicit various verbal responses.

B type: See T TYPE.

bubble concept of personal space an imaginary region around a person that serves as a buffer against potential emotional or physical threats by other individuals. The theoretical private space also serves as a means of determining the distance to be maintained in communicating with others, either verbally or nonverbally. The size of the "bubble" varies with different individuals and the persons with whom they interact and is much smaller for lovemaking than when conducting business with a stranger. For most individuals, the "bubble" extends from about 18 inches to four feet for contacts between close friends, from four to 12 feet for impersonal business contacts, and beyond 12 feet for strangers. The distance also may vary in different cultures; Americans may back away from persons in Europe who are perceived as standing "too close" during conversations. Also see TERRITORIALITY; PROXEMICS.

Buber, Martin /boob'ər/ Austrian philosopher, 1878–1965. See I-IT; I-THOU.

buccal intercourse = OROGENITAL ACTIVITY.

buccal onanism = FELLATIO.

buccal speech a type of phonation which does not depend on laryngeal voice generation (from Latin *bucca*, "cheek"). It is produced by shaping of an air bubble at an optimal place in the cheek pouch. Through contractions of the buccal musculature the air is forced through some narrow opening in the posterior buccal area. It is a difficult mode of speaking and is not encouraged as the method of choice of phonation following laryngectomy.

buccinator one of the cheek muscles that compresses the cheek and retracts the angle of the mouth for eating and speaking. During mastication, the b. helps hold the food between the teeth. In speech, the b. compresses air in the mouth and forces it out between the lips. Contraction of the b. produces a facial feature of a trumpet player, a musical occupation whose name is the Latin source of the b. muscle.

buccolingual masticatory syndrome = BLM.

Buck, J. N. American psychologist, fl. 1948. See HOUSE-TREE-PERSON TECHNIQUE.

Bucy, Paul Clancy American neurologist, 1904—. See KLÜVER-BUCY SYNDROME; EATING BEHAVIOR.

Buddhism the religion and philosophy founded by Gautama Buddha (ca. 566–480 B.C.), which holds that life is suffering and that the way to end suffering is through enlightenment, leading to disappearance in the all, or "nirvana." Of psychological interest is that the self is central yet must be given up as an illusion—a self that does not want to suffer but also does not want to love; that wholly respects others so as not to add to the total suffering in the world; that does not want to act and is ready to forego what non-Buddhists see as the joy of struggling and creating; that wants peace and stillness and the absence of wishing. The true Buddhist is virtuous and compassionate without believing in a Supreme Being or a hereafter where he would be rewarded or punished. Also see NIRVANA PRINCIPLE; MYSTIC UNION; ZEN B.

Buerger, Leo American physician, 1879–1943. See BUERGER'S DISEASE; GANGRENE.

Buerger's disease a chronic progressive condition marked by inflammation of the peripheral blood vessels, mainly the arteries, resulting in gangrene or claudication of the extremities. In some cases, the central nervous system is affected, with lesions of the cerebral hemispheres, paralysis, mental deterioration, personality changes, aphasia, and convulsions. Tobacco-smoking is a contributing factor in development of the disease, and most patients are young adult males. Also called **presenile gangrene; thromboangiitis obliterans; Winiwarter-Buerger syndrome.** Also see GANGRENE.

buffer an interspersed item in a test or experiment. e.g., a question that is not scored and is introduced to separate or to disguise other items.

buffoonery psychosis a type of hyperkinetic catatonia, or hyperkinetic motor psychosis, characterized by awkward and inept buffoon behavior, e.g., pouring water onto the floor instead of into a cup, while otherwise seeming well oriented. B.p. has been described as a flight into disease to escape reality. Also called **faxen psychosis** (from German *Faxen* /fok'sən/, "antics"). Also see FACTITIOUS DISORDERS; GANSER SYNDROME.

bufotenine $C_{12}H_{16}N_2O$—an indolic hallucinogen found in the poison gland of toads as well as in plant sources. It has been reported in the urine of certain schizophrenic patients. B. is chemically related to lysergic acid diethylamide (LSD), psilocybin, and dimethyltryptamine (DMT). Also spelled **bufotenin**. Also see PSYCHEDELICS; TRYPTAMINE DERIVATIVES; INDOLE ALKYLAMINES.

buggery a term sometimes used in legal documents as a synonym for sodomy, or sexual analism. The word is derived from Latin *Bulgarus*, probably because sodomy at one time was associated with ancient Bulgarian heretics.

building-fear = DOMATOPHOBIA.

bulbar pertaining to a bulb or bulblike structure, e.g., the eyeball, but especially the medulla oblongata. Combining form: **-bulb-; -bulbo-**.

bulbar paralysis muscle impairment due to damage in the motor centers of the medulla oblongata. Paralysis and atrophy of the muscles of the lips, tongue, mouth, pharynx, and larynx affect speech.

bulbar poliomyelitis: See POLIOMYELITIS.

bulbocapnine an alkaloid drug obtained from plants of the Fumariaceae family. B. is used in the treatment of parkinsonism, Ménière's disease, vestibular nystagmus, and similar neuromuscular disorders.

bulbocavernosus muscle = BULBOSPONGIOSUS MUSCLE.

bulbospinal poliomyelitis: See POLIOMYELITIS.

bulbospongiosus muscle a urogenital muscle of men and women, serving as a urine accelerator in both sexes, as an ejaculation aid in men, and a weak vaginal sphincter in women. Also called **bulbocavernosus muscle**, or, if in women, **sphincter cunni** or **constrictor vaginae**, or, if in men, **ejaculator seminis**.

bulbotegmental reticular formation the portion of the reticular activating system (RAS) that passes through the medulla oblongata.

bulbourethral glands two mucus-secreting glands located on either side of the male urethra, near the urethral sphincter. The b.g. are homologous to the Bartholin glands in the female reproductive tract. Also called **Cowper's glands**.

bulimia an eating disorder (Greek *boulimia*, "hunger of an ox") involving repeated episodes of uncontrolled consumption of large quantities of food and drink in a short time (binge eating). The episodes are followed by a depressed mood and self-deprecation, and in many cases attempts to lose weight by dieting, vomiting, or the use of cathartics. B. may occasionally be due to endocrinic disturbance, but is more often attributed to psychological factors such as relief of stress, an attempt to recapture childhood feelings of security, or substitution of food for satisfactions presently denied, such as affection or sex. Also called **hyperorexia; polyphagia; eating compulsion; bulimy; boulimia**. Also see HYPERBULIMIA; ACORIA; BINGE-EATING SYNDROME; OBESITY; BULMOREXIA; APPETITIVE BEHAVIOR.

bulla of fornix = MAMMILLARY BODIES.

bulmorexia an eating disorder in which periods of bulimia are followed by self-induced vomiting. See BULIMIA; ANOREXIA.

bumps: See PHRENOLOGY.

Bunsen, Robert Wilhelm Eberhard /bŏŏn'sən/ German chemist, 1811–99. See BUNSEN-ROSCOE LAW.

Bunsen-Roscoe law the principle that the visual threshold for light is a mathematical function expressed as the product of the stimulus intensity and stimulus duration.

bureaucratic leader the type of leader whose responsibilities and leadership style are largely determined by his position in a hierarchical organization, e.g., the church or government. The term may also be used to describe a leader who rigidly adheres to prescribed routine and makes no allowance for extenuating circumstances.

Burkitt, Denis Parsons English physician, 1911—. See EPSTEIN-BARR VIRUS (there: **Burkitt's lymphoma**); LYMPHOMA.

Burkitt's lymphoma: See EPSTEIN-BARR VIRUS; LYMPHOMA.

burn centers and units hospital facilities that are established primarily for the treatment of burn injuries. Burn centers sometimes are identified as hospital facilities that provide research and teaching in the treatment and rehabilitation of burn patients, whereas a burn unit does not offer the research and education support to burn-injury treatment.

burned-out a term applied primarily to chronic schizophrenic patients who have deteriorated to an apathetic, withdrawn, anergic state. Such patients exhibit persistent schizophrenic thought processes, but have few other florid symptoms. Also called **b.-o. schizophrenic; anergic schizophrenic**. Also see ANERGIA; BURN-OUT.

burn injuries tissue damage caused by exposure to flame, intense heat without flame—e.g., contact with high-voltage electricity, redhot metal, or scalding liquids—or ultraviolet (actinic) radiation. Types of b.i. include superficial, or first-degree, burns, characterized by redness, swelling, and peeling of the skin; partial-thickness, or second-degree, burns, marked by penetration of damage beyond the skin layer which can be blistered and dull white to cherry red and streaked with coagulated capillaries; full-thickness, or third-degree, burns, with damage in tissues that are subcutaneous or deeper, including destroyed epithelial tissue, nerve endings, and blood vessels; and fourth-degree burns, usually identified by a distinct odor and visual appearance of charred flesh. Because of sometimes excruciating pain and cosmetic damage b.i. often are mentally traumatic, and psychological or psychiatric help is needed.

burn-out a vogue term for exhaustion or failure, especially in one's job or career. The term is mainly applied to middle-aged persons who perform at a high level until stress and tension take their toll. Also see BURNED-OUT.

Burrow, Trigant American psychoanalyst, 1875–

1951. See PHYLOANALYSIS; THIRD NERVOUS SYSTEM.

bursitis any inflammation of a **bursa**, a fluid-filled sac or cavity that may be found in most body areas where muscles or tendons are likely to produce friction in their movements. Bursa are most commonly found around major joints, e.g., shoulder, hip, elbow, knee. The cause usually is excessive use or exposure to cold, and effects are pain and limited range of motion. Calcium-salt deposits at a joint can result in chronic b. that may require surgery.

bushy cells: See STELLATE CELLS.

business game an industrial training method in which teams of employees compete in solving typical but simulated management problems. The game requires an organized approach, interaction among the participants, and the analysis and application of information appropriate to the problem.

Butazolidin a trademark for a brand of the analgesic **phenylbutazone**, which is prescribed for patients afflicted with acute gout, rheumatoid arthritis, ankylosing spondylitis, and bursitis. In addition to analgesic effects, the drug has antiinflammatory and antipyretic properties. Also see PYRAZOLONES.

butch a slang term for a Lesbian who plays the male role in a homosexual relationship, or whose behavior conveys the impression that she does. The term is used as noun or adjective.

Butler, John S. American psychiatrist, 1803–90. B. was a cofounder of the Association of Medical Superintendents of American Institutions for the Insane, which later evolved into the American Psychiatric Association.

buttonmaker's chorea: See CHOREA.

butylcarbamic acid: See TYBAMATE.

-butyr- a combining form relating to butter or anything butterlike (from Latin *butyrum*, "butter").

butyrophenones a category of neuroleptic drugs administered primarily in the treatment of manic and severely agitated states. B. also are used as alternative medications in the treatment of certain cases of schizophrenia and Gilles de la Tourette's syndrome. Some b. have been developed with pharmacologic effects similar to morphine and the phenothiazines. B. generally are alpha-adrenergic blockers with antidopaminergic actions and minimal autonomic side effects. The prototype drug is **haloperidol**— $C_{21}H_{23}ClFNO_2$. Also see ANTIMANICS.

buzz groups small subdivided groups whose purpose is to involve each member in active discussion to ascertain his feelings or opinions. The results are then conveyed to the main group by a spokesperson. Also called **buzz sessions**.

B-values = METANEEDS.

B wave of electroretinogram a large positive wave pattern that follows a brief negative A wave as part of a complex electrical response to stimulation of an animal's retina by a flash of light. The effect is recorded by microelectrodes placed in either the rods or cones. See ELECTRORETINOGRAM.

by-idea a secondary thought or symbol that displaces a primary or latent thought. According to Kraepelin, the b.-i. is the common feature in dream paraphrasias. Also called **metaphoric paralogia**.

bystander effect the observation that people are more likely to act in an emergency or come to the aid of others when they are alone. Also see DIFFUSION OF RESPONSIBILITY.

C

c̄ an abbreviation used in prescriptions, meaning "with" (Latin *cum*).

C = COCAINE.

CA = CHRONOLOGICAL AGE.

caapi a powerful hallucinogenic beverage made from the stems of a woody vine, Banisteriopsis c., and the leaves of a shrub that has been identified as Prestonia amazonica, both growing in Peru. The pharmacologically active ingredient has been identified as **harmaline**, a psychotomimetic drug. Also called **yagé; ayahuasca**.

CABG: See CORONARY ARTERY BYPASS.

-cac-; -caco- a combining form denoting something bad or unpleasant, such as a disease or a deformity.

cacao a species of tree, Theobroma c., that is indigenous to Brazil and Central America and is the source of cocoa and chocolate. The genus name is derived from a Greek word for "food of the gods." See THEOBROMINE.

cachexia a state of emaciation, extreme weakness, and wasting due to malnutrition associated with a chronic disease such as carcinoma or tuberculosis, or with deterioration or destruction of the anterior lobe of the pituitary gland, called hypophyseal c. A similar condition may occur in anorexia nervosa. See HYPOPHYSEAL C.

cachinnation an unrestrained and inappropriate type of laughter observed in the hebephrenic (disorganized) form of schizophrenia.

cacodemonomania a delusion in which the patient believes he is possessed by a demon, devil, or other evil spirit. C. is occasionally observed in hebephrenic schizophrenia. Also called **cacodaemonia; cacodemonia**. See EXORCISM; SCHIZOPHRENIC DISORDER, DISORGANIZED TYPE.

cacogenic a term that refers to deteriorating factors in heredity, as contrasted with eugenic influences.

cacogeusia a perception of bad taste, as experienced by patients with idiopathic epilepsy, somatic delusional states, and those receiving tranquilizer therapy.

cacolalia = COPROLALIA.

cacophoria a generalized feeling of unhappiness. It is the opposite of euphoria.

Caesarian section a surgical procedure in which an incision is made through the abdominal and uterine walls to deliver a fetus. The name stems from the belief that Gajus Julius Caesar (100–44 B.C.) was delivered in this manner. This belief is refuted by the fact that this operation was never performed on a living woman in antiquity and Caesar's mother was still alive when he was an adult.

cafeteria feeding a technique for studying the hunger drive by offering children (or animals) a variety of foods with freedom to choose any kind or amount. E.g., at one meal, babies might eat all butter or all vegetables, but over a period of weeks will usually try all kinds of food and eat a balanced diet, indicating that the organism possesses a basic physiological wisdom of its own. Also see SELF-SELECTION OF DIET.

caffeine $C_8H_{10}N_4O_2$—an alkaloid which acts as a psychomotor stimulant, found in coffee, tea, cola, cocoa, chocolate, and over-the-counter analgesics, "cold" preparations, and "keep-awake" pills. Also see METHYLXANTHINES; ASPIRIN COMBINATIONS; CAFFEINE EFFECTS.

caffeine effects reactions that involve stimulation of the central nervous system, quickened respiration, increased pulse rate and blood pressure, and reduced feelings of fatigue. Precise effects vary with the size of the caffeine dose and tolerance of the subject; however, moderate doses affect the cerebral areas, producing an improved flow of thought and clearness of ideas. Large doses may make concentration or continued attention difficult. Moderate doses stimulate the medulla, as evidenced by increased respiratory and vasomotor activity. Large doses cause insomnia, headaches, and confusion in some individuals. Because of its CNS effects, caffeine is used in "keep-awake" pills and certain analgesics and cold remedies containing ingredients that usually cause drowsiness in the patient. Also see METHYLXANTHINES.

caffeine intoxication an organic disorder due to recent consumption of over 250 milligram of caffeine (coffee, tea, cola, medications), and involving at least five of the following symptoms, depending on individual reaction: restlessness, nervousness, excitement, insomnia, flushed face, diuresis (increased urination), gastrointestinal complaints, muscle twitching, rambling thought and speech, cardiac arrythmia, periods of inexhaustibility, psychomotor agitation. Coffee contains 100 to 150 milligram of caffeine per cup; tea contains about half, and cola about one-third, that amount. Also called **caffeinism**. (DSM-III).

cafta = KHAT.

CAGE an acronym derived from *c*ut down, *a*nnoyed, *g*uilt feelings, *e*ye-opener—a four-question screening instrument used in detecting alcoholism (Ewing and Rouse): (1) Have you ever felt you should *c*ut down on your drinking? (2) Have people *a*nnoyed you by criticizing your drinking? (3) Have you ever felt bad or *g*uilty about your drinking? (4) have you ever used a drink as an *e*ye-opener?

CAI = COMPUTER-ASSISTED INSTRUCTION.

Cain complex a complex characterized by rivalry, competition, and even destructive impulses directed toward a brother. The term is derived from the Biblical story of Cain and Abel. Also called **brother complex**.

Cain-Levine Social Competency Scale an instrument assessing the competence of trainable mentally retarded children from five to 13 years of age, yielding scores on self-help, social skills, initiative, communication, and total social competency.

Cairns' stupor a condition characterized by stupor, rigidity, postural catatonia, and a lack of spontaneous emotion or movement. Also called **akinetic stupor; diencephalic stupor**. See AKINETIC MUTISM.

Cajal: See RAMON Y C.

CAL: See COMPUTER-ASSISTED INSTRUCTION.

-calc-; -calci-; -calco- a combining form relating to calcium or calcium salts.

calcarine area a spur-shaped projection of the occipital lobe that is a part of the visual projection area.

calcarine cortex: See VISUAL CORTEX.

calcarine fissure a fissure extending from the occipital end of the cerebrum to the parietal-occipital fissure. The c.f. separates the occipital and temporal lobes of the cerebrum and runs along the border between the cunneus and the lingual gyrus. Also called **calcarine sulcus**.

calcitonin a hormone produced by the parafollicular, or "C," cells of the thyroid gland as a normal reaction to elevated blood levels of calcium. C. functions by inhibiting the release and resorption of calcium and phosphorus by bone tissue. A commercial form of c. is administered in the treatment of Paget's disease. Excessive C. secretion is an effect of thyroid cancer.

calcium-deficiency disorders effects of calcium deficiency which commonly include rickets in children, marked by deformed bones and teeth and lax muscles. A lack of vitamin D in the diet is a contributing factor to inadequate absorption of calcium from food. Tetany, or muscle spasms, also is among c.-d.d. In adults, c.-d.d.

may be expressed as osteomalacia, a form of rickets, or osteoporosis, in which calcium is eroded from bone tissue to meet other body needs. Also see OSTEOMALACIA.

calcium regulation maintenance of calcium levels in the blood and other extracellular fluids by secretions of parathormone by the parathyroid glands. The hormone causes release of ionic calcium from the bones in which it is stored. See PARATHORMONE. Also see PARATHYROID GLAND.

calendar age = CHRONOLOGICAL AGE.

calendar calculation the rare ability to identify the day of the week for any given date, such as February 19, 1878, in a matter of seconds. **Calendar calculators** are frequently idiots savants who usually have no mathematical ability but may be able to perform other feats with the calendar, as in answering the question "In what years did April 16 fall on a Sunday?" No fully satisfactory explanation has been found for this skill. Also see IDIOT SAVANT.

calf love = PUPPY LOVE.

California Achievement Tests four batteries of tests (primary, elementary, intermediate, advanced), each measuring the same general areas of school learning: reading vocabulary, arithmetic reasoning, reading comprehension, arithmetic fundamentals, spelling, and mechanics of English and grammar.

California F scale = F SCALE.

California Infant Scale for Motor Development a battery of 76 items used to assess motor development at specific months from birth to three years, e.g., sitting without support, walking alone, walking up and down stairs.

California Psychological Inventory a self-report inventory that draws about half of its 480 items from the MMPI, scored for such personality characteristics as self-control, dominance, sociability, self-acceptance, sense of well-being, and achievement-via-independence. Abbrev.: CPI.

California Tests of Mental Maturity scales designed to measure the same general factors, such as memory and logical reasoning, on five different levels of difficulty, starting with nonverbal materials and progressing to verbal concepts and more complex nonverbal material.

California Tests of Personality a personality inventory of the questionnaire type designed to yield scores on personal worth, self-reliance, sense of freedom, belongingness, various social skills, and total adjustment.

call boys: See MALE HOMOSEXUAL PROSTITUTION.

callosal gyrus = CINGULATE GYRUS.

callosal sulcus a fissure or groove that separates the corpus callosum and the cingulate gyrus along the medial side of the cerebral hemispheres.

calomel electrodes electric cell terminals consisting of mercury in contact with mercurous chloride. C.e. can collect or release chloride ions from neutral or acidic solutions and are used to record electric potentials of brain cells.

-calor-; -calori- a combining form relating to heat (Latin *calor*).

caloric intake the consumption of units of energy in food measured in calories. See CALORIE.

calorie a unit of heat that is equivalent to the amount of energy required to raise the temperature of one kilogram of water by one degree Celsius or one pound of water by four degrees Fahrenheit. Every bodily process requires an expenditure of calories. The brain utilizes approximately 500 calories per day through the metabolism of glucose.

Calvé, Jacques /kälvā'/ French surgeon, 1875–1954. See LEGG-CALVÉ-PERTHES DISEASE.

Cameron: See LEAST-RESTRICTIVE ALTERNATIVE.

camisole in psychiatry, a restraining device consisting of a canvas shirt with long sleeves that can be fastened behind the back of the patient after his arms are folded in front of his body. Also called **straitjacket**.

campimetry the measurement of the visual field of a subject. The normal field of vision is limited by the area that can be seen peripherally while the eye is fixed on a single point. Glaucoma and other visual disorders that cause field defects can be studied by c.

camptocormia a hysterical or conversion symptom in which the back is bent forward at a sharp angle, often accompanied by tremors, lumbar pain, and impotence. The condition is most frequently observed in soldiers. See WAR NEUROSIS.

Camus, Albert /kämē'/ French philosopher and novelist, 1913–60. See EXISTENTIALISM; SUICIDE.

canalization the channeling of needs into specific, fixed patterns of gratification. The term was first used by Janet for substitutive discharges of tension, and later (1946) applied by G. Murphy to food preferences, esthetic interests, friendships, sexual activity, work, and recreational satisfactions.

Canavan, Myrtelle May American neuropathologist, 1879—. See CANAVAN'S DISEASE.

Canavan's disease a degenerative neurologic disorder characterized by macrocephaly and demyelinization. The brain is larger and heavier than normal, but there is widespread vacuolization and myelin deterioration. Infants appear normal for the first months of infancy but then lose the ability to smile, coo, or control the enlarged head. Also called **spongy degeneration of the CNS in infancy**.

cancellation test a test of perceptuomotor speed requiring the subject to cancel out randomly scattered symbols.

cancer a group of cellular-tumor diseases characterized by unregulated growth and invasion of neighboring tissues, and generally capable of spreading to other body areas or organs by the process of metastasis. Noncancerous, or benign, tumors usually are encapsulated and do not spread by metastasizing through blood and lymph vessels. Causes of c. include viruses, hormones, environmental carcinogenic chemicals, radiation from sunlight, X-rays, or radioactive substances. Cancers generally are classified as carcinomas if they involve cells of epithelial origin, e.g., uterus, breast, stomach, or skin, and sarcomas if the affected tissues are of mesenchymal origin, such as bone or muscle. More than 150 different kinds of c. have been identified in humans, based on cells types, rate of growth, and other factors. Because cancers can be disfiguring and life-threatening, psychological counseling often is necessary for c. patients. Also see CARCINOMA; SARCOMA; BLADDER C.; LARYNGEAL C.; SKIN C.

cancer phobia a morbid fear of cancer, particularly in elderly persons but sometimes in younger people as well. Some psychoanalysts relate c.p. to a fear of castration or the dread of being devoured from within.

cancer reactions emotional responses to the presence or possibility of carcinoma, ranging from acceptance of the inevitable and determination to conquer the disease, to pathological reactions such as interpretation of loss of an organ as punishment for a real or fancied infraction. See CANCER PHOBIA.

candida infection; candidiasis: See MONILIASIS.

canes sitting, standing, and mobility aids for persons who are blind or otherwise disabled. C. for patients with neuromuscular handicaps, often designed as orthopedic c., usually are fashioned as sturdy shafts of solid wood or metal with a curved or horizontal handle at the top, a rubber tip at the bottom, and sometimes with three or four feet. They are designed for weight-bearing. C. for blind patients generally are slimmer, lighter, longer, made of metal, and used for orientation.

cannabis: See CANNABIS SATIVA.

cannabis abuse a disorder whose distinguishing features are (a) a pattern of pathological use (intoxication throughout the day, and use nearly every day for at least a month) with episodes of cannabis delusional disorder, and (b) impaired functioning, such as loss of interest in previous activities, loss of friends, absence from work, loss of job, or repeated legal difficulties. (DSM-III)

cannabis-delusional disorder an organic-delusional disorder in which persecutory delusions are most prominent, developing immediately after cannabis use or during cannabis intoxication, and persisting for up to six hours. (DSM-III)

cannabis dependence a disorder characterized by (a) a pattern of pathological use (intoxication throughout the day, with use nearly every day for at least a month, and episodes of cannabis-delusional disorder), (b) impaired social and occupational functioning, such as marked loss of interest in previous activities, loss of friends, absence from work, loss of job, or legal difficulties other than a single arrest, and (c) tolerance, that is, the need for markedly increased amounts to achieve the desired effect or decreased effect from the same amount. (DSM-III)

cannabis intoxication an organic syndrome that develops within a half hour of cannabis use, and characterized by (a) rapid heartbeat (tachycardia), (b) one or more psychological symptoms (euphoria, intensification of perceptions, sensation of slowed time—five minutes seems like an hour—or apathy), (c) one or more physical symptoms (conjunctival injection, increased appetite, dry mouth), and (d) maladapties other than a single arrest, and (e) tolerance, that is, the need for markedly increased amounts to achieve the desired effect or decreased effect from the same amount. (DSM-III)

cannabis organic mental disorders a category that includes cannabis intoxication and cannabis-delusional disorder, stemming from smoking or eating (in food) substances from the cannabis plant, as well as chemically similar substances: marijuana, hashish, and THC (purified delta-9-tetrahydrocannabinol). (DSM-III)

cannabis psychosis a psychotic symptom pattern resulting from use of marijuana, hashish, or THC (tetrahydrocannabinol). See CANNABIS-DELUSIONAL DISORDER; CANNABIS INTOXICATION.

Cannabis sativa /kan'-/ the botanical name of the hemp plant that is the source of marijuana and hashish. The pharmacologically active ingredients of C.s. are cannabinols.

cannibalism in psychiatry, a compulsive urge to devour human flesh. C. is a rare symptom observed in schizophrenic and schizophrenialike psychoses such as witigo. Some psychoanalysts associate cannibalistic impulses with fixation at the oral-biting stage of psychosexual development. C. is not pathological if it is part of a religious ceremonial or if a dead companion is eaten when a group is stranded without access to other food. Also see KURU.

cannibalistic fantasy the fantasy of devouring another person which, according to psychoanalytic theory, goes back to the early period of psychosexual development when the infant "incorporates" the mother's breasts, and perhaps her total being during the process of nursing. See INCORPORATION.

cannibalistic fixation in psychoanalysis, a libido fixation at the late oral or biting stage, marked by fantasies or impulses of biting, eating, swallowing, and thus eliminating, a hated object.

cannibalistic phase the second half of the oral stage in which, according to psychoanalysis, the infant first expresses hostility and aggressiveness by biting the mother's breast, or the nipple of the bottle, during the feeding process. Also called **cannibalistic stage**. See ORAL-BITING PERIOD.

Cannon, Walter B. American physiologist, 1871–1945. Cannon's studies of the digestive system, carried out with A. J. Carlson, led to the theory that hunger is due to contractions of an empty stomach; and his studies of the bodily changes that take place in emotion (increased blood pressure, respiration, and heartbeat) led to the theory that the sympathetic and adrenal systems worked together to put the organism on a "war footing" (and he later theorized, with Phillip Bard, that the thalamus is the actual control center). See CANNON'S THEORY; EMERGENCY THEORY OF EMOTIONS; FIGHT-FLIGHT REACTION; LOCAL THEORY OF THIRST; PAPEZ'S THEORY OF EMOTIONS; TROPHOTROPIC PROCESS; VOODOO DEATH.

Cannon's theory the theory of emotions developed by W. B. Cannon and his pupil Philip Bard, which holds that the thalamus controls the experience of emotion, since it is the station on the way to the cortex, while the hypothalamus controls emotional expression. Since both of these structures are involved when external stimulation occurs, the theory is sometimes referred to as the **thalamic theory of Cannon** and sometimes as the **hypothalamic theory of Cannon**. Also called **Cannon-Bard theory**. Also see PAPEZ'S THEORY OF EMOTIONS.

cannula /kan'-/ a tube that can be inserted into a body cavity to provide a channel for the escape of fluid from the cavity. One type of c. contains two barrels to permit the introduction of an irrigation fluid through one tube and drainage of the fluid through the other.

canonical correlation a correlation coefficient describing the degree of relationship between one combination of variables and a second combination of variables.

cantharides the dried bodies of Spanish or Russian flies that are the source of an irritating drug, **cantharidin**. C. have been used as irritants of the skin in the treatment of arthritis and similar complaints and to remove warts. Taken internally, c. can have fatal effects, but because it may irritate the urethra and induce priapism, the substance has been used as an aphrodisiac. Also see SPANISH FLY.

capacity the maximum ability of an individual to function in mental or physical tasks.

Capgras, Jean Marie Joseph /käpgrä'/ French psychiatrist, 1873–1950. See CAPGRAS' SYNDROME; L'ILLUSION DES SOSIES.

Capgras' syndrome a rare psychotic disorder in which the patient insists that other individuals are not really themselves, but are "doubles" or impostors. This reaction is believed to serve the unconscious purpose of rejecting the individual (the mother, for instance) as indicated by the fact that the double becomes the target for resentment. The C.s. is generally considered to be a special symptom of paranoid schizophrenia, organic disorder, or, less often, affective psychoses. See L'ILLUSION DES SOSIES.

capitalization on chance the process of basing a conclusion on data wholly or partly biased in a particular direction by chance factors. Purely random factors often seem to show interpretable patterns, and c.o.c. involves mistaken inferences from these patterns.

capping techniques methods utilized by a counselor in directing an interview along less painful or threatening lines for the purpose of lessening the client's anxiety, distress, or resistance.

caps. an abbreviation used in prescriptions, meaning "capsule" (Latin *capsula*).

capsula externa = EXTERNAL CAPSULE.

-carb-; -carbo- a combining form relating to carbon.

carbachol a parasympathetic stimulant drug or cholinergic agent with the pharmacologic effects of acetylcholine. It is applied therapeutically to the conjunctiva of the eye to cause the pupil to contract and is used to reduce intraocular pressure in cases of glaucoma.

carbamates pharmacotherapy the use of carbamate drugs, such as carbamazepine, in the treatment of neurologic disorders. Carbamazepine is administered in the United States mainly for the relief of symptoms of trigeminal and glossopharyngeal neuralgia, but in Europe it is used as an anticonvulsant ·in the treatment of epilepsy.

carbamazepine: See CARBAMATES PHARMACOTHERAPY; TRICYCLIC ANTIDEPRESSANTS; ANTIEPILEPTICS.

carbidopa: See SINEMET.

carbohydrate metabolism the utilization by the body tissues of starch and sugar molecules, which are broken down by various enzymes to simple glucose molecules. The glucose molecule is the ultimate source of cellular energy for the brain and other organs.

carbon-dioxide therapy a form of inhalation therapy occasionally applied to neurotic patients with anxiety, conversion, or psychophysiologic symptoms, sometimes in conjunction with psychotherapy. The technique was first used by the Hungarian psychiatrist J. Meduna to induce a brief coma as a means of interrupting pathological brain circuits.

carbon-disulfide intoxication intoxication due to inhalation of **carbon disulfide**—CS_2, a colorless liquid with an ethereal odor used primarily as a solvent or fumigant or in the manufacture of carbon tetrachloride, but sometimes sniffed to obtain a high.

carbonic-anhydrase inhibitors a group of drugs that interfere with the action of an enzyme, **carbonic anhydrase**, in the body. Although the primary role of c.-a.i. is that of improving urine excretion and electrolyte balance, the drugs have been found to function also as antiepileptics. The prototype, **acetazolamide**—$C_4H_6N_4O_3S_2$, inhibits epileptic seizures and decreases the rate of cerebrospinal-fluid formation. A related drug, **sulthiame**—$C_{10}H_{14}N_2O_4S_2$, is a mild anticonvulsant that is sometimes administered with hydantoins because sulthiame interferes with hydantoin metabolism and in effect doubles the amount of time the hydantoin drug is available to CNS tissues.

carbon-monoxide poisoning a toxic disorder resulting from inhalation of carbon monoxide, a colorless, odorless gas. Symptoms are produced by lack of oxygen in the tissues (**anoxia**), and range from headache and light-headedness due to mild exposure to an acute, transient state of confusion and delirium and, in cases of a severe exposure, deep coma followed by permanent brain damage and death by asphyxiation. Also called **carbon-monoxide intoxication**.

carbon tetrachloride: See PSYCHEDELICS.

carbon-tetrachloride poisoning a toxic disorder resulting from inhalation or ingestion of carbon tetrachloride, a cleaning fluid, producing such symptoms as kidney and liver damage and, in some cases, CNS damage involving anorexia, confusion, memory loss, blurred vision, personality change, and unconsciousness.

-carcin-; -carcino- a combining form relating to cancer or carcinoma (from Greek *karkinos*, "crab, cancer").

carcinogen /-sin'ǝjǝn/ any cancer-producing substance. Adjective: **carcinogenic** /-jen'ik/.

carcinoma a malignant tumor derived from epithelial cells that infiltrates surrounding tissues and spreads by metastasis to other areas of the body. Most cancers of the skin, tongue, breast, uterus, and intestinal tract are of the c. type. A c. can occur in many forms, e.g., oat-cell c., composed of tiny oval cells, squamous-cell c., containing cuboid cells, and mucinous c., composed of cells that secrete mucin. See CANCER.

carcinomatous myopathy = EATON-LAMBERT SYNDROME.

car controls special automobile-driving devices for disabled persons, e.g., gearshift extensions, hand controls for brakes, relocated transmission and turn-signal controls, and adjustable seat controls. See DRIVER EDUCATION.

-card-; -cardio- a combining form relating to the heart (Greek *cardia*). Adjectives: **cardiac; cardial**.

cardiac disorders any malfunction or abnormality of the heart as a result of disease, injury, or inherited or congenital defect. Certain infectious diseases, e.g., rheumatic fever and diphtheria, can result in c.d. Congenital defects may include TETRALOGY OF FALLOT. See this entry.

cardiac muscle the muscle of the heart, a specialized type of muscle tissue that consists of involuntary striated fibers.

cardiac neurosis an anxiety reaction precipitated by a heart condition, the suspicion of having a heart condition, or the fear of developing coronary disease. In some cases a c.n. develops when the patient detects a purely functional heart murmur, palpitations, or a chest pain due to emotional stress. In others, it may be caused or aggravated by a physician's examination. See IATROGENIC ILLNESS.

cardiac pacemakers: See PACEMAKERS.

cardiac psychosis a disorganization of thought processes associated with an acute state of fear and anxiety following a heart attack.

cardiac reactions in psychiatry, responses to psychological stimuli that result in abnormal activity of the heart and circulatory system. Anxiety, anger, fear, and excitement are among emotional reactions known to precipitate attacks of angina pectoris. One study found that 30 percent of both men and women suffering a myocardial infarction blamed marital difficulties for the event.

cardiac symptoms symptoms that indicate the presence of angina pectoris, myocardial infarction, congestive heart failure, or some other form of heart disease. C.s. may include chest pains that can extend from the upper abdomen to the jaw, aches or pains involving the inside of one or both arms, pain between the shoulder blades, difficult breathing, or burning or bloating sensations usually associated with indigestion.

cardial: See -CARD-.

cardinal trait a term applied by G. W. Allport to a basic and significant characteristic, such as overweening ambition, that influences an individual's total behavior.

cardiomyopathy a generic diagnostic term for a disease involving the heart-muscle tissues, particularly when the specific cause is uncertain.

cardiospasms: See ACHALASIA.

cardiovascular diseases diseases, congenital or acquired, that affect the heart and blood vessels. Kinds of c.d. include high blood pressure, congestive heart failure, myocardial infarction, arteriosclerotic heart disease, and rheumatic heart disease.

cardiovascular surgery the treatment of heart and blood-vessel disorders by manual or operative methods. C.s. may be performed to install an artificial cardiac pacemaker, to replace defective heart valves, or to perform a heart transplant from a donor. Corrective c.s. may be performed to correct genetic or congenital heart defects, e.g., a fetal circulatory mechanism that failed to adjust to life outside the womb.

card-sorting test a test in which the subject is asked to sort randomly mixed cards into specific categories. The test is used to determine learning ability and discriminatory powers, as well as clerical aptitude.

card-stacking a technique of persuasion in which an attempt is made to influence opinion through deliberate distortions, as in suppressing information, overemphasis on selected facts, manipulation of statistics, and quoting rigged research.

care-and-protection proceedings court intervention on behalf of a child when the parents or caretakers do not adequately provide for the child's welfare.

carebaria a form of headache characterized by distressing sensations of pressure or heaviness.

career choice selection of a vocation, usually on the basis of some or all of the following: parental guidance, vocational counseling, identification with admired figures, trial or part-time jobs, training opportunities, interest, and ability tests.

career conference a vocational program provided by many schools in which a representative of a given occupational field meets with interested students to provide information and answer questions related to the requirements for and opportunities in the field.

career development elements of a person's experience that contribute to the formation of a "work identity," including life experience, education, career choice, on-the-job experience, level of professional achievement, and degree of satisfaction.

career planning a vocational-guidance program designed to assist a client in one or more aspects of his or her decision-making process. A realistic appraisal of the individual's desires and abilities is formulated in relation to existing occupational opportunities. Various tests may be administered to aid a counselor in assessing a client's skills and aptitudes.

career workshop a study group in which occupational opportunities and requirements are discussed and explored.

caregiver any individual involved in the process of identifying, preventing, or treating an illness or disability; in child psychiatry, a person who attends to the needs of an infant or child. Caregivers include, among others, family physicians, pediatricians, nurses, social workers, and indigenous nonprofessionals. See INDIGENOUS WORKER.

care of young a manifestation of parental behavior in animals, usually stimulated by certain hormonal and other physiological changes in the presence of offspring. The influences include the secretion of prolactin which induces broodiness and parental feeding of young and reduced gonadal activity so that reproductive urges are suppressed during c.o.y.

caretaking behavior an expression of attachment in which parents take care of the needs of their children, respond to them when they approach, and protect them from the aggressions of others.

carezza a form of coitus in which the male does not reach orgasm. It is sometimes used for birth control; but if it is combined with meditation, it is similar to the coitus reservatus technique practiced by members of the Oneida Community. C. techniques are derived from principles of Hindu Tantrism, and in this sense were first described by Alice B. Stockham in 1896. Also called **coitus prolongatus; karezza.** See COITUS RESERVATUS.

cargo culture a native religious movement in South Pacific islands which holds that at the millennium the spirits of the dead will return in airplanes with large cargoes of modern goods which will free the adherents from work and from control by the white race.

caricature a drawing or description of an individual in which peculiarities or defects are exaggerated for purposes of ridicule. Psychoanalysts compare caricatures to puns, in which repressed impulses, such as hostility, elude the censor and express themselves. For this reason caricatures often represent someone in authority.

carisoprodol: See PROPANEDIOLS.

Carlson, Anton Julius Swedish-born American physiologist, 1875–1956. See CANNON.

carnosine $C_9H_{14}N_4O_3$—a dipeptide composed of two amino acids, beta-alanine and histidine, found in the skeletal-muscle tissue of vertebrates.

carotene any of a group of yellow to red pigments found in carrots and other dark vegetables, fats such as butterfat, and egg yolk. Several types of c., alpha-c., beta-c., and gamma-c., are provitamins that are converted in the body to vitamin A. One molecule of beta-c. yields two molecules of vitamin A on hydrolytic splitting. Human adults need about 30,000 micrograms of c. daily in their diet.

carotid /kərot′id/ either of the two chief arteries that convey the blood to the head and neck (from Greek *karos*, "stupor"). Also called **c. artery**.

carotid sinus a small swelling or dilation in the common carotid artery, located in the neck. The c.s. contains nervous tissue that when stimulated can alter the heart rate, blood pressure, and lumen of blood vessels.

carotid-sinus syndrome: See AORTIC-ARCH SYNDROME.

carotid syphon a series of sharp turns in the internal carotid artery after it enters the skull on its route upward from the neck. The c.s. forms a shape like that of the letter S and is an anatomical landmark rather than a true syphon.

carotodynia pain in the cheek, neck, and region of the eyes resulting from pressure on the common carotid artery.

-carp-; -carpo- a combining form relation to (a) the wrist (Greek *karpos*, "wrist"), (b) fruit or anything fruitlike (from Latin *carpere*, "to pluck, gather", from Greek *karpos* "fruit").

Carpenter, George Alfred English physician, 1859–1910. See CARPENTER'S SYNDROME.

Carpenter's syndrome an autosomal-recessive hereditary disorder marked by acrocephaly, syndactly of the fingers and toes, subnormal intelligence, and usually obesity. Also called **acrocephalopolysyndactyly**.

-carph-; -carpho- a combining form meaning dried up, withered (from Greek *karphos*, "dry straw").

carphenazine $C_{24}H_{31}N_3O_2S.2C_4H_4O_4$—an antipsychotic drug equal in effectiveness to thioridizine, trifluoperazine, and chlorpromazine. Also called **prochlorperazine**.

car phobia = AMAXOPHOBIA.

carphology = FLOCCILLATION.

Carr, Harvey A. American psychologist, 1873–1954. See FUNCTIONALISM.

carrier a person whose chromosomes contain one or more genes for a dominant or recessive trait that can be expressed as a birth defect in an offspring. More than 2,000 inherited disorders have been identified and more than seven percent of all children born in the United States have defects. The number of birth-defect carriers in the United States is estimated to be 15,000,000.

Cartesian dualism the theory advanced by René Descartes (Renatus Cartesius) that the mind is an unextended, incorporeal substance (**res cogitans**) separate and distinct from the body, which is a material, extended substance (**res extensa**). He held that the rational acts of the soul, or mind, and the mechanical activities of the body can each be studied in their own right, but he also recognized that mind acts upon the body and body on mind, and proposed that the locus for interaction is the point in the pineal body termed the CONARIUM. See this entry.

Cartesius: See DESCARTES.

carunculae small areas of mucous membrane about the vaginal opening that are remnants of the hymen ruptured during sexual intercourse.

Carus, Carl Gustav /kä′rəs/ German physiologist and psychologist, 1789–1868. See CARUS' TYPOLOGY; CONSTITUTIONAL TYPE.

Carus' typology a classification of individuals by body types proposed by Carl Gustav Carus. The categories of types in his system are athletic, phlegmatic, phthisic, cerebral, and sterile.

Casanova, Giovanni Giacomo Italian adventurer and diplomat, 1725–98. C. is the author of 12 volumes of well-written *Memoirs*. As they contain accounts of thousands of his sexual conquests, his name has become synonymous with a skilled seducer and promiscuous lover. Of psychological interest is (a) his pathological fear of any commitment, (b) his habit of tactfully passing his mistresses on to other men when he is "through" with them, and (c) his frequent sexual relations with three or four women simultaneously. C., at ease in his masculinity, truly worshiped women and lived for them, in contrast to the insecure and ruthless DON JUAN. See this entry. Also see EROTOCRAT.

case advocate: See ADVOCATE.

case-finding in psychiatry, methods of identifying individuals who need treatment for mental disorder, e.g., by administering screening tests, locating individuals who contact social agencies or mental-health facilities, obtaining referrals from general practitioners, or triage after a disaster.

case history a record of all available information relating to a person's medical or psychological condition and composed of test results, interviews, professional evaluations, and sociological, occupational, and educational data.

case load in social psychiatry, the number of cases or comparative difficulty of cases assigned to a therapist, social worker, or counselor.

case method an industrial training technique in which a group of management or supervisory personnel are presented with an actual or hypothetical business problem in writing, on film, through recordings, or with individuals playing different roles.

case study in-depth investigation of a single individual, a family, or another social unit. In this process, every type of data (psychological, physiological, biographical, environmental) is assembled in order to throw light on the subject's background, relationships, behavior, and adjustment.

case work = SOCIAL C.W.

cassina leaves foliage of a plant, Ilex cassine, that grows wild in eastern North America, particularly Virginia and the Carolinas. The leaves contain caffeine and are used in an herbal tea known as **Apalache tea, yaupon**, or **youpon**. Members of the Creek nation roasted the leaves and made a decoction from them that presumably contained so many "virtues" that only men were permitted to drink the beverage.

castrating a term that literally refers to the physical removal of the male or female sex organs but which also may be applied to a psychological threat to the masculinity or femininity of an individual.

castrating woman a woman, usually a wife or mother, who emasculates a man or men in the psychological sense through domination, derogation, and insistence on making all the decisions unilaterally.

castration removal of the male testes or female ovaries by surgery, or inactivation of the glands by radiation, parasites, infections, or drugs. C. alters the hormonal function of the individual and generally reduces libido. With psychiatric treatment, major behavioral changes seldom result from c. Also see ORCHIECTOMY; EUNUCH; SKOPTSY.

For the psychoanalytic meaning of c. (focusing on the penis, not the gonads), see C. COMPLEX and ACTIVE C. COMPLEX.

castration anxiety; castration fear: See CASTRATION COMPLEX.

castration complex in psychoanalysis, the unconscious feelings and fantasies associated with being deprived of the sex organs, that is, in males, the loss of the penis, and, in females, the belief that the penis has already been removed. In boys, fear of loss of the penis is associated with punishment for sexual interest in the mother (the Oedipus complex), which is sometimes aggravated by threats of castration as punishment for masturbation, and by the discovery that girls have no penis. In girls, the c.c. takes the form of a fantasy that the penis has already been removed as a punishment, for which they blame their mother. See ELECTRA

COMPLEX; OEDIPUS COMPLEX; PENIS ENVY. Also see ACTIVE C.C.; ANAL CASTRATION ANXIETY; ANTICIPATORY AUTOCASTRATION.

-cat-; -cata-; -cato-; -cath- a combining form meaning (a) downward, going down, beneath, (b) against.

CAT = CHILDREN'S APPERCEPTION TEST.

CAT = COMPUTERIZED AXIAL TOMOGRAPHY.

catabolic: See CATABOLISM.

catabolic phase: See METABOLISM.

catabolism the phase of metabolism marked by the breakdown of tissues and expenditure of energy. Adjective: **catabolic**.

catagelophobia a morbid fear of ridicule.

catalepsy a condition in which the skeletal muscles become semirigid and will remain in any position in which they are placed, however awkward, for long periods of time without evidence of discomfort. C. is most frequently found in catatonic schizophrenics during a stuporous or trancelike state of withdrawal and occasionally observed in hysteria, cerebellar disorders, and epilepsy. Also called **cerea flexibilitas; flexibilitas cerea; waxy flexibility; cataleptic immobility; catalepsia cerea**. Also see EPIDEMIC C.

catalexia a form of dyslexia characterized by a tendency to reread words and phrases.

catalogia the constant repetition of meaningless words or phrases. It is a symptom frequently observed in schizophrenia. Also see CATAPHASIA.

catalytic agent a member of a psychotherapy group who activates emotional reactions in other members.

catamenia = MENSTRUATION.

catamite a boy who participates in pederasty.

catamnesis the medical history of a patient following the onset of a mental or physical disorder. The term is also applied to the history after the initial examination or after discharge from treatment, then also called **follow-up history**.

cataphasia uncontrollable repetition of apparently meaningless words or phrases. It is a language disorder that occurs in catatonic schizophrenia and in patients with brain lesions. Also called **verbigeration**.

cataphora a type of coma that may be interrupted by intervals of partial consciousness. Also called **coma somnolentium**.

cataplexy /kat'-/ a sudden loss of muscle tone resulting in collapse of the entire body. C. is a temporary condition usually precipitated by an uncontrollable fit of laughter or an event that produces overwhelming anxiety or anger. Adjective: **cataplectic** /-plek'-/. See NARCOLEPSY; NARCOLEPSY-CATAPLEXY SYNDROME.

cataract the progressive clouding of the lens of the eye that gradually reduces the passage of light to the retina, eventually causing blindness. A c. frequently is associated with the degenerative processes of aging, but it also may be congenital or due to disease, injury, or exposure to radiation. The only symptom is a gradual dimming of vision marked by the need of the patient for brighter illumination or a peculiar way of holding reading material.

catarrhal ophthalmia: See OPHTHALMIA.

catastrophe theory a psychoanalytic term for the belief that sexual intercourse is destructive to the penis.

catastrophic anxiety a state of overwhelming anxiety and helplessness in patients with organic brain syndromes and aphasia, who, according to K. Goldstein (1939) "become agitated and fearful and more than usually inept when presented with once simple tasks that they can no longer do." See CATASTROPHIC REACTION.

catastrophic behavior a term used by K. Goldstein to denote the efforts of aphasic patients to adapt to their language defects through such defensive reactions as excessive orderliness, disinterest, and aversion. By these means they seek to avoid embarrassment and agitation arising from ineptness in communicating or carrying out simple tasks.

catastrophic expectation according to F. Perls, the fear that accompanies thoughts, wishes, or behavior that contradicts social standards or an internal moral code, e.g., a fantasy of future retribution for one's action. See GESTALT THERAPY.

catastrophic illness an extremely severe or chronic illness with which the patient must cope in his own way and come to terms with such reactions as (a) feeling that he has been cheated, (b) denial of illness, and (c) hesitation to ventilate feelings of shame, guilt, or fear.

catastrophic reaction a breakdown in the ability to cope with a threatening or traumatic situation. The individual experiences acute feelings of inadequancy, insecurity, anxiety, and helplessness and many show signs of pallor, sweating, and incipient collapse, indicating a physical as well as mental shock. C.r. is often observed in patients with dominant-hemisphere lesions. Also see DISASTER SYNDROME.

catastrophic schizophrenia = SCHIZOCARIA.

catathymia a condition in which an unconscious complex becomes so affect-laden that it produces changes in conscious functioning.

catathymic amnesia a loss of memory for a specific event although the individual has a clear memory for all other events.

catathymic crisis = ISOLATED EXPLOSIVE DISORDER.

catatonia = CATATONIC STATE.

catatonia mitis a relatively mild and transient form of catatonia in which stupor and lack of movement are the main symptoms. When the condition is extended and severe, it may be termed **catatonia protracta**.

catatonic cerebral paralysis a rare form of schizophrenia in which a fever of unknown origin is followed by a fatal episode of catatonic excitement or delirium. Also called **Stauder's lethal catatonia**. Also see BELL'S MANIA.

catatonic excitement a symptom of catatonic schizophrenia consisting of periods of extreme restlessness and excessive motor activity. See SCHIZOPHRENIC DISORDER, CATATONIC TYPE.

catatonic negativism; catatonic posturing; catatonic rigidity; catatonic schizophrenia: See SCHIZOPHRENIC DISORDER, CATATONIC TYPE.

catatonic state a state of muscular rigidity or other disturbance of motor behavior such as catalepsy, posturing, or extreme overactivity. It is most frequently observed in catatonic schizophrenia. Also called **catatonia; katatonia**. See SCHIZOPHRENIC DISORDER, CATATONIC TYPE. Also see TRAUMATIC PSEUDOCATATONIA.

catatonic stupor a symptom of catatonic schizophrenia involving inaccessibility to stimuli, waxy flexibility, mutism, extreme negativism, and stereotyped behavior. See SCHIZOPHRENIC DISORDER, CATATONIC TYPE; CATATONIC STATE.

catatonoid attitude catatonialike behavior characterized by stereotyped responses, such as a vacant smile, in all personal or social situations.

catatony /-tat'-/ a rarely used term for catatonic state, or catatonia.

catchment area in community psychiatry, the geographic area that is served by a particular COMMUNITY MENTAL-HEALTH CENTER. See this entry.

catch trials in tests or experiments consisting of several trials, those trials in which the independent variable is surreptitiously withheld by the experimenter while the subject's responses are recorded as usual. E.g., in an experiment in which subjects identify auditory signals, c.t. are those in which no signal is given. Results of c.t. assist the experimenter in determining the subjects' level of accuracy and reliability.

cat-cry syndrome = CRI DU CHAT SYNDROME.

catecholamine hypothesis a theory used to explain affective disorders and the efficacy of antidepressant medications. It hypothesizes that depression is caused by abnormally low concentrations of free catecholamines, as measured in terms of the norepinephrine levels in cerebrospinal fluid. Manic states are marked by excessively high concentrations of free catecholamines. Therapy is directed toward restoring a normal balance of catecholamines.

catecholaminergic neurons nerve cells that act by releasing catecholamine, such as norepinephrine. Also called **adrenergic neurons**.

catecholamines a group of hormones including epinephrine, norepinephrine, and dopamine produced in adrenal glands and cells of the central nervous system and autonomic nerves. A primary function of c. is that of neurotransmission. C. production usually increases in body tissues as emotional stress increases. Drugs with similar effects include amphetamine and ephedrine.

catechol-O-methyltransferase a synaptic enzyme that deactivates catecholamines.

categorical attitude = ABSTRACT ATTITUDE.

categorical imperative the rule of Immanuel Kant (1785) that our behavior should be guided by principles that we would want to be the guiding principles of all humankind. It is the unconditional command of conscience (as opposed to the hypothetical imperative, which is a law relative to further ends).

categorical thought a term used by Piaget for abstract thinking. Such thinking involves the use of general concepts and classifications, and is particularly lacking in schizophrenics, who tend to think concretely. See ABSTRACT ATTITUDE; ABSTRACT THINKING.

category a group of items usually organized by qualitative rather than quantitative factors.

Category Test: See CEREBRAL DYSFUNCTION TESTS.

CAT-H: CHILDREN'S APPERCEPTION TEST.

catharsis the therapeutic release, or discharge, of anxiety, tension, or other symptoms by talking out disturbing feelings and impulses, or, on a deeper level, by bringing to the surface and reliving the unconscious events and experiences that produced these symptoms. The **cathartic method** was introduced by Breuer and developed by Freud. See ABREACTION.

cathected: See CATHEXIS.

cathectic discharge a release of psychic energy or affect, as in weeping or expressing anger. Also called **affective discharge**.

catheter /kath'-/ any flexible tubular instrument used to introduce or remove fluids through a body passageway. A c. may be indwelling, if required for a long period of time, or temporary. A double-current c. contains two parallel tubes so that a fluid can be introduced through one channel and removed through the other. A c. is used to introduce radiopaque substances into an artery for arteriographic studies. Use of a c. is called **catheterization**.

cathexis /-theks'-/ the investment of psychic energy, or drive, in an object of any kind, such as wishes, fantasies, persons, goals, ideas, a social group, or the self (from Greek *cathexo*, "I occupy"). Such objects are said to be **cathected** when we attach emotional significance, or affect (positive or negative), to them. Also called **investment**. See ACATHEXIS; BODY C.; COUNTER-CATHEXIS; DECATHEXIS; EGO C.; ENDOCATHECTION; EXOCATHECTION; FANTASY C.; HYPERCATHEXIS; HYPOCATHEXIS; NEGATIVE C.; OBJECT C.; ORAL-SADISTIC C.; POSITIVE C.; RECATHEXIS.

cation /kat'ī·ən/ an ion carrying a positive charge and therefore attracted to the negatively charged cathode (Greek, "going down"). Also spelled **kation**.

cationic drugs /katī·on'ik/ drugs that are used in complex pharmacological actions because they contain acidic or phenolic ions and can make electrolyte exchanges in solutions with substances possessing a positive electrical charge.

catnip a plant that grows wild and in gardens in Europe, Asia, and North America. The leaves and flowering tops are used as an herb for tea and in medications. Native Americans have smoked the dried leaves, identifying the plant as **shinecock**. The botanical name is Nepeta cataria, and the common name in many languages includes a reference to cat. The volatile oils in c. are related to a substance used by veterinarians to tranquilize lions and other large cats.

cat phobia = AILUROPHOBIA.

cat powder: See METATABI.

CAT scan = COMPUTERIZED AXIAL TOMOGRAPHY.

cat's-eye syndrome a chromosomal disorder caused by a small additional acrocentric bit of chromosome material, resulting in a set of birth defects that include an imperforate anus and a cleft iris that produces a cat's-eye appearance. Most of the children with c.-e.s. have been retarded. Also called **syndrome of extra-small acrocentric chromosome; 47,XX+?G**.

Cattell, James McKeen American psychologist, 1860–1944. C. studied with Wundt in Leipzig and with Galton in England, and at 28 was appointed professor of psychology of the University of Pennsylvania, the first chair of psychology in America. He later transferred to Columbia University and exerted broad influence by editing many scientific publications; by founding the Psychological Corporation; by teaching distinguished contributors such as Woodworth and Thorndike; by carrying out experiments on reaction time, perception, and word association; and by devising the first battery of psychological tests of special ability. Also see GENIUS; BALDWIN; BINET; DEWEY; WOODWORTH.

Cattell, Raymond B. American psychologist, 1905—. See CATTELL'S FACTORIAL THEORY OF PERSONALITY; CATTELL INFANT SCALE; CATTELL INVENTORIES; AUTIA; BOHEMIAN UNCONCERNEDNESS; COMENTION; CORTERIA; DESURGENCY; DYNAMIC-EFFECT LAW; ENVIRONMENTAL-MOLD TRAIT; ERG; FRUSTRATION RESPONSE; HARRIA; L-DATA; LONG-CIRCUITING; MALERG; METAERG; NEUROTIC-PROCESS FACTOR; NEUROTIC-REGRESSIVE DEBILITY; PARMIA; PATHEMIA; PERSONALITY SPHERE; PRAXERNIA; PREMSIA; PROMETHEAN WILL; PROTENSION; SIXTEEN PERSONALITY FACTOR QUESTIONNAIRE; SOURCE TRAITS; SURFACE TRAITS; SURGENCY; SYNTALITY; T-DATA; THRECTIA; ZEPPIA. Also see ERG; FACTOR THEORY OF PERSONALITY; INFANT AND PRESCHOOL TESTS; PERSONALITY STRUCTURE.

Cattell Infant Scale an intelligence and developmental scale for ages two months to 30 months, consisting of developmental items and Stanford-Binet items.

Cattell inventories self-report inventories based on a study of personality traits by factor analysis (R. B. Cattell). The best known inventory stemming from this research is the Sixteen Personality Factor Questionnaire, which yields 16 scores on such traits as trusting versus suspicious, humble versus assertive, and reserved versus outgoing. Similar Cattell inventories include the **High School Personality Questionnaire**, the **Chil-**

dren's Personality Questionnaire, and the **Early School Personality Questionnaire**.

Cattell's Factorial Theory of Personality an approach to personality description based on the identification of traits, their measurement through factor analysis, and their classification into 35 surface traits and 12 source traits which underlie them. See SURFACE TRAITS; SOURCE TRAITS.

-caud- a combining form relating to a tail, to anything tail-shaped, or to the lower or tail end of something. Adjectives: **caudal; caudate**.

caudate nucleus a long arched mass of gray matter that follows the general curvature of the lateral ventricle and terminates in the amygdaloid nucleus. The c.n. is part of the BASAL GANGLIA and CORPUS STRIATUM. See these entries.

causalgia a sensation of intense, burning pain resulting from injury to the peripheral nerves. The condition is most often due to a penetrating wound inflicted by a bullet or knife, and involves swelling, redness, and sweating in addition to almost unbearable pain.

causality the hypothesis that all events are consequences of preceding events. Freud was one of the first to explain mental events in terms of causes (instincts, drives, traumatic experiences) rather than purposes. The causal approach contrasts with the purely descriptive approach of statistical research, and with the introspective method.

causal texture the environment as composed of mutually dependent events. The dependence is conceived in terms of probability rather than certainty (E. C. Tolman, E. Brunswick).

cause-and-effect test an intelligence test that offers alternative causes for different effects and alternative effects for different causes, requiring the examinee to choose the most logical explanations.

CAVD Test an intelligence test developed by E. L. Thorndike consisting of a battery of four types of items: *c*ompletion, *a*rithmetic problems, *v*ocabulary, and following *d*irections.

cebocephaly a type of congenital defect in which the eyes are abnormally close to each other, the nose may be missing or not fully formed, and the facial features resemble those of a monkey. In some cases, the defect pattern may include cyclopia. C. is associated with chromosome-13 trisomy and 18p—syndromes.

CEEB College Level Examination Program: See ADVANCED PLACEMENT EXAMINATIONS.

ceiling the maximum possible score in any test.

ceiling age the maximum level reached on a scaled test such as the Stanford-Binet, that is, the level where all tests are failed and the test is discontinued.

ceiling effect the inability of a test to measure or discriminate above a certain point, usually because its items are too easy. Compare FLOOR EFFECT.

-cele-; -coele- a combining form relating to a swelling, tumor, or hernia.

-celi-; -celio- a combining form relating to to the abdominal region. Adjective: **celiac**.

celibacy a state of being unmarried. The term is generally applied to members of religious orders who take a vow to abstain from marriage. C. is sometimes, but not always, interpreted as abstinence from sexual activity.

cell the basic unit of organized tissue, consisting of an outer membrane, a nuclear control center, and a mass of protoplasm known as cytoplasm. Some primitive cell structures may not possess all of the components; e.g., certain bacteria lack a specific nuclear entity.

cell assembly a group of neurons that develop as a functioning unit through repeated stimulation. The term also applies to a theoretical organization of brain cells that enables a subject to form a complete mental image of an object when only a portion actually may be visible. The c.a. theory, proposed by D. O. Hebb, assumes that perceptual memory depends upon routes of impulses through cell assemblages established when the individual learns to recognize shapes and other details of objects.

cell body the central part of a cell containing the nucleus, which controls its life processes.

cell differentiation a process that involves changes in physical and functional aspects of cells as they become specialized in the embryo in order to form different body structures.

cell division the steps through which a body or somatic cell produces daughter cells. The stages include prophase, metaphase, anaphase, and telophase.

cell nucleus a portion of the cell that controls its metabolic functions, including growth and repair of structures of the cell. It also contains the deoxyribonucleic acid (DNA) which is necessary for cell reproduction.

cellular immunity factors: See IMMUNITY FACTORS.

cellular layers of cortex the six layers of cells that are components of the neocortex. The layers, identified by Roman numerals, are: I, the **plexiform molecular layer of Cajal**, a narrow band of myelinated fibers; II, the **external granular layer**, containing granular cells and shafts of pyramidal cells; III, the **external pyramidal-cell layer**, with medium-size cells in the outer zone and larger pyramidal cells in the inner zone; IV, the **internal granular layer**, which contains synapses of layer-III cells along with small stellate and pyramidal cells; V, the **ganglionic layer**, which includes large pyramidal cells and the giant cells of Betz; and VI, the **polymorphic fusiform layer**, which contains cells of many shapes but mainly spindle-shaped cells. The six layers are characteristics of parietal, temporal, and occipital lobes more than other brain areas.

-cen-: See -COEN-.

cenesthesia; cenesthesis = COENESTHESIA.

cenesthopathy a general feeling of illness or lack of well-being that is not identified with any particular part of the body.

cenophobia = KENOPHOBIA.

cenotrope acquired behavior believed to be a product of hereditary and environmental forces because it appears in all members of a species in the same environment. Also called **coenotrope**.

censor the name figuratively applied by Freud to the components of the personality (ego, superego, and ego-ideal) that determine which of our memories, thoughts, and impulses enter consciousness, and which are banned because they violate conscience, standards, or the reality principle. Also called **endopsychic c.**

censorship in psychoanalysis, the exclusion of unacceptable or forbidden thoughts and impulses from consciousness by the process of selection and repression. Freud held that this process is governed by the rules and prohibitions imposed by parents or other members of society.

census tract a small area, comprising 3,500 to 4,000 residents, whose boundaries are established by the Bureau of the Census. Demographic data on such variables as median age, sex ratio, number of children, foreign-born status, labor force, school enrollment, income characteristics, delinquency, suicide rate, and housing characteristics are frequently used in the assessment of area characteristics and needs, including mental-health needs.

centering a term applied by Kurt Goldstein to a state of perfect integration of the organism with its environment.

center median a large group of nerve cells associated with the thalamus. It is innervated by fibers from the motor cortex, globus pallidus, and putamen areas of the brain and serves as part of the arousal system.

-centesis /-səntē′-/ a combining form relating to a puncture (from Greek *kentein*, "to puncture").

central anticholinergic syndrome a syndrome observed in patients receiving combinations of psychotropic drugs, and due to the additive anticholinergic effects of tricyclic depressants, the weaker phenothiazines, and antiparkinson agents. The symptoms include anxiety, disorientation, short-term-memory loss, hallucinations, and agitation.

central aphasia the term used by Kurt Goldstein (1948) to denote an interiorized loss of language functioning due to brain lesions. It is the loss of an individual's inner language system.

central canal the channel in the spinal cord containing cerebrospinal fluid.

central conflict a term introduced by Horney to describe the intrapsychic struggle between the healthy constructive forces of the real self and the obstructive, neurotic forces of the idealized self.

central deafness a perceptive impairment caused by dysfunction of the inner ear or damage to the eighth nerve between the inner ear and the brainstem. It may be caused by vascular changes in the brain, brain tumor, trauma, or genetic blood incompatibilities.

central fissure = FISSURE OF ROLANDO.

central force a term used to describe the keystone of the individual's total psychic system. C.f. is Jung's primal libido or life force.

central gray the unmyelinated gray nerve fibers that form a generally H-shaped pattern in the central portion of the spinal cord.

central inhibition a CNS process that prevents or interrupts the flow of neural impulses that control behavior.

centralism a concept that behavior is a CNS function mediated by the brain. See CENTRALIST PSYCHOLOGY. Compare PERIPHERALISM.

centralist psychology a psychological approach that focuses on behavior as a function of the higher brain centers, as opposed to peripheralist psychology, which focuses on the effects of the receptors, glands, and muscles on behavior. The term is essentially equivalent to CENTRALISM. See this entry.

central-limit theorem the statistical principle that sample means drawn from a population are normally distributed, whether or not the population they were drawn from was normally distributed.

central motive state a theoretical function of the nervous system that accounts for a persistent level of activity in the absence of external stimuli or a continuation of nervous activity when the original motive no longer exists.

central nervous system the entire complex of nerve cells, fibers, and supporting tissue within the brain and spinal cord. The c.n.s. is primarily involved in the control of mental activities and in coordinating and integrating incoming and outgoing messages. Abbrev.: **CNS**. Also called **cerebrospinal system; voluntary nervous system**.

central pain pain that is caused by a disorder of the central nervous system, such as a brain tumor or spinal-cord infection or injury.

central process a process that occurs in the central nervous system.

central-processing dysfunction a disorder in the analysis, storage, synthesis, and symbolic use of information. Differences in processing styles affect a child's learning ability.

central reflex time = REFLEX LATENCY.

central sulcus = FISSURE OF ROLANDO.

central tegmental nucleus = NUCLEUS OF THE RAPHE.

central tendency the middlemost location or direction in a set of scores, represented by the mean, median, or mode.

central-tendency measure = MEASURE OF CENTRAL TENDENCY.

central traits a term used by Allport for a cluster of traits that comprise the basic pattern of an individual's personality, e.g., "compassionate, ambitious, sociable, helpful."

central vision vision that occurs primarily in the region of the retinal fovea.

centrencephalic epilepsy a form of epilepsy marked by generalized and petit mal seizures that appear to originate near the center of the brain. C.e. is not associated with any particular local anatomical or functional system but is instead radiated outward through both cerebral hemispheres. The EEG reveals a characteristic three-cycles-per-second spike-and-wave pattern in petit mal.

centrencephalic seizure an epileptic seizure involving the centrencephalic system located in the central core of the brainstem.

centrencephalic system a term introduced by Wilder Penfield to identify a central anatomical brain area in which neurons provide a coherent unity for mental processes. The c.s. is believed by some authors to be the reticular activating system.

centrencephalon the center of the encephalon, or brain, a small region of relatively undifferentiated neurons in the subcortical area. The term was introduced by Wilder Penfield as part of his theory of a centrencephalic system or seat of free-will control over human activities.

centrifugal nerve /-trif'-/ a neuron that carries impulses from the central nervous system to the periphery of the body; an efferent or motor nerve.

centrifugal peripheral pathways the routes followed by certain nerve fibers or impulses that move from the center to the periphery.

centripetal /-trip'-/ directed toward the center. In psychiatry, the term is used to characterize treatment or approaches that focus inward on minute changes in feelings and impulses, as in psychoanalysis. The term is also used to characterize nerve fibers and nerve impulses that move from the periphery toward the central nervous system.

centroid an average of a set of data points. The term also refers to a type of factor analysis used before the advent of computers.

centromere /sen'trəmēr/ a portion of a chromosome which is attached to the equatorial plane of the mitotic or meiotic spindle during cell division. The c. of a chromosome occasionally becomes a separate body of genetic material, accounting for certain types of anomalies. See CAT'S-EYE SYNDROME.

centro ritual: See FOLK PSYCHIATRY.

-cephal-; -cephalo- a combining form relating to the head. Adjective: **cephalic.**

cephalalgia an intense headache, such as occurs in infectious diseases or states of tension. Also called **cephalagia; cephalagra.**

cephalic index a measure of the proportions of an individual head calculated by dividing the maximum width by the maximum height and multiplying the result by 100. The average, or medium, c.i. is in the range of 76 to 81 for humans. The longer the head in proportion to its width, the smaller the c.i. number below 76. Likewise, a c.i. figure greater than 81 indicates a shorter- or wider-than-average head proportion. Also called **cephalization index.**

cephalocaudal axis: See AXIS.

cephalocaudal development the head-to-tail

progression of anatomical and motor development, as determined by the anterior-posterior development gradient. The head and its movements develop first, then the upper trunk, arms and hands, followed by the lower trunk and leg, foot, and toe movements. See ANTERIOR-POSTERIOR DEVELOPMENT GRADIENT.

cephalogenesis the stage of embryonic development in which the head begins to form.

cephalometry the scientific measurement of the dimensions of the head. C. is applied in orthodontics to predict and evaluate craniofacial development. **Fetal c.** is determined by the use of ultrasound or X-ray techniques when necessary for planning delivery of the offspring.

cephaloskeletal dysplasia a congenital disorder, believed to be hereditary, marked by low birth weight, skeletal anomalies, microcephaly, and brain malformations. The brains of those patients autopsied were found to be globular in shape and small in size. The patients have been short-lived and severely retarded.

cerea flexibilitas = CATALEPSY.

-cereb-; -cerebri-; -cerebro- a combining form relating to the brain (Latin *cerebrum*). Adjective: **cerebral** /sərēb'-/ or /ser'əbrəl/.

cerebellar: See CEREBELLUM.

cerebellar ataxia lack of muscular coordination due to damage in the neocerebellum. The patient cannot integrate voluntary movements and therefore finds it difficult to stand or walk, feed himself, or perform complex activities such as playing the piano.

cerebellar cortex gray matter, or unmyelinated nerve cells, covering the surface of the cerebellum.

cerebellar fit a type of seizure associated with a tumor of the vermis and marked by sudden loss of consciousness and collapse, cyanosis, and dilated pupils. The posture is OPISTHOTONOS. See this entry.

cerebellar folia the pattern of leaflike structures that subdivide the cerebellar cortex.

cerebellar gait an unsteady, wobbly gait due to lack of coordination between the trunk and legs, so that the trunk lags behind or is thrust forward.

cerebellar rigidity: See EXTENSOR RIGIDITY.

cerebellar speech a type of speech that is jerky, irregular, explosive, and scanning, due to a cerebellar lesion. Also called **asynergic speech; ataxic speech.**

cerebellum a three-lobed portion of the brain located on the back of the brainstem. The c. modulates muscular contractions to reduce jerking or tremors and helps maintain equilibrium by predicting body positions ahead of actual body movements. Adjective: **cerebellar.**

cerebra: See CEREBRUM.

cerebral: See -CEREB-.

cerebral anemia a condition of abnormally low levels of hemoglobin or red blood cells in the blood reaching brain tissues. The disorder can be the cause of cerebral infarction by decreasing the amount of blood reaching the brain. One form of c.a. is associated with sickle-cell anemia which can be a factor in the high incidence of stroke among members of the black population.

cerebral angiography a technique of studying the blood circulation of the brain by injecting a solution of an iodine compound into one of the arteries supplying the brain. X-rays or similar radiological methods of tracing the path of the injected material can reveal areas of blood-vessel rupture, blockage, or tumor. In some European countries, c.a. is used to verify brain death. Also called **cerebral arteriography**.

cerebral angiomatosis a disease characterized by the formation of multiple tumors in the blood vessels that carry blood to brain tissue. A congenital form of the disorder is marked by frequent epileptic seizures and muscular weakness on one side of the body as a result of impaired blood flow to the brain.

cerebral arteriography = CEREBRAL ANGIOGRAPHY.

cerebral arteriosclerosis a hardening of the arteries that provide freshly oxygenated blood to the brain. See ARTERIOSCLEROTIC BRAIN DISORDER.

cerebral beriberi = WERNICKE'S DISEASE.

cerebral-blast syndrome a condition involving diffuse bleeding in the tissues or protective membranes of the brain, resulting from exposure to an explosion that does not produce external skull injury. The bleeding within the skull usually results in loss of consciousness. C.-b.s. is generally associated with military combat.

cerebral blindness = CORTICAL BLINDNESS.

cerebral brain stimulation: See BRAIN STIMULATION.

cerebral compression a head injury, e.g., contusion or concussion, that results in a cerebral hemorrhage. The intracranial hemorrhage may be subdural or extradural.

cerebral contusion an injury to the brain that results in damage to blood vessels without a break in the surrounding membranes that would result in a loss of blood from the affected region. The effect is similar to a bruise in which released blood is trapped beneath the skin. A c.c. often results in epilepsy or other neurologic disorders. It may result from contre coup effects of a head injury.

cerebral cortex the covering of gray cells several layers in thickness on the outside of the cerebral hemispheres of the human brain. Each hemisphere of the c.c. is divided into an occipital, parietal, frontal, and temporal lobe. It functions as the source of conscious nervous activity, including reasoning, memory, learning, intelligence, and interpretation of sensory inputs. See CEREBRAL HEMISPHERES.

cerebral dominance the control of lower brain centers by the cerebrum or cerebral cortex. See LATERAL DOMINANCE; LATERALITY; SPLIT BRAIN.

cerebral dynamic imaging = NUCLEAR IMAGING.

cerebral dysfunctions impaired cerebral processes, especially those associated with organic brain syndromes, e.g., disturbances of memory, verbal ability, numerical ability, psychomotor functioning, and diminished or fluctuating levels of consciousness.

cerebral-dysfunction tests clinical instruments for assessing neuropsychological impairment (organicity; brain damage). Among the functions most sensitive to pathological processes are perception of spatial relations and memory for newly learned material. Examples of tests that measure these functions are the Benton Visual Retention Test and the Bender Gestalt Test. However, since there is a wide variety of organic brain dysfunctions, and it is useful to localize impaired brain areas, two major batteries of tests have been developed: (a) the Halstead-Reitan Neuropsychological Battery, which includes sensorimotor and perceptual tests, an aphasia test, the Category Test (deducing general principles from data); the Trail-Making Test (connecting circles in numerical order), the MMPI, and the WAIS; and (b) the Luria-Nebraska Neuropsychological Battery, comprising 269 items, each representing different aspects of relevant skills such as motor function, memory, expressive speech, and tactile functions.

cerebral dysplasia any abnormality in the development of the brain. Kinds of c.d. may include anencephaly, marked by failure of the cerebral hemispheres to develop; microcephaly, in which the cerebral hemispheres are abnormally small; porencephaly, characterized by development of a hemisphere containing a cavity; and corpus callosum agenesis, in which the nerve tract joining the hemispheres fails to develop.

cerebral dysrhythmia abnormal brain-wave rhythms that are associated with neurologic disease or other pathologic conditions such as a drug overdose. During an attack of epilepsy, a patient's EEG recording may show a diffuse mixture of different rhythms. In some cases of drug intoxication, the EEG rhythm appears as fast activity superimposed on generalized slowing of brain-cell discharges.

cerebral eclipse brief loss of consciousness, perception, and motor functions due to chronic cerebral circulatory insufficiency, but without cardiac arrest or lowered blood pressure.

cerebral edema an abnormal accumulation of fluid in the intercellular spaces of the brain tissues. C.e. may be caused by injury, cerebrovascular accident, or tumor. The condition results in a rise in intracranial pressure and, if uncorrected, may be followed by herniation of cerebral tissue through weakened areas. It may be reversible unless the damage extends to the brainstem, where the effects can be fatal. In adults, the intracranial pressure may result in headaches and visual disorders. C.e. also may be a cause of dementia that recedes when the defect is corrected. Also called **wet brain; water on the brain**.

cerebral electrotherapy application of low-voltage pulses of direct electrical current to the brain. It is occasionally used in the treatment of depression, anxiety, and insomnia. Abbrev.: **C.E.T**. See ELECTRONARCOSIS.

cerebral embolism a small mass of a substance floating in the blood vessels of the brain. The mass of material can be a part of a blood clot, an air bubble, or a fat globule. The c.e. may block or impede the flow of blood to a part of the brain, usually causing only a temporary neurologic deficit and less damage than a cerebrovascular accident.

cerebral gigantism a growth-hormone disorder marked by excessive size and usually a mild degree of mental retardation in childhood, although most patients can function adequately as adults. At birth and during early childhood, the patients generally are above the 90th percentile in height and weight, and the head is unusually large; the hands, feet, and head of the individual grow rapidly for the first five years of life, after which the rate of development slows to a normal pace. The individual lacks normal muscular coordination and often suffers from mental retardation. Except for identical twins and first cousins, the condition rarely occurs as a genetic or familial trait.

cerebral hemispheres the two halves, left and right, of the cerebrum. The hemispheres are separated by a deep longitudinal fissure but the white matter of the left and right sides is connected by commissural, projection, and association fibers so that each side of the brain normally is linked to functions of tissues on either side of the body.

cerebral hemorrhage any bleeding into the brain tissue due to a damaged blood vessel. The cause may be a ruptured aneurysm triggered by hypertension, an injury caused by a blow to the head, or other factors.

cerebral hyperplasia an abnormal increase in the volume of brain tissue, usually due to a proliferation of new, normal cells. Although neurons do not proliferate after CNS maturity is achieved, glial cells do continue to multiply into adulthood, and in some cases glial-cell growth is associated with hydrocephalus.

cerebral hypoplasia the incomplete development of the cerebral hemispheres. C.h. may occur as a result of a congenital defect or because of malnutrition during early childhood. Studies of brain weights of children who have survived severe protein-deficiency diets show they are smaller than those of children of similar ages and similar total body weights.

cerebral infarct the necrosis, or death, of an area of brain tissue due to an interruption of blood flow caused by rupture of a blood vessel, blockage of a blood vessel by a clot, or a narrowing, or stenosis, of a blood vessel. A c.i. is a common cause of stroke symptoms. A c.i. site often can be located by EEG, as shown by a lack of activity in the region, by cerebral angiography, or by motor or other deficits associated with the brain areas affected. Also see STROKE.

cerebral infection the invasion of brain tissues by a pathogenic organism, such as a virus or bacterium. Most cases occur as a complication of a viral infection such as measles or chicken pox. A **viral c.i.** usually is identified as encephalitis; a **bacterial c.i.** is called **cerebritis**.

cerebral injection a psychosurgery technique in which small amounts of frontal-lobe tissue are destroyed by injecting alcohol, formalin, procaine, or other solutions.

cerebral integration the theory that all neural functions of the body are integrated through the cerebrum.

cerebral intermittent claudication a transient spasm of the circulation of the brain caused by an inadequate blood supply. C.i.c. may result from atherosclerosis of the cerebral arteries and result in temporary hemiplegia.

cerebral ischemia a form of local anemia in which an area of tissue is deprived of an adequate blood supply and therefore is in effect starved for oxygen and nutrients. The condition usually is marked by loss of normal function and occasionally other symptoms such confusion and dizziness. A brief interruption in blood supply, which may be due to a change in blood pressure, usually causes no serious damage. An interruption that continues beyond several minutes may result in a cerebral infarction. A sudden brief interruption caused by a circulatory disturbance in the vertebral-basilar or carotid-middle cerebral arteries can be the cause of a **transient ischemic attack (TIA)**, a mild stroke, that may last for a few minutes and in some cases a few hours, the symptoms then receding without loss of consciousness or functional brain tissue by the patient.

cerebral laceration the tearing or cutting of brain tissue due to a severe head injury.

cerebral pacemaker a hypothetical group of CNS tissue cells that are believed to regulate the rhythms of brain waves in both cerebral hemispheres. The c.p. is believed to be located at the base of the brain, in the region of the hypothalamus or in the reticular formation.

cerebral palsy a group of noninherited neuromuscular disorders resulting from damage primarily to the motor region of the brain, causing impairment in control over voluntary muscles. The damage is generally produced by such factors as prenatal infection (e.g., rubella), Rh incompatibility, premature separation of the placenta, marked prematurity, intracerebral hemorrhage, hyperbilirubinemia, toxic disorder, difficult delivery, and, in a few cases, postnatal head injury. Symptoms include spasticity, uncontrolled movements (athetosis), staggering gait, guttural speech, and, in some cases, seizures, visual defects, hearing loss, and mental retardation. Abbrev.: **CP**. Also see FORCEPS INJURY.

cerebral peduncles two cylindrical bundles of motor-neuron white matter that connect the pons with the underside of either of the cerebral hemispheres forming the pyramidal tract. Also called **crura cerebri**.

cerebral syphilis a condition that results when untreated syphilis involves the cerebral cortex and surrounding meningeal membranes, causing general paresis. The condition, which usually develops about ten years after the infection, is marked by irritability, memory deterioration, inability to concentrate, headaches, insomnia, and behavioral deterioration. Also called **meningovascular syphilis; interstitial neurosyphilis**.

cerebral thrombosis: See THROMBUS.

cerebral trauma an impairment of brain functions, temporary or permanent, following a blow to the head of sufficient severity to produce a concussion, contusion, or laceration. See ACUTE TRAUMATIC DISORDERS; CHRONIC TRAUMATIC DISORDER. Also see HEAD TRAUMA.

cerebral-vascular accident = CEREBROVASCULAR ACCIDENT.

cerebral-vascular disease a pathologic condition of the blood vessels of the brain. The condition may manifest itself as symptoms of stroke or a transient ischemic attack, or temporary interruption of blood flow to a brain area. A stroke suggests a rupture of an artery in the brain or a thrombosis that blocks blood flow to a vital area. Depending upon the degree of circulatory failure and the location of the tissues affected, c.-v.d. symptoms may include paralysis, loss of vision or speech ability, headaches, dizziness, lethargy, or personality changes. Signs of progressive c.-v.d. may not be noticed until the condition begins to interfere with work or other daily activities. Also called **cerebrovascular disease**.

cerebral-vascular insufficiency failure of the cardiovascular system to supply adequate levels of oxygenated blood to the brain tissues. The condition is diagnosed with EEG studies while one of the four main sources of blood to the brain, namely the two carotid and two vertebral arteries, is interrupted briefly. Alterations in blood-flow patterns will register as EEG abnormalities. Also called **cerebrovascular insufficiency**.

cerebration a term applied to any kind of conscious thinking such as pondering or problem-solving. Also see UNCONSCIOUS C.

cerebritis: See CEREBRAL INFECTION.

cerebrocranial defect a deformity or dysfunction involving the cerebrum and the eight bones of the skull that form a protective layer around it. Examples include premature closing of the sutures of the skull resulting in a displacement of

cerebral tissues, and hydrocephalus, which is associated with a cranial deformity.

cerebrohepatorenal syndrome a relatively rare hereditary disorder marked by a complex of brain, liver, and kidney anomalies. Specific abnormalities of the organs differ, but all patients have severe muscular hypotonia and slow psychomotor development, and some may have seizures.

cerebromacular referring to an area distinguishable by color or other factors from its surroundings in the brain and other CNS tissue. The term may be used to refer to the macula retinae, a yellowish depression below the optic disk that is involved in color vision, particularly the short wavelengths of visible light.

cerebromacular degeneration a disease of the gray matter of the brain, marked by excessive accumulation of lipids in the neurons, causing them to swell and degenerate. At the same time, a reddish discoloration spreads over the macula of the retina. The effect is progressive blindness and dementia. Kinds of c.d. disorders include Tay-Sachs disease, Bielschowsky's disease, Batten-Spielmeyer-Vogt disease, and Kufs' disease.

cerebroretinal arteriovenous aneurysm = WYBURN-MASON'S SYNDROME.

cerebroside lipidosis = GAUCHER'S DISEASE.

cerebroside a fatty acid compound present in the myelin sheath of nerve fibers that are usually identified as white matter. In certain neurologic disorders, such as Gaucher's disease or Niemann-Pick disease, abnormal metabolism of the c. often is involved.

cerebrospinal fluid the fluid within the central canal of the spinal cord, the four ventricles of the brain, and the subarachnoid space of the brain. The c.f. serves as a watery cushion to protect vital CNS tissues from damage by shock pressure. Abbrev.: **CSF**.

cerebrospinal system = CENTRAL NERVOUS SYSTEM.

cerebrotendinous xanthomatosis an autosomal-recessive disease marked by white-matter lesions and loss of myelin in the cerebellum. The disease has three clinical stages, beginning with mild-to-moderate mental retardation in childhood, followed by dementia and spasticity in early adulthood, then progressive paralysis, bedridden helplessness, loss of ability to speak, and muscular atrophy. Leg tendons show extensive yellowish deposits of cholesterol. Also called **van Bogaert's disease**.

cerebrotonia the personality type which, according to Sheldon, is associated with an ectomorphic (linear, fragile) physique. C. is characterized by a tendency toward introversion, restraint, inhibition, love of privacy and solitude, and sensitivity.

cerebrovascular accident an interruption of arterial blood flow to an area of the cerebrum as a result of a ruptured blood vessel, the blockage of a blood vessel by a clot or other debris, e.g., cellular material, compression of a blood vessel by a tumor or accumulation of trapped fluid, or an arterial spasm. A c.a. that lasts more than a few seconds often results in the death of brain tissue with ensuing neurological damage. Abbrev.: **CVA**. Also called **cerebral-vascular accident**. See STROKE.

cerebrovascular disease = CEREBRAL-VASCULAR DISEASE.

cerebrovascular insufficiency = CEREBRAL-VAS-CULAR INSUFFICIENCY.

cerebrum /ser'-/ or /sərēb'-/ the larger part of the brain in front of and above the cerebellum and consisting of two hemispheres (Latin, "brain"). It includes the forebrain and midbrain. Plurals: **cerebrums; cerebra**. Also called **telencephalon**.

ceremonials: See RITUALS.

Cerletti, Ugo /cherlet'ē/ Italian psychiatrist, 1877–1963. See ELECTROCONVULSIVE TREATMENT.

certification in psychiatry and neurology, official designation of competence by the American Board of Psychiatry and Neurology, including issuance of a diploma which indicates that the candidate has passed the required examinations and has the right to be called a diplomate. C. also applies to the process of reviewing case records to determine whether the health care is necessary in a particular case, and if the level of care provided is appropriate. Also, it applies to the process of completing the necessary documents in commitment proceedings.

certification laws legislation governing the admission of patients to mental institutions, including commitment proceedings as well as a review of case records to determine whether health care is necessary and whether the site and type of care are appropriate. The term also applies to state laws governing the right of an individual to represent himself as a psychologist.

cerumen the waxlike secretion normally present in the external canal of the ear.

cerveau insolé /servō'eNsōlā'/ a detached brain, usually applied to a laboratory animal whose brain has been excised at the level of the mesencephalon for experimental purposes (French, "isolated brain").

-cervic-; -cervico- a combining form relating to the neck of the body or of an organ. See CERVIX.

cervical: See CERVIX.

cervical erosion the loss of the surface layer of cells of the cervix at its junction with the vagina due to irritation. The cervix may appear raw and red to an examining physician, who may recommend a biopsy study if the condition does not respond to treatment.

cervical evaluation an examination of the cervix with laboratory study of cells and secretions removed from the surface in Pap-smear tests.

cervical migraine = BÄRTSCHI-ROCHAIX'S SYN-DROME.

cervical nerves the eight spinal nerves in the neck

area, each with a dorsal root which is sensory in function, and a ventral root which has motor function. The cervical ganglia innervate the blood vessels and sweat glands of the head, the dilator fibers of the pupils, the blood vessels of the heart, and the heart itself.

cervical vertigo syndrome = BÄRTSCHI-ROCHAIX'S SYNDROME.

cervix any necklike part (Latin, "neck"), especially the neck of the uterus, or the portion of the uterus that projects into the vagina. Technically, the c. extends about an inch from the vaginal junction toward the fundus of the uterus and includes the cervical canal. But in most instances, references to the c. apply mainly to the surface facing the vagina. Adjective: **cervical**.

C.E.T. = CEREBRAL ELECTROTHERAPY.

C factor a cleverness factor, marked by quickness in thinking, uncovered in IQ studies.

C fiber an unmyelinated postganglionic fiber of the autonomic nervous system.

Chaddock, Charles Gilbert American neurologist, 1861–1936. See CHADDOCK REFLEX.

Chaddock reflex dorsal extension of the great toe in response to stroking the skin over the outside of the ankle joint. The C.r. is a diagnostic sign of a pyramidal-tract lesion.

Chagas, Carlos Ribeiro Justiniano /chä'gäsh/ Brazilian physician, 1879–1934. See MENINGO-ENCEPHALITIS (there: **Chagas' disease**).

chain behavior an integrated series of responses such that each response acts as the discriminative stimulus for the next response in the sequence; e.g., in reciting the alphabet, A is the cue for B which is the cue for C. Also called **chain reflex**. Also see CHAINING.

chained reinforcement intermittent reinforcement in which the stimulus is changed.

chaining an operant-conditioning technique in which a complex behavior chain is learned by the subject. Rats can be taught to perform relatively elaborate sequences by this method which makes reinforcement contingent on the final response in the series. The final response is taught first. Once established, it becomes a secondary reinforcer for the next response in the chain. The chain is taught backwards, one response at a time. Also called **behavior c.**

chain reflex = CHAIN BEHAVIOR.

chain reproduction the process of relaying material (pictures, ideas, stories) from person to person or group to group. The ultimate product is compared with the original in order to show, e.g., that a picture of a cat gradually becomes that of an owl. The same type of distortion occurs in rumors through the processes of leveling (simplification), sharpening (emphasis on selected details), and assimilation (altering the accounts to suit attitudes, expectations, and prejudices). The same principles apply to gossiping, legends, and court-room testimony.

chance action an action that appears to have no

conscious purpose but may subserve an unconscious intention, e.g., leaving a personal article in another person's bedroom.

chance difference a statistical difference between two measured variables that is ascribed to random elements. That is, a c.d. is not considered the result of systematic error, biased sampling, prejudice, or some other improper experimental procedure.

chance error = RANDOM ERROR.

chance variations changes in hereditary traits due to unknown factors.

change agent in community psychiatry organized on the ecological model, the role of the psychiatrist as an active participant in social-policy planning, social action, and social engineering directed to community mental health. See ECOLOGICAL-SYSTEMS MODEL.

change fear = NEOPHOBIA.

change of environment a technique for eliminating undesirable behavior patterns. A mere change of scene usually produces only temporary results, but if the new environment brings new satisfactions, it is sometimes effective; e.g., Alcoholics Anonymous provides an opportunity to form new friendships and engage in new recreational activities to replace the companionship of the bottle and its devotees.

change of life: See CLIMACTERIC.

channel an information transmission system. E.g., the nervous system transmits coded messages from sense receptors (input) to effectors (output).

channel capacity in information theory, the maximum capacity of information or messages that a given channel can accommodate.

channels of communication channels involved in the source and destination of face-to-face messages, comprising speech (source: vocal track; destination: ear), kinesics (body movement; eye), odor (chemical processes; nose), touch (body surface; skin), observation (body surface; eye), proxemics (body placement; eye).

character the totality of an individual's qualities or traits, particularly his or her characteristic moral, social, and religious attitudes. The term is often used synonymously with personality.

character analysis psychoanalytic treatment focused on character defenses, that is, defensive behavior that has become an integral part of the personality (Wilhelm Reich); also, psychoanalytic treatment of character disorders; also, the study of character traits allegedly revealed by external characteristics, such as the length of the fingers or shape of the jaw. See CHARACTEROLOGY; PHYSIOGNOMY.

character-analytic vegetotherapy a term applied by Wilhelm Reich to the system of character analysis and orgone therapy which he developed in opposition to Freud between 1924 and 1934. See CHARACTER ANALYSIS; CHARACTER ARMOR; ORGONE THERAPY.

character armor a term used by Wilhelm Reich

in his character-analytic approach. He and his followers held that the analyst's first task is to identify the patient's set of character patterns that serve as defenses against anxiety and stand in the way of attempts to penetrate to the deeper, unconscious levels of the personality. Examples of this c.a. are overaggressiveness, cynicism, passivity, and ingratiation. Every available clue—gestures, facial or verbal expressions, posture—were used to reveal these resistances and trace them to their origin.

character defense a defensive pattern, such as overaggressiveness or intellectualization, which has become a personality trait. See CHARACTER ARMOR.

character development the gradual development of moral concepts, conscience, religious values or views, and social attitudes as an essential aspect of personality development.

character disorder a persistent personality pattern characterized by (a) a specific type of maladaptive behavior, such as antisocial, paranoid, or cyclothymic tendencies, (b) emotional instability, (c) marked immaturity, (d) compulsive gambling, (e) sexual deviations, or (f) alcohol or drug addiction. The term is often used interchangeably with personality disorder.

character neurosis a disorder in which neurotic traits, such as overmeticulousness or excessive impulsivity, are part and parcel of the total personality and do not generate intrapsychic conflicts. Other examples are compulsive, antisocial, schizoid, cyclothymic, or passive-aggressive tendencies. A **neurotic character**, as it is sometimes called, is considered more of a personality disorder than a clear-cut neurosis; it occupies a midpoint between emotional health and emotional illness.

characterology a branch of psychology concerned with character and personality; also, a pseudoscience in which character is "read" by external signs such as hair color.

character structure the unique, enduring pattern of attitudes, traits, and reaction patterns that characterize the individual personality.

character traits the characteristic tendencies and behavior patterns on which our personality is built, including our more or less consistent values, attitudes, and motivations. See ALLPORT'S PERSONALITY-TRAIT THEORY; CATTELL'S FACTORIAL THEORY OF PERSONALITY.

character types categories of personality based upon character traits and behavior patterns, e.g., ANAL CHARACTER, EXPLOITATIVE ORIENTATION, ORAL CHARACTER, PARANOIAC CHARACTER. See these entries. Also see PERSONALITY TYPES.

charas one of several forms of Cannabis sativa. C. is a potent cannabis preparation and is consumed as hashish. See PSYCHEDELICS.

Charcot, Jean-Martin /shärkō′/ French physician, 1825–93. C. became head of the Salpêtrière Hospital in Paris in 1862 and held the world's first Chair of Medical Diseases of the

Nervous System, to which he was appointed by the French government in 1882. In the field of clinical neurology, which he founded, he identified causes of cerebral hemorrhage, described the effects of spinal-cord injury, and gave the first accurate description of multiple sclerosis. In the field of psychiatry, he studied the stages of hypnosis and its effect on the nervous system, and was the first to induce and remove hysterical symptoms by this means. See CHARCOT-BOUCHARD ANEURYSM; CHARCOT-MARIE-TOOTH DISEASE; NEUROPATHIC ARTHROPATHY (also called **Charcot joint**); BRAIN ATROPHY; PROGRESSIVE SPINAL-MUSCULAR ATROPHY; SALPÊTRIÈRE; TOE DROP. Also see FREUD; JANET.

Charcot-Bouchard aneurysm a slight dilation of one of the small internal arteries of the brain. C.-B.a. ruptures are frequently a cause of cerebrovascular accidents and occur most frequently among persons who have been diagnosed as hypertensive.

Charcot joint = NEUROPATHIC ARTHROPATHY.

Charcot-Marie-Tooth disease a progressive neuromuscular disorder due to demyelination of peripheral nerves and degeneration of axons and anterior-horn cells of the spinal cord. Symptoms are first observed in muscular atrophy on the outside of the leg, beginning in childhood or early adult years. Pain, paresthesia, and foot drop develop, and stretch reflexes are lost. The disease is not fatal, and patients usually maintain an active though somewhat restricted life. C.-M.-T.d. is inherited as an autosomal-dominant trait and often is associated with other neurologic disorders, e.g., Friedreich's ataxia. Abbrev.: **C-M-T**. Also called **peroneal muscular atrophy**.

charge of affect a form of cathexis in which a part of the instinct is detached from the idea and acquires affective value.

charisma the quality of personal magnetism and the ability to appeal to and win the confidence of large numbers of diverse people as exemplified in outstanding world political, social, religious, and literary leaders.

Charles Bonnet's syndrome a disorder of aging marked by visual hallucinations that are not related to any other expressions of mental disease. Also called **Bonnet's syndrome**.

Charpentier, Pierre Marie Augustin /shärpäNtyä'/ French physician, 1852–1916. See CHARPENTIER'S LAW; AUTOKINETIC EFFECT (also called **Charpentier's illusion**).

Charpentier's law a visual-perception rule that the product of the foveal image area and the intensity of light is constant for threshold stimuli.

chart. an abbreviation used in prescriptions, meaning "paper" (Latin *charta*).

Chaslin, Philippe /shäsleN'/ French physician, 1857—. See CHASLIN'S GLIOSIS.

Chaslin's gliosis a pathologic change in the brain tissue of epilepsy patients marked by sclerosis of the glial fibers beneath the pia mater. Also called **neuroglial sclerosis**.

chat = KHAT.

chatterbox effect a manifestation of the personalities of many hydrocephalus patients with mental retardation. The patient may appear quite fluent and sociable in conversations but is unable to communicate in a meaningful manner, may tend to fabricate information as long as it seems interesting to the listener, but may be unable to recall what was discussed earlier. Also called **cocktail-party conversationalism**.

Chavany, Jean Alfred Emile /shävänē'/ French physician, 1892–1959. See CHAVANY-BRUNHES SYNDROME.

Chavany-Brunhes syndrome a condition caused by calcification of the falx cerebri resulting in persistent headaches and a wide range of mental disorders. The headaches may be triggered by fatigue, anxiety, or stress, or simply by holding the head in a fixed position for a period of time.

CHD = CORONARY HEART DISEASE.

checkerboard patterns: See SMETS-PATTERN RESPONSES.

-cheil-; -cheilo-; -chil-; -chilo- a combining form relating to the lips (from Greek *cheilos*, "lip").

cheilitis: See MELKERSSON-ROSENTHAL SYNDROME.

cheimaphobia = PSYCHROPHOBIA.

-cheir-; -cheiro-: See -CHIR-.

chelating agents: See CHELATION.

chelating ion the ion of a chemical compound that is capable of binding a metal into a molecular complex. A c.i. can, e.g., form an insoluble complex with a heavy metal in the body tissues so that it will be excreted rather than retained. In a case of hemochromomatosis, the technique is used to remove excess iron deposits from human tissues.

chelation the process of binding or attaching chemically, especially bond formation between a metal ion and another molecule. **Chelating agents** such as BAL are used in treating heavy-metal poisoning by forming stable compounds with the metal, which can then be eliminated without exerting toxic effects.

chemical dependence: See SUBSTANCE DEPENDENCE.

chemical senses the senses of taste and smell, which are activated by contact with electrolytes. Taste buds on the tongue and other oral surfaces and olfactory organs in the nasal cavity are part of the system of c.s.

chemical stimulation an activity change in certain types of nerve receptors caused by contact with a specific electrolyte or molecule. The effect usually occurs only in the senses of taste and smell. See CHEMICAL SENSES; CHEMORECEPTORS.

chemical transmitter any substance that participates in the transmission of a nerve impulse. C.t. substances include acetylcoline, norepinephrine, dopamine, serotonin, and gamma-aminobutyric acid (GABA).

chemopallidectomy the injection of alcohol into the globus pallidus portion of the corpus striatum in the treatment of basal-ganglia-hyperkinetic disorders.

chemopsychiatry the use of chemical substances in the treatment of psychiatric disorders.

chemoreceptors sensory nerve endings, such as those in taste buds, which are capable of reacting to certain chemical stimuli. The chemical molecule or electrolyte generally must be in solution to be detected by c. Some c. react only to certain stimuli, such as those producing a bitter taste. Sour taste buds detect the pH of acidic substances.

chemoreceptor trigger zone a cluster of cells in the medulla oblongata that is sensitive to certain toxic chemicals and reacts by causing the individual to vomit. The c.t.z. is particularly sensitive to narcotics and responds to their stimulation by producing dizziness, nausea, and vomiting, the precise effects depending upon the agent and the dosage.

chemotactic; chemotaxis: See TAXES.

chemotherapy = DRUG THERAPY.

chemotropism an involuntary change of orientation of an organism toward or away from a chemical.

chest voice the low register and full tones created by pectoral breathing and chest resonance.

chewing behavior a reflex process related primarily to the ingestion of food. Studies of animals have shown that c.b. is controlled by neurons in the lateral hypothalamus and can be produced by stimulation of the area by electrodes. Conversely, bilateral destruction of the lateral hypothalamic nuclei results in starvation unless the animals are sustained by tube or intravenous feeding. C.b. may also be observed as a manifestation of nervous tension, as in bruxism.

chewing method a nonspecific relaxation method in the treatment of certain types of functional speech and voice disorders such as stuttering. It was originated by Froeschels in 1952.

Cheyne, George Scottish physician, 1671–1743. See CHEYNE'S DISEASE.

Cheyne, John Scottish medical writer, 1777–1836. See CHEYNE-STOKES BREATHING.

Cheyne's disease a form of hypochondriasis first described in 1733 by George Cheyne and marked by morbid anxiety of a patient about his health. Also called **English malady**.

Cheyne-Stokes breathing labored breathing that alternates between increasing and decreasing rates, as in premature infants and individuals with heart disease, senility, or cerebral arteriosclerosis.

chi /kī/ 22nd letter of the Greek alphabet (X, χ).

Chiari, Hans Czech physician, 1851–1916. See ARNOLD-CHIARI MALFORMATION.

chiaroscuro /kē·ärəskyo͞or′ō/ the illusion of depth or distance in a picture produced by the use of light and shade (Italian, "bright-dark").

chiasma; chiasmata: See OPTIC CHIASM.

chicken breast = PECTUS CARINATUM

chicken pox a highly contagious viral infection characterized by skin eruptions with fever, headache, anorexia, and other mild constitutional symptoms. The **varicella-zoster virus** that causes c.p. in children also causes shingles in adults, although children or adults may experience both forms. A common neurologic complication is acute cerebellar ataxia. Cranial-nerve paralysis also may follow a c.p. infection. Also called **varicella**.

-chil-; -chilo-: See -CHEIL-.

child a young boy or girl. Until the 17th century, there were no children in Western cultures; in fact, there was not even a word for "child" in the English language (or in German or French). Children, after infancy, were simply small and inferior adults, sharing the then more limited adult world, also dressing and speaking like adults; and the word c. referred to kinship rather than age. (Medieval paintings depicted even neonates, including the infant Jesus, with adult features and adult head-to-body proportions.) It was only with the evolution of the modern concepts of individuality and personality that children were seen apart from adults, and that the reality of c. development and the need for c. education became recognized.

child abuse: See CHILD MOLESTATION; BATTERED-CHILD SYNDROME.

child analysis the application of psychoanalytic principles to the treatment of children. In his first and most famous case, Freud involved five-year-old Hans in a question-and-answer "game" with his father, since free association proved inappropriate at that age. C.a. became a separate field when Melanie Klein and Anna Freud developed the play technique, in which the patient acts out feelings and relationships through the use of dolls and toys. See PLAY THERAPY.

childbirth fear = MAIEUSIOPHOBIA.

child-care aids any device or system that enables a handicapped parent to care for an infant. C.-c.a. may include cribs with adjustable height and swing sides, infant chairs on wheels, pre-folded diapers, prepared formula in ready-to-use bottles and bottle-holder attachments for cribs, baby dishes and other equipment with suction cups, and special carrying devices for moving or transporting a baby or small child.

child-care facilities day-care centers usually established by government agencies but sometimes by industrial firms, churches, or social agencies with the prime object of enabling disadvantaged mothers to hold jobs. The term also applies to special facilities such as developmental schools for physically handicapped, retarded, or abused children. Also see FAMILY CARE.

child-care worker an individual trained to work with disturbed or neglected children on a day-to-day basis, in collaboration with other members of the treatment team including psychiatrists, psychologists, social workers, and educators.

child-centered referring to a school environment designed to encourage fulfillment of the child's needs, or to a home environment dominated by the children's needs or desires.

child-centered family = CHILD-FOCUSED FAMILY.

child development the sequential changes in the child's behavior patterns and physical characteristics as he matures. See DEVELOPMENTAL TASKS; PSYCHOSEXUAL DEVELOPMENT; GESELL; CHILD.

child-focused family a family in which the children's needs are paramount, sometimes to a point where they dominate the family constellation and the parents' needs become secondary. Also called **child-centered family**.

child guidance a mental-health approach focused on the prevention of possible future disorders by offering didactic and therapeutic aid to the child and his family at a time when intervention may have a prophylactic effect.

child-guidance clinics: See CHILD-GUIDANCE MOVEMENT.

child-guidance movement a trend toward the establishment of clinics, institutes, and organizations devoted to the prevention or active treatment of mental and emotional disorders in children. The major focus is on the application of mental-health principles to behavior and adjustment problems before they become fixed and hard to modify.

childhood fears fears occurring at different stages of childhood. Though no single fear is inevitable, many children tend to fear strangers at about eight months, darkness at about three years, snakes or large animals between three and four, imaginary monsters and ghosts between four and five, punishment during the school years, and death beginning at nine or ten.

childhood Huntington's chorea: See HUNTINGTON'S CHOREA.

childhood land: See LAND OF CHILDHOOD.

childhood motivation: See PROPRIATE STRIVING.

childhood-onset pervasive developmental disorder a rare and atypical but severe, persistent disturbance in social relationships, including lack of emotional response, inappropriate clinging, disinterest in peers. It is accompanied by a number of specific symptoms, such as sudden anxiety and panic attacks, inappropriate affect, unprovoked rage, resistance to slight changes in routine, peculiar posturing or walking on tiptoe, monotonous voice, excessive or diminished sensitivity to sensory stimuli, self-mutilation, or head-banging. (DSM-III)

childhood-onset pervasive developmental disorder, residual state a diagnostic category that comprises individuals who no longer have the full disorder, but who still show some signs of the illness, such as oddities of communication and social awkwardness. (DSM-III)

childhood schizophrenia an inexact term applied to varied reactions of a generally schizophrenic character appearing early in life. Some of the more common symptoms are inability to respond emotionally, extremely narrow interests, failure to relate to other people, disturbed language functions, low frustration tolerance, distorted and autistic thinking, and disordered motor activity. These symptoms take many forms, such as bizarre posture, extreme restlessness, sudden kicking and screaming, refusal to communicate or eat, awkwardness, loss of interest in play, or playing endlessly with the same toy, head-banging, and irregular sleep patterns. The disorder is attributed by some authorities to disturbed mother-child relationships, by others to an extremely frightening or threatening experience early in life, and by still others, such as Bender, to constitutional defect, particularly brain pathology. It is quite possible that c.s. is not a single disorder but a group of disorders with different etiologies.

childhood sensorineural lesions organic disorders of the auditory system that may be a cause of hearing loss in children. The condition may be congenital and due to a failure of the inner ear to develop normally in the fetal stage or the result of an infection. Measles, mumps, and scarlet fever are among infectious causes. C.s.l. also can result from a German-measles infection of the mother during pregnancy.

child molestation a form of child abuse marked by sexual activity. C.m. may take the form of incest involving an older member of the family, rape, fondling, or other erotic behavior between an adult and a person between the periods of infancy and adolescence. Also see BATTERED-CHILD SYNDROME.

child neglect the denial of attention, care, or affection considered essential for the normal development of a child's physical, emotional, and intellectual qualities, usually due to indifference or disregard.

child-parent fixation in psychoanalysis, a strong child-parent relationship that interferes with other relationships.

child-penis wish in psychoanalysis, the replacement of a little girl's wish for a penis by a wish for a child of her own. The girl may associate her own father with the father of the child she wishes to have, thereby initiating an Oedipus-complex situation.

child-placement counseling a form of counseling focused on decisions and problems associated with the placement of an unwanted or handicapped child.

child psychiatry the branch of general psychiatry that deals with the mental and emotional disorders of children and adolescents. These disorders received little attention until (a) Freud and Meyer emphasized the effect of childhood experiences on later adjustment, (b) educators, inspired by Pestalozzi's early work, established remedial programs for learning and behavior problems, (c) the first child-guidance clinics were established in the 1920s, and (d) Leo Kanner published the first modern book on child psychiatry, in 1935. However, the field did not become a specialty certified by the American Board of Psychiatry and Neurology until 1959. For DSM-III categories see ATTENTION-DEFICIT DISORDER, RESIDUAL TYPE; ATTENTION-DEFICIT DISORDER WITH HYPERACTIVITY; ATTENTION-DEFICIT DISORDER WITHOUT HYPERACTIVITY; CONDUCT DISORDER, SOCIALIZED, AGGRESSIVE; CONDUCT DISORDER, SOCIALIZED, NONAGGRESSIVE; CONDUCT DISORDER, UNDERSOCIALIZED, AGGRESSIVE; CONDUCT DISORDER, UNDERSOCIALIZED, NONAGGRESSIVE; ANXIETY DISORDERS OF CHILDHOOD OR ADOLESCENCE; REACTIVE-ATTACHMENT DISORDER OF INFANCY; SCHIZOID DISORDER OF CHILDHOOD OR ADOLESCENCE; ELECTIVE MUTISM; OPPOSITIONAL DISORDER; IDENTITY DISORDER; STUTTERING; FUNCTIONAL ENURESIS; FUNCTIONAL ENCOPRESIS; SLEEPWALKING DISORDER; SLEEP-TERROR DISORDER; PERVASIVE DEVELOPMENTAL DISORDERS; SPECIFIC DEVELOPMENTAL DISORDERS. Also see INFANT PSYCHIATRY; STEREOTYPY; EATING BEHAVIOR.

child psychology the branch of psychology concerned with the systematic study of behavior, adjustment, and growth from birth to maturity. Typical areas investigated are cognitive and emotional processes, the developmental "timetable," emotional and behavioral disorders, parent-child relations, psychosexual development, and peer relationships. Also see CHILD.

child-rearing practices child-raising patterns viewed as an expression of a particular society, subculture, family, or period in cultural history. The patterns are concerned with such areas as methods of discipline, expression of affection, toilet-training, breast-versus-bottle-feeding—all of which are believed to have a profound effect on character and personality formation, mental and physical health, and interpersonal relationships.

Children's Apperception Test a projective test developed by L. Bellak and S. S. Bellak for three-to-11-year olds based on the same principles as the Thematic Apperception Test. In one form the pictured situations involve animal characters, and in a second version, the CAT-H (Bellak and Hurvich), human characters are used. Abbrev.: **CAT**.

Children's Personality Questionnaire: See CATTELL INVENTORIES.

chill factor: See WIND-CHILL INDEX.

chimeric stimulation a technique used by Sperry in split-brain experiments: E.g., a **chimeric face** consisting of the left half of one person's face joined to the right half of another person's face, and shown to the subject, has led to the finding that one hemisphere perceived one face while the other hemisphere perceived the other. The subject, however, was unaware of anything peculiar about the stimuli, which indicates that there are two separate spheres of conscious awareness running parallel in each of the two hemispheres.

China Syndrome syndrome a form of nuclear neurosis in which concern is directed toward a possible catastrophic meltdown of a nuclear reactor core. The term is derived from the folk fantasy in which the melting down of a runaway nuclear-reactor core would burn a hole all the way through the earth, and presumably to China on the other side, while producing a massive fallout of radioactive debris on the countryside. See NUCLEAR NEUROSIS.

chionophobia a morbid fear of snow.

chipping controlled, often long-term, use of heroin or other opiates.

-chir-; -chiro-; -cheir-; -cheiro- a combining form relating to the hands (from Greek *cheir*, "hand").

chi-square /kī/ a statistic indicating the likelihood that a result is due to chance. C.-s. compares the frequency of occurrence actually observed with the frequency expected by chance. Symbol: χ^2 = Σ $(o-e)^2/e$, where o = observed frequency and e = expected frequency.

-chlor-; -chloro- a combining form (a) meaning light green, (b) denoting the presence of chlorine.

chloral derivatives a group of sedative-hypnotic drugs first synthesized in the 19th century and introduced as substitutes for alcohol and opium, which were then used to induce sleep. The prototype of the c.d., **chloral hydrate**—$C_2H_3Cl_3O_2$—was originally and erroneously believed to produce anesthesia by being converted by the body's chemistry into chloroform. C.d. function by depressing sensory and reducing motor activity of the central nervous system. Other c.d. include **chloral betaine**—$C_7H_{14}Cl_3NO_4$—and **triclofos sodium**—$C_2H_3Cl_3NaO_4P$.

chloral hydrate: See CHLORAL DERIVATIVES.

chlorazepate dipotassium; chlorazepate monopotassium; chlordiazepoxide; chlordiazepoxide hydrochloride: See BENZODIAZEPINES.

chlorimipramine a drug administered in the treatment of narcolepsy. C. is a powerful antidepressant and usually is prescribed for severe cases because of potential adverse effects and withdrawal symptoms.

chlormezanone $C_{11}H_{12}ClNO_3S$—an anxiolytic that resembles meprobamate in its pharmacologic activity and is administered for treatment of anxiety and tension states associated- with psychoneurotic disorders. Also called **chlormethazanone**.

chlorphenoxamine: See ANTIHISTAMINES.

chlorphentermine hydrochloride: See ADRENERGIC DRUGS.

chlorpromazine $C_{17}H_{19}ClN_2S$—a neuroleptic drug of the phenothiazine class. Its effects include a slowing of motor activity and reduction in emotionality. C. also is an antihistamine, anticholinergic, and antispasmodic agent. It is used mainly in the treatment of schizophrenia and natural and drug-induced manic states. Also see PHENOTHIAZINES.

chlorpromazine hydrochloride: See PHENO-THIAZINES.

chlorprothixene: See THIOXANTHINES.

choc an uncoordinated response elicited by an unexpected sudden stimulus (French, "shock").

chocolatl an Aztec name for beans of the cacao plant. According to historians, cloistered nuns at Chiapas, Mexico, invented hot chocolate in 1550 by grinding c. and adding sugar, vanilla, and hot water.

choice of a neurosis = SYMPTOM CHOICE.

choice point a place in a test, e.g., a maze, where the subject must make a choice of direction or response.

choice reaction a test or situation that requires different responses to different stimuli, as in braking at a red light and accelerating at a green light.

choked disk = PAPILLEDEMA.

chokes: See DECOMPRESSION SICKNESS.

choking-fear = PNIGOPHOBIA.

-chol-; -chole-; -cholo- a combining form relating to bile or gall (Greek *chole*).

cholecystitis; cholelithiasis: See GALLBLADDER DISEASE.

choleric type a type of temperament characterized by irritability and quick temper, which Hippocrates and Galen attributed to an excess of yellow bile.

cholesterol $C_{27}H_{45}OH$—a substance, technically an alcohol, that is present in animal fats and many kinds of animal tissues, e.g., brain tissues and myelinated nerve fibers, milk, egg yolk, and blood. C. is a precursor of all the steroid hormones and also of vitamin D. It is associated with circulatory disorders because of high levels of the substance in obese persons and individuals afflicted by stress, tension, high blood pressure, and atherosclerosis. However, a causative link between c. and heart attacks has not been established. See ALCOHOL.

choline a water-soluble vitamin involved in the metabolism of fat and a precursor of the neurotransmitter acetylcholine. C. has the same pharmacologic actions as acetylcholine but is much less potent. It is converted to acetylcholine by the influence of acetyl-coenzyme A. It occurs as a component of lecithin in foods but can be synthesized in the body from serine, an amino acid. The average adult diet provides about 700 milligrams of c. per day from many foods containing phospholipids, such as eggs, meats, whole grains, and legumes. C. has vitaminlike activity and sometimes is included in the vitamin-B complex.

choline acetylase an enzyme that is involved in the production of the neurotransmitter acetylcholine from choline and acetyl-coenzyme. Also called **choline acetyltransferase.**

cholinergic pertaining to nerve cells and organs that are activated by the neurotransmitter acetylcholine.

cholinergic drugs agents that increase the activity of acetylcholine or have effects similar to acetylcholine. C.d. are used as acetylcholine substitutes in research and therapy because they resist destruction by enzymes that deactivate acetylcholine. Kinds of c.d. include plant alkaloids such as nicotine and pilocarpine. Also called **parasympathetic drugs.** See CHOLINESTERASE.

cholinergic synapses synapses that utilize acetylcholine as a transmitter substance to mediate a neural activity. They are found in postganglionic parasympathetic fibers, autonomic preganglionic fibers, preganglionic fibers to the adrenal medulla, somatic motor nerves to the skeletal muscles, and fibers to certain parts of the skin, e.g., the sweat glands.

cholinergic system the part of the autonomic nervous system that reacts to cholinergic drugs, such as acetylcholine. C.s. activities are inhibited by cholinergic blocking drugs, such as atropine.

cholinesterase an enzyme that destroys acetylcholine. C. occurs in two forms, acetylcholinesterase, found in nerve tissue and red blood cells, and pseudocholinesterase, found in blood plasma and tissues other than neurons. The enzyme cleaves the acetylcholine molecule after it has been released so the choline unit can be recycled into a new acetylcholine molecule. See ACETYLCHOLINE; CHOLINERGIC DRUGS.

Chomsky, Noam American educator and linguistic theorist, 1928—. See ORIGIN-OF-LANGUAGE THEORIES; TRANSFORMATIONAL GRAMMAR.

-chondr-; -chondrio-; -chondro- a combining form relating to cartilage (from Greek *chondros*, "corn, grain, cartilage").

chondrodystrophia calcificans congenita = CONRADI'S DISEASE.

chondroectodermal dysplasia = ELLIS-VAN CREVELD SYNDROME.

chondroosteodystrophy = MORQUIO'S SYNDROME.

chondroosteomyelitis an acute infection of developing bone and the surrounding cartilage. The infection usually involves the long bones of children and is a complication of a local infection in another body area, e.g., the lungs or middle ear. If the infection invades the mastoid bone cells or those of the ethmoid or sphenoid sinuses, the disease can break through into the brain tissue.

chondroplasia: See METAPHYSIAL C.

chorda tympani a branch of the facial nerve which passes downward and in back of the tympanic membrane. It contains taste sensation and sublingual salivary-gland fibers.

chorditis tuberosa a small whitish node on one or both vocal chords caused by vocal abuse and resulting in a low pitch and hoarse voice.

chorea /kərē'ə/ a motor-nerve disorder with irregular and involuntary jerky movements of the limbs and facial muscles (Greek *choreia*, "dance"). Kinds of c. include **buttonmakers's c.**, which develops in hands and arms of buttonmakers; **electric c.**, a Mediterranean form associated with malaria; Huntington's c., a hereditary, progressive disease; and **Sydenham's c.**, an infective or toxic form associated with rheumatism and formerly known as **Saint Vitus' dance**. Various kinds of c. also have been known historically as **Saint Anthony's dance, Saint John's dance**, or **Saint With's dance**. Also SEE HUNTINGTON'S C.; VARIABLE C. OF BRISSAUD.

chorea nutans a symptom of hysteria consisting of a rhythmical nodding. When the entire body is involved in rhythmical hysterical movements, the condition is called **chorea oscillatoria**.

chorea saltatoria a type of chorea marked by involuntary jumping, which may be rhythmical or irregular.

choreiform /kôrā'ē-/ any condition involving involuntary movement that resembles chorea.

choreoathetosis a form of chorea in which the patient is unable to sustain any group of muscles in a fixed position. The effort is interrupted by slow, sinuous, purposeless movements. The condition is most often found in the hands and fingers but also may occur in such muscles as those of the tongue.

choreomania an uncontrollable impulse to dance, as in the epidemics of frenzied, convulsive dancing that occurred in tenth-century Italy, spreading to Germany and the Flemish countries in the 13th and 14th centuries. Also called **dancing mania**. See MASS HYSTERIA; TARANTISM.

chorion the outermost membranes of the sac that surrounds and protects the developing fertilized ovum.

choroid layer one of three coats, or tunics, covering the eyeball. C.l. is located between the retina and sclera layers, covering almost 85 percent of the globe of the eyeball. It contains blood vessels that supply the retina and a pigment that prevents extraneous light from affecting the retina. Also called **choroid coat**.

choroid plexus a wormlike fringe of blood vessels in the pia mater layer of the meninges of the central nervous system, and a source of cerebrospinal fluid. The c.p. folds extend through the third, fourth, and lateral ventricles of the brain.

Chotzen's syndrome a form of craniosynostosis usually involving the coronal suture of the skull and accompanied by syndactyly of the soft tissues, which may appear merely as webbing. Subnormal intelligence may be associated with the disorder. The trait is transmitted by an autosomal-dominant gene. Also called **acrocephalosyndactyly, Type III**.

chrematophobia a morbid fear of handling money or of the sight of money (from Greek *chremata*, "goods, money").

Christian, Henry Asbury American internist, 1876–1951. See HAND-CHRISTIAN-SCHÜLLER SYNDROME.

Christmas disease a hereditary bleeding disease similar to hemophilia but due to a different genetic defect, a deficiency of clotting factor IX. (Classic hemophilia is due to a deficiency of clotting factor VIII.) The disease is named for the first patient studied in detail, rather than the religious holiday. Also called **hemophilia B**.

-chrom-; -chromato-; -chromo- a combining form relating to color (Greek *chroma*).

chroma the saturation or depth of color or hue in the Munsell color system.

chromatic colors all colors other than black, white, and gray, that is, those colors that possess saturation and hue. Compare ACHROMATIC COLORS.

chromatic contrast = COLOR CONTRAST.

chromatic dimming an apparent decrease in color saturation when light intensity is suddenly decreased.

chromatic flicker a flicker sensation caused by rapid periodic changes in hue or saturation.

chromaticity a color-stimulus quality determined by its purity and wavelength.

chromatic response a category used in the evaluation of certain tests in which one or more colors may be included in addition to shapes or forms, such as in the Rorschach ink-blot test. See RORSCHACH TEST.

chromatic scale the sequence of musical tones in semitone steps through an octave.

chromatid in cell division, one of the two spiral filaments joined at the centromere which make up a chromosome and which then separate, each going to a different pole of the dividing cell to become a new chromosome in one of the daughter cells.

chromatin a substance present in chromosomes and cell nuclei which accepts the stains of certain identifying dyes. The substance is composed of DNA material and proteins.

chromatin-negative pertaining to the absence of a substance in the nuclei of human tissue cells that would indicate the presence of an XX, or female, complement of sex chromosomes. A c.-n. cell, therefore, would identify the tissue as being from a male individual. See CHROMATIN-POSITIVE.

chromatin-positive pertaining to the presence in a human tissue cell of a nuclear substance that identifies the cell as being from a female. The substance, sometimes called a Barr body, represents X chromosome material not observed in the tissue cells of normal males. See CHROMATIN-NEGATIVE.

chromatography a method of chemical analysis in which different molecules in a mixture of chemicals are separated according to their solubility, absorptive properties, or other factors. Kinds of c. include **column c., paper c.**, and gas c. Column c. and paper c. depend upon gravity to move a solvent through a substance as the components separate into predictable zones or areas. Also see GAS C.

chromatophobia = CHROMOPHOBIA.

chromatopsia a visual aberration caused by drugs, intense stimulation, or other abnormal conditions, e.g., snow blindness.

chromesthesia a type of synesthesia or crossed perception in which sounds, and sometimes tastes, odors, and sensations of heat and cold or pain are accompanied by color sensations. Strictly, c. is not a conscious juxtaposition of two different sense perceptions; the two perceptions coincide as responses to the same stimulus; e.g., the note G may be consistently experienced as blue. When c. involves sounds, it is also called COLOR HEARING. See this entry.

chromic myopia: See **myopia.**

chromophil substance = TIGROID BODIES.

chromophobia a morbid fear of color or colors. Also called **chromatophobia; color phobia.**

chromosomal aberration an abnormal chromosome or a congenital defect that can be attributed to an abnormal chromosome. Also see SEX-C.A.

chromosome a usually invisible strand or filament of DNA, RNA, and other molecules that carries the genetic or hereditary traits of an individual. A c. is located in the cell nucleus and visible, through a microscope, only during cell division. The normal human complement of chromosomes totals 46, or 23 pairs, which contain more than 30,000 genes for specific hereditary traits.

chromosome 18, deletion of long arm a chromosomal disorder characterized by microcephaly, deafness, and mental retardation associated with the absence of part of the long arm of chromosome 18. Hypotonia and nystagmus are other neurologic effects observed in patients. Also called **46,XX18q—.**

chromosome-18 trisomy a chromosomal disorder involving an extra E-group chromosome (chromosomes 16, 17 or 18), resulting in offspring with a short neck with webbing, congenital heart disease, hernias, and neonatal jaundice. Neurologic effects include deafness, marked psychomotor retardation, jitteriness, seizures, and CNS defects. Also called **47,XX+18.** See PSEUDOTRISOMY 18.

chromosome 5, deletion of short arm = CRI DU CHAT SYNDROME.

chromosome 4, deletion of short arm a chromosomal disorder involving absence of a portion of chromosome 4, resulting in microcephaly, visual defects, severe retardation, and indifference to painful stimuli. Until 1965, the condition was considered a variation of cri du chat syndrome, involving chromosome 5, although the cat-cry effect was rarely noted. Also called **46XX4p—.**

chromosome number the number of chromosomes present in the tissue cells of an individual. All members of a species normally have the same number of chromosomes. The normal number for humans is 46. The chromosome number of a gamete, or reproductive cell, of a human is half the somatic chromosome number, or 23. See DELETION.

chromosome 13, deletion of long arm a chromosomal disorder involving an abnormal chromosome-13 condition and resulting in offspring with microcephaly, microphthalmos, iris colobomas, cataracts, retinoblastomas, pelvic-girdle and lower-spine defects, and missing thumbs. Also called **46,XX13q—; 46,XX13r; ring-D syndrome.**

chromosome-13 trisomy a chromosomal syndrome involving an extra chromosome 13, resulting in the birth of an infant with a variety of defects including mental retardation, cleft lip and palate, polydactyly, cerebral anomalies, and visual abnormalities such as anophthalmia, microphthalmia, cataracts, and iris colobomas. Also called **D trisomy; 47,XX+13; trisomy 13-15; Patau's syndrome.**

chromosome-21 trisomy = TRISOMY 21.

chromotherapy: See PHOTOBIOLOGY.

-chron-; -chrono- a combining form relating to time (Greek *chronos*).

chronic alcoholism habitual, long-term dependence on alcohol, usually of the gamma type. See ALCOHOL DEPENDENCE; GAMMA ALCOHOLISM.

chronic anxiety a persistent, pervasive state of apprehension not targeted to specific situations or objects. See ANXIETY.

chronic brain disorders a group of disorders caused by or associated with brain damage, and producing permanent impairment of intellectual and emotional functions. C.b.d. result from such conditions as cranial anomalies, lead or carbon-monoxide poisoning, cerebral arteriosclerosis, head injury, intracranial neoplasm, and senile brain disease. See BRAIN DISORDERS.

chronic bronchitis Type B: See BLUE BLOATER.

chronic cryptococcal meningitis: See MONILIASIS.

chronic delusional state of negation = COTARD'S SYNDROME.

chronic factitious disorder with physical symptoms a disorder characterized by plausible physical symptoms that are apparently under voluntary control but severe enough to require hospitalizations, e.g., rashes, abscesses, fevers, and blacking out. The individual's goal is apparently to become a patient, not in one but in many hospitals; and to achieve this goal, he or she may exaggerate or fabricate dramatic symptoms (pseudologia fantastica), even through other symptoms appear to be real. See MUNCHAUSEN SYNDROME. (DSM-III)

chronic granulocytic leukemia: See LEUKEMIA.

chronic idiopathic xanthomatosis = HAND-CHRISTIAN-SCHULLER SYNDROME.

chronicity = SOCIAL-BREAKDOWN SYNDROME.

chronic lymphocytic leukemia: See LEUKEMIA.

chronic mania a manic state that persists for an indefinite period or permanently.

chronic motor-tic disorder a disorder that consists of recurrent, rapid involuntary movements involving no more than three muscle groups at any one time. The condition lasts at least a year, but can be voluntarily suppressed for a short period of time. (DSM-III)

chronic-obstructive pulmonary disease a term applied to any of several related respiratory diseases, including emphysema, chronic bronchitis, and asthma. The symptoms are chronic cough, wheezing, particularly after exertion or during a respiratory infection, and either constant or periodic periods of breathlessness. Abbrev.: **COPD.**

chronic or delayed posttraumatic stress disorder: See POSTTRAUMATIC STRESS DISORDER.

chronic peritonitis: See PERITONITIS.

chronic progressive ophthalmoplegia = GRÄFE'S DISEASE.

chronic schizophrenia schizophrenia of any type —paranoid, disorganized, catatonic, residual, undifferentiated—in which the symptoms are persistent but relatively mild, in contrast to acute episodes in which the symptoms are florid and extreme..

chronic-traumatic disorder a long-lasting or permanent impairment of brain functions resulting from a blow to the head that is severe enough to cause brain damage. Common symptoms are persistent headaches, dizziness, fatigue, impaired memory, anxiety, and difficulty in concentrating; also, if the damage is extensive, there may be a general loss of intellectual ability, personality change, paralysis, aphasia, and, in some cases, seizures. See POSTCONCUSSION SYNDROME; POSTTRAUMATIC PERSONALITY DISORDER.

chronic undifferentiated schizophrenia a persistent, mixed form of schizophrenia in which symptoms develop insidiously and there is no acute attack. The patient becomes apathetic, poorly adjusted, and develops mild changes in thought, behavior, and affect that are sometimes termed latent, borderline, incipient, or prepsychotic schizophrenia.

chronological age the age from birth; the actual age of an individual in years. Abbrev.: **CA.** Also called **calendar age; life age.**

chronophobia a neurotic fear based on preoccupation with time, particularly among prison inmates. The major features of this reaction, which is often called **prison neurosis**, are feelings of panic, restlessness, dissatisfaction with life, and claustrophobia arising out of contemplation of the length of the sentence and the idea of confinement.

chronotaraxis a condition of time confusion in which the individual tends to underestimate or overestimate the passage of time or expresses confusion about the time of day or day of the week. The disorder is associated with bilateral lesions of the thalamic nuclei.

chunk a unit of information. According to G. Miller, short-term memory holds seven plus or minus two chunks, that is, between five and nine. The capacity of short-term memory is thus believed to be constant for the number of individual units it can store; but the units themselves can range from simple chunks, such as individual letters or numbers to complex chunks, e.g., words or phrases. Thus, short-term memory can hold seven words as easily as seven letters, because both types of information are encoded as units.

Chvostek, Franz Austrian surgeon, 1835–84. See CHVOSTEK'S TREMOR.

Chvostek's tremor a disorder involving the facial nerve and marked by facial muscle spasms when the muscles or branches of the facial nerve are tapped. Also called **Chvostek's sign; Weiss' sign.**

cibophobia = SITOPHOBIA.

-cicatr- a combining form relating to a scar or the formation or healing of a scar (Latin *cicatrix*).

cicatrization the formation of a scar, or **cicatrix**, following a wound; also, deliberate scarring of some part of the body for cosmetic or religious purposes, especially in non-Western societies.

-cide a combining form relating to a killer or killing.

CIDS: See INTERPERSONAL DISTANCE.

cigarette-smoke pollution the contribution to air pollution by tobacco-smoking, especially cigarette-smoking. Studies show that nonsmokers who inhale air polluted by cigarette smoke experience a higher incidence of heart and respiratory disorders than nonsmokers who are not exposed to cigarette smoke of others. Nonsmokers also tend to increase their "bubble" of personal space when interacting with cigarette smokers.

cilia; ciliary: See CILIUM.

ciliary muscles muscles that change the shape of the lens of the eye automatically in order to focus on objects near or far. When viewing a near object, the c.m. contract, relaxing the suspensory ligament to give the lens a more convex shape, in effect increasing the power of the lens.

cilium an eyelash or eyelid; also, any hairlike structure. Plural: **cilia.** Adjective: **ciliary.**

Cinderella complex: See DEPENDENCY SYNDROME.

Cinderella syndrome a form of childhood behavior marked by (a) the belief that the individual is a victim of parental rejection or neglect or (b) the simulation of such rejection or neglect. The C.s. is often a cry for help. (The term is derived from the little "cinder girl" who in the literature of many cultures was forced to perform the undesirable household chores while her siblings attended parties).

cineplasty /sin'-/ a surgical technique used in restoring limb function following an amputation by attaching a prosthetic connection to a part of the remaining muscle tissue. The prosthesis can then be attached to the connecting device so that voluntary control of the muscle will in turn produce movement of the prosthesis.

cineseismography a photographic method of recording and measuring abnormal movements of an involuntary nature. The movements remain spontaneous and uninhibited, since no devices are attached to the subject.

-cingul- a combining form relating to a girdlelike zone (from Latin *cingulum*, "girdle, zone"; plural: *cingula*).

cingulate cortex the portion of the cortex that includes the cingulate gyrus, a component of the brain's limbic system.

cingulate gyrus a long convolution on the medial surface of the cerebral hemisphere containing association fibers. The c.g. arches over and generally outlines the location of the corpus callosum. Experimental lesions of the c.g. in animals result in impaired learning ability. The c.g. may also play a role in hunger. Also called **gyrus cinguli; callosal gyrus**.

cingulate sulcus the fissure that separates the cingulate gyrus from the superior frontal gyrus. The c.s. follows the curve of the corpus callosum along the medial surface of the hemisphere, then turns upward near the central fissure.

cingulotomy a procedure in the treatment of chronic psychosis in which portions of the cingulum bundle are coagulated bilaterally. C. may be performed when a psychosis, chronic-alcoholism, or drug-dependency case has failed to respond to other treatments. Also called **cingulumotomy**.

circadian rhythms biological activities that follow cycles that repeat at approximately 24-hour intervals. Also see BIOLOGICAL RHYTHM.

circle: See COMMUNICATION NETWORKS.

circle of Willis = ARTERIAL CIRCLE.

circular illness = CYCLIC ILLNESS.

circular insanity = FALRET'S DISEASE.

circular-pattern responses responses given by subjects viewing circles that contain varying color patterns. As the uncertainty level increases, based on the number of colors per pattern, responses of pleasure, interestingness, and complexity judgments increase while judgments of orderliness decrease. The test was devised by D. E. Berlyne.

circular psychosis an alternative term for manic-depressive psychosis, or bipolar psychosis.

circular reaction a voluntary act or a reflex that generates its own repetition, sometimes without apparent motive or reward, e.g., Piaget's observation that infants may go on sucking after the nipple is withdrawn. Also called **circular response**.

circulatory psychosis a confused mental state associated with a disorder of the cardiovascular system, e.g. a stroke.

circumcision the surgical removal of the prepuce, or foreskin, of the penis. C. is performed for hygienic, medical, or religious reasons. It usually is performed in infancy, on the eighth day after the birth for a boy born into the Jewish faith. In some cultures, it is a puberty rite and a requirement for marriage. Also see CLITORIDECTOMY.

circumlocution a manifestation of nominal aphasia caused by left-sided posterior temporal lesions. The subject perceives an object and recognizes its function but has difficulty in finding the right words to identify or explain it. The resulting "roundabout" way of describing things is often used as a means of evading a damaging or threatening revelation, or as a substitute for a lapse of memory. In some cases c. is an indication of disorganized thought processes, as in schizophrenia. See CIRCUMSTANTIALITY.

circumscribed amnesia = LOCALIZED AMNESIA.

circumstantial evidence in forensic psychology, evidence based on inference or coincidence.

circumstantiality circuitous, "labyrinthine" speech in which the patient digresses to give unnecessary and often irrelevant details before arriving at the main point. The disorder is far more extreme and bizarre than ordinary small-mindedness, and arises from disorganized associative processes. It occurs primarily in schizophrenic patients, but is also found in obsessional disorders, epileptic dementia, and senile brain disease. See OVERINCLUSION; TANGENTIAL THINKING.

CIRCUS a series of instruments with a circus theme developed by the Educational Testing Service for use by teachers from kindergarten through high school. Among the areas covered (at appropriate levels) are the meaning of words, quantitative concepts, and prereading, reading, mathematics, and writing skills. In addition, two questionnaires are included for teacher ratings of the children's classroom behavior and familial educational background.

cirrhosis a liver disease marked by widespread fibrosis and development of nodules, leading to cellular disorganization of the liver tissues and loss of normal function. It is the fourth leading cause of death in the United States and in most cases an effect of chronic alcohol abuse. C. also may be due to congenital defects involving metabolic deficiencies, exposure to toxic chemicals, and infections, e.g., hepatitis.

cisterna cerebellomedullaris = CISTERNA MAGNA.

cisternal-block syndrome = ZANGE-KINDLER SYNDROME.

cisterna magna an enlarged space between the lower surface of the cerebellum and the rear surface of the medulla oblongata, serving as a reservoir of cerebrospinal fluid. Also called **posterior subarachnoidean space; cisterna cerebellomedullaris**.

cistern puncture = SUBOCCIPITAL PUNCTURE.

cisvestitism the wearing of clothing that is of the appropriate sex but otherwise improper, such as an adult dressing as a child or a layman wearing the clothing of a priest.

Citelli, Salvatore /chētel'ē/ Italian laryngologist, 1875–1947. See CITELLI'S SYNDROME.

Citelli's syndrome a disorder characterized by obstruction of the nasopharynx by adenoid tissue, and such symptoms as drowsiness, loss of concentration, frequent sinus infections, and mental retardation.

citric-acid cycle = KREBS CYCLE.

cittosis an alternative term for pica. Also called **citta; sissa**. See PICA.

civil commitment a legal procedure that permits a person to be certified as mentally ill and to be institutionalized against his will.

civil disobedience nonviolent opposition, on the grounds of conscience, to certain government laws or policies by such tactics as picketing, boycotting, refusal to obey orders by police or other government organs, or refusal to pay taxes.

civilian-catastrophe reaction transient situational personality disorders resulting from severely traumatic experiences in civilian life, and classified under the heading of "gross stress reactions" in DSM-I. Typical experiences are automobile accidents, earthquakes, plane crashes, near drownings, fires, tornados, and sexual assault. A typical reaction is a temporary personality disorganization characterized by confusion or disorientation, inability to cope, intense anxiety, and, in some cases, temporary amnesia for the event and feelings of guilt and depression. The most acute reactions are experienced by individuals with a history of immaturity and instability, or when the catastrophe occurs with little or no warning or preparation. See DISASTER SYNDROME; POSTTRAUMATIC STRESS DISORDER.

civilization the highest level of human development, consisting of the sum total of our arts, sciences, laws, religions, moral values, and philosophical concepts. In *Civilization and Its Discontents* (1930) Freud described civilization as "the whole sum of the achievements and regulations which distinguish our lives from those of our animal ancestors," and maintained that it provides increased security and control of our aggressive and sexual instincts, and also permits us to gratify our needs for beauty and order through the process of sublimation.

CJD = CREUTZFELDT-JAKOB DISEASE.

claiming type of depression a term applied by S. Arieti to a depression in which the anguished patient clings to others and demands their pity and help: "It is in your power to relieve me."

claims review evaluation of the appropriateness of a claim for payment for a medical service rendered, including a determination of whether the claimant is eligible for reimbursement, whether the charges are consistent with customary fees or published institutional rates, and whether the service was necessary.

clairaudience a parapsychology term for the alleged ability to hear sounds without use of the ears.

clairvoyance alleged extrasensory perception of external objects or events in the past, present, or future.

clan a group of families that claims common ancestry. As an anthropological term, c. refers either to the unit of tribal society (with descent usually calculated through the maternal line) or to a group believed to have descended from a common ancestor. Also see SEPT.

clang association an association of words by similarity of sound rather than meaning. C.a. is pathological disturbance occurring in manic states and schizophrenia, and a normal tendency of young children, expressed, e.g., in nonsense rhymes. Also called **clanging**.

clarification a counselor's formulation of a client's statement or expression of feelings in clearer terms without indicating approval or disapproval. C. goes further than RESTATEMENT and REFLECTION OF FEELING but stops short of INTERPRETATION. See these entries.

Clarke, Jacob Augustus Lockhart English anatomist, 1817–80. See CLARKE'S COLUMN.

Clarke's column a group of nerve cells at the base of the posterior horn of the spinal cord, extending from the eighth cervical nerve to the second lumbar nerve. The column contains the dorsal spinocerebellar tract. Also called **Clarke's posterior vesicular column; Stlling's nucleus; nucleus thoracicus**.

clasp-knife effect a disorder of the motor nerves controlling the extensor muscles which contract and relax in more or less continuous spasms. The cause is a lesion at a pre-pontine level of the brain.

class: See MIDDLE C.; SOCIAL C.; CORPORATE C.

class advocate: See ADVOCATE.

classical analysis psychoanalysis in which major emphasis is placed on the libido, psychosexual development, the irrational (id) instincts, the rules of free association and abstinence, dream interpretation, and unconscious conflicts. Later developments, such as the dual-instinct theory (Eros versus Thanatos), the transference neurosis, the analysis of the resistance, and ego psychology, are not considered classical. See ORTHODOX PSYCHOANALYSIS.

classical conditioning = PAVLOVIAN CONDITIONING.

classical depression in general, according to S. Arieti, a depression characterized by (a) a pervading feeling of melancholia, (b) disordered thought processes with retardation and unusual content such as delusions of poverty and sin, (c) psychomotor retardation, and (d) accessory somatic dysfunctions such as decreased appetite, insomnia, backache, and loss of weight. For details and types, see DEPRESSION.

classical paranoia a rare disorder characterized by elaborate, fixed, systematic delusions usually of a persecutory, grandiose, or erotic character. See PARANOIA.

classicism factor the role of traditional values of artistic style, particularly those associated with the art and architecture of ancient Greece and Rome, in evaluation of any artistic endeavor. Classicism sometimes is used as a term to distinguish formal art forms from art forms that are influenced by imagination, or the **romanticism factor**.

classification: See PSYCHIATRIC C.; DSM-III; INTERNATIONAL C. OF DISEASES.

classification method in industrial psychology, a system of establishing a table of organization in which job categories are classified along a hypothetical scale. An example is the General Schedule system of the United States Civil Service System.

classification test a test in which objects or people are sorted into specific categories.

class inclusion the term used by Piaget to describe the operation of assigning an object to the several categories to which it simultaneously belongs. Children progress from classifications based on personal factors, perceptual features, and common function to classifications based on hierarchical relationships; e.g., a monkey is a primate, a mammal, and a vertebrate animal. See CONCRETE OPERATIONS.

class interval the range of scores or numerical values that constitute one segment or class in a quantitative series or frequency distribution; e.g., weights might be grouped in class intervals of ten pounds each. Also called **class; class size; interval; step interval**.

class limits the limits of a class interval; the lowest and uppermost values that define the boundaries of a particular interval or range. Also called **class range**.

Classroom Environment Scale: See ENVIRONMENTAL ASSESSMENT.

classroom test a test constructed by a teacher for use in his or her own classes in contrast to a standardized test.

class size = CLASS INTERVAL.

class structure the composition, organization, and interrelationship of social classes within a society. The term encompasses the makeup of individual classes as well as their economic role, political power, and social dynamics. Also see SOCIAL CLASS.

claudication literally, limping; also, a certain cramping pain in the muscles. Also see MENTAL C.; CEREBRAL INTERMITTENT C.

Clausius, Rudolf Julius Emanuel /klous'ē-ōōs/ German physicist, 1822–88. See ENTROPY.

-claustr-; -claustro- a combining form relating to a barrier, a cage, or anything that encloses (from Latin *claudere*, "to shut, restrict, lock up").

claustral complex a complex, such as desire for security, attributed to an unconscious effect of prenatal or paranatal events.

claustrophilia the abnormal desire to be enclosed within a small place. Compare CLAUSTROPHOBIA.

claustrophobia a morbid fear of being confined. It is a common anxiety symptom that may rise to panic proportions. Adjective: **claustrophobic**. Compare CLAUSTROPHILIA; AGORAPHOBIA.

claustrum a thin layer of gray matter on the outer surface of the external capsule of the cerebral cortex and a part of the basal ganglia. Its cells are small and spindle-shaped, like those found deep in the cortex. Some anatomists believe the c. is gray matter that has become detached from the central lobe and separated from it by a layer of white matter. C. lesions result in a loss of taste sensation in some animals.

clava = GRACILE TUBERCLE.

clavus a sharp, severe headache, as if a nail (Latin *clavus*) were being driven into the head. It is usually a conversion symptom.

clawfoot = PES CAVUS.

clawhand a physical abnormality of the hand in which there is flexion and atrophy of the hand and fingers as a result of a lesion of the ulnar nerve. C. is observed in cases of leprosy and syringomyelia. Also called **main en griffe** /men'äNgrif'/.

clawing attacks a form of aggressive behavior marked by the use of the nails in scratching or clawing an opponent. C.a. are a normal defensive action taken by some animals but regarded as improper among normal older children and adults. See BITING ATTACK.

clay-modeling equipment recreational- and physical-therapy-training devices and facilities to aid disabled persons in eye-hand coordination and development of neuromuscular abilities of the upper extremities. C.-m.e. may include potter's wheels, mortar and pestle, sieve, scale, kilns, wedging table, and glaze applicators.

clay-modeling therapy a form of therapy for children often used in physical rehabilitation, in stimulating the mentally retarded, and in treating speech disorders. Playing with clay provides substitute satisfactions, the acting out of hostile emotions and "messing" impulses, as well as opportunities for gratification, achievement, and acceptance.

cleaning-fluid inhalation: See CARBON TETRACHLORIDE POISONING.

clear sensorium normal functioning of all the senses enabling the individual to know who and where he is and what he is doing; unimpaired perception of the environment. Compare CLOUDED SENSORIUM.

clear twilight-state a type of twilight state that may occur in an epilepsy patient in lieu of a grand mal attack. The patient may experience the c.t.-s. as a vivid dream state in which he may live briefly in another world without cognizance of his true self.

cleft lip = HARELIP.

cleft palate a congenital disorder characterized by a fissure or split in the roof of the mouth because of a failure of bones of the head to fuse properly during prenatal development. If the defect is not corrected by surgery in the first few months of life, the child may develop a speech defect. The defect is not related to mental retardation, although it is not unusual for c.p. to be associated with other birth defects. Also called **uranoschisis**. Also see URANISCOLALIA.

cleft-palate speech a speech impairment caused by a congenital fissure of the soft palate and roof of the mouth which allows air and speech sounds to be emitted through the nose without control. The resulting speech has a nasal quality.

Clérambault, G. G. de /kläräNbō'/ French psychiatrist, 1872–1934. See CLÉRAMBAULT'S SYNDROME; CLÉRAMBAULT-KANDINSKY COMPLEX.

Clérambault-Kandinsky complex a psychotic syndrome in which the patient believes his mind is controlled by an outside power or another person.

Clérambault's syndrome a psychotic form of erotomania, usually in females, consisting of the fixed delusion that a person of high status is in love with them. The disorder is variously interpreted as a projection of self-love, a narcissistic defense against feeling unloved, and a means of denying homosexual tendencies. G. G. de Clérambault first described it in 1922. Also called **psychose passionnelle; de C.s.**

clerical-aptitude tests tests designed to measure specific skills needed in office work, such as perceptual speed (comparing names or numbers), speed in tapping (for typing), learning shorthand, alphabetizing, error location, and vocabulary.

Clever Hans /huns/ the famous "thinking horse" (Berlin, around 1900) that was reputed to be able to solve mathematical problems, spell words, distinguish colors, and identify coins by tapping its foot. By using experimental methods, the psychologist Oskar Pfungst proved that C.H. was responding to "minimal cues" in the form of involuntary movements on the part of its owner. C.H. was one of the ELBERFELD HORSES. See this entry.

cliché /klishā'/ a stereotyped expression that takes the place of genuine thinking or judgment. Most racial, religious, and nationality prejudices are disseminated by clichés.

client the term frequently used by social workers, counselors, and counseling psychologists to refer to the individual receiving treatment or services. The term **patient** is usually employed by psychiatrists, psychoanalysts, and many clinical psychologists.

client-centered psychotherapy the nondirective approach developed by C. Rogers, in which psychotherapy is viewed as an opportunity for the individual to realize his own inner potentialities. The therapist is a warm, accepting person who sets the stage for personality growth by reflecting and restating the client's ideas in such a way that the client sees himself more clearly and comes into closer touch with his real self. As this process continues, the client gradually arrives at his own interpretations, resolves his own conflicts, and reorganizes his own values and approach to life.

-climac-; -climax- a combining form meaning stairs, a ladder, a step, or a high point (from Greek *klimas*, "ladder").

climacophobia a morbid fear of stairs or ladders. Also called **stair phobia**.

climacteric /-ter'-/ the period of life in which reproductive capacity declines and finally ceases. In women this period is known as menopause (popularly, change of life), which occurs between 40 and 55 years of age, lasting two or three years. During this time, menstrual flow gradually decreases and finally ceases altogether, and such symptoms as hot flashes, chills, irritability, mood swings, palpitations, fatigue, joint pains, and depression occur in varying combinations and degrees. Sometimes men undergo a similar period about ten years later, characterized by noctural frequency, fatigue, flushes, indecision, decreased sexual desire and potency, and in some cases depression and a desperate attempt to prove their sexual vigor. In rare instances and both sexes, a full-blown psychosis may develop. Also called **climacterium**. See INVOLUTIONAL PSYCHOTIC REACTION. Also see MALE C.

climacteric melancholia a term sometimes used to identify a form of depression that develops during the menopause.

climacteric psychosis = INVOLUTIONAL PSYCHOTIC REACTION.

climacterium = CLIMACTERIC.

climate conformance the design and construction of a physical environment to insure comfortable temperature and humidity levels for those who use the area.

climax = ORGASM.

clinging behavior a form of attachment behavior in which a child from six months onward clings to the mother or mother figure and becomes acutely distressed when left alone. C.b. reaches a maximum in the second and third years, and then slowly subsides.

clinical counseling counseling that addresses a client's personal or emotional difficulties, encompassing general goals for the client such as greater self-acceptance, better reality orientation, improved decision-making ability, and greater effectiveness in interpersonal relationships. The counselor's responsibilities include the gathering and interpretation of data, identification of the client's major problems, and the formulation of a treatment plan.

clinical diagnosis in psychiatry, diagnosis of mental disorder through the study of the symptom pattern, investigation of background factors, analysis of significant relationships, psychiatric examination, and, where indicated, administration of psychological tests.

clinical grouping the classification of patients into groups according to their behavioral symptoms.

clinical prediction the process of matching such factors as signs and symptoms with personality profiles and case history to determine the psychiatric diagnosis and progress of patients.

clinical psychiatry psychiatry concerned primarily with the diagnosis and treatment of organic and psychogenic mental disorders.

clinical psychology the branch of psychology that specializes in the study, diagnosis, and treatment of behavior disorders.

clinical psychopharmacology a branch of pharmacology concerned with the clinical evaluation of drugs developed for the treatment of disorders of the central nervous system. The clinical evaluation may be carried out by private physicians or hospitals or clinics, recording all effects on individual patients, and comparing results with alternative drugs or with drugless therapies.

clinical sociology a term sometimes applied to the study of the influence of a culture on the mental health of members of that culture.

clinical study an in-depth psychological or psychiatric study of an individual or group, utilizing such techniques as diagnostic observation, psychiatric examination, psychological testing, depth interviewing, questionnaires, and a case-history approach.

clinical teaching a method of teaching which is geared to the individualized needs of a particular and usually atypical child.

clinodactyly a permanent deflection of one or more of the fingers (from Greek *klinein*, "to bend," and *daktylos*, "finger"). This is a rather common physical trait associated with genetic or chromosomal disorders that also may be related to mental retardation.

clipping the shortening of a word in such a way that the new word is used with the same meaning, e.g., "exam" from "examination." In general, adults prefer **back-c.**, e.g., "prof" for "professor," while children prefer **front-c.**, e.g., "fessor" for "professor." The clipped word has the same part of speech as the full form, unlike a BACK-FORMATION. See this entry. Also see PEAK C.

clithrophobia a morbid fear of being enclosed (perhaps from Greek *kleithria*, "keyhole"). Also see CLAUSTROPHOBIA.

clitoral hood the prepuce that covers the clitoris when it is flaccid. The c.h. is homologous to the foreskin of the male penis.

clitoridectomy the surgical removal of the clitoris. As recently as the early 20th century, the procedure was performed on sexually active female children of the Western world in the mistaken belief that a c. would reduce the risk of an unwanted pregnancy. C. is still a regular practice in Muslim and other male-dominated societies in the (largely mistaken) belief that the absence of the clitoris will prevent a woman from experiencing the pleasures of orgasm, which is the male prerogative. A popular, and somewhat euphemistic, term for c. is **female circumcision**.

clitoris a small body of erectile tissue situated above the vaginal opening. It is homologous to the male penis but usually much smaller. Girls born with an abnormally large clitoris have been mistakenly identified as boys and raised as male children. Also see PHALLUS.

cloaca /klō·ā′kə/ the common cavity into which the intestinal, urinary, and reproductive canals open during the course of development. The proxim-

ity of these functions and the pleasure involved in them are a major factor in Freud's psychosexual theory.

cloaca theory the fantasy among young children that birth takes place through the anus and is a form of defecation. Freud theorized that this fantasy may be a source of bisexuality.

clofazimine an antibiotic developed in the 1950s that is particularly effective in treating leprosy, or Hansen's disease. In addition to being leprostatic, c. is antiinflammatory. However, c. causes a reddish-brown skin pigmentation that many patients find objectionable. In most cases, two leprosy drugs are used together to reduce the risk of bacterial resistance. Thus, c. often is combined with DAPSONE. See this entry.

cloisonnism = SYNTHETISM.

-clon- a combining form relating to a spasm. Adjective: **clonic.** See CLONUS.

clone two or more organisms originating from a single individual as a result of asexual reproduction (Greek *klon*, "twig"). Since they have the same heredity, any observable differences in their features are assumed to be the result of environmental influences.

clonic: See -CLON-.

clonic phase the phase of a grand mal seizure following the tonic, or rigid, phase. It is characterized by rapidly alternating contraction and relaxation of the jaw and skeletal muscles.

clonic spasm: See SPASM.

clonidine an antihypertensive drug that functions by direct action on alpha receptors in the brainstem to restrict the flow of impulses in peripheral sympathetic nerves. Most of the other commonly prescribed antihypertensive drugs act as beta blockers or as diuretics.

clonus involuntary contractions and relaxations of the muscles in alternate rapid succession (Greek *klonos*, "turmoil"). Some forms of c., such as hiccups or jactitations that may occur when falling asleep, are considered normal. C. also may be a part of an epileptic convulsion. More severe forms are associated with spinal-cord damage, poisoning as from strychnine, or an infection, such as syphilis. Clonic wrist movements can be induced in some patients by forcibly extending the hand at the wrist.

closed-class word = FUNCTION WORD.

closed-ended question in an examination, survey, or interview, a question that provides the student, subject, or respondent with alternative answers from which he selects his response, e.g., a multiple-choice item. Also called **fixed alternative.** Compare OPEN-ENDED QUESTION.

closed group a counseling or therapy group comprised only of those members who constituted the original group. New members may not join during the course of therapy. Compare OPEN GROUP.

closed-loop feedback system a self-contained reflex system in which a physiological need stimulates a neuromuscular portion of the body to satisfy the need. An example is the autonomic activity of thirst that induces the subject to seek water to satisfy the desire.

closesightedness: See MYOPIA.

Clos-O-Mat a trademark for an automatic toilet designed for handicapped patients. The device, which fits over a toilet seat, automatically cleans the anal area following a bowel movement with jets of warm water and dry air.

closure the Gestalt concept that the mind synthesizes the missing parts of a perceived image and, in effect, closes the gap between the reality and the desired "picture." If an occasional note is deleted from a popular song, the listener may unconsciously supply the missing notes from his mind. C. also may refer to a grouping of things enclosing a space. Also see GOODNESS OF CONFIGURATION; LAW OF PRÄGNANZ; AUDITORY C.; VISUAL C.

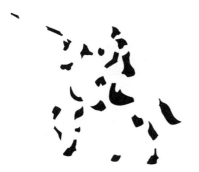

CLOSURE. Did you immediately see a horseman with a lance?

clotting factor any of a dozen substances involved in the blood-clotting process. The various factors are assigned Roman numerals I to V and VII to XIII; the substance originally designated as factor VI was deleted after careful studies indicated it was not essential to the clotting process. A deficiency of any of the factors results in increased risk of hemorrhage when a blood vessel breaks. See BLOOD DISORDER; CHRISTMAS DISEASE.

clouded sensorium a state of consciousness in which the ability to perceive and understand the environment is impaired and the patient is confused and disoriented as to time, place, circumstances, and his own identity. A c.s. occurs most strikingly in toxic psychoses and acute alcoholism, but is also found in schizophrenic and manic-depressive states. Compare CLEAR SENSORIUM.

clouding of consciousness a disturbance in which the patient is in a **mental fog** and in which sensory, perceptual, and thought processes are impaired to such an extent that it is hard or impossible to "get through" to him. The condition is most often associated with infectious or toxic disorders, and less often with extreme tension and anxiety.

cloverleaf skull = KLEEBLATTSCHÄDEL SYNDROME.

cloze procedure a technique used in testing and teaching reading and comprehension by deleting words from a text and leaving blank spaces. Measurement is made by rating the number of blanks that are filled in correctly. The c.p. is based on the Gestalt principle of closure.

clubfoot a type of foot deformity in which the foot is twisted out of normal position and, in most cases, in more than one positional distortion. E.g., the foot may be turned inward and downward, outward and upward, or in some other variation. The cause may be congenital or the condition may be due to injury or a disease, e.g., poliomyelitis. C. often is associated with another anomaly, such as meningomyelocele. Also called **talipes** /tal'əpēz/.

clumsy-child syndrome one of the many equivalent terms for MINIMAL BRAIN DYSFUNCTION. See this entry. Also see LEARNING DISABILITIES.

cluster analysis a method of identifying factors underlying an intercorrelation matrix by grouping together correlations of similar magnitude.

cluster approach in evaluation research, a strategy for accumulating information concerned with combining and reconciling studies from which conflicting conclusions have been drawn. This approach suggests criteria for determining when data from dissimilar studies can be pooled.

cluster headaches headaches that typically occur for a period of up to three months night after night, followed by a headache-free period of months or years. Usually c.h. set in two or three hours after falling asleep, and usually they are limited to the area of one of the eyes. C.h. may be a special case of migraine; and just as the cause of migraine is unknown, no cause has been determined for c.h.

cluster marriage a nontraditional sexual style in which two or three married couples live together.

cluttering a rapid, nervous speech pattern resulting in confused, jumbled, and imprecise speech. The term is essentially equivalent to TACHYPHEMIA. See this entry.

Clytemnestra complex the obsessive impulse of a wife to kill her husband so that she can possess one of his male relatives. The term was derived from the classical myth of the wife and murderess of Agamemnon.

CM = COCHLEAR MICROPHONICS.

CME = CONTINUING MEDICAL EDUCATION.

C-M-T = CHARCOT-MARIE-TOOTH DISEASE.

CNS = CENTRAL NERVOUS SYSTEM.

CNS abnormality any defect in structure or function of the tissues of the brain and spinal cord. Examples include glial insufficiency, cerebral-vascular disease, disorders that affect the fatty protective covering of white matter as in Tay-Sachs disease, or congenital anomalies marked by failure of tissues or neural connections to develop normally.

CNV = CONTINGENT NEGATIVE VARIATION.

coaching specialized instruction, training, and practice for taking psychological tests. Studies indicate that these methods have a more positive effect on students with deficient educational background than on those with superior educational opportunities. The College Entrance Examination Board attempts to choose items that are not readily amenable to c.

coacting group a group that works together on a mutual problem or project with minimal interpersonal exchange or communication; that is, the group's attention is not diverted to interpersonal processes but is focused on the work, e.g., organizing a fund-raising campaign.

coarse tremor: See TREMOR.

cobalt treatment a type of radiation treatment for cancers in which radioisotopes of cobalt, e.g., cobalt 60, are implanted in or about the site of the malignancy.

coca a tree of the species Erythroxylon coca that is indigenous to Peru, Bolivia, and other South American countries. It has been introduced as a commercial plant in India, Sri Lanka, and Indonesia. The leaves have been used for centuries as the source of an alkaloid, cocaine, which is a CNS stimulant.

cocaine $C_{17}H_{21}NO_4$—an alkaloid obtained from leaves of the coca tree. C. was isolated in 1855 but its therapeutic uses were not investigated until the 1880s. In 1884, Freud experimented with c. as a possible antidote for morphine addiction; the experiment failed, but Freud observed that the drug had the effect of a topical anesthetic. C. acts by paralyzing sensory-nerve terminals and stimulates adrenergic nerves by inhibiting the uptake of norepinephrine. The stimulating effect on the cerebrum is similar to that of alcohol in that the user feels excited, experiences an absence of fatigue, and becomes garrulous, followed by a period of depression as the effects diminish. C. is rapidly detoxified by the liver and excreted through the urinary tract, some of the chemical remaining unchanged. The toxicity of c. varies in different users, and there is some evidence that tolerance develops, with increasingly larger doses required to achieve equivalent effects. Among the many street names for c. are **C, coke, snow, blow,** and **toot.** Also see PSYCHO-STIMULANTS; ANALEPTICS; C. ABUSE.

cocaine abuse a disorder with the following criteria: (a) pathological use of cocaine, as indicated by inability to reduce or stop intake, (b) intoxication throughout the day, (c) episodes of overdose with hallucinations and delusions, (d) impaired functioning, as shown by fights, loss of friends, absence from work, loss of job, and legal difficulties beyond a single arrest for possession, purchase, or sale of cocaine, and (e) at least a month's duration. (DSM-III)

cocaine bug a symptom occurring among cocaine users, who experience itching and biting sensations and feel as if insects are crawling on or under their skin. See FORMICATION.

cocaine habituation psychological dependence on cocaine resulting in habitual use. See COCAINE ABUSE.

cocaine intoxication a disorder that involves a pattern of reactions starting within one hour and consisting of (a) two or more psychological symptoms (agitation, elation, grandiosity, loquacity, hypervigilance, that is, extreme wakefulness), (b) two or more physical symptoms (rapid heartbeat, dilated pupils, elevated blood pressure, perspiration or chills, nausea and vomiting), and (c) such behavioral effects as fighting, impaired judgment, or poor social or occupational functioning. Large doses, especially when taken intravenously, may produce confusion, incoherence, apprehension, transient paranoid ideas, increased sexual interest, and formication (sensation of insects crawling on the skin: the "cocaine bug"). An hour or so after these effects subside, the user may experience tremulousness, anxiety, irritability, fatigue, and depression. (DMS-III)

coccygeal /koksij′ē·əl/ pertaining to the **coccyx** /kok′siks/, the last bone of the spinal column (plural: **coccyges** /koksī′jēz/).

coccygeal nerve: See SPINAL NERVES.

coccyges; coccyx: See COCCYGEAL.

cochlea the labyrinthine portion of the inner ear, shaped like two and a half turns of a snail shell. Its membranous interior contains the organ of Corti, the small hair-cell units that transmit the sensation of sound to the eighth cranial nerve. The c. is filled with fluid and separated from the middle ear by two membrane-covered windows, one of which relays sound vibrations from the tympanic membrane via the ossicles, or tiny bones, in the middle ear.

cochleagram a recording of the electrical activity of the hair cells in the organ of Corti in response to sound stimuli of different frequencies and intensities. The data obtained may help in diagnosing suspected nerve deafness due to a disorder of the retrocochlear nerve or the end organ of the cochlea.

cochlear aplasia the clinical absence or defective development of the cochlea.

cochlear microphonics neural potentials generated by cochlear hair cells in the inner ear that have the same wave forms as the sounds producing the stimulus. A strong sound burst at a frequency of 5,000 cycles per second will produce a cochlear-microphonic wave form of the same frequency. Abbrev.: **CM.** See COCHLEA.

cochlear nerve a part of the eighth cranial nerve concerned with the sense of hearing.

cochlear nuclei nerve cells located in the floor of the cochlea where they receive incoming fibers from the cochlear portion of the inner ear and serve as the point of origin of the auditory nerve.

cochlear recruitment the recruitment of neurons in the cochlea to aid in the spread of response to a stimulus of prolonged intensity. The recruitment is needed sometimes to replace the participation of neurons that have dropped out of the response because of fatigue.

cochleopalpebral-reflex test a hearing test in

which a sudden noise is sounded near the ear. It is used to measure contraction of the orbicularis palpebrarum muscle.

Cockayne, Edward Alfred English physician, 1880–1956. See COCKAYNE'S SYNDROME.

Cockayne's syndrome a hereditary disorder involving dwarfism, microcephaly, mental retardation, visual disorders, actinic dermatitis, and progressive neurologic deterioration. Early psychomotor development is slow and most patients show an IQ of less than 50. The patients become blind, deaf, and helpless by age 20. Also called **Cockayne-Neill dwarfism**.

cocktail-party conversationalism = CHATTERBOX EFFECT.

cocoa a product of the cacao plant manufactured by roasting and grinding the beans and removing the oils. The pharmacologically active ingredients are theobromine and caffeine. Theobromine content of c. varies from about one to three percent of dry weight, with the highest values observed in South American c. and the lowest in Nigerian c.

co-conscious personality a term used by M. Prince for a personality that is "split-off and independently acting," as in cases of MULTIPLE PERSONALITY. See this entry.

code a set of symbols used to represent information items in a convenient form, e.g., for computer use.

code capacity the maximum amount of coded data a channel can transmit in a fixed time period.

codeine; codeine phosphate: See OPIUM ALKALOIDS.

code of ethics a set of standards and principles of professional conduct. The **American Psychiatric Association code** deals with such issues as confidentiality, soliciting of patients, seeking consultation upon request, not disposing of services under terms that interfere with medical judgment, and responsibility to society as well as to the individual patient. The **American Psychological Association code** includes statements on professional responsibility, professional competence, moral and legal standards, confidentiality, welfare of the consumer, public statements, professional relationships, assessment techniques, and research with human and animal subjects.

code test a test that requires translating one set of symbols into another, e.g., writing "California" in numbers that stand for letters according to the code A = 3, B = 4, C = 5, etc. Also called **coding test; symbol-substitution test**.

codification the act of classifying items into identifiable categories; also, the conversion of data or other information into a code that can be translated by others. Also called **coding**.

codification-of-rules stage the attitude displayed by children age 11 and 12 toward rules. In the c.-o.-r.s., according to Piaget, children view rules as binding once they are agreed to, and games are seen as a system of interconnecting laws. Although the awareness of rules emerges at an earlier age, systematic adherence is not manifested until the c.-o.-r.s.

coding = CODIFICATION.

coding test = CODE TEST.

codominance a sharing of rank or peck-order positions in certain animal populations. Wild macaque monkeys control their colonies through a small group of dominant males, rather than through a linear hierarchy. Studies indicate that codominance is more common among arboreal animals while linear dominance is characteristic of ground-living species who are exposed to greater threats from predators.

coefficient of alienation a measure of the amount of unexplained variance or error in prediction. Symbol: $k = \sqrt{1 - r^2}$.

coefficient of concordance a measure of the correlation among three or more sets of ranks. It is a generalization of the rank-order correlation. Symbol: **W**. Also called **Kendall c.o.c.**

coefficient of determination a statistic indicating the percentage of variance two variables have in common, and equal to r^2. Therefore, a correlation of .70 would indicate the two variables have 49 percent of their variance in common.

coefficient of stability a reliability-test measure based on the use of the same type of measuring instrument administered at two points in time to a sample of people. It is one of three kinds of reliability checks recognized by the American Psychological Association. Also called **test-retest method; test-retest coefficient**. Also see TEST-RETEST RELIABILITY.

-coel- a combining form relating to something hollow, as a cavity (from Greek *koilos*, "hollow").

-coen-; -coene-; -cene- a combining form meaning common, general, or sharing (from Greek *koinos*, "common, public").

coenesthesia general body feeling including the sense of being alive, and of well-being or discomfort. C. is believed to be derived from internal sensations often occurring below the level of consciousness. Also called **cenesthesia; cenesthesis**.

coenotrope = CENOTROPE.

coenzyme a nonprotein organic compound that functions with the protein portion of an enzyme called an apoenzyme. Most enzymes fail to function in the absence of a specific c., which in many cases is a vitamin. Niacin, riboflavin, and thiamine are examples of coenzymes. **C.A** contains, among other molecules, pantothenic acid, a B-complex vitamin; it is essential for carbohydrate and fat metabolism and in the activity of steroid hormones and acetylcholine.

coercive behavior behavior designed to force others to do one's bidding, often masked as filial devotion or marital or parental concern, and sometimes expressed in undisguised form: "If you don't do what I say, I'll kill myself."

coercive persuasion systematic, intensive indoctrination of political or military prisoners who have been "softened up" by such methods as threats, punishments, bribes, isolation, continuous interrogation, and repetitious "instruction." See BRAINWASHING.

coercive treatment = FORCED TREATMENT.

coexperimenter an experimenter who assists the main experimenter, especially by maintaining double-blind conditions or in some other way keeping the main experimenter uninformed and therefore unbiased.

coffee the common name of an evergreen tree that grows wild and is cultivated in mild tropical climates throughout the world. Of more than 100 species, two are commercially important sources of the coffee bean, a seed of the cherrylike fruit, used in caffeine beverages. They are Coffea arabica and Coffea robusta whose beans contain about one and two percent caffeine respectively. C. beverage was introduced into Europe from the Arabian countries about 1615.

cofigurative culture a society or culture in which children learn chiefly from other children while adults learn from other adults. Also see POST-FIGURATIVE CULTURE; PREFIGURATIVE CULTURE.

Cogan, David Glendenning American physician, 1908—. See COGAN'S SYNDROME.

Cogan's syndrome a condition described by D. G. Cogan in 1945 in patients with keratitis (inflammation of the cornea). Attacks of vertigo, tinnitus, and deafness are experienced, with pain in the eyes and reduced vision. As the symptom of vertigo subsides, the patient becomes deaf. Also called **nonsyphilitic interstitial keratitis.**

cognition a general term for all forms of knowing and awareness, such as perceiving, conceiving, reasoning, judging, and imagining. Cognitive processes are often contrasted with conative processes (striving, willing) and emotive processes (feeling, affect). Also see PRIMARY C.

cognition disorder impaired thought processes; inability to know and be aware of people, stimuli, or events, or to perform such cognitive functions as perceiving, conceiving, and reasoning.

Cognitive Abilities Test a group of tests for the elementary grades—kindergarten through third grade, and grades 3 through 12. The latter comprises eight levels which contain the same ten subtests grouped into three batteries: (1) verbal—vocabulary, sentence completion, verbal classification, verbal analogies; (2) quantitative—quantitative relations, number series, equation-building; and (3) nonverbal—figure classification, figure analogies, figure synthesis.

cognitive-awareness level the level at which a diagnostic-therapeutic concept is effective.

cognitive behavior modification a recently-developed behavior-therapy approach based on the assumption that clinical disorders are the result of maladaptive or faulty thought patterns, and that the task of therapy is to identify these patterns and replace them with more adaptive

cognitions, a process known as **cognitive restructuring.** For other details, see COGNITIVE THERAPY. Also see RATIONAL PSYCHOTHERAPY.

cognitive behavior therapy = COGNITIVE THERAPY.

cognitive conditioning a type of behavior therapy in which an aversive stimulus is paired with thoughts of the behavior to be modified. E.g., the subject imagines he is smoking a cigarette and gives himself an electric shock; the procedure is repeated until the thought produces the effect of discouraging the behavior. Also see COGNITIVE REHEARSAL.

cognitive control the aspect of cognitive style having to do with the extent to which a person differentiates objects or ideas into either a few broad categories or into several smaller carefully defined categories. As children develop, they tend to progress from general to specific groupings. See COGNITIVE STYLE.

cognitive defects symptoms involving difficulty in knowing, understanding, and interpreting reality, including impairment (a) in recognizing and identifying objects or individuals, (b) in reasoning and judging, (c) in thinking abstractly, (d) in remembering, (e) in comprehending or using language, and (f) in performing practical calculations. If c.d. are pervasive and the result of organic brain disorder, the condition may be termed dementia.

cognitive derailment the shifting of thoughts or associations so that they do not follow one another in a logical sequence. C.d. is a symptom of schizophrenia. Also called **slippage.** The term is essentially equivalent to COGNITIVE SLIPPAGE. See this entry.

cognitive development the development of thinking processes of all kinds, such as perceiving, remembering, concept formation, problem-solving, imagining, and reasoning. For the stages of c.d., see PIAGET.

cognitive dissonance a term applied by L. Festinger to a state of conflict and discomfort occurring when existing beliefs or assumptions are challenged or contradicted by new evidence. The individual usually seeks to relieve the discomfort by such means as denying the existence or importance of the conflict, reconciling the differences, altering one of the dissident elements, or demanding more and more information, as frequently occurs among smokers who are faced with evidence that cigarettes are hazardous to health.

cognitive flexibility a term in educational psychology referring to the teacher's capacity for objective appraisal of and appropriate, flexible action within the teaching setting. C.f. involves adaptability, objectivity, and fair-mindedness.

cognitive growth: See COGNITIVE DEVELOPMENT.

cognitive map a theoretical map, or pattern, formed in the mind of a subject for solving problems such as a maze. The concept is based on an assumption that an individual seeks and collects clues, such as environmental relationships, rather than being a passive receptor of information needed to achieve a goal.

cognitive mediation the thought processes that occur in the mind between arrival of the stimulus and initiation of the response.

cognitive need a curiosity-exploratory drive to observe and comprehend the environment.

cognitive-physiological theory a concept that emotion is bodily function that interfaces with cognitive processes. Also see JAMES-LANGE THEORY.

cognitive processes the mental functions assumed to be involved in perception, learning, and thinking. See COGNITION.

cognitive psychology a fast-growing and relatively new branch of psychology that explores the cognitive processes, mainly through inference from behavior—in contrast to the past approaches of either studying the mind through introspection or studying behavior while setting the mind aside. C.p. is largely based on Piaget's innovative theories but is advancing beyond them into areas such as computer science. Among related branches is **cognitive psychophysiology**. Also see COGNITIVE SCIENCE.

cognitive rehearsal a behavior-modification technique in which the client rehearses those situations that tend to produce anxiety or self-defeating behavior while practicing positive coping statements designed to reduce the anxiety. E.g., if public speaking is the target situation, the individual envisions the setting of the speech and repeats statements such as "One thought at a time; speak slowly and clearly; it's going fine."

cognitive restructuring: See COGNITIVE BEHAVIOR MODIFICATION.

cognitive schema a perceptual pattern used as a reference for future experiences, as in a Gestalt configuration based on proximity, or a concept of socialism.

cognitive science a blend of psychology, philosophy, psychobiology, anthropology, psycholinguistics, and computer science. C.s. consists mainly of COGNITIVE PSYCHOLOGY. See this entry.

cognitive slippage a term coined by P. E. Meehl for the disconnected thought processes that are characteristic of schizophrenia. See LOOSENING OF ASSOCIATIONS. Also see COGNITIVE DERAILMENT; THOUGHT DERAILMENT.

cognitive structure a mental framework, pattern, or scheme that maintains and organizes the informational elements of a body of facts in any learning situation. When a need arises for the c.s., as in a test, the individual is thought to engage in a memory search in which the stored c.s. is retrieved and applied to the present requirements. The term is also used for a unified structure of beliefs and attitudes about the world or society.

cognitive style the characteristic manner in which a person thinks about a problem and then conceives and implements his solution, e.g., an analytical, methodical, cautious style in contrast to intuition and impetuousness. According to some theorists, one's degree of field dependence or independence is a major component of c.s. Also see COGNITIVE CONTROL; CONCEPTUAL TEMPO.

cognitive theory of learning the concept that learning requires central constructs and new ways of perceiving events.

cognitive therapy a psychotherapeutic approach based on the concept that emotional problems are the result of faulty ways of thinking and distorted attitudes toward oneself and others. The therapist takes the role of an active guide who helps the patient correct and revise his perceptions and attitudes by citing evidence to the contrary or eliciting it from the patient himself. Also called **cognitive behavior therapy**. Also see COGNITIVE BEHAVIOR MODIFICATION.

cognitivist a theorist who is primarily concerned with describing intellectual development (Jean Piaget, Jerome Bruner) or early language behavior (Roger Brown).

cognizance need the drive to acquire knowledge through questions, exploration, and study (Murray).

cohabitation the act of living together as husband and wife, regardless of the marital status of the partners. The term may also apply to a homosexual relationship.

cohesion in psychiatry, the emotional bonds that hold a group together. Such bonds arise out of interactions among the members as well as mutual interests, activities, and purposes. Group cohesion is frequently considered essential to effective group psychotherapy. Also called **cohesiveness; group c.**

cohesion law: See LAW OF COHESION.

cohesiveness = COHESION.

cohort a group of individuals sharing a common attribute. This term is often used in epidemiological literature to classify, e.g., groups at risk or not at risk for a disease, or those born in a certain year.

cohort effects the effects attributed to being a member of a group born at a particular time and influenced by pressures and challenges of the era of development.

coil: See INTRAUTERINE DEVICE.

coin test a test involving estimation of the size of coins. Underestimation has been considered indicative of a lesion in the pyramidal system. However, the test is controversial since 70 percent of normals are unable to make accurate estimates, and 90 percent underestimate the size of the coins.

coital positions various postures that may be assumed by sexual partners during intercourse. C.p. commonly used are face-to-face, with the man above the woman; face-to-face, with the woman above the man; face-to-face, with the partners lying on their sides; rear-entry, with the man facing the woman's back "doggy"-style or lying down, or the woman sitting on the man's lap, either facing toward or away from the man.

coition = COITUS.

coitophobia a morbid fear of sexual intercourse.

coitus an act of sexual intercourse, usually the union of the male and female genitals (from Latin *coire*, "to go together"). Examples of variations are **c. a tergo**, or c. from the rear, and **c. inter femora**, or c. in which the penis is inserted between the pressed thighs of the female. C. is also called **coition; intercourse; sexual intercourse**. Also see COPULATION; PRIMAL SCENE; PAINFUL INTERCOURSE; CAREZZA; FELLATIO; ANAL INTERCOURSE; SODOMY.

coitus à la vache /äläväsh'/ a form of coitus a tergo in which the female is in the knee-chest position (French, "coitus like a cow").

coitus analis = ANAL INTERCOURSE.

coitus a tergo: See COITUS.

coitus condomatus sexual intercourse performed with the penis enclosed in a condom or sheath.

coitus fear = COITOPHOBIA.

coitus in ano = ANAL INTERCOURSE.

coitus in axilla coitus in which the penis is inserted "in the armpit" of the partner.

coitus inter femora: See COITUS.

coitus interruptus the withdrawal of the penis during intercourse, mainly to reduce the likelihood of conception. See ONANISM.

coitus intra mammas coitus in which the penis is inserted "between the breasts" of the female.

coitus prolongatus = CAREZZA.

coitus representation the symbolic representation of sexual intercourse through symptoms or other mechanisms, e.g., the use of the voice in a manner that allows the tongue to represent the movements of coitus.

coitus reservatus sexual intercourse in which the male suppresses the ejaculation of semen. C.r. has been practiced for generations in the Orient by men who sometimes apply opium paste to the glans penis to reduce its sensitivity. In the Oneida community of the United States, in the 19th century, young men were encouraged to practice c.r. with menopausal women until they were able to achieve a state of "male continence." See CAREZZA.

coitus sine ejaculatione /sē'nā/ or /sī nē/ sexual intercourse in which ejaculation does not occur despite adequate erection. The absence of ejaculation is due mainly to involuntary factors, as opposed to coitus reservatus in which ejaculation is deliberately suppressed. Also called **ejaculatory incompetence; ejaculatio deficiens; dry orgasm**. See COITUS; IMPOTENCE; INHIBITED MALE ORGASM.

coke = COCAINE.

-col-; -coli-; -colo- a combining form relating to the colon.

cola nut = KOLA NUT.

colchicine an alkaloid derived from the meadow saffron plant Colchicum autumnale, which has been used in the treatment of gout for more than 1,500 years. The name is derived from the Greek community Colchis, where the plant flourishes, but the therapeutic value was discovered by fifth-century Arabian physicians. C. apparently acts by inhibiting the formation of uric-acid crystals. C. can cause birth defects of offspring in women using the drug. C. also can interfere with the normal absorption of vitamin B_{12}, a deficiency of which can result in mental disorders.

cold-blooded animals = POIKILOTHERMS.

cold effects effects of cold temperatures on physical and mental health. Research on cold stress indicates that reaction time, tracking proficiency, tactile discrimination, and other types of performance begin to deteriorate at temperatures of 55°F (13°C) or below. Studies of cold effects on social behavior have produced conflicting evidence of both increased and decreased aggression. Criminal activity generally declines in cold weather.

cold-fear = PSYCHROPHOBIA.

cold-pack treatment the use of ice packs or sheets wrung out in cold water as a sedative in the control of delirious or excited states. Sometimes ice packs are applied to the back of the neck and hot packs to the feet. See PACKS.

cold spot any point on a body surface containing nerve receptors sensitive to low-temperature stimuli.

cold turkey the abrupt cessation in the use of narcotic drugs without cushioning the impact with methadone or tranquilizers. It is a popular term referring to the combination of chills and goose flesh experienced during the withdrawal period.

colitis a term applied to two principal diseases of the large intestine, or colon, each of which may be caused or aggravated by emotional tension. In **mucous c.**, or **spastic c.**, the bowels become highly sensitive and irritable, with constipation, mucus in the stool, abdominal distention, and poor appetite. According to many psychiatrists, the symptoms are usually associated with guilt, anxiety, and resentment in individuals who are oversensitive and overconscientious. In **ulcerative c.** an actual inflammation produces lesions in the intestinal wall, which can cause diarrhea, blood in the stool, intense abdominal pain, and anemia. The condition is believed to be associated with such factors as a strong dependency need and a cold, dominating mother who frustrated the normal need for care, resulting in feelings of rage, fear of retaliation, overconcern with security, and inability to handle stress or failure.

colla = KOLA NUT.

collaboration a specialized term used by H.S. Sullivan for an interpersonal relationship that combines cooperation with sensitivity to the needs of another person.

collaborative therapy marriage therapy conducted by two therapists, each seeing one spouse but conferring from time to time.

collagen: See EVERSION THEORY OF AGING.

collapse delirium a severe and dangerous form of delirium observed most frequently in patients who have suffered prostration and exhaustion during the febrile or postfebrile stage of systemic infectious disease such as pneumonia, diphtheria, or typhoid fever. The delirium is characterized by disorientation, confusion, transient delusions, and emotional lability, and is followed by physical collapse. The term is essentially equivalent to HYPERMANIA. See this entry.

collateral sulcus a fissure that runs along the lower medial surface of the hemisphere from approximately the occipital pole to the temporal pole.

collative properties the structural properties of such stimulus patterns in art forms as complexity and novelty. Studies indicate that mind processes tend to favor these c.p., which may have hedonic value.

colleague-centered consultation: See PSYCHIATRIC CONSULTATION.

collecting mania a morbid, compulsive preoccupation with indiscriminate collecting, usually of useless articles or trash. The condition is most frequently found in chronic schizophrenia and senile dementia. Psychoanalytic theory associates it with anal eroticism. See ANAL CHARACTER; HOARDING.

collective behavior a general term for group or mass behavior and the characteristic actions and reactions of various kinds of "collectivities," such as audiences, crowds, mobs, clubs, and therapeutic groups. Social psychologists have studied c.b. in such situations as bank runs, lynchings, strikes, revival meetings, race riots, food stampedes, and special events such as the Mardi Gras, Woodstock, and the Florida real-estate boom of the 1920s. Also see CROWD BEHAVIOR; MASS HYSTERIA.

collective experience a phrase used by S. R. Slavson for the common body of emotional experience which develops in therapeutic groups out of identification with each others problems, mutual support and empathy, and putting aside ego defenses.

collective hypnotization the act of hypnotizing a group of people at the same time.

collective hysteria = MASS HYSTERIA.

collective monologue: See PSEUDOCONVERSATION.

collective neurosis neurotic behavior, usually transient, on the part of a group of people, as in disaster syndrome, mass hysteria, and panic disorder.

collective psychosis grossly distorted reactions of an entire group of people. Examples are the belief in time of war that the enemy is the incarnation of evil, and the epidemic of lycanthropy that occurred in 16th-century France and Italy in which hundreds of people experienced the illusion that they had been transformed to wolves.

The term c.p. has also been mistakenly applied to mass-hysterical reactions, which would be more appropriately described as neuroses. See MASS HYSTERIA.

collective suicide a term sometimes applied to mass-suicidal behavior, as in large numbers of people jumping off a sinking ship to certain death; stampeding for exits, as in the Coconut Grove fire; or the mass suicide of more than 900 by poisoning that occurred in Jonestown, Guyana, in 1978.

collective unconscious the division of the unconscious that, according to Jung, is common to all humankind: "All those psychic contents I term collective that are peculiar not to one individual, but to many at the same time, that is, either to a society, a people, or to mankind in general. Such contents are the 'mystical collective ideas'...of the primitive. They include also the general concepts of right, the state, religion, science, etc., current among civilized men." (*Contributions to Analytical Psychology*, 1928) See PERSONAL UNCONSCIOUS; RACIAL UNCONSCIOUS; ARCHETYPE.

college admission tests tests for admission, placement, and counseling of college students. The SAT (Scholastic Aptitude Test) provides separate scores for the verbal and mathematical sections, including such items as antonyms, sentence completions, analogies, reading comprehension, as well as multiple-choice questions and quantitative comparisons in the mathematical portion. For another widely used college admission test, see ACT ASSESSMENT.

College Entrance Examination Board Advanced Placement Program: See ADVANCED PLACEMENT EXAMINATIONS.

college psychiatry a form of community psychiatry in which mental-health services are provided in colleges through a more or less comprehensive psychiatric service which provides professional diagnosis, counseling, short-term psychotherapy, and referral where needed. Typical problems dealt with are depression, anxiety, psychosomatic symptoms, suicidal impulses, drug abuse, alcoholism, apathy, psychosexual problems, student unrest or violence, and dropouts.

Colles, Abraham Irish surgeon, 1773–1843. See SILVER-FORK DEFORMITY (there: **Colles' fracture**).

colliculus an elevated or raised area or prominence on an organ or section of body tissue. In physiological psychology, c. usually refers to masses of nerve tissue at the back of the midbrain that are associated with auditory and other reflexes.

Collins, Edward Treacher English ophthalmologist, 1862–1919. See TREACHER COLLINS' SYNDROME; CRANIOFACIAL ANOMALIES; DISFIGUREMENT; DYSOSTOSIS.

collyr. an abbreviation used in prescriptions, meaning "eyewash" (Latin *collyrium*).

coloboma: See IRIS C.

color the quality of light which corresponds to

wavelength as perceived through retinal receptors. C. is divided into chromatic c. (analyzable into hue brightness and saturation) and achromatic c. (varying in brightness alone). See CHROMATIC COLORS; ACHROMATIC COLORS. Also see FILM C.; FLIGHT OF COLORS; NEUTRAL C.; OSWALD COLORS; SPECTRAL C.; SUBJECTIVE COLORS; SURFACE C.

color attribute any of the basic characteristics of color: hue, saturation, brightness.

color blindness the inability to discriminate between certain colors. The most common form of the disorder involves the green or red receptors of the cone cells in the retina, causing a red-green confusion. About six percent of males and one-half of a percent of females are affected. Total c.b. is rare, affecting about three out of one million persons. C.b. may be caused by disease, drugs, or injury, but most often is an inherited trait. Also see DEUTAN C.B.

color cells the three types of cone cells in the retina each of which is sensitive to one of the visual primary colors, red, green, and violet. Some investigators believe there are four types of retinal c.c. in humans. The three-c.c., or trichromatic, theory is based on patterns of color blindness. The four-cell, or opponent-process, theory assumes the fourth cell is a luminosity receptor. See COLOR BLINDNESS.

color circle an array of chromatic colors around the circumference of a circle. The colors are arranged in the order in which they are seen in the spectrum, but nonspectral purples and reds are also included. Complementary colors are opposite each other.

color cone = COLOR SOLID.

color constancy the tendency to experience a familiar object as having the same color under different conditions of illumination. That is, the object appears the same although its stimulus properties are modified. C.c. is one of the perceptual constancies. Also see OBJECT CONSTANCY.

color contrast the effect of one color upon another when they are perceived in close proximity. In **simultaneous contrast**, complementary colors such as yellow and blue are enhanced by each other: the yellow appears yellower and the blue bluer. In **successive contrast**, the complement of a fixated color is perceived when the fixation is shifted to a neutral surface. Also called **chromatic contrast**.

color dreams dream images in color, which are believed to serve definite psychological functions. Eidelberg (*Encyclopedia of Psychoanalysis*, 1968) cities "camouflage or communication," and states that "repetitive color dreams may be related to traumatic events with visual shock, in which color was involved or defensively incorporated as a screen." Though dreaming in color is usually normal, it is also common in epilepsy, migraine, and substance use (especially LSD or other hallucinogens).

color fusion: See FUSION.

color hearing a type of color sensation experienced by some individuals when sounds are heard. In schizophrenics, the effect may accompany voices rather than tones or other sounds. Also see CHROMESTHESIA.

colorimeter an instrument used to measure or identify colors by comparison with a known mixture.

color mixture a fusion effect produced by combining pigments (subtractive mixture), projecting lights simultaneously (additive mixture), or rapid rotation in a color mixer (retinal mixture).

color-mixture primaries the primary colors, usually red, green, and blue, which by their additive mixture produce a total range of hues.

color phobia = CHROMOPHOBIA.

color preference: See LAWS OF C.P.

color pyramid = COLOR SOLID.

color scotoma: See SCOTOMA.

color shades colors of a specified hue and saturation which vary only in brightness.

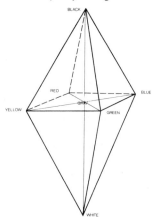

COLOR SOLID

color solid a three-dimensional representation of all dimensions of color, including the various degrees and combinations of hue, brightness, and saturation. Also called **color cone; color pyramid; color spindle**.

color sorting test: See HOLMGREN TEST.

color spindle = COLOR SOLID.

color surface a plane made by cutting through a color pyramid or color triangle to show all possible hues and saturations at a specific level of brightness.

color system: See RIDGWAY C.S.

color theories theories constructed to explain color phenomena, especially those proposed by Hering, Ladd-Franklin, and Young-Helmholtz. See HERING THEORY OF COLOR VISION; LADD-FRANKLIN THEORY; YOUNG-HELMHOLTZ THEORY OF COLOR VISION; GRANIT THEORY OF COLOR VISION; LAND THEORY OF COLOR VISION.

color triangle a triangular representation of the relationships of hues, brightness, and saturation.

color vision: See COLOR THEORIES.

color weakness an impaired ability to perceive hues accurately. The term is often used interchangeably with color blindness.

color zones retinal areas that respond differently to various colors. All colors are perceived in the fovea; blues, yellows, and grays in the middle zone; and (with some overlap) achromatic colors in the periphery.

colostomy a surgical procedure in which an opening is made through the abdomen in order to divert the flow of feces through the opening rather than through the rectum. The fecal matter is collected in a plastic disposal bag. The procedure may be performed to permit healing of the bowel following an injury, such as a gunshot wound in the abdomen, or when a section of the bowel must be removed because of an invasive or obstructive tumor. Various kinds of c. include **transverse c.,** or **double-barreled c.,** in which both ends of the colon are brought to the margins of the skin incision, **loop c.,** in which a loop of transverse colon is brought to the abdominal surface, and **ileostomy,** in which the ileum portion of the intestine is brought to the surface rather than the colon. A c. may be temporary or permanent.

colostrum the first milk secreted by a mother immediately after termination of a pregnancy. The milk is thin, opalescent, and different in nutrients from milk secreted during the normal nursing period. The term is derived from Latin words meaning "foremilk."

-colp-; -colpo- a combining form relating to the womb or the vagina (from Greek *kolpos*, "womb").

Columbia Mental Maturity Scale a test of general ability for children aged three to 12, including the cerebral palsied. The materials consist of a colored set of cards with several drawings on each, and the child is required to point to or nod toward the item that does not belong with the others.

column a group of identical or similar neurons that extend together in a longitudinal bundle. In statistics, a c. is a vertical row of values.

columnar organization of cortex the vertical stacking of processes (that is, projections) of the neurons in the several layers of cortex gray matter.

column chromatography: See CHROMATOGRAPHY.

coma a profound state of unconsciousness characterized by little or no response to stimuli, absence of reflexes, and suspension of voluntary activity. The condition occurs primarily in cases of brain injury, intracranial tumor, encephalitis, cerebral hemorrhage or embolism, diabetes, drug or alcoholic intoxication, and catatonic schizophrenia. Also called **comatose state.**

coma somnolentium = CATAPHORA.

comatose state = COMA.

coma-vigil coma with the eyes open, occurring in patients with acute brain syndromes resulting from systemic infection, exhaustion, ingestion of drugs, or other toxic conditions. Also called **agrypnocoma.**

combat fatigue a state of physical and emotional exhaustion precipitated by the stresses and anxieties of combat. Also called **combat exhaustion; operational fatigue.** Also see COMBAT REACTIONS.

combat hysteria a functional disorder manifested by some soldiers in combat as a means of avoiding further exposure to danger. See SHELL SHOCK; COMBAT REACTIONS.

combat neurosis: See COMBAT FATIGUE.

combat reactions traumatic reactions to combat conditions in war, classified in DSM-I as "gross stress reactions," under the heading of "transient situational personality disorders," and placed in the category of "posttraumatic stress disorders" in DSM-III. See COMBAT FATIGUE.

combination (in genetics) = MIXOVARIATION.

combination law: See LAW OF COMBINATION.

combination tone a third tone produced by simultaneous sounding of two tones of similar timbre.

combined therapy psychotherapy in which the patient is engaged in both individual and group treatment with the same or different therapists. Various combinations are employed in marriage therapy particularly, such as group therapy with several couples in addition to individual therapy or conjoint therapy with each pair.

combined transcortical aphasia a form of aphasia resulting from lesions in both the anterior speech areas (**transcortical motor aphasia,** or **TMA**) and the posterior speech areas (**transcortical sensory aphasia,** or **TSA**), producing the "isolation" syndrome characterized by echolalia in the context of impaired speech and impaired comprehension. Abbrev: **CTA.** See ECHOLALIA.

comention the trait of conformity to cultural standards and obedience to authority (Cattell).

cometophobia a morbid fear of comets.

Comfortable Interpersonal Distance Scale: See INTERPERSONAL DISTANCE.

comic a word meaning laughable or amusing, but a concept that is not easy to define. Kant emphasized the element of surprise: "the sudden transformation of a strained expectation to nothing." Bergson asserted that we never laugh at things, but only at people when they behave like things or automata, as they do when they slip and fall. Freud agreed with another statement of Bergson's, that "a situation . . . is always comic when . . . it can be interpreted simultaneously in two quite different senses," as in a double entendre or a slip of the tongue. See HUMOR; WIT.

comical nonsense: See EXAGGERATION IN WIT.

command automatism mechanical obedience to any orders, no matter how inappropriate or even dangerous. It is a form of heightened suggestibility most frequently seen in catatonic schizophrenia.

command negativism = NEGATIVISM.

command style in education, a highly structured,

authoritarian instruction method dominated by the teacher and excluding student participation. Compare INDIVIDUAL PROGRAM.

commissura cinera: See INTERTHALAMIC ADHESIONS.

commissural fibers nerve fibers consisting of myelinated axons of nerve cells that connect the same or equivalent structures in the left and right hemispheres. Also called **intercerebral fibers**. See ASSOCIATION FIBERS.

commissure a body-tissue structure that forms a bridge or junction between two anatomical areas. Kinds of commissures include the **anterior c.**, which joins parts of the two cerebral hemispheres, the **middle c.**, which joins the optic thalami, and the **hippocampal c.**, which joins the posterior columns of the fornix.

commissurotomy the disruption of the components of a commissure by surgery. A c. may be performed to control intractable seizures. In laboratory animals, c. may be performed in the course of experiments involving hemispheric asymmetry.

commitment in psychiatry, confinement to a mental institution by court order, often against the individual's will, following certification by appropriate authorities. See CERTIFICATION LAWS. Also see OBSERVATIONAL C.; TEMPORARY C.; VOLUNTARY ADMISSION; CIVIL C.; CRIMINAL C.

commitment laws in psychiatry, laws governing the involuntary commitment of a patient to a mental hospital upon certification by one or more physicians. See CERTIFICATION LAWS.

common cold a viral infection of the respiratory passages resulting in persistent mucus secretion, general malaise, and sometimes a low-grade fever. Some studies have shown that susceptibility to colds is increased not only by fatigue, drafts, and contagion, but by emotional stress. Psychoanalysts, including Alexander and Saul (1940) have noted that colds and other respiratory ailments often develop while the patient is working through significant conflicts or while repressing feelings of rage. The c.c. is sometimes called **coryza** /kərī′zə/, also **upper respiratory infection (URI)**.

common-fate law: See LAW OF COMMON FATE.

common phobias: See UNIVERSAL PHOBIAS; PHOBIA.

common sense: See SENSUS COMMUNIS.

common traits according to G. W. Allport, those traits that are shared by all persons in a specific culture. While a common trait is said to exist to some extent in all culture members, it will vary in the degree to which it is manifested.

communal feeling a feeling of closeness, neighborliness, and mutual interest directed toward the community, as opposed to individualistic, competitive drives. C.f. was termed **community feeling** by Adler. Also called **communal spirit; community spirit**.

communality common factor variance, as measured by the sum of the squares of factor loadings for a particular test or item. A test with high c. is loaded on several factors. Symbol: $h^2 = a^2 + b^2 + \ldots + n^2$.

communal spirit = COMMUNAL FEELING.

commune a shared living arrangement among individuals of both sexes which has developed as an alternative to marriage and the nuclear family. In most communes the sharing includes household chores, building or improving a dwelling, working together in the fields or at odd jobs, lengthy existential discussions, sexual activities, child-rearing, alienation from prevailing cultural norms, and the sense that the members are developing a counterculture.

communicated psychosis = FOLIE À DEUX.

communication the process by which one person transmits an idea to another person by means of spoken or written words, pictures, sign language, gestures, and body language.

communication channels: See CHANNELS OF COMMUNICATION.

communication disorder an impaired ability to transmit thoughts and feelings through speech or writing at a normal rate and without distortion of content or form. Examples are tachylogia, circumstantiality, and perseveration.

communication engineering the application of scientific principles to the development of technical systems for communication, such as telephone, radio, television, and computer programing.

communication magic the naive assumption that if we tell and share everything, our problems will be solved automatically.

communication networks diagrams that represent alternative "communication paths" between individuals in an organization. Among the various possibilities are the **wheel**, associated with central control of information and greater efficiency, and the **circle**, associated with free exchange of information and higher group morale and flexibility.

communication skills abilities that make for effective communication; general language proficiency including appropriate vocabulary, syntax, and speech patterns. Additional skills are the ability to order communications logically, adjust to the listener's level, and anticipate the connotative impact of words.

communications theory the study of the interchange of signs and signals that constitutes communication; the branch of science concerned with all aspects of exchange of information, mechanical, psychological, social, and physiological.

communications unit a combination of (a) sender or encoder, (b) channel, and (c) receiver or decoder, e.g., a hearing aid.

communicology an area covering the theory and practice of audiology, speech pathology, and improvement in communication by such methods as exchange of ideas, relating experiences, and giving voice to feelings.

communion in psychoanalytic theory, the unconscious feeling of magical or mystical union with objects or people through the process of incorporation. This feeling is believed to apply to the sharing of ideas and emotions with others, as well as to sharing food and drink, the primitive ritual of mixing bloods as an expression of friendship, and the religious rite of the Eucharist. Also called **magical c.** Also see MYSTIC UNION.

communion principle a principle of the organismic approach, which holds that the first requisite of individual and group therapy is a sense of unity and mutuality between patient and therapist, on which is based the feeling that they are engaged in a common enterprise which will bring about a higher degree of self-realization for the patient.

communiscope a tachistoscopic device that gives the subject a brief glimpse of printed material, such as an advertisement. The subject is then questioned about what he saw in the material. A c. may be used as an aided-recall technique in readership studies of advertising effectiveness.

communities for the retarded facilities that consist of clusters of houses in which retarded adults who are able to live and work with some degree of independence can function in a dignified setting. With the help of staff members, the retarded adults manage each of the houses independently, planning meals and purchasing and preparing food, participating in household-maintenance chores, and enjoying leisure activities with their peers.

community according to I. T. Sanders (1966), "a territorially organized system coextensive with a settlement pattern in which (1) an effective communication network operates; (2) people share common facilities and services . . ., and (3) people develop a psychological identification with a 'locality symbol' (the name)." R. L. Warren (1972) defines a c. as a "combination of social units and systems which perform the major social functions having locality relevance," that is, production-distribution-consumption, socialization, social control, social participation, and mutual support.

community-action group a dynamic group of citizens specifically organized to attack social problems within the community, e.g., slum conditions, inadequate delivery of health services, gun control, crime in the streets, and establishment of residences for the retarded.

community care in psychiatry and rehabilitation, community-based care of the mentally or physically disabled through such services and facilities as halfway houses, adult homes, sheltered workshops, supervised residences for the multihandicapped and retarded, schools for the developmentally disabled, home treatment, cooperative apartments, and satellite clinics.

community-centered approach a concerted, coordinated attack on such problems as mental disorder, delinquency, and alcoholism on the part of agencies and facilities in the local community or catchment area. The c.-c. a. holds that since these problems developed in the community, efforts at prevention and treatment should be community-based rather than the province primarily of state institutions or federal agencies. See COMMUNITY MENTAL-HEALTH CENTER; COMMUNITY PSYCHIATRY; COMMUNITY PSYCHOLOGY; COMMUNITY SERVICES; COMMUNITY PROGRAM.

community competence: See COMPETENCE.

community feeling: See COMMUNAL FEELING.

community intervention organized efforts by mental-health professionals, paraprofessionals, indigenous nonprofessionals, and others with special competence, to deal actively and constructively with community problems such as drug abuse, alcoholism, homelessness, child abuse, air and water pollution, juvenile delinquency, inadequate housing, or a high suicide rate. Intervention is probably most effective where the residents are themselves involved in coping with such problems through neighborhood councils, block committees, and service groups; social and fraternal organizations; and community educational and self-help programs.

community mental health as described by Bernard L. Bloom (*Community Mental Health; a General Introduction*, 1977), "all activities undertaken in the community in the name of mental health . . . as opposed to practice in institutional settings." The community approach focuses primarily on the total population of a single catchment area rather than on individual patients; emphasizes preventive services as distinguished from therapeutic services; seeks to provide a continuous, comprehensive system of services designed to meet all mental-health-related needs in the community; approaches mental health indirectly through consultation and education; emphasizes innovative strategies such as brief psychotherapy and crisis intervention; involves overall planning and demographic analyses; utilizes new types of workers, such as paraprofessionals and indigenous mental-health workers; and seeks to identify sources of stress within the community.

community mental-health center a community-based facility or group of facilities providing a full range of prevention, treatment, and rehabilitation services, organized as a practical alternative to the largely custodial care given in mental hospitals that are located far from the patient's home and community. Typical services are .full diagnostic evaluation; out-patient individual and group psychotherapy; emergency in-patient treatment; day, night, and weekend hospital treatment; specialized clinics for alcoholics and disturbed children and families; aftercare (foster homes, halfway houses, home visiting); rehabilitation programs (vocational, educational, social) for current and former patients; consultation to physicians, clergymen, courts, schools, health departments, welfare agencies; training for all types of mental-health personnel. Also called **comprehensive mental-health center**.

community mental-health program an integrated program designed to meet the overall
psychiatric needs of a particular community, including in-patient, out-patient, and emergency
treatment; special facilities for alcoholics, drug
addicts, and children; educational, rehabilitation, research, and training programs. See COM-
MUNITY MENTAL-HEALTH CENTER; COMMUNITY
PROGRAM; COMMUNITY SERVICES; COMMUNITY-
CENTERED APPROACH.

community needs assessment: See NEEDS ASSESS-
MENT.

community-of-content theory the principle that
complex situations have stimuli common to
other situations, resulting in consistent responses to different situations.

Community Outreach Program a service founded by the Mental Retardation Institute of New
York Medical College to provide health care to
retarded individuals and their families. The
C.O.P. sends interdisciplinary health-professional teams to day-care centers, Head Start
facilities, clinics, and public schools where the
retarded can be given physical examinations, developmental evaluation and laboratory tests,
and specialist consultations. Abbrev.: **COP.**

community program in community psychiatry, an
organized, planned approach to a specific problem such as public education or mental illness,
aftercare and rehabilitation of ex-mental patients, early case finding, reeducation of mental
patients, epidemiological studies, and counseling programs on such problems as alcohol, child
abuse, and drug abuse. Also see COMMUNITY-
CENTERED APPROACH.

community psychiatry the branch of psychiatry
defined by Hume (1966) as "the maximum utilization of community resources in the identification, treatment, or rehabilitation of the mentally
ill or retarded..." It is "simultaneously treatment-oriented, prevention-oriented, and com-
munity-oriented." Its major objectives are the
development of comprehensive clinical services
within the community; coordination of all nonpsychiatric organizations that have a bearing on
mental health, such as schools, courts, family
agencies, labor unions, industry, churches, and
hospitals; promotion of epidemiological research on mental disorders; and development of
a corps of psychiatrists to serve as mental-health
consultants and specialists for community mental-health services. See COMMUNITY SERVICES;
COMMUNITY-CENTERED APPROACH; SOCIAL PSY-
CHIATRY.

community psychology the application of psychological methods (in collaboration with psychiatry, sociology, and social work) to problems
of mental health, education, group relationships,
delinquency, crime, alcoholism, family planning, and social welfare arising in a community
setting and soluble only through a community-
wide approach. See COMMUNITY-CENTERED
APPROACH; COMMUNITY SERVICES.

community services in community psychiatry and

psychology, the complex of community-based
services and facilities designed to maintain
health and welfare, including mental-health clinics, methadone and alcohol centers; public-
health and adoption services; family services;
vocational-training facilities; rehabilitation centers; psychiatric emergency services; and living
facilities such as halfway houses, home care, and
foster-family care. Also see COMMUNITY-
CENTERED APPROACH.

community social worker a person who functions
in an advocacy role to maintain liaison between
government officials and the public on matters
affecting the physical and psychological health
of the community. E.g., the c.s.w. may try to
raise the social consciousness of the community
regarding recreational facilities, adequate housing, local employment problems, and environmental obstacles to the mobility of handicapped
citizens.

community speech-and-hearing centers local
facilities that provide speech and hearing evaluation and rehabilitation for children and adults.
The c.s.-a.-h.c. also assist in the treatment of
learning problems associated with speech and
hearing deficiencies. Because the United States
alone has 8,000,000 persons with speech and
hearing deficiencies, community centers are
needed to handle cases that may not require hospital or institutional care.

community spirit = COMMUNAL FEELING.

companion-therapist a nonprofessional who is
trained to work in an area of community mental
health, usually in collaboration with or under
the supervision of a professional worker. This
term may be specifically applied to a nonprofessional who works with a disturbed child or
adult in a one-to-one long-term relationship
characterized by friendly, informal camaraderie.

comparable groups two or more representative
samples drawn from the same population for the
purpose of observation or experiment.

comparative judgment a judgment by a subject of
how two or more stimuli are similar or different.

comparative psychiatry = CROSS-CULTURAL
PSYCHIATRY.

comparative psychology the study of animal behavior, conducted in the natural habitat and in
the laboratory, with the double objective of
understanding lower organisms in their own
right, and of furthering the understanding of human behavior. See YERKES.

compartmentalization the defense mechanism in
which particular types of thoughts and feelings
that seem to conflict or to be incompatible are
isolated from each other in what has been called
impermeable psychic compartments. C. involves
fragmentation where ideally there might exist
toleration of ambiguity and ambivalence. Isolation is a closely related term.

Compass Diagnostic Test of Arithmetic: See DI-
AGNOSTIC EDUCATIONAL TESTS.

compassion a strong feeling of sympathy with
another person's feelings, or a strong feeling of

sympathy with the human condition and humanity in it's joyful-sorrowful and comic-tragic aspects. C. presupposes understanding and acceptance of one's own emotions to the extent that one can draw upon one's emotional experience to enter into the meaning of another's feelings, whether joyful or sorrowful.

compelled behavior a behavior that generally is expected of an individual living in any of a large variety of cultures. Kinds of c.b. may include concealing parts of the body, expressing grief, being fertile, avoiding bad luck, being industrious, obeying others, respecting others, naming others, and self-cleansing or self-purifying. Compare PROHIBITED BEHAVIOR.

compensating error an error that cancels another error.

compensation the development of strength in one area to offset real or imagined deficiency in another. C. is a conscious or often unconscious defense mechanism. Examples include not only the boasting of a braggart, the pomposity of a petty bureaucrat, but the more constructive efforts of the timid boy who becomes a chess expert or the quadriplegic who develops a successful mail-order business. Also called **compensatory mechanism**. See ADLER; OVERCOMPENSATION.

compensation neurosis a psychoneurotic reaction associated with a real or presumed disability involving the question of financial compensation. There is disagreement on the nature of the neurosis (traumatic, anxiety, conversion, or hypochondriacal) and on the underlying factors involved (self-deception, malingering, financial benefits, unconscious exaggeration). In many cases there appears to be a mixture of motives and a mingling of different levels of consciousness. Interestingly, a c.n. is more likely to develop after slight than after obvious and detectable injuries, and tends to clear up with startling rapidity when compensation is won. Also called **accident neurosis; indemnity neurosis**.

compensatory education educational programs that are specially designed to enhance the intellectual and social skills of disadvantaged children, e.g., Head Start, a program initiated in the United States in 1965.

compensatory mechanism = COMPENSATION.

compensatory nystagmus = BEKHTEREV'S NYSTAGMUS.

compensatory scoliosis: See SCOLIOSIS.

compensatory trait a trait that serves to compensate for another trait possessed in low degree.

competence the ability to exert control over one's life, to cope with specific problems effectively, and to modify oneself and one's environment, as contrasted with the mere ability to adjust or adapt to circumstances as they are. Similarly, **community c.** consists of the utilization and development of resources, including human beings, that help the community cope with its problems. In the legal sense, c. is the capacity to comprehend the nature of a transaction and to assume legal responsibility for one's actions.

competence knowledge in social psychology, self-esteem and self-worth based on appraisals of one's competence made by others. C.k. is the component of self-image that derives from an individual's unique gifts and accomplishments in contrast to legitimacy knowledge which derives from acceptable and worthwhile group identifications.

competence motivation the drive to develop personal skill and capability in one or more fields.

competency-based instruction a teaching method in which students work at their own pace toward individual goals in a noncompetitive setting. The teacher works with students in identifying appropriate goals and monitoring progress.

competency to stand trial capacity to be tried in court, as determined by ability to understand the nature of the charge and the potential consequences of conviction, as well as ability to assist the attorney in one's defense. See DURHAM RULE; M'NAGHTEN RULES. Also see INCOMPETENCY PLEA.

competition intense rivalry between individuals or groups struggling toward the same goal, such as victory on the playing field, advancement in business, or the attainment of academic honors. Psychologically speaking, c. may be healthy or unhealthy, benign or bitter, controlled or uncontrolled, a stimulus for achievement or an expression of hostility. In any case it is important and realistic to develop a degree of **c. tolerance** in a society that is highly competitive.

competitive motive a type of motivation that influences an individual to advance himself while exceeding or frustrating the progress of others. Compare COOPERATIVE MOTIVE; INDIVIDUALISTIC MOTIVE.

competitive reward structure in group situations, a condition that restricts the number of members who can achieve the highest reward such that the success of one member reduces the success of others, e.g., an examination graded on a curve. In many cases, the c.r.s. is found to reduce group trust, communication, and possibly achievement. Compare COOPERATIVE REWARD STRUCTURE; INDIVIDUALISTIC REWARD STRUCTURE.

complementarity in any dyadic relationship, the existence of different personal qualities in each of the partners that contribute a sense of completeness to the other person and provide balance in the relationship.

complementarity of interaction the concept that each individual in a dynamic situation plays both a provocation role and a responsive role. It places emphasis on interaction as opposed to reaction.

complementary instinct the tendency of infantile sexual instincts with an active aim to be integrated with antithetical instincts with a passive aim. E.g., the childhood wish to beat and to be beaten may be complementary infantile sexual instincts.

complementary role a social-behavior pattern

that conforms to the expectations and demands of other people. See ROLE. Compare NONCOMPLEMENTARY ROLE.

complete-learning method the presentation of material repeatedly until it is learned error-free.

complete mother the ideal mother sought by the schizophrenic in fantasy and real life—a mother who loves the child for himself alone and not as a means of gratifying her own needs (Federn).

complete Oedipus the presence in an individual of both the positive and negative Oedipus complexes at the same time, e.g., mother-love with father-identification and father-love with mother-identification.

complete spinal transection: See SPINAL TRANSECTION.

completion, arithmetic, vocabulary, direction-following = CAVD.

completion test the type of test in which the subject must supply a missing phrase, word, or letter in a written text. On a nonverbal test, a missing number, symbol, or representation must be supplied.

complex a group or system of related ideas or impulses that have a common emotional tone and exert a strong but usually unconscious influence on our attitudes and behavior. The term was introduced in psychiatry by Jung. Primary examples are Jung's POWER C., Freud's CASTRATION C. and OEDIPUS C., and Adler's INFERIORITY C. See these entries. Also see CAIN C.; CLYTEMNESTRA C.; DEMOSTHENES C.; DIANA C.; ELECTRA C.; GRISELDA C.; JOCASTA C.; MEDEA C.; ORESTES C.; PHAEDRA C.; POLYCRATES C.; QUASIMODO C.; ACTIVE CASTRATION C.; APPRENTICE C.; AUTHORITY C.; BREAST C.; CLAUSTRAL C.; CLÉRAMBAULT-KANDINSKI C.; EGO C.; FEMININITY C.; GRANDFATHER C.; INVERTED OEDIPUS C.; MOTHER C.; NUCLEAR C.; OBSCENITY-PURITY C.; PARTICULAR C.; REPRESSED C.; SMALL-PENIS C.; URETHRAL C.; COMPLETE OEDIPUS; CULTURE C.; GOD C.

complexity-curvilinearity factor an art-judgment factor that combines simple-complex and curved-angular factors. The term is applied to descriptions of paintings that receive high positive ratings for simple-complex, emotions, and surface judgments and high negative ratings for curved-angular, disorderly, orderly, and line judgments from subjects asked to evaluate the artistic work.

complexity factor in psychological esthetics, a property of a work of art that has light and complexity as principal components of its stylistic ratings. The c.f. may represent an information overload in a painting, such as the *Guernica* by Picasso, and a reflection of the artist's feelings of tension. By contrast, a simple work of art may convey a feeling of tranquillity.

complex of ideas a system of ideas closely associated with emotions and other psychic factors so that when one of the ideas is recalled, the associated experience is recalled with it.

complex tone the sound one hears in a musical tone that is a mixture of the fundamental tone plus halves, thirds, quarters, fifths, or other frequency overtones.

complex type: See AGGRESSIVE TYPES.

compliance in general, submission to the wishes or suggestions of others. In psychiatry, c. is a compulsion to yield to the desires and demands of other people; neurotic oversubmissiveness. C. is a defensive reaction frequently observed in obsessive-compulsive neurosis. Also see SOCIAL C.

compliant character an overly self-effacing person with a strong tendency to move toward people (Horney).

complication the effect of simultaneous stimuli from different senses, e.g., the taste and smell of an apple. The term also applies to a second disease that develops during the course of another disease.

complication experiment the attempted perception of two or more events simultaneously, resulting in one being perceived in the focus of attention and the other in the margin. See LAW OF PRIOR ENTRY.

component impulse an impulse derived from a component instinct, e.g., sucking, biting, touching, or other libidinal-drive factors that become subservient to the adult genital organization.

component instinct in psychoanalysis, an instinct associated with an organ or zone (e.g., mouth or anus), which gave pleasure during the pregenital period and continues to be a source of gratification, or forepleasure, when these organs become subordinated to the genital zone. An individual may, however, become fixated on one of the component instincts and develop neurotic symptoms such as exhibitionism or sadism. Also called **part-instinct; partial instinct.** See SEXUALITY.

components-of-variance model = RANDOM MODEL.

composite person an image or dream figure that has been created from the images of two or more persons. The c.p. usually cannot be identified by the dreamer but psychoanalytic interpretation may reveal the identities of the individuals forming the composite that has been formed by the process of condensation in dream-making. Also called **composite figure.**

composite score an average score derived from several other scores, including weighted scores.

composition of movement the sequence and pattern of neuromuscular activity, as in walking, including the integration of signals in the premotor and cerebellar areas of the brain.

compos mentis a forensic term meaning mentally competent; neither mentally deficient nor legally insane. See COMPETENCE. Compare NON C.M.

compound eye the type of eye found in certain lower forms of animals, such as insects, that is composed of a number of separate visual units.

compound fracture: See FRACTURE.

compound reaction a reaction-time test in which

the subject must make a decision before responding, e.g., reacting to nouns but not verbs. Also called **disjunctive reaction**.

comprehension test a test requiring the subject to state how he would deal with a given practical situation; also, a reading-ability test in which understanding is assessed by asking questions about the passages read.

comprehensive mental-health center = COMMUNITY MENTAL-HEALTH CENTER.

comprehensive solution a Horney term for the resolution of a conflict by identifying the real with the idealized self.

compression pressure on the brain, spinal cord or nerve fibers (exerted by a tumor), head injury, fracture, blood clot, or other pathological entity, producing such symptoms as pain, motor disorders, and disturbances of sensation, memory, or consciousness.

The term c. also refers to the use of one symbol to convey more than one meaning or represent more than one thing at the same time; e.g., a national flag compresses many feelings and attitudes into one symbol. In this sense, c. can be equivalent to CONDENSATION. See this entry.

compromise distortion a Freudian term used to describe the distortion of a repressed idea into a delusion or hallucination that results from a compromise between ego resistance and the strength of the idea repressed. Also see COMPROMISE FORMATION.

compromise formation in psychoanalysis, the release of a repressed impulse or conflict in disguised or modified form as a means of avoiding censorship. An action of this kind is therefore a compromise between expression and repression, that is, a way of gaining expression without giving up one's ego defenses. Also see COMPROMISE DISTORTION.

compromiser a group member who, having previously advocated a specific policy, accedes to the opposing or majority viewpoint to facilitate group progress.

compulsion a persistent, uncontrollable impulse to perform a stereotyped, irrational act, such as washing the hands 50 times a day. The act serves an unconscious purpose, such as a means of warding off anxiety, avoiding unacceptable impulses, or relieving a sense of guilt. Also see OBSESSIVE-COMPULSIVE DISORDER; COUNTERCOMPULSION.

compulsion neurosis = COMPULSIVE NEUROSIS.

compulsive behavior inappropriate, irrational actions, such as counting, repeatedly performed as a result of an irresistible impulse.

compulsive ceremonial a term applied to the retualistic behavior of the obsessive-compulsive patient. See RITUALS.

compulsive changing a compulsion-neurotic symptom in which the patient continuously changes various aspects of his world, e.g., job, dress, or personal habits, in an effort to make the world conform to his own life-style.

compulsive character a personality pattern char-

acterized by rigid, perfectionistic standards, an exaggerated sense of duty, and meticulous, obsessive attention to order and detail. Individuals of this type are usually humorless, parsimonious, stubborn, inhibited, rigid, and unable to relax. Also called **compulsive personality**. Also see ANANCASTIC PERSONALITY.

compulsive coercion = COMPULSIVE RESTRAINT.

compulsive disorders disorders in which the individual feels forced to perform acts that are against his own conscious wishes or better judgment, e.g., compulsive gambling, drinking, or drug-taking. See ALCOHOL ABUSE; PATHOLOGICAL GAMBLING; SUBSTANCE ABUSE; OBSESSIVE-COMPULSIVE DISORDER.

compulsive drinker an alcoholic, or alcohol addict; an individual in the grip of an uncontrollable drive to drink excessively ("One drink is too many, a thousand are not enough").

compulsive eating an irresistible drive to overeat, in some cases as a reaction to frustration or disappointment, a substitute for denied satisfactions, or an unconscious attempt to recapture the love and acceptance experienced in infancy when the mother provided food and love at the same time. See BULIMIA.

compulsive gambling: See PATHOLOGICAL GAMBLING.

compulsive laughter a common symptom of the hebephrenic (disorganized) type of schizophrenia in the form of compulsive, inappropriate laughter. The c.l. in some cases appears to be automatic in that even the patient seems to be unaware of the activity.

compulsive magic an uncontrollable urge to perform a ritual act or utter a prayer or incantation as a means of warding off anxiety or attempting to control events such as the roll of dice or the alleviation of illness.

compulsive masturbation habitual, obsessive masturbation performed without pleasure or adequate sexual feeling. It may serve such unrecognized purposes as an attempt to relieve tension or depression, to avoid "perverse" sexual impulses, or to substitute for social satisfactions when the individual is too shy or inhibited to establish interpersonal relationships.

compulsive neurosis a mental disorder marked by an uncontrollable impulse to perform stereotyped, irrational acts. Also called **compulsion neurosis**. See OBSESSIVE-COMPULSIVE DISORDER.

compulsive orderliness overconcern with everyday arrangements, such as a "clean desk" or dust-free house, with unbearable anxiety if there is any variation.

compulsive personality = COMPULSIVE CHARACTER.

compulsive-personality disorder a personality disorder involving a long-standing disruptive pattern manifested in such behavior as difficulty in expressing warm emotions, stilted attitudes, stinginess, perfectionism and preoccupation with details and schedules, emphasis on work to the exclusion of pleasure, and avoidance or postponement of decisions for fear of making a mistake. (DSM-III)

compulsive repetition the irresistible need to perform needless acts such as checking and rechecking a door to see whether it has been locked.

compulsive restraint the uncontrollable need to hold oneself or others in check by demanding complete devotion to routine or detail. Also called **compulsive coercion** (especially when applied to controlling others).

compulsive sexual activity an insatiable, irresistible drive for sexual activity, sometimes without full gratification. See EROTOMANIA; NYMPHOMANIA; SATYRIASIS; COMPULSIVE MASTURBATION.

compulsive stealing: See KLEPTOMANIA.

computer anxiety: See COMPUTER ILLITERACY.

computer-assisted instruction a sophisticated offshoot of programed learning, in which the memory-storage and retrieval capabilities of the computer are utilized to provide drill and practice, problem-solving, simulation, and gaming forms of instruction, as well as relatively individualized tutorial instruction. Abbrev.: **CAI.** Also called **computer-assisted learning (CAL).** Also see COMPUTER-MANAGED INSTRUCTION.

computer illiteracy the condition of being culturally handicapped by not knowing how to use a computer as an aid in thought processes or, at least, in gaining access to information. The concept assumes that in the near future no one who has no skill with this tool can be considered truly literate, regardless of his knowledge and intelligence, and regardless of his field of endeavor. (He must overcome "kilobytophobia," or "computer anxiety.") C.i. is related to the broader concept of **technological illiteracy**, which refers to an inability to function in an increasingly technical society.

computerized axial tomography a radiographic technique for producing detailed cross sections of the brain or other organs very quickly by feeding X-ray images into a computer rather than projecting them onto a piece of film. An electronic device called a **scintillator** receives the X-ray images in terms of tissue density so that bone is white and air and water are black on the computer pictures; organs and tissues are gray. Because c.a.t. produces may slice-by-slice pictures of the head, chest, or abdomen, it is possible to locate defects such as lesions or tumors without exploratory surgery. The system sometimes is called **transaxial** because it produces images, which can be projected on a television screen or printed as photographs, across the long axis of the body. C.a.t. is currently the most accurate method for determining organ pathology and represents a great milestone in medical diagnosis. Abbrev.: **CAT** /kat/; **CAT scan.**

computerized diagnosis the use of electronic computers for cataloging, storing, comparing, and evaluating medical or psychiatric data as an aid in the diagnosis. In view of the many possible variables involved in a particular type of dis-

order, c.d. utilizes information based on thousands of similar or related sets of signs and symptoms of previous patients, along with information on diagnoses and effective treatments, stored in data banks or data bases. See PROBLEM-ORIENTED RECORD; DATA BASE.

computerized therapy the use of a specially programed computer as a therapist or trainer, as in giving audiotape instructions for systematic desensitization, for administering positive or negative reinforcement, or for developing language function in nonspeaking children, and in applying nondirective therapy by having the client converse with a computer.

computer-managed instruction a method of instruction in which the learner does not interact directly with the computer; rather, the computer is used to assist the teacher in carrying out a plan of individualized instruction by processing the mass of daily data regarding the performance of each student, and by utilizing these data in prescribing the next instructional step for each student.

computer model a computer program that is designed to simulate psychological functioning. A c.m. may be designed, e.g., to enable a computer to simulate the decision-making processes of a human playing a game of chess.

computer thought: See ARTIFICIAL INTELLIGENCE.

Comrey Personality Scales a recently developed multitrait personality inventory constructed primarily through factor analysis, and yielding scores in eight personality scales: trust versus defensiveness, orderliness versus lack of compulsion, social conformity versus rebelliousness, activity versus lack of energy, emotional stability versus neuroticism, extraversion versus introversion, masculinity versus femininity, and empathy versus egocentrism.

Comte, August /kôNt/ French philosopher, founder of positivism, 1798–1857. See ALTRUISM.

conarium in Descartes' theory, the point of contact between mind (**res cogitans**) and body (**res extensa**) in the centrally located pineal body. According to some authorities, Freud's id represents the same concept. Also see CARTESIAN DUALISM.

conation mental processes concerned with striving and purposive action. C. comprises drives, desires, instincts, and motives of all kinds. Adjective: **conative** /kon′ətiv/.

concealed antisocial activity a form of antisocial behavior that is derived from socially acceptable drives, e.g., cheating on income-tax returns.

conceived values a set of ideal values as conceived by an individual.

concentration a term applied to any act of bringing together at a central point several or more components of a process or thing. Examples include the focusing of thinking processes on a central problem or subject, and the act of increasing the bulk of a dissolved substance by reducing the proportion of the solvent.

concentration-camp syndrome persistent stress symptoms in concentration-camp victims consisting of severe anxiety, defenses against anxiety, an obsessive ruminative state, psychosomatic reactions, depression, and "survival guilt" produced by remaining alive while so many others died. One of the self-protective responses experienced by young survivors has been a lack of affective response—which Minkowski termed "emotional anesthesia"—toward those who died, including close relatives. See SURVIVAL GUILT; SURVIVOR SYNDROME.

concentration difficulty: See MENTAL ASTHENIA.

concept an idea that is not the direct result of sensory inputs but is produced by the manipulation of various sensory impressions; also, a general idea.

concept-attainment model a term sometimes applied to Jerome Bruner's orientation to teaching characterized by an emphasis on the development of concepts through inductive reasoning.

concept formation the development of concepts, that is, ideas based on the common properties of a group of objects, events, or qualities. Some concepts, such as truth or causality, are more abstract; some, such as apple or table, are more concrete; but all tend to be formed by the two processes of abstraction and generalization. Educational psychologists have also identified four other processes involved in forming concepts: discrimination, context clues, definition, and classification.

concept-formation tests tests used in studying the process of concept formation and in assessing the level of concept formation achieved by a specific subject. See WEIGL-GOLDSTEIN-SCHEERER TEST; VIGOTSKY TEST; HANFMANN-KASANIN CONCEPT FORMATION TEST.

conception a union of the spermatozoon and the ovum (fertilization), which marks the beginning of life; also, the process of forming a concept (conceptualization), as well as a general concept or group of ideas, such as democracy.

concept learning = CONCEPTUAL LEARNING.

Concept Mastery Test a test that provides sufficient ceiling for the examination of highly gifted adults. It consists of analogies and synonym-antonym items, drawing on many fields: mathematics, history, geography, physical and biological sciences, literature, music, and others.

conceptual disorder a disturbance in the thinking process or in the ability to formulate abstract ideas from generalized concepts.

conceptual disorganization one of the major marks of psychotic thought processes, consisting of irrelevant, rambling, or incoherent verbalizations, frequently including neologisms and stereotyped expressions.

conceptual disturbances impaired thought processes comprising such symptoms as difficulty in forming associations, discriminating differences, summoning of images, using words as symbols

for meaning, and thinking abstractly. The condition is due to inability to perceive similarities and to generalize from specific instances, and is characteristic of patients with brain damage and schizophrenia.

conceptualization the process of using thought processes and verbalization in forming concepts, particularly of an abstract nature, such as hypotheses, theories, and ideologies.

conceptual learning the acquisition of new concepts or modification of existing concepts. Also called **concept learning**.

conceptually guided control a stage of human information-processing that is controlled by higher-level constructs. C.g.c. functions primarily to direct thinking processes toward certain goals.

conceptual model a concept presented in the form of a diagram or other illustration.

conceptual nervous system a hypothetical model of the neurological and physiological functions of the nervous system that can be manipulated to provide analogies of behavioral activities. It is intended primarily for the development of concepts and theories rather than as a standard representation of the human nervous system.

conceptual replication: See REPLICATION.

conceptual system a term sometimes used to denote the organization of a person's cognitive achievement, emotional awareness, experience, and philosophical or religious orientation.

conceptual tempo the pace that is typical of a person's approach to cognitive tasks, e.g., a hasty versus deliberate approach to observing, thinking, and responding. C.t. is an aspect of COGNITIVE STYLE. See this entry.

concinnity the quality of an artistic design that features a harmonious arrangement of the various parts to each other and to the whole design.

concomitant variation the concept that when two phenomena vary together they are causally related; also, a correlation between variables.

concordance a term used in studies of twins to denote the degree to which both members of a pair of twins have the same trait or disorder. See TWIN STUDIES.

concordance coefficient: See COEFFICIENT OF CONCORDANCE.

concordance rate the percentage of twin pairs or other blood relatives that exhibit the same trait or disorder. Also called **concordance ratio**. See TWIN STUDIES.

concrete attitude a way of thinking that is directed to a specific object or immediate situation. A person who exhibits the c.a. tends not to make abstract comparisons and will not usually respond to abstract qualities, concepts, or categories. Compare ABSTRACT ATTITUDE.

concrete image a memory image that is recalled in terms of sense qualities such as the taste of a particular kind of cheese or the sound of a ship's bell.

concrete intelligence the ability to handle concrete, practical relationships and situations. Compare ABSTRACT INTELLIGENCE.

concreteness the quality of being concrete, that is, specific and particular, as opposed to general and abstract.

concrete operational stage Piaget's third stage of cognitive development (from seven to 11 years) during which the child becomes capable of logical thinking and developing conservation concepts.

concrete operations a term applied by Piaget to the mental representations of time, space, and quantity with which the growing child begins to deal with the physical elements of everyday life, such as pieces of clay or glasses of milk, as contrasted with more abstract entities such as words or mathematical symbols.

concrete picture a term used to identify primitive thinking and to distinguish it from abstract thoughts. It is assumed that primitive humans thought in concrete pictures rather than abstract ideas.

concrete thinking thought processes focused on immediate experiences and specific objects or events, as contrasted with thinking that involves abstractions, generalizations, and totalities. C.t. is characteristic of young children, schizophrenics, and brain-injured individuals, especially those with frontal-lobe damage. Also called **concretistic thinking**.

concretism in Jung's analytic psychology, a form of thought and feeling that represents concrete concepts and views that are related to sensation, as opposed to abstraction.

concretistic thinking = CONCRETE THINKING.

concretization the process of being specific, or giving an example of a concept or relationship. E.g., to the question "What is democracy?" one may answer "It's America." In psychiatry, c. is an associative disturbance in which there is an overemphasis on detail and immediate experience, that is, seeing the trees rather than the forest.

concretizing attitude a symptom of schizophrenia manifested by conversion of an abstract idea into a concrete representation, as in transforming the belief that one's wife is unfaithful into the delusion that she is secretly married to another man.

concurrent medical audit: See MEDICAL AUDIT.

concurrent reinforcement in operant conditioning, two or more separate reinforcement schedules running simultaneously.

concurrent review an analysis of admissions, or utilization review, carried out while care is being provided, and comprising certification of the necessity for admission (admission certification) and assessment of the need for care to be continued (continued-stay review).

concurrent therapy the simultaneous treatment of spouses or other family members in marriage and family therapy, either by the same or different therapists.

concurrent validity the extent of correspondence between two variables at about the same time; specifically, the measure of one test's validity by comparison of its results with a separate but related test, such as a standardized test. Also see CONTENT VALIDITY; CRITERION VALIDITY.

concussion: See HEAD TRAUMA.

condensation the fusion of several meanings into one image, word, or event. C. is particularly common in dreams, where one person may exhibit characteristics of several, and in schizophrenic neologisms, such as "gruesor," which is apparently a combination of "gruesome" and "sorrowful" (Bleuler). Also see COMPRESSION.

Condillac, Étienne Bonnet de /kôNdēyäk'/ French philosopher, 1715–80. C. was a leading advocate of sensationalism. See STATUE OF CONDILLAC.

condition the antecedent circumstance on which an event is dependent.

conditionability the capability of a person to acquire and maintain conditioned responses. The studies by H. J. Eysenck indicate that introverts acquire conditioned responses more easily and retain them longer than extroverts.

conditionalism the viewpoint that one can predict an effect by knowing the cause and that an effect can be explained in terms of its cause.

conditional positive regard a term applied by C. Rogers to an attitude of acceptance and esteem which is expressed by others on a conditional basis, that is, depending on the acceptability of the individual's behavior. Rogers assumes that the need for positive regard, whether conditional or unconditional, is universal. Every person needs it not only from others but from his own self.

conditional probability the probability of one event's taking place, given the occurrence of another event.

conditioned avoidance response a conditioned response that anticipates and averts the occurrence of a harmful or unpleasant stimulus. In the c.a.r. the organism successfully avoids exposure to the painful stimulus, whereas in the conditioned escape response the organism is already exposed but maneuvers away from the stimulus or finds a way to stop it.

conditioned emotion a feeling or affective state acquired as a result of conditioning, that is, an emotional response (e.g., fear) elicited by a previously ineffective stimulus (a buzzer) that has come to be effective by virtue of its association with an unconditioned stimulus.

conditioned escape response a conditioned response by means of which an organism ends its exposure to a harmful or unpleasant stimulus, either by flight or by managing to stop the stimulus. Also see CONDITIONED AVOIDANCE RESPONSE.

conditioned inhibition the suppression of a conditioned response by pairing it with a nonreinforced, indifferent stimulus.

conditioned reflex = CONDITIONED RESPONSE.

conditioned-reflex therapy a form of behavior therapy developed by A. Salter, based on the idea that the core of life is excitation, and the core of neurosis is overinhibition. According to this approach, emotional health consists in behaving spontaneously, and therefore clients are encouraged to act on the basis of feeling rather than thinking and planning, to say what they feel ("feeling-talk"), and show emotions on their face ("facial talk"), since emotional release is the first step toward emotional health.

conditioned reinforcers stimuli that require the capacity to reinforce by being paired with primary reinforcers; e.g., food may be paired with a token, which then becomes the conditioned reinforcer. See REINFORCEMENT; SECONDARY REINFORCEMENT.

conditioned response in classical conditioning, the learned or acquired response to a conditioned stimulus, that is, to a stimulus that did not elicit the response originally. Abbrev.: **CR**. Also called **conditioned reflex**.

conditioned stimulus a previously neutral stimulus repeatedly associated with an unconditioned stimulus to the extent that it comes to acquire the power of the unconditioned stimulus to elicit the same response or some aspect of that response. E.g., in Pavlov's experiment, the tone associated with the food is the c.s. Abbrev.: **CS**. Also see UNCONDITIONED STIMULUS.

conditioned suppression a combination of painful and neutral stimuli that decreases the strength of the neutral stimulus acting alone.

conditioning the process by which a conditioned response is learned, that is, a response to a stimulus that did not originally evoke it. For details, see PAVLOVIAN C.; INSTRUMENTAL C.; OPERANT C.

conditioning therapy a descriptive term sometimes applied to behavior therapy.

conditions not attributable to a mental disorder a group of conditions that become the focus of psychiatric attention or treatment even though they are not due to a mental disorder (but a mental disorder may also exist). The term is a DSM-III category that includes malingering, borderline intellectual functioning, adult antisocial behavior, childhood or adolescent antisocial behavior, academic problem, occupational problem, uncomplicated bereavement, noncompliance with medical treatment, phase-of-life problem, marital problem, parent-child problem, other specified family circumstances, and other interpersonal problems. (DSM-III)

conditions of worth as used by C. Rogers, the specific conditions under which a child feels worthy of love, or the state in which a child experiences love as conditional. According to C. Rogers, the establishment of c.o.w. leads the child to believe that his self-worth is contingent upon behaving in accord with another's wishes. See CONDITIONAL POSITIVE REGARD.

condom a sheath, usually made of rubber, that fits over the penis during intercourse, serving both as a contraceptive device and a means of preventing the spread of venereal disease. The term is of unknown origin; it is popularly associated with a fictitious 18th-century doctor named Condom or Conton as the inventor of the device. Sexual intercourse with use of a c. is sometimes called coitus condomatus. A c. is also called **prophylactic** or **rubber**.

conduct the behavior of the total individual as expressed in psychological as well as physical activity; also, behavior that conforms to (or violates) the standards established by the person's social group.

conduct disorder, socialized, aggressive a conduct disorder marked by repetitive, persistent aggressive conduct in which the basic rights of others are violated, as manifested in physical violence against persons or property (vandalism, rape, breaking and entering, fire-setting, mugging, assault) or thefts involving confrontation with the victim (extortion, purse-snatching, gas-station robbery), with evidence of personal attachment, such as establishing lasting friendships or showing concern for others. (DSM-III)

conduct disorder, socialized, nonaggressive a conduct disorder involving repetitive, persistent nonaggressive conduct in which the basic rights of others or major social norms or rules are violated (persistent truancy, drug abuse, running away from home overnight, serious lying, stealing without confrontation with a victim), with evidence of personal attachment, as in lasting friendships and extending one's self for others. (DSM-III)

conduct disorder, undersocialized, aggressive a conduct disorder involving repetitive, persistent aggressive conduct in which the basic rights of others are violated, as manifested by physical violence against persons or property (vandalism, rape, breaking and entering, fire-setting, mugging, assault) or thefts involving confrontation with the victim (extortion, purse-snatching, gas-station robbery), with failure to establish a normal degree of affection, empathy, or bond with others. (DSM-III)

conduct disorder, undersocialized, nonaggressive a conduct disorder characterized by repetitive, persistent nonaggressive conduct in which the basic rights of others or major social norms or rules are violated (persistent truancy, drug abuse, running away from home overnight, serious lying, stealing without confrontation with the victim), with failure to establish a normal degree of affection, empathy, or bond with others. (DSM-III)

conduction: See EXCITATION AND C.

conduction aphasia a form of aphasia associated with lesions in the postcentral cortical areas, and characterized by difficulty in differentiating speech sounds and repeating them accurately, even though spontaneous articulation may be intact.

conduction deafness the loss of hearing due to a disorder in the auditory structures associated with the transmission of sound vibrations between the tympanic membrane and the inner ear. The cause may be an injury or disease that interferes with the normal functioning of the middle-ear ossicles. There is a uniform loss of sensitivity to all frequencies and an altering of the sound-intensity threshold. Also called **conductive deafness**.

cones any objects with a circular base and a body that tapers to a point, such as the retinal c.

confabulation the falsification of memory in which gaps in recall are filled by fabrications which the patient accepts as fact. C. is often interpreted as an unconscious attempt to conceal embarrassment due to actual memory loss or confusion. It occurs most frequently in Korsakoff's syndrome, and to a lesser extent in other organic psychoses such as senile dementia, general paresis, lead poisoning, Wernicke's encephalopathy, and head-injury cases.

confabulosis a condition that occurs at the recovery stage of acute brain syndrome and is characterized by systematized confabulations against a background of otherwise relatively clear consciousness.

confederates in an experimental situation, the aides of the experimenter who pose as subjects but whose behavior is rehearsed prior to the experiment. The real subjects are sometimes termed **naive subjects**.

conference method a personnel-development technique in which participants develop problem-solving and decision-making abilities, acquire new information, and modify their attitudes by pooling ideas, testing assumptions, discussing new approaches, and drawing inferences and conclusions on business problems and issues.

confession in psychiatry, the first or cathartic stage of Jung's analytic therapy, in which the patient describes everything that is troubling him.

confidence limits the limits on either side of a measure of variability such as central tendency beyond which a statistic is not expected to occur except by chance alone in more than a stated percentage of the time. The term also refers specifically to a paired set of numbers within which a parameter probably falls; if the 95 percent c.l. on a mean are "five" and "ten," then we can be confident that 95 percent of the time the true mean falls between these two numbers. Also called **confidence interval; fiducial limits**.

confidentiality a principle of medical ethics requiring the physician to hold secret all information given to him by the patient, as well as test scores and other research data concerning the patient. Certain states do not recognize this principle and can require the physician to divulge such information if needed in a legal proceeding.

configuration: See GOODNESS OF C.; WORD C.

confinement effects effects of restricting an individual's freedom of action. C.e. generally result in a higher-than-usual incidence of maladaptive behavior, even though inmates of prisons and patients in nursing homes and mental hospitals may find ways to adapt to their restricted environments. Loss of perceived control and helplessness are forms of maladaptive behavior observed. Loss of privacy, which produces similar behaviors, often complicates c.e.

confinement fear = CLAUSTROPHOBIA.

confirmation Tolman's term for the fulfillment of an expectancy. That is, the behavior in question leads to the expected goal, which tends to reinforce the process.

confirming reaction a presumed reaction that occurs in a subject when an objective is reached.

conflict in psychiatry, the clash of opposing or incompatible emotional or motivational forces, such as drives, impulses, or wishes. In psychoanalytic terms, c. is a struggle taking place between conscious and unconscious forces, especially between the id, ego, and superego, and may be a major source of neuroses. See EXTRAPSYCHIC C.; INTRAPSYCHIC C.

conflict-free area an aspect of the personality that is so well-integrated that it does not give rise to internal conflict, maladjustment, or neurotic symptoms.

conflict of interest in general, the pursuit of goals that ethically conflict, such as using a political position to further one's business interests. In psychiatry, c.o.i. may be a conflict generated by being employed in a court, in the army, or in a government agency: Is the psychiatrist's obligation primarily to the patient or to the organization? Under what conditions, if any, can the rule of confidentiality be set aside?

Conflict Resolution Inventory a test designed to measure self-assertiveness, by presenting 35 situations in which the individual is asked to do something unreasonable such as letting a casual acquaintance interrupt last-minute study for an examination. The test is sometimes used in assessing the effects of ASSERTIVENESS TRAINING. See this entry.

confluence the fusion of several instincts, motives, or perceptual elements.

confluence model a controversial and probably untenable theory that intelligence of siblings is correlated with family size. According to this model, average intelligence declines as the number of children in a family increase. Thus, the greater the number of children, the less intelligent they would be expected to be. Intelligence is also held to decline with birth order. However, many variables, e.g., spacing of children, could affect and reverse such generalizations. Also see BIRTH ORDER.

conformance in environmental psychology, a criterion of design of a living or working area. Kinds of c. include functional, spatial, climate, and sensory. E.g., sensory c. requires a perceptual environment that includes lighting designed to meet the optimum needs for specific visual tasks. Also see BEHAVIORAL FACILITATION.

conformity the tendency, often unwitting, to adopt

the opinions, norms, or behavior of a particular social group such as a peer group or religious group. C. may be demanded in certain situations, or it may represent an inner need of the individual. Compare ANTICONFORMITY.

confounding the weakening of an experimental design by introducing one or more unintended variables that could account for the results.

confounds the variables that may enter into an experiment unintentionally and become so difficult to define, measure, or separate as to render the study results doubtful or invalid.

confrontation the act of directly facing, or being required to face, one's own attitudes or shortcomings, as well as the way one is perceived by others or the possible consequences of one's behavior. Confrontational techniques are used primarily in group therapy, existential psychotherapy, and encounter groups. They must be employed judiciously since they are extremely powerful tools which have a potential for disruptive as well as constructive effects. C. is also the first step in psychoanalytic therapy, in which the patient must recognize the psychiatric phenomenon to be analyzed. In Adlerian therapy, c. is a statement or question calculated to motivate the patient to make a decision or face the reality of a situation. Also, c. with authorities has been used by student protest groups, particularly in the 1960s.

confrontational methods a technique of attitude and behavior change used, e.g., in residential drug programs staffed by ex-addicts (Day Top, Crossroads, Phoenix House): The group forces the addict to confront his weaknesses and failures by aggressively putting him "on the spot." Similar but less aggressive c.m. are used in encounter groups as a means of increasing awareness and modifying behavior.

confusion a pervasive disturbance of consciousness characterized by bewilderment, inability to think clearly, and disorientation for time, place, and person. C. occurs in extreme form in cases of extensive brain damage due to infection, head injury, toxic agents, or senile brain disease, and in less extreme and persistent form in certain cases of schizophrenia, depression, and mental retardation. Also called **mental c.**

confusional automatism: See AUTOMATISM.

congenital present at birth. The term refers to noninherited disorders, constitutional tendencies and predispositions, as well as defects due to injury incurred during gestation or birth. Some apply the term only to noninherited disorders; others also include genetic disorders as long as they are present at birth. Also called **connate**.

congenital acromicria = DOWN'S SYNDROME.

congenital alexia a form of word blindness due to organic brain damage present at birth, as distinguished from acquired alexia which represents the loss of a skill previously established.

congenital anomalies any defects in body structure that are present at birth. C.a. may result from genetic factors, as in Down's syndrome, or

be due to teratogenic agents, e.g., rubella virus, drugs taken by the mother during pregnancy, or maternal illness. Radiation is a suspected cause, but proof of radioactivity as a factor in human c.a. has not been established. C.a. are found in about seven percent of all children.

congenital aphasia any disorder of written or spoken communication ability due to a defect present at birth.

congenital cytomegalovirus infection a viral infection that affects perhaps three percent of pregnant mothers. Infants born with signs of viruria may show subsequent deafness, cerebral palsy, mental retardation, motor retardation, hyperactivity, seizures, or other abnormalities involving the nervous system. One study found that nearly half of newborns with signs of cytomegalovirus infection later experienced neurologic abnormalities.

congenital deafness deafness that existed at birth, regardless of the cause. Compare ADVENTITIOUS DEAFNESS.

congenital defect any deformity present at birth regardless of the cause, e.g., genetic or teratogenic. A c.d. may occur as a deformity in body structure, called an anomaly, or as a deficiency that may not be discovered until several years after birth, e.g., mental retardation, an allergy, or a metabolic disorder. A few inborn defects, e.g., Huntington's chorea, do not present symptoms until after the patient has reached adulthood.

congenital deformity: See CONGENITAL DEFECT.

congenital facial diplegia = MÖBIUS' SYNDROME.

congenital hip subluxation a form of congenital hip dislocation that is a partial rather than total dislocation. The condition may not be noticeable until a child begins to walk. If not treated early, the condition usually requires surgical reconstruction of the child's hip joint. Also see HIP DYSPLASIA.

congenital hypothyroidism a condition of motor and mental retardation associated with a deficiency of thyroid hormone. More than a dozen causes, mostly hereditary metabolic defects, have been identified with the disorder. The prognosis varies with the degree of thyroid deficiency during fetal and early infant life, but early and adequate thyroid-hormone therapy generally reverses the signs and symptoms. See CRETINISM.

congenital malformation any deformity or abnormal function of the body that was present at birth. The term may be applied regardless of the cause, which could be hereditary, the result of an injury during labor, or the effect of a viral infection or use of alcohol or other drugs by the mother during fetal development.

congenital orthopedic condition any abnormal musculoskeletal condition present in a child at birth, regardless of whether the cause was genetic or acquired as an embryo or fetus. A few kinds of c.o.c., such as collar-bone fracture and epiphyseal separation, can occur as a result of delivery complications. Clubfoot and scoliosis usually are hereditary but torticollis may result from abnormal pressure of the neck muscles during the fetal stage.

congenital-rubella syndrome a complex of congenital defects in infants whose mothers were infected by the rubella virus early in the pregnancy. The defects may include deaf-mutism, cataracts, heart disease, cerebral palsy, microcephaly, and mental retardation. Neurologic abnormalities occur in about 80 percent of the cases, and the brain weight is usually subnormal. Psychomotor retardation, marked by general lack of response to stimuli, and intellectual impairment are common. Also see GERMAN MEASLES.

congenital sensory neuropathy with anhidrosis a disorder marked by the absence of pain perception. Patients experience severe injuries such as multiple fractures and wounds from self-inflicted bites which may go untreated because they cause no pain. All patients studied had IQs below 80. Skin biopsies show normal but nonfunctional sweat glands.

congenital syphilis infection with the syphilitic treponema organism by a pregnant mother. The organism is transmitted to the fetus through the placenta. The precise effects vary with the age of the fetus and the stage of infection of the mother. A recent infection carries a higher risk than an earlier infection of the mother who may have had time to develop immunizing antibodies. The fetus usually is not affected until after the fourth month of pregnancy. Neurologic effects in a surviving infant include seizures, organic dementia, and abnormal behavior such as delusions or hallucinations.

congenital toxoplasmosis an infectious disease caused by a protozoan parasite, Toxoplasma gondii, which is acquired by a pregnant mother and transmitted through the placenta to the fetus. If the fetus survives the intrauterine infection, it may be expected to suffer severe brain damage. Hydrocephalus or microcephaly, seizures, deafness, and mental retardation are common effects. Treatment with drugs such as sulfadiazine improves the prognosis.

congestive dysmenorrhea: See DYSMENORRHEA.

congophilic material a substance with an affinity for Congo red dye, used for diagnostic purposes. C.m. includes protein substances such as amyloid and the intracellular neurofilbrils that are found in the senile plaques of the brains of victims of Alzheimer's disease. The senile plaques also are argentophilic. Amyloid levels in the body can be measured by injecting Congo red dye into the bloodstream of one arm and removing blood samples from the other. Any amyloid deposits in the blood will be tagged with the dye, which is specific for the protein molecule of amyloid, which is involved in a metabolic disease of the spinal cord and peripheral nerves.

congruence in general, mutual agreement or point-by-point conformity, as with two matching geometrical figures or a well-matched couple. Also, C. Rogers uses the term in two senses: the need for the therapist to act in accordance with his true feelings rather than a stylized image ("genuineness"), and the conscious integration of an experience into the self.

congruent points points on the two retinas that normally are involved in perception of the same stimulus.

congruity theory a theory concerned with the direction of attitude change, holding that "when change in evaluation or attitude occurs, it always occurs as increased congruity with the prevailing frame of reference" (R. B. Zajonc, 1960); that is, one's attitude changes in the direction of reducing inconsistency or ambiguity.

conjoint counseling a therapeutic technique commonly applied in solving marital disputes with the spouses meeting together with the therapist or a team of therapists or social workers, as opposed to counseling the individuals separately. C.c. may be used also in resolving disputes involving multigeneration family problems.

conjoint interviewing in marital and sex therapy, an interview with the husband and wife together, in order to observe their reactions to each other through facial expressions, body movements, and expressions of feeling.

conjoint therapy a type of marriage therapy in which the two partners meet with the therapist in joint sessions. Family therapy in which the members meet with the therapist as a group is another form of c.t. Also called **triadic therapy; triangular therapy; conjoint marital therapy**. Also see MARRIAGE THERAPY.

conjugal paranoia paranoia involving a delusion of jealousy and the belief, on unfounded "evidence," that the partner has been unfaithful. See PARANOID DISORDERS.

conjugate movements coordinated movements of the two eyes functioning together.

conjunctiva the mucous membrane covering the anterior surface of the eyeball.

conjunctival reflex the automatic closing of the eyelid when the cornea is stimulated.

conjunctive concept a concept that is based on the joint presence of a group of attributes, as in the concepts of house and personality.

conjunctive motivation the drive to achieve true and lasting, not temporary or substitute, satisfactions.

conjunctive reinforcement a type of intermittent reinforcement using two interval schedules: fixed interval and fixed ratio.

conjunctivity the coordination of motives with actions.

Conn, Jerome W. American physician, 1907—. See ALDOSTERONISM (also called **Conn's syndrome**); ADRENAL-CORTICAL HYPERFUNCTION.

connate = CONGENITAL.

connectionism Thorndike's concept that neural

links, inherited or acquired, bond stimulus and response.

connector neurons; connectors = INTERNUNCIAL NEURONS.

connotative meaning elements of word meaning that convey affect, suggest additional associations, or express value judgments; all subjective aspects of a word's potential impact; everything that deviates from a literal, objective definition. Also called **connotation**. Compare DENOTATIVE MEANING.

Conn's syndrome = ALDOSTERONISM.

Conolly, John British psychiatrist, ca. 1794–1866. C. introduced the principle of nonrestraint in the care of patients at the insane asylum of Hanwell, and was generally influential with his humanitarian approach.

conquering-hero daydream: See DAYDREAM.

Conradi, Erich /kônrä′dē/ German physician, 1882—. See CONRADI'S DISEASE.

Conradi's disease a congenital disorder marked by short limbs, craniofacial anomalies, cataracts, dry skin, and, in some cases, degenerating cartilage at the ends of the long bones. In patients of one phenotype, rhizomelic, mental retardation is common. However, it is rarely present in the Conradi-Hünermann form of the disease. Also called **chondrodystrophia calcificans congenita**.

consanguineous matings marriage or sexual intercourse between persons who are closely related or descended from the same ancestor. See INCEST.

consanguinity a biological relationship between two or more individuals who are descended from a common ancestor. See AFFINITY.

conscience the individual's pattern of moral values and sense of right and wrong. In psychoanalysis, c. is the superego, or ethical component, of personality, which acts as judge and critic of our actions and attitudes. See SUPEREGO. Also see HUMANISTIC C.; AUTHORITARIAN C.

conscious being aware, or being able to respond to stimulation. As a noun, the c. is the portion of the mind that is immediately aware of the environment at any given time, and is synonymous with consciousness. Also see PRECONSCIOUS; SUBCONSCIOUS.

consciousness the *state* of awareness as well as the *content* of the mind—the everchanging stream of immediate experience, comprising our perceptions, feelings, sensations, images, and ideas. C. is also defined as that which is observable by introspection, or the current totality of experience. Also see ALTERED STATES OF C.; CLOUDING OF C.; COSMIC C.; CROWD C.; DIVIDED C.; DOUBLE C.; EXPANDED C.; FIELD OF C.; GROUP C.; HEAD C.; MARGINAL C.; PERCEPTUAL C.; SELF-C.; SOCIAL C.; STREAM OF C.; SUBLIMINAL C.

consciousness disturbances disorders of consciousness that are symptomatic of mental illness, including clouding, confusion, delirium, fugue states, dream states; also, disturbances produced by hallucinogens or other consciousness-altering drugs.

consciousness expansion: See EXPANDED CONSCIOUSNESS.

consciousness-raising a group-discussion process directed toward greater awareness (a) of one's condition, needs, values, and goals as a means of achieving one's full potential as a person, or (b) of discrimination against a particular group of people. A member of one group has described the process as opening the door to the mind: What is happening? Why is it happening? Does it have to happen that way? Also see RAP GROUP.

conscious processes the combination of active and passive mental activities. An **active mode of consciousness** may include planning and carrying out an activity. A **passive mode of consciousness** may be represented by watching a sports event on television.

conscious resistance a Freudian term for the deliberate withholding of information by a patient because of shame, fear of rejection, or distrust of the analyst.

conscious state the condition of being mentally aware and mentally active.

consensual eye reflex a phenomenon in which the pupil of a shaded eye contracts when the other eye is stimulated by a bright light.

consensual validation a term used by H. S. Sullivan for the process by which a therapist helps the patient recognize and modify his distorted thoughts and feelings by comparing them with the thoughts and feelings of others. See PARATAXIC DISTORTION.

consent: See INFORMED C.

conservation Piaget's term for the awareness that physical quantities do not change in amount when they are altered in appearance. In Piaget's famous c. experiment, all the water from one beaker is poured into a taller, thinner beaker, whereupon the child is asked whether the amount of water has changed. By age seven or eight, children will give the correct answer as well as understand the underlying principles. C. is also a seldom-used term for **memory retention**. Also called **c. theory**. Also see REVERSIBILITY; PERCEPTUAL CONSTANCY; CONSTANCY.

conservation-withdrawal the tendency of a patient to withdraw from family and friends and want to be left alone during the second week after surgery, as a means of recouping his psychological and physical strength.

conservator an individual appointed by a court to protect the interests and property of a person who cannot be declared incompetent, but who is too infirm by reason of a physical or mental condition to take full responsibility for managing his own affairs.

consideration in social psychology, an important component of the group leader's role, consisting in his ability to foster and sustain productive group spirit and cooperation through even-handed and sympathetic interaction with group members.

consistency theory a theory of work behavior introduced by Korman in 1970 and based on a two-point premise: a balance notion and a self-image standard. The theory states that workers will engage in and find satisfying behaviors that maximize their sense of cognitive balance and they will be motivated to perform in a manner consistent with their self-image.

consolation dream a dream that contains an expression of encouragement or reassurance.

consonance the quality of harmony between elements, e.g., in music. In communication, c. refers to harmony between content (denotative meaning) and intent (connotative meaning); e.g., if a talk on the subject of peace is uttered in peaceful tones, content and intent agree and the communication is said to possess c. (G. S. Belkin and J. L. Gray, *Educational Psychology*, 1977). In social psychology, c. is the extent to which the components of an attitude are internally consistent or in agreement with each other.

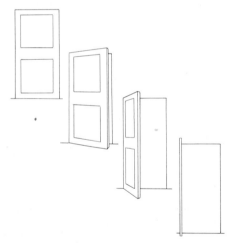

CONSTANCY. Example of perceptual constancy.

constancy the tendency of perceptions to remain unchanged despite variations in the external conditions of observation. See BRIGHTNESS C.; COLOR C.; OBJECT C.; SIZE C.; SHAPE C.; PERCEPTUAL C.; WHITENESS C. Also see CONSERVATION.

constancy hypothesis the principle that a given stimulus will always produce a given response.

constancy law: See LAW OF CONSTANCY.

constancy of internal environment the tendency of the internal state of an organism to remain in equilibrium. See HOMEOSTASIS.

constancy of the IQ a tendency for IQ results to remain approximately the same when the same or similar test is administered.

constant an aspect of an experiment that does not change from one condition to another; also, a mathematical expression whose value is fixed; also, the opposite of a variable.

constant error a systematic bias in some particular direction; an observational error that is repeated by most subjects given the same test. Compare RANDOM ERROR.

constant-stimuli method: See METHOD OF CONSTANT STIMULI.

constellation a group of separate ideas with a common theme or association.

constellatory construct a concept or construct that holds together a group of concepts, e.g., the concept of democratic society.

constipation difficult or infrequent excretion of feces. The normal frequency of human bowel movements varies from three times a day to once every three days. In addition to diseases and mechanical obstructions, c. may be caused by psychogenic factors. **Psychogenic c.** is observed in obsessive-compulsive persons who assign such importance to "regularity" that abnormal amounts of time and effort are devoted to daily bowel movements.

constitution the basic psychological and physical makeup of an individual, in part due to heredity and in part to life experience and environmental factors. Some authors, however, limit the term to the individual's innate, genetically determined, characteristics, or **endowment**.

constitutional depressive disposition the ingrained "melancholic mood" (Bleuler) of an individual who appears consistently depressed and pessimistic, lacks self-confidence, and has difficulty in making decisions.

constitutional factors basic physiological tendencies that are believed to contribute to personality, temperament, and the etiology of specific mental and physical disorders. These factors include, e.g., body build, hereditary predispositions, and physiological characteristics (circulatory, musculoskeletal, glandular, etc.).

constitutional insanity a term that may be applied to mental disorders caused by genetic factors. The original, 19th-century, meaning suggested congenital, hereditary, or constitutional defects or deviant trends.

constitutional manic disposition a personality type characterized by an impulsive and thoughtless manner representative of the manic temperament. According to Bleuler, the "manic mood" may also be expressed in a sunny disposition and tireless energy as well as in snobbish, inconsiderate, or quarrelsome manners.

constitutional medicine a branch of medicine that deals with hereditary factors involved in resistance or susceptibility to disease and the possible associations between susceptibility factors and body builds.

constitutional psychopath an obsolete term for antisocial personality disorder, based on the idea that the condition is congenital. Also see CONSTITUTIONAL PSYCHOPATHIC INFERIOR; PSYCHOPATHY.

constitutional psychopathic inferior an obsolete term for what is now called antisocial personality disorder. The term psychopathic inferior was introduced by Koch in 1888 and included in Kraepelin's classification of mental disorders. Meyer added the word constitutional in the sense of deep-seated, but not in the sense of congenital.

constitutional type a classification of individuals based on physique and other biological characteristics or a hypothetical relationship between physical and psychological characteristics such as temperament, personality, and a tendency to develop a specific type of mental disorder. For examples of typologies, see KRETSCHMER TYPOLOGY; SHELDON'S CONSTITUTIONAL THEORY OF PERSONALITY; CARUS' TYPOLOGY; HIPPOCRATES.

constrained association = CONTROLLED ASSOCIATION.

constraint of thought a belief, particularly among schizophrenic patients, that their thoughts are controlled or influenced by other persons. A related effect is **constraint of movement**, in which the patient believes his movements are controlled by others.

constrictor vaginae = BULBOSPONGIOSUS MUSCLE.

construct a concept based on relationships between empirically verifiable and measurable events or processes—an **empirical c.**— or on processes inferred from data of this kind—a HYPOTHETICAL C. See this entry.

constructional apraxia an inability because of brain damage to assemble parts of an object so that it is a complete structure or device. Tests include drawing from a model, reconstructions of puzzles, and building with wooden sticks or blocks toward a particular structure. Also called **constructive apraxia**. See APRAXIA.

constructional praxis the ability to draw, copy, or manipulate spatial patterns or designs.

constructionism the theory, advanced by Piaget, that the child constructs his understanding of reality out of his actions on objects in the environment, which produce both a knowledge of the effects of his actions, and the properties of the objects.

construction need H. A. Murray's term for the need to create and build.

constructive approach: See PSYCHOSYNTHESIS.

constructive apraxia = CONSTRUCTIONAL APRAXIA.

constructive memory the use of general knowledge stored in one's memory to construct a more complete and detailed account of an event or experience.

construct validity an accurate reflection or assessment of a specific theoretical concept.

consultant a specialist called upon to advise an attending physician on questions of psychiatric or psychological diagnosis, treatment, or rehabilitation. Although the advice of the c. is patient-oriented, he does not ordinarily meet directly with the patient.

consultation: See PSYCHIATRIC C.

consultation-liaison psychiatry clinical psychiatry carried out in nonpsychiatric units of a general hospital, in close collaboration with nonpsychiatric physicians primarily concerned with the medical or surgical treatment of the patient.

consulting psychologist a psychologist who provides professional guidance to individuals on their emotional, vocational, marital, or educational problems either on a private basis or an organizational basis, as in a business organization or health agency.

consulting psychology expert psychological guidance mainly to business and industry, federal and state agencies, the armed forces, or educational and scientific groups.

consumer behavior as defined by J. F. Engel, R. D. Blackwell, and David T. Kollat (*Consumer Behavior*, 1978), "the acts of individuals directly involved in obtaining and using economic goods and services, including decision processes that precede and determine these acts."

consumer characteristics personality traits of consumers that can be used in planning advertising campaigns. Most sophisticated studies of c.c. go beyond area, sex, income, and neighborhood of residence and use established psychologic techniques of analyzing motives behind buying decisions, which may be psychosexual or emotional rather than of a practical nature.

consumer education educational programs directed primarily to (a) the criteria by which to evaluate complex technical products and services, (b) decision-making skills, (c) increased consumer knowledge of the workings of business, government, and the marketplace, (d) techniques for judging advertising and selling claims, and (e) insight into money-saving buying strategies.

consumerism a movement to protect the rights of the consumer with regard to the quality and safety of medical care, as well as products and services in the marketplace. C. has resulted in the legally enforced rights of patients to have access to treatment or to refuse treatment. Also included is the patient's right not to be administered experimental, unusual, or hazardous treatment without informed consent.

consumer-jury technique a method of testing advertising appeals before an actual product-promotion campaign is started in a test market. "Jury" members usually consist of typical consumers of the product category. They are shown a selection of different proposed advertisements and asked to evaluate them in terms of which ad, or TV commercial, would be most likely to induce them to purchase the product. The c.-j.t. has been found to be an accurate predictor of advertising effectiveness. Also see CONTINUOUS PANEL.

consumer psychology the branch of psychology that specializes in the behavior of individuals as consumers and the techniques of communicating information that will influence consumer decisions to purchase a manufacturer's product.

Words, symbols, colors, and cultural backgrounds are among factors considered in marketing a single product, such as cigarettes. A picture of a cowboy on horseback smoking a cigarette might influence Americans to think the product is associated with masculinity, but in another part of the world consumers might reject the product on the ground that anybody who rides around in the hot sun on horseback may be mentally retarded. Tea-drinking, once avoided in the United States by men who regarded tea as a "sissy drink," increased after the Tea Council of the U.S.A. hired professional athletes to pose as tea drinkers in advertising pictures.

consumer research the application of clinical, scientific, and statistical research techniques in the study of consumer behavior. C.r. may include studies of consumer tastes and preferences, package-design influences, and personality traits of a target audience. C.r. could, e.g., find that while housewives may prefer convenience food packaging, they may avoid products that might suggest they are lazy. Also called **market research**. See MOTIVATION RESEARCH.

consumer surveys surveys of consumer likes and dislikes in certain product categories, e.g., beverages, that may yield information that can be used to design and package a product the consumer will find attractive. C.s. may be conducted by questionnaires, in-depth interviews, group interviews, visualization, and similar techniques.

consummatory act the final stage of a complex response to a stimulus or learning experience. A c.a. might be the fertilization of the eggs of a female fish by the male after the innate sequence of nest establishment and courtship to entice the female to the nest. In human sex, the c.a. is the act of coitus. The term also applies to the fulfillment of any other drive, such as thirst. Also called **consummatory response**.

consummatory communication a message that conveys the sender's ideas or feelings and does not require feedback.

consummatory response = CONSUMMATORY ACT.

contact behavior actions and interactions occurring during an intimate, **personal relationship** (e.g., sexual contact) or a relatively **impersonal relationship** (e.g., buying or selling).

contact dermatitis any acute or chronic skin disorder caused by an agent that damages normal skin surfaces or aggravates an existing skin sensitivity. C.d. agents include plants, e.g., poison ivy or ragweed; soaps or detergents; chemicals used in the manufacture of shoes and clothing; cosmetics; and industrial and household chemicals. Some medications, e.g., antihistamines, can be either a causative factor or a therapeutic agent for c.d.

contact desensitization in behavior therapy, a desensitizing method involving physical contact between therapist and patient.

contact lens a corrective-eyeglass lens that fits

directly over the eye although separated from the eye surface by a thin layer of fluid. A c.l. is made of glass or plastic, molded to the exact shape of the individual corneas of the patient. Like conventional eyeglasses, the c.l. is designed to correct for refractive errors in the patient's natural lens.

contagion in psychiatry, the dissemination of behavior, attitudes, or emotional reactions through suggestion, imitation, or the words and gestures of a charismatic leader. Generally in psychology, c. is the transmission of ideas, feelings, or mental disorders from person to person or group to group by psychological forces such as suggestion, propaganda, rumor, imitation, or sympathy. See BITING MANIA; CHOREOMANIA; FOLIE À DEUX; LYCANTHROPY; MASS HYSTERIA; SHARED PARANOID DISORDER.

contamination in psychiatry, the creation of neologisms by amalgamating a part of one word with a part of another, usually resulting in a word that is unintelligible. In testing and experimentation, c. means the process of permitting knowledge about the variable to be validated to influence the variable used for validation.

contamination fear = MYSOPHOBIA; MOLYSOPHOBIA.

contamination obsession an obsession with disease, dirt, germs, mud, excrement, sputum, and the like, based according to E. W. Straus on an absence of pleasurable emotions and a feeling that the world is disgusting, decaying, and dying. An extreme c.o. of this kind is regarded as a symptom of schizophrenia.

contemplation = MEDITATION.

contemporaneity in psychotherapy, the principle of focusing on immediate experience, the here-and-now. See HERE-AND-NOW APPROACH.

contemporaneous-explanation principle the concept that only present events can influence behavior.

content analysis a systematic, quantitative procedure for coding the themes in qualitative material, such as projective-test responses, propaganda, or fiction; a systematic, quantitative study of verbally communicated material (articles, speeches, films) by determining the frequency of specific ideas, concepts, or terms. Called **quantitative semantics** by H. D. Lasswell.

contentiousness quarrelsomeness observed in manic syndromes and the early stages of paranoid reactions when patients feel they are being treated unfairly.

contentive = CONTENT WORD.

content psychology a branch of psychology that is concerned with the role of conscious experience. See PHENOMENOLOGY; STRUCTURALISM.

content-thought disorder a type of thought disturbance typically found in schizophrenia, and characterized by multiple, fragmented, bizarre delusions.

content validity an aspect of test validity having to do with the extent to which a test measures a representative sample of the subject matter or behavior in question That is, c.v. deals with the question of how well the test covers a designated area of investigation. E.g., if a test is designed to survey arithmetic skills on a third-grade level, how well does it represent the range of arithmetic operations possible at that level? Also called **content validation**.

content word a word that has a full lexical or semantic meaning, such as a noun, verb, or adjective (in contrast to a function word such as a preposition or conjunction). Also called **full word; lexical word; notional word; vocabulary word; autonomous word; semanteme; contentive; open-class word**. Compare FUNCTION WORD.

context clues clues permitting the recognition of words in the context of the sentence, or paragraph, in which they appear.

context-shifting a term applied to the schizophrenic's tendency to change the subject abruptly and irrelevantly in order to avoid an anxiety-laden idea. D. L. Burnham cites the following example. Interviewer: "You seem to feel that if you develop any close friends, they will desert you"; patient: "I wonder what's for dessert today."

context theory of meaning E. B. Titchener's theory that meaning depends upon the mental images associated with a specific body of sensations, as in the concept of fire.

contextualism the theory that the memory of experiences is not the result merely of linkages between events, as in the associationist doctrine, but is due to the quality of the experiences themselves.

contiguity of associations the concept that an internal connection, or association, is usually established between two objects, experiences, or behaviors that are close together in space or time. Also see LAW OF CONTIGUITY.

continence the ability to control sexual urges or the urge to defecate or urinate.

contingency a dependency relationship between events, as between response and reward.

contingency awareness awareness of a relationship or connection between two occurrences; awareness of the dependence of one variable upon another.

contingency coefficient a nonparametric measure of correlation, useful with nominal (categorical) data. Symbol: $C = \sqrt{\chi^2/(N + \chi^2)}$.

contingency contract = CONTRACT.

contingency management the regulation of management of reinforcement with reference to such questions as: *Who* does the reinforcing? *How much* reinforcement for how much work? *When* is reinforcement to be delivered? *What* does it consist of?

contingency model a leadership concept of industrial psychology based on the generalization that management or supervisory personnel are either task-oriented or person-oriented.

contingency reinforcement a behavior-therapy technique in which a reinforcement, or reward, is given each time the desired behavior is performed, that is, the reward is contingent, or dependent, on the behavior.

contingency table a table of data showing relationships among variables.

contingency theory of leadership a theory of leadership stating that a leader's efficacy is contingent not only on the leader's own qualities, but also on elements of the group situation. According to F. Fiedler, a leader's effectiveness is influenced by (a) his or her personal relationships with group members, (b) the extent of the leader's actual authority or power, and (c) the nature of the group task, e.g., the degree to which it is structured or vague.

contingent negative variation a form of evoked potential (EP) consisting of a slow negative D.C. wave recorded from the forehead, produced when a subject attends to a task but not produced by electromyogram (EMG) activity. The cerebral processes represented by the c.n.v. are not fully known. Abbrev.: **CNV**.

continued-stay review in psychiatry, an aspect of utilization review which focuses on the duration of stay within a mental hospital or hospital unit. C.-s.r. consists largely of a comparison of cases under review with regional norms which are usually expressed in terms of average length of stay for each diagnostic category. Abbrev.: **CSR**. Also see EXTENDED-STAY REVIEW.

continuing-care unit a hospital unit to which a patient with a catastrophic or chronic illness is transferred for additional care after the acute hospitalization period.

continuing medical education a postdoctoral educational program on a continuing basis, and in some cases coupled with evaluation, licensing, and certification in a particular specialty. Courses and seminars are usually provided by university medical centers. In psychiatry, the term refers to a specified number of hours of additional medical education (150 hours in any consecutive three-year period) for professional growth and continued membership in the American Psychiatric Association, at least 75 hours of which are directly related to psychiatry. Individual programs can be selected from such areas as medical education with or without sponsorship by an accredited institution; medical teaching; papers, publications, books, presentations, exhibits; nonsupervised individual education, such as self-instruction, self-assessment, and specialty-board preparation; and other meritorious learning experiences individually submitted for credit. Abbrev.: **CME**.

continuity hypothesis the assumption that discrimination learning or problem-solving results from a progressive, incremental, continuous process of trial and error. Responses that prove unproductive are extinguished while responses that yield results are strengthened. Problem-solving is conceived as a step-by-step learning process in which the correct response is discovered, practiced, and reinforced. The c.h. is an associationist position. Compare DISCONTINUITY HYPOTHESIS.

continuity of germ-plasm theory the principle that all germ cells are derived from other germ cells, and not from other tissues.

continuity theory of learning the concept that in discrimination learning every reinforced response results in an increase.

continuous amnesia: See PSYCHOGENIC AMNESIA.

continuous-bath treatment a method of calming excited, delirious, or agitated patients by placing them in a continuously flowing tub of warm water kept at body temperature. Also see HYDROTHERAPY.

continuous group = OPEN GROUP.

continuous narcosis a type of manic therapy introduced in the 1920s that prescribed 20 hours of sleep daily under sedation for up to three weeks. The treatment has been replaced by other therapies, e.g., tranquilizers or electroshock treatments. See SLEEP TREATMENT; DAUERSCHLAF.

continuous panel a form of consumer jury in which members serve on a more or less permanent basis so that consumer psychologists can detect shifts in attitudes, values, or behavior. The c.p. members are carefully selected to represent the demographic or psychographic characteristics of a population, and they are tested periodically for signs of psychic mobility that may also represent attitude changes in the general population.

continuous positive-airway pressure a technique employed to increase oxygenation of the blood and other tissues of newborn infants suffering from hyaline-membrane disease, also called respiratory-distress syndrome. C.p.-a.p. is applied by endotracheal tube, nasal prongs, a sealed head chamber, or a face mask. The principle of c.p.-a.p. is to provide a back pressure in the infant's lungs so that total exhalation is prevented. The respiratory gases are directed through the endotracheal tube with a reservoir bag on the end and a pressure manometer attached to monitor the amount of air pressure. The back pressure prevents pressure within the lungs from falling to below-normal levels at the end of an expiration, a frequent cause of brain damage in infants. Abbrev.: **CPAP.**

continuous reinforcement in operant conditioning, the modification of a subject's behavior by providing a reinforcement, or reward, for each correct response, as compared with partial reinforcement in which the behavior is reinforced intermittently rather than continuously.

continuous scale a scale in which increments are assumed or known to be continuous.

continuous-sleep therapy the use of prolonged sleep as treatment for certain psychiatric disorders. Also called **prolonged-sleep treatment.** For details, see SLEEP TREATMENT.

continuous variable a variable that can assume any value, e.g., length or weight. Compare DISCRETE VARIABLE.

continuum any scale, series, or graph that extends continuously without gaps or other interruptions.

-contr-; -contra- a combining form meaning opposed in direction or function.

contra. an abbreviation of "contraindication."

contraception the prevention of conception, or planned prevention of the natural fertilization of the female ovum by the male spermatozoa. See BIRTH CONTROL.

contraceptives: See BIRTH CONTROL.

contract an explicit agreement used by behavior therapists in treating such conditions as drug abuse, obesity, and smoking problems as well as family relationships. The c. states, usually in writing, what the patient and the therapist are to do (patient and therapist obligations), as well as provisions for benefits or privileges to be gained through specific performances, specified consequences of failure to meet the terms of a c. (e.g., skipping sessions), and bonuses for complying with its terms. Also called **contingency c.; behavioral c.**

contractibility the capacity of living tissue, particularly muscle, to contract in response to a stimulus. Also called **contractility.**

contracture an abnormal shortening of a muscle, a condition that can result in permanent disability due to difficulty in stretching the muscle. Causes include fibrosis of the involved tissues, arthritis, injury, inadequate exercise, and muscle-fiber disorders. A c. often follows a disorder or injury that makes movement painful, resulting in muscle shortening due to lack of exercise. A c. may be congenital, due to fetal pressures in the uterus.

contralateral referring to something on the other side. The term is used, e.g., in neurology to identify a physical effect, such as paralysis, that occurs on the side of the body opposite to the side on which a brain lesion is found. Compare IPSILATERAL.

contralateral hearing aid: See HEARING AID.

contrasexual a term introduced by Jacobi to describe the repressed side of the male-female elements assumed by Jung to be present in all individuals, regardless of their sex.

contrast an intensification of differences between stimuli caused by contiguous presentations, either simultaneous or successive.

For a different meaning of the term, see PRINCIPLE OF MAXIMUM C.

contrast effect the perception of an intensified or heightened difference between two stimuli or sensations when they are juxtaposed (simultaneous contrast) or when one immediately follows the other (successive contrast), e.g., when a trombone precedes a violin or when bright yellow and red are viewed simultaneously. In social psychology, contrast effects are said to occur when there is a shift in judgment away from an anchor. Also see ASSIMILATION EFFECT.

contrast effects in interviewing in industrial psychology, a generalization that an interviewer's judgment of an applicant will be affected by a previous interview of another person. Thus, a good average candidate may seem very good if the previous applicant was rated as below average. But a good average candidate may appear a poor choice when a previous candidate was very good.

contre coup /kôNtrəkoo'/ an effect in which an external injury to an area on one side of the head causes a brain injury on the opposite side of the head. The c.c. effect is caused by pressure waves traveling to the right and left around the skull from the point of impact and producing a summation of force 180 degrees away. C.c. explains why an injury to the left side of the head may disrupt motor functions on the left rather than right side.

contrectation touching or fondling another person, usually involving genital stimulation. The term is derived from the Latin word *contrectare*, meaning "to handle" or "to take hold of."

control in psychiatry and psychoanalysis, the process of restraining or regulating impulses, which Freud believed to be the major function of the ego. Also, c. is the regulation of the conditions of an experiment in such a way that the effects will be due solely to the experimental or independent variable and not to any extraneous factor.

control adoptees offspring of normal parents reared by normal adopting parents, selected for comparison with **index adoptees**. See CROSS FOSTERING.

control analysis = CONTROLLED ANALYSIS.

control-devices research the study of devices used to control machines, in terms of (a) correct identification through shape, size, color, or texture coding, in order to reduce errors, (b) specific design features of knobs, levers, push buttons most suitable for different purposes, and (c) location, as in the relative location of the brake and accelerator in motor vehicles.

control experiment a repetition of an experiment for the purpose of gathering information about or increasing the validity of the original experiment. The experimental conditions may be duplicated exactly to provide another measure of the dependent variable, or to assess the impact of a variable that experimenters suspect was not previously controlled.

control group a group of subjects exposed to all the aspects of an experiment except for the experimental variable. Also see EXPERIMENTAL GROUP.

controlled analysis psychoanalysis conducted by a trainee under the supervision of a qualified analyst. Also called **control analysis**.

controlled association in an association experiment, a constraint imposed on the subject's responses such that the given response relates to the stimulus word in accordance with the experimenter's directions; e.g., the c.a. may be a synonym or antonym. Also called **constrained association**. Compare FREE ASSOCIATION.

controlled attention the ability to attend selectively to what is significant in the environment; the capacity to distinguish important stimuli from peripheral, incidental stimuli. Also called **selective attention**.

controlled drinking a term sometimes applied to a pattern of drinking alcoholic beverages that tends toward moderation and away from the extremes of abuse and abstinence.

controlled-drinking therapy a type of behavioral therapy designed to reduce a patient's tendency to excessive consumption of alcoholic beverages by self-control techniques.

controlled-exposure technique a method of pre-testing advertising effectiveness by presenting advertisements to a limited audience in the setting of a magazine display or radio or television broadcast. Several variations of the advertising appeal may be used and tested by tachistoscopes, hidden cameras, or GSR equipment to detect physiological reactions, in addition to questionnaire surveys of the potential consumer responses.

controlled sampling a sampling technique in which the risk of chance effects is eliminated.

controlled variable a variable controlled by the experimenter; the independent variable.

contusion: See HEAD TRAUMA; CEREBRAL C.; ACUTE TRAUMATIC DISORDER.

convalescent centers extended care facilities for patients whose recovery from disease or injury has reached a stage where full-time hospital inpatient services are no longer required. C.c. generally provide professional personnel, including an available physician and 24-hour nursing service, rehabilitation services, and an authorized system of dispensing medications. Licensure standards for c.c. may vary according to local laws.

convenience dreams a Freudian term for dreams that appear to solve a practical problem, e.g., a dream that one has started the day's routine while the person actually is sleeping later than usual.

convention a rule of social conduct that is generally accepted but seldom enforced.

conventionalism a personality trait marked by excessive concern with and inflexible adherence to social customs and middle-class values and standards of behavior. The term is also used to refer specifically to one of the traits associated with the authoritarian personality. See AUTHORITARIANISM.

conventional level Kohlberg's second and intermediate level of moral reasoning characterized by identification with and conformity to the moral rules of family and society. Stage 3 of this level is marked by approval-seeking behavior and evaluation of underlying intentions. Stage 4 of this level is marked by the emphasis on fixed rules, duty, obedience to authority, and defense of the existing social order. Also see PRECONVENTIONAL LEVEL; POSTCONVENTIONAL LEVEL.

conventional virus viruses that persist in host cells for long periods and produce a wide variety of chronic and degenerative diseases such as subacute herpetoviral encephalitis of herpes simplex, cytomegalovirus brain infection, progressive congenital rubella togavirus, and possibly multiple sclerosis, Parkinson's disease, amyotrophic lateral sclerosis, and some forms of schizophrenic dementia. The infections believed to be involved in these conditions are called **conventional-slow-virus infections**. Compare UN-CONVENTIONAL VIRUS.

convergence the rotation of the two eyes inward toward the source of light so that the image will fall on corresponding points in the foveas. C. enables the slightly different images of an object seen by each eye to come together and form a single image. The muscular tension exerted is also one of the cues to the distance of the object from the eyes.

convergent evolution a tendency of unrelated animals in a particular environment to acquire similar body structures that enable them to adapt effectively to the habitat. Aquatic animals generally acquire external features that include smooth surfaces for rapid movement through a watery medium.

convergent strabismus = CROSS-EYE.

convergent thinking an aspect of critical thinking characterized by the search for a problem's best answer. In c.t., the possible solutions are given and the task is one of analyzing the alternatives to determine the most logical answer. Compare DIVERGENT THINKING.

conversational catharsis the release of repressed or suppressed thoughts and feelings through verbal interchange in group or individual psychotherapy.

conversion an unconscious psychological process in which repressed material (impulses, memories, fantasies) are transformed into bodily (somatic) symptoms. The symptoms have the common purpose of protection against anxiety, and may be either a direct expression (e.g., a violinist may develop a stiff arm just before a dreaded concert) or a symbolic representation (e.g., an intensely hostile person may develop a paralysis of the arm just before going into the boss' office). The corresponding DSM-III term is C. DISORDER. See this entry.

conversion disorder a somatoform disorder involving a loss or alteration in physical functioning that suggests physical disorder, but for which there is instead evidence of psychological involvement or need. The symptoms of c.d. are not under voluntary control, and include paralysis, loss of voice, seizures, blindness, tunnel vision, and disturbance in coordination or balance. Examples of psychological factors involved in these symptoms are losing one's voice when there is a conflict over expressing anger, developing a paralyzed arm as a means of avoiding killing in combat, and developing an inability to walk or stand (astasia-abasia) to gain emotional support and attention. Also called **hysterical neurosis, conversion type**. See PRIMARY GAINS; SECONDARY GAINS. (DSM-III)

conversion hysteria a psychoneurosis in which repressed inner conflicts are unconsciously transformed into physical symptoms that have no organic basis, e.g., paralysis, blindness, or loss of sensation. See CONVERSION DISORDER.

conversion of emotion a psychosomatic disturbance in which a functional conflict involving one organ is expressed, usually symbolically, through the energizing of another part of the body. An example is the displacement of tumescence of the penis or clitoris to the head area where the reaction is expressed in the form of blushing.

conversion paralysis = HYSTERICAL PARALYSIS.

conversion reaction the DSM-I term for the DSM-III diagnostic category "conversion disorder (or hysterical neurosis, conversion type)".

conversion seizures = HYSTERICAL CONVULSIONS.

conversion symptoms symptoms developed by patients with hysteria, or conversion disorder, for such unconscious purposes as screening out feelings of anxiety arising from intrapsychic conflicts, and obtaining such "secondary gains" as sympathy, attention, and control over others. Though physical, these symptoms are functional in nature, and fall into two major categories: **sensory c.s.** (tunnel vision, anesthesias, impairment of taste or smell) and **motor c.s.** (paralyses, tics, unsteady gait), though practically any other body system may be involved, as indicated by such symptoms as headache, loss of appetite, coughing spells, and false pregnancy.

convulsant any substance that causes or otherwise results in convulsions. An example of a c. drug is pentylenetetrazol which has been used in the past as a c. analeptic in the treatment of patients suffering from severe depression.

convulsion an involuntary, generalized, violent muscular contraction, in some cases tonic (contractions without relaxation), in others clonic (alternating contractions and relaxations of skeletal muscles). For epileptic convulsions the term SEIZURE is preferred. See this entry. Also see PSEUDOCONVULSION.

convulsive disorders disorders involving generalized seizures, as in grand mal and petit mal, or focal seizures, as in Jacksonian and psychomotor epilepsy. Also called **epileptic disorders; seizure disorders**.

convulsive therapy a form of psychiatric therapy based on the induction of a generalized seizure by electrical or chemical means. For details, see METRAZOL SHOCK TREATMENT; ELECTROCONVULSIVE TREATMENT.

Cooley, Thomas Benton American pediatrician, 1871–1945. See COOLEY'S ANEMIA; ANEMIA; BLOOD DISORDER; BONE-MARROW DISEASES; DESFERRIOXAMINE; HEMOGLOBINOPATHIES; HYPERTRANSFUSION TREATMENT; IRON OVERLOADING; THALASSEMIA; TRANSFUSIONAL HEMOSIDEROSIS.

Cooley's anemia one of a group of hereditary anemias, thalassemia, characterized by a deficiency in the synthesis of one or more hemoglobin components. C.a. is a homozygous form of beta-chain hemoglobin deficiency that appears in the newborn and often is accompanied by skeletal deformation, mongoloid features, and enlarged heart. An estimated 200,000 persons in the United States are afflicted with the disorder, which is believed to have originated in the Mediterranean basin in prehistoric times. See THALASSEMIA.

cooling of affect the tendency to become emotionally cold. It is a disturbance of affectivity occurring in schizophrenia and in presenile and senile brain disorders.

cooperation working together to produce a common result. Early studies (Crawford, Tsai) indicate that chimpanzees as well as rats reared together performed cooperative food-getting activities. The human infant soon learns to hold still while being dressed, and begins to play with other children at two and a half to three years of age, but team play and group activities do not usually begin until six or seven. Among adults cooperation and competition often exist together, as in football. In industry, workers frequently become more cooperative and more productive if they are encouraged to discuss and set up group goals.

cooperative education a school-administered program that combines study with employment. In higher education, the program especially seeks to enrich academic studies by supplementing them with practical field experience, ideally in responsible jobs in the student's field of interest. Periods of full-time study alternate with periods of full-time employment at intervals of three or six months.

cooperative motive a type of motivation that influences an individual to advance all the members of his group through behavior that is cooperative and neither competitive nor individualistic. Compare COMPETITIVE MOTIVE; INDIVIDUALISTIC MOTIVE.

cooperative reward structure in group situations, a condition in which rewards are assigned on the basis of group rather than individual achievement, and the success of each member promotes the success of the group as a whole. In most cases, the c.r.s. is found to improve group trust, communication, and possibly achievement. Compare COMPETITIVE REWARD STRUCTURE; INDIVIDUALISTIC REWARD STRUCTURE.

cooperative therapy = MULTIPLE THERAPY.

cooperative training a vocational program for high-school students who are placed in jobs related to the occupational fields of their choice. A program coordinator provides classroom instruction that supplements the job experience while monitoring the students' progress on the job by consulting with employers.

cooperative urban house a halfway house in the form of a small residence for ten to 30 ex-mental patients, usually of the same sex, who need minimum supervision and are potentially employable or ready to enroll in an academic program. The residents assume certain responsibilities such as household chores, and participate in group meetings to discuss personal and vocational problems.

cooperators a descriptive term for parents who try to work out a relationship with their children that is based on mutual respect, favoring the use of reason and avoiding strong authoritarian measures that elicit submissive obedience. (Lafore, 1945) Also see APPEASERS; DICTATORS; TEMPORIZERS.

coordination the capacity of various body parts to function together, especially the muscles, as in playing tennis, or the eyes and hands, as in writing shorthand.

coordination of secondary schemes according to Piaget, the increasingly adept and purposeful combination of secondary circular (that is, repetitive) reactions to achieve a desired aim, e.g., picking up a pillow to get a toy placed underneath. This behavior usually emerges near the end of an infant's first year and is distinguished from earlier behavior by the child's ability to choose and coordinate previous schemes that are logically related to the requirements of new situations. This occurs in the latter part of the sensorimotor stage. See SECONDARY CIRCULAR REACTION; SCHEMES. Also see PRIMARY CIRCULAR REACTION; TERTIARY CIRCULAR REACTION.

COP = COMMUNITY OUTREACH PROGRAM.

COPD = CHRONIC-OBSTRUCTIVE PULMONARY DISEASE.

coping behavior any conscious or unconscious adaptation that lowers tension in a stressful experience or situation. Examples of c.b. range from a simple detour around a crowded city street to elaborate defense mechanisms employed to ward off anxiety. Also called **coping mechanisms**.

coping strategy an action, series of actions, or thought process utilized in meeting a stressful or unpleasant situation or in modifying one's reaction to such a situation. Usually, the term implies a conscious and direct approach to problems, in contrast to defense mechanisms. Also see COPING BEHAVIOR.

cop-out a slang expression for quitting or refusing to take responsibility. It is used in transactional analysis for a pattern of exonerating oneself, as in saying "But I couldn't help it."

-copr-; -copro-; -kopr-; -kopro- a combining form relating to feces or filth (from Greek *kopros*, "dung, excrement, filth").

coprolagnia a type of paraphilia in which the sight, or even the thought, of excrement may result in sexual pleasure. Also spelled **koprolagnia**.

coprolalia an uncontrollable impulse to use obscene words and expressions, particularly those related to feces (Greek, "fecal speech"). It is a symptom observed in some chronic schizophrenics, and in patients with Tourette's disorder or latah. Also called **coprophrasia; cacolalia; koprolalia**.

coprophagia /-fā′jē·ə/ eating of feces. It is a symptom occasionally found in chronic, deteriorated schizophrenics, which some psychoanalysts attribute to "an attempt to stimulate the erogenous zone of the mouth with the same pleasurable substance that previously stimulated the erogenous zone of the rectum" (Fenichel, *Psychoanalytic Theory of Neurosis*, 1945). Also called **coprophagy** /-prof′-/; **koprophagia**.

coprophemia the use of obscenities as a paraphilia, e.g., to stimulate sexual excitement. Also spelled **koprophemia**. See SCATALOGIA.

coprophilia an excessive or pathological preoccupation with excreta or filth, or with objects and words that represent feces. Examples are constant jokes or obscene expressions involving defecation; hoarding of feces; sexual excitement only when thinking about feces; and smearing excrement (a symptom found in some hebephrenic patients). In psychoanalytic theory, these tendencies represent a fixation at the second phase of the anal stage, in which the child exhibits interest in fecal material. Also spelled **koprophilia**. See HOARDING; ANAL EROTISM.

coprophobia a morbid fear of excrement, often symbolically expressed as fear of dirt or contamination, and interpreted psychoanalytically as a defense against anal erotism (coprophilia). Also called **scatophobia; koprophobia**.

coprophrasia = COPROLALIA.

copulation coitus, or sexual intercourse. The term usually is applied to the nonhuman procreative act. See COITUS.

copulatory behavior behavior patterns associated with sexual intercourse. C.b. patterns may include species-specific courting activities with peck order or dominance playing a significant role in some animals. Studies of rhesus monkeys show that 20 percent of the males perform 80 percent of the copulations. A female baboon abandons her infant during monthly estrus periods and presents herself to dominant males.

copying mania a morbid, obsessive impulse to imitate the speech or actions of other people, observed in catatonic schizophrenia (echolalia, echopraxia) and certain culture-specific disorders such as AMURAKH and MIRYACHIT. See these entries.

-cor-; -cord- a combining form relating to the heart or any heartlike structure (from Latin *cor*, "heart").

core construct a concept that determines the way a person maintains himself in his environment.

core gender identity physical identity as male or female, which begins to emerge in late infancy and early childhood as a result of the influence of sex chromosomes, development of the fetal gonads, hormones secreted by the fetal gonads, and the development of the external genitals under the influence of hormonal differentiation—all of which affects the body image and gender behavior of a boy or a girl. See GENDER IDENTITY.

core hours: See FLEXIBLE WORK HOURS.

core temperature = DEEP BODY TEMPERATURE.

Cori, Gerty Theresa Radnitz Czech-born American biochemist, 1896–1957. See CORI'S DISEASE.

Cori-Forbes disease = CORI'S DISEASE.

Corino de Andrade: See ANDRADE.

Corino de Andrade's paramyloidosis = ANDRADE'S SYNDROME.

Cori's disease a glycogen-storage disorder with involvement of the heart and muscles. There may be enlargement of the heart and progressive loss of muscle strength. Also called **Type III glycogenosis; Cori-Forbes disease**.

corneal reflection technique a method of studying eye movements with light reflected from the cornea.

corneal transplant an operative procedure in which the opaque cornea of a living patient is removed from the eye and replaced by a clear healthy cornea from a donor. The donor is usually a deceased person who bequeathed his corneas to an eye bank. A c.t. is a relatively safe and simple type of tissue graft because the cornea does not contain blood vessels and there is no risk of rejection of the transplant because of an immune reaction.

Cornelia de Lange's syndrome = DE LANGE'S SYNDROME.

Cornell, William Mason American psychiatrist, 1802–95. C. is remembered mainly for his contributions to mental hygiene.

Cornell Medical Index a psychological test system that was designed originally during World War II for screening potentially unstable military personnel and later adapted for other purposes, such as diagnosing psychosomatic disorders on the basis of pathological mood and anxiety.

Cornell Word Form a modified word-association technique used primarily in industrial psychology to reveal psychiatric and psychosomatic disorders. Each stimulus word is followed by two response words from which the subject is required to select the one that seems to be most closely related to the stimulus, e.g., father—boss, man.

corona glandis: See SMEGMA; TYSON'S GLANDS.

coronary artery bypass a surgical procedure for relief of deficient blood flow to the myocardium by grafting a vein from the patient's own body to portions of the coronary artery that still have a normal blood flow. The graft, usually made with a portion of the saphenous vein of the leg, then bypasses the coronary artery section in which blood flow is restricted. Also called **c.a.b. graft (CABG)**.

coronary heart disease a cardiovascular disorder characterized by restricted flow of blood through the coronary arteries supplying the heart muscle. The cause usually is due to atherosclerosis of the coronary arteries and often leads to fatal myocardial infarction. Behavioral and psychosocial factors frequently are involved in the development and prognosis of the disease. Abbrev.: **CHD**.

coronary occlusion the obstruction or closing of a coronary artery, an event that usually is due to a gradual narrowing of the bore of the artery by atherosclerotic processes or to the formation of a clot, or thrombus. See CORONARY THROMBOSIS.

coronary thrombosis the occlusion of one of the coronary arteries of the heart by the formation of a clot in the artery. The clot, a thrombus, usually results from atherosclerotic changes in the lining of the artery wall and causes a myocardial infarction. C.t. occurs in about one-fourth of all cases of fatal heart attacks. Also see THROMBUS; CORONARY OCCLUSION.

-corp- a combining form relating to a body, a substance, or a structure (from Latin *corpus*, "body, matter, person, framework"; plural: *corpora*).

corpora cavernosa two columns of erectile tissue that form the upper portion of the body of the penis. During erection, the penis acquires the general shape of an inverted prism with the c.c. forming the base of the triangle and a third column of tissue, the corpus spongiosum, beneath the c.c., forming the apex of the prism.

corpora quadrigemina the four rounded prominences on the surface of the midbrain, identified as the left and right superior colliculi and the left and right inferior colliculi.

corporate class a social class comprising, in the United States, the major owners and controllers of wealth, and constituting, according to H. Waitzkin (1978), the one percent of the population who own 80 percent of all corporate stock and who, in 1975, had a median annual income of $114,000 to $142,000.

corpse phobia = NECROPHOBIA.

corpus callosum a bundle of white-matter fibers running through the longitudinal fissure of the brain and connecting the cerebral hemispheres. It is the principal connection between the two sides of the brain. See COMMISSURAL FIBERS.

corpus cavernosum urethrae = CORPUS SPONGIOSUM.

corpuscle any of a group of small bodies distributed throughout the body and containing nerve endings or cells. Kinds of corpuscles include Krause's, Purkinje's, and tactile.

corpuscula lamellosa = PACINIAN CORPUSCLE.

corpus luteum a yellowish glandular mass in the ovary that remains after a follicle has ruptured and released an ovum. The development of the c.l. is stimulated by secretions of the luteinizing hormone of the pituitary gland. The c.l. in turn becomes a transient endocrine gland, secreting estrogen and progesterone.

corpus mamillare = MAMMILLARY BODIES.

corpus spongiosum a column of erectile tissue on the lower side of the body of the penis containing the urethra. The two columns of the corpora cavernosa lie above the c.s., and the three col-

umns are bound together by skin and connective tissue. Also called **corpus cavernosum urethrae**. Also see CORPORA CAVERNOSA.

corpus striatum a mass of gray and white nerve fibers beneath the cortex and in front of the thalamus in each cerebral hemisphere. It contains projection fibers passing in both directions between the thalamus and cortex, as well as cell bodies, giving the c.s. a striped (Latin *striatus*) appearance.

correction in statistics, the elimination or reduction of chance or observational errors. The term applies also specifically to the rectification of visual defects through the use of lenses.

correctional psychology a branch of psychology concerned with the application of counseling and clinical techniques to delinquents and criminals in penal and correctional institutions (reformatories, training schools, penitentiaries). **Correctional psychologists** also participate professionally in court activities, probation departments, parole boards, prison administration, supervision of inmate behavior, and programs for the rehabilitation of offenders. Also see FORENSIC PSYCHOLOGY.

correction for continuity: See YATES CORRECTION.

corrective emotional experience a technique of short-term psychotherapy advocated by Franz Alexander. It consists of reviving an experience the patient could not handle in the past, with the therapist playing a significant role in discussing that experience in order to facilitate insight and change.

corrective therapist an adjunctive health professional who directs therapeutic exercises and physical-education activities in the treatment of mentally or physically ill patients. The c.t. programs are supervised and reviewed by physicians. In addition to improving coordination, strength, and agility, the exercise routines are intended to build morale, self-confidence, and resocialization interests of the patient.

correlate a variable that is related to another variable.

correlated axes: See ORTHOGONAL.

correlation any relationship between two variables, especially a concomitant variation.

correlational method a research method used to establish relationships between two or more variables.

correlational redundancy: See DISTRIBUTIONAL REDUNDANCY.

correlational studies the studies of acts or processes in which two or more variables co-vary, usually with the objective of establishing an orderly relationship between the variables or of considering them together in order to find relationships.

correlation coefficient a statistical index of the magnitude of a relationship between two variables, ranging in value between $+1$ and -1. Also see PRODUCT-MOMENT CORRELATION.

correlation matrix an intercorrelation table,

showing all possible relationships among a set of variables. E.g., the correlations between Variable 1 and Variables 2, 3, 4, and 5 are given, then the correlations between Variable 2 and Variables 3, 4, and 5, etc.

correlation ratio a measure of the magnitude of a curvilinear or nonlinear relationship. Also called **eta** (η).

correspondence the extent to which an observed behavior, such as cutting in on a telephone line, is attributed to a general personality trait, e.g., rudeness or aggressiveness.

corteria the factor of cortical alertness and arousal as displayed on objective tests such as reaction time and flicker-fusion speed (Cattell).

cortex the outer or superficial layer (Greek *kortex*, "bark, rind") of a structure, as distinguished from the central core. The bark of a tree is an example of a c. In the human body, the c. of a structure is identified with the name of the gland or organ, as adrenal c., cerebellar c., cerebral c., or renal c. See ADRENAL-CORTICAL HYPERFUNCTION; ADRENAL C.; AGRANULAR C.; ALLOCORTEX; ARCHICORTEX; ASSOCIATION C.; AUDITORY C.; CELLULAR LAYERS OF C.; CEREBELLAR C.; CEREBRAL C.; CINGULATE C.; COLUMNAR ORGANIZATION OF C.; ENTORHINAL-C. LESION; EXTRINSIC C.; GRANULAR C.; HEMIDECORTICATION; INFEROTEMPORAL C.; INTRINSIC C.; LIMBIC C.; NEOCORTEX; NONSTRIATE VISUAL C.; ORBITOFRONTAL C.; PALEOCORTEX; PERIAMYGDALOID C.; PREMOTOR C.; PRESTRIATE C.; PRIMARY C.; SENSORY C.; STRIATE C.; TERTIARY C.; TRANSITIONAL C.; VISUAL C.; SOMATIC SENSORY AREAS.

Corti, Alfonso Giacomo Gaspare /kôr′tē/ Italian anatomist, 1822–76. See ORGAN OF CORTI; RODS OF CORTI; TECTORIAL MEMBRANE (also called **Corti's membrane**); BASILAR MEMBRANE; COCHLEA; COCHLEAGRAM; EAR; EXTERNAL HAIR CELLS OF EAR; HAIR CELLS; INTERNAL HAIR CELLS; OSSICLES; SCALA MEDIA; SPIRAL GANGLION.

-cortic-; -cortico- a combining form relating to the cortex.

cortical amnesia a form of amnesia due to organic causes, such as a stroke or brain injury.

cortical-arousal factor a term introduced by D. E. Berlyne to identify a humor-evaluative factor. The c.-a.f. is related to ratings that are high on the drowsy-alert and weak-powerful scales, as judged by subjects asked to respond to random adjective-noun combinations.

cortical blindness a condition of complete or partial blindness caused by ischemia, or inadequate blood flow to occipital lobes, in the posterior areas of the cerebrum. The defect usually involves the vessels of the vertebrobasilar arterial network. In most cases of c.b. the condition is accompanied by other neurological deficits usually associated with strokes. Also called **cerebral blindness**.

cortical center areas of the cortex where sensory fibers terminate or motor fibers originate.

cortical deafness deafness that is caused by damage to auditory-nerve tissue in the cortex.

cortical-evoked response = EVOKED POTENTIAL.

corticalization the increased cerebral control of neural functions in higher animals. See ENCEPHALIZATION.

cortical lesions pathological changes in tissues of the cortex of the brain. C.l. may be caused by congenital defects such as hypoplasia, tumor development, cerebral infarction, primary or secondary viral infections, or injury. The sites of c.l. generally determine the type of sensory and/or motor-function effects.

cortical localization of function = LOCALIZATION OF FUNCTION.

cortical motor aphasia = EXPRESSIVE APHASIA.

cortical potentials effects of firing small electrical currents across cortical cells. The procedure generally has been limited to experiments in enhancing consolidation or reinforcing learning experiences or recall of memorized information.

cortical sensory aphasia = WERNICKE'S APHASIA.

cortical undercutting one of a number of types of prefrontal lobotomy used in controlling severe emotional and mental disturbance. In this procedure the skull is opened and long association fibers are severed. The object is to prevent frontal-lobe damage, which affects thinking processes.

cortical zones three types of of cortical regions behind the central sulcus defined by function. They include the **primary c.z.**, consisting of specific-sense primary projection areas, **secondary c.z.**, concerned with perception, and **tertiary c.z.**, with cells that integrate information areas. The c.z. are associated with specific layers of the cortex, layer IV predominating in the primary zones and layers II and III in the secondary zones.

corticobulbar fibers = CORTICONUCLEAR FIBERS.

corticobulbar nucleus a nerve-cell body in the medulla that links neurons of the cortex and the motor system. It is associated with the corticoreticular fibers that terminate in the reticular formation of the rhombencephalon and corticonuclear fibers that innvervate muscles of the face, tongue, and jaws.

corticofugal nerve fibers: See AROUSAL.

corticofusimotor system nerve pathways that involve gamma motoneurons extending from the cerebral cortex to the intrafusal fibers of the muscle spindles. It is part of a feedback loop of the body's motor-control system, and dysfunction of the c.s. results in movement disorders.

corticoids: See GENERAL ADAPTATION SYNDROME.

corticoid therapy the use of a natural adrenal-cortex hormone, or synthetic compound with similar activity, in the treatment of a variety of disorders. Uses include control of bronchial asthma, stimulating the appetite in celiac disease, and relieving the painful symptoms of rheumatoid arthritis. Nearly every organ and function of the body is influenced by one or more of the 50 known corticoid agents.

corticonuclear fibers longitudinal-pyramidal-tract fibers that extend from the cerebral cortex to the mesencephalon, pons, and medulla oblongata. Also called **corticobulbar fibers**.

corticopontine nucleus a neural-cell body in the pathway connecting the cerebral cortex and the pons. The c.n. is a collecting point for numerous fibers from all parts of the cerebral cortex. The individual fibers usually are further labeled as to their origin in the cortex, as **parietopontinus, occipitopontinus**, and so on.

corticoreticular nucleus a nerve-cell body of fibers extending from the cerebral cortex to the reticular formation of the mesencephalon and rhombencephalon.

corticospinal tract nerve fibers that connect the cerebral cortex with the spinal cord. The c.t. contains motor-control fibers that are excitatory for flexor action. The **rubrospinal tract** duplicates much of the c.t. pathway except that it passes through the red nucleus.

corticosteroids any of the steroid hormones produced by the adrenal cortex. Kinds of c. include cortisol, which is involved in carbohydrate metabolism, aldosterone, which has a role in electrolyte balance and sodium retention, and corticosterone, which is active in both functions.

corticosteroid therapy medical treatment that involves the use of corticosteroid drugs to replace or supplement action of the hormones normally secreted by the cortex of the adrenal gland. Following surgery to remove one or both adrenal glands, c.t. may involve intravenous doses of hormones to maintain normal blood pressure, blood sugar, and electrolyte levels. Other forms of c.t. may be employed in the treatment of arthritis, herpes simplex, bronchitis, and pemphigus.

corticosterone a steroid hormone secreted by the adrenal cortex. It is a glucocorticoid hormone with functions that include metabolism of proteins, fats, and carbohydrates into energy sources for body cells.

corticotropin = ADRENOCORTICOTROPHIC HORMONE.

corticotropin-releasing factor a substance produced by the hypothalamus that stimulates the release of the corticotropin hormone by the pituitary gland. The corticotropin hormone in turn stimulates growth and function of the adrenal cortex.

corticovisceral control mechanisms the brain centers that regulate autonomic and hormonal body functions. An example of c.c.m. is the lateral-hypothalamus control of the desire to eat.

cortin a complex of several hormones secreted by the adrenal cortex, including cortisone. C. is important in control of salt intake, regulation of the gonads, and reaction to prolonged stress.

Corti's membrane = TECTORIAL MEMBRANE.

cortisol one of the glucocorticoid hormones secreted by the adrenal cortex. Since 1963, c. and its synthetic analogs have been administered in the treatment of rheumatoid arthritis. Blood levels of c. in humans vary according to wake-sleep cycles, being highest around 9 A.M. and lowest at midnight, and according to other factors, e.g., increasing during pregnancy but decreasing during diseases of the liver and kidneys. Also called **hydrocortisone**.

cortisone a hormone produced by the adrenal cortex, or synthetically.

Corybantic rites in classical mythology, the rites performed in celebration of Cybele, a nature goddess of Phrygia and Asia Minor. The rites included frenzied dancing, which was believed to have a therapeutic effect. See CHOREOMANIA.

coryza: See COMMON COLD.

cosmic consciousness a sense of awareness of the universe as a whole, which appears to be achieved in some cases through hallucinogenic drugs, "peak" experiences, religious ecstasy, or metaphysical disciplines such as yoga exercises and Zen meditation. Also see MYSTIC UNION.

cosmic identification the feeling of identification with the universe: "I am the whole world." In psychiatry, in contradistinction to religion, c.i. is most frequently observed in disorganized (hebephrenic) schizophrenia, and is explained psychoanalytically in terms of regression to the stage of infantile incorporation, when there was no distinction between the self and the outside world. Also see MYSTIC UNION.

cosmic sensitivity the feeling of unity with the entire universe arising out of meditation, religious or mystical experiences, and in some cases body exercises such as yoga, or hallucinogenic drugs. Also see MYSTIC UNION.

cosmology the philosophic study of the basic structure, origin, and evolution of the universe.

-cost- a combining form relating to the ribs (from Latin *costa*, "side, rib"). Adjective: **costal**.

costal stigma = STILLER'S SIGN.

cost-benefit analysis in evaluation research, "an attempt to compare the costs and benefits of a single program by translating each into dollar values and comparing the resulting figures; cost in dollars is compared to benefits in dollars." (W. R. Meyers, *The Evaluation Enterprise*, 1981)

cost containment: See REVIEW.

cost-effectiveness analysis in evaluation research, "an attempt to compare the costs of various programs for attaining a goal or objective that is known or assumed to be worthwhile." (W. R. Meyers, *The Evaluation Enterprise*, 1981)

cost-reward analysis in social psychology, a model that attempts to explain helping behavior according to the reinforcements and costs associated with any specific helping action. That is, a helping act that possesses either high reinforcement value or very low cost value is more likely to be performed than a low-reinforcement, high-cost act.

cost-reward model in environmental psychology, an approach based on an analysis of the potential costs and benefits of different environments. Individuals and companies are likely to choose the environment with the highest reward-to-cost ratio.

Cotard, Jules /kôtär'/ French neurologist, 1840–87. See COTARD'S SYNDROME; VON DOMARUS PRINCIPLE; INSANITY OF NEGATION.

Cotard's syndrome a psychotic state first reported in 1880 by the French neurologist Jules Cotard, characterized by anxious depression, suicidal tendencies, and nihilistic delusions in which the patient insists that his body, and in some cases the whole of reality, has ceased to exist. This symptom pattern most often occurs in women of involutional age. Also called **délire de négation; chronic delusional state of negation**.

cot death = CRIB DEATH.

cotherapy = MULTIPLE THERAPY.

cottage plan decentralized organization of a mental institution or training school, with the patients living in separate, supervised units according to their symptomatology or level of mental retardation.

co-twin control an experimental method in which the relative effects of maturation and learning are gauged by subjecting one twin to special experiences or training while the other serves as a control.

couch in psychoanalysis, the c. on which the patient reclines, on the theory that this posture will facilitate free association, encourage the patient to direct attention to his inward world of feeling and fantasy, and enable him to recover childhood experiences. Also called **analytic c**.

Coué, Emile /kwā/ French pharmacist and psychotherapist, 1857–1926. C. was the originator of a psychotherapeutic system called **Couéism** /kōō·ā'izəm/. See AUTOSUGGESTION.

coumarin derivatives a series of drugs, including sodium warfarin and phenprocoumon, that have anticoagulant activity by inhibiting the formation of prothrombin and clotting factors VII, IX, and X by the liver. C.d. are antivitamins to vitamin K.

counseling professional assistance in coping with emotional, vocational, marital, educational, rehabilitation, retirement, and other personal problems. The counselor makes use of such techniques as guidance, advice, discussion, and administration and interpretaion of tests.

counseling interview an interview that has the purpose of providing psychological guidance or counseling.

counseling ladder the succession of techniques employed by a counselor while guiding the course of treatment.

counseling process the process engaged in by counselor and client as they attempt to define, address, and resolve specific client problems in face-to-face interviews. See COUNSELING.

counseling psychologist a psychologist who has received professional education and training in one or more counseling areas such as education, vocational, employee, old-age, personal, marriage, or rehabilitation counseling. In contrast to a clinical psychologist who usually emphasizes underlying motivation and unconscious factors, a c.p. emphasizes adaptation, adjustment, and more efficient use of the individual's available resources.

counseling relationship the interaction between counselor and client. The c.r. is an affective, personal, yet professional relationship in which the counselor brings his or her professional training, experience, and personal insight to bear on the problems revealed by the client. The relationship in and of itself is considered to be of central importance in effecting desired modifications in the individual.

counseling services a government agency that provides counseling to families with problems associated with social conflicts, e.g., drug addiction or alcoholism. C.s. generally are a subdivision of a state-funded Department of Social Services.

counselor a psychologist or professionally trained individual who specializes in one or more counseling areas such as psychological counseling, geriatric counseling, sex counseling, vocational or career counseling, rehabilitation counseling, educational counseling, marriage and family counseling, or drug counseling. A c. provides professional evaluations, information, and suggestions designed to enhance the client's ability to make decisions and effect desired changes in attitude and behavior.

counselor-centered therapy = DIRECTIVE COUNSELING.

counteraction need a need to overcome difficult challenges rather than accept defeat (Murray).

counterbalancing the process of arranging a series of experimental treatments in such a way as to minimize practice effects, fatigue, or other order effects. A simple form of c. would be to administer experimental conditions in the order ABBA.

countercathexis in psychoanalysis, the psychic energy used by the unconscious to block the entrance of id impulses into consciousness. E.g., an obsessive impulse to wash may block the desire to play with feces; philanthropy may neutralize a concealed tendency to hoard (reaction formation); also, if the love feelings of a child toward a parent (cathexis) are thwarted and repressed, then the psychic energy attached to ideas, fantasies, or persons related to the repressed feelings is spoken of as c. Also called **counterinvestment; anticathexis**. See CATHEXIS.

countercompulsion a compulsion that is secondarily developed to resist the original compulsion when it cannot be continued. The new compulsion then replaces the original so that compulsive behavior can continue.

counterconditioning the extinction of a particular response, such as a fear, through conditioning an incompatible response to the same stimulus. C. is a behavior-therapy technique used in eliminating unwanted behavior and replacing it with a more desirable response. See SYSTEMATIC DESENSITIZATION.

counterconformity a behavioral pattern in conflict with socially approved or group standards.

counterculture a social movement, such as the hippie or drug "cultures," which maintains its own mores and values in opposition to the prevailing cultural norms. Also see YOUTH CULTURE.

counterego the part of the unconscious self that is antagonistic to the ego.

counteridentification a form of countertransference in which the analyst identifies with the patient.

counterinvestment = COUNTERCATHEXIS.

counterirritant an agent that produces a superficial irritation which has the effect of relieving symptoms of another irritation. The effect is based on the gate-control theory of sensory-receptor stimulation. The specific c. depends upon the type and site of the original irritation and may be relieved by heat, cold, various forms of touch, or medications, such as the application of oil of clove as a c. for a toothache.

countermeasure-intervention programs = SOCIAL-REFORM PROGRAMS.

counterphobia the attempt of some phobic individuals to overcome their anxiety and terror by facing and defying the feared object or situation.

countershock mild electrical stimulation administered to an electroconvulsive-shock patient for one minute after the convulsive shock. The purpose of the c. is to relieve some of the common aftereffects of the ECT treatment, e.g., postconvulsion confusion or amnesia.

countertransference in psychoanalysis, the arousal of the analyst's own repressed feelings through identification with the patient's experiences and problems, or through responding in kind to the patient's expressions of love or hostility toward him. This tendency runs counter to the objective attitude of the therapist, but it may also be a source of insight into the patient: The analyst understands the patient by understanding himself. In any case, he must be aware of the c. if it occurs, and analyze it (or have someone else analyze it), so that it does not interfere with the therapeutic process. See DIDACTIC ANALYSIS.

countertransference neurosis in psychoanalysis, neurotic reactions in the analyst precipitated by the patient's reactions to him, or by an unconscious reaction to the patient's neurotic tendencies; e.g., the analyst's repressed paranoid or masochistic tendencies may be aroused.

counterwill: See WILL THERAPY.

counter-wish dream a Freudian term for a dream in which the content is the opposite of what the dreamer wants, though it may conceal a real wish. E.g., an impotent man may dream he has syphilis, since this is likely to imply that he is potent.

counting obsession an obsessive-compulsive impulse to count. See ARITHMOMANIA.

couples therapy = MARRIAGE THERAPY.

coupling in genetics, the association, or linkage, of different hereditary characteristics for several generations, in contrast to the Mendelian principle of independent assortment. See LINKAGE.

coupon-return technique a method of testing advertising effectiveness in a printed medium, e.g., magazine or newspaper, by inducing the consumer to mail a coupon. The c.-r.t. may be utilized on a split-run basis in which the coupon may be offered to only a part of the publication's audience, or several variations may be tested in different demographic areas of the publication's circulation. Some publications cooperate with advertisers using the c.-r.t. by charging for advertising space on a per-inquiry, or p.i., basis, each coupon returned counting as an inquiry.

courtesan fantasy = HETAERAL FANTASY.

courtroom psychology the psychological study of courtroom procedure such as the evaluation and presentation of testimony, methods of interrogation, examination of defendants, guilt-detection techniques, and the functions of an expert witness in commitment, adoption, or criminal proceedings. See FORENSIC PSYCHOLOGY.

courtship behavior the behavior of different species of animals and human beings in different societies or social strata during the courtship period. E.g., in Western societies courtship and engagement are generally regarded as a testing period when the couple should have a full opportunity to become acquainted, explore interests and values, discover areas of agreement and disagreement, and test their responsiveness to each other.

couvade /kōōväd′/ a custom among several non-Western peoples in which the father takes to bed before or after his child is born, as if he himself suffered the pangs of birth. Often he must enact the birth experience in detail, usually subjecting himself to elaborate taboos. (The term is French, derived from Latin *cubare*, "to lie down.")

covariate a correlated variable that is controlled or held constant through the analysis of covariance. E.g., apparently significant differences in means across groups might need to be adjusted for the effects of a c., which could be any variable systematically related to the means.

cover memory = SCREEN MEMORY.

covert denoting anything that is not directly observable, often because it is disguised or concealed.

covert reinforcement a behavioral-therapy technique in which the reinforcement is imagined.

covert response any unobservable response such as a thought, image, emotion, or internal physiological reaction. There are, however, instruments designed to measure covert responses, e.g., polygraphs. The study of covert behavior or "subjective" experience is rejected by behaviorists. Compare OVERT RESPONSE.

covert sensitization a form of aversive conditioning in which noxious mental images are associated in the patient's mind with an undesirable behavior that needs to be eliminated.

Cowper, William English anatomist, 1666–1709. See BULBOURETHRAL GLANDS (also called **Cowper's glands**).

coxa vara a deformity of the hip joint in which the neck of the femur is situated at a right angle. C.v. is one of the forms of orthopedic pathology associated with dwarfism.

Coxsackie infection an enteric virus infection by any of the approximately 30 different Coxsackie viruses responsible for a wide range of diseases, such as childhood respiratory ailments. Other disorders caused by a C.i. include herpangina, aseptic meningitis, epidemic pleurodynia, and paralytic disease. The disease category is named for Coxsackie, New York, where the virus was first isolated.

CP = CEREBRAL PALSY.

CPAP = CONTINUOUS POSITIVE-AIRWAY PRESSURE.

CPI = CALIFORNIA PSYCHOLOGICAL INVENTORY.

CPK = CREATINE PHOSPHOKINASE.

CR = CONDITIONED RESPONSE.

Craig's Wife compulsion: See HOUSEWIFE'S SYNDROME.

cramp a painful, involuntary contraction of a muscle or muscle group. See OCCUPATIONAL C. Also see WERNICKE'S C.

cramp neurosis = WERNICKE'S CRAMP.

-cran-; -crani-; -cranio- a combining form relating to the cranium. Adjective: **cranial**.

cranial anomaly an abnormal head due to a congenital defect that often is related to a chromosomal error. The effect may be manifested as abnormally large, as in cases of hydrocephalus, or abnormally small, as in microcephaly, square-shaped, as in some cases of osteopetrosis, or with sutures that fail to close. Chromosome 17 and 18 often are involved through trisomy or other aberrations.

cranial arteritis: See ARTERITIS.

cranial bifida a congenital disorder manifested by a horseshoe-shaped depression of the medial plane of the forehead. The subject also has a median-cleft palate, a cleft of the nose ranging from a notch to complete division, and eyes that are widely separated. Because of a failure of the two sides of the head to fuse normally during prenatal development, the corpus callosum may be defective. Mental retardation is common.

cranial nerves the 12 pairs of nerves that come directly from the brain and are distributed mainly to structures in the head and neck. Some of the c.n. are sensory, some are motor, and some are both sensory and motor. One mixed nerve, the vagus, innervates organs as far away as the large intestine. C.n. are numbered as follows: I, OLFACTORY NERVE; II, OPTIC NERVE; III, OCULOMOTOR NERVE; IV, TROCHLEAR NERVE; V, TRIGEMINAL NERVE; VI, ABDUCENS NERVE; VII, FACIAL NERVE; VIII, STATOACOUSTIC NERVE; IX, GLOSSOPHARYNGEAL NERVE; X, VAGUS NERVE; XI, ACCESSORY NERVE; XII, HYPOGLOSSAL NERVE. See these entries.

cranial pia mater: See PIA MATER.

craniofacial anomalies structural deformities that involve the face and cranium. C.a. usually are congenital disorders. Examples include Treacher Collins' syndrome, hypertelorism, Crouzon's disease, microcephaly, and Hurler's syndrome.

craniofacial dysostosis = CROUZON'S DISEASE.

craniograph a chart or photograph of the skull; also, an instrument for measuring skulls.

craniology the scientific study of size, shape, and other characteristics of the human skull. The term is also applied to F. J. Gall's and J. K. Spurzheim's pseudoscience of PHRENOLOGY. See this entry. Also see CRANIOSCOPY.

craniometry the measurement of the skull. See CRANIOLOGY.

craniosacral system the parasympathetic nerve network that runs through the spinal cord but extends branches only through four cranial and three spinal nerves. The cranial nerves of the system are the oculomotor, facial, glossopharyngeal, and vagus nerves. The spinal nerves are those of the pelvic plexus.

cranioscopy a technique employed by phrenologists, who palpated the various prominences of the skull in order to learn the strengths and weaknesses of the brain areas beneath. This unscientific method originated with the notion that the skull is larger above cranial areas associated with highly developed mental functions, thereby indicating where an individual's superior talents are centered. See PHRENOLOGY.

craniosinus fistula: See FISTULA.

craniostenosis a skull deformity caused by premature closing of the cranial sutures. The condition restricts normal development of brain structures and usually results in mental retardation.

craniosynostosis syndrome a condition caused by premature fusion of cranial bones, resulting in a skull deformity. The sagittal suture along the top of the skull is most often involved. Premature closing of one suture is unlikely to affect brain growth or intelligence, but premature fusion of multiple sutures increases the risk of neurologic disorders.

craniotelencephalic dysplasia a type of craniosynostosis accompanied by protrusion of the frontal skull bone, mental retardation, and with or without encephalocele (brain herniation through the skull). The disorder does not appear to be familial or hereditary, and chromosomes of the patients do not show abnormalities.

craniotomy the surgical opening of the skull. The practice of c. represents one of the oldest types of surgery, as evidence of c. has been found in prehistoric skulls in every part of the world except southern Asia. C. is a common procedure for diagnosis and therapy of many types of brain injury and disease, such as brain abscess, brain tumor, and brain hemorrhage. Also see TREPHINATION.

cranium bifidum with encephalocele a CNS disorder involving a skull-fusion defect that permits a herniation of the meninges through the opening. If the herniation contains neural tissue, it is identified as an encephalocele. The most common site for the defect is the occiput. About half the persons born with the disorder have less-than-normal intelligence. Also see MENINGO-CELE.

crashing withdrawal symptoms, usually dominated by severe feelings of depression, that occur at the end of a run with an amphetamine drug. During a c. phase, the drug abuser may sleep for several days more or less continuously, displaying signs of exhaustion and irritation during waking periods. Tolerance to the drug is lost during withdrawal. The term applies also to the period following the "rush" or "high" produced by taking cocaine intravenously. As feelings of euphoria wear off, they are replaced by irritability, depression, or anxiety, along with a strong urge for another dose. Also called **crash period**.

Crawford Small Parts Dexterity Test a psychomotor test involving several manipulative skills: use of tweezers in inserting pins in holes and placing a collar over each pin, and placing small screws in threaded holes and screwing them down with a screwdriver.

craze a widespread and enthusiastic adoption of an unusual behavior or FAD. See this entry.

craze of why = FOLIE DU POURQUOI.

crazy-chick disease: See LEUKOENCEPHALOMALA-CIA.

creatine phosphokinase an enzyme present in heart muscle, skeletal muscle, and brain tissues. High levels of c.p. in the blood generally are a sign of disease or tissue damage, e.g., muscular dystrophy or myocardial infarction. Electrophoresis techniques can identify the sources as myocardial (MB), heart or skeletal muscle (MM), and brain (BB); the MB form is usually specific for myocardial infarction. Abbrev.: **CPK**.

creative imagination a process whereby dormant unconscious elements are organized with conscious thoughts to produce new ideas.

creative self a concept proposed by Adler to emphasize the dynamic aspects of human development. The c.s. was never fully defined, but was described as the "first cause" of all behavior and the "active principle of life," comparable to the concept of soul. Its function was to guide each individual in his quest for experiences that would enable him to realize his unique style of life.

creative thinking the mental processes leading to a new invention, solution, or synthesis in any area. A creative solution may use preexisting objects or ideas but creates a new relationship between the elements it utilizes. New mechanical inventions, social techniques, scientific theories, and artistic creations are examples of c.t. Compare FUNCTIONAL FIXEDNESS.

creativity the ability to apply original ideas to the solution of problems; the development of theories, techniques, or devices; or the production of novel forms of art, literature, philosophy, or science. In psychoanalytic theory, c. is attributed to sublimation, or transformed expres-

sion, of unconscious impulses (usually erotic or hostile), which might otherwise lead to neurosis. In psychological studies, attempts have been made to analyze the process of creative thinking, though no full answer has been found to the question why one individual or group is creative and another is not. See CREATIVE THINKING; CREATIVITY TEST.

creativity test a psychological test designed to identify creative ability, or "divergent thinking," which is believed to be as essential in the sciences as in the arts. Existing tests focus on a variety of factors, such as word and ideational fluency, original associations, solutions to practical problems, suggesting different endings to stories, and listing unusual uses for objects.

creeping and crawling aids devices that can aid a handicapped child in gaining mobility while exercising the muscles and neural circuits involved in normal movements. Examples include wheeled creepers, wheeled crawlers, beach balls, plastic barrels, and scooterlike carts that can be propelled by the arm muscles.

cremasteric reflex the contraction of the cremaster muscle, which extends in loops over the spermatic cord as far as the testes. The c.r. is demonstrated by stroking the skin on the inside of the male thigh, causing the testes to be drawn upward toward the abdomen.

cremaster muscle a muscle composed of fibers extending from the internal abdominal muscle with a function of suspending the testis.

cremnophobia a morbid fear of precipices. Also see BATHOPHOBIA.

crenated notched or scalloped. E.g., red blood cells become c. in a hypertonic medium that reduces the fluid content of the cells.

-crepusc- a combining form relating to twilight (Latin *crepusculum*).

crepuscular animals animals that are most active in a dimly lighted environment, such as the outdoors at twilight. Bats are c.a.

Crespi effect an increase in learning or response strength disproportionate to the reinforcement.

cretinism a thyroid-deficiency condition first described in 1657 by the Austrian physician Wolfgang Hoefer. The term is derived from an Old French word, *chrétien*, "Christian," because many early victims were children of a European Christian sect that lived in isolated valleys on iodine-deficient food. See CONGENITAL HYPO-THYROIDISM; ATHYREOSIS.

Creutzfeldt, Hans Gerhard /kroits'felt/ German psychiatrist, 1885–1964. See CREUTZFELDT-JAKOB DISEASE; SLOW VIRUS; UNCONVENTIONAL VIRUS.

Creutzfeldt-Jakob disease a form of rapidly progressive dementia that occurs world-wide in certain individuals past the age of 40. Vacuoles form in the neurons, giving the brain a spongy appearance. Myoclonic jerks are an early sign of the disease, which is believed to be caused by a slow virus that may not produce symptoms until many years after exposure. Abbrev.: **CJD**. Also called **Jakob-Creutzfeldt disease; Heidenheim's disease**.

Creveld, Simon van Dutch pediatrician, 1894—. See ELLIS-VAN CREVELD SYNDROME.

crib death the sudden, unanticipated death of an infant with no apparent reason. The victim usually is a child between the ages of one and 12 months who dies quietly during sleep with no signs of a struggle or sounds of distress. Autopsy often shows the cause to be infant botulism acquired by the ingestion of botulinal spores from unwashed toys or other objects placed in the mouth. Others show signs of an unsuspected heart or nervous-system disorder. Still another cause may be a respiratory-system inflammation, hypoxia, or a temporary obstruction of the breathing passages. Also called **cot death; sudden-infant-death syndrome (SIDS)**.

cribiform plate a sievelike layer in the skull that supports the olfactory bulb which has olfactory-receptor fibers that extend through the holes to the olfactory epithelium.

cricoid cartilage a ring-shaped cartilage. The term is usually applied to any of about 20 horseshoe-shaped cartilaginous rings that hold the trachea (windpipe) open.

cri du chat syndrome /krēdēshä'/ a chromosomal disorder involving a chromosome 5 defect resulting in severe mental retardation, walking and talking difficulty or inability, and an anomaly of the epiglottis and larynx that causes a high-pitched wailing cry like that of a cat (French, "cat's cry"). Almost all patients are microcephalic. The defect seems to be hereditary. Also called **chromosome 5, deletion of short arm; 46,XX5p—; cat-cry syndrome; crying-cat syndrome**.

Crigler, John Fielding, Jr. American physician, 1919—. See CRIGLER-NAJJAR SYNDROME.

Crigler-Najjar syndrome an autosomal-recessive disorder involving a deficiency of the enzyme gluconyl transferase. The condition is marked by severe brain damage and excessive bilirubin in the tissues. Most of the patients die within 15 months after birth.

crime from sense of guilt the commission of a crime by an individual with an unconscious need for punishment. According to psychoanalysts, this need is related to repressed oedipal wishes.

criminal commitment the confinement of a person in a mental institution either because he has been found not guilty by reason of insanity or in order to establish his competency to be tried as a responsible defendant.

criminal intent a legal term indicating a conscious disregard of the law, which is presumed to be known by the defendant.

criminality a fixed pattern of illegal antisocial behavior such as stealing, rape, or assault.

criminally insane characterizing a defendant who is judged to be insane and therefore not responsible for the criminal act he is alleged to have committed.

criminal psychiatry the branch of criminology that studies the psychological aspects of crime and the criminal personality. In addition to personality factors, social environment and heredity may also be investigated.

criminal psychology a branch of psychology that specializes in criminal behavior. See CRIMINAL PSYCHIATRY.

criminal responsibility a legal term meaning that before a person charged with a crime can be convicted, it must be proved in court that he possessed the ability to formulate a criminal intent at the time of the alleged crime. The court may appoint a psychiatrist or psychiatrists to help determine whether he had that ability or lacked criminal responsibility by reason of insanity. See COMPETENCY TO STAND TRIAL; DURHAM RULE; M'NAGHTEN RULES; IRRESISTIBLE IMPULSE.

criminology the science of the causes, effects, and sociopsychologic aspects of crime, including penology and rehabilitation.

crisis a situation or event that produces stress and precipitates marked disorganization of behavior or affect; also, a turning point or period in which a decisive change for the better or worse occurs (Greek *krisis*, "decision, putting apart"). See CRITICAL PERIOD.

crisis center in psychiatry, a facility established for emergency therapy or referral.

crisis effect the fact that direct action to study and prevent disasters tends to be undertaken only during or immediately after a crisis. E.g., an imminent drought may induce officials to enact water-conservation measures whereas the potential of a future drought is far less likely to stimulate action.

crisis groups groups organized by a mental-health facility to explore and resolve crisis situations, such as loss of a job, arrest of a child for shoplifting, a bad LSD trip, or withdrawal of financial support for a patient.

crisis intervention the administration of psychotherapy when a highly disruptive experience taxes an individual's coping skills, such as the sudden death of a loved one. By c.i. techniques, more serious consequences of the experience are avoided.

crisis-intervention group psychotherapy group therapy directed to alleviating emotional disturbances resulting from situational crises, such as civilian or military disasters, or other situations involving overwhelming stress.

crisis team a group of professionals and paraprofessionals trained and prepared to handle psychiatric emergencies such as suicide threats or attempts, situations involving danger to the individual or others, or sudden decompensation, that is, breakdown.

crisis theory the body of concepts that deals with the nature of a crisis, crisis behavior, crisis precipitants, crisis prevention, crisis intervention, and crisis resolution.

crisis therapy psychiatric or psychological intervention provided on an emergency, "drop-in," basis for such crises as psychotic break, suicidal threats, acute alcoholism, drug intoxication, continuous seizures, or family crises.

crispation = DYSPHORIA NERVOSA.

crista = CRYSTA.

criteria-referenced testing an approach to testing based on the comparison of a subject's performance with an established standard or criterion. The criterion is fixed; that is, each subject's score is measured against the same criterion and does not influence the relative standing of others. C.-r.t. is associated with the assessment of mastery of subject content, e.g., the score reveals what percentage of items the testee can answer correctly. Compare NORM-REFERENCED TESTING.

criterion a standard by which a judgment can be made; a test or score against which other tests, scores, or items are tested. E.g., a well-validated test of creativity might be used as the c. to select new tests of creativity.

criterion behavior a response, aspect of behavior, score, or value that represents the standard or model used to evaluate other responses, types of behavior, scores, or values.

criterion data information obtained from personnel appraisals or other sources that may be used in measuring job-related behavior.

criterion dimensions in industrial psychology, the use of multiple criteria for evaluating overall job performance of an employee. The c.d. may include such aspects as productivity, effectiveness, absences, errors, and accidents. Multiple criteria are considered especially reliable because an individual may be outstanding in one aspect of job performance but below average in another.

criterion group a group tested for traits it is already known to possess, usually for the purpose of validating a test. E.g., a group of children with diagnosed visual disabilities may be given a visual test to assess its reliability in relation to the specific dimension.

criterion validity an index of how well a test predicts a criterion; the ability of a test to predict behavior accurately. Also called **predictive validity**.

critical common-sense approach: See DISTRIBUTIVE ANALYSIS AND SYNTHESIS.

critical flicker frequency the rate at which a periodic change, or flicker, in an intense visual stimulus fuses into a smooth, continuous stimulus. A similar phenomenon can occur with rapidly changing auditory stimuli. Also called **fusion frequency**.

critical-incident technique a method of studying job performance through descriptions of specific instances of job behavior that are characteristic of either satisfactory or unsatisfactory workers.

critical period a definite stage when an organism is especially "ripe" or open to specific learning, emotional, or socializing experiences that are necessary for healthy development and will not

occur in a later stage. E.g., according to Lorenz, the first three days of life constitute a c.p. for imprinting in ducks; and, according to Caldwell, infants exhibit increasingly severe emotional reactions to adoption between three and twelve months of age. See SENSITIVE PERIOD.

critical point a point in psychotherapy when the patient sees his problem clearly and decides on an appropriate course of action to deal with it.

critical ratio a mean difference or coefficient of correlation divided by its standard error. The c.r. is used in tests of significance or data reliability.

critical region the area under a portion of a statistical curve within which the null hypothesis will be rejected.

critical score a score used as a dividing line between groups or categories, e.g., a passing score.

critical thinking a form of directed thinking which includes such purposeful mental activities as examining the validity of a hypothesis, interpreting the meaning of a poem, or comparing the effectiveness of different types of psychotherapy.

critical value a number above or below which a statistic is significant.

criticizing faculty an expression used by Freud to characterize conscience, or the superego. He pointed out that healthy individuals may be more or less severe with themselves, but that in depressives, the superego may become overcritical, abusive, reproachful, and humiliating toward the ego, or self.

Crocodile Man a term applied to the forensically intriguing case of Charles Decker (1974) whose sudden murderous assaults had no apparent reason and did not seem to be in keeping with his personality. The defense focused on the issue of brain chemistry and criminal violence, arguing that Decker suffered from a dysfunction or lesion of the limbic system that released impulses that might be comparable to those of a crocodile. Also see ISOLATED EXPLOSIVE DISORDER.

crocodile tears = BOGORAD'S SYNDROME.

Crohn, Burrill Bernard American physician, 1884—. See CROHN'S DISEASE.

Crohn's disease an inflammation of the small intestine characterized by the development of cobblestonelike ulcers on the interior surface and a thickening of the intestinal wall. The cause is unknown, but C.d. is most likely to affect persons in their 20s. Because of the symptoms of abdominal pain and cramps, fever, and diarrhea, C.d. often is mistaken for appendicitis. It is treated with antibiotics and anticholinergic drugs.

crop milk a fluid secreted in the crops of doves which is fed to the squabs, or offspring, for several weeks until they are able to provide their own food. The c.m. is provided by both the parents.

cross adaptation the change in sensitivity to one stimulus by adaptation to another.

cross addiction = CROSS TOLERANCE.

cross breaks = CROSS TABULATIONS.

cross conditioning conditioning to a stimulus that is coincidental to an unconditioned stimulus, e.g., a postural reflex.

cross-correlation mechanism the auditory mechanism that permits sound localization by an individual through the brief time difference required by sound to reach auditory nerves in both ears and summate effectively.

cross correspondence in psychic research, messages in automatic writing by one medium that are interpreted by another.

cross-cultural approach the observation, study, or comparison of a specific practice or behavioral pattern in persons of different cultures, e.g., the comparison of diverse sexual patterns, child-rearing practices, or therapeutic attitudes and techniques. Also called **cross-cultural method**.

cross-cultural psychiatry the comparative study of mental illness and mental health among various societies around the world, including data on the incidence of disorders and variations in symptomatology. Also called **comparative psychiatry; cultural psychiatry; ethnopsychiatry; transcultural psychiatry**. Also see CULTURE-SPECIFIC SYNDROMES.

cross-cultural testing testing of individuals with diverse cultural backgrounds and experiences, including people in the newly developing nations, and those associated with subcultures, minority cultures, and the disadvantaged within a dominant culture. The need for cross-cultural tests is due to the demand for increasing educational and work opportunities among all segments of the world's population. Typically, such tests are nonverbal in instructions and content, avoid objects indigenous to a particular culture, and usually deemphasize speed. Specific examples are the Leiter International Performance Test, the Culture-Fair Intelligence Test, the Progressive Matrices, the Goodenough Draw-a-Man test, and the Goodenough-Harris Drawing Test.

cross dependence of hallucinogens a temporary tolerance effect that develops in the use of alkylamine-derived psychedelic drugs. E.g., a user of lysergic acid diethylamide (LSD), which is a substituted indole alkylamine, tends to have a similar tolerance for mescaline, a substituted phenyl alkylamine. A similar kind of cross dependence occurs in users of barbiturates and other sedatives, e.g., alcohol.

cross dressing the process or habit of putting on the clothes of the opposite sex, (a) by heterosexual males or females with the purpose of achieving sexual excitement (fetishistic c.d.), (b) as part of a performance in which women are mimicked or mocked by a man (effeminate homosexuality), or (c) as one attempt at transformation into the opposite sex (transsexualism). See TRANSVESTITISM; TRANSVESTISM.

crossed dominance the tendency for some right-handed persons to have a stronger or dominant left eye, and vice versa for the left-handed.

crossed-extension reflex a reflexive action by a contralateral limb to compensate for loss of support by an injured limb. The reflex, which helps shift the burden of body weight, also is associated with the coordination of legs in walking by flexing muscles on the left side when those on the right are extending, and vice versa.

crossed-nerve experiments studies which found that although nerves in mammals can be transferred to different muscles, the muscles then act as would those to which the nerves were originally connected. E.g., when nerves to leg muscles are crossed, the animal extends when it should flex, and vice versa.

crossed perception = SYNESTHESIA.

cross-eye a type of squint or strabismus in which there is a deviation of one or both eyes toward the other. The condition usually begins in infancy and is caused by a deficiency in the activity of one or more extraocular muscles. Uncorrected c.-e. results in double visual images or amblyopia, a type of blindness caused by unconscious suppression of the visual imputs of one of the eyes. C.-e. can be treated surgically in most cases. Also called **esotropia; convergent strabismus**.

cross fostering a technique for investigating the effect of genetic factors in the development of a disorder by having offspring of normal biologic parents reared by adopting parents who manifest the disorder being studied, or having offspring of parents with the disorder reared by normal adopting parents. Offspring that are cross-fostered in this manner are called **index adoptees**. See CONTROL ADOPTEES.

cross-gender behavior the process or habit of assuming the role of the opposite sex by adopting the clothes, hair design, manner of speaking and gesturing that society considers characteristic of the opposite sex. See CROSS DRESSING.

cross-linkage theory = EVERSION THEORY OF AGING.

cross-modal association the coordination of sensory inputs involving both cerebral hemispheres. C.-m.a. usually is required in matching tasks that involve auditory and visual, tactual and visual, or a similar combination of cognitive functions. Lesions in temporal, parietal, or occipital lobes may be diagnosed by c.-m.a. testing.

cross-modal transfer the transfer of information from one sensory source into an association area where it can be integrated with information from another sensory source. C.-m.t. is required in tasks that coordinate two or more sensory-motor activities, such as playing a musical instrument according to the pattern of notes on a page of sheet music. Also called **cross-modal perception; intersensory perception**.

crossover (in genetics): See RECOMBINATION.

crossover design an experimental procedure in which a treatment is introduced and withdrawn, and often introduced and withdrawn again, with assessment of behavior before and after these treatments. Also called **reversal design**.

cross-parental identification a strong emotional attachment for a parent of the opposite sex.

Crossroads: See CONFRONTATIONAL METHODS.

cross-sectional study a research project conducted at one point in time, and therefore one that does not study development or changes over time. Also called **cross-sectional method**. Compare LONGITUDINAL STUDY.

cross tabulations arrangement of data in tables to show the influence of one or more variables. Also called **cross breaks**.

cross tolerance the ability of one drug to produce effects of another when the body has developed a tissue tolerance for effects of the first substance. A person who has developed a dependence upon alcohol can substitute barbiturates to prevent withdrawal symptoms, and vice versa. Similarly, a c.t. can develop between mescaline and lysergic acid diethylamide (LSD) even though they have different molecular characteristics. Also called **cross addiction**.

cross validation the process of reestablishing a test's validity on a new sample, to check the correctness of the initial validation. C.v. is necessary because chance and other factors may have inflated or biased the original validation.

Crouzon, Octave /krōōzôN′/ French neurologist, 1874–1938. See CROUZON'S DISEASE; CRANIOFACIAL ANOMALIES; DISFIGUREMENT; DYSOSTOSIS.

Crouzon's disease a form of craniosynostosis characterized by a wide skull with a protrusion near the anterior fontanel, a beaked nose, and ocular abnormalities. The visual anomalies may include optic atrophy, divergent strabismus, and blindness. Mild-to-moderate mental retardation is typical. Other neurologic disorders may result from intracranial pressure. Also called **craniofacial dysostosis**.

crowd behavior the characteristic behavior of an unorganized group of people who congregate temporarily when their attention is focused on the same object or event. Typically, an **audience** is a relatively passive crowd that may smile, laugh, or applaud; a **milling crowd** on New Year's Eve is likely to shout, jostle, and sing; and a mob is even more active since it may stampede and perform irrational acts such as lynching or bomb-throwing. Also see MOB; COLLECTIVE BEHAVIOR; CROWD CONSCIOUSNESS; MOB PSYCHOLOGY; MASS HYSTERIA.

crowd consciousness the mentality of a crowd or mob. Mobs are usually distinguished from crowds by their activity, irrationality, and potential for violence. The tendency for people in crowds to act emotionally and sometimes do what they would ordinarily condemn was attributed by Le Bon to the loss of personal responsibility engendered by a temporary suspension of identity or merging with the crowd's "unitary consciousness." Also see CROWD BEHAVIOR.

crowd fear = DEMOPHOBIA.

crowding in learning, a situation that contains too many items or tasks for the time allowed, e.g., an exam requiring the student to respond to 20 in-depth essay questions in one hour. In social psychology, c. refers to psychological tension produced in environments of high population density.

crucial experiment an experiment that is decisive in determining whether a given hypothesis is to be accepted or rejected.

crude score = RAW SCORE.

crura: See CRUS.

crura cerebri: See CEREBRAL PEDUNCLES.

crus a leglike part of the body (Latin, "leg, shin"), such as the ventral portion of the cerebral peduncle, called the c. cerebri. When used without a modifying term, c. generally identifies the portion of the leg between the knee and the foot. Plural: **crura**.

crus communis a part of the superior semicircular canal that joins with the posterior semicircular canal to form a common passageway into the vestibule of the bony labyrinthe.

crus penis the posterior portion of the corpora cavernosa, in the area where these columns are attached to the internal supporting tissues of the pelvis.

crutches devices, usually made of wood or metal, designed to aid handicapped individuals in walking by providing support for the upper limbs. A standard wood crutch consists of two vertical pieces with a thick horizontal bar at the top that fits under the armpit and a smaller horizontal bar at the hand level. The vertical pieces are attached at the bottom to a thick rubber-tipped shaft. Types of metal c. include the Lofstrand, an aluminum tube with a forearm cuff and a handbar, and the Canadian elbow-extensor model, which is similar to the Lofstrand crutch but is designed to fit on the upper arm rather than the forearm.

-cry-; -cryo- a combining form relating to cold or freezing (from Greek *kryos*, "icy cold, frost").

crying weeping, shedding tears, sobbing, which may be elicited by a variety of experiences and needs: frustration, defeat, sadness, pain, shame, or a need for help. C. may also be employed by hysterical or histrionic individuals, consciously or unconsciously, for secondary gain (sympathy; power over others).

crying-cat syndrome = CRI DU CHAT SYNDROME.

cryogenic methods the use of extremely cold temperatures in diagnostic, therapeutic, or investigational procedures. Certain immunoglobulins associated with a variety of diseases are detected in the blood by reducing the temperature of a blood sample to 4°C (39°F), at which point the substances separate from the blood serum. C.m. are used to freeze tissue samples to be sliced for microscope slides. **Cryogenic surgery** is employed in the destruction of thalamic lesions responsible for symptoms of Parkinson's disease, and **supercold surgery** may be used in operations for cataracts and retinal detachment.

cryophobia = PSYCHROPHOBIA.

cryoprobe a surgical instrument sometimes used in the treatment of neurologic disorders such as Parkinson's disease. The c., containing liquid nitrogen, may be applied to the globus pallidus to destroy cells associated with the rigidity symptoms and/or the thalamus to destroy cells responsible for tremor.

cryothalamectomy the therapeutic destruction of groups of neurons in the thalamus by the application of extreme cold. C. is used in the treatment of a variety of neuromuscular disorders, e.g., torticollis and spastic hemiparesis, that fail to respond to more conservative measures.

-crypt-; -crypto- a combining form meaning concealed (Greek *kryptos*).

cryptesthesia the experience of clairvoyance, clairaudience, or similar forms of paranormal cognition that cannot be associated with any known sensory stimulus.

Cryptococcus a genus of fungus that can cause meningitis infections and CNS lesions. The specific agent, Cryptococcus neoformans, occurs world-wide, but in North America it is encountered most often in the southeastern United States, where men between the ages of 40 and 60 are most frequently the victims. Primary target organs are the lungs and kidneys, but CNS effects include, in addition to meningitis, meningeal granulomas, infarcts, glial-tissue increase and general tissue destruction. Symptoms include headaches, blurred vision, confusion, depression, and behavioral abnormalities such as improper speech or dress. Also called **Torula**.

cryptogenic symbolism the use of mental imagery to represent mental functions (Silberer).

cryptomnesia the memories of repressed or forgotten experiences that appear as new and sometimes creative ideas.

cryptophoric symbolism a form of indirect or hidden representation; a pictorial representation based on a metaphor. C.s. is sometimes called **metaphoric symbolism**.

cryptophthalmos syndrome a familial or hereditary disorder in which a child is born with skin covering the eyes. The anomaly may occur on one side or both. The eyes usually are present under the facial skin, which lacks eyelids, eyelashes, and, usually, tear ducts, and the patient may be able to discern light and colors. Hearing loss is common as are ear anomalies. The patients are often mentally retarded.

cryptorchid a male whose testes have not descended into the scrotum. The condition (**cryptorchidism**) is not unusual and does not interfere with male hormonal function, but sperma-

togenesis is unlikely if the c. is not treated in childhood. The untreated c. also has an increased incidence of testicular cancer in later life. See ARRESTED TESTIS; HYPERMOBILE TESTES.

crysta an enlargement at the end of each semicircular canal in which an encapsulated group of sensory-hair cells is embedded in a gelatinous material. As the fluid in the canals moves with the movement of the head, the sensory hairs also are moved, firing neurons that transmit signals to the brain indicating the position of the head in the external environment. Also spelled **crista**. Plurals: **crystae; cristas**.

crystal: See PHENCYCLIDINE.

crystal gazing a hypnotherapy technique in which a hypnotized subject is instructed to visualize significant experiences, or produce associations, while staring into a glass ball, light bulb, or mirror. C.g. is used also by mediums to produce what they claim to be extrasensory perception of events in the lives of their clients. Also called **scrying**.

crystallization in general, the process of assuming definite form, as with one's attitudes, values, or goals. More specifically, according to E. Ginzberg, c. is the emergence of a career direction or the decision to enter a given field. He holds that c. in this sense typically occurs during the "realistic stage" of adolescence, a period characterized by realistic examination of career options based on individual interest, abilities, and educational opportunities. Also see EXPLORATION; FANTASY PERIOD.

crystallized abilities those abilities, such as vocabulary, mechanical knowledge, and logical reasoning, that are a function of learning and experience in a specific culture. C.a. are believed to depend somewhat less than fluid abilities on physiological condition; thus, they may be better sustained in old age. Compare FLUID ABILITIES.

crystallized intelligence: See CRYSTALLIZED ABILITIES.

crystallophobia = HYELOPHOBIA.

Cs: See SYSTEMATIC APPROACH.

CS = CONDITIONED STIMULUS.

CSF = CEREBROSPINAL FLUID.

CSR = CONTINUED-STAY REVIEW.

CT computerized *tomography* scan. See COMPUTERIZED AXIAL TOMOGRAPHY.

CTA = COMBINED TRANSCORTICAL APHASIA.

cuckoo theory: See ORIGIN-OF-LANGUAGE THEORIES.

cuddling behavior a form of attachment behavior initiated by the mother or sometimes by the child as a means of allaying feelings of fear, fatigue, or strangeness. "Noncuddlers" are not necessarily detached, but may be so active that they resist close and confining physical contact.

cue reduction the ability of a portion of a stimulus to elicit a total response. E.g., a two-year-old child will reach for a kitten when he only sees the end of its tail. See MINIMAL CUE; REDUCED CUE.

cues to localization auditory signals that indicate the source of a sound. Cues may include intensity (which should be greater in the ear nearest the source), phase (which is more easily detectable at frequencies below 800 cycles per second), and time difference between the arrival of the sound at one ear and, a small fraction of a second later, at the other ear.

cul-de-sac: See BLIND ALLEY.

Cullen, William Scottish physician and chemist, 1710–90. C. was the first to use "neurosis" for all types of mental disorders (melancholia, convulsions, anxiety attacks, etc.), which he attributed to physiological disturbances and treated with diet, purging, blistering, and bloodletting.

cult a group of individuals bound together by a set of strongly felt beliefs, often of a dogmatic or esoteric nature. The term also applies to the ideology and related rituals that may be used for such purposes as worship, exorcism, or the treatment of mental or physical disease.

cult of personality a group of individuals bound together by devotion to a charismatic political, religious, literary, or other leader. Also called **personality cult.**

cultural absolutism the view that values, concepts, and achievements of diverse cultures can be understood and judged according to a universal standard; also, the idea that a psychological theory developed in one culture has equal validity in a different cultural setting. Compare CULTURAL RELATIVISM.

cultural adaptability the ability of individuals or groups to adapt to the culture of a new community to which they have migrated.

cultural anthropology: See ANTHROPOLOGY.

cultural area = CULTURE AREA.

cultural assimilation the learning and adoption of customs of another culture in order to merge with it. The term is also used for ACCULTURATION. See this entry.

cultural deprivation lack of opportunity to participate in the culture of the larger society due to such factors as economic deprivation, substandard living conditions, or discrimination. See CULTURALLY DEPRIVED. Also see PSEUDORETARDATION.

cultural determinism the theory or premise that character patterns are largely influenced by culture, that is, the combined features of a given society's economic, social, political, and religious organization. C.d. is aligned with the view that environment and learning influence personality to a greater extent than biological or hereditary factors. **Social determinism** usually refers to the view that history is primarily influenced by broad social forces. Also see DETERMINISM.

cultural-familial mental retardation a term applied to mental retardation that develops in the absence of any organic cause and is therefore attributed to hereditary or environmental factors.

culturalists a term used to refer to therapists who

—in contrast to Freud—are not content with primary emphasis on the individual and who prefer instead to look at the overall social context in dealing with personality. Examples are Horney and E. Fromm. Also see NEO-FREUDIAN.

cultural items test questions that cannot be correctly answered unless the testee is sufficiently familiar with their cultural or subcultural meanings. C.i. constitute bias in favor of the group or social class from whose experience they are drawn. See CULTURE-FAIR TESTS.

cultural lag the tendency of one aspect of a culture to change at a slower rate than another, resulting in a retention of dated or obsolete beliefs, customs, and values.

culturally deprived disadvantaged persons, usually children, who are members of a minority group or subculture in which early family and social environment is inadequate preparation for successful adjustment, specifically in school. Deprivation may include physical, social, intellectual, and emotional aspects. Also see CULTURALLY DISADVANTAGED; CULTURAL DEPRIVATION.

culturally different persons or children who are members of a minority group or subculture that differs substantially from the larger society and is, frequently, economically disadvantaged. The term may merely indicate different racial, national, or ethnic background, but more commonly it is used as a nonpejorative term equivalent to CULTURALLY DEPRIVED. See this entry.

culturally disadvantaged children whose culturally deprived environments hinder their social and intellectual development. Such children show low personal motivation and inadequate language skills. They are poorly prepared to succeed in school, especially if curriculum and methods are not adjusted to their needs. See CULTURALLY DEPRIVED. Also see SIX-HOUR RETARDED CHILD.

cultural parallelism an anthropological term for the development of analogous cultural patterns, such as sun worship, in geographically separate groups assumed to have had no communication with each other.

cultural process the process by which ethnic and social values are transmitted through the generations and modified by prevailing influences of each generation.

cultural psychiatry = CROSS-C.P.

cultural relativism the view that attitudes, values, concepts, and achievements must be understood in light of their specific cultural milieu and not judged according to an alien culture's standards. In psychology, the relativist position questions the universal application of psychological techniques or insights since theories developed in one culture may not apply to another. Compare CULTURAL ABSOLUTISM.

cultural transmission the processes by which customs, beliefs, rites, and knowledge are imparted to successive generations.

culture the distinctive customs, manners, values,

religious behavior and other social and intellectual aspects of a society. Also see POSTFIGURATIVE C.; COFIGURATIVE C.; PREFIGURATIVE C.; COUNTERCULTURE; YOUTH C.

culture area a geographical area in which the indigenous groups exhibit significant correspondence in cultural patterns. Also called **cultural area**.

culture-bound syndromes = CULTURE-SPECIFIC SYNDROMES.

culture complex in a specific culture, the activities, beliefs, rites, and traditions that, taken as a whole, distinguish one central feature of life in that culture, e.g., the cluster of activities, ceremonies, folklore, songs, and stories associated with the hunting and use of the buffalo by Native American nations.

culture conflict the competition or antagonism between neighboring but different cultures; also, conflicting loyalties experienced by immigrants.

Culture-Fair Intelligence Test: See CROSS-CULTURAL TESTING.

culture-fair tests mental-ability tests based on common human experience and relatively free of special cultural influences. Unlike the standard intelligence tests, which reflect predominantly middle-class experience, these tests are designed to apply across social lines and to permit fair comparisons between people from different cultures. Nonverbal, nonacademic items are used, such as matching identical forms, selecting a design that completes a given series, or drawing human figures. Studies have shown, however, that even these items may be culture-bound: "a circle in one place may be associated with the sun, in another with a copper coin, and [in] still another with a wheel" (D. Wechsler, 1966). The term has replaced culture-free tests. An example of c.-f.t. is the Culture Fair Intelligence Test. Also see CROSS-CULTURAL TESTING; IQ; SIX-HOUR RETARDED CHILD.

culture-free tests intelligence tests designed to completely eliminate cultural bias by constructing questions that contain either no environmental influences or no environmental influences that reflect any specific culture. However, the creation of such a test is probably impossible. See CULTURE-FAIR TESTS.

culture shock feelings of inner tension or conflict experienced by an individual or group who have been suddenly thrust into an alien culture or who experience divided loyalties to two different cultures.

culture-specific psychological motives: See PSYCHOLOGICAL MOTIVE.

culture-specific syndromes atypical psychological or psychiatric disorders that are peculiar to a small ethnic or cultural population. The disorders generally involve a belief in spirit possession, black magic, or acceptance of mythology as reality. Members of the culture may accept the abnormal behavior of the patient as a manifestation of the spirit world. While these symptom patterns are observed in societies in nearly all parts of the world, they are not included in Western classifications such as DSM-III. Also called **culture-bound syndromes**. See AMOK; AMURAKH; ARCTIC HYSTERIA; BANGUNGUT; BERSERK; DELAHARA; ECHUL; HSIEH-PING; IMU; JUMPING FRENCHMEN OF MAINE SYNDROME; JURAMENTADO; KIMILUE; KORO; LATAH; MENERIK; MIRYACHIT; PIBLOKTO; PSEUDOAMOK SYNDROME; PUERTO RICAN SYNDROME; SUSTO; TOURETTE'S DISORDER; TROPENKOLLER; VOODOO DEATH; WINDIGO. Also see CROSS-CULTURAL PSYCHIATRY; FOLK PSYCHIATRY.

culture trait any basic belief, practice, technique, or object that can be said to identify a given culture in some aspect of its economic, political, social, or religious organization, e.g. a specific agricultural practice, legal system, ritual, belief about child-rearing, or architectural design.

cumulative frequency distribution a statistical chart in which each new observation is added to the previous one. Areas of the chart with no new observations appear as a flat horizontal line, while areas with observations present are shown with a line sloping upwards.

cumulative record a continuous record in which new data are added, as in operant-conditioning records.

cumulative response curve a method of measuring responses, widely used in operant conditioning, in which each response steps a pen up one unit along a moving sheet of paper. Lack of response, therefore, is indicated by a flat horizontal line, while faster responses are indicated by steeper slopes away from the horizontal.

cumulative scale an attitude scale in which a positive response to one item indicates agreement with all items lower in the scale. Also called **Guttman scale; scalogram**.

cumulative tests tests that measure abilities and traits which can be expected to increase with age. Scoring is usually done by establishing a criterion and determining the subject's deviation from it.

cuneate wedge-shaped, such as the portion of the occipital lobe above the posterior calcarine fissure.

cuneate funiculus a dorsal-column tract which carries A fibers from the skin and deep tissues to the cuneate nuclei. See A FIBER.

cuneate nuclei dorsal-column nuclei located in the medulla, and the terminal point for tracts carrying fibers from the skin and deep tissues. See DORSAL COLUMNS.

cuneate tubercle a swelling on the fasciculus cuneatus that contains the nucleus cuneatus, which receives posterior-root fibers from sensory nerves of the arm and hand. The c.t. is the largest of the three nuclei swellings on the dorsal surface of the medulla oblongata and with the gracile tubercle forms the origin of the medial lemniscus.

cunnilinctio; cunnilinction; cunnilingam = CUNNILINGUS.

cunnilinguist a male or female who performs cunnilingus.

cunnilingus stimulation of the external female genital organs (vulva, clitoris) with the mouth or tongue (from Latin *cunnus*, "vulva, vagina," and *lingua*, "tongue," or *lingere*, "to lick up"). Also called **cunnilingam; cunnilinction; cunnilinctio**. Also see OROGENITAL ACTIVITY.

cunnus = VULVA.

cupula a gelatinous flap that fits over the ampulla at the end of a semicircular canal. The c. contains the crysta, with hair cells that monitor the sense of balance. See AMPULLA; CRYSTA.

curare /kyo͞orär′ē/ any of a variety of toxic plant extracts used as arrow poisons, such as the Strychnos genus plants used for that purpose in Latin America. A skeletal-muscle relaxant is prepared from a Chondodendron shrub as a source of c. C. is administered in the treatment of tetanus spasms and spastic paralysis, and to relax muscles during certain surgical procedures.

curiosity the impulse to investigate, observe, or gather information, particularly when the material is novel or interesting. This drive appears spontaneously in animals and in young children who inspect, bite, handle, taste, or smell practically everything in the immediate environment (sensory exploration and motor manipulation). C. is a prime method for learning and takes the form of asking myriad questions from the nursery-school period onward. Because of its early appearance, many psychologists believe it is an inborn, unlearned drive. Some psychoanalysts, on the other hand, regard intellectual c. as a sublimation of the scopophilic impulse, which was originally aroused by the primal scene. See EXPLORATION DRIVE; MANIPULATORY DRIVE; QUESTION STAGE. Also see SEXUAL C.

curiosity instinct: See EPISTEMOPHILIA.

current material data from present feelings and interpersonal relationships used in understanding individual psychodynamics, as contrasted with data from past experience. See GENETIC MATERIAL.

Curschmann, Hans /ko͞orsh′män/ German neurologist, 1875–1950. See CURSCHMANN-BATTENSTEINERT SYNDROME.

Curschmann-Batten-Steinert syndrome a familial disorder with neurologic effects that include atrophy of the face and shoulder muscles, retarded motor and speech development, and mental retardation. Atrophy of muscles of the face cause a hatchet-face appearance. The onset of symptoms may occur at any time from puberty into middle age. Also called **Batten-Steinert syndrome**.

curse: See PREMENSTRUAL DISORDERS.

cursing magic the idea that one can bring misfortune to another by reciting a formula or uttering an imprecation. It is based upon a belief in MAGICAL THINKING. See this entry. Also see VOODOO DEATH; WITCHCRAFT.

curvilinear regression a curved line fitted to a set of data points, and describing the trend of the data more closely than a straight line does. Also called **curvilinear relationship**.

Cushing, Harvey Williams American neurosurgeon, 1869–1939. See CUSHING'S ANGLE-TUMOR SYNDROME; CUSHING'S SYNDROME; ADRENAL-CORTICAL HYPERFUNCTION; BASOPHILE ADENOMA.

Cushing's angle-tumor syndrome a condition usually caused by an acoustic neuroma affecting the fifth, sixth, seventh, eighth, ninth, and tenth cranial nerves, and the brainstem. Symptoms include nystagmus, tinnitus, deafness, facial-nerve paralysis, loss of corneal reflex, hiccups, vomiting, and headaches.

Cushing's syndrome a group of signs and symptoms related to a chronic overproduction of corticosteroid hormones, mainly cortisol, by the adrenal cortex. The condition occurs most commonly in women and usually is associated with a cancer of the adrenal gland. C.s. is characterized by a "moon-shaped" face due to fat deposits, "buffalo hump" fat pads on the trunk, hypertension glucose intolerance, and psychiatric disturbances.

custodial care minimal maintenance care for institutionalized patients; hospitalization without treatment. C.c. service was once commonly provided for mentally retarded, deaf, or otherwise handicapped individuals by placing them in institutions which offered meals and sleeping facilities for a lifetime, but little if any rehabilitation. The objective of c.c. was to remove the handicapped from the mainstream of society, the patients being regarded as generally incurable. They often were denied other rights, e.g., marriage or voting privileges.

-cut-; -cuti- a combining form relating to skin (Latin *cutis*).

cutaneous albinism: See ALBINISM.

cutaneous anesthesia impairment or loss of sensitivity in an area of the skin, resulting from medications, from nerve damage, or from psychogenic factors, as in conversion disorder. In the latter case the anesthesia does not correspond to the distribution of the nerve fibers, e.g., in glove, stocking, trunk, girdle, or garter anesthesia.

cutaneous experience sensations resulting from stimulation of receptors in the skin. Kinds of c.e. include warmth, cold, tickle, itch, pin prick, sharp pain, and dull pain.

cutaneous perception = DERMO-OPTICAL PERCEPTION.

cutaneous sense = TOUCH SENSE.

Cutter, Nehemiah American psychiatrist, 1787–1859. C. was a cofounder of the Association of Medical Superintendents of American Institutions for the Insane, which later evolved into the American Psychiatric Association.

cutting a form of self-multilation consisting of repeatedly cutting the wrists. Most "slashers," as they are called, feel little if any pain and seem to be fascinated by the sight of oozing blood, which some authors interpret as autoerotic activity.

Others, noting that c. occurs most frequently in women, associate it with physical trauma in childhood, menstrual irregularities, difficulty in sexual identification, and depression.

cutting score a critical score that serves as a dividing point for score distributions.

CVA = CEREBROVASCULAR ACCIDENT.

-cyan-; -cyano- a combining form meaning blue.

cyanates any salt of cyanic acid that contains the chemical radical CNO.

cyanopsin a bluish retinal pigment composed of photopsin and retinene$_2$ and important for vision. See IODOPSIN; OPSIN; RHODOPSIN; SCOTOPSIN; PHOTOPSIN.

cyanosis /sī·ənō′sis/ a purplish discoloration of the skin caused by a lack of oxygen in the blood. Also see HYPOXEMIA.

cyanotic syndrome of Scheid a theory proposed by Scheid to explain sudden death among manic or catatonic patients in terms of a feverish or toxic condition resulting from the psychosis itself. The view has been challenged by other investigators who hold that the sudden deaths are related to physiologic exhaustion resulting from pathologic hyperactivity.

cybernetics a term coined by Norbert Wiener in 1948 (from Greek *kybernetes*, "steersman") for the scientific study of communication and control as applied to machines and living organisms. It includes the concept of self-regulation mechanisms, as in thermostats or feedback circuits in the nervous system, as well as transmission and self-correction of information not only in computers but in persons who are communicating with each other.

cybernetic theory of aging the concept that aging is related to a loss of ability to handle information-transfer functions from environmental inputs. The loss is related to the rate at which neurons and neural activity gradually decrease with advancing age. Also see EVERSION THEORY OF AGING.

cyclazocine: See NARCOTIC ANTAGONISTS.

cyclencephaly a birth defect marked by the partial or complete fusion of the two cerebral hemispheres during the fetal stage of development. Cyclopia and various malformations may be associated with the condition.

cyclic AMP a natural substance formed from a common cellular chemical, adenosine triphosphate, with a role of mediating many hormonal activities in body tissues. C.AMP translates various hormones into specific cellular actions, e.g., the release of insulin. C.AMP also is involved in functions of epinephrine. High levels of c.AMP are found in the brain. Also called **adenosine 3′, 5′-monophosphate.**

cyclic GMP a substance in the body that is associated with acetylcholine activity. Acetylcholine increases concentrations of c. GMP in a manner similar to the effect of other neurotransmitters. It has been postulated that certain physiological

actions depend upon a ratio between levels of c.GMP and cyclic AMP. Also called **cyclic guanosine monophosphate.**

cyclic illness any mental disorder characterized by alternating phases. The term is most frequently applied to the minority of cases of manic-depressive, or bipolar, disorder in which alternation between manic and depressive phases occurs. Also called **circular illness.** See CYCLOTHYMIC DISORDER.

cyclic insanity = FALRET'S DISEASE.

cyclic nucleotides substances in physiological systems that function as "second-messenger" hormonal accessories to translate the original hormone code into specific activity within a cell. The cyclic nucleotide cyclic AMP (adenosine 3′, 5′-monophosphate), e.g., can translate the antidiuretic hormone message into a change in the water permeability of tissues in the kidney.

cyclobarbital a short-acting barbiturate drug administered as a CNS depressant for its hypnotic or sedative effects.

cycloheximide an antibiotic substance that does not affect bacteria but is an effective agricultural fungicide. It also is used as a rat repellent; rats can detect as little as one part per million of c. in food or water and will die of thirst or starve rather than ingest the substance.

cycloid a ring-shaped object or process, such as an organic molecule. The term also applies to a personality type that is characterized by alternating states of psychic and motor activity and well-being on the one hand and diminished activity and malaise on the other. The condition is similar to manic-depressive (bipolar) psychosis except that the symptoms occur in an otherwise normal person. (The term is used as noun or adjective.)

cycloid psychoses: See ACUTE DELUSIONAL PSYCHOSIS.

cyclophoria an eye-muscle imbalance in which one eye deviates when not focused on an object.

cyclopia a birth defect characterized by the merging of the two eye orbits into a single cavity that contains one eye. The anomaly sometimes is a part of a pattern that includes cyclencephaly. The pituitary gland usually is absent. C. occurs with chromosome-13 trisomy, monosomy G, and 18p— syndromes.

cyclopropane an inhalation anesthetic that can be administered in small doses because of its potent effects as a CNS depressant. Surgical anesthesia is induced in less than three minutes with c. However, c. is highly explosive and flammable, as well as expensive, and requires a closed system of respiration for the patient.

cyclothymia a tendency to relatively mild and uneven fluctuations of mood, from periods of elation and excitement to periods of depression and underactivity. Also called **cyclothemia.**

cyclothymic-depressive behavior the behavior of bipolar II patients who experience periods of mildly increased activity or euphoria, frequently at the end of a depressive episode or during treatment with antidepressants or ECT.

cyclothymic disorder a chronic mood disturbance lasting at least two years and characterized by numerous periods of depression and hypomania in which the symptoms are as severe as in full affective syndromes. The periods may be separated by intervals of normal mood lasting for months, and may be intermixed or alternate. See MANIC EPISODE; MAJOR DEPRESSIVE EPISODE. (DSM-III)

cyclothymic-personality disorder in DSM-II, a personality-pattern disturbance characterized by frequently alternating moods of elation and dejection, usually occurring spontaneously and not related to external circumstances. In DSM-III the term has been changed to CYCLOTHYMIC DIS-ORDER and is subsumed under AFFECTIVE DISORDERS. See these entries.

cycrimine hydrochloride: See ANTICHOLINERGICS.

cyesis = PREGNANCY.

-cyn-; -cyno- a combining form relating to a dog (from Greek *kyon, kynos,* "dog").

cynanthropy a delusion in which the patient believes he is a dog. It is a rare symptom occurring in disorganized (hebephrenic) schizophrenia.

cynophobia /sinō-/ or /sīnə-/ a morbid fear of dogs; also, a fear of rabies. In the latter sense, c. is also called **pseudohydrophobia**. Also see HYDROPHOBOPHOBIA.

cyophoria = PREGNANCY.

cypriphobia a morbid fear of contracting a venereal disease (from *Cypris,* a name for Venus). Also called **cypridophobia**.

cyproheptadine $C_{21}H_{21}N$—a migraine remedy that has antihistaminic and antiserotonergic effects. Because of its antagonistic action against histamine and histaminelike substances, c. also is employed in drugs designed to relieve the symptoms of allergic skin disorders. Also see ANTIHISTAMINES; MIGRAINE-NEURALGIA ANALGESICS.

cyproterone $C_{22}H_{27}ClO_3$—a substance which in acetate form functions as a steroid with antiandrogenic action.

-cyst-; -cysto- /-sist-/ a combining form relating to a bladderlike structure, e.g., the urinary bladder (from Greek *kystis,* "bladder, sac").

cystathionine synthetase deficiency = HOMOCYS-TINURIA.

cystathioninuria an inherited disorder of amino-acid metabolism marked by a failure of the genetic material to produce the enzyme cystathionase. The effects include vascular, skeletal, and ocular abnormalities. Mental retardation occurs in less than half the cases, often accompanied by behavioral disorders. The incidence of c. is about five times as high in Ireland as in other countries.

cystic fibrosis an autosomal-recessive hereditary disease marked by generalized exocrine-gland dysfunctions and excessive accumulation of mucus in the bronchioles, the pancreatic duct,

and other body passageways. The patients also experience excessive secretion of sweat and saliva. Common complications are respiratory infections and malnutrition. Psychological counseling frequently is required for patients and families of the patients.

cystinuria the occurrence of **cystine**, an amino acid, in the urine.

-cyt-; -cyto-; -cyte /-sīt-/ a combining form relating to cells (from Greek *kytos,* "hollow place, container, vessel").

cytoarchitectonics a system of organizing information about the structure of cells, their occurrence and arrangement, in an organ such as the brain. Various neuron maps dividing the cerebral cortex into from 20 to 200 areas have been drawn. One of the commonly used c. maps, prepared by Brodmann, divides the cortex into 50 different numbered areas. Also called **architectonic structure**.

cytoarchitecture the arrangement of the various cells of the cerebral cortex, particularly those in the neocortex. The different types of cells are organized in layers and cortical zones. The number of layers varies in different brain areas, but a typical section of cortex shows six rather distinct layers. See CELLULAR LAYERS OF CORTEX; CORTICAL ZONES.

cytology: See CYTOTECHNOLOGIST.

cytomegalic disease an infection caused by a virus of the herpes group that can be identified by its production of large intranuclear and cytoplasmic inclusion bodies. The c.d. agent originally was called a salivary-gland virus because it was first found in salivary-gland infections. It is now known to be a cause of mononucleosis and infections of endocrine glands, the central nervous system, and other tissues. Also see SALIVARY-GLAND VIRUS.

cytomegalic inclusion disease a disease due to an infection of **cytomegalic virus**, resulting in enlarged spleen and liver, microcephaly, and neurologic damage that may include both mental retardation and neuromuscular deficiencies. C.i.d. may be acquired at any time in life, including *in utero* as evidenced by the high incidence of congenital defects and stillbirths associated with the infection.

cytoplasm the protoplasm of a cell, excluding the material within the nucleus. Adjectives: **cytoplastic; cytoplasmic**.

cytosine $C_4H_5N_3O$—one of the base components of DNA molecules.

cytotechnologist a health professional employed in a clinical laboratory in the preparation of tissue-cell components for study by pathologists. The work is particularly important in the diagnosis of cancers. Qualifications for a c. include two years of college plus six months in an approved **cytology** training course and six months in an approved clinical laboratory, followed by a certifying examination administered by the American Society for Clinical Pathologists.

D

d. an abbreviation of "daily," used, e.g., in prescriptions.

DA = DEVELOPMENTAL AGE.

Da Costa, Jacob Méndez American surgeon, 1833–1900. See DA COSTA'S SYNDROME; IRRITABLE HEART OF SOLDIERS.

Da Costa's syndrome a condition observed in soldiers during the stress of combat and marked by fatigue, heart palpitations, chest pain, and breathing difficulty. It is a form of cardiac neurosis. Also called **neurocirculatory asthenia; soldier's heart.** Also see CARDIAC NEUROSIS; EFFORT SYNDROME; IRRITABLE HEART OF SOLDIERS.

D'Acosta's syndrome = ACOSTA'S SYNDROME.

-dacry-; -dacryo- a combining form relating to tears or to lacrimal glands.

-dactyl-; -dactylo- a combining form relating to fingers or toes (from Greek *daktylos*, "finger").

dactylology a technique of communicating by symbols made with the fingers, usually using one hand. D. is generally employed by deaf-mutes.

DAD = DEVICE FOR AUTOMATED DESENSITIZATION.

daemonophobia a morbid fear of spirits, ghosts, devils, and the like. Also called **phasmophobia; demonophobia.** Also see SATANOPHOBIA.

DAH test: See MACHOVER DRAW-A-PERSON TEST.

daily living: See ACTIVITIES OF D.L.

daily-living aids any objects, mechanisms, or techniques that enable a handicapped person to function as a more normal individual. D.-l.a. can include eating and drinking utensils, clothing and personal grooming aids, furniture, electronic communication equipment, automatic book-page turners, head or chin sticks for pushing typewriter keys, canes, crutches, walkers, and special kitchen and household cleaning devices.

Dalton, John English chemist, 1766–1844. See DALTONISM.

Daltonism an obsolete term for red-green color blindness. It was named after the British chemist John Dalton, who was himself color-blind and gave the first accurate description of the condition in 1794.

dammed-up libido in psychoanalysis, a situation in which the erotic forces are frustrated or inhibited by such factors as superego prohibitions, lack of opportunity for sexual expression, inability to achieve excitement (impotence, frigidity), or, in the latency stage, the building of what Freud called "dams" which divert sexual impulses to the development of various organized, constructive activities.

damming up: See FRUSTRATION.

damping the attenuation of vibrations, e.g., of sound, by the use of external pressure or internal friction.

damping effect the diminution of the amplitude of vibrations because of the absorption of energy by the surrounding medium. In speech, this refers to the tension and elongation of the vocal cords beyond maximal level to reach still higher tones on the ascending scale.

dampness fear = HYGROPHOBIA.

Dana, Charles Loomis American physician, 1852–1935. See DANA'S SYNDROME.

Dana's syndrome a degenerative disease with neurologic effects, involving demyelinization of lateral and posterior columns of the spinal cord associated with pernicious anemia. Symptoms include headaches, recurrent mental disorders and hallucinations, and weakness or paralysis of the limbs. Also called **funicular myelitis.**

dance education in psychiatry, professional training in dance and rhythmic movement for therapeutic and rehabilitative purposes. See DANCE THERAPY.

dance epidemics the rapid spread of "dancing madness" among the masses during the period of the Black Death (bubonic plague) in 14th- and 15th-century Europe. See CHOREOMANIA.

dance therapy the use of various forms of rhythmic movement—folk dancing, ballroom dancing, exercises to music—in the treatment and rehabilitation of psychiatric patients. This nonverbal technique was pioneered by Marian Chase in 1942.

dancing eyes: See OPSOCLONUS.

dancing madness: See DANCE EPIDEMICS.

dancing mania = CHOREOMANIA.

Dandy, Walter Edward American surgeon, 1886–1946. See DANDY-WALKER SYNDROME; DYSMORPHOGENESIS OF BRAIN, JOINTS, AND PALATE.

Dandy-Walker syndrome a form of hydrocephalus caused by a cystic enlargement of the fourth ventricle. Macrocephaly may be present at birth or develop a few weeks after. The fourth ventricle expands posteriorly, laterally, and occasionally into the spinal canal. If detected and corrected early, the prognosis for normal psychomotor development is good.

dangerousness in psychiatry, a state in which a patient becomes so agitated and hostile, either toward himself or toward others, that he cannot control his harmful impulses and becomes a threat to his own or other persons' safety. Today, the use of chemical restraints (tranquilizing or sedative drugs) is usually effective in such cases, in addition to constant observation and placement of the patient in an isolation room, or "quiet room," until the episode has subsided.

danger situation: See DREAD.

Danielssen, Daniel Cornelius Norwegian physician, 1815–94. See DANIELSSEN-BOECK DISEASE.

Danielssen-Boeck disease a form of leprosy involving hyperesthesia followed by anesthesia and paralysis. Also called **anesthetic leprosy.**

Dantrium a trademark for the sodium salt of dantrolene. See DANTROLENE SODIUM.

dantrolene sodium a skeletal-muscle relaxant whose primary effect is on the synaptic junctions between the muscle tissue and the neural innervations of the muscle fibers. D.s. also affects the central nervous system as a secondary action.

dapsone a sulfone drug administered orally or by injection in the treatment of leprosy, or Hansen's disease. D. frequently is administered with another leprostatic medication, e.g., clofazimine, to prevent the bacillus, Mycobacterium leprae, from becoming resistant to d.

DAP test = MACHOVER DRAW-A-PERSON TEST.

dark adaptation the ability of the eye to adjust to conditions of low illumination through an increased sensitivity to light. The process takes roughly a half hour and involves expansion of the pupils and retinal alterations, specifically the regeneration of rhodopsin and iodopsin.

darkness fear = ACHLUOPHOBIA; FEAR OF DARKNESS.

dart and dome a term used to describe the spike and wave EEG pattern recorded in cases of petit mal epilepsy.

Darwin, Charles English naturalist, 1809–82. A by-product of Darwin's studies of plant and animal species, which gave rise to his theory of adaptation and evolution, was his influence on the field of psychology in five significant ways: (a) functionalism, in which mental processes are looked upon as adaptive measures, became the dominant approach; (b) comparative psychology, the study of animal behavior, became an important field; (c) studies of expressive behavior were stimulated by his book *Expressions of Emotions in Man and Animals*; (d) genetic and developmental psychology became a major area

of research; and (e) the concept of survival of the fittest focused attention on individual differences, hereditary tendencies, and the measurement of human capacities through psychological tests. See SOCIOBIOLOGY (there: **Darwinian psychology**); EVOLUTION THEORY; FACIAL DISPLAY; NATURAL SELECTION; PANGENESIS.

Dasein analysis /dä′zīn/ a philosophic and psychological approach which emphasizes the need for recognizing not only where we are (German *Dasein*, "existence," literally, "being there"), but what we can become. Its objective is not to adapt to others or eliminate anxiety, since that type of "cure" tends to submerge individuality and encourage outer conformity. Rather, its goal is to help people to be themselves and realize their potential. See EXISTENTIALISM; HEIDEGGER.

DAT: See MULTIPLE-APTITUDE TEST.

data base a computerized word bank or data file, that is, data stored in a computer or on magnetic disks or tapes, from which information can be instantly retrieved by issuing the proper commands. E.g., commands may be typed on the keyboard of a terminal to obtain data via telephone and review them on a screen or record them through a high-speed printer. In medical charting, the term d.b. refers specifically to one of five parts of a problem-oriented medical record, consisting of a standardized collection of pertinent information from the patient's history, physical examination, laboratory and X-ray studies, social history, mental-status examination and psychologic evaluation, and observation of the patient's behavior. For the other four parts, see PROBLEM-ORIENTED RECORD. Also see COMPUTERIZED DIAGNOSIS.

data collection scientific methods of gathering facts for research or practical purposes. Examples are consumer surveys, consumer panels, rating methods, structured interviews, and preference-recording devices in market research.

data snooping looking for unpredicted, post hoc effects in a body of data; also, examining data before an experiment is over, sometimes resulting in premature conclusions.

Dauerschlaf /dou′ərshläf/ a type of therapy in which prolonged sleep is induced with drugs, e.g., barbiturates (German, "perpetual sleep"). D. is employed in the treatment of chemical dependence, status epilepticus, and acute psychotic episodes. Also see CONTINUOUS NARCOSIS.

dawn fear = EOSOPHOBIA.

Dawson, James Robertson American pathologist, 1908—. See PANENCEPHALITIS (also called **Dawson's encephalitis**).

Day, Richard Lawrence American pediatrician, 1905—. See FAMILIAL DYSAUTONOMIA (also called **Riley-Day syndrome**); NEUROPATHIC ARTHROPATHY.

day blindness an abnormal sensitivity of the retinal fovea to bright light.

day camps in rehabilitation, facilities that provide educational, recreational, and rehabilitation services for disabled persons, mainly children, on a short-term, day-by-day basis, as opposed to long-term camp experiences that require overnight accommodations. D.c. usually are organized by local social, civic, or church groups, or health agencies, using facilities of schools, churches, parks, private estates, country clubs, or private or public recreation centers.

day-care program an activity and treatment program provided for the mentally ill, physically disabled, or mentally retarded during the day. The physically disabled and mentally retarded may engage in vocational training, adjustment programs, and, where possible, gainful work in sheltered workshops. For mental-patient programs, see DAY HOSPITAL.

daydream a waking fantasy, or reverie, in which conscious or unconscious wishes are fulfilled in imagination. Among these are the wish for self-enhancement and recognition (the "conquering-hero" d.), the wish for pity and compassion (the "suffering-hero" d.), and daydreams that express social, sexual, romantic, and vocational interests. In moderation, **daydreaming** is considered a healthy and sometimes inspiring outlet for emotions; in excess, it may be an unhealthy form of escape or retreat from reality. Also see FANTASY.

day hospital a hospital program organized on a daytime basis. Patients receive a full range of treatment services and return to their homes at the end of the day. The concept was introduced by D. E. Cameron in 1946 and is now used in rehabilitation as well as psychiatric care. Also see DAY-CARE PROGRAM; NIGHT HOSPITAL; COMMUNITY PSYCHIATRY.

daylight fear = PHENGOPHOBIA.

daymare an attack of acute anxiety precipitated by waking-state fantasies.

day residues a psychoanalytic term for remnants of experiences that play a part in determining the manifest content of a dream. Freud believed it is always possible to find a point of contact between any dream and events of the preceding day.

Day Top: See CONFRONTATIONAL METHODS.

db = DECIBEL.

DC amplifier *d*irect *c*urrent devices used to amplify the potential difference across a neural membrane so that the cortical current can be recorded and studied.

DC potentials *d*irect *c*urrent electrical sources used to sensitize or stimulate the cortex. In experiments with animals, small DC p. of a few microamperes have been used to polarize areas of the cortex so that any stimulus, e.g., visual or auditory, might result in a motor response such as a limb movement.

dead end = BLIND ALLEY.

deadly catatonia = BELL'S MANIA.

deadly nightshade: See BELLADONNA ALKALOIDS; NIGHTSHADE POISONING.

deaf-blind having neither vision nor hearing. The d.-b. individual encounters special communication and learning difficulties; a deaf person usually learns by depending upon vision, and the blind person depends heavily upon the sense of hearing. D.-b. individuals sometimes can be trained in special sheltered workshops or schools with facilities and professional personnel prepared to assist persons with the double handicap.

deaf-mute a person who can neither hear nor speak, usually one who has been born deaf.

deafness the partial or complete absence or loss of the sense of hearing. The condition may be hereditary, because of a genetic defect, or acquired by injury or disease at any stage of life, including *in utero*. The major kinds of d. are conduction d., due to a disruption in sound vibrations before they reach the nerve endings of the inner ear, and sensorineural, or nerve d., caused by a failure of the nerves or brain centers associated with the sense of hearing to transmit or interpret properly the impulses from the inner ear. Some patients experience both conduction and sensorineural d., a form called mixed d. Conduction d. responds more easily to medical or surgical treatment because of accessibility of the malfunctioning areas, whereas it is virtually impossible to perform surgery on auditory nerves or brain centers. Also see ADVENTITIOUS D.; BOILERMAKERS D.; CENTRAL D.; CONDUCTION D.; CONGENITAL D.; CORTICAL D.; EXPOSURE D.; FUNCTIONAL D.; HYSTERICAL D.; PERCEPTION D.; SENSORINEURAL HEARING LOSS.

deaggressivization the neutralization of the aggressive drive so that its energy can be diverted to various tasks and wishes of the ego.

deanalize to transfer instincts from the anal region to another form of expression or object, such as mud, money, and cleanliness.

deanol acetamidobenzoate = DIETHYLAMINOETHANOL.

death technically, the cessation of physical and mental processes in an organism, sometimes determined in humans by two flat encephalograph readings taken 24 hours apart. Among schizophrenics, "d." may signify the end of the patient's life in a particular environment as a step toward rebirth in another, without actual cessation of physical or mental functions. Also see AUTOPSY-NEGATIVE D.; BELL'S MANIA; BRAIN D.; CRIB D.; DYING-PROCESS; PHENOTHIAZINE D.; THANATOLOGY; VOODOO D.

death anxiety a depressive state in which anxiety over dying and fear of death (thanatophobia) are the salient symptoms.

death expectation the expectation of death, and the psychological response to that expectation. E. Kübler-Ross in her book *On Death and Dying* cites five major stages in this response—(a) denial: "It can't be true"; (b) anger: "Why me?"; (c) bargaining: being amiable and cooperative; (d) depression, either reactive to loss of body parts or preparatory for ultimate loss of life; and (e) acceptance, with increasing detachment. Hope, however, persists through all these phases.

death-feigning the act of becoming immobile, or "playing dead," when threatened.

death instinct a universal impulse for death, destruction, self-destruction, and aggression. This instinct, or drive, which is not widely accepted, was first proposed by Freud in 1920 (*Beyond the Pleasure Principle*). He believed the d.i. is under control of the repetition-compulsion principle, which impels us to repeat earlier experiences regardless of pleasure or pain, and ultimately to return the organism to the inorganic state. According to some analysts, the d.i. is first manifested in the oral, "cannibalistic" stage, and takes the form of defiance during the anal-retention stage, and of penetration fantasies and sadistic impulses during the genital stage. Ostow (1958) believes this concept was suggested not only by the cruelty so widely manifested in human behavior but by the destructiveness of World War I. As a consequence, Freud pictured human life as a theater of operations in which two ultimate forces, the life instinct (Eros) and the death instinct (Thanatos) battle for supremacy. See DESTRUDO; THANATOS.

death neurosis a term suggested by E. M. Pattison for neurotic defenses against awareness of death and neurotic depression arising out of unresolved grief. Preventive measures have been suggested such as "orthonasia," or teaching children about death as a part of life; the Widow-to-Widow Program, in which widows are contacted by local mental-health teams; Parents Without Partners; and Big Brothers and Big Sisters Programs.

death phobia = THANATOPHOBIA.

death-trance a state of apparent suspended animation of a patient during an episode of hysteria or catatonia.

death wish in psychoanalysis, a conscious or unconscious wish that another person, particularly a parent, will die. According to Freud, such wishes are a major source of guilt, desire for self-punishment, and depression. The d.w. is usually related to oedipal rivalry for the affections of the other parent. Guilt and depression over such wishes may in some cases direct the d.w. inwardly.

Debré, Robert /debrã'/ French physician, 1882—. See KOCHER-DEBRÉ-SEMELAIGNE SYNDROME.

Debré-Semelaigne syndrome = KOCHER-D.-S. SYNDROME.

debriefing at the conclusion of an experiment, a complete disclosure to the subjects of full details of the experimental process including the reasons for any emotional manipulation or deception. D. is an ethical responsibility of the experimenter if deception or induced stress constitute part of the experimental design. The term has its roots in military jargon.

decadence the deterioration of an individual or group as a result of social changes rather than physical or biological factors.

decathexis in psychoanalysis, withdrawal of libido from objects in the external world; retreat from reality in schizophrenic patients, usually resulting in delusions and hallucinations as an attempt to recover the lost objects.

decay theory the idea that learned material leaves in the brain a trace or impression which eventually recedes and disappears unless it is practiced and used. D.t. is a theory of forgetting. Also called **trace-d.t.**

decenter to be able to recognize another person's thoughts and feelings even if they differ from one's own. According to Piaget, the capacity to d. develops as the child moves away from a predominantly egocentric mode of thinking at around seven or eight years of age.

decentralization the trend toward modifying the centralization of living conditions, care, and administration inherent in the massive mental hospitals designed according to the Kirkbride plan. As a result, most patients now live and are treated in smaller units with a more intimate and homelike atmosphere, and these units are given semiautonomous administrative status. See COTTAGE PLAN; KIRKBRIDE.

decentration a term used by Piaget to describe the child's gradual progress away from egocentrism toward a reality shared with others. D. includes understanding how others perceive the world, knowing in what ways one's own perceptions differ, and recognizing that people have motivations and feelings different from one's own. See EGOCENTRIC.

decerebrate: See DECEREBRATION.

decerebrate plasticity a form of motor-function reaction in which the limbs of a decerebrate animal can be "molded" in various positions by lengthening or shortening the degree of contraction of the extensor muscles. Depending upon location of the lesion, plasticity may be controlled by stimulation of appropriate reflexes.

decerebration the surgical removal of the cerebrum, the largest part of the brain, resulting in loss of ability to discriminate, learn, and control movements. A **decerebrate** is an animal whose cerebrum has been removed. **Decerebrate rigidity** or **decerebrate posture** is the condition following removal of the cerebrum in which the four limbs are spastic.

decibel the smallest difference in loudness that can be detected by a person of normal hearing ability; a quantitative unit equal to the logarithm of the ratio of two levels of intensity. Ten decibels equal one bel (named in honor of Alexander Graham Bell). Abbrev.: **db.**

decile the tenth part of a statistical distribution. The first ten percent of cases comprises the first decile, the second ten percent is the second decile, and so on.

decision-making the ability to make independent and intelligent decisions, a process which counselors seek to enhance. Counselor and client explore and evaluate practical courses of action considered in relation to the client's goals.

Some writers view the facilitation of effective client d.-m. as central to the counseling role.

decision-theoretic approach = BAYESIAN APPROACH.

de Clérambault's syndrome = CLÉRAMBAULT'S SYNDROME.

decoding in information theory, the process in which a receiver (the brain, or a device such as a teletype machine) translates signals (electrical impulses, sounds, writing, gestures) into readable or audible messages.

decompensation a gradual or abrupt breakdown in the individual's psychological defenses, resulting in neurotic symptoms, such as depression or anxiety, or in psychotic symptoms, such as thought disorder (delusions, hallucinations, feelings of unreality).

decompensative neurosis a neurosis in which the patient's defense system breaks down and he experiences, as a result, a flood of incapacitating anxiety.

decomposition in psychiatry, the tendency of a paranoid schizophrenic to split himself or his persecutor into separate personalities.

decompression sickness an adverse effect of exposure of the body to extremely high air pressure, resulting in the formation of nitrogen bubbles in the body tissues. The circulatory system is particularly sensitive to the effect. D.s. develops as one rapidly moves from an environment of high pressure to one of lower air pressure, causing dissolved gases to form bubbles. Neurological effects may include loss of consciousness, convulsions, paresthesias, and damage to the brain and spinal cord. A form of d.s. that affects the heart-lung systems and may lead to circulatory collapse is called **chokes**, and is characterized by discomfort underneath the sternum and coughing on deep inspiration. When d.s. affects mainly the bones and joints, the disorder is called BENDS. See this entry.

deconditioning a behavior-therapy technique in which learned responses such as phobias are "unlearned," or deconditioned. E.g., a person with a phobic reaction to water following a near drowning might be desensitized by going wading with a trusted friend. See DESENSITIZATION.

decorticate conditioning a conditioned reflex that is learned without involvement of the cerebrum.

decortication removal by surgery of the outer layer of the brain while allowing brain tissues below that level to remain functional. A d. effect may occur in the form of cortical damage as a result of anoxia.

decubiti a type of skin ulceration produced by body pressure on a bedridden patient, that is, pressure sores or body sores. (D. is the plural of *decubitus*, meaning a recumbent or horizontal position.) The term is essentially equivalent to BEDSORES. See this entry.

decussation an X-like intercrossing of structures or parts of structures, as in the d. of pyramids of the medulla oblongata and of the fibers of optic nerves from the right and left eyes in the optic chiasm. See MEDULLA OBLONGATA; OPTIC NERVE; OPTIC CHIASM.

dedifferentiation a process in which ordinarily differentiated psychic contents are confused, as in the obliteration of the difference between concrete and abstract concepts, and confusion of symbols with their referents. D. is a form of thought disorganization and primitivization that most characteristically occurs in schizophrenia.

deduction a conclusion or inference derived by reasoning from formal premises or propositions. See DEDUCTIVE REASONING. Compare INDUCTION.

deductive reasoning the form of logical reasoning in which conclusions are drawn or derived from propositions or premises that stand for known facts or agreed-upon data, e.g., reasoning by means of a syllogism. D.r. underlies the process of deriving predictions from theories; it is reasoning from the general to the particular. Compare INDUCTIVE REASONING.

deep body temperature the body's internal temperature. Also called **core temperature**.

deep depression a depression that has progressed to the point where the facial expression is hopeless, the mouth sags, the eyes are directed downward, initiative is lost, questions are answered in a halting manner, and the patient becomes preoccupied with ideas of guilt and unworthiness, spending hour after hour recounting his faults and mistakes. Delusions of sin are also common, and suicidal thoughts are entertained and may be acted out.

deep-pressure sensitivity a sensitivity of tactile receptors in subcutaneous tissues.

deep reflex a reflex of one of the tendon systems, e.g., the knee-jerk or jaw-jerk reflexes.

deep side: See VISUAL CLIFF.

deep structure any organ or tissue that is located beneath the surface layers of the body. Examples of deep structures include the heart, liver, and kidneys.

In linguistics, d.s. is the meaning of a sentence, that is, the grammatical relationship inherent in the words of a sentence which is not immediately apparent from the formal order of the words alone—in contrast to the SURFACE STRUCTURE. See this entry.

deep trance: See TRANCE.

de-erotize to eliminate the sexual emotional investment (libidinal cathexis) from the psychic representation of an object.

defaulter an individual who does not follow the recommended dosages of prescribed drugs. Also called **drug d.**

defecation reflex an action that causes emptying of the rectum and lower portion of the colon by movement or pressure of fecal material. As the rectum fills, receptors send impulses to the spinal cord. Motor nerve impulses are transmitted through the sacral parasympathetic nerves to the descending colon, causing relaxation of the inner anal sphincter and contraction of muscles of the abdominal wall. In order for the act to be completed, however, the external sphincter muscle which is controlled by voluntary, skeletal muscle nerves, must also be relaxed. The voluntary nervous system can override the reflex and, under normal conditions, prevent automatic defecation. Also see ANAL PHASE; TOILET TRAINING.

defective referring to anything, person or object, that is incomplete or lacking a significant quality, as in "mentally d."

defective children a general term applied to children who are physically or mentally impaired due to hereditary or congenital disorder, severe illness, or trauma. The term is sometimes limited to the mentally retarded, who are often termed "mentally defective".

defect theorist a term applied to an individual who believes that cognitive processes of mentally retarded persons are qualitatively different from those of normal individuals. Compare DEVELOPMENTAL THEORIST.

defendance a term used by Murray for the need to defend one's actions or to respond to blame or criticism.

defense hysteria a term employed by Freud to indicate that the dissociation which frequently occurs after traumatic experiences is due to the fact that unacceptable ideas and affects are expelled from consciousness and form the focus for hysterical symptoms. This concept was in direct opposition to Breuer's explanation in terms of a hypnoid state.

defense interpretation an interpretation of the ego and superego that helps the therapist understand the defensive resistances of the patient.

defense mechanism a reaction pattern, usually unconscious, which serves the purpose of protecting an individual from anxiety, guilt, unacceptable impulses, internal conflicts, or other threats to the ego. Defensive behavior is a common, normal means of coping with problems, but excessive use of any mechanism, such as displacement or repression, is considered pathological. The term was first used by Freud in *The Neuro-Psychoses of Defense* (1894), and various types were described by Anna Freud in *The Ego and the Mechanisms of Defense* (1936). Also called **ego-d.m.; defense strategies.** For examples of individual mechanisms, see AGGRESSION; AVOIDANCE; COMPENSATION; DENIAL; DISPLACEMENT; EMOTIONAL INSULATION; FANTASY; FLIGHT INTO REALITY; IDEALIZATION; IDENTIFICATION; INCORPORATION; INTELLECTUALIZATION; INTROJECTION; ISOLATION; PROJECTION; RATIONALIZATION; REACTION FORMATION; REGRESSION; REPRESSION; SUBSTITUTION; SYMPATHISM; UNDOING. Also see DYNAMISM.

defense psychoneurosis a Freudian term for neuroses or psychoses derived from a painful experience that may have been repressed to become an unconscious source of a mental disorder.

defense strategies = DEFENSE MECHANISM.

defensible space a term primarily used in connection with large multiple-family dwellings whose design permits residents to closely observe movements of nonresidents on the premises.

defensive avoidance reaction: See FEAR APPEAL.

defensive behavior behavior characterized by the use or overuse of defense mechanisms operating on an unconscious level; a pattern of responses to real or imagined threats of bodily harm or ego damage. E.g., a cat may exhibit d.b. by spitting and hissing, arching its back, and raising the hair along the back of the neck. Also see DEFENSE MECHANISM. Compare ATTACK BEHAVIOR.

defensive emotion an expression of one intense emotion, such as anger, as a means of screening out a more threatening or anxiety-provoking feeling, such as fear.

defensiveness a behavioral trait consisting of being sensitive to criticism or about one's deficiencies.

defensive reaction any activity, such as over-aggressiveness or the use of a defense mechanism, that is adopted either consciously or unconsciously by the individual for protection against threat, loss of self-esteem, embarrassment, or anxiety.

deference /def'-/ a need to follow a leader and serve under him (Murray).

deferred obedience according to Freud, a command that is not obeyed immediately but may be repressed for a period extending into years before it is finally obeyed, usually after the onset of a neurotic illness. Examples include commands or prohibitions by parents made early in life.

deferred reaction a later response to an experience that had little effect at the time of its occurrence. Freud cites the case of the Wolf Man, who viewed the primal scene (parental intercourse) when he was a year and a half old, but reacted to it in disguised form in a dream about a wolf at age four.

deficiency love according to A. Maslow, a type of love characterized by dependency, possessiveness, lack of concern for mutuality, and diminished caring for another's welfare. Also called **D love.** Compare BEING LOVE.

deficiency motivation according to A. Maslow, the type of motivation operating on the lower four levels of his hierarchy of needs. D.m. is characterized by the striving to correct a deficit that may be physiological or psychological in nature. Also see NEED-HIERARCHY THEORY. Compare METAMOTIVATION.

deficiency motive the tendency to strive only for the degree of gratification required to fill a particular need, e.g., eating only the amount of food required to reduce physical tension. Compare ABUNDANCY MOTIVE.

deflection a defensive act in which attention is diverted from an unpleasant thought or idea.

defloration the rupture of the hymen, or membrane that covers the opening of the vagina, usually during the woman's initial coital experience.

The concept that a female is **deflowered**, or deprived of her "bloom," by the act is not found in all cultures. Also see VIRGINITY; WEDDING NIGHT; JUS PRIMAE NOCTIS; HYMEN.

deflowering = DEFLORATION.

deformation fear = DYSMORPHOPHOBIA.

deformation of the self a term applied by S. Arieti to a negative effect upon the self of the modern overemphasis on science and technology in the form of mass production, consumerism, emphasis on numbers rather than feelings, and manipulation of the public through advertising and publicity.

deformity any malformation or distortion or disfiguration of any part of the body. Also see ANOMALY.

defusion in psychoanalysis, the separation of instincts that usually operate together. This occurs in regressed patients, and is best illustrated by the separation of the destructive or aggressive instinct from the constructive, sexual instincts, which in some cases leads to self-destruction.

degeneracy a state characterized by absence of moral and social standards. D. is often popularly used with special reference to sexual offenses. Adjective, noun: **degenerate**.

degeneracy theory the physiognomic theory advanced toward the end of the 19th century by the Italian sociologist Cesare Lombroso, who maintained that criminals can be identified by certain "stigmata of degeneracy," such as low foreheads, closely-set eyes, and small, pointed ears. The theory was later revived by the anthropologist Ernest Hooton, who attributed such hypothetical characteristics to organic inferiority and primitivism. In either form the theory is considered invalid today.

degenerate: See DEGENERACY.

degenerating axons axons that have been injured or killed, leaving a residue that absorbs a particular dye. A degenerating myelinated nerve fiber releases myelin which absorbs osmium, producing a black trail where the live or healthy fiber had been.

degeneration a general term denoting deterioration or decline in any of a number of contexts, e.g., in the quality of organic, intellectual, emotional, or moral functioning.

degenerative psychoses an obsolete term for psychoses in which the patient regresses to earlier, sometimes infantile, behavior. The term is also applied to psychoses involving irreversible intellectual deterioration (dementia).

degenerative status a constitutional body type marked by an accumulation of deviations from what is considered normal, although a single deviant feature would have no particular pathological significance.

degrees of freedom the number of elements that are free to vary in a statistical calculation, or the number of scores less the number of mathematical restrictions. If the mean of a set of scores is fixed, then d.o.f. means one less than the number of scores. E.g., if we know that four individuals have a mean IQ of 100, then we have three d.o.f. because knowing three of the IQs determines the fourth IQ. Abbrev.: **df**.

dehoaxing following an experiment, the disclosure of deceptions carried out during the experiment, for the purpose of informing naive subjects as to the precise nature of the experiment.

dehumanization the process of reducing human beings, particularly in the older mental institutions, to an animal-like existence by depriving them of freedom, personal care, and cultural and recreational activity. Also see OPEN HOSPITAL; THERAPEUTIC COMMUNITY.

dehydration the lack of water in the body tissues. D. may be absolute as measured in terms of the difference from normal body-water content, or relative as considered in terms of fluid needed to maintain effective osmotic pressure. The physiologic lag between water loss through excretion and the development of thirst sensations that would stimulate replacement of the water may be called **voluntary d.** Compare HYDRATION.

dehydration reactions metabolic and psychological disturbances occurring when the body's water supply falls far below its normal quota, as in patients with cholera or third-degree burns, as well as in survivors of shipwrecks and persons lost in the desert. Early symptoms are apathy, irritability, drowsiness, inability to concentrate, and anxiety; d.r. may progress to delirium, spasticity, blindness, deafness, stupor, and death if more than ten percent of body weight is lost.

deindividuation in social psychology, the condition of comparative anonymity in a group. It is characterized by the lessening of members' feelings of individuality, reduction of self-consciousness, and the weakening of group members' internal restraints. To induce this state experimentally, subjects may be asked to wear identical laboratory coats over their clothes and sit in a partially darkened room.

deinstinctualization: See NEUTRALIZATION.

deinstitutionalization the process of transferring care of persons who are mentally retarded or mentally ill from the structured institutional facilities of a community to homes and workplaces that are part of the social mainstream of the community. See COMMUNITIES FOR THE RETARDED.

Deiters, Otto Friedrich Karl /dī′tərs/ German anatomist, 1834–63. See BONNIER'S SYNDROME (also called **Deiter's nucleus syndrome**).

deity fear = THEOPHOBIA.

déjà entendu /dāzhä′äNtäNdē′/ the feeling that what is now being heard has a familiar ring, even though it has not been heard before (French, "already heard"). D.e. is a distortion of memory, or false recognition. See PARAMNESIA.

déjà pensé /dāzhä′päNsā′/ the feeling that one has had the same thoughts before when this is not the case (French, "already thought"). D.p. is a distortion of memory, or false recognition. See PARAMNESIA.

déjà raconté /dāzhä′räcôNtā′/ a patient's feeling that a long-forgotten event which he now recalls has been told to him before (French, "already told"). In psychoanalysis, the term is applied to a patient's belief that he has already related an experience when he had not done so. The illusion is believed to arise from the need for reassurance that a threatening experience was previously mastered and could therefore be mastered again. See PARAMNESIA.

déjà vécu /dāzhä′vākē′/ a form of paramnesia in which the individual feels he has lived previously (French, "already lived"); a déjà vu experience in which feelings of familiarity in novel situations are attributed to recollection of experiences from another life. See PARAMNESIA.

déjà vu /dāzhävē′/ the uncanny conviction that a newly experienced event has already been experienced (French, "already seen") or that the same scene has been witnessed before. The feeling of familiarity may be due to resemblance between the present and the past scenes, or to the fact that a similar scene has been pictured in a daydream or night dream. Though usually normal in nature, such experiences are also found in epileptic and hysteric patients. See PARAMNESIA. Also see DÉJÀ VÉCU.

Déjérine, Jules Joseph /dāzhārēn′/ Swiss-born French neurologist, 1849–1917. See DÉJÉRINE-THOMAS SYNDROME; LANDOUZY-DÉJÉRINE DYSTROPHY; PERSUASION THERAPY; SPLIT BRAIN.

Déjérine-Klumpke, Augusta French neurologist, 1859–1927. See DÉJÉRINE-KLUMPKE'S SYNDROME.

Déjérine-Klumpke's syndrome paralysis and atrophy of the forearm and small muscles of the hand, together with paralysis of the cervical sympathetic. It is often due to birth injury. Also called **Klumpke's paralysis**.

Déjérine-Thomas syndrome a usually slowly progressive form of cortical cerebellar degeneration, characterized by ataxia of the trunk and extremities, unsteady gait, loss of normal ability to speak and write, and general mental deterioration. The disorder usually begins in adulthood, and the period of degeneration may extend for as much as 20 years before the patient is completely incapacitated.

delahara a culture-specific syndrome occurring among Philippine women and occasionally among men. D. bears a resemblance to amok, but is somewhat less violent.

de Lange: See LANGE.

de Lange's syndrome a congenital disorder that occurs in two forms, both of which include moderate-to-severe mental retardation and appear to be familial although the genetic factors are uncertain. One form, the **Bruck-de Lange type**, features a short broad neck, broad shoulders, short and thick extremities, and muscular hypertrophy which gives the child the appearance of a small professional wrestler. The other, **Brachman-de Lange type**, is characterized by retarded bone maturation, visual problems, microbrachycephaly, syndactyly, and short arms and fingers. It also is known as the **Amsterdam type of retardation** and **Amsterdam dwarf disease**, because the disorder was identified among patients in the Amsterdam area. Also called **Cornelia d.L.s.**

delayed-alternation test a variation of the delayed-response test in which the reward is alternated from side to side with a delay between trials. The subject must learn that a cup containing food is always on the opposite side from the previous trial. The d.-a.t. is used in the study of lesions in various brain areas and their effects on memory or related functions.

delayed auditory feedback: See AUDITORY FEEDBACK.

delayed conditioned response a response to a slowly presented stimulus with delayed reinforcement.

delayed discharge in psychoanalysis, a major function of the ego, consisting of postponement of immediate gratification of instinctual drives, such as sex or hostility. The delay gives the individual time to master any danger that may be involved, especially by trying different ways of dealing with the situation in thought rather than action.

delayed-matching test a test in which the subject is rewarded for pressing an illuminated colored panel that matches the color of a sample. Scoring is based on the amount of time required to match the color. Subjects with frontal-lobe lesions often have difficulty in making the proper choices in the allotted time.

delayed reaction = DELAYED RESPONSE.

delayed recall the ability to recollect information acquired earlier. D.r. is used sometimes in neuropsychological examinations at the end of sessions to determine the rate of loss of information presented earlier, compared with persons believed to be normal.

delayed reinforcement an adaptation mechanism whereby a subject may acquire a new behavior pattern through discriminative conditioning. The reward or punishment may occur after a delay following introduction of a new stimulus. D.r. usually is demonstrated with relatively simple neural circuits, such as taste or smell sensations, in which new information can be stored for long periods of time. An example of d.r. is bait shyness.

delayed response a conditioned response marked by a lapse of several seconds after a stimulus. In d.r. animal experiments, a subject may be shown a piece of food hidden under one of several cups. After a measured delay, the animal is allowed to choose one of the cups. Performance in d.r. tasks usually is impaired by frontal-lobe lesions. A similar technique is used in studying thinking processes and learning ability in young children. Their ability is enhanced by the use of language, but chimpanzees can apparently use a nonlinguistic form of "symbolic activity." Also called **delayed reaction**.

delayed reward a reward that is not given immediately after the required response but is administered following a designated interval.

delayed speech the failure of speech to develop at the expected age. D.s. may be due to lags in maturation, hearing impairment, brain injury, mental retardation, or emotional disturbance.

delay of gratification the ability to contain tension arising from an unsatisfied urge, desire, or drive, especially the ability to postpone satisfaction until an appropriate time. D.o.g. is an aspect of FRUSTRATION TOLERANCE. See this entry.

delay-of-reward gradient a concept that rewards and punishments are less effective when separated in time from the response.

delay therapy a type of behavior therapy employed in treating obsessive-compulsive patients by placing them in situations that ordinarily would provoke their rituals—but preventing them from carrying out the behavior. Also called **response prevention**.

deletion in genetics, the loss of genetic material from a chromosome. A deleted arm of a chromosome may become reorganized in a small circle, known as a ring chromosome. A d. usually is associated with physical and mental retardation, e.g., cri du chat syndrome. A d. syndrome usually is identified with the chromosome number and a minus sign, such as 46,XX13q—, the q denoting a d. of the long arm of chromosome number 13. If the d. results in a ring, the symbol is 46,XX13r.

delibidinization in psychoanalysis, elimination or neutralization of a sexual aim. Examples are expression of the oral-sadistic wish to devour in terms of the need to acquire knowledge, or the diversion of a scopophilic impulse (voyeurism) to curiosity about intellectual matters. Also called **desexualization**.

Delilah syndrome female promiscuity associated with an unsatisfactory relationship with the father, who is dominating and exploitative in the manner of Samson and the Philistines. The female feels impelled to take over this role and render her partners, who represent the father, weak and helpless by seducing them (as in the story of Samson and Delilah).

delimination: See PROBLEM-SOLVING BEHAVIOR.

délire d'emblée /dālēr'däNblä'/ a delusion that is fully developed when it first appears (French, "delirium at one blow"). See AUTOCHTHONOUS DELUSION.

délire de négation = COTARD'S SYNDROME.

délire du toucher /dālēr'dētooshä'/ a compulsion to touch objects (French).

deliriant confusion: See SUNDOWNER.

delirious mania a term used in DSM-I for the most severe type of manic reaction, in which the patient becomes totally disoriented and incoherent, develops vivid auditory and visual hallucinations, and engages in constant overactivity that includes screaming, gesticulating, shouting, and pacing up and down. The patient's eyes have a peculiar glare, and he may smear excreta,

and may at one time eat voraciously and at another refuse to eat and have to be tube-fed. The administration of psychotropic drugs has made this condition extremely rare. Also see BELL'S MANIA; HYPERMANIA.

delirious states clinical states exhibiting the essential features of delirium. D.s. develop during amphetamine, barbiturate, or phencyclidine intoxication, alcohol withdrawal, or as a result of other toxic conditions, systemic infections, hypoxia, head trauma, thiamine deficiency, postoperative conditions, or seizures. See DELIRIUM.

delirium a state of clouded consciousness in which attention cannot be sustained, the environment is misperceived, and the stream of thought is disordered. The individual experiences hallucinations, illusions, and misinterpretation of sounds or sights and may become incoherent, disoriented, agitated, and extremely restless. The episode is usually brief and may be precipitated by such factors as infection, insufficient oxygen supply, renal disease, substance intoxication and withdrawal, head trauma, or seizures. Also see ALCOHOL-WITHDRAWAL D.; AMPHETAMINE OR SIMILARLY ACTING SYMPATHOMIMETIC D.; BARBITURATE OR SIMILARLY ACTING SEDATIVE OR HYPNOTIC WITHDRAWAL D.; BELLADONNA D.; COLLAPSE D.; EXHAUSTION D.; MUTTERING D.; PHENCYCLIDINE (PCP) OR SIMILARLY ACTING ARYLCYCLOHEXYLAMINE D.; RHYMING D.; SENILE D.; SUBDELIRIOUS STATE; TOXIC D.; TRAUMATIC D. (DSM-III)

delirium grave = HYPERMANIA.

delirium of metamorphosis the belief that one can transform oneself or others into a wolf or other animal. The delusion is rare today but was not uncommon during the medieval period. See LYCANTHROPY.

delirium tremens = ALCOHOL WITHDRAWAL DELIRIUM.

delirium verborum a delirious state in which the patient is excessively loquacious (Latin, "delirium of words").

Delphi technique in evaluation research, a method of developing and improving group consensus which originated at the RAND Corporation. It attempts reliable predictions about the future of technology. The D.t. is now often used in many kinds of situations where convergence of opinion is desirable, e.g., for arriving at goal definition, setting standards, or identifying and ranking needs and priorities. (The term is derived from the Delphic oracle at the temple of Apollo at Delphi.)

delta fourth letter of the Greek alphabet (Δ, δ).

delta alcoholism according to E. M. Jellinek, a type of alcoholism characterized by daily consumption, increased tolerance, cellular adaptation, and withdrawal symptoms if the patient goes "on the wagon" for even one or two days. There is, however, no compulsive craving, and control over intake is not completely lost. Also called **inveterate drinking**.

delta movement a form of apparent movement in which a brighter stimulus appears to move toward a darker stimulus, provided certain conditions of stimulus size, distance, and time between stimuli obtain.

delta-9-tetrahydrocannabinol: See HASHISH.

delta waves the slowest of the different kinds of brain-wave patterns recorded with EEG equipment. They are large, regular-shaped waves that have a frequency of one to three cycles per second. D.w. are associated with deep sleep and indicate a synchronization of cells of the cerebral cortex as if all parts of the higher brain were functioning in a single coordinated activity. Also called **slow waves**.

delta-wave sleep periods of deep, usually dreamless, sleep in which delta waves (one to three cycles per second) predominate. Such periods occur at irregular intervals, and the waves appear to arise from the deeper regions of the brain. See SLEEP STAGES; NREM SLEEP.

delusion a false belief or system of beliefs arising from unconscious sources and maintained in spite of irrationality or evidence to the contrary. Delusions may be transient and fragmentary, as in delirium, or highly systematized and superficially convincing, as in paranoid states, though most of them fall between these two extremes. Though logically absurd, and a symptom of psychosis, they appear to serve such purposes and needs as emotional support, relief of anxiety or guilt, blaming others for one's failures, or counteracting feelings of inferiority or insecurity. Also see AUTOCHTHONOUS D.; AUTOPSYCHIC D.; BIZARRE D.; COTARD'S SYNDROME; DOUBLE ORIENTATION; ENCAPSULATED D.; EROTIC D.; EXPANSIVE D.; FRAGMENTARY D.; HALLUCINOGEN-DELUSIONAL DISORDER; HYPOCHONDRIACAL D.; MIGNON D.; MISIDENTIFICATION; MULTIPLE DELUSIONS; NIHILISM; ORGANIC-DELUSIONAL SYNDROME; RELIGIOUS DELUSIONS; SEXUAL D.; SOMATIC D.; SYSTEMATIZED D.

delusional jealousy a paranoid jealousy reaction characterized by a fixed delusion that the spouse or other loved one is unfaithful. The patient is constantly on the watch for indications that this suspicion is justified, manufactures evidence if it is not to be found, and is completely blind to facts that contravene the conviction. The condition was once called AMOROUS PARANOIA. See this entry.

delusional mania a term applied by Kraepelin to a subtype of acute mania characterized by grandiose delusions similar to those in the expansive type of general paresis.

delusional misidentification inability of a patient to identify a known person or object because of a delusion that the person or object has been changed or transformed.

delusional system = DELUSION SYSTEM.

delusion of being controlled the false belief that machines or people are controlling one's thoughts or actions. The reaction is one type of delusion of influence, and is often associated with delusions of persecution. See DELUSION OF INFLUENCE.

delusion of impoverishment a false belief in which the patient, usually elderly, insists that his money has run out or will soon run out. Some investigators suggest that the delusion originates in the patient's feeling that he has lost his social or personal worth, or has committed a sin that will be punished by poverty.

delusion of influence the false belief, often associated with delusions of persecution, that other people are exerting secret control over one's thoughts and behavior, e.g., that one is being subjected to harmful radio waves, or that enemies are "pouring filth" into one's mind. Also called **idea of influence**.

delusion of negation = NIHILISM.

delusion of observation = DELUSION OF REFERENCE.

delusion of orientation = DOUBLE ORIENTATION.

delusion of persecution the false conviction that others are threatening or conspiring against the individual. This type of delusion is believed to originate in the patient's feelings of guilt or self-dissatisfaction, which he disowns by shifting (projecting) them to others. Also called **persecutory delusion**.

delusion of reference a pathological misinterpretation in which the patient feels that others are whispering, talking, or smiling about him, or are referring to him in newspaper articles, films, or plays, or that events which occur in the external world have some special relation to him. The symptom occurs frequently in paranoid schizophrenia. Also called **idea of reference; delusion of observation**.

delusion of sin and guilt a delusion in which the patient becomes convinced that he has committed unpardonable sins, is the incarnation of all evil, and is to blame for wars, depressions, droughts, and other catastrophes. Delusions of this kind are often believed to be exaggerations of guilt feelings generated by hostile attitudes and wishes. They are frequently accompanied by intense fear of punishment.

delusions of grandeur a grossly exaggerated belief in one's own importance, power, wealth, or mission in life. The patient feels he is a brilliant scientist, a powerful military leader, a descendant of a historical character such as the Genghis Khan, or the savior of mankind. These delusions, which are believed to be reactions to feelings of insecurity or guilt, tend to be transient and confused in paranoid schizophrenia, but more organized and persistent in paranoia and general paresis. Also called **grandiose delusions; grandiose ideas**. Also see MEGALOMANIA.

delusion system a pattern of delusions that is internally coherent and systematized. Also called **delusional system**.

demand any internal or external condition that arouses a drive in an organism.

demand character a Gestalt term for the need-arousing attribute of a stimulus.

demand characteristics features of a situation that indicate the expected behavior; e.g., a theater and a curtain call elicit applause. In an experiment, d.c. are those **perceptual cues** in the environment or in the experimenter's attitude and behavior that may suggest to a subject the response expected. Also see EXPERIMENTER EFFECT.

demand feeding = SELF-DEMAND SCHEDULE.

demandingness insistence upon attention from others. It is a common symptom found in hypomania.

Demby, Emanuel H. American psychologist, 1919—. See PSYCHOGRAPHICS.

démence précoce: See DEMENTIA PRAECOX.

dementia a generalized deterioration of intellectual and emotional functions, such as memory, judgment, understanding, and affective response, due to organic brain disease. The pervasive loss of intellectual abilities usually does not involve clouding of consciousness, but is severe enough to interfere with social and occupational activity. The condition commonly occurs in senile dementia, cerebral arteriosclerosis, encephalitis, and syphilitic infection, and less commonly in Alzheimer's disease, Pick's disease, Huntington's chorea, Korsakoff's psychosis, and Wernicke's disease. In some cases it may be associated with brain tumor, hypothyroidism, hematoma, or other specific factors which may be treated. Specific symptoms include impairment of memory, abstract thinking, and judgment and, in some cases, aphasia or apraxia and personality changes. Also see ALCOHOLIC D.; ARTERIOSCLEROTIC D.; ATROPHIC D.; BINSWANGER'S DISEASE; BOXER'S D.; EPILEPTIC DETERIORATION; IDIOTISM; MULTIINFARCT D.; MYOCLONIC D.; ORGANIC D.; PRESBYOPHRENIA; PRIMARY DEGENERATIVE D.; SEMANTIC D.; SUBCORTICAL D. (DSM-III)

dementia associated with alcoholism a disorder associated with prolonged heavy use of alcohol, rarely occurring before age 35. Diagnosis is made only if all other causes of dementia have been excluded. The disorder takes three forms: mild, moderate, and severe, depending on the degree of social, occupational, and personality impairment. The severe form replaces the DSM-II category "alcoholic deterioration." (DSM-III)

dementia dialytica an aluminum-induced encephalopathy in patients undergoing dialysis. Major symptoms are progressive mental deterioration, paranoid ideas and psychotic behavior, with such neurologic signs as seizures, dysarthria, dysnomia, and dyspraxia.

dementia paralytica = GENERAL PARESIS.

dementia paranoides an obsolete term for "schizophrenic disorder, paranoid type" (DSM-III). Kraepelin, who first used the term, distinguished two types: **d.p. gravis**, which begins with simple delusions and terminates in severe deterioration, and **d.p. mitis**, a milder form in which the personality is less seriously damaged.

dementia praecox Kraepelin's Latin translation (1896) of the Belgian psychiatrist François Morel's earlier term (1857) **démence précoce**, "early deterioration of the mind." These terms were applied to what is now called schizophrenia since both Morel and Kraepelin held that the symptoms of the disorder arose in adolescence or before, and involved incurable degeneration. Bleuler questioned both of these views and renamed the disorder schizophrenia (1911). Also see PREDEMENTIA PRAECOX.

dementia pugilistica = BOXER'S DEMENTIA.

demineralization an excessive loss of mineral components from the body tissues, particularly the skeletal tissues. D. may be associated with certain disorders; e.g., iron and zinc levels usually decline at the onset of an infection, calcium and phosphorus losses occur with osteomalacia, rickets, and tuberculosis, and diarrhea can cause life-threatening losses of sodium, chloride, potassium, and phosphorus.

-demo- a combining form relating to people or population (from Greek *demos*, "district, land, people").

democratic atmosphere a nonauthoritarian situation in which group members participate in planning and are encouraged to give their opinions (K. Lewin).

democratic leader the type of leader who participates with group members in developing goals and procedures. A d.l. stimulates group participation by making but not imposing suggestions. In studies by Lewin, Lippitt, and White, groups with democratic leaders showed greater originality and higher morale, and less anxiety, aggression, and apathy than groups with authoritarian leaders. See LAISSEZ-FAIRE LEADER.

demographic analysis: See DEMOGRAPHY; DEMOGRAPHIC PATTERNS.

demographic patterns statistical patterns revealed by a study of population variables such as marriages, births, infant mortality, income, and geographical distribution of mental retardation or mental illness.

demography the statistical study of human populations in regard to various factors including geographical distribution, sex and age distribution, size, and population-growth trends. Such **demographic analyses** are utilized in epidemiological studies. Also see DEMOGRAPHIC PATTERNS.

demon fear = DAEMONOPHOBIA.

demonic character a self-destructive trait in the personality of a masochistic individual who repeats actions that are damaging to himself. It is an expression of the death instinct (Freud).

demonic possession invasion of the body by an evil spirit or devil that controls the soul and produces madness, disease, or criminal behavior. See DEMONOLOGY.

demonolatry /-nol'-/ the worship of a devil or demon.

demonologic concept of illness the view that mental and physical disease are caused by an evil spirit that has gained possession of the soul and must be exorcised if the victim is to recover.

demonology the systematic study of the belief in invisible demons and evil spirits, frequently pictured in folklore and mythology as invading the mind, gaining possession of the soul, and producing disordered behavior. See EXORCISM; INCUBUS; SUCCUBUS; WITCHCRAFT.

demonomania a morbid preoccupation with demons and demonic possession; the belief that one is possessed by or under the control of an evil spirit or demon.

demonophobia = DAEMONOPHOBIA.

demophobia a morbid fear of crowds. Also called **ochlophobia**.

demoralization a breakdown of values, standards and mores in an individual or group, such as occurs in periods of rapid social change, extended crises including war and economic depression, or personal traumas. A **demoralized** person is disorganized and feels lost, bewildered, and insecure.

Demosthenes complex a form of neurotic behavior marked by an impulse to overcome feelings of inferiority through the use of spoken language (named for the Athenian orator of the fourth century B.C.).

demyelinating diseases pathologic conditions resulting from destruction of the fatty myelin sheath covering the fibers of nerves generally outside the central nervous system. Kinds of d.d. include acute disseminated encephalomyelitis following an acute infection and genetic disorders such as amaurotic familial idiocy.

demyelinating encephalopathy = BINSWANGER'S DISEASE.

demyelination the loss of the myelin sheath that covers the nerve fibers of white matter. The condition is associated with several kinds of diseases and inborn errors of lipid metabolism.

demyelination plaque: See PLAQUE.

denasality the voice quality associated with obstructed nasal passages which prevent adequate nasal resonance during speech.

dendrite any of the threadlike extensions of the receptive surface of a neuron. The d. contains a cytoplasmic communication with the perikaryon, or cell body. The number and length of d. processes may vary with the specific function of the neuron.

dendritic zone any part of a receptive surface of a neuron, including the membrane of the nerve-cell nucleus, or perikaryon. For some neurons, the d.z. may extend several feet from the perikaryon.

dendrophilia a paraphilia in which the person is sexually attracted to trees. The subject may have actual sexual contact with trees or venerate them as phallic symbols, or both. Also called **dendrophily** /-drof'-/.

denervation hypersensitivity a condition in which neurons that have not fired for a while become hypersensitive and require less stimula-tion to fire. The condition of d.h. is observed in cases of spinal shock.

denial a defense mechanism in which painful, anxiety-provoking thoughts, wishes, or events are screened out. D. operates on an unconscious level and consists, e.g., in failure to perceive homosexual or hostile urges, physical or mental defects in one's children, or the existence of a terminal illness. In catatonic schizophrenia the patient may deny his own existence or the whole of reality (nihilism). Also called **d. of reality; disavowal; negation**.

denial visual hallucination syndrome = ANTON'S SYNDROME.

denotative meaning the object, event, or process signified by a word; the objective, explicit, or literal meaning. Also called **denotation**. Compare CONNOTATIVE MEANING.

density a stimulus quality, e.g., a tonal characteristic of solidity distinct from pitch, volume, or timbre.

density function the probability of a continuous variable where the area under the curve is equal to one and the function is zero or greater.

-dent-; -denti-; -dento- a combining form relating to the teeth.

dental a loosely used, alternative term for ALVEOLAR. See this entry.

dental age a measure of childhood dental development based on the number of permanent teeth.

dental-patient reactions responses of individuals with differing behavioral patterns to dental care. Studies show pleasure, pain, and sexuality associations with the oral cavity and some transference to the dentist in the form of sexual attraction by certain patients. Other d.-p.r. may be manifested by ambivalence and an association of pain and money with dental care. But most patients are aware of the need to maintain an attractive, healthy set of teeth.

dental phobia a morbid fear of dental treatment usually traceable to at least one traumatic dental experience in childhood, but also associated in many cases with a lower-than-normal pain threshold and in some cases with a neurotic predisposition.

dental plaque: See PLAQUE.

dentate gyrus a brain convolution that interlocks with Ammon's horn in the hippocampal system. The d.g. is a narrow strip of cortical tissue that lies in the hippocampal sulcus and is named for its surface which resembles a set of teeth.

dentate nucleus a semicircle of cerebellar cell bodies believed to be associated with emotions.

dentolabial = LABIODENTAL.

deorality the transfer of instinctual drives from the oral region to some other region or agency. In psychoanalysis, d. may be interpreted as a transfer of breast-feeding pleasure to dependency on a maternal person.

deoxyribonucleic acid = DNA.

dependence = DEPENDENCY. Also see PSYCHOLOGICAL D.

dependence on combination of opioid and other nonalcoholic substance a diagnostic category comprising dependence on an opioid substance such as heroin and a nonopioid such as barbiturates, or on nonopioid substances that cannot be identified, or when the combination involves so many substances that the clinician prefers not to list each one. (DSM-III)

dependence on combination of substances, excluding opioids and alcohol a diagnostic category comprising dependence on two or more nonopioid-nonalcoholic substances such as both amphetamines and barbiturates, or on such a combination that cannot be identified or involves so many substances that the clinician prefers to indicate a combination rather than list each substance. (DSM-III)

dependence on therapy the pathological conviction on the part of some patients that they cannot survive without psychotherapy.

dependency a state in which assistance from others is expected or actively sought for emotional or financial support, protection, security, or daily care. The dependent person leans on others for guidance, decision-making, and nurturance. In psychoanalysis, this tendency dates from the oral stage, in which the infant is totally dependent on the mother for sustenance. Also called **dependence**.

dependency needs personal needs that must be satisfied by others, including the need for affection, love, shelter, physical care, food, warmth, protection, and security. Such needs are considered universal and normal for both sexes and at all ages, but it is also recognized that dependence can be excessive, and overencouraged, as often happens in immature or disabled individuals or those who exhibit a compulsive need to efface themselves and surrender to a stronger person (a condition termed **morbid dependency** by Horney).

dependency syndrome the tendency of women of many cultures, including the Anglo-Saxon cultures, to identify themselves in terms of a mated relationship, usually involving a hidden fear of independence. **Cinderella complex** has been used with a similar meaning (but note the unrelated meaning of the term Cinderella syndrome).

dependent model = INTEGRATED MODEL.

dependent-personality disorder a personality disorder manifested in a long-term pattern of passively allowing others to take responsibility for major areas of life, and of subordinating personal needs to the needs of others due to lack of self-confidence and self-dependence. (DSM-III)

dependent variable the variable, usually a facet of behavior or experience, that is observed and measured, e.g., a subject's reaction. The d.v. is the response or behavior sequence predicted to change as a result of and in relation to manipulations of the independent variable by the experimenter. If other variables are held constant, variations in the d.v. are assumed to occur as a result of variations in the application of the independent variable. Abbrev.: **DV**. Compare INDEPENDENT VARIABLE.

depersonalization a state of mind in which the self appears unreal. The individual feels estranged from himself and usually also from the external world, and thoughts and experiences have a distant, dreamlike character. Transient feelings of unreality are not uncommon, but in its persistent form d. is observed in such disorders as depression, hypochondriasis, dissociative states, temporal-lobe epilepsy, and early schizophrenia. It is often interpreted as an unconscious attempt to escape from threatening situations. The extreme form is called **d. syndrome**. The corresponding DSM-III term is D. DISORDER. See this entry.

Also, the term d. was suggested by Morton Prince to replace hypnosis.

depersonalization disorder a dissociative disorder characterized by one or more episodes of depersonalization (that is, a sense of unreality of the self) that is severe enough to impair social and occupational functioning. Onset of depersonalization is rapid and usually manifested in a sensation of self-estrangement, a feeling that one's extremities are changed in size, a sense of being mechanical, perceiving oneself at a distance, and, in some cases, a feeling that the external world is unreal (derealization). Also called **depersonalization neurosis**. (DSM-III)

depersonalization syndrome: See DEPERSONALIZATION.

depersonification an inability to achieve independence and individuation, e.g., a failure to separate from the parents that may be reflected in distorted family relationships.

depletive treatment a type of treatment based on the concept of driving out mental disorders by weakening the organism through such means as bleeding, purging, blistering, and making the patient vomit. D.p. originated in the time of Hippocrates, and held sway for one thousand years.

depolarization the electrical activity within the neuron as a nerve impulse is transmitted. Before the impulse, the cell is in polar equilibrium with negative ions inside the cell and positive ions outside the membrane. When stimulated, or irritated, the membrane lowers its barrier and allows the positive ions to enter, thereby depolarizing the cell in a wavelike movement lasting a few milliseconds.

depressants agents that diminish or retard any function or activity of a body system or organ. Kinds of d. include alcohol, barbiturates, and tranquilizers.

depression an emotional state of persistent dejection, ranging from relatively mild discouragement and gloominess to feelings of extreme despondency and despair. These feelings are usually accompanied by loss of initiative, listlessness, insomnia, loss of appetite, and difficulty in concentrating and making decisions. For different types and degrees, see ACUTE D.; AGITATED D.; ANACLITIC D.; AUTONOMOUS D.; ANXIOUS D.; BIPOLAR DISORDER, DEPRESSED; CLAIMING TYPE OF D.; CLASSICAL D.; CONSTITUTIONAL DEPRESSIVE DISPOSITION; DEEP D.; ENDOGENOUS D.; MAJOR D.; MAJOR DEPRESSIVE EPISODE; MANIC-DEPRESSIVE ILLNESS; MANIC-DEPRESSIVE REACTION; MASKED D.; MENOPAUSAL D.; MILD D.; MODERATE D.; MONOPOLAR D.; POSTICAL D.; POSTSCHIZOPHRENIC D.; PRIMAL D.; PSYCHOTIC-DEPRESSIVE REACTION; REACTIVE D.; RETARDED D.; SELF-BLAMING D.; UNIPOLAR MANIC-DEPRESSIVE PSYCHOSIS.

depressive character: See MELANCHOLIC PERSONALITY.

depressive hebephrenia a type of depression usually associated with manic-depressive psychosis but observed periodically in hebephrenic (disorganized) schizophrenia patients.

depressive mania a mixed state described by Kraepelin, characterized by a combination of manic and depressive symptoms.

depressive neurosis = DYSTHYMIC DISORDER.

depressive position a term applied by Melanie Klein and her school to the stage of development that reaches its peak at about the sixth month of life. The infant begins to fear destroying and losing the beloved object, but the object does not appear as persecutor, as in the preceding paranoid-schizoid position, but as a love object which the infant wants to appease. See PARANOID-SCHIZOID POSITION.

depressive psychosis a psychosis whose major feature is a severe depression. See MAJOR DEPRESSIVE EPISODE; BIPOLAR DISORDER, DEPRESSED; PSYCHOTIC-DEPRESSIVE REACTION; INVOLUTIONAL PSYCHOTIC REACTION; MANIC-DEPRESSIVE REACTION.

depressive reaction = REACTIVE DEPRESSION.

depressive stupor the most severe form of the depressive phase of bipolar (manic-depressive) disorder. Spontaneous activity and response to stimuli are practically nonexistent, and the patient usually is mute, is disoriented, wears an anxious or masklike expression, is constipated, refuses food, and is at the same time preoccupied with hallucinations, delusions, and fantasies involving sin, death, and rebirth.

depressor nerve an afferent nerve that depresses motor or glandular activity when stimulated.

deprivation dwarfism in children, a state of retarded physical growth believed to represent the physiological result of insufficient emotional nurturance. Studies of children from emotionally aloof homes recorded increases in weight and height when the children were temporarily withdrawn from the home environments; however, these children again failed to thrive when restored to their homes. A hypothetical connection between emotional deprivation and decreased production of pituitary and growth

hormones has been proposed. Studies of infant rats provide evidence for a link between maternal deprivation and the suppression of growth hormones.

deprivation experiments experiments in which the subject is deprived of something desired or expected in order to study the subject's reaction. When an animal is deprived of food, the result may be the substitution of drinking for eating.

deprivation index a measure of the degree of inadequacy of a child's intellectual environment with respect to such variables as achievement expectations, incentives to explore and understand the environment, provision for general learning, emphasis on language development, and communication and interaction with significant adult role models.

deprivative amentia an obsolete term for a form of mental retardation due to a lack of social stimuli or due to an organic disorder, e.g., cretinism.

deprograming the use of rational argument, persuasion, manipulation, and reindoctrination in the effort to "win back" an individual who has adopted a new system of values or beliefs under duress or undue influence. If d. is successful, the individual will repudiate the imposed values and embrace the original belief system. Also see BRAINWASHING.

depth a perception of distance based on visual or auditory receptor stimulation.

depth fear = BATHOPHOBIA. Also see ACROPHOBIA.

depth interview an interview designed to reveal deep-seated feelings, opinions, and motives by encouraging the subject to express himself freely without fear of disapproval or concern about the interviewer's attitudes. In consumer psychology, **depth interviewing** is a motivation-research interviewing technique in which the subject is encouraged to express himself freely rather than answer a structured questionnaire. This kind of interview may utilize free-association psychoanalytic methods to reveal, e.g., psychosexual attitudes that determine product choices among automobile styles. Such answers probably would not be elicited by direct questions.

depth perception awareness of three-dimensionality, solidity, and the distance between observer and objects observed. D.p. is gradually achieved through various cues such as linear perspective, atmospheric perspective, chiaroscuro, motion parallax, visual accommodation, retinal disparity, and convergence. (The two eyes, being set apart, see the object or objects from slightly different angles.) Also called **stereoscopic vision; stereopsis.** Also see RETINAL DISPARITY; VISUAL CLIFF.

depth psychology a general approach to psychology and psychotherapy that focuses on unconscious mental processes as the source of emotional disturbance and symptoms, as well as personality, attitudes, creativity, and style of life. A classic example is Freudian psychoanalysis, but others, notably Jung, Adler, Horney, and Sullivan, employed a depth approach. The techniques of psychodrama, hypnoanalysis, and narcosynthesis are also designed to explore the unconscious.

depth therapy any form of psychotherapy, brief or extended, that involves uncovering and working through unconscious conflicts and repressed experiences that interfere with behavior and adjustment. Its focus may be on symptomatic relief lief and immediate improvement, as in narcosynthesis; on reconstruction of the total personality, as in psychoanalysis; or on objectives that lie between these two approaches, as in hypnoanalysis. See DEPTH PSYCHOLOGY.

derailment a type of thought disorder in which the patient, usually a schizophrenic, constantly interrupts himself and jumps from one idea to a totally unrelated and irrelevant idea. See D. OF VOLITION; SPEECH D.; THOUGHT D.; COGNITIVE D.

derailment of volition a type of indecisiveness observed in schizophrenics in which consistency of goals and purposes is replaced by tangential and irrelevant impulses, contradictory wishes, and short-lived causes.

Dercum, Francis Xavier American neurologist, 1856–1931. See DERCUM'S SYNDROME.

Dercum's syndrome a neurologic condition affecting mainly menopausal women and resulting from pressure and subcutaneous fat deposits on cutaneous nerves. The symptoms include paresthesia, pain, tenderness, depression, and mental deterioration.

derealization a defense mechanism in which people, events, and surroundings appear changed and unreal. Its purpose, according to Freud, is to ward off danger and feelings of helplessness. In its extreme form d. may be a symptom of schizophrenia. See DEPERSONALIZATION DISORDER; DEPERSONALIZATION; DEREISM.

dereism mental activity that is not in accord with reality, experience, or logic. Normal daydreams are sometimes dereistic, but the most striking cases are found in the irrational fantasies of the schizophrenic, who may, e.g., maintain that he can cure all disease with a gesture. D. is similar to autistic thinking. Also called **dereistic thinking**.

derepressor in genetics, a substance that can react with operator genes to influence a DNA molecule to develop a particular type of tissue cell. It is believed the d. in effect removes a mask from part of a DNA molecule so it can serve as an RNA pattern needed to direct a basic cell toward becoming a neuron or bone cell or some other kind of specialized cell.

derivative in psychoanalysis, behavior disguised by the ego to permit expression without anxiety.

derivative insight an insight into a problem achieved by the patient without interpretation by the therapist.

derived property a Gestalt term for parts of a perception derived from the whole.

-derm-; -derma-; -dermo-; -dermato- a combining form relating to the skin.

dermal sensitivity the cutaneous sensations detected by nerve receptors in the skin.

dermal-sweating response: See PSYCHOGALVANIC SKIN-RESISTANCE AUDIOMETRY.

dermatitis: See CONTACT D.

dermatoglyphics a technique employed in the diagnosis of certain kinds of chromosomal abnormalities. The method is based on a theory that patterns of finger-, palm-, and footprints are associated with certain types of birth defects. E.g., Down's-syndrome patients have a simian crease across the palm and a single crease on the skin of the fifth, or smallest, finger.

dermatome an area of skin that runs around the body like a belt. Each d. is innervated by sensory-nerve fibers extending from the spinal cord. Each d. also is overlapped by the d. above and the d. below it, providing double protection for any of the skin-surface areas.

dermatopathic lymphadenopathy: See LYMPHADENOPATHY.

dermatophobia a morbid fear of injury to the skin.

dermatosiophobia a morbid fear of contracting a skin disease.

dermatozoic pertaining to the sensation that some form of insect or animal life has invaded the skin, as in cases of formication that are caused by toxic psychosis.

dermo-optical perception a rare but apparently subtantiated ability to identify the color of objects with the fingers, with vision excluded. R. P. Youtz, who has performed many experiments on d.-o.p., has hypothesized that the subjects detect colors by means of temperature differences due to reflection of hand heat or other heat from the object. Abbrev.: **DOP**. Also called **cutaneous perception**.

DES: See MORNING-AFTER PILL.

de Sade: See SADE.

Descartes, René (Renatus Cartesius) /dekärt'/ French philosopher and mathematician, 1596–1650. D. had a profound influence on philosophical psychology in several ways: In his celebrated statement "cogito, ergo sum" (I think, therefore I am), he focused on the self and its cognitive powers; in his theory that mind and body are distinct substances, he held that thought and emotion (that is, psychological factors) and bodily mechanisms (that is, physiological factors) can each be studied in their own right; and in his recognition that mind acts on body as well body on mind, he paved the way to the holistic, psychophysiological approach of today. Adjective: **Cartesian**. See CARTESIAN DUALISM; ANIMAL SPIRITS; CONARIUM; HYDRAULIC MODEL; MECHANISTIC APPROACH; PINEAL GLAND.

descending pathways sensory nerves that appear to carry impulses away from the central nervous system rather than from sense organs to the brain or spinal cord. The efferent sensory fibers function as inhibitors or suppressors that in fact have an effect of improving the clear transmission of signals from a receptor. See EFFERENT.

descending reticular system a part of a closed-loop reticular-transmission mechanism in which signals are sent downward from the cortex to the spinal cord as well as along ascending pathways from the spinal cord to the cortex. See RETICULAR ACTIVATING SYSTEM.

descriptive approach = SYSTEMATIC APPROACH.

descriptive average an approximate, rough estimate of the average calculated on the basis of imprecise or partial data.

descriptive behaviorism an early characterization of behaviorism by B. F. Skinner when he was experimenting with the effects of reinforcement on learning.

descriptive era the period in psychiatry during the latter part of the 19th century when the nosological approach was carried to the extreme, and greater emphasis was placed on describing symptoms and naming and classifying diseases as separate and distinct entities than on a search for all possible causal factors and on an attempt to probe the specific meaning of the symptoms for the particular patient.

descriptive principle a generalized description and classification of a phenomenon without cause-and-effect explanation. See DESCRIPTIVE PSYCHIATRY.

descriptive psychiatry a systematic approach based on the observation, study, and classification of directly observable symptoms and clinical entities, or syndromes. This contrasts with the dynamic approach, which focuses on the conscious and unconscious factors that produce the symptoms and disorders. D.p. arose out of the conviction of Kraepelin and others, such as Broca and Alzheimer, that each type of mental disorder is a distinct disease, like pneumonia or typhoid fever, and that the course and outcome are as predictable as in any physical illness.

descriptive responsibility in forensic psychology, the judgment that a defendant has performed a criminal act, as distinguished from ASCRIPTIVE RESPONSIBILITY. See this entry.

descriptive statistics quantitative information that describes and summarizes specific measures, such as correlation coefficient, central tendency, and variability collected on samples of a population. Usually the term is used only in reference to the samples and not in reference to general conclusions regarding the population. Compare INFERENTIAL STATISTICS.

desensitization a reduction of the emotional effect of disturbing experiences or thoughts through such means as gaining insight into their nature or origin, catharsis, or deconditioning techniques. See DECONDITIONING. Also see DEVICE FOR AUTOMATED D.; SYSTEMATIC D.; CONTACT D.

deserpidine one of the alkaloids isolated from a Rauwolfia plant and used clinically in the treatment of mental disorders because of its tranquilizing effects. It is somewhat less potent than reserpine but seems to act in a similar manner, by depleting stores of neurotransmitters. See RAUWOLFIA DERIVATIVES.

desexualization = DELIBIDINIZATION.

desferrioxamine another name for **desferoxamine**, an iron-chelating drug used in the treatment of Cooley's anemia. D. causes the iron to form a chemical complex that is easily excreted. See COOLEY'S ANEMIA.

design cycle in environmental psychology, a concept for the improvement of building designs by utilizing information gained from existing buildings in the design and construction of future buildings. The d.c. concept, introduced by J. Zeisel in 1975, includes five steps: programing, or analysis; design, or synthesis; construction, or realization; use, or reality testing; and diagnostic evaluation, or review.

design-judgment test: See GRAVES DESIGN JUDGMENT TEST.

desipramine hydrochloride: See TRICYCLIC ANTIDEPRESSANTS.

desmethylamitryptyline a chemical name for an antidepressant that is closely related to imipramine drugs which are also used to treat depression. It has been suggested that d. functions as an anticholinergic drug to counter the effects of excessive cholinergic activity in the brain that is associated with depressive states.

desocialization gradual withdrawal from social contacts and interpersonal communication, with absorption in private thought processes and adoption of idiosyncratic and often bizarre behavior, as frequently observed in chronic schizophrenics. See AUTISM.

despair: See EGO INTEGRITY VERSUS D.

destination in information theory, the place where messages arrive; the recipient of messages.

destiny neurosis in psychoanalysis, a compulsive unconscious need to arrange life experiences in such a way that failure and defeat are bound to occur. Neurotics of this type blame an unkind fate for their reverses and are unaware that they are themselves responsible or that they are "paying the piper" for guilty impulses or behavior. Also called **fate neurosis; neurosis of destiny**. See MASOCHISM.

destructive behavior a tendency to express anger, hostility, or aggression by damaging or destroying external objects or oneself (self-destructiveness).

destructive drive the impulse to destroy; in psychoanalysis, the DEATH INSTINCT, or THANATOS. See these entries. Also see DESTRUDO. Also called **destructive instinct**.

destructiveness the expression of aggressive behavior by destroying or defacing objects.

destructive obedience behavior that violates moral standards when associated with submission to or identification with an authority figure. In one of Milgram's follow-up experiments, obedient subjects who administered "lethal" doses scored significantly higher on authoritarian measures than did subjects who refused to obey. See AUTHORITARIANISM; OBEDIENCE.

Destrudo a term coined by the psychoanalyst Edoardo Weiss for the energy associated with

Freud's death or destructive instinct (Thanatos). D. contrasts with libido, the energy of Eros, the life instinct. See THANATOS.

desubjectivization of the self a term used by S. Arieti for diminishing the intensity and content of subjective experience by such processes as blunting of affect, denial, undoing, reaction formation, suppression, and repression.

desurgency a term applied by R. B. Cattell to a personality trait characterized by anxiety, brooding, and seclusion.

desymbolization the process of depriving symbols, especially words, of their accepted meaning and substituting distorted, neologistic, autistic, or concrete ideas for them. D. is one of the most prominent symptoms of schizophrenia.

desynchronization a blocking or disruption of a brain-wave pattern, or EEG recording, usually because of a stimulus that alters the rhythm. A stimulus that disrupts a normal alpha-wave pattern of EEG tracings sometimes is called an alpha block. The stimulus is usually one that alerts or arouses or otherwise changes the cortical activity of the subject.

desynchronized sleep sleep stages that are characterized by interruption or deprivation of periods of slow-wave EEGs which are associated with restoration of the body's physical resources. Repeated d.s. results in psychological disturbances.

detached affect an affect that is separated from the generating idea but attached to a second idea that is less threatening, such as an obsession or compulsion (Freud).

detached retina the separation of the inner layer of the retina, or neural retina, from the pigment epithelium layer of the choroid portion. The onset of symptoms, depending upon the size and site of the detachment, may include flashes of light followed later by a clouding of vision, the appearance of floaters (spots or visual artifacts before the eye), or a sudden complete loss of vision. D.r. usually is treated by surgery. Also see DIABETIC RETINOPATHY.

detachment lack of social or emotional involvement; also, objectivity, and the ability to consider a problem on its merits alone (that is, intellectual d.). When used as a defense mechanism, d. is termed emotional insulation. Horney characterizes extreme self-sufficiency and lack of feeling for others as a neurotic need. In developmental psychology, the term is used for the child's desire to have new experiences and develop new skills; this occurs at about two years of age, as he begins to outgrow the period of total attachment and dependence. See EMOTIONAL INSULATION.

detection theory a body of concepts relating to the perception of signals on a background of noise —an outgrowth of studies on the detection of targets by radar in World War II. Experiments indicate that the process is more complex than it appears to be, for it depends on such factors as internal noise (from the individual's body processes) as well as external noise, the ability to make a decision based on probabilities when the signal is faint, personality factors such as the tendency to be cautious or daring, and motivational factors (detection is often improved when rewards are offered). Also called **signal-d.t.**

detection threshold = ABSOLUTE THRESHOLD.

deterioration in psychiatry, progressive impairment or loss of basic psychological functions such as impulse control, emotional reaction, and personality integration.

deterioration effect in abnormal psychology, an adverse effect that is attributed to the psychotherapeutic technique applied in a particular case.

deterioration index a term introduced in 1944 by Wechsler in measuring the degree of reduced performance that could be attributed to aging. The "don't hold" functions that usually show loss with age are digit span, digit symbol, block design, and similarities; the "hold" functions are vocabulary, information, object assembly, and picture completion. Also called **deterioration quotient.**

deterioration of attention a primary symptom of schizophrenia in Bleuler's categories, marked by inconstant and shifting attention and impaired ability to concentrate on external reality.

deterioration quotient = DETERIORATION INDEX.

deteriorative psychosis a severe mental illness characterized by increasing impairment of such psychological functions as memory, emotional and social response, judgment, and reality testing.

determinant an internal or external condition that is antecedent to and the cause of an event.

determinant need: See AFFILIATIVE NEED.

determination coefficient: See COEFFICIENT OF DETERMINATION.

determinative idea the goal or objective of a thought system which is achieved by focusing attention toward the end-result, an ability which is lacking in many schizophrenics.

determining quality a Freudian term introduced for the evaluation of factors involved in the etiology of a case of hysteria. The d.q. (a disturbing memory) and the traumatic power (of a disturbing event) were considered the two conditions needed to explain a symptom of hysteria.

determining tendency the role of a goal direction or set in arousing and maintaining a behavior sequence. Also see AUFGABE; WURZBURG SCHOOL.

determinism the doctrine that all events, physical or mental, including all forms of behavior, are the result of specific causal factors. In psychology, these factors may be either in the individual's environment or within himself. **Hard d.**, as in psychoanalysis, allows no room for freedom of choice or indeterminism; **soft d.**, as in existentialism, holds that within the limitations of one's constitution and past experience, it is possible to determine one's own goals, type of life, and future. Also see RECIPROCAL D.; BIOLOGICAL D.; CULTURAL D.

deterrence in forensic psychology, the belief that punishing a criminal will deter that offender and others from perpetrating criminal acts in the future.

deterrent therapy therapeutic techniques aimed at actively discouraging and preventing faulty behavior. Examples are the administration of Antabuse in cases of alcoholism; ringing a bell or automatically administering a mild electric shock in cases of enuresis; and painting the nails with a bitter substance in cases of nail-biting. See AVERSIVE THERAPY.

detour problem any problem that must be solved indirectly or circuitously; any goal that requires an indirect approach because direct access is blocked.

detoxification any therapeutic procedure designed to reduce or eliminate the presence of toxic substances in the body tissues of a patient. D. procedures may be metabolic, e.g., converting the toxic substance to a less harmful agent that is easily excreted, induced vomiting, gastric lavage, and dialysis, depending upon the nature of the poison and other factors. Concrete examples are the use of methadone in opiate intoxication, tranquilizers in alcoholism, and lavage and artificial respiration in barbiturate poisoning. A popular abbreviation of d. is **detox**.

detoxification center a clinic or hospital unit organized to alleviate the toxic effects of drug or alcohol overdose, and to treat acute withdrawal symptoms. Prior to discharge from the center, arrangements are usually made for long-term treatment. See METHADONE CENTER; ALCOHOL WITHDRAWAL; ALCOHOLICS ANONYMOUS.

detumescence the reduction or subsidence of a swelling, especially in the genital organs of either sex following sexual excitement. Adjective: **detumescent**. Compare TUMESCENCE.

-deut-; -deuter-; -deuto- /-dyo͞ot-/ a combining form meaning two, second, secondary.

deutan color blindness a type of color blindness in which green hues are perceived imperfectly or green is confused with red. In some cases, the condition results from an ability to perceive only two distinct hues, blue and yellow.

deuteranomaly a form of color blindness in which the green part of the spectrum is perceived inadequately. In testing for d., an unusual amount of green would be required in a red-green mixture to match a given yellow.

deuteranopia a type of red-green color blindness in which the color-perception deficiency is due to a fusion of red and green receptor processes with green-sensitivity loss. The condition may be unilateral in that an individual may have normal color vision in one eye. Also see PROTANOPIA.

deuterophallic phase according to Ernest Jones, the second stage of the phallic phase (between ages three and seven), when the child first suspects that the world of people is divided into male and female, each with a different type of genital organ. See PROTOPHALLIC PHASE.

Deutsch, Felix /doitsh/ Polish-born American

psychologist, 1884–1964. See ASSOCIATIVE ANAMNESIS; SECTOR THERAPY.

Deutsch, Helene /doitsh/ Polish-born American psychologist, 1884–1982. See AS-IF-PERSONALITY.

development the progressive changes in shape, organization, and behavior patterns of an organism from birth to death.

developmental acceleration an abnormal or precocious growth in one or more functions, e.g., language.

developmental age a measure of development expressed in an age unit or age equivalent; e.g., a four-year-old may have a d.a. of six in verbal skills. The term is also used to mean an average measure of maturation derived from several tests in several developmental areas. Abbrev.: **DA**.

developmental amentia an obsolete term for mental retardation associated with a combination of heredity and environmental factors.

developmental aphasia = DEVELOPMENTAL DYSPHASIA.

developmental arithmetic disorder marked impairment in arithmetic skills not due to chronological age, mental retardation, or inadequate schooling. The diagnosis is made only by individual IQ tests and academic achievement tests. (DSM-III)

developmental articulation disorder failure to develop consistent pronunciation of the later-acquired speech sounds, such as /r/, /sh/, /th/, /f/, /z/, /l/, or /ch/. Though grammar and vocabulary are up to par, and the child is not mentally retarded, "baby talk" persists and is characterized by misarticulation of /s/ and /z/ sounds (lisping) or /l/ and /n/ sounds (lalling). (DSM-III)

developmental assessment the evaluation of a child's level of development in terms of such factors as developmental tasks, maturity tests (e.g., the Vineland Social Maturity Scale), and observation of his peer relationships, activities, intellectual status, and academic adjustment.

developmental counseling a term sometimes applied to a counseling approach that is directed to helping clients develop more effective behavior in personal and social relationships through a process of learning about the self and testing out new patterns of behavior. Emphasis is placed on the client's mastery of social and emotional goals that were not achieved in earlier stages.

developmental crisis = MATURATIONAL CRISIS.

developmental disability a mental or physical disorder originating before the age of 18, which will probably continue indefinitely and constitute a substantial handicap to normal functioning (Developmental Disabilities Act, 1975). Examples are cerebral palsy, epilepsy, autism, blindness, deafness, mutism, muscular dystrophy, osteogenesis imperfecta, familial dysautonomia, and mental retardation. Also called **developmental disorder**. DSM-III categories are ATYPICAL PERVASIVE D.D.; CHILDHOOD-ONSET PERVASIVE D.D.; CHILDHOOD-ONSET PERVASIVE D.D., RESIDUAL STATE; DEVELOPMENTAL ARITHMETIC DIS-

ORDER; DEVELOPMENTAL ARTICULATION DISORDER; DEVELOPMENTAL LANGUAGE DISORDER; DEVELOPMENTAL READING DISORDER; MIXED SPECIFIC D.D.; PERVASIVE DEVELOPMENTAL DISORDERS; SPECIFIC DEVELOPMENTAL DISORDERS. See these entries.

developmental dysphasia language retardation believed to be associated with brain damage or cerebral maturation lag, and characterized by defects in expressive language and articulation (expressive dysphasia) and in more severe cases by defects in comprehension of language (receptive dysphasia). Also called **developmental aphasia**.

developmental factors in child psychology, the conditions that influence emotional, intellectual, social, and physical development from conception to maturity. Examples are parental attitudes and stimulation, peer relationships, learning experiences, recreational activities, and hereditary predispositions.

developmental hyperactivity a term applied to children who are within or above the normal range intellectually but show high activity levels as an integral part of their personality.

developmental imbalance a disparity in the normal developmental patterns of cognitive and perceptual skills.

developmental language disorder a diagnostic category that comprises two types: (a) an expressive type consisting of failure to develop vocal expression (encoding) despite relatively normal comprehension (decoding), that is, vocabulary is seriously restricted and articulation is immature; and (b) a receptive type consisting of failure to develop both comprehension and vocal expression, with defective recognition of sounds and pictures, defective recall of auditory and visual sequences, and reading and spelling difficulties. (DSM-III)

developmental levels a chronological division of the life span: (a) neonatal, from birth to one month, (b) infancy, from birth to one year, (c) preschool childhood, from one to six years, (d) midchildhood, from six to 11 years, (e) late childhood or preadolescence, from ten to 12 years, (f) adolescence, from 12 to 21 years, (g) adulthood or maturity, from 21 years to old age or from 21 to (h) the involutional period, or climacterium, which is 40 to 55 for women and 50 to 65 for men, and (i) old age, or senium, beginning at 65 or 70.

developmental norms the typical skills and expected levels of achievement associated with the successive stages of development. D.n. are derived from extensive testing and observation; they reflect the average growth trends of children in many areas of development, e.g., perception, motor skills, and language acquisition.

developmental psycholinguistics an area of psycholinguistics that concentrates on the development of language ability in children. Observations are made of young children learning to speak to discover the steps by which they progress in their comprehension of language and

in their ability to speak in syntactically correct constructions. D.p. focuses on the evolution of language as a functioning system with special emphasis on the relationships that link overall cognitive development with the development of language. Also see PSYCHOLINGUISTICS.

developmental psychology the branch of psychology that deals with all phases and stages of growth and maturation of behavior from conception to the end of adulthood.

developmental quotient the developmental age, or a substitute measure of development, divided by the chronological age. Abbrev.: **DQ**. See DEVELOPMENTAL AGE.

developmental readiness in education, the student's state of psychological and intellectual preparedness for a given task, subject, or grade level. See READINESS.

developmental reading the acquisition and growth of skills in a child normally learning the sequential stages of the reading process.

developmental reading disorder a language disorder characterized by marked impairment in reading skills and in school tasks involving reading, but not due to chronological age, mental retardation, or inadequate schooling. Tests indicate that the child's performance in this area is significantly below intellectual capacity, and involves faulty oral reading. slow reading, and often reduced comprehension. (DSM-III)

developmental retardation abnormally slow growth in any or all areas—intellectual, motor, perceptual, linguistic, social.

developmental scale an inventory of developmental norms used to evaluate an individual's developmental stage. See DEVELOPMENTAL NORMS.

developmental school an educational facility for retarded children of preschool age. A typical d.s. may be sponsored by local voluntary organizations to provide early growth and learning experiences, helping the individual participate in and adjust as much as possible to the mainstream of society at a very early age.

developmental sequence the order in which changes in structure or function occur during the process of development of an organism. For examples, see CEPHALOCAUDAL DEVELOPMENT; COGNITIVE DEVELOPMENT; PSYCHOSEXUAL DEVELOPMENT; MOTOR MILESTONES.

developmental stage a stage of life in which specific traits or behavior patterns appear.

developmental tasks the fundamental physical, social, intellectual, and emotional achievements and abilities that must be acquired at each stage of life for normal and healthy development, e.g., talking in early childhood or achieving independence during adolescence. Since development is largely cumulative, the inability to master d.t. at one stage is likely to inhibit development in later stages. Also see DEVELOPMENTAL SEQUENCE.

developmental teaching model a general approach in education based on the work of

Piaget and others: Cognitive, social, and moral development are considered to advance in discrete and distinctive stages. In the area of cognitive development, the emphasis is on logical reasoning and the enhancement of intellectual development. There is a concern with orienting school curricula toward an emphasis on operative knowledge. See PIAGET; KOHLBERG.

Developmental Test of Visual Perception: See FROSTIG D.T.O.V.P.

developmental theories theories based on the continuity of human development and the importance of early experiences in shaping the personality. Examples are the psychoanalytic theory of psychosexual development; Erikson's eight stages of personality development; learning theories that stress early conditioning; and role theories that focus on the gradual acquisition of different roles in life.

developmental theorist a person who believes that mental retardation is merely due to a slower-than-normal development of cognitive processes and is not qualitatively different from the cognitive processes of normal persons. Compare DEFECT THEORIST.

developmental zero the starting point or base line; the moment when a new organism begins to develop, usually considered to be the time of union between ovum and sperm cell.

deviant behavior any behavior that deviates significantly from what is considered normal for a social group. Also called **deviance.** Also see SECONDARY DEVIANCE; SEXUAL DEVIANCY.

deviate an individual whose behavior differs markedly from normal or standard conduct.

deviation-amplification feedback positive feedback in which the output is fed back into the system with the effect of increasing or decreasing its output, a method in which small variations may lead to major changes, as seems to occur frequently in brief psychotherapy.

deviation IQ a standard score on an IQ test that has a mean of 100 and a standard deviation specific to that of the test administered.

deviation score a raw score subtracted from the mean, indicating the score's value relative to the mean.

Devic, M. Eugène French physician, died 1930. See DEVIC'S DISEASE.

device for automated desensitization a computerized system for applying desensitization therapy to the treatment of focused-phobic behavior. The device administers audiotape instructions for muscle relaxation and visualization of fear stimuli arranged in a hierarchical order. Abbrev.: **DAD.** See SYSTEMATIC DESENSITIZATION.

Devic's disease a form of encephalomyelopathy accompanied by demyelination of the optic nerves and spinal cord. Loss of optic-nerve myelin results in progressive blindness. Demyelination of the brain occurs mainly in the occipital lobes. The protein content of cerebrospinal fluid increases, and there is a rapid growth of astrocytes and fat-containing phagocytes in the CNS tissues. Also called **neuromyelitis optica; disseminated myelitis with optical neuritis; ophthalmoneuromyelitis.**

devil fear = DAEMONOPHOBIA; SATANOPHOBIA.

devil's advocate: See ADVERSARY MODEL.

Dewey, John American philosopher, 1859–1952. Author of the first scientific text on psychology in America (*Psychology*, 1886), D. went on to develop the functionalist, or instrumentalist, approach, in conjunction with James Cattell and others, which defined psychology as the study of the total adjustment of the individual to the environment and to the practical problems of life, in contrast to the then current overemphasis on reflex arcs and other isolated units of behavior. Similarly, he held that education must be related to the child's own experience, evoke the child's participation, and develop a spirit of inquiry that would lead to the solution of real rather than merely academic problems. See FUNCTIONALISM; INSTRUMENTALISM; PROGRESSIVE EDUCATION; PROBLEM-SOLVING BEHAVIOR. Also see ANGELL.

dexamethasone a synthetic analogue of cortisol, an adrenocortical steroid, with similar biological action. The empirical formula is $C_{22}H_{29}FO_5$. See CORTISOL.

dexamethasone suppression test a laboratory test which is positive in 67 percent of patients with a major depressive disorder. Hypersecretion of cortisol is demonstrated, and failure to suppress cortisol after dexamethasone administration. While the sensitivity of the test is 67 percent, its specificity is 96 percent (very few false positives), making the d.s.t. an excellent predictor of endogenous depression.

Dexedrine a trademark for a formulation of dextroamphetamine sulfate, a CNS stimulant.

-dexter-: See -DEXTR-.

dexterity test a manual test of speed and accuracy. For an example see CRAWFORD SMALL PARTS DEXTERITY TEST.

-dextr-; -dextro-; -dexter- a combining form relating to the right-hand side.

dextrad toward the right side.

dextrality a tendency or preference to be right-handed or to use the right side of the body in motor activities. Also see RIGHT-HANDEDNESS; D.-SINISTRALITY.

dextrality-sinistrality the phenomenon by which an uninfluenced child will spontaneously develop right-handedness (dextrality) or left-handedness (sinistrality).

dextroamphetamine a form of amphetamine with a greater stimulating effect than the same dosage of an alternative form, levamphetamine. It has a temporary effect of increasing energy output and mental alertness and has been used in treatment of mental depression, alcoholism, encephalitis, narcolepsy, and obesity. See AMPHETAMINES.

dextroamphetamine sulfate: See AMPHETAMINES.

dextromoramide: See SYNTHETIC NARCOTICS.

dextrophobia a morbid fear of anything situated to the right. Compare LEVOPHOBIA.

dextropropoxyphene: See SYNTHETIC NARCOTICS.

dextrosinistral referring to a person who was originally left-handed but was retrained to be right-handed.

df = DEGREES OF FREEDOM.

d'Hout, Alfred Belgian magnetizer, 1845–1900. He was known under the pseudonym **Donato.** See DONATISM.

-di- a combining form meaning two or double.

-dia- a combining form meaning (a) through, (b) apart, (c) completely.

diabetes insipidus a metabolic disorder marked by a deficiency of posterior pituitary-gland hormones that normally control the excretion of water through the kidneys. The hormones are the antidiuretic hormone and vasopressin, which promotes the reabsorption of water from kidney tubules. The patient experiences excessive thirst and excretes large amounts of urine, but without the high level of sugar found in the urine of diabetes mellitus patients. Also see NEPHROGENIC D.I.

diabetes mellitus a metabolic disorder caused by ineffective production or utilization of the hormone insulin secreted by the pancreas gland. Because of the insulin disruption, the patient is unable to oxidize and utilize carbohydrates in food. Glucose accumulates in the blood, causing weakness, fatigue, and a spillover of sugar into the urine. Fat metabolism also is disrupted so that end-products of fat metabolism accumulate in the blood. Also see MATERNAL DIABETES; MATURITY-ONSET DIABETES.

diabetic enteropathy a gastrointestinal complication of diabetes mellitus, marked by intermittent occurrence of nocturnal fecal incontinence. The condition often is associated with autonomic and peripheral neuropathy and is regarded as one of several manifestations of visceral neuropathy in the diabetes patient. Also see DIABETIC GASTROPATHY; GASTRIC NEUROPATHY.

diabetic gastropathy any disorders of the stomach and related digestive organs that are due primarily to autonomic-nervous-system effects of diabetes. See GASTRIC NEUROPATHY; DIABETIC ENTEROPATHY.

diabetic reactions psychophysical symptoms occurring in diabetics, such as a rise in blood-sugar level during periods of emotional stress, a state of acidosis or insulin coma precipitated by a life crisis, and the tendency of some depressed and suicidal patients to give up their diet or neglect to take their insulin.

diabetic retinopathy the deterioration of the retina marked by tiny aneurysms of the retinal capillaries. D.r. first appears as small venous dilations and red dots, observed during ophthalmologic examination; they progress to retinal hemorrhages and exudates that impair vision. New vessels may form in the vitreous cavity and also hemorrhage. Detached retina is a complica-

tion. Treatment includes control of diabetes and hypertension and photocoagulation by argon laser.

diabetogenic factor literally, an agent that causes diabetes. However, the term also is used to identify a substance released from the anterior pituitary gland that controls the release of insulin from cells of the pancreas gland.

diacetylmorphine $C_{21}H_{23}NO_5$—a variation of the morphine molecule that is produced by substituting acetyl radicals for hydroxyl radicals at two positions on the molecule. Many narcotics, e.g., codeine, and narcotic antagonists are produced by changing radicals at one or two positions of the morphine molecule. Also called **heroin.** Also see OPIUM ALKALOIDS.

diad = DYAD.

diadochokinesis the ability to rapidly perform repetitive muscular movements such as finger-tapping, pursing, and retracting lips.

diagnosis the determination of the type of disorder afflicting an individual, on the basis of symptoms and signs, or tests and examinations; also, the classification of individuals on the basis of a disease, abnormality, or set of characteristics. See PATHOGNOMONIC SIGNS.

Diagnostic and Statistical Manual of Mental Disorders: See DSM-III.

diagnostic audiometry: See AUDIOMETRY.

diagnostic center a facility designed and equipped with skilled personnel and appropriate laboratory and other equipment for evaluating the condition of a patient and determining the cause of the patient's physical or psychological disorder. The d.c. may be a part of a larger health-care facility or a separate institution.

diagnostic educational tests tests designed to identify and measure academic deficiencies. Examples are the Iowa Silent Reading Tests, the Gray Oral Reading Test, the Peabody Picture Vocabulary Test, the Iowa Tests of Basic Skills, the Nelson-Denny Reading Test, the Durrell Analysis of Reading Difficulty, the Compass Diagnostic Test of Arithmetic, the Stanford Diagnostic Reading Tests, and the Stanford Diagnostic Arithmetic Test.

diagnostic formulation in psychiatry, a comprehensive evaluation of a patient, including a summary of his behavioral, emotional, and psychophysiological disturbances. D.f. includes the most significant features of the patient's total history; the results of medical and psychological examinations; a tentative explanation of the origin and development of his disorder; the diagnostic classification of the disorder; a therapeutic plan, including basic and adjunctive treatments; and a prognostic evaluation based on carrying out this plan.

diagnostic interview an interview in which a psychologist or a psychiatrist explores the patient's presenting problem, current situation, and background, with the aim of formulating a diagnosis and prognosis, as well as developing a treatment program.

diagnostic-prescriptive educational approach the concept that effectiveness of classroom teaching of disabled children depends upon the teacher's understanding of the medical model of the disability. E.g., the more the teacher and educational administrators know about hydrocephalus, the more effectively they can diagnose and prescribe an appropriate educational program for the patients.

diagnostic test any test that may help reveal the nature and source of a person's problems.

diagnostic X-ray technologist a radiologic technologist trained in the preparation and interpretation of various types of radiologic recordings used for diagnostic purposes, as opposed to personnel who use radiologic equipment for therapeutic purposes. The d.X-r.t. usually is trained in a hospital-based school that provides from 24 months to four years of education and experience; the four-year program leads to a Bachelor of Science degree.

dialectic = DIALECTICAL REASONING.

dialectical method = DIALECTICAL TEACHING.

dialectical reasoning a logical process involving a series of deductions leading to a conclusion. Also called **dialectic**.

dialectical teaching a method that engages students in a critical examination of their reasoning through repeated questioning of their answers, much as Socrates is portrayed doing in the Platonic dialogues. Also called **dialectical method**.

dialogue an exchange of ideas between two or more persons. In Gestalt therapy, one of the "exercises" is to engage in an imaginary dialogue (a) with a body part to which the patient feels alienated, (b) with a person such as the mother or father, who is pictured as sitting in an empty chair, or (c) with an object associated with a dream. The technique often elicits strong feelings.

dialysis /dī·al′-/ a natural process whereby a diffusion of molecules in solution pass through a semipermeable membrane from the side with the highest concentration to the side with the lower concentration. Membranes of most body cells utilize d. for exchange of nutrients and waste products. The principle is used in **artificial-kidney d.** See KIDNEY FAILURE; PERITONEAL D.

Diana complex the repressed desire of a woman to be a man. (Diana was conceived to be goddess of hunting and protectress of women.)

dianetics "an amalgam of vulgarized notions lifted from psychoanalysis and a mumbo jumbo potpourri of terms common in cybernetics... offered as a cheap method of psychotherapy guaranteed not only to cure mental and emotional disorders but also to raise the intelligence of consumers to genius levels." (A. Rapoport, in *American Handbook of Psychiatry*, 1974)

diaphragm a contraceptive vaginal device made from a layer of thick latex rubber fitted over a round or spiral spring. The cup-shaped d. is filled with a contraceptive jelly and inserted in the vagina so that it forms a barrier between the cervix and any spermatozoa that enter the vagina during coitus. The spring holds the d. in place during coitus. The d. has been used by women since 1882.

diary method a technique for compiling child-development data by recording daily observations.

diaschisis /dī·as′kisis/ a functional deficiency that occurs in a part of the body that is distant from the site of a lesion. The term sometimes is applied to conditions in which a lesion in one hemisphere produces effects on both sides of the body instead of just the opposite side. Also, the term d. is used to describe a type of vascular failure possibly due to sudden release of sympathetic-vasomotor tone (spinal shock). Adjective: **diaschistic** /dī·əskis′tik/.

diastolic blood pressure the pressure of blood in a major artery when the blood is flowing into the ventricles while the heart rests briefly between contractions. On blood-pressure recordings, the d.b.p. is the smaller number, usually noted to the right side of the systolic blood pressure. See BLOOD PRESSURE.

diastrophic dwarfism: See BONE DISEASE.

diathermy the use of high-frequency electrical current to deliver heat to the body's deep tissues. D. may be applied in the form of shortwave, ultrasound, or microwave radiation for a variety of therapies, e.g., to cauterize blood vessels, destroy tumors, or decrease muscle spasms. The term is derived from the Greek words *dia*, "through," and *thermainein*, "to heat"—a "heating through."

diathesis /dī·ath′-/ an inherited susceptibility to certain diseases, e.g., arthritic d.

diathesis-stress paradigm a generalization that an individual predisposed toward a particular mental disorder will be particularly affected by stress and will then exhibit abnormal behavior.

diazepam: See BENZODIAZEPINES.

dichotic listening a form of perception in the absence of sustained attention. A subject can hear and retrieve information from different but simultaneous inputs of material in the left and right ears. In d.l., attention is shifted alternately from left to right for a few seconds, and vice versa.

dichotomous thinking either-or thinking; the tendency to think in terms of bipolar opposites, which has been found to be especially common among depressed individuals.

dichotomy in statistics, the division of scores into two units, e.g., above versus below the median.

dichromatism a form of partial color blindness in which the subject identifies colors on the basis of two wavelengths of light, rather than the three required for normal color perception. Red-green color blindness is observed fairly frequently, whereas the blue-yellow variety is quite rare. A **dichromat** is an individual who exhibits d. Also called **dichromacy; dichromatic vision; dichromatopsia**. Also see ANOMALOUS TRICHROMATISM; ACHROMATISM.

dichromic distinguishing only two colors.

Dickens, Charles English novelist, 1812–70. See PICKWICKIAN SYNDROME.

dictators in child psychology, a descriptive term for parents who stress the role of obedience and authority in their relationships with their children (Lafore, 1945). Also see APPEASERS; COOPERATORS; TEMPORIZERS.

didactic analysis psychoanalysis of an analytic candidate with the purpose not only of providing training in the concepts and techniques of psychoanalysis, but also to increase insight into personal sensitivities or other emotional reactions that might interfere with the process of analyzing patients. Also called **tuitional analysis; training analysis**. See COUNTERTRANSFERENCE.

didactic group therapy an early form of group psychotherapy based on the theory that institutionalized patients will respond most effectively to the active guidance of a professional leader. In one form of d.g.t. the patients bring up their own problems and the therapist leads the discussion, often giving his own interpretations; in another form, the therapist presents a short lecture based on printed material designed to stimulate the patients to break through their resistances and express themselves. The didactic approach is also used in therapeutic social clubs, such as Recovery, Inc., founded by Abraham Low.

-didym-; -didymo- a combining form relating to the testicles.

diencephalic stupor = CAIRNS' STUPOR.

diencephalon an interbrain group of neural structures that include the thalamus and hypothalamus, the geniculate bodies, and the pineal gland. Also called **betweenbrain**. Also see POSTERIOR D.

diet: See SELF-SELECTION OF D.

diethylaminoethanol a chemical that is a precursor of acetylcholine. D. is administered in some cases of mental disorders to enhance the body's rate of production of acetylcholine leading in turn to a remission of symptoms. Also called **deanol acetamidobenzoate**.

diethylpropion: See ADRENERGIC DRUGS; ANALEPTICS.

diethylstilbesterol: See MORNING-AFTER PILL.

diethyltryptamine: See PSYCHEDELICS; TRIPTAMINE DERIVATIVES.

difference limen minimum change in a stimulus that can be detected as a change. Abbrev.: **DL**. Also see ABSOLUTE THRESHOLD.

difference threshold the smallest perceptible difference between two stimuli that can be consistently and accurately detected on 75 percent of trials. Also called **differential threshold; just-noticeable difference (j.n.d.); least-noticeable difference**. Also see ABSOLUTE THRESHOLD; WEBER'S LAW.

difference tone a third tone heard when two tones of similar timbre and pitch are sounded together. Its frequency is the difference between the frequencies of the two tones. Also called **Tartini's tone**.

differential accuracy the ability to determine accurately in what way a person's traits differ from a stereotype associated with his group, e.g., to determine in what way Kim differs from the stereotype of her teen-age group. Compare STEREOTYPE ACCURACY.

differential amplifier an electrical device that amplifies the voltage difference between two input leads. In neural research, potential changes may be as small as one microvolt, and electrical resistances and sources of interference may be greater than the voltages being studied. Thus, complex electronic equipment, such as a d.a., is required.

Differential Aptitude Test: See MULTIPLE-APTITUDE TEST.

differential conditioning a conditioning program in which two stimuli are employed, one positive and one negative. An animal may thus be conditioned to lift a leg in response to the positive stimulus and not to lift its leg as a response to the negative stimulus. D.c. is employed mainly in experimental studies.

differential diagnosis the process of determining which of two or more diseases with overlapping symptoms applies to a particular patient; also, the distinction between two similar diseases by identifying critical symptoms that are present in one but not the other.

differential extinction the extinction of one or more responses established through conditioning while other related conditioned responses are not extinguished.

differential growth the growth rate of an organ at a rate different from other organs in the body.

differential inhibition a decreased tendency to respond to stimuli resembling the original conditioning stimulus.

differential psychology a branch of psychology that studies the nature, magnitude, cause, and consequences of psychological differences among individuals and groups.

differential reinforcement the selective reinforcement of desirable behavior by rewarding that behavior while extinguishing undesirable behavior by punishing or failing to reward it.

differential reinforcement of high rate = DRH.

differential reinforcement of low rate = DRL.

differential relaxation a relaxation technique which involves reduction in the contraction of muscles directly employed in an activity, and at the same time relaxation of the muscles that are not involved, e.g., relaxing the left hand while writing with the right.

differential response a response limited to a specific stimulus among a variety of stimuli.

differential scoring a method of scoring tests in more than one way to obtain different data, as in scoring an interest test for different occupations.

differential threshold = DIFFERENCE THRESHOLD.

differential validity an indication of the value of a test or test battery for decision-making. D.v. is a function of the test and the criterion to be predicted. Selection is best when the d.v. is highest.

differentiation in psychology, (a) sensory discrimination between stimuli, (b) a conditioning process in which discrimination is achieved through selective reinforcement of successive approximations, and (c) a change from homogeneity to heterogeneity in the psychological field. In mathematics, the term is used for the process of obtaining a differential coefficient, and in biology, for the transformation of cells from an undifferentiated mass into specialized tissue.

differentiation of cells a process whereby daughter cells of a developing embryo undergo the changes necessary to become specialized in structure and function, such as heart-muscle tissue, a neuron, or a part of a bone. See DEREPRESSOR.

differentiation theory the theory that perception can be understood as an incremental sifting or filtering process whereby environmental "noise" (dispensable, incidental, peripheral information) is screened out while one learns to distinguish the hallmarks or essential characteristics of sensory patterns.

difficulty scale a test organized with items in order of increasing difficulty.

difficulty value the difficulty of a test item as measured by the percentage of subjects or students in a designated class, age level, or experimental group who respond to the item correctly.

diffuse sclerosis a group of neurological disorders involving extensive demyelination in the cerebral hemispheres. Symptoms vary from case to case since different areas may be affected, and may include hemianopsia, optic atrophy, various motor and sensory disturbances, headache, vertigo, convulsions, memory defect, and, in the terminal stage, confusion, disorientation, dementia, and paralysis of all limbs. The etiology is unknown, and there is no effective treatment.

diffuse thalamic projection system a set of thalamic nuclei that project diffusely into the cerebral cortex. The d.t.p.s. has arousal and activation functions similar to those of the reticular activating system but with less intensity in most instances and with more transient effects. Abbrev.: **DTPS**.

diffusion of responsibility the observation that an individual's acknowledgment of personal responsibility diminishes in a group. Apparently, willingness to accept responsibility decreases as group size increases. Also see BYSTANDER EFFECT; CROWD BEHAVIOR.

diffusion process in consumer psychology, the technique employed in gaining general acceptance by the public of a new concept or product. The term is based on the analogy of a stone dropped in the water, producing waves that spread outward to reach the entire pond. The d.p. depends upon acceptance by an initial core of people who influence those around them, the effect rippling outward through the entire population.

digestive epilepsy a form of visceral epilepsy in which the symptoms include nausea, vomiting, epigastric distention, diarrhea, flatulence, and difficulty in urinating or defecating.

digestive type a constitutional body type in which the alimentary system dominates other systems. It corresponds to Kretschmer's PYKNIC TYPE. See this entry.

digital representing information in binary form (yes-no, 0-1), in contrast to analog representation, which is graded or continuous.

digital angiography a new radiologic technique to visualize the intra- and extracranial vasculations and the aortic arch using a venous injection. Repetitive subtraction by the machine results in a clear set of images and will account for this technique replacing arterial catheterization.

digit-span test a test of the ability of a subject to repeat a random series of digits. It is a test of immediate memory.

digraph a combination of two letters or symbols representing a single speech sound, e.g., *ph* in "digraph" or *ou* in "house," also the phonetic transcription /ks/ for the *x* in "explain." The corresponding term **trigraph** refers to three letters or symbols, e.g., *tth* in "Matthew."

dihydrocodeine; dihydromorphine: See OPIUM ALKALOIDS.

dikephobia /dēkā-/ a morbid fear of justice, of seeing justice applied (from Greek *dike*, "justice").

Dilantin a trademark for a form of **phenytoin**, an anticonvulsant and antiepileptic drug.

dilapidation deterioration of chronic mental patients to a point where they cannot feed themselves, may not control eliminative processes, and completely lose interest in their appearance. The condition is most frequently observed in regressed schizophrenics and senile-brain-disease patients. See VEGETATIVE STATE.

dildo an artificial penis, usually made of rubber or plastic but also occasionally manufactured of wood or other materials. A d. usually is used by a female in autoerotic practices but also may be employed as a sexual stimulation device in heterosexual or Lesbian activities. Also called **olisbos; lingam; godemiche** /gōdəmēsh'/. Also see VIBRATOR.

dimenhydrinate: See ANTIHISTAMINES.

dimercaprol = BRITISH ANTI-LEWISITE.

dimethyl ketone = ACETONE.

dimethyltryptamine: See TRYPTAMINE DERIVATIVES.

diminishing-returns law: See LAW OF DIMINISHING RETURNS.

diminutive visual hallucination = LILLIPUTIAN HALLUCINATION.

ding-dong theory: See ORIGIN-OF-LANGUAGE THEORIES.

Dionysian attitude a state of mind that is irrational, sensuous, frenzied, and disordered (from Dionysus, Greek god of wine, orgiastic religion, and fertility). Friedrich Nietzsche, in 1872, introduced Dionysian with the meaning of creative-passionate in contrast to Apollonian, or critical-rational. Compare APOLLONIAN ATTITUDE.

diphenhydromine hydrochloride: See ANTIHISTAMINES.

diphenylhydantoin: See HYDANTOINS; MIGRAINE-NEURALGIA ANALGESICS.

diphenylmethanes a category of anxiolytics that produce sedative, antihistaminic, cardiac antifibrillatory, and local anesthetic effects. The prototype drug of the d. is **hydroxyzine hydrochloride**—$C_{21}H_{29}Cl_3N_2O_2$. Other d. include **hydroxyzine** (trademark: **Atarax**)—$C_{21}H_{27}ClN_2O_2$—and **benactyzine hydrochloride**—$C_{20}H_{26}ClNO_3$.

diphtheria an acute contagious disease caused by a toxin-producing bacterium, Corynebacterium d. The disease occurs in several biotypes, or strains, with varying degrees of severity. The effects include formation of a fibrous membrane on the lining of the respiratory tract and damage to heart and neural tissues, e.g., anterior horn cells of the spinal cord and anterior and posterior nerve roots.

dipipanone: See SYNTHETIC NARCOTICS.

-dipl-; -diplo- a combining form meaning double or doubled.

diplacusis a condition whereby low and high tones are heard with an altered relationship in one ear due to abnormal stiffness or resonance in its conductive system.

diplegia a paralysis that affects like parts on both sides of the body, e.g., facial d.

diploid pertaining to the normal number of human chromosomes, which is 22 pairs of homologous chromosomes plus the male or female set of XY or XX sex chromosomes. Also see HAPLOID.

diploid mode the normal number of human chromosomes. See DIPLOID.

diplopia double vision, usually due to weak or paralyzed eye muscles resulting in a failure of coordination and focus. D. may also be a conversion symptom. The term is essentially equivalent to DOUBLE VISION. See this entry.

dippoldism the flogging of children, particularly school children. The term is derived from the name of a German schoolteacher, Dippold, who was convicted of manslaughter in the fatal flagellation of a schoolchild.

dipsomania an alcoholic mental disorder involving periodic drinking bouts or "binges." Behavior during these episodes is highly individualized, and may include such reactions as shyness, exuberance, belligerence, and paranoid trends. Between the drinking bouts are periods of sobriety that can last months, and thus d. should be distinguished from chronic alcoholism. The condition is believed to be indicative of a more serious underlying disturbance, e.g., epilepsy or

schizophrenia. D. is essentially equivalent to EPSILON ALCOHOLISM. See this entry.

direct aggression aggressive behavior directed toward the source of the frustration or anger. Compare DISPLACED AGGRESSION.

direct analysis a modification of psychoanalytic techniques developed by J. Rosen, based on an attempt to communicate directly with the psychotic patient's unconscious. In this process, the therapist makes a head-on attack on the patient's delusions and fantasies by helping him understand their origin and meaning, by interpreting the patient's bizarre behavior or verbalizations, by encouraging him to relive early traumatic experiences involving emotional deprivation, and by providing "emotional nutriment" needed to alleviate their harmful effects. Also called **direct psychoanalysis**.

direct-contact group = FACE-TO-FACE GROUP.

directed analysis = FOCUSED ANALYSIS.

directedness G. W. Allport's descriptive term for the sense of unified purpose that provides the mature individual with enduring motivation, continuity, and orientation to the future.

directed thinking thought processes that display control and purpose; thinking that is focused on a specific goal and guided by the requirements of that goal, e.g., creative or critical thinking. See CREATIVE THINKING; CRITICAL THINKING.

directional confusion difficulty in distinguishing left from right and in some cases other directions as well, such as uptown from downtown. Some d.c. is to be expected up to age six or seven, especially during the beginning stages of reading, writing, and spelling and in cases of mixed dominance. Persistent d.c. may involve minimal brain damage or forced conversion from the left to the right hand. See HARRIS TESTS OF LATERAL DOMINANCE.

directionality problem in correlational studies, a problem in which it is known that two variables are related but it is not known which is the cause and which is the effect.

directional test of hypothesis a statistical test that specifies direction of an effect or a relationship. The null hypothesis is rejected only if statistical significance is achieved in a particular direction. Compare NONDIRECTIONAL TEST OF HYPOTHESIS.

direction prognosis a term used by Bleuler to identify the course of development a patient's case, e.g., schizophrenia, might be expected to follow, as distinguished from **extent prognosis**, which predicts the progress of the case.

directions test an intelligence test which measures the subject's ability to follow verbal instructions on a series of tasks.

directive counseling an approach that utilizes active advice-giving and direction of the therapeutic process along lines considered relevant by the therapist. D.c. is based on the assumption that superior training and experience equip the counselor to control the therapeutic process and to actively guide the patient's behavior. Therapy is considered to progress along primarily intellectual lines in contrast to psychodynamic approaches that emphasize unconscious motivation. Also called **directive therapy; counselor-centered therapy**.

directive fiction an Adlerian term for a concept of superiority, fantasized as an absolute truth, to compensate for a feeling of inferiority.

directive group psychotherapy a type of group therapy designed to help group members adjust to their environment through didactic educational tasks, group guidance, group counseling, and therapeutic recreation (S. R. Slavson).

directive-play therapy a controlled approach in which the therapist structures the child's activities by providing selected dolls or figurines which represent significant individuals in the child's life, and by encouraging him to use them in enacting "pretend" situations. The therapist also encourages the child to express his feelings of guilt or hostility, after which he may offer direct guidance such as "You needn't feel badly about that."

directive therapy = DIRECTIVE COUNSELING.

direct measurement a measurement that can be made directly, without conversion to another scale.

direct psychoanalysis = DIRECT ANALYSIS.

direct reflex a reflex involving a receptor and effector on the same side of the body.

direct suggestion supportive therapy in which attempts are made to alleviate emotional distress and disturbance through reassurance, encouragement, hypnotic and posthypnotic suggestion, as well as direct instructions (e.g., instructing a patient with a hysterical paralysis to move the affected limb slowly and without intense effort).

dirt phobia a morbid fear of dirt often accompanied by a fear of contamination (mysophobia) and a hand-washing compulsion (ablutomania). Also called **rhyphobia; rupophobia**. Also see MYSOPHOBIA; ABLUTOMANIA.

disability a lasting physical or mental impairment which significantly interferes with functioning in major areas of life, such as self-care, ambulation, communication, social intercourse, sexual expression, or ability to work inside the home or to engage in substantial gainful activity outside. Also see HANDICAPPED.

disability syndrome an institutional neurosis consisting primarily of apathy, withdrawal, and resignation, occurring in long-term institutionalized patients with physical or psychiatric disabilities. See SOCIAL-BREAKDOWN SYNDROME.

disadvantaged in social psychiatry, a term used to identify individuals or families who lack the advantages of economic or cultural assets. Also see CULTURALLY D.

disarranged-sentence test a test or test item in which the object is to put a scrambled sentence in proper order.

disaster adaptation a form of adaptive behavior assumed by most of the population of a community following earthquakes, floods, hurri-

canes, tornadoes, or other natural cataclysms. D.a. activities include establishment of communications, and organization of the survivors into self-help work units. A common d.a. phenomenon is rejection of recovery assistance from outside the community except in extreme cases.

disaster syndrome a three-stage symptom pattern observed by Raker and colleagues (1956) in civilian catastrophes: (a) In the shock stage the victim is so dazed, stunned, and disorganized by overpowering anxiety that he does little to help himself or others; (b) in the suggestible stage he regresses to a state of dependence and passively accepts directions from others, but is highly inefficient even in performing routine tasks; and (c) in the recovery stage he gradually regains control, but remains somewhat tense and apprehensive, talks incessantly about the disaster and the rescue efforts, and may relive the experience in nightmares. Also see POSTDISASTER ADAPTATION.

disavowal = DENIAL.

discharge in neurophysiology, the firing or excitation of a neuron or group of neurons. In psychiatry, d. means the abrupt reduction in psychic tension that occurs in symptomatic acts, dreams, or fantasies. In hospital administration, the term applies to the dismissal of a patient from treatment or other services. In industrial psychology, d. is an alternative term for the dismissal of an employee.

discharge of affect the reduction of an emotion by giving it active expression, e.g., by crying.

discharge procedure in psychiatry, the process of discharging a patient from a mental hospital or psychiatric unit. Common steps in the process are participation in a discharge group, final interview and evaluation by the attending psychiatrist, instruction of the patient about prescribed maintenance medication, and a final interview with the psychiatric social worker concerning personal and practical problems.

discharge rate the ratio of the number of patients discharged from a hospital or other institution in a given period to the number admitted.

discipline in child psychology, the gradual process whereby a child learns to behave in a way that fulfills the requirements of his social group or society. "D. arises from the need to bring about a balance between what an individual wants to do, what he wants of others, and the limitations and restrictions demanded by society or by the hazards in the physical environment" (Jersild, 1960). "The child cannot be counted on to teach himself to curb his impulses...He has to be taught by others. This teaching, however, satisfies many of his own inner needs. It helps him learn what is expected of him, it protects him from his own destructive urges, and it gives him a sense of security by letting him know how far he can go and what he must do to win the approval of others...Good discipline cultivates inner growth, understanding, and self-discipline. It is scaled to the child's level of maturity...

Poor discipline . . . rests entirely on external authority and restraint. It utilizes disapproval more than approval and coercion more than education" (R. M. Goldenson, *The Encyclopedia of Human Behavior*, 1970). Also see BONDAGE AND D.

disclosure of deceptions: See DEHOAXING.

discomfort-relief quotient = DISTRESS-RELIEF QUOTIENT.

disconnection syndrome the neurologic condition resulting from a break in the transmission of impulses required to complete a response. The term is usually applied to situations in which there is a failure to complete execution of a command due to parietal lesions. The apraxias, e.g., dressing apraxia, are manifestations of a d.s.

discontinuity hypothesis the Gestalt viewpoint that emphasizes the role of sudden insight and perceptual reorganization in discrimination learning and problem-solving. According to this view, a correct answer is recognized when its relation to the issue as a whole is discovered. This approach is in contrast to the associationist emphasis on step-by-step trial-and-error learning. Compare CONTINUITY HYPOTHESIS.

discontinuity theory of learning a concept that discrimination learning cannot succeed until the subject relates the discrimination to the total situation.

discordance a research term used in twin studies to indicate dissimilarity with respect to a particular trait or disease. See TWIN STUDIES.

discovery method in education, the teaching method that seeks to provide students with experience of the *processes* of science through inductive reasoning and active experimentation with minimal teacher supervision. Students are encouraged to organize data, develop and test hypotheses, and formulate conclusions or general principles. The d.m. is associated with the cognitivist school, e.g., Piaget and Bruner.

discovery risk: See ETHICAL-RISK HYPOTHESIS.

discrepancy evaluation in evaluation research, the search for differences between two or more elements or variables of an education-training program that should be in agreement. Reconciling differences may then become a major objective.

discrepant stimulus a term primarily encountered in studies of perception in childhood, referring to a stimulus that varies moderately from a known stimulus or schematic image. E.g., a stranger's face represents a d.s. for an infant.

discrete measure a measure taken from values that are discrete, or discontinuous, e.g., the number of people who patronize a given store.

discrete variable a variable that can only take on a limited set of values, e.g. the whole numbers between one and ten, or the number of questions on a specific psychological test. Compare CONTINUOUS VARIABLE.

discrimen a sensory difference whether experienced as such or not (Latin, "division, distinction").

discriminal dispersion the distribution of discriminated responses around a given mean.

discriminant function a statistical technique for classifying individuals into one of two groups, based on a combination of predictors. E.g., a number of signs suggesting organic brain damage could be combined into a regression equation and used to predict either "organic" or "not organic." Also called **discriminant analysis.**

discriminant validation a type of concurrent validity in which test scores of different groups are compared. If mechanics score higher on a test of mechanical ability than clerks, then this provides additional d.v. for the test.

discriminated operant a conditioned operant to a generalized stimulus associated with the original reinforced stimulus.

discriminating power the ability of a test to discriminate between two groups being measured.

discrimination the ability to distinguish between different but sometimes similar stimuli. (Detection of differences is considered more advanced than detection of similarities.) In social psychology, d. is an act of exclusion or hostility directed against members of an ethnic, religious, nationality, or other group. In conditioning, d. is the act of identifying and responding to pertinent stimuli while suppressing a response to irrelevant stimuli. Also see SEX D.

discrimination index: See INDEX OF DISCRIMINATION.

discrimination learning a conditioning or learning experience in which the subject must learn to make choices between seemingly identical or similar alternatives in order to reach a goal. A cat may have to learn to find food under a white cup on the left side of an area in which there are white and black cups on both sides. Also called **discriminative learning.**

discrimination range the range of scores within which a test has discriminating power.

discrimination-reaction time reaction time involving a choice between stimuli that is, a differential or disjunctive response, as in a pitcher responding to the catcher's signals.

discrimination value = D VALUE.

discriminative learning = DISCRIMINATION LEARNING.

discriminative stimulus in operant conditioning, the stimulus that an organism learns to associate with a specific response and reinforcer; the stimulus that signals the organism to perform the associated response or sequence that leads to reinforcement. Abbrev.: S^D. See REINFORCEMENT.

discussion group a term applied to a range of groups that explore problems and questions in a variety of vocational, educational, guidance, therapeutic, and community settings. In schools, a d.g. is usually an instructional technique; in psychiatric and other therapeutic settings, the focus is emotional and interpersonal; in vocational, guidance, and community settings, the objective may be to stimulate decision-making processes and to channel recommendations to a study or action group.

discussion leader the member of a small group who is responsible for stimulating and guiding discussions.

discussion method a teaching method in which both teacher and students actively contribute to the instructional process through classroom dialogue.

disease a definite pathological process marked by a characteristic set of symptoms and which may affect the entire body or a part of the body. The cause, cure, and prognosis of a d. may be known or unknown.

disease-fast: See ANETHOPATHY.

disease fear = NOSOPHOBIA.

disease model an alternative term for medical model, the physiological paradigm of abnormal behavior.

disease narcissism a reaction to disease or injury in which an unaffected body area is overvalued, perhaps as compensation for the defect.

diseases of adaptation a term applied to the psychosomatic disorders, such as peptic ulcers, that are associated with stress-adaptation patterns.

disengagement theory the view that retirement involves a sharp decline in social interaction, a reduced life space, and loss of social esteem and morale, as contrasted with the view that such withdrawal is not a necessary concomitant of retirement, but, rather, that the individual shifts from one set of activities and social roles to others that may be equally or even more satisfying. See RETIREMENT NEUROSIS.

disequilibrium a loss of physical balance, as in Parkinson's disease and ataxias due to cerebellar disorder or injury. The term also denotes emotional imbalance, as in patients with extreme mood swings and lability. In developmental psychology, d. is a state of tension between cognitive processes competing against each other. Some theorists believe, in contrast to Piaget, that d. is the optimal state for significant cognitive advances to occur. See EQUILIBRATION.

disfigurement a blemish or deformity that mars the appearance of the face or body, e.g., a severe burn scar, mutilation due to a wound, accident, or radical cancer surgery, and a wide variety of congenital anomalies, some of which are at least partially reparable: HYDROCEPHALUS; MACROCEPHALY; MICROCEPHALY; CRETINISM; ROMBERG'S DISEASE; DOWN'S SYNDROME; ACROCEPHALY; APERT'S SYNDROME; GARGOYLISM; HYPERTELORISM; CROUZON'S DISEASE; TREACHER COLLINS' SYNDROME; MICROGNATHIA. See these entries.

The psychological effects of d. are often devastating, especially since they are due in part to the negative and often humiliating reactions of others in a society that places a high value on physical attractiveness. Among these effects are damage to the self-image, loss of self-esteem,

feelings of inferiority, self-consciousness, shame, resentment, hypersensitivity, withdrawal, antisocial behavior, and paranoid reactions. Also see FACIAL D.

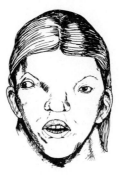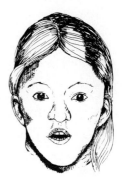

DISFIGUREMENT. Improvement of self-image through corrective surgery in a case involving hypertelorism.

disgust a feeling of revulsion, loathing, and in some cases nausea.

dishabituation the elimination of a response to which an animal or human being has become habituated, as in altering the gill-withdrawal reflex in the marine mollusk Aplysia by applying a strong stimulus to the head or tail. A human example may be toilet training.

disillusioning process a term used by Horney to describe the first stage of therapy, which consists of undermining two of the neurotic patient's pervasive illusions—that he is his idealized self, and that he is his despised self. In the process of **disillusionment**, he becomes increasingly aware of the compulsive, insatiable nature of his drives and their effects on his behavior and relationships, and begins to reorient his values. See HORNEY.

disincentive as used primarily in industrial psychology, an obstacle to productivity or worker motivation, such as excessive overtime or unpleasant working conditions. In business, high taxes may also act as a d.

disinhibition a loss of cortical control; unrestrained emotions or actions often due to alcohol, drugs, or brain injuries. In conditioning experiments, d. means response to a new stimulus, e.g., a buzzer that is unexpectedly introduced after the animal no longer responds to the original conditioned stimulus, such as a bell.

disintegration a disorganization of psychic and behavioral functions due to a loss of control by the higher mental processes, as in schizophrenia.

disintegration of personality a fragmentation of the personality to such an extent that the individual no longer presents a unified, predictable set of beliefs, attitudes, traits, and behavioral responses. The most extreme examples of disintegrated, disorganized personality are found in the schizophrenias.

disjoint sets a term applied to two sets that have no elements in common. The intersection of the sets is empty, and they are mutually exclusive.

disjunctive concept a concept possessing some but not necessarily all the elements of a particular category. E.g., a car can be described as a four-wheeled vehicle, a self-propelled vehicle, or an automobile.

disjunctive reaction = COMPOUND REACTION.

dismantling-treatment strategy in behavior therapy, the identification of the effective components of a treatment package by comparing groups that receive the entire package with groups that receive the package minus different components.

dismemberment complex = FEAR OF DISMEMBERMENT.

disorders of impulse control not elsewhere classified a residual class for impulse-control disorders not classified in other categories (such as substance-abuse disorder), and including pathological gambling, kleptomania, pyromania, intermittent explosive disorder, isolated explosive disorder, and atypical impulse-control disorder. These disorders have the following common features: failure to resist an impulse or a drive or a temptation to perform an act that is harmful to the individual or others, with or without resistance or premeditation; mounting tension before committing the act; and pleasure or relief during the act, with or without regret and self-reproach afterward. See the individual disorders. Also see IMPULSE-CONTROL DISORDER. (DSM-III)

disorders of the self Heinz Kohut's term for narcissistic problems.

disorganization in psychiatry, inability to integrate thought processes, emotions, and volition in meeting the demands of life. D., in extreme form, is a fragmentation or disintegration of the personality such as occurs in advanced schizophrenia. See DISINTEGRATION; SCHIZOPHRENIC DISORDER, DISORGANIZED TYPE.

disorganized behavior behavior that is self-contradictory and marked by extreme emotional reaction, as in laughing after a catastrophe.

disorganized schizophrenia = SCHIZOPHRENIC DISORDER, DISORGANIZED TYPE.

disorientation the impaired ability to identify time, place, or persons. It occurs most frequently in acute and chronic brain disorders (toxic psychoses, delirious states, advanced senile brain disease, cerebral arteriosclerosis), but also in advanced schizophrenia and, more transiently, in situations of acute stress such as fires or earthquakes. Also see ORIENTATION; TIME D.; TOPOGRAPHICAL D.

disparation a double visual image seen when the object is behind or in front of the fixation point.

dispersion the extent to which scores vary from a reference point or among themselves.

displaceability of libido the substitution or replacement of partial impulses related to the four libidinal phases, that is, oral, anal, phallic, and genital, for each other in sexual arousal, particularly in foreplay or perversions.

displaced aggression the direction of hostility away from the source of frustration and toward either the self or a different person or object. This type of aggression tends to occur when circumstances preclude an attack on the real source of frustration; e.g., the responsible person or institution may be perceived as too powerful to attack without fear of reprisal. See DISPLACEMENT. Compare DIRECT AGGRESSION.

displaced-child syndrome a pattern consisting of sibling jealousy, irritability, discouragement, and feelings of rejection that may be precipitated by the birth of another child in the family.

displacement a defense mechanism in which we discharge tensions or express hostility by taking it out on a neutral, nonthreatening target; e.g., an angry child might hurt a brother instead of attacking the father, a frustrated employee might criticize his wife instead of the boss, or a man who fears his own hostile impulses might transfer that fear to knives, guns, or other objects that might be used as a weapon. Also see DISPLACED AGGRESSION; DRIVE D.

displacement behavior a form of behavior in which a subject substitutes one type of action for another when the first fails to answer a need adequately. An animal that is frustrated by servings of food that are small and delivered slowly may express d.b. by drinking instead of eating. Also called **displacement activity**.

displacement of affect = TRANSPOSITION OF AFFECT.

display behavior actions that are intended to effect a response by another animal or individual. D.b. may be verbal or nonverbal, usually involving stimulation of the visual or auditory senses. It may include body language that would convey a message of courtship to a member of the opposite sex (such as a show of plumage or color) or a suggestion that would be interpreted by an opponent as threatening (such as bared teeth or hissing noises). Also see DISPLAY RULES.

display design in industrial psychology, the design of displays for effective transmission of information in different situations. Examples are numerical scales with moving pointers versus moving scales with a fixed pointer, circular versus linear displays, horizontal versus vertical scales, pictorial signs versus word signs, simple versus detailed signs. Displays may be static devices (such as signs, labels, and diagrams) or dynamic devices (such as speedometers, clocks, radios) designed to convey information in auditory and/or visual form—as equipment dials, directions and instructions, safety messages, and auditory or visual devices on biofeedback instruments.

display rules the socially learned standards or guidelines that control and inhibit the expression of emotion. D.r. vary from culture to culture; e.g., direct expression of anger may be socially appropriate in one culture but unacceptable in another. Also see DISPLAY BEHAVIOR.

disposition the sum total of the individual's characteristic tendencies, such as basic temperament, attitudes, inclinations, and drives.

dispositional attribution the ascription of internal or psychological causes to one's own or another's behavior. Also called **personal attribution**. See ATTRIBUTION THEORY. Compare SITUATIONAL ATTRIBUTION.

disruption a sudden loss of personality organization that is similar to disintegration but which occurs at a more rapid pace.

disseminated myelitis with optical neuritis = DEVIC'S DISEASE.

dissociated learning = STATE-DEPENDENT LEARNING.

dissociation an unconscious defense mechanism in which conflicting impulses are kept apart, or threatening ideas and feelings are separated from the rest of the psyche. For examples, see DISSOCIATIVE DISORDERS.

dissociative amnesia a sudden failure to recall one's own identity and, in some cases, one's past life, but without forgetting basic habits and skills. Recovery of memory often occurs spontaneously within a few hours, but in resistant cases hypnosis or sodium Amytal may be used. See PSYCHOGENIC AMNESIA.

dissociative disorders a group of disorders characterized by a sudden, temporary alteration (a) in the normal integrative functions of consciousness, e.g., PSYCHOGENIC AMNESIA, (b) in identity, e.g., MULTIPLE PERSONALITY and DEPERSONALIZATION DISORDER, and (c) in motor behavior, e.g., PSYCHOGENIC FUGUE and SLEEPWALKING DISORDER. See these entries. Also see ATYPICAL DISSOCIATIVE DISORDER. D.d. are also called **hysterical neuroses, dissociative type**. (DSM-III)

dissociative group a group with which one wishes not to be associated. Compare ASPIRATIONAL GROUP.

dissociative hysteria an obsolete term for dissociative disorders, in contrast to a second type of hysteria termed conversion hysteria or conversion reaction. See DISSOCIATIVE DISORDERS.

dissociative reaction a DSM-I and DSM-II term replaced in DSM-III by DISSOCIATIVE DISORDERS. See this entry.

dissociative syndrome any of the dissociative disorders described under the DSM-III term DISSOCIATIVE DISORDERS. See this entry.

distal farther away from an area such as a body organ, or from the center of the area. The toe is d. from the hip. Compare PROXIMAL.

distal dystrophy a rare type of muscular dystrophy characterized by initial and primary involvement of the muscles of the extremities and often confused with other disorders, e.g., peroneal muscle atrophy, a nervous-system disease. See MUSCULAR DYSTROPHY.

distal response a response that occurs away from the body or boundaries of an organism and produces an effect in the environment. A d.r. is related to a proximal response; e.g., in playing the piano, the proximal response is the action of the fingers on the keyboard whereas the d.r. is the chord produced. Also see PROXIMAL RESPONSE.

distal stimulus the actual object or physical energy in the environment that stimulates or acts on a sense organ. Compare PROXIMAL STIMULUS.

distal variable a stimulus source (e.g., a bell) that acts indirectly on a receptor through a proximal variable (the sound waves striking the ear).

distance cues the auditory or visual cues that enable the subject to judge the distance of the source. Auditory d.c. include the time difference, however brief, between the arrival of a sound at the left and at the right ears.

distance perception: See DEPTH PERCEPTION.

distance receptors sensory organs that can detect stimuli from a distance, e.g., visual and auditory receptors. Some authors believe that schizophrenic children avoid the use of d.r., accounting in part for their vacant gaze.

distance vision vision that permits discrimination of objects more than 20 feet (six meters) away.

distance zones in social psychology, the areas of interpersonal physical distance most commonly adopted between persons in intimate, personal, business and social, or public and formal interactions. Interpersonal distance usually increases in proportion to the formality of the relationship, the setting, and the interaction's function.

distorted room an experimental room constructed by A. Ames, Jr., so that sizes and shapes appear distorted even though the room itself appears to be rectilinear when viewed with one eye. Also called **Ames distortion room**.

distortion in psychoanalysis, the modification of forbidden thoughts, impulses, or experiences to make them more acceptable to the ego. In dreams, e.g., forbidden wishes are frequently expressed in disguised or symbolic form: The innocent act of walking upstairs is more likely to pass the censor set up by the superego than the guilt-laden act of intercourse which it represents. D., however, can take other forms: Many people give a warped account of experiences that would otherwise put them in a bad light, usually without realizing they are doing so. On a more pathological level, many psychiatric symptoms (delusions, hallucinations, feelings of unreality, flattened affect, neologism) may be described as distortions of mental or emotional processes.

distortion by transference a misperception of the analytic situation or the analyst due to transference.

distractibility an inability to maintain attention; a tendency to be easily diverted from the matter at hand. Excessive d. is frequently found in children with learning disorders, and in manic patients who shift rapidly from topic to topic. Also see FLIGHT OF IDEAS.

distractible speech a speech pattern in which the patient shifts rapidly from topic to topic in response to external or internal stimuli. It is a common symptom in mania. Also see FLIGHT OF IDEAS.

distress-relief quotient the ratio of verbal expressions of distress to those of relief, used as an index of improvement in counseling and psychotherapy. Also called **discomfort-relief quotient**.

distributed practice the learning procedure in which practice periods are separated by time intervals that are as long as practical. In many learning situations, d.p. is found more effective than massed practice. Also called **distributed learning**. Compare MASSED PRACTICE.

distributional redundancy in psychological esthetics, the development of uncertainty in an artistic pattern by making some kinds of elements occur more frequently than others. D.r. is one of two kinds of internal restraint in pattern variation, the other being **correlational redundancy**, in which certain combinations of elements are made to occur more frequently than others.

distribution curve a plot showing values on the base line and frequency on the vertical axis.

distribution-free statistics statistics that make no a priori assumption about the shape of the frequency distribution under study; statistics that are applicable even in the absence of a normal distribution. Also see NONPARAMETRIC STATISTICS.

distribution-free tests tests of statistical significance that make relatively few assumptions about the underlying distribution of scores. E.g., the chi-square test does not assume that observations are normally distributed.

distributive analysis and synthesis Adolf Meyer's "critical common-sense" approach to psychotherapy, in which (a) a systematic analysis is made of the patient's past and present experience, including his symptoms and complaints, assets and liabilities, and pathological or immature reactions, (b) this study, or anamnesis, is used as a prelude to a constructive synthesis built on the patient's own strengths, goals, and abilities. See MEYER; PSYCHOBIOLOGY.

distributive justice Piaget's term for the older child's belief that rules can be changed and punishments and rewards distributed according to relative standards, specifically according to "equality" and "equity." In the **equality stage** (age eight to ten), children demand that everyone be treated in the same way. In the **equity stage** (age 11 and older), children make allowances for subjective considerations, personal circumstances, and motive. Compare IMMANENT JUSTICE.

disturbances of associations according to Bleuler, one of the basic symptoms of schizophrenia, in which interruptions of thought associations lead to haphazard, confused, bizarre thinking.

disturbing event; disturbing memory: See DETERMINING QUALITY.

disulfiram an organic sulfide that interferes with normal metabolism of alcohol. The substance rarely produces pharmacologic effects by itself. But when small amounts of alcohol are ingested after certain blood levels of d. are established through administration of the medical form of d., a toxic reaction occurs as long as the alcohol is being metabolized. Individual reactions may vary from discomfort to death. See ANTABUSE.

disuse principle the assumption that responses not practiced will weaken and disappear.

disynaptic arc a nerve circuit in which there is one neuron between a motoneuron and a sensory neuron, requiring a nerve impulse to cross two synapses to complete the arc.

Ditran: See PSYCHEDELICS.

diuretics substances that increase the flow of urine. D. may be naturally occurring body agents, e.g., dopamine, or prescription or nonprescription drugs, e.g., caffeine. D. generally act by increasing the blood flow through the kidneys while increasing the rate of filtration by kidney tissues or by altering the osmolality of kidney function, as by inhibiting the reabsorption of sodium which in turn reduces the amount of fluid required by the tissues. Some d. may produce adverse effects with psychological implications, e.g., lassitude, weakness, vertigo, sexual impotence, headaches, polydipsia, irritability, excitability.

diurnal cycles patterns of activity or behavior that follow the day-night cycles. Most humans and many other species, e.g., wild birds, often follow predictable patterns of daylight activity in seeking food and water. Other animals may be crepuscular or nocturnal in their 24-hour activity cycles. A number of species undergo diurnal color changes that persist even in a controlled environment of continuous light or darkness. See CIRCADIAN RHYTHMS.

diurnality the daily repetition of an activity, such as the opening of a flower each morning.

diurnal rhythm an activity or series of activities occurring each day during the day, e.g., eating and digesting three meals at fairly regular intervals, or the common energy changes that occur every day. See BIOLOGICAL RHYTHM; DIURNAL CYCLES.

divagation rambling, digressive speech and thought.

divergence the tendency for the eyes to turn outward when shifting from near to far fixation. A permanent d. ("walleye") of one eye is termed EXOTROPIA. See this entry.

divergent strabismus: See GRIEG'S DISEASE.

divergent thinking an aspect of creative thinking characterized by the formulation of alternative solutions to problems. In d.t. the task is to generate answers, whereas in convergent thinking the task is to logically analyze solutions that have already been formulated. Compare CONVERGENT THINKING.

diversive exploration a form of behavior that may result from boredom or a lack of stimulation, causing the individual to seek arousing stimuli in his environment. E.g., a bored adolescent may seek excitement in street-gang activities if his life at home provides inadequate stimulation. Also see RESTLESSNESS; BOREDOM.

divided brain = SPLIT BRAIN.

divided consciousness a state of consciousness in which two or more mental activities are carried out at the same time, e.g., listening, planning questions, and taking notes during an interview. The view that two activities can be performed simultaneously is in accord with parallel-processing theory. Serial-processing theory, however, holds that the ability to attend to two things at once is a misconception, and that there is only a rapid shifting between information sources.

divination a paranormal process in which future events are alleged to be foretold, or hidden knowledge is discovered, by means of (a) a spiritualistic medium's supernatural powers, as in crystal-gazing, or (b) augury, that is, the interpretation of omens or portents such as the flight of birds or the entrails of a sacrificed animal.

divorce the legal dissolution of marriage. A d. may be granted in some jurisdictions if the spouse can be proved to be mentally incompetent. Also see EMOTIONAL D.

divorce counseling the counseling process applied to divorced individuals, usually on a group basis in order to provide group support and to encourage a sense of belonging and identity during the transitional period. Members of the group are also encouraged to let go of the past, to learn through the experiences of others what types of behavior contributed to the breakup, and to learn to deal with their present emotions such as mood swings and vindictiveness.

Dix, Dorothea Lynde American educator, 1802–87. After witnessing the cruel and inhuman treatment of "lunatics" during a visit to an East Cambridge house of correction, Miss D., a former school teacher, launched a 25-year crusade in which she investigated conditions in no less than 500 almshouses, 300 houses of detention, and 18 penitentiaries, in addition to innumerable asylums and hospitals. She presented her findings forcibly and insistently in the press and before government officials and legislatures, and was instrumental in improving conditions for the mentally ill not only in the United States, but in England, France, Scandinavia, Holland, and Russia.

dizygotic twins twins that have developed from separate fertilized ova. Three-fourths of all twins are dizygotic, or fraternal, and may be of the same or different sexes. D.t. also tend to be larger and to have fewer congenital defects than identical twins. Although d.t. are genetically no more closely related than siblings, their being born at the same time and place reduces the number of possible factors that might influence their psychological development. Thus, dizygotic-twin studies are useful in providing data regarding genetic and environmental influences on child development. Also called **fraternal twins; biovular twins**. See MONOZYGOTIC TWINS; TWIN STUDIES.

dizziness a whirling sensation, often with nausea and a fear of fainting. See VERTIGO.

DL = DIFFERENCE LIMEN.

D love = DEFICIENCY LOVE.

DMPEA: See PINK SPOT.

DMT: See TRYPTAMINE DERIVATIVES.

DNA *d*eoxyribo*n*ucleic *a*cid; a complex molecule that occurs in all body-cell nuclei as a pair of helix-shaped strands of smaller molecules called bases, or basic nucleotides. The bases, adenine, guanine, thymine, and cytosine, are linked through molecules of phosphoric acid and a sugar, deoxyribose. The DNA molecule is the primary structural unit of genetic material for all living organisms, including viruses. The DNA is self-replicating, or able to reproduce itself from other substances in the environment, and contains the template or formula for building any living organism from a bacterium to a human from the other molecules in the external environment. Also see RECOMBINANT DNA.

doctor game a sex game involving the touching and examination of the genitals of girls by boys, or of the boy's genital by the girl who plays the role of a "nurse." In certain cultures, children's sex games may include simulated sexual intercourse.

doctor-patient relationship the interpersonal relationship which develops between doctor and patient. If this relationship is characterized by warmth, cooperation, patience, and mutual esteem, it can have a positive effect on the outcome of both physical and psychological treatment.

Doctrine of Signatures: See salicylates.

Doerfler, Leo G. American audiologist, 1919—. See DOERFLER-STEWART TEST.

Doerfler-Stewart test a test originated for screening for functional hearing loss during World War II. It is used to examine a person's ability to respond to selected two-syllable words in the presence of a masking noise.

Dogiel, Alexander Stanislavovic Russian histologist, 1852–1922. See DOGIEL'S CORPUSCLES.

Dogiel's corpuscles sensory end organs found in the mucous membranes of the genitals and other body organs. D.c. are Krause-type end bulbs which in the penis and clitoris have a distinct mulberrylike appearance at the end of their attached nerve fibers. Also called **genital corpuscles**.

dog phobia = CYNOPHOBIA.

-dolich-; -dolicho- /-dōl'ik-/ a combining form meaning long.

dolichocephalic characterizing a head that is long and narrow, with a cephalic index below 75.

dolichomorphic characterizing a body that is tall and thin.

Dollard, John American psychologist, 1900–80. See AGGRESSION; FRUSTRATION-AGGRESSION HYPOTHESIS.

doll fear = PEDIOPHOBIA.

Dollinger, Albert German physician, 1888—. See DOLLINGER-BIELSCHOWSKY SYNDROME.

Dollinger-Bielschowsky syndrome a form of amaurotic familial idiocy in which the onset of symptoms occurs between the ages of three and four years. The effects include cerebroretinal degeneration with cerebellar ataxia, defective hearing, convulsions, ocular disorders, and mental deterioration. Pathology shows a high concentration of gangliosides in the brain. See TAY-SACHS DISEASE. Also see GANGLIOSIDOSIS.

doll play in psychiatry and mental hygiene, the use of dolls and figurines representing familiar individuals in playing out such feelings as anger, rejection, and anxiety (**permissive d.p.**); also, their use in telling or enacting "stories" that express emotional needs or reveal significant family relationships (**projective d.p.**). See PLAY THERAPY.

-dom- a combining form relating to a house or abode (from Latin *domus*, "house").

DOM: See PSYCHEDELICS; PHENYLETHYLAMINE DERIVATIVES; AMPHETAMINES.

domal sampling a survey in which a specific member of a predetermined household is interviewed.

Doman, Glenn Joseph American child-development worker, 1919—. See PATTERNING EXERCISES.

domatophobia a morbid fear of being inside a building. Also see OIKOPHOBIA.

domesticated pride: See PRIDE.

domicile in psychiatry, a residential setting in which continued care is given to deinstitutionalized patients according to need. These settings include chronic-care hospitals, skilled-nursing facilities, health-related facilities, intermediate-care facilities, halfway houses, residential facilities or homes, social-rehabilitation facilities, and satellite housing.

domiciliary care in psychiatry, residential care of chronic mental patients. Some settings, such as chronic-care hospitals and skilled nursing facilities, provide full supervision and nursing care; others, such as health-related and intermediate-care facilities, provide less supervision and only occasional nursing care; still others, such as halfway houses, residential-care facilities, social-rehabilitation facilities, and satellite housing, actively promote independence and provide only temporary or minimal assistance and supervision.

dominance ascendance, or assertion of control over others; also, the tendency for one hemisphere of the brain to exert greater influence than the other over certain functions, such as language and handedness. The term also applies to the prepotency of one response over another; e.g., flexion is dominant over extension in withdrawing the hand from a hot stove. In genetics, d. is the tendency for one trait to predominate over another, such as a gene for brown eyes over a gene for blue eyes. Also see LATERAL D.; HANDEDNESS.

dominance aggression: See ANIMAL AGGRESSION.

dominance hierarchy in behavior, the ordering of responses in terms of their priority or importance; e.g., a sneeze takes precedence over feeding the cat. In social psychology, d.h. denotes

the classification of group members in relation to their power or prestige; e.g., a captain takes precedence over a corporal, a cardinal over a bishop.

dominance need the need to dominate, lead, or otherwise control others (Murray).

dominance-submission = ASCENDANCE-SUBMISSION.

dominance-subordination relationships the tendency of animal communities to organize in social patterns with a leader or dominant member who imposes his will on the other, subordinate members of the community. The d.-s.r. are highly organized in troops of baboons, where dominant males and subordinate females and offspring form affectionate but protective clusters to insure survival of the species.

dominant gene a gene or hereditary trait that manifests itself in the offspring. The d.g. will express itself even when it occurs on only one of the two inherited chromosomes. See RECESSIVE GENE; GENE.

dominant genotype: See GENOTYPE.

dominant hemisphere: See LATERALITY; LATERAL DOMINANCE; DOMINANCE; SPLIT BRAIN.

dominant inheritance a category of genetic disorders based on single-gene defects, which may be autosomal or sex-linked. **Autosomal-d.i.** persons must have at least one affected parent, and a union between an affected parent and a normal person will produce on the average an equal number of affected and normal children. Because of the presence of other genes, the defect may be expressed in various ways in different offspring.

dominant trait in genetics, the member of a gene (allele) pair that is expressed and produces an observable effect (phenotype) in the organism.

dominant wavelength a color wavelength which when mixed with white will match a given hue.

dominator-modulator theory the theory that chromatic vision depends upon a modulator that mediates the dominant receptor for brightness.

dominators visual receptors that react to peaks of brightness at certain color frequencies although they respond to a broad band of the spectrum and produce ganglion-cell responses.

donatism a term used to identify a form of hypnosis in which imitation plays an important role. The term is derived from Donato, the professional name of Alfred d'Hout of Belgium, who first demonstrated this role.

Donato: See D'HOUT.

Donders, Franciscus Cornelius Dutch ophthalmologist, 1818–89. See DONDERS' LAW.

Donders' law the principle that the position of the eyes in looking at an object is independent of their movement to that position.

Don Juan a legendary Spanish libertine, the subject of literature and Mozart's opera *Don Giovanni*. The name has become synonymous with a ruthless seducer, who is concerned only with sexual conquest, after which he abruptly loses interest in his victim (**Don Juanism**). In contrast to Casanova, who adored women with male confidence, a D. J. thinks of women as prey, is insecure as a man, and therefore is obsessed with the need to prove his masculinity. See CASANOVA. Also see SATYRIASIS; EROTOMANIA.

Don Juan syndrome = SATYRIASIS. Also see DON JUAN.

Donohue, William Leslie Canadian pathologist, 1906—. See LEPRECHAUNISM (also called **Donohue's syndrome**).

'don't hold' functions: See DETERIORATION INDEX.

door-in-the-face effect in social-psychology experiments, the finding that an individual who denies a substantial request is more likely to accede later to a lesser request. Also see FOOT-IN-THE-DOOR EFFECT.

DOP = DERMO-OPTICAL PERCEPTION.

DOPA /dō′pə/ an acronym for the chemical name of a naturally occurring substance that is a precursor of the catecholamines. The chemical name is *di*hydr*o*xyphenyl*a*lanine, which is derived from the amino acid phenylalanine. DOPA is converted by the body to dopamine, which, in turn, is a precursor of epinephrine and norepinephrine.

dopamine the precursor of epinephrine and norepinephrine. D. is derived from DOPA and is a primary form in which catecholamines are stored in tissues outside the nervous system. Almost all of the catecholamine of the liver and portions of the digestive tract occurs as d. A deficiency of d. in the brain is a diagnostic sign of parkinsonism.

dopamine hypothesis the concept that schizophrenia is caused by an excess of dopamine in the brain. The excess may be due either to an overproduction of dopamine or a deficiency of the enzyme needed to convert dopamine to norepinephrine (adrenaline).

dopamine receptors receptors sensitive to dopamine and chemically related compounds. D.r. are located in blood vessels of the kidneys and mesentery, where the dopaminergic effect results in artery dilation, and also in nervous-system tissue, e.g., the striatum, where subnormal levels may result in parkinsonism.

dopaminergic neurons nerve cells of the sympathetic system and ganglia and of the central nervous system that are influenced by the adrenergic drug dopamine. D.n. that appear most sensitive to dopamine are located in the abdominal region where the drug produces dilation of blood vessels. See DOPAMINERGICS.

dopaminergics drugs or other agents that affect the production or utilization of the catecholamine dopamine, a precursor of norepinephrine. Because of evidence that parkinsonism is caused by a dysfunction of dopaminergic neurons in the brain, drugs that enhance the maintenance of adequate levels of dopamine have therapeutic value in the treatment of the disorder. A commonly used dopaminergic drug is **levodopa (L-dopa)**—$C_9H_{11}NO_4$. See DOPAMINERGIC NEURONS.

Doppelgänger phenomenon /dô′pəlgangər/ the fantasy or delusion that one has a double, twin, or alter ego, who looks and acts the same as oneself (German, "double walker"). See AUTOSCOPIC SYNDROME.

Doppler, Johann Christian /dôp′lər/ Austrian physicist and mathematician, 1803–53. See DOPPLER EFFECT.

Doppler effect the increase or decrease in wave length when a source of light or sound recedes or approaches the observer, producing a change in hue or pitch.

Dora Case one of Freud's earliest and most celebrated cases, reported in *Fragment of an Analysis of a Case of Hysteria* (1905). The study of this woman's multiple symptoms (headaches, aphonia, suicidal ideation, amnesic episodes) contributed to his theory of repression and the use of dream interpretation as an analytic tool.

doraphobia a morbid fear of touching or seeing the skin of animals (from Greek *dora*, "skin, fur").

Dorian love a term referring to male homosexuality, particularly pederasty (as probably practiced among the Dorians, a prehistoric Greek tribe).

Doriden: See PIPERIDINEDIONES.

-dors-; -dorsi-; -dorso- a combining form relating to the back.

dorsal pertaining to the back or posterior side. Compare VENTRAL.

dorsal columns tracts of nerve fibers that run through the spinal cord on its dorsal side. See A FIBER; LEMNISCAL SYSTEM.

dorsal roots the stalks of sensory-nerve fibers that enter the spinal cord on the dorsal sides of the cord.

dorsomedial nucleus a mass of nerve tissue projecting from the thalamus to the frontal lobes. It is associated with the emotional expressions of anxiety and fear.

Doryl a commercial form of carbachol, a cholinergic drug, used as a stimulant of the parasympathetic system.

dose-response relationship a principle that the pharmacological effect of a drug is generally dependent upon the size of the dose. The d.-r.r. is modified in practice to accommodate a number of variables, e.g., the body weight, skin-surface area, and rate of metabolic activity, of individual subjects. With variables adjusted, the d.-r.r. of a drug usually plots as a straight-line curve.

dotting test a pencil-and-paper motor test in which the subject makes as many dots as possible in a given time period, either randomly (tapping test) or in small circles (aiming test).

double-agentry an ethical term applied to a conflict of interest that exists when a psychiatrist examines a patient and is at the same time employed by a hospital, government agency, court, or other authority—a situation that should be made clear to the individual under examination.

double approach-avoidance conflict a complex

conflict situation arising when a person is confronted with two goals that both contain equally significant attractive and repellent features. Also see APPROACH-AVOIDANCE CONFLICT.

double-approach conflict = APPROACH-APPROACH CONFLICT.

double-aspect theory: See BODY-MIND PROBLEM.

double-avoidance conflict = AVOIDANCE-AVOIDANCE CONFLICT.

double-barreled colostomy: See COLOSTOMY.

double bind a situation in which a child receives contradictory messages from one or both parents, and is therefore torn between conflicting feelings and demands; e.g., the mother may complain that the child is not affectionate, yet turn a cold shoulder when he tries to put his arm around her. The anthropologist Gregory Bateson, who proposed the term, claimed that this type of situation is a major cause of schizophrenia.

double blind an experimental condition in which both experimenter and subject, or both physician and patient, are unaware of the nature of the experiment, manipulation, or drug administered. Also see SINGLE BLIND.

double consciousness a term occasionally used in describing the state of mind of a dual or alternating personality. See MULTIPLE PERSONALITY.

double dissociation the association between anatomical lesions and behavioral disturbances. D.d. involves processes for demonstrating possible multiple sites of brain lesions to account for multiple symptoms in syndromes of neurologic defects.

double entendre: See PUN.

double heterozygousness a situation in which an individual has both dominant and recessive alleles for two linked genes.

double images duplicate retinal images that occur as a result of eye defects; also, doubling of images in the distance when fixating on near objects, and of near images when fixating on far objects.

double insanity = FOLIE À DEUX.

double meaning: See PUN.

double orientation a term used by Bleuler to describe the ability of some schizophrenic patients to function normally in the real world while maintaining a fantastic delusion. E.g., a woman may be a satisfactory restaurant worker but sincerely believe she is a daughter of Czar Nicholas of Russia. Also called **delusion of orientation**.

double personality: See DUAL PERSONALITY; MULTIPLE PERSONALITY.

double representation the perception of two hues or brightnesses when an object is illuminated by light of a different color.

double sampling the use of two or more methods of selecting samples for surveys or studies of a population. Also called **mixed sampling**.

double-simultaneous stimulation a test used in studies of parietal-lobe lesions by presenting two stimuli simultaneously. Various types of inattention are seen visually, tactually, and so on. See DOUBLE-SIMULTANEOUS TACTILE SENSATION.

double-simultaneous tactile sensation the ability of a person to perceive that he has received two tactile sensations in different areas at the same time. In one test of the ability, the **Fink-Green-Bender test**, the person is touched on the face and hand at the same time. Normal individuals can perceive the d.-s.t.s. by the age of six, but the ability often is impaired in persons with certain neurologic disorders, including childhood schizophrenia. Also see FACE-HAND TEST.

double standard the general concept that a code of behavior is permissible for one group or one individual but not for another; in particular, the concept that free sexual expression is acceptable for males but not for females, as exemplified in the father who insists on his daughter's virginity while encouraging, or winking at, his son's escapades.

double superego the existence of two consciences in cases of psychic dualism. One conscience usually is masculine and the other feminine, and each is antagonistic toward the other.

double vision the perception of a single object as a separate image by each eye. D.v. may be caused by strabismus in which the image perceived by the right eye may appear to the left of the image perceived by the left eye, as a binocular effect of two separate parallel images, or in vertical displacement in which one image appears above the other. D.v. may occur only in certain visual fields, e.g., when looking to the left rather than straight ahead. The term is essentially equivalent to DIPLOPIA. See this entry.

double-Y condition a genetic disorder involving an abnormality of the male sex chromosome. Individuals born with this condition have a XYY complement of sex chromosomes rather than the normal male set of XY. Because early studies found a high proportion of XYY cases among violent, aggressive men in prisons and mental institutions, it was believed the extra Y chromosome might be a causal factor.

doubt: See AUTONOMY VERSUS D.

doubting mania extreme and obsessive doubting; a feeling of uncertainty about even the most obvious matters, such as the names of one's children. It is a common symptom of obsessive-compulsive neurosis. The individual may feel compelled to check and double-check to see whether the gas has been turned off, the door has been locked, or a column of figures has been added up correctly. The condition has long been recognized, and was named by Jean-Pierre Falret (French, *folie du doute*). Also called **folie du doute** /fōlē'dēdo͞ot'/; **doubting madness; maladie du doute** /mälädē'dēdo͞ot'/.

dowager's hump: See KYPHOSIS.

Down, John Langdon Haydon English physician, 1828–96. See DOWN'S SYNDROME; ACROMICRIA; AMNIOCENTESIS; AUTOSOMAL ABERRATIONS; BIRTH DEFECT; CONGENITAL ANOMALIES; DERMATOGLYPHICS; DISFIGUREMENT; FRAGILE X CHROMO-

SOME; GROUP G MONOSOMY; INFANT-STIMULATION PROGRAM; KALMUK IDIOCY; LEUKEMIA; MONGOLIAN IDIOT; MOSAICISM; SYNCHRONISM; TARTAR TYPE; TERATOLOGICAL DEFECTS; TRISOMY 21.

downers a colloquial term for DEPRESSANTS. See this entry.

Downey, June Etta American psychologist, 1875–1932. See DOWNEY'S WILL-TEMPERAMENT TESTS.

Downey's Will-Temperament Tests an early attempt (1924) to measure personality and temperamental differences primarily through controlled handwriting tasks.

Down's syndrome a chromosomal disorder, characterized by an extra chromosome 21—in some cases, 22—and manifested by so-called mongoloid features, a round flat face, and eyes that seem to slant. Brain size and weight are below average, and the patients usually are mildly to severely retarded and have docile, agreeable dispositions. Muscular movements tend to be slow, clumsy, and uncoordinated. In many cases growth is retarded, the tongue is thick, and the fingers are stubby. Also called **mongolism; Langdon Down's disease; congenital acromicria; autosomal trisomy of Group G**. Also see TRISOMY 21; MONGOLIAN IDIOT.

downward mobility the movement of a person or group from one social class to a lower social class. Also see SOCIAL MOBILITY. Compare UPWARD MOBILITY.

dowsing the use of a divining rod or forked stick to allegedly locate underground water or minerals. Also see RHABDOMANCY.

doxapram: See PSYCHOSTIMULANTS.

doxepin hydrochloride: See TRICYCLIC ANTIDEPRESSANTS.

D-penicillamine = PENICILLAMINE.

DQ = DEVELOPMENTAL QUOTIENT.

drama therapy: See PSYCHODRAMA.

dramatic personality: See HISTRIONIC PERSONALITY DISORDER.

dramatics the use of drama as a rehabilitation technique, using published or original scripts with patients as performers. Therapists may use special puppet-show scripts in the rehabilitation of disabled children. Also see PSYCHODRAMA.

dramatization the use of attention-getting behavior as a defense against anxiety. An example of d. is the exaggeration or d. of the symptoms of an illness to make it appear more important than the occurrence of the same illness in another person. In psychoanalysis, d. is the expression (as in dreams) of repressed wishes or impulses.

Draw-a-House Test; Draw-a-Person Test: See MACHOVER DRAW-A-PERSON TEST.

drawing disability: See DYSGRAPHIA.

dread anxiety elicited by a specific threat, or "danger-situation" (Freud), such as going out on a dark night, as contrasted to anxiety that does not have a specific object.

dream: See DREAMS.

dream anxiety attacks = NIGHTMARE.

dream censorship the disguise of unconscious impulses in dreams. According to Freud, the thoroughness of dream disguise varies directly with the strictness of the censorship.

dream content in psychoanalysis, the images, ideas, and impulses expressed in dreams. See LATENT CONTENT; MANIFEST CONTENT.

dream ego a term introduced by Jung to identify a fragment of the conscious ego that is active during the dream state.

dream function the view that, (a) according to Freud, the dream is a disguised fulfillment of a repressed wish, and (b) according to Jung, that it is a reflection of fundamental personality tendencies with either a transient or continuous importance.

dream induction the production of a dream through hypnosis, either by command or as a posthypnotic suggestion. D.i. is a technique used in hypnoanalysis.

dream interpretation in psychoanalysis, the deciphering and understanding of the unconscious meanings of dreams and dream symbols, primarily through free association.

dream pain = HYPNALGIA.

dreams a fleeting sequence of images, more or less structured, occurring spontaneously and with a sense of reality during sleep. In nature, d. may be echoes of past experiences, anticipations of future events, attempts to solve problems, wish-fulfilling fantasies, expressions of inner conflict, and dramatizations of anxieties that plague the dreamer in waking life. They also appear to serve many functions: as outlets for tension, guardians of sleep, or safety valves in preventing emotional disorder. In the psychoanalytic process, Freud has described d. as "the royal road to the unconscious" and as expressing repressed impulses and ideas that exert so much influence on our behavior. Also see ARTIFICIAL DREAM; COLOR D.; CONSOLATION D.; CONVENIENCE D.; COUNTER-WISH D.; EMBARRASSMENT DREAM; EXAMINATION DREAM; INSOMNIUM DREAM; MASOCHISTIC WISH-DREAM; PARALLEL DREAM; PERENNIAL DREAM; PRODROMIC DREAM; PROPHETIC D.; RECURRENT D.; TELEPATHIC DREAM; WET DREAM.

dream screen a term used by K. Lewin (1946) for a surface, or screen, on which dreams sometimes seem to be projected. Eidelberg quotes a patient as saying, "While lying here looking at my dream, it turned over and away from me, rolled up and away from me, over and over like two tumblers." See ISAKOWER PHENOMENON.

dream state the D-state or REM state during which dreaming takes place. The d.s. usually occurs four or five times during the night and is physiologically distinct from the ordinary sleep state (S-state) and the waking state (W-state), since rapid eye movements (REM) can be detected and EEG patterns resemble those of wakefulness. Studies indicate that about 20 percent of sleeping time is spent in the d.s. and that there is probably a basic need for dreaming. The pons appears to be the area most involved in the d.s., which is therefore often referred to as **pontine sleep**. Also see TWILIGHT STATE.

dream stimulus any of the stimuli that may initiate a dream, e.g., external stimulation, internal sensory stimulation, internal organic or physical stimulation, or stimulation by the psyche.

dream suggestion a specialized hypnotic technique in which the subject is instructed to dream about his problems or their source either during the hypnotic state or posthypnotically, during natural sleep. The technique is sometimes used as an aid in hypnotherapy.

dream within a dream a part of a dream that is regarded during the dream state as having been dreamed, an event that is interpreted as a repudiation of that part by the dreamer.

dream work in psychoanalysis, the transformation of the latent dream content into the manifest content which the dreamer experiences. Involved in this transformation are CONDENSATION, SYMBOLIZATION, DISPLACEMENT, DRAMATIZATION, and SECONDARY ELABORATION. See these entries.

dreamy state a brief altered state of consciousness similar to a dream, during which the patient experiences visual, olfactory or auditory hallucinations, but no convulsions. It is most commonly associated with temporal-lobe lesions. Marijuana-smoking produces a similar state in some individuals.

dressing a daily-living aspect of occupational therapy for disabled persons, who may require training in the use of special clothing fasteners, e.g., Velcro shoe closures, zippers that close or open by pulling on a ring, or devices to aid in pulling up stockings or pants.

dressing apraxia a brain-damage disorder manifested by an inability to clothe oneself properly. In a typical case, a patient may put his clothing on so that it covers only the right side of the body, neglecting the left side. The cause is believed to be a parietal lesion of the nondominant hemisphere.

dressing behavior in psychiatry, dressing in accordance with one's sex as an important factor in gender identity. Studies of transvestites and transsexuals indicate that they usually cross-dressed (or were cross-dressed) in childhood. See CROSS DRESSING.

DRH differential *r*einforcement of *h*igh rate, a schedule in which faster responding brings about more frequent reinforcement. Also see DRL.

Driesch, Hans /drēsh/ German biologist and philosopher, 1867–1941. D. opposed the strict mechanistic approach of the time and postulated an irreducible purposive force, or "vital energy," which gives form and direction to all living organisms. See VITALISM.

drift hypothesis a concept purporting to explain the higher incidence of schizophrenia in the center of an urban area than in the outskirts, suggesting that during the preclinical phase, people tend to drift into the anonymous environment of the central city.

drifting attention a tendency to maintain attention for a few moments, when alerted, but to drift back to a somnolent state. The condition is a disorder of the subcortical alerting system which usually indicates pathological involvement of the midbrain or thalamic portion of the reticular activating system. Also see WANDERING ATTENTION.

drill the methodical repetition or systematic practice of a physical or mental response or response sequence for the purpose of learning. D. may be necessary when the material to be learned does not yet represent to the student an integrated or internally coherent entity; e.g., an American learning the Arabic alphabet may need to employ d.

drinking aids daily-living aids that permit a disabled individual to ingest liquids without the aid of another person. D.a. may include terry-cloth tumbler jackets, wooden or metal glass holders, various built-in and flexible sipping straws, coasters with suction-cup attachments, and cups designed for drinking when the patient is in a supine position.

drinking behavior (Jellinek's categories): See ALPHA ALCOHOLISM; BETA ALCOHOLISM; GAMMA ALCOHOLISM; DELTA ALCOHOLISM; EPSILON ALCOHOLISM.

drinking bouts: See DIPSOMANIA.

drive a state of organic tension, as in hunger, sex, or pain, which motivates the individual to perform actions that will alleviate the tension. The distinction is sometimes made between primary drives, which are directly based on physiological needs, and secondary or acquired drives, such as competition, which are indirectly based on these needs. The term d. was introduced by R. S. Woodworth in 1918. See INSTINCT; MOTIVATION.

drive arousal the activation of a drive by any internal or external stimulus, or a combination of both.

drive displacement the replacement of a frustrated drive by one more easily gratified, e.g., "raiding the icebox" when disappointed.

driver education in rehabilitation, the training of disabled persons to operate an automobile, which may be equipped with appropriate special controls. E.g., a previously trained driver may have to learn to operate a vehicle with hand-operated accelerator and brakes, or a gearshift extension for left-hand rather than right-hand use. See CAR CONTROLS.

drive-reduction theory a theory that motivated behavior depends on drives, and that drive-satisfying responses tend to be reinforced or strengthened (Hull, Thorndike).

drive state an internal condition, e.g., hunger, that activates drive behavior.

DRL differential *r*einforcement of *l*ow rate, a schedule in which slower responses bring about more frequent reinforcements, while faster responses postpone reinforcement. The concept was proposed by B. F. Skinner. Also see DRH.

droit du seigneur = JUS PRIMAE NOCTIS.

-drom-; -dromo- a combining form relating to movement, e.g., traveling (from Greek *dromos*, "running, course").

dromolepsy a short spurt of running that may precede an epileptic seizure and usually ends in the seizure. Also called **procursive epilepsy**.

dromomania the abnormal drive or desire to travel. Also called **vagabond neurosis**.

dromophobia a morbid fear of crossing a street or road; also, a morbid fear of traveling.

drop foot an abnormal condition in which the foot, due to damage to the peroneal nerve, hangs in a plantar-flexed (toes-downward) position. The condition can be corrected by an electronic prosthesis that dorsiflexes the foot (toes upward) on a signal triggered by lifting the heel when taking a step. When the heel strikes the ground again, the stimulus is terminated until the heel is raised the next time.

drop-in center a mental-health facility, such as a methadone clinic, in which treatment can be obtained without an advance appointment.

dropout in education, a student who leaves school before graduating; in psychiatry, a patient who terminates treatment before it is completed.

drowsiness: See SOMNOLENCE; TWILIGHT SLEEP.

drug abuse: See SUBSTANCE ABUSE; SUBSTANCE-USE DISORDER.

drug culture a population group whose members utilize one or more kinds of drugs of abuse, usually illicit drugs such as marijuana, hashish, cocaine, heroin, LSD, or other agents known to produce altered states of consciousness. The term d.c. usually is not applied to accepted religious groups, such as the Native American Church, whose members use mind-altering drugs in their ceremonies and rituals.

drug defaulter = DEFAULTER.

drug dependence: See SUBSTANCE DEPENDENCE.

drug education the process of informing individuals or groups of persons about the effects of various chemical agents on the human body, usually with special emphasis on effects of mind-altering substances.

drug holiday discontinuance of a psychoactive drug for a limited period in order to control dosage and side effects, and to evaluate the patient's behavior with and without it.

drug-induced parkinsonism: See PARKINSONISM.

drug-induced psychosis a psychotic state resulting from heavy doses of therapeutic drugs such as thiocyanate, belladonna, chloral hydrate, paraldehyde, isoniazid, cortisone, or ACTH. The term also applies to psychotic states resulting from substance abuse or substance use. For the latter disorders, see ALCOHOL ABUSE; COCAINE ABUSE; HALLUCINOGEN ABUSE; OPIOID ABUSE; PHENCYCLIDINE; AMPHETAMINE OR SIMILARLY ACTING SYMPATHOMIMETIC DEPENDENCE; BARBITURATE OR SIMILARLY ACTING SEDATIVE OR HYPNOTIC DEPENDENCE.

drug interaction the effects of the administration of two or more pharmacologically active agents within the same time period. Phenobarbital accelerates the metabolism of steroid hormones while salicylates increase the concentration of coumarin derivatives in the body. Drugs most likely to cause d.i. include hypnotics, CNS stimulants, antidepressants, tranquilizers, muscle relaxants, and antihistamines. Barbiturates can cause d.i. by altering liver enzymes so that other drugs administered later are rendered less effective.

drug of choice the drug that is preferred or recommended over alternative medications because of clinical, or bedside, evidence that it is the most effective for most patients. Because of individual factors, e.g., allergies or possible interactions with other drugs being administered, the d.o.c. may not be the medication chosen.

drug therapy the use of chemical agents in the treatment of physical or psychological disorder. Also called **chemotherapy**. See PSYCHOPHARMACOLOGY; MAINTENANCE DRUGS.

drug tolerance: See TOLERANCE.

dry mouth an autonomic-nervous-system effect associated with intense emotion and caused by sympathetic changes that restrict or inhibit salivation. The condition also can be a symptom of thirst or the result of a drug, e.g., the thiazide medications which increase the excretion of sodium and water.

dry orgasm = COITUS SINE EJACULATIONE.

DSM-III the third edition (1980) of the **Diagnostic and Statistical Manual of Mental Disorders**, prepared by the Task Force on Nomenclature and Statistics of the American Psychiatric Association. The classification presents descriptions of diagnostic categories (which appear as entries in this dictionary) without favoring any particular theory of etiology. It is largely modeled after the *International Classification of Diseases*, 9th Edition, 1978, developed by the World Health Organization, and modified for use in the United States (ICD-9-CM), but contains greater detail and recent changes, as well as a method of coding on different axes (multiaxial classification). Previous editions were published in 1952 (**DSM-I**) and 1968 (**DSM-II**). Also see INTERNATIONAL CLASSIFICATION OF DISEASES, and see the Appendix DSM-III CLASSIFICATION.

D-state: See DREAM STATE; W-STATE.

DT: See ALCOHOL-WITHDRAWAL DELIRIUM.

d.t.d. an abbreviation used in prescriptions, meaning "give of such doses" (Latin *dentur tales doses*).

DTPS = DIFFUSE THALAMIC PROJECTION SYSTEM.

D trisomy = CHROMOSOME-13 TRISOMY.

DTVP: See FROSTIG DEVELOPMENTAL TEST OF VISUAL PERCEPTION.

dual ambivalence the conflicting emotions of adolescents and parents that characterize their changing relationship as the adolescent strives for independence while still wanting and needing guidance and support.

dual-arousal model a plan for explanation of the physiological relationships between sleep and wakefulness. It is based on evidence that the arousal function involves two nerve pathways, the diffuse thalamic system and the reticular activating system. The two systems, according to the plan, allow the brain to operate in two modes, one a stimulus-processing and the other a response-executing function.

dual-instinct theory the view that human life is governed by two antagonistic forces, the life instinct, or Eros, and the death instinct, or Thanatos. This was a late and controversial contribution of Freud, who held that "the interaction of the two basic instincts with or against each other gives rise to the whole variegation of the phenomena of life" (*Beyond the Pleasure Principle*, 1920).

dualism: See BODY-MIND PROBLEM; CARTESIAN D.

dual-leadership therapy = MULTIPLE THERAPY.

dual masturbation: See MUTUAL MASTURBATION.

dual-memory theory the concept that memory is a two-stage process, namely, a short-term memory, which allows retention of certain information for a few seconds to a few hours, and long-term memory, which permits the retention of information for hours to many years.

dual personality a dissociative disorder in which the personality is divided into two relatively independent and generally contrasting systems. The primary personality is usually unaware of the existence of the secondary, or "co-conscious," personality. See MULTIPLE PERSONALITY.

dual-process theory the concept that the response taken by an individual to a stimulus that permits behavioral control involves two stages, a decision as to whether or not to respond and a decision as to the choice of alternative methods of response.

dual-sex therapy a form of psychotherapy for sexual disorders developed by William Masters and Virginia Johnson. Treatment is focused on a specific sexual problem, and consists largely of a round-table session with a couple in which the male-and-female therapy team suggest special exercises that will improve sexual performance, alleviate inhibitions and anxieties, and facilitate communication both in sexual and nonsexual areas.

dual-transference therapy treatment of the same patient by two therapists, used primarily when the patient needs both support and confrontation with reality and cannot accept both from the same therapist.

Dubini, Angelo Italian physician, 1813–1902. See DUBINI'S DISEASE.

Dubini's disease a usually fatal form of chorea caused by an infection of the central nervous system. The onset of symptoms is sudden and violent. Also called **electrolepsy**.

Dubois, Paul-Charles /dēbô·ä'/ French psychiatrist, 1848–1918. See PERSUASION THERAPY.

Duchenne, Guillaume Benjamin Amand /dēshen'/ French physician, 1806–75. See DUCHENNE'S PSEUDOHYPERTROPHIC MUSCULAR DYSTROPHY; ARAN-DUCHENNE DISEASE; PROGRESSIVE SPINAL-MUSCULAR ATROPHY.

Duchenne's pseudohypertrophic muscular dystrophy one of several kinds of inherited diseases marked by weakness and degeneration of the muscle fibers, but without degeneration of motor neurons as found in other muscular-atrophy disorders. It affects young boys after the age of three years with loss of muscle strength first in the pelvic girdle, followed by weakness in the shoulder girdle. The patients have a waddling gait, have difficulty in rising to a standing position, and often fall. They usually are confined to bed or a wheelchair by the age of 12 and frequently die from obesity and other complications before the age of 20. Blood enzymes are enormously high before the onset of observable symptoms. About one-third of the children have IQs below 75. Also called **Duchenne's muscular dystrophy**.

ductless gland a gland that secretes a substance directly, or without a duct, into the bloodstream, such as the pituitary or thyroid. Also called **endocrine gland**.

ductus deferens /def'-/ the excretory testis duct and a continuation of the epididymis canal. Spermatozoa travel through the d.d. from the epididymis to a junction with the seminal-vesicle duct emptying into the urethra. Also called **seminal duct; spermatic duct; vas deferens**.

dull normal pertaining to an individual whose intelligence is just below normal, roughly between 80 and 90 on the IQ scale.

dummy = PLACEBO.

Duncan, David Beattie Australian-born American statistician, 1916—. See DUNCAN MULTIPLE-RANGE TEST.

Duncan multiple-range test a nonparametric test for comparing several means.

duos the word pairs uttered by children, usually by 24 months or earlier. D. express children's ideas of cause and action as well as their understanding of relationships between people and objects; e.g., recurrence may be verbalized as "more milk," possession as "my milk," and quantity as "little milk." See TELEGRAPHIC SPEECH; HOLOPHRASES. Also see ACTION-INSTRUMENT; ACTION-LOCATION; ACTION-RECIPIENT; AGENT, ACTION, AND OBJECT; ATTRIBUTION; IDENTIFICATION; NEGATION; NONEXISTENCE; POSSESSION; QUESTION STAGE; RECURRENCE.

duplicative reaction a perceptual manifestation observed in some schizophrenic children who encounter the same person at different times or places and believe they are seeing different persons.

duplicity theory the concept that the human eye contains two separate types of light receptors, cone cells that detect color and rod cells that detect variations in light intensity, or brightness. Also see COLOR BLINDNESS; COLOR CELLS.

dura mater the outermost of the three layers of membranes covering the brain and spinal cord, extending as far down the body as the second sacral vertebra. The d.m. is the thickest and strongest of the three membranes. Also called **pachymeninx**. Also see MENINGES.

durance a unit of time within which a life activity occurs (Murray).

Durante's disease = OSTEOGENESIS IMPERFECTA.

Durham rule a 1954 ruling by the United Sates Court of Appeals, that "an accused is not criminally responsible if his unlawful act was the product of mental disease or mental defect." (Durham was the name of a defendent.) This rule has since been replaced by the American Law Institute formulation of INSANITY. See this entry. Also called **Durham test; Durham decision**.

Durkheim, Emile French sociologist, 1858–1917. See ALTRUISTIC SUICIDE; ANOMIC SUICIDE.

Durrell, Donald Dewitt American educator, 1903—. See DIAGNOSTIC EDUCATIONAL TESTS (there: **Durrell Analysis of Reading Difficulty**).

Duso program an educational program developed by the American Guidance Services to provide therapy for emotionally disturbed children. The program is one of several similar methods of providing a curriculum milieu in which the child can explore and understand his feelings, and how they affect his friends and family.

dust fear = AMATHOPHOBIA.

duty fear = HYPENGYOPHOBIA.

DV = DEPENDENT VARIABLE.

D value the *di*scrimination value of test results displayed in a statistical index that shows the relationship of individual items to the total scores.

dwarfism a condition of underdeveloped body structure due to a development defect, a hereditary trait, hormonal or nutritional deficiencies, or diseases. The proportions of the body to the head and limbs may be normal or abnormal. A perfectly formed but undersized dwarf is called a **midget**. Some forms of d., such as **thyroxine-hormone-deficient dwarfs**, are likely to be mentally retarded. Achondroplastic dwarfs usually have normal mentality. Also see ACHONDROPLASIA; PSEUDOACHONDROPLASTIC SPONDYLOEPIPHYSIAL DYSPLASIA; BONE DISEASE; PSYCHOSOCIAL D.; NANISM; PYGMYISM.

Dx an abbreviation of "diagnosis."

dyad a pair of persons in an interpersonal situation, such as mother and infant, husband and wife, mother and father, cotherapists, or patient and therapist; also, two individuals who are so closely knit and interdependent that they would become emotionally disturbed if either one were replaced, e.g., twins reared together, mother and infant, or a closely attached husband and wife. Also see SOCIAL D.

dyadic relationship in psychotherapy or counseling, the working relationship between therapist and patient, or counselor and client.

dyadic session a psychotherapeutic session involving only the therapist and patient.

dyadic therapy = INDIVIDUAL THERAPY.

dying-phobia = THANATOPHOBIA.

dying-process psychological processes taking place in the dying patient, usually involving feelings of fear, anger, shame, and sadness. Psychotherapy includes an opportunity to ventilate these feelings, to grieve for lost functions, and if possible to plan or delegate responsibility for the care of others left behind, and to regress to a more dependent state without feeling guilty. See DEATH EXPECTATION.

Dyke Davidoff syndrome hemiatrophy of the brain, with seizures, mental retardation, facial asymmetry, and contralateral hemiplegia.

Dymphna, Saint Irish princess, fl. seventh century. She was a Christian martyr and became the patron saint of the insane. See SAINT DYMPHNA'S DISEASE; GHEEL COLONY.

-dyn-; -dynia a combining form relating to pain.

-dyna-; -dynam- a combining form relating to power (Greek *dynamis*).

dynamical-system theory the interpretation of events and relationships—including homeostasis, personality, and psychopathology—in terms of mutual interactions and feedback mechanisms. Psychopathology, e.g., is described in terms of a total or molar system disturbance rather than a loss of single, or molecular, functions such as individual sensations, drives, and isolated symptoms. Schizophrenia is therefore attributed to a disorganization of many essential functions, including symbolic processes, ego integration, and emotional activities.

dynamic approach the psychological and psychiatric approach that views human behavior from the standpoint of underlying and often unconscious forces that mold the personality, influence attitudes, and produce emotional disorder. The emphasis is on tracing behavior to its origins, as contrasted with the systematic or descriptive approach, which concentrates on overt events, personality characteristics, and symptoms. See DYNAMIC PSYCHOLOGY. Compare SYSTEMATIC APPROACH; NOSOLOGICAL APPROACH.

dynamic apraxia impairment of the ability to perform purposeful, continuous movements due to lesions in the premotor cortex.

dynamic-effect law a theory that goal-directed behaviors become habitualized as they effectively attain the goal (R. B. Cattell).

dynamic equilibrium a concept of energy stabilization in which an energy-level change at one point results in redistribution of total energy.

dynamic formulation the integration of diverse and seemingly conflicting pieces of information about a patient's behavior, traits, attitudes, and symptoms into a consistent and meaningful picture.

dynamic psychiatry a system of psychiatry that deals with internal, unconscious drives associated with behavior patterns, as opposed to the observable, objective factors of descriptive psychiatry.

dynamic psychology in general, a psychological approach based on the study of motivation and causation; in particular, the approach developed by R. S. Woodworth, which focuses on the inner forces (drives, needs, purposes, emotions, wishes) that motivate behavior. His objective was to explain the "whys" of human behavior and to "put the organism back into the picture." He therefore changed the traditional S-R (stimulus-response) formula to S-O-R (stimulus-organism-response).

dynamic psychotherapy any form or technique of psychotherapy that focuses on the underlying, often unconscious, factors (drives, experiences) that determine our behavior and adjustment. See DEPTH THERAPY; DYNAMIC APPROACH.

dynamic reasoning a term employed by Franz Alexander for the process of reconstructing the patient's developmental history based on clinical evidence gathered from the patient's own account, or ANAMNESIS. See this entry.

dynamics = PSYCHODYNAMICS.

dynamic-situations principle a concept that any stimulus pattern undergoes continuous changes due to such factors as uncontrolled variables, visceral change, and responses.

dynamic system a system in which a change in one part influences all interrelated parts.

dynamic theory a concept of Wolfgang Köhler that brain activity is determined by constant energy changes which do not correspond point-for-point with environmental stimuli.

dynamism a psychological device employed to protect the ego. The term was preferred by H. S. Sullivan to defense mechanism, since it implies an active, adaptive process rather than an automatic reaction. The specific dynamisms are, however, basically the same as defense mechanisms.

dynamogenesis the principle that motor responses are proportional to sensory activities.

-dys- a combining form meaning difficult, abnormal, painful, impaired.

dysacusis a distressing subjective, rarely objective, sensation of tones or noises of peripheral origin, e.g., tinnitus from cochlear or tympanic disease. Also called **dysacousia; dyacusia.** Adjective: **dysacusic.**

dysarthria /disär'thrē·ə/ an inability to use the voice effectively in speaking because of an emotional or organic disorder affecting the muscles used for speech. Kinds of d. include **d. literalis,** which is marked by stammering, and **d. syllabaris spasmodica,** which is characterized by stuttering. Also see ATAXIC D.; ATHETOID D.; APRAXIC D.; ATHETOTIC D.

dysautonomia: See FAMILIAL D.

dysbasia distorted or difficult walking that may be of either organic or psychic origin.

dysbulia a difficulty in thinking or maintaining attention or a train of thought, also described as a disturbance of will.

dyscalculia = ACALCULIA.

dyscontrol syndrome a pattern of abnormal social behavior, which may be characterized by sex offenses, assaults, or recurrent traffic accidents,

that results from diseases of the limbic system or the temporal lobe of the brain.

dyscrasia a pathologic condition associated with an imbalance of normal constituents or the presence of abnormal materials in a tissue. The term is most commonly applied to a blood disorder marked by a proliferation of immunoglobulin cells or antibodies in the absence of an antigenic stimulus. A d. also may be caused by the presence of tumor or cancer cells, a chronic infectious agent such as tuberculous bacteria, or a reaction to a medication. Also see BLOOD D.

dysdiadochokinesis /-ōkō-/ an impairment in the ability to perform rapid alternating movements, as in fanning onself, due to cerebellar disorder. Also see ADIADOCHOKINESIS.

dysencephalia splanchnocystia: See MECKEL'S SYNDROME.

dyseneia a deafness-caused articulation difficulty.

dysergasia a term introduced by Adolf Meyer for psychiatric syndromes caused by toxic psychoses or similar brain dysfunctions. Delirium is a common symptom.

dysfluencies: See PRIMARY STUTTERING; SECONDARY STUTTERING; STUTTERING.

dysfunction a term used to describe any impairment, disturbance, or deficiency in the functioning of an organ or body system.

dysgenic a term applied to influences that may be detrimental to heredity. D. is the opposite of eugenic.

dysgeusia an impairment or perversion of the sense of taste. Occasionally hysterical patients eat such substances as ashes, salt, or vinegar; schizophrenics sometimes complain of peculiar tastes in their mouths; and strange tastes may be experienced as an aura, or warning signal, before an epileptic attack. For other examples, see PICA.

dysgrammatism a persistent use of incorrect grammar not due to educational impoverishment. It is a symptom of aphasia. See AGRAMMATISM.

dysgraphia an imprecise term, not much used today, for an inability to perform motor movements needed for handwriting. D. is a type of aphasia, usually associated with a lesion between the temporal and occipital lobes. The patient (the **dysgraphic**) is able to copy a drawing of an object but is unable to draw the same object, e.g., a clock, when asked to do so. The auditory input fails to evoke the visual image needed to carry out the task.

dysidentity a characteristic of childhood schizophrenia in which the patient is unable to perceive boundaries, limits, or other distinguishing features of identities including his or her own.

dyskinesia a distortion of voluntary movement, as in cerebral palsy; also, involuntary muscular activities such as tics, spasms, or sudden "myoclonic" contractions of the limbs, body, or face that frequently occur in petit mal or grand mal. See TARDIVE D.; EXTRAPYRAMIDAL D.; OROFACIAL D.

dyslalia errors of articulation due to functional causes, especially errors of omission, distortion, and substitution that often accompany delayed speech in children.

dyslexia a mild or severe reading disorder consisting of impaired ability to understand the written word due to minimal brain dysfunction or gross brain damage. The condition is often aggravated by emotional disturbance or environmental deprivation, but the term is not applied in cases of mental retardation. D. usually is unrelated to disorders of speech and vision. The patient may be able to read numbers but not letters or words, letters but not numbers or words, or some other variation. He also may be able to read only by tracing letters with a finger. See READING DISABILITY; PARALEXIA; CONGENITAL ALEXIA.

dyslexia with dysorthographia = LEGATHENIA.

dyslogia a speech defect associated with mental retardation, manifested as inability to express oneself clearly.

dysmenorrhea difficult or painful menstruation. The cause may be an obstruction in the cervix or vagina that traps menstrual blood, or the condition may be secondary to an infection or tumor. More than three-fourths of d. cases are a primary, or functional, form of the disorder for which no organic cause can be found. Some studies show the patients to have unresolved emotional conflicts or psychosexual conflicts such as resentment of their female status. D. may be characterized by cramplike pains in the lower abdomen, headache, irritability, depression, and fatigue. Kinds of d. include **congestive d.**, marked by congestion of the uterus, **inflammatory d.**, associated with inflammation, **membranous d.**, marked by loss of membrane tissue from the uterus, **obstructive d.**, associated with mechanical interference of menstrual flow, and **essential d.**, for which there is no obvious cause.

dysmentia a form of pseudoretardation in which the subject shows impaired performance that is due to psychological factors rather than true mental retardation.

dysmetria an impaired ability to gauge distance of body movements. It can be tested, e.g., by having the patient raise both arms to a horizontal level with his eyes closed.

dysmnesia an impairment of memory, as in acute and chronic brain disorders.

dysmnesic syndrome a disorder that frequently develops after an acute delirious episode. It is characterized by amnesia for the episode, with faulty orientation and difficulty in retaining recent events. The condition usually clears up within a few days, but in some cases takes weeks or months to abate.

dysmorphogenesis of brain, joints, and palate a familial or hereditary disease marked by joint contractures, cleft or narrow palate, and a Dandy-Walker form of hydrocephalus. See DANDY-WALKER SYNDROME.

dysmorphophobia a morbid fear of being or

appearing physically deformed; also, the illusion of being thus deformed.

dysnisophrenia a general term for psychopathic disorders including antisocial personality.

dysnomia = ANOMIA.

dysontogenetic = DYSRHAPHIC.

dysorexia an appetite that is impaired or perverted. See PICA.

dysostosis the defective development of the skeleton of an individual, either because of hereditary factors or because of improper care following birth. The genetic causes usually are expressed in faulty development of the bones of the face and skull. Examples of d. include Crouzon's disease, Franceschetti's syndrome, and Treacher Collins' syndrome.

dyspareunia painful sexual intercourse, particularly in women. It is usually due to intense aversion to sexual relations or fear of pregnancy or disease. The term is sometimes used for inability to enjoy intercourse. The corresponding DSM-III term is FUNCTIONAL **d**. See this entry.

dysperception any impairment or abnormality in perceptual functions.

dysphagia impaired ability to swallow, usually due to a physical condition, as in some cases of cerebral palsy. But in other instances d. may be a hysterical symptom involving spasms of the throat muscles. See D. SPASTICA.

dysphagia spastica a somatic or, more often, functional symptom in which the act of swallowing is painful or difficult because of throat muscle spasms. In functional cases, it is classified as a hysterical symptom.

dysphasia an inability to communicate clearly with speech, usually because of cortical damage. The d. patient often is identified by his difficulty in arranging a series of spoken words in a meaningful or understandable pattern. The term is sometimes used as an alternative for aphasia. Also see DYSARTHRIA.

dysphemia a nervous disorder of speech associated with psychological disturbance and, frequently, a neurological predispositon. It includes such disorders as STUTTERING and TACHYPHEMIA. See these entries.

dysphonia a defect in phonation or vocalization. Also see FUNCTIONAL VOICE DISORDER; SPASTIC D.

dysphoria an unpleasant mood characterized by discontent, depression, anxiety, and restlessness. Also called **dysphoric mood**. Compare EUPHORIA.

dysphoria nervosa fidgets; mild convulsive or spasmodic muscle contractions. Also called **crispation**.

dysphoric mood = DYSPHORIA.

dysphrasia a difficulty in speaking or writing due to a CNS or intellectual defect.

dysplastic type the disproportioned type of an individual who, according to E. Kretschmer, presents a combination of traits but frequently tends toward the introversive, schizothymic temperament (from Greek *dys-* and *plastos*, "formed"). See CONSTITUTIONAL TYPE.

dyspnea shortness of breath or difficult breathing that often has subjective overtones. The patient has an awareness of increased breathing efforts or a feeling of inadequate breathing. D. may be a hysterical symptom, or associated with heart or lung disease.

dysponesis a faulty or misdirected effort. The term is used in biofeedback work to describe a state of unconscious and habitual tension that generates hypertension, migraine headaches, bruxism, or related disorders.

dyspraxia an impaired ability to perform skilled, coordinated movements. D. is usually due to cerebral lesions and not to muscular defect. Also see SYMPATHETIC D.

dysprosody an altered melodic speech pattern often associated with brain injury.

dysrhaphic pertaining to a developmental disorder, particularly one involving the central nervous system. Also called **dysontogenetic**. For an example see ARNOLD-CHIARI MALFORMATION.

dysrhythmia an abnormality in speech rhythm due to defects in breathing, inflection, and placement of stress.

dyssocial behavior delinquent or criminal activities such as gangsterism, racketeering, prostitution, or illegal gambling. It is usually attributed to distorted moral and social influences, frequently aggravated by a broken home or a deprived environment. It was formerly termed sociopathic behavior. See ANTISOCIAL-PERSONALITY DISORDER.

dyssocial drinking = ALPHA ALCOHOLISM.

dyssocial reaction a DSM-I term for a type of sociopathic-personality disorder in which a delinquent or criminal way of life is adopted as a result of distorted environmental influences such as juvenile gangs or adult models in the family or neighborhood. In contrast to the extreme egocentricity of antisocial personalities, dyssocial individuals are capable of strong loyalties, at least within the delinquent subculture, and the condition is therefore sometimes called **adaptive delinquency**.

dyssomnia a form of insomnia characterized by wide fluctuations in depth of sleep, and such disturbances as nightmares, teeth-grinding, and sleepwalking.

dyssymbiosis pathological symbiosis between mother and child in which the child uses psychotic defenses to control the mother. Symbiotic relationship must be maintained by the child since separation is experienced as annihilation, yet he must seek that the relationship is not too close, since he fears engulfment by the mother.

dyssymboly an inability to discriminate among gradations of personal emotions in language that can be comprehended by others. The condition may be due to either a semantic or emotional deficiency of the patient, and is frequently observed in schiophrenics. Also called **dyssymbolia**.

dyssynergia cerebellaris = HUNT'S SYNDROME.

dystaxia a mild degree of ataxia; difficulty in performing coordinated muscular movements.

dysthymia a depressive mood that is less severe than observed in cases of manic-depressive psychosis. The depression may be accompanied by neurasthenic-hypochondriacal symptoms.

dysthymic disorder a chronic mood disturbance lasting at least two years in adults and one year in children, and characterized by persistent or recurrent periods in which relatively mild depressive symptoms predominate: depressed mood or marked loss of interest or pleasure, with such specific symptoms as insomnia or hypersomnia, low energy levels, loss of self-esteem, decreased productivity, social withdrawal, irritability, unresponsiveness, tearfulness, pessimistic attitude, and thoughts of death or suicide. Also called **depressive neurosis**. (DSM III)

dystonia an abnormal tension or spasms in the muscles resulting in uncoordinated or spasmodic movements, such as twisting of the neck or arching of the back. See EXTRAPYRAMIDAL SYMPTOMS; TARDIVE DYSKINESIA; TORTICOLLIS.

dystonia musculorum deformans a progressive disorder of muscular atrophy marked by twisting of the muscles and associated bones into bizarre postures. The condition is believed to be due to lesions in the extrapyramidal system although pathological evidence is lacking. The limbs and spinal column are progressively involved. Two genetic types are known, one autosomal-dominant and one autosomal-recessive. Also called **torsion dystonia; torsion spasm; Oppenheim's disease**.

dystrophia myotonica = MYOTONIC DYSTROPHY.

dystychia = ANHEDONIA.

dysuria difficult or painful urination. A frequent cause is a bacterial infection that produces irritation or inflammation of the urethra or the neck of the bladder.

E

Eagle, Harry American physician, 1905—. See WASSERMANN TEST (there: **Eagle test**).

ear the auditory organ of the body. In humans and other mammals, the ear usually has three main divisions, an external, middle, and inner ear. The inner ear contains receptors for two different functions, the maculae and crystae cells to help maintain equilibrium and the organ-of-Corti cells, which translate sound vibrations into impulses for the sense of hearing. Also see OSSICLES; INNER EAR; MIDDLE EAR; EXTERNAL EAR.

eardrum = TYMPANIC MEMBRANE.

Earle, Pliny American psychiatrist, 1809–92. E. was a reformer in hospital administration and the author of *The Curability of Insanity*, 1877.

early infantile autism L. Kanner's original name for what is now known as INFANTILE AUTISM. See this entry.

Early School Personality Questionnaire: See CATTELL INVENTORIES.

earphone: See HEARING AID.

ear pulling a habit that has been interpreted variously as a substitute for thumb-sucking or masturbation.

eastern equine encephalitis: See EQUINE ENCEPHALITIS.

Eastman, Max American editor and writer, 1883—. See HUMOR.

eating aids daily-living aids that can be utilized by disabled persons who might not otherwise be able to feed themselves. E.a. include metal or plastic devices for holding sandwiches, nonslip place mats, bowls, and dishes with suction cups attached to the bottom, handles that can swivel or are designed at angles or with extensions, and combination eating devices, e.g., knife-fork or fork-spoon combinations.

eating behavior in psychiatry, types of behavior that include the pathological forms ANOREXIA NERVOSA, BULIMIA, HYPERPHAGIA, PICA, RUMINATION DISORDER OF INFANCY, VOMITING, and, in DSM-III, ATYPICAL EATING DISORDER. See these entries. Also see FEEDING BEHAVIOR; KLEINE-LEVIN SYNDROME; KLÜVER-BUCY SYNDROME.

eating compulsion = BULIMIA.

eating-fear = PHAGOPHOBIA.

Eaton, Leades McKendree (Lee M.) American physician, 1905–58. See EATON-LAMBERT SYNDROME.

Eaton-Lambert syndrome a form of carcinomatous muscle weakness in which myotatic reflexes are frequently depressed and the patient appears to become increasingly stronger during repeated tests. The action potential of the muscle, as measured by electromyography, increases with repetitions to more than three times its initial value. Limbs may be painful and movements slow. The cause is impaired acetylcholine release at the nerve terminals. Also called **Lambert-Eaton syndrome; myasthenic syndrome of Lambert-Eaton; carcinomatous myopathy**.

Ebbinghaus, Hermann /eb'inghous/ German psychologist, 1850–1909. E. was the first to apply quantitative, psychophysiological methods to the higher mental processes. His experiments, frequently employing nonsense syllables, involved systematic studies of memory span, overlearning, spaced versus massed learning, and the curve of forgetting, and had a lasting effect in establishing experimental psychology as a scientific discipline. See EBBINGHAUS' CURVE OF RETENTION; NONSENSE SYLLABLE.

Ebbinghaus' curve of retention a curve that measures the rate of loss of nonsense material immediately after learning it. The curve shows a sudden drop followed by a gradual decline.

EBV = EPSTEIN-BARR VIRUS.

-ec-; -ect-; -ecto- a combining form meaning outer, external, outside, out of.

ecbolics = OXYTOCICS.

eccentric projection the location of a sensation as an object in space rather than in the sense organ, as in vision and hearing.

ecchymosis a small purple or bluish patch similar to a bruise and caused by the extrusion of blood into the skin or another membrane of the body. Ecchymoses are found in areas of the heart and chest in infants that have strangled or suffocated while in the mother's uterus. Similar patches of e. are found in tissues of persons who have been strangled.

eccyesis = ECTOPIC PREGNANCY.

ecdemomania a morbid desire to wander or travel. Also called **ecdemonomania**.

ecdysiasm /-diz'-/ a morbid impulse to disrobe in

order to arouse sexual excitement in a member of the opposite sex (from Greek *ekdysis*, "shedding, getting out of"). (H. L. Mencken coined the word **ecdysiast** for stripteaser.)

ECG: See ELECTROCARDIOGRAM.

echocardiography an ultrasound device that uses sonarlike reflections to produce images of the internal structures of a patient's heart. E. permits the visualization and measurement of all of the chambers and valves of the heart. Because the ultrasound impulses do not traverse air and bone as well as soft tissues, the images help differentiate areas that are heart structures from the rib cage and air sacs of the lungs.

écho des pensées /ākō′depäNsā′/ an auditory hallucination in which the patient hears his own thoughts repeated in spoken form. Also called **thought-echoing**.

echoencephalograph a method of mapping the inside of the head for diagnostic purposes by using ultrasonic waves. The waves are beamed through the head from both sides, and echoes of the waves from midline structures are recorded as visual images. Any variation in reflections from the midline may indicate an abnormality in the brain structure. The recording is called an **echoencephalogram**.

echolalia mechanical repetition of words and phrases uttered by another individual. E. is a symptom of catatonic schizophrenia or latah and, in some patients, of Tourette's disorder, Pick's disease, Alzheimer's disease, and diffuse sclerosis. Also called **echophrasia; echo-speech**.

echolocation the ability to judge the direction and distance of large objects or obstacles from reflected echos made, e.g., by one's footsteps, the tapping of a cane, or traffic noises. The phenomenon, often highly developed in blind people, is similar to "bat radar," that is, bats' ability to locate objects by emitting high-pitched sounds that bounce back to them from walls or even wires. Dolphins have also been found to judge their distance from objects by the same means. E. was once described as **facial vision** on the mistaken theory that blind people develop unusual facial sensitivity to air currents.

echomatism; echomimia = ECHOPRAXIA.

echopathy /ekop′-/ a pathological, automatic copying and repetition of another's movements and speech. It is a common symptom of catatonic schizophrenia. E. is a combination of echopraxia and echolalia. See ECHOPRAXIA; ECHOLALIA; ECHO PHENOMENON.

echo phenomenon a term used by Kraepelin for echolalia and echopraxia. Also see ECHOPATHY.

echophrasia = ECHOLALIA.

echopraxia automatic imitation of another person's movements or gestures. E. is a common symptom of catatonic schizophrenia, sometimes in association with echolalia. Also called **echomatism; echomimia**. See AUTOMATIC OBEDIENCE.

echo principle an assumption that one animal will imitate the behavior of another if they have been involved in the same act simultaneously; also, the tendency of children to imitate the behavior or linguistic patterns of their parents.

echo-speech = ECHOLALIA.

ECHO virus /ek′ō/ any of more than 30 types of small viruses that tend to produce respiratory, gastrointestinal, and poliolike symptoms during the summer and autumn. ECHO is an acronym for *e*nteric *c*ytopathic *h*uman *o*rphan; and the word orphan is used because the viruses, when first discovered, were not a part of any known family of infectious agents. The viruses are found in cerebrospinal fluid and CNS tissues.

echul a culture-specific syndrome observed among the Native American Diegueno of lower California, characterized by sexual anxiety and convulsions which reach a peak during severe crises such as divorce or death of a spouse or child.

eclampsia: See TOXEMIA OF PREGNANCY.

eclampsia nutans = WEST'S SYNDROME.

eclampsic amentia a term formerly applied to cases of mental retardation associated with a brief period of epilepsylike seizures during infancy.

eclamptic symptoms convulsions that occur in patients who have experienced preeclampsia, with signs of edema, hypertension, headaches, dizziness, and nervous irritability. It is a condition peculiar to pregnant women and is not associated with epilepsy or other cerebral disorders. E.s. are sometimes classified as **prepartal e.s., intrapartal e.s.,** or **postpartal e.s.**, depending on whether they occur before, during, or after delivery of the child. Also see TOXEMIA OF PREGNANCY.

eclectic behaviorism a behavior-therapy approach that does not adhere to one theoretical model, but applies, as needed, any of several techniques, including classical conditioning, modeling, operant conditioning, self-control mechanisms, cognitive restructuring, and psychodynamic concepts of personality.

eclectic counseling any counseling theory or practice that incorporates and combines doctrines, findings, and techniques selected from diverse theoretical systems.

eclecticism a theoretical and practical approach which blends, or attempts to blend, diverse conceptual formulations or techniques into an integrated approach.

ECM = EXTERNAL CHEMICAL MESSENGER.

ecmnesia a rarely used term for ANTEROGRADE AMNESIA. See this entry.

ecnoia a fear reaction in children provoked as a normal fright event but continuing for days or weeks with adverse effects on sleep and appetite.

ecological perception the individual's view of the environment in terms of reciprocal adjustments between physical, social, and individual influences. J. J. Gibson has proposed that e.p. is holistic, that environmental properties are perceived as meaningful entities, and that perceptual patterns may be direct rather than concepts that require interpretation by higher brain centers from visual or other cues. Thus, e.p. is not necessarily a matter of human judgment but a reaction of any organism that may interpret environmental features in terms of affordances. See AFFORDANCE.

ecological perspective a concept of community psychology in which a community (or other social entity) is viewed in terms of the interrelations between persons, roles, organizations, local events, resources, and problems to be handled by these resources. As J. G. Kelly (1971) states, the premise of the e.p. is that intervention should contribute to the development of the entire community.

ecological psychiatry; ecological psychology: See ECOLOGICAL-SYSTEMS MODEL.

ecological studies research on the mutual relations between organisms and their environment. Examples relating to animal behavior are studies of eating habits, formation of groups, and building of shelters. Examples relating to human behavior are studies of occupants of trailer camps, the geographical and social class distribution of mental disorders, voting patterns in different areas or among different social groups, and the comparative incidence of criminal behavior in urban versus rural areas. Also see ECOLOGICAL-SYSTEMS MODEL.

ecological-systems model in ecological psychiatry (ecopsychiatry) and ecological psychology (ecopsychology), the concept that mental disorders are reflections not merely of personal imbalance but of environmental disequilibrium, and can be effectively prevented and treated only by studying and modifying the environmental forces that impinge on the individual. According to this model, the mental-health worker must be a social therapist engaged in community action. Also see ECOLOGICAL STUDIES.

ecological validity sampling of the typical environment in the design of psychological research, with the goal of more general applicability of findings. The term was originated by Egon Brunswik.

ecology the study of relationships between organisms and their physical and social environments (from Greek *oikos*, "house").

ecomania irritable, domineering behavior directed toward members of one's own family. Also called **oikomania**.

economic approach in psychoanalysis, a study of the amount and distribution of psychic energy used in maintaining the mental economy, that is, the force exerted by our drives, both unconscious and conscious.

economically disadvantaged: See CULTURALLY DIFFERENT.

Economo, Constantin Alexander /ekôn′-/ Austrian neurologist, 1876–1931. See ECONOMO'S DISEASE; POSTENCEPHALITIS SYNDROME.

Economo's disease a CNS infection, believed to be caused by a virus, resulting in clonic and choreiform movements, delirium, stupor, reversal of sleep patterns, parkinsonism, and personality changes. Also called **Redlich's encephalitis; African sleeping sickness; encephalitis lethargica; hypersomnic encephalitis; epidemic encephalitis**.

economy principle: See OCCAM'S RAZOR.

ecopharmacology a branch of pharmacology that is concerned with the relationships between drugs and the external environment, including the role of the individual patient in his ecological background. The identification of a person as a psychoneurotic may be influenced by the attitudes of members of a community or social or economic pressures of the patient's community.

ecophobia = OIKOPHOBIA.

ecopsychiatry; ecopsychology: See ECOLOGICAL-SYSTEMS MODEL.

ecosystem a continuing balance maintained among competing and mixed components within a group or society, requiring that a change in any one component be followed by commensurate changes in the other components.

écouteur /āko͞otœr′/ an individual who derives sexual excitement from listening to sexual accounts or sounds produced during sexual encounters.

ECS an abbreviation of *e*lectroconvulsive *s*hock. See ELECTROCONVULSIVE TREATMENT.

ecstasy in psychiatry, a state of exaltation or extreme euphoria sometimes experienced in epileptic or hypomanic states. In sexology, e. is the peak of sexual excitement and pleasure at the moment of orgasm. In religion, e. is the rapturous, trancelike experience of union with the cosmos (mystic union). Adjective: **ecstatic**.

ECT = ELECTROCONVULSIVE TREATMENT.

-ecto-: See -EC-.

ectoderm the outer layer of cells of a developing embryo after the primary germ layers for various types of tissues have become established (literally, "outer skin"). The e. layer eventually evolves into the skin and its nails, hair, and glands, the mucous membranes, and the nervous system and external sense organs such as the ears and eyes. Adjective: **ectodermal**. See EMBRYONIC PERIOD.

ectodermosis erosiva pluriorificialis = STEVENS-JOHNSON SYNDROME.

ectomorph one of W. H. Sheldon's constitutional types, or somatotypes, characterized by a thin, long, fragile physique (from Greek *ektomorphe*, "outer form"), which he found to be highly correlated with a cerebrotonic temperament (tendency toward introversion, inhibition, and love of solitude). Also called **ectomorphic body type**. See CEREBROTONIA.

-ectomy /-ek′-/ a combining form relating to the surgical removal of a part of the body.

ectopic pregnancy a pregnancy that develops outside the uterus. Also called **extrauterine pregnancy; eccyesis** (eksī·ē′sis/; **paracyesis**. Also see PREGNANCY.

ectopic testis a testis that descended improperly from the abdominal cavity and became lodged outside the scrotum. An e.t. may be located beneath the outer tissue layers of the thigh or in the perineum.

ectoplasm the outer layer of a cell or of a one-cell organism; also, a parapsychology term for a substance said to emanate from a medium's body.

EDC: See GESTATION PERIOD.

edema an excess accumulation of fluid in body cells, organs, or cavities. The cause may be a loss of fluid through the walls of the blood vessels as a symptom of a circulatory disorder or the interruption of flow of cerebrospinal fluid due to blockage of a passageway or failure of tissues to absorb the excess. Also see CEREBRAL E.

Edinger, Ludwig German anatomist, 1855–1918. See EDINGER-WESTPHAL nucleus.

Edinger-Westphal nucleus a collection of small nerve cells comprising the parasympathetic pathway to the ciliary muscle and the pupillary sphincter of the eye, which play a role in visual accommodation.

edipism = OEDIPISM.

EDR: See GALVANIC SKIN RESPONSE.

edrophonium a cholinomimetic drug that has a short duration of action and is used as an anti-curare agent and in the diagnosis of myasthenia disorders. As a cholinomimetic drug, it produces effects similar to those of acetylcholine, although often with less potency. It is antagonistic to acetylcholinesterase and seems to act directly on the motor end-plate of neuromuscular junctions. Also called **Tensilon**.

educability the potential for academic learning.

educable a term applied to mentally retarded individuals who test in the mild category, with IQs of 50 to 70, and are capable of achieving approximately a fifth-grade academic level. See MILD MENTAL RETARDATION. Also see TRAINABLE.

educational acceleration educational progress at a rate faster than usual through a variety of measures such as strengthening curriculum, combining two years' work into one, or grade-skipping. These measures are designed to provide the intellectually gifted with work better suited to their abilities. Grade-skipping is thought by some to represent a potential disadvantage if the student's social and emotional development is lagging behind his or her intellectual development. Also called **scholastic acceleration**.

educational age the level of a child's performance on school subjects as measured by academic achievement tests scored in terms of age.

educational counseling the counseling specialty concerned with guiding students in their choice of educational program and choice of college or technical school. It may also be concerned with school-related problems that interfere with performance, e.g., learning disabilities. E.c. is closely associated with vocational counseling because of the relationship between educational training and occupational choice. Also see COUNSELING PSYCHOLOGIST; VOCATIONAL COUNSELING.

educationally subnormal: See ESN.

educational measurement the development and application of tests used to measure student abilities.

educational programs in rehabilitation, services for disabled children that may adapt standard teaching materials and methods to the type of handicap in order to achieve the optimum level of training for the individual. Kinds of e.p. include diagnostic-descriptive approach, cross-categorical approach, and individually prescribed curriculum.

educational psychology a branch of psychology that deals with the principles and theories of psychology that can be applied to methods of learning and psychological problems arising in the educational system.

educational quotient a ratio of educational age to chronological age times 100. Abbrev.: **EQ**.

educational tests: See DIAGNOSTIC E.T.

educational therapist a rehabilitation professional who specializes in the application of teaching techniques to persons with emotional or physical handicaps. The courses are usually on a high-school level and may lead to a high-school-equivalency diploma. The objective of **educational therapy** is helping to build self-esteem and confidence in the patients while keeping them in touch with the world of people and ideas.

education stage the stage of Jung's analytic therapy in which the patient achieves a more effective adaptation to environmental and social demands.

Edwards, Allen L. American psychologist, 1914—. See EDWARDS PERSONAL PREFERENCE SCHEDULE.

Edwards, John Hilton English geneticist, 1928—. See TRISOMY 17-18 (also called **Edward's syndrome**).

Edwards Personal Preference Schedule a personality inventory for college students and adults in which the strength of 15 of the needs listed by H. A. Murray is assessed on a forced-choice basis: achievement, order, deference, autonomy, exhibition, affection, succorance, sympathy, change, endurance, heterosexuality, aggression, intraception, abasement, and affiliation.

Edward's syndrome = TRISOMY 17-18.

EE = EXPRESSED EMOTIONS.

EEG: See ELECTROENCE-PHALOGRAPH.

EEG examination a method of diagnosing the normal or abnormal functioning of the living brain by evaluating the recording of EEG fluctuations. The EEG e. enables the neurologist to determine whether there are any variations from normal in waking or sleeping brain-wave patterns that could be due to tumors, epileptic foci, or other types of brain lesions. See BRAIN WAVES; ELECTROENCEPHALOGRAPH.

effectance motive the motivation in childhood to develop competence, to initiate projects, and to find effective ways of coping with the environment. Several major theorists (e.g., Adler and

Erikson) believe that children's need to master inferiority feelings contributes to the motivation to develop competence.

effect gradient: See GRADIENT OF EFFECT.

effective-habit strength the strength of a learned reaction established by a reinforcement process and determined by the number of reinforcements (Hull).

effective-reaction potential the reaction-potential strength minus any inhibitory tendencies.

effective stimulus a stimulus that produces a response.

effective temperature an index of ambient temperature obtained by considering both the temperature and humidity levels.

effect law: See LAW OF EFFECT.

effector a motor-nerve ending that triggers activity in neighboring tissue cells, such as causing a muscle to contract or a gland to secrete.

effect spread: See SPREAD OF EFFECT.

effeminate homosexuality: See CROSS DRESSING.

efferent /ef′-/ conducting or conveying (nervous-system impulses) away from the central nervous system and toward effector units in muscles or glands. Noun: **efference.** Compare AFFERENT.

efferent motor aphasia a form of expressive aphasia marked by difficulty in articulating sound and speech sequences due to lesions in the lower part of the left premotor area.

effort-shape technique a technique used in dance and movement therapy (as well as systematic observation of human movement in general), based on an analysis of such factors as the flow of muscular tension between bound and free, movement that flows toward or away from the body, exertion related to attitudes toward space, time, and force, and a relationship between gesture and posture. See LABANANALYSIS.

effort syndrome an anxiety reaction associated with excessive exertion or tension, characterized by such somatic symptoms as heart palpitations, fatigue, shortness of breath, and neurocirculatory weakness, all of which are out of proportion to the exertion. Also see DA COSTA'S SYNDROME.

efficient cause the total of the antecedent factors leading to a given effect or event.

E-F scale a MMPI subscale of 30 items designed to measure ethnocentric and authoritarian factors.

ego in psychoanalysis, the component of the personality that deals with the external world and its practical demands. More specifically, the ego enables us to perceive, reason, solve problems, test reality, and adjust our instinctual impulses (the id) to the behests of conscience (the superego). Also see ALTER E.; ALTER-EGOISM ANTILIBIDINAL EGO; AUXILIARY EGO; BODILY EGO FEELING; BODY EGO; BODY-EGO CONCEPT; COUNTEREGO; DOUBLE SUPEREGO; DREAM EGO; EXISTENTIAL EGO FUNCTION; EXTINCTION OF EGO; GROUP SUPEREGO; HETERONOMOUS SUPEREGO; ID-EGO; INTEREGO; PARASITIC EGO; PLEASURE EGO; PRESCHIZOPHRENIC EGO; PRESUPEREGO PHASE; PRIMITIVE SUPEREGO; REACTIVE EGO ALTERATION; REALITY LIFE OF EGO; REWARD BY THE SUPEREGO; SUPEREGO; SUPEREGO ANXIETY; SUPEREGO LACUNAE; SUPEREGO RESISTANCE; SUPEREGO SADISM; SUPPORTIVE EGO; TRANSIENT EGO IDEAL; WEAK E.

ego-alien = EGO-DYSTONIC.

ego-alter theory the concept that social interaction is controlled by the individual's perception of himself in relation to others (alters); also, the theory that social institutions are based on self-interest.

ego analysis psychoanalytic techniques directed toward discovering the ego's strengths and weaknesses, and toward uncovering defenses against unacceptable impulses. E.a. is a shorter form of psychoanalysis; it does not attempt to penetrate to the ultimate origin of impulses and repressions. See EGO STRENGTH.

ego anxiety the anxiety caused by conflicting demands of the ego, id, and superego.

ego boundaries the flexible boundaries that, according to the psychoanalyst Paul Federn, exist between the ego and the unconscious (inner or internal boundary) and between the ego and the outside world (outer or external boundary). If the inner boundary is blurred, as in falling asleep, repressed material may enter consciousness; if the outer boundary is blurred, the individual experiences a feeling of unreality.

ego-boundary loss a condition in schizophrenia in which the parameters of the ego are lost as the ego is unable to test reality and merges with the nonego or with the cosmic identity of the entire world.

ego cathexis in psychoanalysis, concentration of psychic energy in the conscious ego and its executive function of integrating the id, ego, and superego in the process of adjusting to reality. E.c. is a form of narcissism. Also called **ego libido.** Compare OBJECT CATHEXIS.

egocentric self-centered; overconcerned with one's own needs, wishes, and feelings, and usually insensitive to the rights or interests of others. In Piaget the term characterizes a type of thinking that is directed by the needs and concerns of the self. See EGOMANIA. Also see EGOCENTRISM; DECENTRATION.

egocentric speech speech in which there is no attempt to exchange thoughts or take into account another person's point of view. According to Piaget, e.s. prevails until the seventh or eighth year, but other observers, such as McCarthy, have found that children are capable of socialized speech as early as three or four. According to Vigotsky, e.s. develops into inner speech, or INNER LANGUAGE. See this entry.

egocentrism in cognitive development, the tendency to think that others see things from the same point of view as oneself, and that they elicit the same thoughts, feelings, and behavior in others as in oneself. Also see EGOCENTRIC.

ego complex a term used by Jung for concentration of psychic energy in the ego or self.

ego-coping skills adaptive techniques developed by an individual to deal with personal problems and environmental stresses.

ego decomposition the division of the ego in dreams into various tendencies represented by different events, localities, individuals, or objects.

ego defense in psychoanalysis, protection of the ego from threatening impulses and conflicts through the use of defense mechanisms. See DEFENSE MECHANISM.

ego-defense mechanism: See DEFENSE MECHANISM.

ego development in psychoanalysis, the gradual transformation of a part of the id into the ego as a result of environmental demands. E.d. goes through a preconscious stage, in which ego cathexis is partly developed, to the conscious stage, in which ego functions such as reasoning, judging, and reality-testing come to fruition and help to protect the individual from internal and external threats. Also called **ego formation**.

ego-dystonic a term used to describe impulses, wishes or thoughts that are unacceptable or repugnant to the ego or self. Also called **ego-alien**. Compare EGO-SYNTONIC.

ego-dystonic homosexuality a psychosexual disorder in which the individual complains that he or she cannot, or cannot fully, be aroused by the other sex and therefore cannot initiate or maintain heterosexual relationships that are desired, and in which there is a sustained pattern of homosexual arousal that he or she explicitly states has been unwanted and persistently distressing. The condition is frequently accompanied by feelings of loneliness, shame, anxiety, and depression. (DSM-III)

ego formation = EGO DEVELOPMENT.

ego functions in psychoanalysis, the various activities of the ego, including perception of the external world, self-awareness, problem-solving, control of motor functions, adaptation to reality, memory, and reconciliation of conflicting impulses and ideas. The ego is frequently described as the executive agency of the personality, working in the interest of the reality principle.

ego ideal in psychoanalysis, the part of the ego that is the repository of introjected positive identifications with parental goals and values the child genuinely admires and wants to emulate, such as integrity and loyalty. The e.i. acts as a model of how one wishes to be. As new identifications are incorporated in later life, it may develop and change. Also called **self ideal**. Also see INTROJECTION; SUPEREGO.

ego identity in psychoanalysis, the experience of the self as a recognizable, persistent entity resulting from the integration of one's unique ego ideal, life roles, and ways of adjusting to reality. In Erikson, e.i. is the gradual acquisition of a sense of continuity, worth, and integration which he believed to be the essential process in personality development.

ego instincts in psychoanalysis, the nonsexual instincts, such as eating, defecating, and urinating, which are directed toward self-preservation. The e.i. may, however, become eroticized. See EROTIZATION.

ego integration the process of organizing the various aspects of the personality (drives, attitudes, aims) into a balanced whole.

ego integrity versus despair stage eight of Erikson's eight stages of man. In old age, the individual may look back in despair, seeing his life as a series of missed opportunities and irretrievable mistakes; or he may have what Erikson calls integrity, looking back on life with satisfaction, continuing to enjoy his grandchildren, and generally taking a positive view. See ERIKSON'S EIGHT STAGES OF MAN.

ego involvement the relative degree of involvement, commitment, or concern manifested by an individual with respect to any problem or goal; the extent to which an individual cares about and identifies with a given task, event, or situation. The areas in which an individual is **ego-involved** are determined by that person's goals and sources of self-esteem. High e.i. situations lead to arousal and, in some cases, stress.

egoism a personality characteristic marked by selfishness and behavior based on self-interest with disregard for the needs of others. Adjective: **egoistic**. Also see EGOTISM.

egoistic suicide a type of suicide that is the result of the individual's feelings of extreme alienation from others and from society in general.

ego libido = EGO CATHEXIS.

egomania extreme, pathological preoccupation with one's self; the tendency to be totally self-centered, selfish, callous to the needs of others, and interested only in the gratification of one's own impulses and desires.

ego model a person on whom an individual patterns his ego or ego ideal; a person he admires, identifies with, and tries to emulate.

egomorphism the interpretation of the behavior of others in terms of one's own motives, needs, and desires.

ego needs: See NEED-HIERARCHY THEORY.

ego nuclei the first components of the ego, arising during the oral and anal stages (M. Klein). The term is also used in the singular by E. Weiss, who held that the **ego nucleus** integrates new experiences with old ones by relating them to already acquired knowledge.

egopathy hostile attitudes and actions stemming from an exaggerated sense of self-importance, often manifested by a compulsion to deprecate others.

ego psychology in psychoanalysis, an emphasis on the functions of the ego in controlling impulses and dealing with the external environment, in contrast to id psychology, which focuses on the primitive instincts of sex and hostility. In Adler's theory, the term e.p. is used to characterize his view that human beings are governed by a conscious drive to express and create a unique style of life, instead of being controlled by "blind," irrational impulses acting on an unconscious level.

ego psychotherapy an approach developed by

Paul Federn and Edoardo Weiss primarily for treatment of psychotic and schizoid disorders. E.p. is based on the concept that mental disturbance involves a weakening of the integrating capacity of the ego, and a blurring of the boundaries between the ego and the outer reality or between the ego and the id. Therapy is largely a question of redirecting the ego cathexis (or integrating force), repressing id impulses, increasing reality-testing ability, and solving current problems of adjustment.

ego resistance = REPRESSION-RESISTANCE.

ego-splitting according to M. Klein, a mechanism in which the infant defends his ego against the death instinct by making a distinction between good and bad objects. E.-s. is also a tendency that runs counter to the synthesizing function of the psyche; and a pathological coexistence of different personality systems such as occurs in multiple personality.

ego state an integrated state of mind which determines our relationships to the environment and to other people. In Paul Federn's and Edoardo Weiss' ego psychotherapy there are two basic ego states: one that establishes boundaries separating the ego from the id, and the other that separates the ego from external reality. In Eric Berne's transactional analysis, our behavior patterns are based on the interactions between three ego states: parent, adult, and child. See EGO PSYCHOTHERAPY; TRANSACTIONAL ANALYSIS.

ego strength the ability of the conscious self to maintain an effective balance between inner impulses and outer reality. In Freudian terms, e.s. is the capacity of the ego to mediate effectively between the id, the superego, and the demands of life. An individual with a strong ego can tolerate frustration and stress, postpone gratification, modify selfish desires when necessary, and resolve internal conflicts and emotional problems before they lead to neurosis.

ego stress any situation, external or internal, producing stress that requires adaptation by the ego, often expressed as unusual defensive reactions, such as dissociation, somatization, or panic.

ego structure a continuing pattern of personality traits that influence ego processes.

ego suffering in psychoanalysis, the guilt feelings produced in the ego by the aggressive forces in the superego when it disapproves of the ego.

ego-syntonic compatible with the ego or conscious self-concept. Thoughts, wishes, impulses, and behavior are said to be e.-s. when they form no threat to the ego and can be acted upon without interference from the superego. Homosexuality may also be e.-s. Compare EGO-DYSTONIC.

egotism excessive conceit or excessive preoccupation with one's importance. Adjective: **egotistic**. Also see EGOISM.

ego transcendence a term sometimes used to refer to the feeling, experienced mainly during altered states of consciousness, that one is beyond a concern with self and thus able to perceive reality with less anthropocentric bias and greater objectivity.

ego weakness inability to control impulses and tolerate frustration, disappointment, or stress. The individual with a weak ego suffers from anxiety and conflicts, makes excessive use of defense mechanisms, and is likely to develop character defects or neurotic symptoms.

Egyptian ophthalmia: See TRACHOMA.

EGY test = KENT SERIES OF EMERGENCY SKILLS.

Ehret, Heinrich /ā′ret/ German physician, 1870—. See EHRET'S SYNDROME.

Ehret's syndrome a form of paralysis that is an effect of neuromuscular conditioning by a patient in an effort to compensate for a painful injury. By constantly assuming the least painful posture, muscular atrophy and contractures develop. Some authors consider the disorder a type of hysterical paralysis.

Ehrlich, Paul /ār′lish/ German bacteriologist, 1854–1915. See ADDISON-BIERMER ANEMIA (also called **Biermer-Ehrlich anemia**).

Eidelberg, Ludwig /īd′-/ Austrian-born American psychoanalyst, 1898–1970. See ACTING IN; AUTO-SYMBOLISM; BARRIER; COLOR DREAMS; DREAM SCREEN; FANATICISM; HYSTERICAL MATERIALIZATION; INFLUENCING MACHINE; LAUGHTER; PROGERISM.

eidetic image mental imagery, usually visual but occasionally auditory, which closely resembles actual perception; unusually vivid and detailed memory images. A form of **eidetic imagery** may occur in patients with tetany or Basedow's disease (hyperthyroidism). But it mainly occurs in children. Roughly ten percent show strong eidetic imagery, and perhaps 50 percent or more show some degree of it. In a few cases, eidetic imagery may continue beyond adolescence, e.g., in those who exhibit photographic memory or in artists. Also called **primary memory image**.

eidetic type a constitutional body type in which a major feature is eidetic imagery. See EIDETIC IMAGE.

Eigenwelt /ī′gənvelt/ an existentialist term meaning man's relationship to himself (German, "own world"), as contrasted to UMWELT and MITWELT. See these entries.

8-azaguanine a nucleic-acid antagonist used in certain learning experiments. If injected into a cerebrospinal-fluid reservoir of the rat brain, the substance, an analog of the nucleic acid guanine, is incorporated into the RNA of the brain tissue, producing an impaired learning effect. 8-a. also can control certain mouse tumors because of its antimetabolic action. See RNA.

eighth cranial nerve = STATOACOUSTIC NERVE.

Einstellung /īn′shteloong/ a mental set or relatively inflexible attitude (German, "attitude"); a propensity to react to or perceive a situation in an established way, e.g., the tendency to apply formerly successful techniques to the solution of a new problem.

eisoptrophobia a morbid fear of mirrors or of seeing one's reflection. Aso called **spectrophobia**.

either-or situation a condition of doubt and vacillation, usually manifested in an inability to make a choice between two different things desired at the same time. The situation frequently is expressed in dreams of a neurotic person.

either-or thinking: See DICHOTOMOUS THINKING.

ejaculatio deficiens = COITUS SINE EJACULATIONE.

ejaculation the automatic expulsion of semen and seminal fluid through the penis resulting from involuntary and voluntary contractions of various muscle groups. See ORGASM. Also see FEMALE E.; PREMATURE E.; RETROGRADE E.

ejaculation physiology the activity of the nervous, muscular, circulatory, and other organ systems associated with the forceful emission of semen through the penis. Ejaculation is initiated by a subjective signal that the act is inevitable, triggering motor impulses that cause rhythmic spasms of the prostate, seminal vesicles, vas deferens, and urethra, along with contractions of skeletal-muscle groups.

ejaculatio praecox = PREMATURE EJACULATION.

ejaculatio retardata excessively delayed ejaculation during sexual intercourse, usually due to psychogenic factors, aging, or use of drugs, but also voluntary. Also called MALE CONTINENCE.

ejaculator seminis = BULBOSPONGIOSUS MUSCLE.

ejaculatory duct a passageway on either side of the prostate gland, formed by a union of the ductus deferens and the seminal-vesicle duct. The ejaculatory ducts on either side converge in the prostate and empty into the urethra at a point below the urinary bladder.

ejaculatory incompetence = COITUS SINE EJACULATIONE.

Ekbom, Karl-Axel Swedish physician, 1907—. See EKBOM'S SYNDROME.

Ekbom's syndrome a sense of uneasiness, twitching, or restlessness that occurs in the legs after retiring for the night. It is believed to be caused by a circulation impairment but also appears to be more common in neurotic patients. Also called **restless-legs syndrome; jimmy-legs syndrome; tachyathetosis; Wittmaack-Ekbom syndrome.**

EKG: See ELECTROCARDIOGRAM.

elaboration the conscious or unconscious process of developing an idea and incorporating details or relationships that amplify the original concept. See SECONDARY E.

élan vital: See VITALISM.

elation a state of extreme joy, exaggerated optimism, and restless excitement. E. is a major symptom of acute mania, but is also found in general paresis, schizophrenic excitement, and psychosis with brain tumor.

Elberfeld horses horses trained around 1900 in Elberfeld, Germany, to react to trainer cues and thus appear to be able to solve mathematical problems. Also see CLEVER HANS.

elective anorexia loss of appetite associated with a conscious effort to limit the amount of food consumed accompanied by a revulsion to food.

elective mutism a rare childhood disorder characterized by (a) persistent refusal to talk in most social situations, including school, in spite of ability to speak and understand language, (b) absence of any other mental or physical disorder. Maternal overprotection, hospitalization, or entering school may be predisposing factors. (DSM-III)

Electra complex in psychoanalysis, the female counterpart of the Oedipus complex in the male, involving the daughter's love for her father, jealousy toward the mother, and blaming the mother for depriving her of a penis. The term, which is now all but obsolete, was derived from the story of Electra, daughter of Agamemnon, who induced her brother Orestes to kill their mother Clytemnestra and Aegisthus after they had murdered their father and married each other. See OEDIPUS COMPLEX.

electrical activity of brain spontaneous electrical discharges observed in the brain cells of humans and lower animals. E.a.o.b. was discovered by R. Caton and others around 1875 but not explored in detail until the development of sophisticated electronic recording devices in the 1930s. E.a.o.b. oscillations may vary from one to more than 50 cycles per second in frequency and from 50 to 200 microvolts in amplitude, as recorded by electrodes attached to the human scalp. See BRAIN WAVES; ELECTROENCEPHALOGRAPH.

electrical habituation the use of EEG recordings to study evoked potentials associated with conditioned and unconditioned stimuli. A novel stimulus, e.g., desynchronizes cortical alpha rhythms while evoking potentials that are recorded as EEG variations.

electrical intracranial stimulation: See INTRACRANIAL STIMULATION.

electrical stimulation in neuropsychology, the use of electrical or electronic devices to initiate sensations and responses of various sensory and motor neurons. E.s. also has been employed to study brain areas associated with memory traces and to follow pathways of impulses through various brain structures.

electrical stimulation of cortex the use of electrical charges introduced through electrodes implanted in the brain cells to produce a desired effect. In animal experiments, a reward or punishment effect depends upon the site of the electrodes and the intensity of the stimulation (Penfield). E.s.o.c. also has been used to promote recall and as therapy.

electrical transcranial stimulation: See ELECTROSLEEP THERAPY.

electric chorea: See CHOREA.

electric ophthalmia: See OPHTHALMIA.

electric senses nervous-system receptors or other organs in certain animals that enable them to detect or generate electric currents. Certain jaw-bearing fish, e.g., trout and salmon, will avoid an electric current produced by a wire hung in a stream and can be separated from other aquatic creatures that do not detect the electric effect. Sea lampreys generate an electric current that is used to detect and disable their prey.

electrocardiogram a wavelike tracing that represents the electrical action of the heart-muscle tissue as it goes through a typical cycle of contraction and relaxation. The electrical currents are detected by electrodes on the patient's chest and amplified more than 3,000 times in an **electrocardiograph (ECG, EKG)**, the device used to make the e. The e. wave patterns reveal the condition of the various heart chambers and valves. Abbrev.: **ECG; EKG** (from German *Elektrokardiogramm*).

electrocardiographic effect a change in the recording of the electrical activity of the heart. It frequently occurs as a side effect of phenothiazines, particularly thioridazine (Mellaril) prescribed for tranquilization.

electrocardiograph technician a medical technician who uses electrocardiograph (ECG, or EKG) equipment to record the electrical impulses produced by contractions of the heart muscle. Interpretation of the recordings is a responsibility of a physician, usually a cardiologist. An e.t. must have at least a high-school education and is trained by the hospital or other medical facility in use of the equipment.

electroconvulsive treatment a painless form of electric therapy introduced in 1938 by two Italian psychiatrists, U. Cerletti and L. Bini, and applied primarily to patients with depressive and schizophrenic disorders. The patient is prepared by administration of barbiturate anesthesia and injection of a chemical relaxant. An electric current is then applied for a fraction of a second through electrodes placed on the temples, and immediately produces a two-stage seizure (tonic and clonic). The usual treatment is bilateral, but unilateral stimulation of a nondominant hemisphere has been introduced in order to shorten the period of memory loss which follows the treatment. Abbr.: **ECT**. Also called **electroshock therapy (EST)**. See CONVULSIVE THERAPY; METRAZOL SHOCK TREATMENT; SHOCK TREATMENT.

electrode placement the positioning of electrodes on the scalp or in neurons to record changes of electrical potential caused by neural activity. For diagnostic work with humans, 16 electrodes are placed in standard locations over the scalp, and reference electrodes are placed on the ears and the vertex of the skull. In animal research studies, and certain human studies, needlelike microelectrodes are placed in specific brain cells.

electrodermal response: See GALVANIC SKIN RESPONSE.

electrodiagnosis the use of electrical instruments, such as the electroencephalograph and electromyograph, as diagnostic tools. The term also denotes application of electric current to nerves and muscles for diagnostic purposes.

electroencephalic audiometry the measurement of hearing sensitivity with use of electroencephalography. Gross measures are obtained from changes in brain-wave patterns when above-threshold sound stimuli are introduced.

electroencephalograph an instrument that amplifies and records the electrical activity of the cerebral cortex through electrodes placed at various points on the skull. The resulting record, or **electroencephalogram (EEG)**, of the brain-wave patterns, or Berger rhythms, is frequently used in studies of waking activities, the stages of sleep, drowsiness, and dreaming, and in the detection and diagnosis of brain lesions, tumors, and epilepsy. Abbrev.: **EEG**. See ELECTRICAL ACTIVITY OF BRAIN.

electroencephalograph technician a member of a staff of a hospital, clinic, or other medical facility who uses an electroencephalograph (EEG) to record a patient's brain waves by the use of electrodes attached to the patient's head. The recordings are interpreted by a physician, usually a neurologist or psychiatrist, to detect brain abnormalities. The e.t. usually has a high-school education and receives on-the-job training in use of EEG equipment.

electrolepsy = DUBINI'S DISEASE.

electrolyte imbalance abnormal levels of one or more **electrolytes**, or ions of chemicals that play a vital role in fluid balance, acid-base balance, and other functions of body cells. Electrolytes that may be involved in e.i. include sodium, which is needed for water regulation and normal nerve and muscle function; potassium, which is necessary for acid-base balance; and calcium, which is essential for normal blood and muscle functions. Also see THIRST.

electromyograph an instrument, that records the electrical potential of the muscles through electrodes placed in or on different muscle groups when they are relaxed or during various activities. The instrument is used in sensory-feedback therapy, and in the study of diseases involving the musculature, such as muscular dystrophy, myasthenia gravis, and spasmodic torticollis. Abbrev.: **EMG**.

electronarcosis application of a subconvulsive electric shock to the brain, producing an initial tonic phase and a clonic phase that is limited or avoided by continued stimulation. E. is a generally less effective alternative to standard electroconvulsive treatment (ECT). The technique has also been used to induce relaxation and sleep. See ELECTRO-SLEEP THERAPY.

electronic aids electronic devices that enable a handicapped person to achieve independent living. E.a. may include tape recorders, portable intercom equipment, walkie-talkie radios, and devices that turn on lights, open doors, and operate a wheelchair.

electrooculogram a graphic representation of the movements of the eyes over a constant distance between two fixation points. The e. is made in the form of electroencephalographic tracings. Abbrev.: **EOG**.

electroolfactogram a recording of the response of olfactory-nerve endings to various stimulating odors. The e. also can be used to diagnose disorders such as anosmia, or loss of the sense of smell, after injury or disease affecting the olfactory receptors. Abbrev.: **EOG**.

electrophobia a morbid fear of electricity.

electrophoresis a method of chemical analysis in which various molecules of a mixture are separated by the influence of an electric field. The substances are dissolved in a liquid and a sample is placed on a paper, gel, or other medium while an electric current is applied. The molecules are identified by the direction and speed exhibited in moving toward the anode or cathode. Also see CHROMATOGRAPHY.

electrophysiology the study of the role of electricity in the physiology of organism functions. The classical concept of e. assumes that a nerve impulse is a traveling wave of depolarization, moving at a constant velocity along a nerve pathway, with an accompanying pattern of circulating currents around and outside the pathway.

electroretinogram a recording of the electrical activity of retinal-nerve endings when stimulated by a pulse of light. The response is detected by a galvanometer attached to leads placed on the surface of the eyeball. Abbrev.: **ERG**.

electroshock therapy = ELECTROCONVULSIVE TREATMENT. Also see REGRESSIVE E.T.

electro-sleep therapy treatment of depression, chronic anxiety, and insomnia by inducing a state of relaxation or sleep through low-voltage **electrical transcranial stimulation (ETS)**, a technique developed in Russia in the 1940s, in which an instrument termed an **electrosone** was used.

electrostimulation an aversion, or negative reinforcement, technique involving administration of an electric shock. See AVERSIVE THERAPY.

electrotherapy a general term for the use of an electrical current on the central nervous system as a therapeutic measure. See ELECTROCONVULSIVE TREATMENT.

electrotonic conduction a type of nerve-impulse transmission that may occur in some nerve and muscle fibers over short distances in addition to or instead of the usual core-conduction properties of fibers. E.c. is related to electrical energy that leaks through the insulating sheath of a nerve fiber. Also called **tonic conduction**.

electrotonus the change in the condition of a nerve or muscle following application of an electric current.

element the simplest unit of analysis; the basic subunit of a sensation, image, or affective state; that which cannot be reduced further. In set theory, an e. is anything that belongs to a set.

elementarism = ATOMISM.

elementary anxiety = PRIMORDIAL PANIC.

elementary hallucination simple sensations without direct external stimuli, usually involving the visual or auditory senses, and consisting of sparks or amorphous darkenings, murmurs, or knocks.

Elephant Man's disease = VON RECKLINGHAUSEN'S DISEASE.

elevation the overall level or trend of an individual's test profile. Compare SCATTER.

elevator phobia a morbid fear of elevators, which may represent fear of height (acrophobia), sexualized sensations of equilibrium and space, or a fear of being shut in (claustrophobia).

eleventh cranial nerve = ACCESSORY NERVE.

elfin facies a disease complex that includes failure to thrive, hypercalcemia, elfin facial appearance, and mental retardation. Supravalvular aortic stenosis occurs in most cases. Some patients have normal intelligence, but most patients have IQs between 40 and 70. Muscular hypotonia in infancy occurs in some cases. Also called **hypercalcemia syndrome**.

Elgin check list a list of behavior patterns associated with psychoses.

elicited behavior = RESPONDENT BEHAVIOR.

elimination drives the urge to expel feces and urine from the body. Psychological factors have considerable effects on these drives: In small children, defecation can be stimulated by cuddling; and if emotional warmth is lacking, as in institutions, they usually become constipated. It is also a well-known fact that tension and fright may precipitate involuntary voiding of both the bladder and intestines. See ANAL EROTISM; ANAL CHARACTER; BLADDER CONTROL; BOWEL CONTROL; FUNCTIONAL ENURESIS; FUNCTIONAL ENCOPRESIS; TOILET TRAINING; DEFECATION REFLEX; MICTURITION REFLEXES.

Elithorn maze a paper-and-pencil maze which requires that the subject trace a path along a pattern made of dotted lines that form a mosaic of diamond shapes. An apparent random scattering of heavy dots along the dotted lines forms an overlapping pattern the pencil trace must pass through. The E.m. test is superior to many others in detecting signs of brain damage.

ellipsis the omission of words in writing or speaking, or of significant ideas in free association or dreams. In psychoanalysis, efforts are made to recover these ideas.

Ellis, Albert American psychologist, 1913—. See INTERNALIZED SPEECH; RATIONAL PSYCHOTHERAPY; SELF-TALK.

Ellis, Havelock English anthropologist, 1859–1939. E. is noted for altering public attitudes toward sexual problems (*Studies in the Psychology of Sex*, seven volumes, 1897–1928) and for his view that eminent individuals tend to come from professional families who have an extremely low incidence of insanity, contrary to the prevailing theory at that time (*The Study of British Genius*, 1904). See AUTOEROTICISM.

Ellis, Richard White Bernard English physician, 1902—. See ELLIS-VAN CREVELD SYNDROME.

Ellison, Edwin Homer American surgeon, 1918–70. See ZOLLINGER-ELLISON SYNDROME; WERMER'S SYNDROME.

Ellis-van Creveld syndrome an autosomal-recessive disorder marked by polydactyly, poorly formed hair, teeth, and nails, and skeletal anomalies. Adult patients are unable to make a tight fist. About half of the cases studied were Old Order Amish, who were abnormally short but had normal intelligence. About ten percent of the other patients were found to be retarded. Also called **chondroectodermal dysplasia**.

elopement in psychiatry, departure of a patient from a psychiatric hospital or unit without permission.

elucidation the second stage of Jung's analytic approach in which the therapist focuses on interpretation of the patient's individual and collective unconscious.

-em-: See -EN-.

emancipated minor the legal term for a minor who has asserted his or her independence and exercises general control over his or her life, and hence may claim the legal rights of an adult.

emancipation disorder a psychiatric problem of early adulthood in which the patient experiences conflicts between a desire for freedom from parental control and the responsibilities of independence. The symptoms include indecisiveness, homesickness, excessive dependence on peers, and paradoxical overdependence on parental advice.

emancipatory strivings attempts to free oneself from the influence or domination of parents and to achieve a sense of independence and self-dependence. E.s. are particularly evident during adolescence, and may take positive form when the young person embarks on constructive new experiences or educational opportunities, or may take negative form such as defiance of school rules, vandalism, sexual acting out, drug abuse, or participation in a gang subculture.

embarrassment dream a dream in which the person feels shame or embarrassment, e.g., appearing naked in public.

Embedded Figures Test a test that consists of finding and tracing a simple form in a complex figure, in some cases further complicated by an irregular colored background (Ammons and Ammons). The test has been used to demonstrate a relationship between personality characteristics and a perceptual task, particularly as a means of showing that field-independent persons tend to follow active, participant approaches to learning, while field-dependent persons more often use spectator approaches and are also more open and responsive to other people's behavior.

emblem a nonverbal body gesture that replaces a spoken word or phrase and communicates a message that can be readily comprehended by most individuals in a culture, e.g., shaking the head back and forth to signify "no" or nodding the head up and down to indicate "yes." Also SEE ILLUSTRATOR.

embolalia a speech disorder in which meaningless words or sounds are interpolated in a sentence. E. often is associated with stuttering. Also called **embololalia**.

embolism the interruption of blood flow by the blockage of a vessel by an **embolus**, or obstructing material, carried by the bloodstream. The embolus may be a blood clot, air bubble, fat drop-

let, or other substance such as a clump of bacteria or tissue cells. An e. usually occurs at a point where a blood vessel branches or narrows. The symptoms are those associated with a disruption of the normal flow of fresh blood to a part of an organ, including pain, numbness, and loss of body warmth in the affected area. An e. in a coronary artery may cause a fatal heart attack, while in the brain the result is a stroke, which also may be fatal depending upon the tissues deprived of blood.

embracing behavior a form of contact-seeking behavior in children, adults, and higher animals (chimpanzees) in stressful or frightening situations. Embracing of this kind (as contrasted with embracing as a form of sexual or affectional expression) is a primary means of seeking comfort and relief from anxiety.

embryo in human prenatal development, the growing organism during the first eight weeks after conception. Following this period, the term **fetus** is used. Adjective: **embryonic**. See EMBRYONIC PERIOD.

embryonic period in human prenatal development, the roughly six-week period in which the endoderm, mesoderm, and ectoderm develop. During this time, the embryo is believed to increase in size by approximately two million percent. The e.p. follows the two-week germinal period and precedes the fetal period beginning in the third month.

emergence: See EPIGENETIC THEORY.

emergency contagion a process whereby emotional reactions by one individual to a presumed emergency stimulate similar reactions in other individuals who sense or observe the emergency function but not the precipitating cause.

emergency dyscontrol a term used by S. Rado for a tendency to overreact emotionally in emergency situations, and inability to use available means of handling them effectively.

emergency intervention in social psychology, an action taken on behalf of another person or persons under stressful and possibly dangerous conditions with little or no expectation of reward. See BYSTANDER EFFECT.

emergency psychotherapy active psychological treatment of patients who have undergone a traumatic experience or period of decompensation and are in a state of acute anxiety, panic, shock, or suicidal ideation. The specific methods depend on the immediate needs of the patient, but may include ventilation of feeling, relaxation with or without hypnotic suggestion, reassurance, catharsis by reliving the experience, and emotional support in which the therapist sits quietly with the patient.

emergency services services provided by a community mental-health center or other facility such as a clinic or general hospital, in emergency situations, as in disasters affecting the entire population, or crises affecting individuals or families. For details, see CRISIS INTERVENTION. Also see PSYCHIATRIC EMERGENCY.

emergency theory of emotions Cannon's theory that emotional and visceral changes controlled by the autonomic system prepare us for fight or flight during an emergency.

emergent evolution the theory that new or unpredictable phenomena evolve from an interaction of simpler factors.

-emet- a combining form relating to vomiting (from Greek *emein*, "to vomit").

emetomania a morbid desire to vomit, which usually is a symptom of hysteria.

emetophobia a morbid fear of vomiting. It is a common hysterical (conversion) reaction.

EMG = ELECTROMYOGRAPH.

-emia; -aemia a combining form relating to blood.

emic pertaining to concepts or constructs that possess meaning only in a designated cultural context; pertaining to concepts that are not universal, e.g., future shock. Compare ETIC.

emitted behavior responses or response sequences that do not depend for their arousal on external stimuli but arise as a result of the organism's internal state. Compare RESPONDENT BEHAVIOR.

Emmert's law the principle that the size of an afterimage or eidetic image increases with the distance between the image and the ground on which it is projected.

emotion a complex reaction pattern of changes in nervous, visceral, and skeletal-muscle tissues in response to a stimulus. The type and intensity of the reaction is appropriate to the stimulus which may be of a pleasurable, threatening, or other nature. As a strong feeling, e. is usually directed toward a specific person or event and involves widespread physiological changes, such as increased heart rate and inhibition of peristalsis. In psychoanalysis, emotions are states of tension associated with instinctual drives, such as sex and hostility. Also see UNCANNY EMOTIONS.

emotional acrescentism = EMOTIONAL DEPRIVATION.

emotional adjustment the ability to maintain a balance in one's emotional life, to exert reasonable control over emotions, and to express emotions that are appropriate to the situation.

emotional anesthesia a mourning reaction consisting of inability to react emotionally. See CONCENTRATION-CAMP SYNDROME.

emotional beggar a term used to describe a person who is unable to detach himself emotionally from his parents or other people, a condition that is attributed to a failure in physical and emotional weaning during infancy.

emotional bias prejudice based on emotional factors.

emotional blocking = BLOCKING.

emotional conflict a clash between intense emotions or affect-laden impulses of approximately equal strength, e.g., ambivalent feelings such as love and hate, affection and hostility, or the conflict between a strong desire for success and a fear of failure.

emotional dependence a dependence on others for support, comfort, and nurturance.

emotional deprivation lack of adequate warmth, affection, and interest, especially on the part of the mother or mother figure during the child's developmental years. It is common in situations involving separation from the mother, child neglect, child abuse, and institutionalization. Also called **emotional acrescentism**. See MATERNAL DEPRIVATION.

emotional deterioration an emotional state observed in chronic institutionalized schizophrenics, characterized by carelessness toward themselves, indifference to their surroundings, including other people, and inappropriate emotional reactions.

emotional development a gradual increase in the capacity to experience and express the full gamut of emotions, beginning with the diffuse excitement of the infant in response to intense stimulation or loss of support, and continuing with pleasure expressed by relaxation of the body and displeasure by crying—to smiles and frowns at about eight weeks; expressions of delight, fear, anger, and disgust by six months; fear of strangers from six to eight months; expressions of affection and jealousy between one and two years; and expressions of rage in the form of temper tantrums a year or so later. From there on, cortical control, imitation of others, glandular influences, home atmosphere, and conditioning play a major role.

emotional disorder = EMOTIONAL ILLNESS.

emotional divorce a marital relationship in which the husband and wife live in separate worlds, with an absence of normal interaction between the partners.

emotional expression the behavioral display of emotions by such means as smiling, laughing, and gesturing; also, the somatic changes such as rapid heartbeat and muscular tension that constitute an integral aspect of emotional reactions.

emotional flatness = FLAT AFFECT.

emotional flooding uncontrolled and uncontrollable emotional expression, such as continuous weeping, sometimes used by hysterical patients as an appeal for sympathy or help in escaping a distasteful situation.

emotional handicap in educational psychology, a learning or behavioral disorder that prevents a child from functioning normally in a regular classroom either socially or academically.

emotional illness a psychological disorder characterized by maladjustive emotional reactions such as irrational or uncontrollable fears, persistent anxiety, or extreme hostility. E.i. is also a lay term often used euphemistically for any type of mental disorder, neurotic or psychotic. Also called **emotional disorder**.

emotional immaturity a tendency to express emotions without restraint or in ways that are characteristic of children. E.i. is also a popular term for maladjustment.

emotional inoculation the prior imagining, practicing, or "cognitive rehearsal" of an anxiety-producing experience. Rehearsal tempers anxiety in allowing the individual to anticipate reactions and plan responses.

emotional insight an awareness of the emotional reactions of oneself or others. In psychotherapy, the term applies to the patient's awareness of the emotional forces, such as internal conflicts or traumatic experiences, that underlie his or her symptoms. Freud and others consider this form of insight a prerequisite to therapeutic change.

emotional insulation a defense mechanism consisting of indifference and detachment in response to frustrating situations or disappointing events. The extreme of e.i. is found in states of complete apathy and catatonic stupor.

emotional instability a tendency to exhibit unpredictable and rapid changes in emotions.

emotionally handicapped child an educational-psychology term for a child who is neurologically normal, and of average or superior intelligence, but who cannot function in a regular classroom as a result of a learning disability or behavioral disorder.

emotionally unstable personality a DSM-I term used to designate a personality-trait disturbance characterized by immaturity and lack of control over emotions, resulting in such reactions as frequent outbursts of anger over minor irritations, poor tolerance for frustration and stress, sulking, quarrelsomeness, and stubbornness.

emotional maturity an adult level of emotional control and expression as opposed to childish emotional behavior.

emotional nutriment: See DIRECT ANALYSIS.

emotional reeducation psychotherapy focused on the modification of the patient's attitudes, feelings, and reactions by helping him gain greater insight into his emotional conflicts and self-defeating behavior. Typical objectives are an increase in self-confidence, sociability, and self-reliance; and typical reeducational methods are group discussions, personal counseling, relationship therapy, and a study of the patient's attitudes toward himself as well as his faulty methods of dealing with life problems.

emotional release the catharsis or sudden outpouring of emotions that have been pent up or suppressed.

emotional response an emotional reaction to people or events. Spitz (1947) has shown that the first signs of e.r. appear in the first few weeks of life when signs of anxiety occur and the mother seeks to alleviate them by holding or caressing the child. If the child is placed in an institution, e.r. is usually curtailed and the child becomes apathetic.

emotional security the feeling of safety, confidence, and freedom from apprehension. In Horney's approach, the need for e.s. is the underlying determinant of behavior, and in H. S. Sullivan's approach, e.s. is itself determined primarily by our interpersonal relations. See SECURITY OPERATIONS.

emotional storm a sudden, intense, uncontrolled flood of emotion, sometimes experienced by individuals with temporal-lobe epilepsy or explosive disorders. See INTERMITTENT EXPLOSIVE DISORDER.

emotional stress: See EMOTIONAL TENSION.

emotional stupor a form of affective stupor marked by depression or intense anxiety and accompanied by mutism.

emotional supplies: See PRIMAL DEPRESSION.

emotional support reassurance, encouragement, and approval received from an individual or group. It is a major factor in maintaining morale, and in inspirational approaches such as Alcoholics Anonymous.

emotional tension the feeling of psychological strain and uneasiness produced by facing situations of danger, threat, and loss of personal security, as well as stresses produced by internal conflicts, frustrations, loss of self-esteem, and grief.

emotive imagery a variation of systematic desensitization used by A. A. Lazarus with phobic children. The child's fears are listed in order of severity, and the therapist tells one of the child's favorite stories, but centers his account on the least fearful characters and events. He then progresses step by step to the most fearful in further story variations.

emotive processes: See COGNITION.

emotive therapy a psychotherapeutic approach based on the evocation of the patient's habitual and often self-defeating attitudes and emotional reactions. See RATIONAL PSYCHOTHERAPY.

empathic understanding insight into the feelings, thoughts, or attitudes of another person achieved by projecting oneself into his situation, that is, by "putting oneself into his shoes."

empathy the objective awareness of another person's thoughts and feelings and their possible meanings. One who empathizes sustains his objectivity and separate feelings even when confronted with disturbing psychological material.

empirical relating to observation, measurement, or experimentation, in contrast to theoretical or explanatory.

empirical construct: See CONSTRUCT.

empirical-criterion keying a method employed in selecting questions for personality inventories, in which the items are chosen and weighted according to an external criterion such as the responses of mental patients or ratings made by a large standardization sample.

empirical law a law based on facts or observations and expressing a general relationship between variables.

empirical-rational strategy in social psychology, the idea that societal and institutional change can be brought about if the public receives enough convincing factual evidence. The concept holds that reason alone can motivate people to change their attitudes. However, this approach seems to be doubtful; e.g., the Surgeon General's warning of medical risk to smokers does not appear to be an effective deterrent. Also see NORMATIVE-REEDUCATIVE STRATEGY; POWER-COERCIVE STRATEGY.

empirical test the test of a hypothesis through experiments or observational data.

empirical validity accurate measurement or prediction of performance, as demonstrated by research. The term refers to a test that has more than mere face validity.

empiricism the philosophic theory advanced by John Locke that the mind is a tabula rasa (Latin, "blank sheet") at birth and all knowledge is derived from sensory experience. This theory led to the view that all science, including psychology, must be based on objective, empirical facts discovered through naturalistic observation and experimentation.

empiric-risk figure in genetic counseling, a percentage representing the risk for common disorders such as schizophrenia and depression where there is evidence of genetic factors of unknown mechanism. The figure is based upon reports of frequency of occurrence in large series of families (in addition to the approximately three-percent risk of mental retardation or birth defects that every couple takes when having a child).

employee evaluation in industrial psychology, the judgment of employee behavior and certain related personal characteristics, which may be exhibited in their work; a judgmental process whereby a superior or consultant evaluates the job-related behavior of a subordinate. Also called **employee appraisal**.

employment interview an interview with an applicant for a job, in which a personnel worker, executive, or supervisor (a) imparts information and answers questions about the company, including its products, working conditions, and benefits offered, (b) describes available jobs in which the applicant shows an interest, and (c) obtains information about the applicant which will make possible at least a preliminary judgment of his or her suitability for a particular job or jobs. Also called **job interview**.

employment workshop: See TRANSITIONAL E.W.

emprosthotonos /-thot'-/ a condition of tetanic contraction of the flexor muscles causing the back to curve with a forward concavity. The resulting body posture is the opposite of opisthotonos. Also called **tetanus anticus**.

emptiness fear = KENOPHOBIA.

empty-chair technique a Gestalt-therapy "exercise" in which the patient conducts an emotional dialogue with some aspect of himself or some significant person in his life, such as a mother, who is imagined to sit in an empty chair, and then exchanges chairs and becomes that aspect or person himself.

empty nest a popular term for the parental home of a family after the children have reached maturity and have established homes or families of their own.

empty organism a term sometimes applied to the stimulus-response approach in psychology,

which, it is charged, neglects the internal drives and activities of the organism.

empty set a set with no elements; a null set.

empty word = FUNCTION WORD.

EMR an abbreviation of *e*ducable *m*entally *r*etarded. See EDUCABLE.

emylcamate /-kam'-/ an anxiolytic and mild CNS depressant. It may be used as a minor tranquilizer. Its pharmacologic action resembles meprobamate and other sedatives. E. is not effective in the treatment of psychoses.

-en-; -endo-; -ento-; -em- a combining form meaning inside, internal.

enabler a member of the community who assists in the deinstitutionalization of mental patients by helping them adjust to normal daily-living routines. The e. may accept patients in his own home or help them manage their own independent homes.

enactive mode J. Bruner's term for the way a child first comes to know his environment through physical interactions, e.g., in crawling. The e.m. is knowing through doing; the iconic mode is knowing through mental images; the symbolic mode is knowing through language and logic. See ICONIC MODE; SYMBOLIC MODE.

enactive period a term introduced by Bruner to identify the period of child development in which the infant gains control over environmental objects and events. See ENACTIVE MODE.

enantiodromia Heraclitus' conception that all things eventually turn into their opposites. As used by Jung, however, e. refers to the "necessary opposition" that governs psychic life, as in the interplay between conscious and unconscious, introversive and extraversive tendencies, or ego and shadow. Jung stresses the need for man to recognize his inner polarities and unite them in awareness.

encapsulated delusion a delusional system that is sealed off from the rest of life, so that it does not have any significant effect on everyday behavior.

encapsulated end organ the terminal portion of a sensory nerve fiber, usually located in peripheral tissue such as the skin, and enclosed in a membranous sheath. Kinds of encapsulated end organs include Meissner's corpuscles in smooth skin, which detect tactile sensations, and Pacinian corpuscles, in deep fibrous structures, sensitive to pressure sensations.

encapsulation in psychiatry, the tendency of a schizophrenic patient to keep his delusional life separated from the routine of the real world.

encéphale isolé /äNsäfäl'izōlā'/ literally, isolated brain (French). The term pertains to a midbrain that has been transected so that the subject is alive but permanently in an unconscious or sleep state. The condition is sometimes produced experimentally in laboratory animals.

encephalitis an inflammation of the brain caused by many agents, including heavy metals as in lead e. Most cases, however, are caused by viruses, which may be transmitted by ticks, mosquitoes, or other biting insects, or through contact with infected people. The symptoms may be mild, with influenzalike characteristics, or very serious, with fever, delirium, convulsions, coma, and death. Also see BICKERSTAFF'S E.; ECONOMO'S DISEASE; EQUINE E.; HERPES SIMPLEX E.; HYPERSOMNIA; JAPANESE B E.; LEAD E.; LEUKOENCEPHALITIS; MENINGOENCEPHALITIS; METABOLIC E.; PANENCEPHALITIS; PARANEOPLASTIC LIMBIC E.; POLIOENCEPHALITIS; WERNICKE'S E.

encephalitis lethargica = ECONOMO'S DISEASE.

encephalization the corticalization or transfer of mental functions from phylogenetically primitive brain areas to cerebral centers as steps in the evolution of the mind.

encephalocele /-sef'-/ a congenital hernia of the brain which protrudes through a cleft in the skull.

encephalofacial angiomatosis = STURGE-WEBER SYNDROME.

encephalogram an X-ray photograph of the skull following the injection of air into areas of the brain normally occupied by cerebrospinal fluid.

encephalomalacia a softening of the brain, usually due to tissue deterioration resulting from an inadequate blood supply to the area.

encephalomyelitis an inflammation of the central nervous system, involving the tissues of both the brain and the spinal cord. The infectious agents generally are the same as those causing encephalitis, but the precipitating factor may be a vaccination with smallpox vaccine. More than a dozen viruses, including herpes simplex as well as syphilis and tuberculosis may be causative agents.

encephalon = BRAIN.

encephalopathy: See ANTIRABIC SERUM-INDUCED DEMYELINATING E.; BILIRUBIN E.; BINSWANGER'S E.; BOXER'S DEMENTIA; EPILEPTOGENIC E.; HYPERKINETIC E.; LEAD E.; MERCURY E.; PORTAL-SYSTEMIC E.; PROGRESSIVE DEGENERATIVE SUBCORTICAL E.; PROGRESSIVE-MULTIFOCAL LEUKOENCEPHALOPATHY; SCHISTOSOMIASIS; TRAUMATIC E.

encephalosis a degenerative brain disorder caused by an infection and characterized by headaches, irritability, apathy, stupor, and convulsions. Brain tissues usually show small hemorrhages, infarcts, and other types of damage to blood vessels, as well as degeneration of ganglia.

encoding the conversion of a sensory input into a form capable of being processed and deposited in memory. Similarly, in communications, e. is the conversion of messages or data into codes or signals capable of being conveyed by a communication channel.

encopresis = FUNCTIONAL E.

encounter direct confrontation or other involvement of one individual with another, or between members of a group, on an emotional level.

encounter group a form of small-group dynamics in which constructive insight, sensitivity to others, and personal growth are promoted through interactions on an emotional level. The

leader functions as a catalyst and facilitator rather than a therapist, and focuses on here-and-now feelings and interaction. The approach is an outgrowth of K. Lewin's training groups, and the term was coined by J. L. Moreno.

encounter movement a trend toward the formation of small groups in which various techniques such as confrontation, games, "stroking", and reenactment are used to stimulate awareness, personality growth, and productive interactions.

enculturation the process involved in modifying attitudes, behavior, and language while attempting to adjust to a different culture.

endarterectomy a surgical procedure in which atherosclerotic plaque is removed from the lumen of a cerebral artery. By removing the plaque accumulation, the bore of the artery is enlarged, allowing a greater flow of blood to the brain tissues. This most commonly involves the carotid arteries at the level of bifurcation. The diagnosis of local arterial-plaque disease is made by carotid sonography (ultrasound) or angiography.

end brush the finely branched terminal of an axon.

end buttons = SYNAPTIC KNOBS.

endemic peculiar to a specific region, nation, or people. The term denotes usually a disease, but is also applied to customs or folkways. Compare EPIDEMIC; PANDEMIC.

-endo-: See -EN-.

endocarditis an inflammation of the **endocardium**, or inner lining of the heart. The valves are often involved in e. Causes include infections of bacteria or fungi, e.g., syphilis, tuberculosis, staphylococcus, and occasionally a rickettsial invasion of the heart valves following an infection of Q fever. Also see BACTERIAL E.

endocathection Murray's term for the inward focusing of psychic energy and withdrawal from external pursuits. Compare EXOCATHECTION.

endocept a term used in the cognitive-volitional school for a nonrepresentational, preverbal mental construct occurring between the phantasmic stage of inner reality toward the end of the first year of life, and later stages when mental constructs are representational and lead to action. Endocepts are feeling states, comparable to Freud's oceanic feeling, and are forerunners of esthetic and empathic states. See OCEANIC FEELING.

endocratic power in the cognitive-volitional school, transformation of the commands, or "imperative attitude," of parents and other authorities into an inner power over one's actions and thoughts. If this introjection is excessive (**endocratic surplus**), it may lead to blind obedience and acceptance of tyranny.

endocrine gland = DUCTLESS GLAND.

endocrinological and metabolic disorders any abnormal mental condition caused or aggravated by a hormonal or metabolic dysfunction, or both. Many inherited forms of mental retardation or neurological deficits are due to inborn errors of metabolism. Endocrinological disorders may also include functional problems due to abnormally high or low levels of pituitary, thyroid, adrenal, or sex hormones. Also see BE-HAVIORAL ENDOCRINOLOGY.

endoderm the embryo's innermost layer of cells from which the gastrointestinal tract, liver, lungs, and other vital organs, and some glands develop (literally, "inner skin"). The other two layers are the ectoderm and mesoderm. Adjective: **endodermal**. Also called **entoderm**. See EMBRYONIC PERIOD.

endogamy /-dog'-/ the practice of limiting marriage to members of a kinship, caste, or religious or social group. Adjective: **endogamous**. Compare EXOGAMY.

endogenetic factors; endogenic factors = EN-DOGENOUS FACTORS.

endogenous /-doj'-/ pertaining to an event or effect that originates within the organism, as in e. depression or genetically determined mental retardation. Also called **endogenic; endogenetic**.

endogenous depression a depression that originates within the psyche, e.g., from ambivalent or hostile impulses operating on an unconscious level. Such impulses generate the feelings of guilt and sin that are frequently observed in e.d. Compare REACTIVE DEPRESSION.

endogenous factors causal factors that arise within the organism, including hereditary factors that give rise to some cases of mental retardation, constitutional factors that many investigators believe to be at the root of schizophrenia and manic-depressive (bipolar) psychosis, and psychological factors such as intrapsychic conflicts. Also called **endogenic factors; endogenetic factors**.

endogenous rhythm = BIOLOGICAL RHYTHM.

endogenous stimulation stimulation that originates within the organism, as in arousal during REM sleep. Compare EXOGENOUS STIMULATION.

endogenous thyrotoxicosis: See THYROTOXICOSIS.

endolymph a fluid contained in the membranous labyrinth of the inner ear. The e. helps translate sound vibrations transmitted through the middle ear into the nerve impulses carried to the sense of hearing by the auditory, or acoustic, nerve.

endolymphatic potential one of several electric potentials measurable with electrodes inserted into the cochlear region of the ear. Endolymph potentials are determined in part by a chemical composition that has a high potassium and low sodium concentration. A potential difference of from 160 to 180 millivolts has been recorded between the perilymph surrounding the hair cells and the endolymph in the chamber immediately above.

endometrial cycle the pattern of proliferation and loss of endometrial tissue during the female reproductive cycle. The e.c. follows the rhythm of the monthly release of an ovum from an ovary, the endometrium becoming thicker and richer in anticipation of implantation of a fertilized ovum. If the ovum is not fertilized, the endometrium sloughs off, becoming the bloody debris of the menses. The e.c. begins again at the end of the period.

endometritis an inflammation of the endometrium, or mucous membrane lining of the uterus. E. may develop as an infection following childbirth or as a result of a benign tumorlike lesion called a syncytioma.

endometrium the layer of cells lining the uterus. The e. varies in thickness during the menstrual cycle, reaching a peak of cellular proliferation approximately one week after ovulation, sloughing off as menstrual flow two weeks after ovulation if the ovum is not fertilized. Also see ENDOMETRIAL CYCLE.

endomorph one of W. H. Sheldon's constitutional types, or somatotypes, characterized by a soft, round physique (from Greek *endomorphe*, "inner form"), which he found to be highly correlated with a **viscerotonic temperament** (tendency toward love of comfort, love of food, relaxation, and sociability). Also called **endomorphic body type**.

endoplasmic reticulum a network of tubular and vesicular structures extending from the nucleus to the outer membrane of a typical body cell. Functions of the e.r. include secretion of proteins and lipids, release of glucose, and transport of substances. The e.r. exists in different forms in different types of cells.

endopsychic pertaining to unconscious material or intrapsychic processes. Compare EXOPSYCHIC.

endopsychic censor = CENSOR.

endopsychic perception a perception, or insight, arising from within the mind, particularly from unconscious sources.

endopsychic structure in psychoanalysis, the internal psychic structure of the mind: the division into the conscious, preconscious, and unconscious, and, in later Freudian theory, the division into the id, ego, and superego.

end organ the terminal structure of a nerve ending. Also see ENCAPSULATED E.O.

endorphin a short chain of amino acids that has the chemical structure of a portion of a pituitary-gland hormone. Several kinds of e. are known, each of which has a neurologic effect. **Alpha-e.** acts as a mild analgesic and tranquilizer, **beta-e.** causes aggressive behavior, and **gamma-e.** causes a catatonialike state. The effects are blocked by morphine-antagonist drugs, indicating they are a natural form of analgesic. Also see ENKEPHALIN.

endowment: See CONSTITUTION.

end plate a specialized motor-nerve fiber terminal that forms a junction with a muscle cell.

end pleasure a psychoanalytic term for the pleasurable release of tension during an orgasm.

end spurt the increased productivity or gain in performance frequently noted near the end of a task, series of trials, or day's work. It is also commonly observed in relation to athletic endeavors, e.g., in long-distance running. Compare INITIAL SPURT.

end-stage renal disease a chronic kidney disease associated with renal failure. Kinds of e.-s.r.d. include glomerulonephritis, genetic renal diseases, pyelonephritis, uncorrected obstructive urinary-tract disorders, hypertensive renal disease, metabolic disorders, anomalies, and tumors. E.-s.r.d. usually has psychological implications since treatment requires disruption of employment, marriage, and family relationships and numerous life-style changes.

end state a thorough, detailed description of the characteristics that define a given behavior in its developed form, e.g., a description of the aspects and characteristics of individuation as the final result of the separation-individuation process (M. S. Mahler). The e.s. is the goal or culmination of progressive stages of development. Once a given e.s. is defined, interest then centers on precise description of the stages that lead to it. The concept of the e.s. is important in developmental psychology.

enelicomorphism the attribution of adult traits or motives to children; the interpretation of children's behavior in terms appropriate to adults. Also called **adultomorphism**.

enema addiction a dependence upon the use of enemas to empty the bowel. E.a. may develop through the use of enemas and laxatives repeatedly, a self-treatment process which in turn reduces normal rectal sensitivity to the presence of feces in the bowel. The condition occurs most frequently among persons with obsessive-compulsive personalities who feel "unclean" if normal bowel movements are irregular. Also see LAXATIVE ADDICTION; KLISMAPHILIA.

enema drug administration: See ADMINISTRATION.

energizer an antidepressant drug which has the effect of restoring or producing a flow of psychic energy in a patient. See PSYCHOTROPIC DRUG.

enforced treatment = FORCED TREATMENT.

Engelmann, Guido Austrian physician, 1876—. See ENGELMANN'S DISEASE.

Engelmann's disease an inherited progressive skeletal disorder marked by a thickening of the midshaft region of the long bones accompanied by small, weak muscles. Puberty and secondary sexual characteristics may be retarded, and there may be loss of special sense-organ functions, such as vision, smell, or hearing. About ten percent of one group of patients had subnormal intelligence. Also called **progressive diaphyseal dysplasia**.

engineering model: See MEDICAL MODEL.

engineering psychologist a psychologist who specializes in the design of the equipment and environment of the workplace so that humans can function more effectively at their tasks. The design of space capsules for astronauts is a responsibility of the e.p.

engineering psychology a psychological field concerned with "research, development, application, and evaluation of psychological principles relating human behavior to the characteristics, design, and use of the environments and systems within which human beings work and live" (Society of Engineering Psychologists, 1974). From an e.p. viewpoint, a computer, e.g., should not be designed for engineering efficiency alone, but some of its features, such as the keyboard, should be adapted to the physical and psychological needs of the user. Also see EQUIPMENT DESIGN; HUMAN ENGINEERING.

English as a second language = ESL.

English malady = CHEYNE'S DISEASE.

English Usage Test: See ACT ASSESSMENT.

engram a hypothetical recording of learned information, based on the assumption that retention and recall processes require an electrical, chemical, or other unit of information storage in the brain or central nervous system. The term was introduced by K. S. Lashley in 1950. Also called **memory trace; mnemonic trace; mneme**.

engrossment intimate involvement of the father with his newborn expressed by touching, holding, and admiring the infant. The bond between father and child generates feelings of elation and self-esteem in the father, and greater recognition of his worth within the family.

enkephalin any of several peptide molecules found in the brain that produce a narcoticlike analgesic effect. **Met-e.** and **leu-e.** are found in brain areas that produce analgesia when stimulated by electricity. It is believed the enkephalins interact with another brain peptide, Substance P, to switch on and off neurons involved in pain control. Also see ENDORPHIN.

enosiophobia a morbid fear of having committed an unpardonable sin. Also see HAMARTOPHOBIA; PECCATOPHOBIA.

enriched environment: See ENVIRONMENTAL ENRICHMENT.

enrichment program an educational program designed to develop the potential and forestall the boredom of very bright or gifted children by providing them with an expanded curriculum. The e.p may be individually applied to students in regular classes or applied to an entire class of gifted students.

entelechy: See VITALISM.

-enter-; -entero- a combining form relating to the intestine. Adjective: **enteric**.

enteric cytopathic human orphan: See ECHO VIRUS.

enteric virus infection a disease produced by one of the polio, Cocksackie, or ECHO viruses, which are members of the picorna-virus family. An e.v.i. may be poliomyelitis, aseptic meningitis, herpangina, myocarditis, or one of the exanthematas. More than 70 viruses have been classed as enteric because they multiply in the gastrointestinal tract of humans. Also called **enteroviral infection**.

entitlement an unreasonable claim to special consideration on the part of narcissistic individuals, including paranoid patients who believe they are President, or important enough to be involved in international intrigue.

entitlement programs programs of the United States government that provide financial assistance and welfare benefits to persons who are mentally or physically disabled. The e.p. are administered through Medicare, Medicaid, Social Security disability insurance, and similar funding sources.

-ento-: See -EN-.

entoderm = ENDODERM.

-entom-; -entomo- a combining form relating to an insect (Greek *entomon*).

entomophobia a morbid fear of insects. Also see ACAROPHOBIA; PARASITOPHOBIA.

entorhinal-cortex lesion an area of tissue damage in a portion of the brain immediately behind the olfactory nerves of the rhinencephalon. The lesion has been induced in wild marsupials to eliminate aggressiveness. The entorhinal cortex sometimes is identified as Brodmann's cytoarchitectural field No. 28.

entropy /en'trəpē/ in thermodynamics, the amount of energy that cannot be converted into work; the tendency of the energy in the universe to reach a state of inertia. (The term was first used by R. J. E. Clausius in 1850, on analogy with *en*—"in"—of "*en*ergy" and Greek *tropos*, "turn, direction.") In psychiatry, e. is the inability to convert psychic energy into active adjustment to reality, e.g., the tendency of elderly people to "turn inward" and become rigid and stodgy. In information theory, e. is a measure of the number of possible outcomes a given event might have.

entry behavior in educational psychology, the equivalent of READINESS. See this entry.

enuresis: See FUNCTIONAL E; NOCTURNAL E.

environment the aggregate of external agents or conditions—physical, biological, social, cultural—that influence the functions of the organism. The physical e. may be measured in terms of temperature, air pressure, noise, vibration, atmosphere, or sources of nutrients, which in turn may be specified by a range of values, e.g., a temperature scale. See ECOLOGY.

environmental approach a therapeutic approach in which efforts are directed toward reducing external pressures, e.g., employment or financial problems, that contribute to emotional conflicts.

environmental assessment the evaluation of situational and environmental variables that have an influence on behavior on the theory that disordered functioning may be rooted, at least in part, in the social system rather than in the individual and his personal characteristics. Examples of instruments used in e.a. are the Classroom Environment Scale (measuring, e.g., teacher support and teacher control) and the Ward Atmosphere Scale (measuring such factors as staff support, patient autonomy, and patient involvement).

environmental attribution = SITUATIONAL ATTRIBUTION.

environmental change: See CHANGE OF ENVIRONMENT.

environmental deprivation an absence of conditions that stimulate personality growth and development, such as educational, recreational, and social opportunities. E.d. is usually associated with social isolation, poverty, and slums, and may be so severe that it causes PSEUDORETARDATION. See this entry.

environmental design the creative planning of living and working areas to enhance their habitability. E.d. also may be applied to the enhancement of recreational areas. Habitability factors may range from simple shelter needs to complex and sophisticated environmental esthetics and conformance factors, e.g., the use of paint colors or specific wavelengths of illumination that elicit optimum performance of tasks.

environmental education the study of the physical environment in its relation to natural resources, energy, economics, social organization, and basic ecology.

environmental enrichment a term denoting an environment enriched by social contacts, play materials, and stimulating activities which has been shown to enhance normal emotional, cerebral, sexual, and activity development in both animals and children, as compared with animals and children reared in an **isolated** or **impoverished environment**.

environmental esthetics one of the factors contributing to the quality of the environment. E.e. may include visual attractiveness of the landscape, noise, traffic, air pollution, and maintenance of the area. E.e. may be influenced by hedonic values of the observer, who may regard an industrial park as a suburban blight or as an attractive working environment.

environmental hazards environmental factors that pose some danger to an organism or community. E.h. in a home or workplace would include exposed electrical wiring; for a community, e.h. would include nuclear reactors or lead smelters; for aquatic animals, e.h. would include factories that dump toxic chemicals or hot water into fresh-water streams.

environmentalist one who maintains that environment and learning are the chief determinants of behavior and thus the major cause of interpersonal variations in ability and adjustment. The e. position holds that behavior is largely modifiable in contrast to the hereditarian position which emphasizes the role of genetic inheritance in determining ability, intelligence, and personality. See NATURE-NURTURE CONTROVERSY.

environmental-learning theory = LEARNING MODEL.

environmental-load theory the concept that humans have a limited ability to handle environmental-stress factors. The limited capacity is determined by the amount of information inputs that can be processed by the central nervous system. When the environmental load exceeds the individual's capacity for processing, the central nervous system reacts by ignoring some of inputs. See INFORMATION OVERLOAD.

environmental manipulation a method of improving the well-being of mental patients by changing their living conditions, as by placing a child in a foster home when the family situation is intolerable, or transferring an adult patient to an adult home or halfway house.

environmental modification: See ENVIRONMENTAL MANIPULATION.

environmental-mold trait a personality trait that results from environmental influences (Cattell).

environmental noise: See DIFFERENTIATION THEORY.

environmental press a term applied by H. A. Murray to an environmental situation or circumstance ("press") that arouses a need. E.g., a person faced with a bear experiences a need to escape, or a child whose brother or sister has just been born is faced with the need to adjust to the newcomer.

environmental psychology a branch of psychology that emphasizes the effects of environmental influences on behavior. The environmental influences may include noise pollution, air pollution, poor illumination, and natural atmospheric conditions such as stormy weather.

environmental stress a condition of tension and strain provoked by an external situation such as a POW camp or crop failure that puts a special burden on the individual's adaptive mechanisms.

environmental-stress theory the concept that autonomic and cognitive factors combine to form a individual's appraisal of environmental-stress factors as threatening or nonthreatening. E.g., a native Alaskan and a Sahara-desert camel driver would have similar autonomic body responses to a blizzard or a heat wave, but their cognition of the environmental stressors would result in different adaptation behaviors. See ENVIRONMENTAL STRESS.

environmental therapy organization of the patient's entire surroundings, especially in a mental hospital, as a means of promoting recovery. Also called **situational therapy**. For details, see MILIEU THERAPY; THERAPEUTIC COMMUNITY.

environment-centered services a term frequently used in industrial psychiatry, but applicable elsewhere, for maintaining the mental and physical health of workers through an improvement of the physical environment (eliminating unnecessary noise, toxic substances, or air pollution) and through an improvement of the psychosocial environment—establishing constructive relationships and attitudes on all levels by (a) applying a knowledge of group dynamics, (b) maintaining group morale, and (c) giving the workers an opportunity to ventilate grievances. Also see PATIENT-CENTERED SERVICES.

envy an unpleasant feeling generated by the desire to possess what someone else possesses, such as wealth, beauty, or status. E. appears to be compounded of frustration, greed, anger, and self-pity, and is probably first experienced in SIBLING RIVALRY or possible in PENIS E. See these entries. Also see VAGINAL E.; WOMB E.

enzygotic twins = MONOZYGOTIC TWINS.

enzyme genes hereditary units that affect enzyme systems. An enzyme deficiency caused by a genetic defect often results in mental retardation.

enzyme induction an effect of some drugs on the liver marked by increased activity of enzymes capable of metabolizing the same drug and other drugs. A barbiturate may induce the liver to activate enzymes that are capable of metabolizing a wide range of drugs, thereby decreasing the duration and effectiveness of any drugs that might be destroyed by the enzymes.

enzymes protein molecules that serve as catalysts in bodily functions, causing chemical activity in other substances without becoming a part of the end product. E. are, with a few exceptions, identified by their role in physiology, such as glucosidases, which convert glucosides to glucose, or acetycholinesterase, which splits the acetylcholine molecule as soon as it has completed a neurotransmitter task.

-eo-; -eos- a combining form relating to dawn or daybreak, also to any beginning (from Greek *eos*, "dawn").

EOG = ELECTROOCULOGRAM.

EOG = ELECTROOLFACTOGRAM.

eonism the adoption by a male of a female role, or vice versa, as in transvestism (named for Charles Eon de Beaumont, French political adventurer, who died 1810, after posing as a woman for many years).

eosinopenia an abnormally small proportion of **eosinophils**, or granular leukocytes, circulating in the blood or other body fluids. E. may be associated with certain types of bacterial or viral infections.

eosinophilia an abnormally high level of **eosinophils**, or granular leukocytes, in the blood or other body fluids. The presence of eosinophils usually is an indication of an allergic reaction or an infection. Sputum smears or nasal-secretion samples obtained from a patient experiencing asthmatic attacks or allergic rhinitis may contain body cells that are mostly eosinophils.

eosophobia a morbid fear of dawn and sunrise.

EP = EVOKED POTENTIAL.

epena a hallucinogenic snuff prepared from a red resinous bark of Virola trees that grow in South America. Also called **nyakwana; parica; yakee**. See PSYCHEDELICS.

epencephalon = METENCEPHALON.

ependyma /əpen'-/ the membrane lining the brain ventricles and the central canal of the spinal cord.

ephebiatrics the branch of medicine concerned with the development and pathology of adolescence; the specialty of diseases of adolescents.

ephedrine: See PSYCHOSTIMULANTS.

ephemeral mania = MANIA TRANSITORIA.

-epi- a combining form meaning upon, above, over.

EPI *e*x*t*ra*p*yramidal *i*n*v*olvement. The term refers primarily to symptoms such as tremors and other parkinsonian side effects induced by phenothiazine compounds.

epicritic sensation a cutaneous sensation, such as pressure or temperature, which the subject detects at a very low threshold of sensitivity. It was proposed by Henry Head in 1920 that lower animals may be less sensitive than humans to cutaneous stimuli. Also see PROTOPATHIC SYSTEM.

epicritic sensibility = GNOSTIC FUNCTION.

epicritic system one of the two subsystems of the sensory-nerve network. The e.s. has receptors that are sensitive to joint movement, light touch, and deep pressure. Impulses from the receptors feed into the somatosensory cortex of the brain. Also see PROTOPATHIC SYSTEM.

epidemic generally prevalent, widespread, e.g., a disease (from Greek *epi-* and *demos*, "people"). Also see PANDEMIC. Compare ENDEMIC.

epidemic catalepsy a condition in which catalepsy occurs in a number of subjects at the same time as a result of identification or imitation.

epidemic encephalitis = ECONOMO'S DISEASE.

epidemic hysteria = MASS HYSTERIA.

epidemiology the science of the incidence of various pathologic conditions and their distribution or other relationship to such factors as heredity, environment, nutrition, or age at onset. Results of e. studies are intended to find clues rather than to show causal relationships. Also see INCIDENCE; RELATIVE RISK IN E.

epididymis /-did′-/ an elongated tubule along the top and back of the testis with the function of storing spermatozoa. The e. receives spermatozoa from coiled tubules within the testis. It is quite convoluted and if uncoiled would be about 20 feet long. It empties into the ductus deferens.

epididymitis an inflammation of the epididymis, marked by severe pain, swelling, and tenderness of the testes and scrotum. The cause usually is an infection in the prostate or urinary tract that spreads to the epididymis. Mumps, tuberculosis, and gonorrhea may be associated with e. Treatment includes antibiotics, rest, and avoidance of alcoholic beverages, spiced food, and sexual activity.

epigenesis the theory that new characteristics not determined by the original fertilized egg can emerge in the process of embryonic development; also, the hypothesis that consciousness emerges when living matter has reached a certain level of complexity. In addition, the term has been used by Erik Erikson for the emergence of different goals and risks at each stage of ego and social development. Also see EPIGENETIC THEORY.

epigenetic theory the concept that mind and consciousness developed unpredictably from living matter that in the course of evolution has reached a high level of complexity. Also called **emergence**.

epilepsia cursiva an obsolete term for aimlessly running about in a state of clouded consciousness during an attack of psychomotor epilepsy,

and occasionally after a grand mal seizure.

epilepsy a group of disorders associated with disturbances in the electrical discharges of brain cells, and characterized by transient, recurrent episodes of clouding or loss of consciousness, often accompanied by convulsive seizures or automatic behavior (from Greek *epilepsia*, "seizure"). The condition may be (a) symptomatic, that is, due to known conditions such as brain inflammation, high fever, brain tumor, vascular disturbances, structural abnormality, brain injury, or degenerative disease, or (b) idiopathic, that is, of unknown origin or due to nonspecific brain defect. Genetic predisposition can be found in many but not all cases. Also called **falling sickness**. For types of seizures, see GRAND MAL; PETIT MAL; PSYCHOMOTOR E.; JACKSONIAN E.; EPILEPSIA CURSIVA; AUTONOMIC SEIZURE; NARCOLEPSY; CATAPLEXY. Also see ABDOMINAL E.; AKINETIC SEIZURE; ANTIEPILEPTICS; CENTRENCEPHALIC E.; DIGESTIVE E.; DROMOLEPSY; FUROR; HALLUCINATORY E.; HYSTEROEPILEPSY; IDIOPATHIC E; LAUGHTER; MUSICOGENIC E.; MYOCLONUS E.; ORTHOSTATIC EPILEPTOID; PHOTOGENIC E.; POSTTRAUMATIC E.; PSYCHOMOTOR E.; PYKNOLEPSY; READING E.; REFLEX E.; RETROPULSIVE E.; RUM FITS; SACRED DISEASE; SENSORY E.; SHORTSTARE E.; SLEEP E.; STATUS EPILEPTICUS; SUBICTAL E.; SYMPTOMATIC E.; TONIC E.; VISCERAL E.

epilepsy fear = HYLEPHOBIA.

epileptic absence a type of petit mal episode in which the patient experiences a brief lapse of mental functions and has retrograde amnesia for the event. The absences usually last from five to 15 seconds. During the e.a., the patient is simply unresponsive, and any activity in which the patient may be engaged is interrupted. This can easily be identified on EEG by a spike-and-wave burst.

epileptic aura a manifestation of nervous or physiological activity that precedes an epileptic convulsion. The aura may include a strange visceral sensation accompanied by a focal effect that is determined by the location of the brain lesion associated with the disorder. Involuntary chewing movements before an attack indicate a lesion in the anterior temporal lobe, an aura of olfactory hallucinations is a manifestation of an approaching convulsion caused by a lesion in the posterior temporal lobe, and so on. Also see MIGRAINE AURA; AURA.

epileptic cephalea a type of epilepsy occurring most frequently in children and characterized by a severe headache as the main symptom.

epileptic character = EPILEPTIC PERSONALITY.

epileptic clouded states a condition in which psychotic symptoms, e.g., hallucinations and bewilderment, occur before or after a convulsive attack.

epileptic cry a momentary cry produced by sudden contraction of the chest and laryngeal muscles during the tonic phase of a grand mal seizure. Also called **initial cry**.

epileptic deterioration a progressive mental deterioration occurring in five percent of, or fewer, epileptic patients, especially those who have had seizures all their lives. E.d. is possibly due to nerve-cell degeneration caused by circulatory disturbances during the attacks. Also called **epileptic dementia**.

epileptic disorders = CONVULSIVE DISORDERS.

epileptic equivalent an epileptic attack or state that is neither petit mal nor grand mal, and that is believed to take the place of seizures of these types, e.g., twilight sleep or a fugue state. Some investigators apply the term to psychomotor epilepsy.

epileptic furor: See FUROR.

epileptic personality a personality pattern observed in a minority of individuals with epilepsy, and probably due to a reaction to the frustrations and anxieties this disease engenders, rather than to constitutional tendencies. These individuals are described as irritable, stubborn, egocentric, uncooperative, and aggressive. Also called **epileptic character**.

epileptiform seizures hysterical (conversion) convulsions that resemble epileptic seizures. The term also applies to convulsions caused by brain injury or by an infectious disease involving a high fever. See HYSTERICAL CONVULSIONS.

epileptogenic encephalopathy a brain disease that results from epilepsy seizures. Repeated epileptic convulsions can cause progressive severe damage to brain tissues beyond the original focus.

epileptogenic foci sites within the brain that are the sources of abnormal electrical discharges associated with epileptic seizures. Petit mal seizures, e.g., are associated with a focus in the thalamus, while psychomotor-epilepsy behavior is accompanied by an abnormal focus in the temporal lobe. Hallucinatory seizures are related to foci in the visual or auditory cortex.

epileptogenic lesion an area of tissue damage in the brain that results in epileptic seizures. Signs of epilepsy may occur immediately after a head injury or, in some cases, months or years later. A depressed fracture of the skull resulting in penetration or infection of brain tissues often give rise to an e.l. Other causes may include a brain tumor, birth injury, or physiological disorder.

epiloia = TUBEROUS SCLEROSIS.

epimenorrhagia = MENORRHAGIA.

epinephrine a hormone secreted by the medulla portion of the adrenal gland. E. also can be produced synthetically. It is secreted in large amounts when an individual is stimulated by fear, anger, or a similar stressful situation. E. is the primary stimulant of both alpha and beta receptors of the adrenergic nerves. It increases the heart rate and force of heart contractions, relaxes bronchiolar and intestinal smooth muscle, and produces varying effects on blood pressure as it acts both as a vasodilator and vasoconstrictor. E. is a catecholamine and technically an alcohol. Also called **adrenaline**. See ADRENAL GLAND; CATECHOLAMINES.

epinosic gain in psychoanalysis, indirect advantages obtained from illness, such as extra sympathy, pity, or power over others. Also called **epinosis**. For details, see SECONDARY GAINS. Also See ADVANTAGE BY ILLNESS.

epiphenomenalism: See BODY-MIND PROBLEM.

epiphenomenon a secondary occurrence that coincides with or accompanies but does not directly result from another occurrence, e.g., an emotional complication that emerges during a patient's pneumonia.

epiphysis; epiphysis cerebri = PINEAL BODY.

-episio- a combining form relating to the vulva.

episodic amnesia a loss of memory only for certain significant events.

episodic-behavior disorder a mental disorder characterized by sudden, usually brief, periods of behavior that is out of character for the individual and inappropriate for the situation, such as periods of impulsive and uncontrolled behavior. Such disorders may be due to psychological factors or, in some cases, to an undetected brain syndrome. Also called **episodic disorder**.

episodic dyscontrol: See IMPULSE NEUROSIS.

epispadias a congenital defect of the penis with the urethra opening through the top or dorsal surface of the penis rather than through the center of the glans. A similar defect may occur in the female urethra as a fissure of the upper wall of the urethra.

epistemic pertaining to the need to know, which is widely considered to be a fundamental drive (from Greek *episteme*, "knowledge").

epistemophilia the love of knowledge; the impulse to investigate and inquire. In psychoanalysis, this impulse is believed to develop out of an interest in the sex organs, particularly during the phallic phase.

epithalamus the area of brain tissue that is immediately above and behind the thalamus. It includes the pineal gland and the posterior commissure. Because of progressive calcification of the pineal gland, the gland serves as a landmark for location of the e. in macroscopic or X-ray examination of the e. The e. contains fibers of cranial nerves and the superior colliculi, but its functions are uncertain.

epithelioma any tumor that originated in cells of the **epithelium**, the type of tissue that lines the internal and external surfaces of the body. E.g, a skin cancer may begin as an e.

epochal amnesia the loss of memory for a certain epoch of one's past, covering a period of days to years after a severe shock.

EPSDT an abbreviation for *e*arly and *p*eriodic *s*creening, *d*iagnosis, and *t*reatment, which is increasingly subject to rigid limitations. E.g., subjects must be told what is being done to and for them as part of informed consent.

epsilon /ep'silon/ fifth letter of the Greek alphabet (E, ε).

epsilon alcoholism according to E. M. Jellinek, periodic drinking bouts interspersed with dry periods lasting weeks or months. During the bouts, the alcoholic drinks heavily day after day until he collapses. Also called **paroxysmal drinking; periodic drinking; binge drinking**. E.a. is essentially equivalent to DIPSOMANIA. See this entry.

epsilon movement the perception of motion when a white line on a black ground is changed to black on white.

EPSP = EXCITATORY-POSTSYNAPTIC POTENTIAL.

Epstein, Michael Anthony English physician, 1921—. See EPSTEIN-BARR VIRUS; INFECTIOUS MONONUCLEOSIS.

Epstein-Barr virus a herpes virus that is the disease agent of infectious mononucleosis. It is commonly found in the extracellular oral fluids of persons who have been exposed to the disease. The virus also has been isolated from cells cultured from **Burkitt's lymphoma** and in certain cases of nasopharyngeal cancer. Abbrev.: **EBV**.

EQ = EDUCATIONAL QUOTIENT.

equal-and-unequal-cases method a constant-stimulus method requiring judgment of paired stimuli as equal or unequal.

equal-appearing-intervals method in psychophysics, a technique in which magnitudes between pairs of stimuli are adjusted so that the sensed differences are equal. Also called **mean-gradation method**.

equal-interval scale a scale marked in equal intervals from a zero-base point.

equality stage: See DISTRIBUTIVE JUSTICE.

equality law: See LAW OF EQUALITY.

equalization of excitation the tendency for nervous excitation to spread evenly throughout a functional system.

equated scores the scores from two tests that have been weighted to form a common basis for comparison.

equatorial plane: See METAPHASE.

equilibration in Piaget's theory of development, the principle that an organism constantly tends toward an ideal stage of biological and psychological balance, which is never fully achieved. An example is the modification, or accommodation, of existing cognitive structures when new information is assimilated. Also see DISEQUILIBRIUM.

equilibratory senses the sense organs that regulate orientation of the body in space and are responsible for body position and the adjustment of parts of the body in relation to each other. The systems that regulate equilibrium are the semicircular canals and the vestibular sacs in the inner ear.

equilibrium maintenance of balance in one's posture, body processes, or psychological adjustment. Also see SENSE OF E.; EQUILIBRATION; DYNAMIC E.

equine encephalitis an arbor-virus infection transmitted through the bite of a mosquito, producing neurologic symptoms that may include drowsiness, disorientation, somnolence, coma, headache, abnormal reflexes, spastic paralyses,

tremors, and hallucinations. E.e. occurs in three main types, **eastern e.e., western e.e.**, and **Venezuelan e.e.**, each transmitted by a different species of mosquito and each type being prevalent in a different geographic area. They are identified as equine because the viruses were first recovered from horses, which also are affected. The viruses are called arbor viruses because arbor is a contraction of the word *ar*thropod-*bor*ne, a term applied to about 250 viruses.

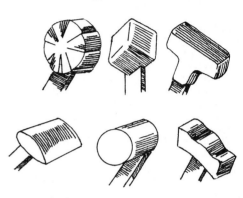

EQUIPMENT DESIGN. Example: Airplane control knobs designed to be identified by touch alone.

equipment design an area of human engineering or engineering psychology concerned with the efficient arrangement of the work space and design of tools, indicators (displays), and controls, as well as home appliances, roads, road signs, vehicles of all kinds, and all types of machines from typewriters to spot welders. The psychologist serves as a "human engineer" whose major function is to see that the equipment is designed with human factors in mind, such as safety, fatigue, convenience, comfort, and efficiency. See ENGINEERING PSYCHOLOGY; TOOL DESIGN; TIME-MOTION STUDY.

equipotentiality equal potential, or the ability to develop or achieve equal power, such as the capacity of one part of the brain to be trained or conditioned to perform a function previously performed by another part of the brain. Also see LAW OF E.

equipotentiality law = LAW OF EQUIPOTENTIALITY.

equity stage: See DISTRIBUTIVE JUSTICE.

equity theory the view that interpersonal interactions are influenced by the desire of involved parties to strike a balance between what is given and what is received. In industrial psychology, the term e.t. denotes the subjective judgment of an employee that the ratio between his or her total outcome from a job (that is, pay, fringe benefits, status, intrinsic interest) to the total input (that is, qualifications, skills, educational level, effort) compares favorably or unfavorably to that of other persons doing the same job.

equivalence a relationship between stimuli or variables that permits one to replace another.

equivalence coefficient the correlation coefficient between results of two equivalent forms of the same test given to the same subjects, indicating the degree of reliability of the test.

equivalent form an alternate form of a test, with similar items, for use in retesting.

equivalent groups two or more groups that have been matched for all significant variables.

equivalents method an average-error technique in which a subject adjusts a variable stimulus until it appears equivalent to a standard.

ER: See EVOKED POTENTIAL.

Erb, Wilhelm Heinrich German neurologist, 1840–1921. See ERB-GOLDFLAM SYNDROME; ERB'S PALSY.

Erb-Goldflam syndrome a form of myasthenia gravis due to faulty transmission of nerve impulses at junctions with muscle tissues. Affected muscles are easily fatigued and may become paralyzed. Muscles involved in eating may fail to function normally toward the end of a meal, or speech may become slurred and the voice weak after a period of talking. The disease is progressive, eventually affecting muscles throughout the body.

Erb's palsy a partial paralysis of the muscles of the upper arm, usually due to a birth injury.

erect: See POSTURE.

erectile dysfunction the lack or loss of ability to achieve an erection. Causes of e.d. may be psychological or physical, including the effects of medications or drugs of abuse. If a man normally experiences a nocturnal erection or is able to induce an erection by masturbation, the dysfunction is assumed to be psychic in nature. See PRIMARY E.D; SECONDARY E.D.

eremiophobia; eremophobia: See AUTOPHOBIA.

eremophilia a morbid desire to be alone.

erethism excessive sensitivity or irritability in some or all parts of the body.

ereuthophobia = ERYTHROPHOBIA.

erg in psychology, a specific innate unitary drive directed toward a goal such as self-assertion, fear, or sex (Cattell).

-erg-; -ergo-; -ergas- a combining form relating to activity, work (from Greek *ergon*, "work").

ERG = ELECTRORETINOGRAM.

ERG; ERG theory = EXISTENCE, RELATEDNESS, AND GROWTH THEORY.

ergasia a term coined by Adolf Meyer for the totality of activities—psychological, biological, and social—that constitute the human personality. See PSYCHOBIOLOGY. Also see THYMERGASIA.

ergasiatry a term introduced by Adolf Meyer as the equivalent of psychiatry.

ergasiology a term introduced by Adolf Meyer as the equivalent of psychology. He conceived e. as a study of the functioning of the personality as a whole. See PSYCHOBIOLOGY.

ergasiophobia a morbid fear of functioning or moving, with the illusion that one's movements would disastrously affect the surrounding world.

ergastoplasm a substance found in the cytoplasm of the cells of glands and the nervous system. E. contains ribonucleic-acid molecules which may be involved in the synthesis of proteins.

ergic trait a dynamic trait that motivates the subject to achieve an objective.

ergograph a recording device for muscular action, usually employed in fatigue experiments.

ergonomics = ENGINEERING PSYCHOLOGY.

ergonovine: See ERGOT DERIVATIVES.

ergot alkaloids pharmacologically active substances derived from a parasitic fungus that grows naturally on rye and other grains. E.a. have been used for centuries by midwives to induce abortion or labor although e.a. are highly toxic. A number of e.a. have been isolated, including lysergic acid, and the compounds are sometimes utilized as adrenergic blocking agents. E.a. can cause hallucinations and "visions," such as those experienced by women tried for witchcraft in 17th-century New England. The accused witches are believed to have consumed grains contaminated with e.a. Because of the pharmacological relationship between ergot and the psychedelic drug LSD, the hallucinogenic effects are similar to those of LSD. Also see ERGOTISM.

ergotamine $C_{33}H_{35}N_5O_5$—an alkaloid drug obtained from ergot, a fungus that infests rye plants. E. is administered in the treatment of migraine attacks. The exact nature of its action is unknown, but e. is believed to constrict the dilated cranial blood vessels responsible for the headache symptoms. It also is employed in enhancing uterine contractions during labor. Also see ERGOT DERIVATIVES.

ergot derivatives a group of adrenergic blocking agents with selective inhibitory activity, derived from ergot fungus alkaloids. E.d. act on the central nervous system to induce sedation and, in various forms and doses, can both stimulate and depress higher brain centers. A circulatory effect is the constriction of cerebral arteries by certain e.d., such as **ergonovine**—$C_{19}H_{23}N_3O_2$—and ERGOTAMINE (see this entry), favoring their use in the control of migraine headaches. The e.d. may be combined with other drugs, e.g., caffeine, producing similar vasoconstrictive effects. The e.d. are related chemically to lysergic acid compounds, which also are among ergot alkaloids.

ergotism the toxic effects of a substance in the fungus Claviceps purpurea, which infests rye and other grain plants. The symptoms include a weak, rapid pulse; tingling, itching, and cold feelings in the skin; intense thirst; vomiting and diarrhea; hemorrhage; gangrene; confusion; and coma. **Spasmodic e.** may be marked by depression, weakness, drowsiness, epilepsylike convulsions, hallucinations, and formication of the skin. E. was not uncommon in the past when large populations were afflicted with the symptoms as a result of eating bread made with fungus-infested grains. E. also was a common risk when the toxic substance ergot, extracted from the fungus, was used to induce abortions. An essentially equivalent term is SAINT ANTHONY'S FIRE. See this entry. Also see ERGOT ALKALOIDS.

ergotropic having the effect of producing action or excitement by stimulating the brain cells, as when an e. agent such as norepinephrine or amphetamine increases brain activity.

ergotropic process the mechanism whereby the sympathetic division of the autonomic nervous system performs functions that are related to the expenditure of energy, e.g., the increased physiologic activity that follows intake of stimulants. Compare TROPHOTROPIC PROCESS.

ergotropic system any system that is marked by a strong drive or arousal factor.

Erhard, Werner American foundation executive, 1935—. See EST.

Erichsen, John Eric English surgeon, 1818–96. See ERICHSEN'S DISEASE.

Erichsen's disease a form of neurosis that sometimes follows a spinal injury regardless of the presence or absence of evidence of tissue damage. E.d. usually follows a concussion and is marked by backache complaints. Also called **railway spine**.

Erikson, Erik H. German-born American psychoanalyst, 1902—. E. revised the standard psychoanalytic account of ego development to relate his eight stages of man to cultural influences and a search for an ego identity in a changing world. See ERIKSON'S EIGHT STAGES OF MAN; ADAPTIVE APPROACH; AUTONOMY; BASIC MISTRUST; BASIC TRUST; DEVELOPMENTAL THEORIES; EFFECTANCE MOTIVE; EGO IDENTITY; EPIGENESIS; HUMANISTIC THEORY; IDENTITY; IDENTITY CRISIS; MORAL JUDGMENT; MORATORIUM; MUTUALITY; ROLE DIFFUSION; TOTALISM.

Erikson's eight stages of man Erik Erikson's theory based on the concept of psychosocial development, in which "ego identity" is gradually achieved by facing positive goals and negative risks at each of eight stages of life—(1) infancy: TRUST VERSUS MISTRUST, (2) toddler: AUTONOMY VERSUS DOUBT, (3) preschool age: INITIATIVE VERSUS GUILT, (4) school age: INDUSTRY VERSUS INFERIORITY, (5) adolescence: IDENTITY VERSUS ROLE CONFUSION, (6) young adulthood: INTIMACY VERSUS ISOLATION, (7) middle age: GENERATIVITY VERSUS SELF-ABSORPTION, and (8) mature age: EGO INTEGRITY VERSUS DESPAIR. See these entries. Also see ERIKSON.

erogenous zone = EROTOGENIC ZONE.

Eros in psychoanalysis, the drive that comprises the instinct for self-preservation, which is aimed at individual survival; and the sexual instinct, which is aimed at the survival of the species. Also called **life instinct**.

erosion in environmental psychology, the deterioration or corrosion of a physical setting from climatic effects and from use by human beings. E.g, the degree of wear evident in footpaths in a park may be taken as an indication of their degree of use. Compare ACCRETION.

erotic invested with sexual sensations, or feelings of love; also, pertaining to stimuli that give rise to sexual excitement.

erotica literature, illustrations, motion-picture films or other artistic material likely to arouse sexual response. The term is sometimes used interchangeably with PORNOGRAPHY. See this entry.

erotic-arousal pattern the sequence of actions or stimuli that produces sexual response. The actions or stimuli vary with different species and in humans may involve such stimuli as dress, perfume, music, and foreplay.

erotic character the specific physical features that make an individual sexually attractive, e.g., hair, figure, skin, or voice.

erotic delusion the false perception that one is secretly loved by or has had a sexual affair with a public figure or other individual he or she has never met. See CLÉRAMBAULT'S SYNDROME. Also see EROTIC PARANOIA.

erotic instinct in psychoanalysis, the sex drive or libido; also, the equivalent of Eros, the life instinct.

eroticism a tendency to experience sexual excitement, usually from stimulation of the genitals, but also, in psychoanalytic theory, from nongenital parts of the body such as the mouth or anus. E. is also a preoccupation with sexual excitement, erotic photographs, and written erotic material. Also called **erotism**. Also see ALLOEROTICISM; AMPHIEROTISM; ANAL EROTISM; AUTOEROTISM; GENITAL E.; HETEROEROTICISM; LIP E.; OLFACTORY E.; ORAL E.; ORAL-E. PHASE; ORGAN E.; PARANOID EROTISM; RESPIRATORY E.; SKIN E.; TEMPERATURE E.; URETHRAL E.

eroticization = EROTIZATION.

erotic paranoia a paranoid disorder in which the patient experiences erotic delusions. E.g., a male patient may claim that a woman of great wealth or high status is in love with him, and find disguised evidence in newspaper photographs or even in the flight of birds. Also see EROTIC DELUSION.

erotic pyromania = PYROLAGNIA.

erotic transference the transference of erotic feelings from one individual to another, e.g., from an individual in the person's past to one in the person's present life.

erotic type: See LIBIDINAL TYPES.

erotism = EROTICISM.

erotization the investment of bodily organs and biological functions or other activities with sexual pleasure and gratification. Examples are the zones (oral, anal); organs, such as the nipple and skin; functions, such as sucking, defecation, urination, scopophilic activities (looking at nudity or sexual activity); and olfactory sensations associated with sex. Various interests and acivities, such as collecting objects that have sexual connotations, pursuing activities such as dancing, and even scientific research may be eroticized. Also called **libidinization; eroticization**.

erotized anxiety a method of dealing with anxiety

by moving toward its source and apparently enjoying it.

erotized hanging a form of sexual perversion in which an individual hangs himself or has his sex partner hang him in order to produce neck constriction and cerebral hypoxia as a means of sexual arousal. Numerous accidental hanging deaths each year are attributed to e.h.

erotocrat a man of great sexual power, a natural sense of his virility, and a strong effect on women. See CASANOVA.

erotogenesis in psychoanalysis, the origination of erotic impulses whose sources may include the anal, oral, and phallic zones.

erotogenic pertaining to any stimulus that evokes or excites sexual feelings or responses. Also called **erotogenetic**.

erotogenic masochism = PRIMARY MASOCHISM.

erotogenic zone in psychoanalysis, an area or part of the body, such as the mouth, anus, urethra, and genitals, through which the sexual instinct, or libido, expresses itself. In addition to these primary areas, the breasts (especially the nipples), the region around the genital organs, other orifices of the body (nose, ears), and the surface of the skin (especially close to the primary zones) are susceptible to erotic stimulation. Also called **erogenous zone** /iroj'-/.

erotographomania a pathological urge to write love letters, usually anonymously.

erotolalia speech that contains sexual obscenities, particularly as used to enhance gratification during sexual intercourse.

erotomania a preoccupation with sexual activities, thoughts, and fantasies; also, compulsive, insatiable sexual activity with the opposite sex, which is believed to arise from latent homosexual tendencies or unrecognized doubts about sexual adequacy. Also called **aidoiomania**. See NYMPHOMANIA; SATYRIASIS; DON JUAN.

error a deviation from true or accurate information, e.g., a wrong response, a mistaken belief. In experimental psychology, an e. is any change in a dependent variable not attributable to the independent variable. In statistics, the term means deviation from a true score.

error analysis in industrial psychology, the study of human factors and engineering-design factors that may result in production errors.

error of measurement any deviation or departure of a measurement from its true value.

error variance score variability that is not systematic or controlled, or not produced by the independent variable.

eructation = BELCHING.

-eryth-; -erythr-; -erythro- /-irith-/ a combining form meaning red (Greek *erythros*).

erythema multiforme major = STEVENS-JOHNSON SYNDROME.

erythema nodosum leprosum an acute inflammatory skin disease with tender red nodules that develop under the skin during an acute attack of leprosy, or Hansen's disease. E.n.l. is regarded

as an emergency situation that if not promptly treated can result in irreversible deformities of the body within hours.

erythredema = ACRODYNIA.

erythrocytes: See BLOOD VOLUME.

erythroleukoblastosis = ICTERUS GRAVIS NEONATORUM.

erythromelalgia = ACRODYNIA.

erythrophobia a persistent, pathological fear of the color red in general, and of blood in particular. E. is also the fear of objects or activities associated with red, such as red flags or blushing. Also called **ereuthophobia**. Fear of blood is also called HEMATOPHOBIA. See this entry. Also see BLUSHING.

erythropoietin a hormone that is involved in the production of red blood cells. Because the kidneys, even when damaged by disease, are a source of e., consideration must be given to the patient's needs for e. when surgical removal of a kidney is proposed as a therapeutic measure or as a transplant donation.

ESB an abbreviation of *electric stimulation of the brain*. See ELECTROCONVULSIVE TREATMENT. Also see EVOKED POTENTIAL.

E scale an attitude scale used in *ethnocentrism* measurement.

escape behavior any behavior directed toward escape of the subject from a painful or otherwise unpleasant situation. E.b. may be a mental form of escape through fantasy or daydreams, avoiding a noxious stimulus by providing a conditioned response, or taking some action to retreat from the perceived threat. Also see ESCAPE LEARNING.

escape conditioning the training of an organism to terminate an aversive stimulus.

escape drinking: See ALPHA ALCOHOLISM.

escape from freedom: See IDENTITY NEED.

escape from reality behavior that enables a person to substitute fantasy for conflicts and problems of daily living.

escape into illness = FLIGHT INTO ILLNESS.

escape learning a conditioning or learning experience in which the subject is exposed to a painful or threatening situation and acquires the proper response behavior for avoiding the noxious stimulus. E.g., by accidentally pressing a wheel or bar that terminates shock, a rat may come to acquire the bar-pressing response as a learned escape mechanism. The principle is identical to that of negative reinforcement. Also see AVOIDANCE CONDITIONING; ESCAPE BEHAVIOR.

escape mechanism a behavioral pattern or device unconsciously adopted as a means of avoiding or freeing oneself from a threatening or anxiety-laden situation, e.g., flight into illness, daydreaming, detachment, or amnesia.

escape training a learning process in which a subject is trained to avoid an unpleasant stimulus, e.g., a shock.

escapism in psychoanalysis, the tendency to escape from the real world to the security of childhood, ordinarily accompanied by symptoms of neurosis. E. is usually a form of resistance.

escutcheon the shieldlike pattern of pubic-hair distribution that develops after puberty.

eserine: See PHYSOSTIGMINE.

ESL /es'əl/ or /ē'es'el'/ an abbreviation of *E*nglish as a *s*econd *l*anguage. In preference to "English as a foreign language," the term ESL is used mainly to refer to English instruction (often remedial lessons) for children from non-English-speaking families in the United States.

ESN *e*ducationally *s*ub*n*ormal. The term was introduced in Great Britain in 1944 in legislation designed to authorize special education programs outside the standard school curriculum for the benefit of children regarded as consistently retarded in scholastic progress. Previously, **ESN children** were covered by an earlier Mental Deficiency Act. **ESN schools** are operated as residential, or in-patient, as well as out-patient facilities.

esophageal fistula an abnormal tubelike passage in the esophagus. An e.f. often occurs as a communication between the esophagus and trachea or a bronchus and may be a congenital defect or acquired as a result of a tumor or infection. Pathological effects depend upon the location and route of the fistula.

esophageal neurosis a difficulty in swallowing or the sensation of an object lodged in the upper esophagus (globus hystericus), usually attributed to an unconscious-guilty oral-aggressive wish. Also see GLOBUS HYSTERICUS.

esophageal voice the low-frequency vibrations produced by the narrow upper portion of the esophagus when swallowed air is belched out. It is associated with laryngectomy.

esophoria an inward deviation of one eye due to muscular imbalance, interfering with binocular vision. E. is a form of heterophoria.

esotropia = CROSS-EYE.

ESP = EXTRASENSORY PERCEPTION.

espanto: See SUSTO.

Esquirol, Jean /zhäN eskērol'/ French psychiatrist, 1772–1840. As director of Salpêtrière Hospital in Paris, and then of the Royal Sanitarium at Charenton, E. expanded Pinel's approach, which resulted in passage of a humane-treatment law and the construction of ten new mental hospitals. Equally important were his systematic studies of patients, which gave rise to his theory that emotionally disturbing experiences are the primary cause of mental illness, in contrast to the prevailing medical view that it was caused by organic factors, and to the lay view that it was due to possession by the devil. See AFFECTIVE MONOMANIA; LYPEMANIA; MORAL TREATMENT.

essay test: See OBJECTIVE EXAMINATION.

essence the real character or important quality of something; a concentrated substance that has the characteristics of the original substance; also, the contribution made by the individual in determining his fate in his given existence.

essential alcoholism = GAMMA ALCOHOLISM.

essential dysmenorrhea: See DYSMENORRHEA.

essential hypertension hypertension, or high blood pressure, that is not secondary to another disease, e.g., adrenal-gland tumor or constricted renal artery. E.h. accounts for at least 85 percent of all cases of hypertension, and causes include obesity, excessive ingestion of table salt, cigarette-smoking, genetic factors, and psychologic influences, e.g., aggressive personality or stressful environment. See TYPE A PERSONALITY.

essential tremor a fine tremor of the hands, head, and voice that appears to be hereditary and is not associated with any findings of nervous-system pathology. Symptoms usually appear during adolescence and may be aggravated by movement or emotion. Also called **benign hereditary tremor**.

EST an abbreviation for Erhard Seminar Training, a controversial training system developed in the 1970s by Werner Erhard. EST is supposedly consciousness-expanding, borrowing from business-world motivation techniques and assorted theories of psychology. Also spelled **est**.

EST: See ELECTROCONVULSIVE TREATMENT.

establishment a term used by Murray for the ego, id, and superego factors modified along functional lines to serve as basic components, or "establishments," of personality.

esteem needs the fourth level in A. Maslow's hierarchy of needs, characterized by the striving for a sense of personal value as derived from achievement, reputation, or prestige. See NEED-HIERARCHY THEORY; MASLOW.

esthetic pleasure a term used by Freud to denote enjoyment of an experience, such as a sexual joke or a painting of a nude woman, for its own sake, without instinctual gratification (sexual excitement).

esthetics the study of the psychological or philosophical components and aspects of beauty, in nature and art. See PSYCHOLOGICAL E. Also see EXPERIMENTAL E.; ENVIRONMENTAL E.

esthetic value the emotional or spiritual value imparted to an observer or participant by the beauty of a work of art or nature.

estimation inference from sample statistics to population parameters, e.g., determination of the size of an effect from its occurrence in one or more samples.

estimators a term applied by R. Gelman to the mental processes involved in judging quantity, as in the child's ability to recognize that a given set contains six elements rather than five or seven. Also see OPERATORS.

estradiol a naturally occurring steroid hormone of the estrogen category. It is produced by the ovary and placenta and also in the testes. E. is found in the adrenal cortex and may be produced there. The 17 Beta form of e. is the most biologically active natural estrogen occurring in mammals. See ESTROGEN.

estrangement: See ALIENATION.

estriol: See SEX HORMONES.

estrogen a generic name for a group of hormones

that may occur naturally in animals or be produced synthetically and that have a general effect of inducing estrus in female animals and secondary female sexual characteristics in humans. The forms of e. occurring naturally in humans are estradiol, estrone, and estriol, secreted by the ovarian follicle, corpus luteum, placenta, testes, and adrenal cortex. E. also is produced by certain plants which may be used in the manufacture of synthetic steroid hormones. In addition to their role in reproductive functions, various forms of e. are used to affect growth and long-bone development in abnormally tall or short people, to control ovulation and lactation, and to treat cases of breast and prostate cancers.

estrone a follicular hormone and metabolite of 17 Beta-estradiol. E. is used therapeutically in the treatment of menopausal and other estrogen-deficiency disorders and in certain cases of vaginitis. See ESTRADIOL; ESTROGEN.

estrous behavior a behavior pattern observed in animals during the phase of their sexual cycle when the female expresses a willingness to mate. Estrous cycles range from as short as two weeks in sheep to as long as six months in a dog while the period of e.b. may last only 12 hours in sheep and cows to a week or more in cats and dogs. Also called **heat; rut**. Also see ESTRUS.

estrus the reproductive cycle of animals as manifested by periods of sexual desire or mating, particularly in the female of the species. Animals that experience one e. cycle per year are called **monestrous**, those that have multiple e. cycles annually are **polyestrous**. Some birds ovulate once every 24 hours until a nest of eggs is filled. Also called **estrum; oestrus**. Also see ESTROUS BEHAVIOR.

et the Latin word for "and," used, e.g., in prescriptions.

eta /ēt′ə/ or /āt′ə/ seventh letter of the Greek alphabet (H, η).

eta = CORRELATION RATIO.

eternal suckling a Freudian term for the type of individual who expects to be cared for, supported, and protected throughout life by somebody else.

eternity fear = FEAR OF ETERNITY.

ethambutol $C_{10}H_{24}N_2O_2$—a drug used in the control of tuberculosis. The drug also affects the vision of patients, producing a loss of visual acuity and red-green perception.

ethanol C_2H_5OH—a substance formed naturally by the fermentation of glucose and produced synthetically by a similar method. E. is of pharmacological interest mainly because of its widespread use in alcoholic beverages, such as beers, wines, and distilled liquors. The e. content of beverages generally ranges from as low as two percent in beers to as much as 60 percent in some distilled products. The effects of e. differ considerably in various individuals and in the same person at different times. In small doses, e. can produce feelings of warmth, well-being, and confidence in one's mental and physical powers.

As dosage is increased, there is a gradual loss of self-control, excitement is increased, speech and control of limbs become difficult, followed by nausea and vomiting, loss of consciousness, and fatal respiratory arrest. E. is a depressant and a narcotic, and has been used as an anesthetic. (Moderate doses reduce reflex actions, endurance, and performance of tasks requiring skill.) E. has been mistakenly identified as a stimulant since the stimulating effect is an illusion association with loss of cortical inhibition. The depressant effect begins in the cortex and gradually spreads to lower centers as dosage increases. Also called **ethyl alcohol**.

ethanolism the psychological and physical dependence upon ETHANOL. See this entry.

ethchlorvynol: See ALCOHOL DERIVATIVES.

ether effects a progressive series of physical and psychological reactions, beginning with a feeling of asphyxia, bodily warmth, visual and auditory aberrations, and a feeling of stiffness and inability to move the limbs. A second stage may be marked by some resistance to the sense of suffocation of the anesthetic, but the muscles relax, blood pressure and pulse increase, and pupils dilate. In the third state, pulse and blood pressure return to normal, pupils contract, and reflexes are absent. If additional ether is administered beyond the third stage, there is danger of paralysis of the medullary centers, followed by shock and death.

ethical approach a term used by Freud to denote the therapeutic goal of helping the patient to achieve high individual standards without blind comformity to the conventional demands of society.

ethical conflict: See CONFLICT OF INTEREST.

ethical highbrow a category of American male personalities described by W. D. Wells in his study of psychographics (1975). The e.h., who is said to represent 14 percent of American men, is described as "very concerned, sensitive to people's needs ... basically a puritan, content with family life, friends, and work, and interested in culture, religion, and social reform." Other psychographic categories include the **he-man** (19 percent of total males), and the **traditionalist** (16 percent). See PSYCHOGRAPHICS.

ethical imperative the commanding influence of moral principles on mental life and behavior; the moral consciousness of the individual. Also see CATEGORICAL IMPERATIVE.

ethical-risk hypothesis the theory that moral or immoral behavior depends on a child's evaluation of the risk involved (getting caught). That is, as the possibility of discovery increases, the occurrence of the behavior diminishes. Some early social-learning theorists viewed this theory as essential in understanding the process of moral judgment in children.

ethics the branch of philosophy that deals with moral values and systems of beliefs focused on the differences between right and wrong; generally, a person's or group's principles of morally right conduct. Also see CATEGORICAL IMPERATIVE; CODE OF E.

ethinamate $C_9H_{13}NO_2$—a mild CNS sedative used to induce sleep in certain cases of insomnia. It may be prescribed for patients who are sensitive to barbiturates. Hypnotic aftereffects are minimal, but e. has the potential of becoming a drug of abuse. Also see ALCOHOL DERIVATIVES.

ethmocephaly a birth defect involving the olfactory system and often marked by a rudimentary proboscis-shaped nose which may have imperforate nostrils. The condition sometimes is associated with cebocephaly, and tends to occur as part of CHROMOSOME-13 TRISOMY. See this entry. Also see **cebocephaly**.

ethmoid fossa: See FOSSA.

ethnic factors the common traits and customs that form the basis of a division of people who are biologically, socially, or politically related.

ethnic group any major social group that possesses a common history, culture, language, and, often, religion. Members are likely to be biologically related, yet an e.g. is not equivalent to a race.

ethnocentrism the attitude that one's own ethnic or national group is superior to other groups, and the tendency to make invidious and prejudicial distinctions based on this attitude. Also see SOCIOCENTRISM.

ethnocentrism scale: See E SCALE.

ethnographic approach a strategy for studying a community as a way of life. The method, which is frequently used by anthropologists, involves extensive residence in the community, fluency in the local languages and active participation in community life in order to develop insight into its total culture.

ethnography the division of anthropology that studies the origin, history, geography, distribution, culture, and social institutions and relationships within and between ethnic groups. Also called **ethnology**.

ethnopsychiatry = CROSS-CULTURAL PSYCHIATRY.

ethnopsychopharmacology the branch of pharmacology that deals with the use of psychotropic drugs in ethnic or subcultural populations. An example is the use of ginseng as a stimulant and aphrodisiac by members of certain Oriental communities.

ethogram an account or chronicle of the behavior of an animal in its natural habitat. See ETHOLOGY.

ethological models of personal space patterns of personal-space use that have presumably evolved in a phylogenetic process. The theory of e.m. argues that personal space "bubbles" have been used by various species throughout evolutionary history to protect the individual organism against intraspecies aggression and against threats to personal autonomy. Because human personal-space use varies with different cultures, some investigators contend that e.m. represent a

learned behavior. See BUBBLE CONCEPT OF PERSONAL SPACE; PROXEMICS.

ethology the comparative study of the behavior of animals in their natural habitat; also, the sociological investigation of human mores and folkways; and the scientific study of ethical systems among different groups.

ethopropazine: See PHENOTHIAZINES.

ethos the character or spirit of an ethnic group, culture, or nation (Greek, "custom, usage").

ethosuximide: See SUCCINIMIDES.

ethyl alcohol = ETHANOL.

ethylphenacemide: See ACETYLUREAS.

etic pertaining to concepts or constructs that are believed to be universal and have been found to exist in all known cultures. Compare EMIC.

etiological validity a validity that is based on the same historical antecedents as the cause of a phenomenon, such as a mental disorder.

etiology the systematic study of the causes of mental and physical disorders, or the causal factors that account for a particular disorder.

E trisomy = TRISOMY 17-18.

etryptamine $C_{12}H_{16}N_2$—a CNS stimulant, not widely used because of toxic effects.

ETS: See ELECTRO-SLEEP THERAPY.

Etzioni, Amitai Werner German-born American educator and sociologist, 1929—. See NORMATIVE COMPLIANCE.

-eu- a combining form meaning normal, well, good, easy.

EUCD an abbreviation of *e*motionally-*u*nstable-character *d*isorder. See EMOTIONALLY UNSTABLE PERSONALITY.

euergasia a term used by Adolf Meyer to denote normal mental functioning.

eugenics the study and control of reproduction of the species as a means of improving hereditary characteristics. **Positive e.** would be directed toward promoting reproduction by individuals with superior traits, while **negative e.** would prevent reproduction by individuals with undesirable traits.

Euler, Leonhard /oil'ər/ Swiss mathematician and physicist, 1707–83. See VENN DIAGRAMS (there: **Euler diagrams**).

eumorphic pertaining to a constitutional body type characterized by normal shape and structure, and roughly equivalent to the normosplanchnic type.

eunuch a male who has been castrated before puberty, and who therefore develops the secondary sex characteristics of a female, such as a higher voice and absence of a beard. (The literal meaning is "guardian of the bed," from Greek *eune*, "couch, bed.") See SECONDARY SEX CHARACTERISTICS; CASTRATION

euphoria in psychiatry, an exaggerated, abnormal, often pathological feeling, sense, or mood of well-being. The patient may experience feelings of boundless strength, happiness, and optimism that do not correspond to his real condition. E. is characteristic of manic states and is also noted in general paresis and certain drug-induced states.

euphoric apathy a Jungian term for a state of happy indifference, equivalent to la belle indifférence.

euphorohallucinogen a substance, such as mescaline, that is capable of producing euphoric hallucinations.

eurotophobia a morbid fear of the female genitals.

eurymorph: See BODY-BUILD INDEX.

euryplastic pertaining to a constitutional body type that is roughly equivalent to Kretschmer's pyknic type and Pende's megosplanchnic hypervegetative type.

Eustachian tube a slender tube extending from the middle ear to the pharynx, with the primary function of equalizing air pressure on both sides of the ear drum.

Eustachio, Bartolommeo /ā·ōstä′kyō/ Italian anatomist, 1524–74. Adjective: **Eustachian** /yōōstak′ē·ən/. See EUSTACHIAN TUBE; AUTOPHONIC RESPONSE; MIDDLE EAR; SALPINGITIS; SEROUS OTITIS MEDIA.

eusthenic pertaining to a constitutional body type that is equivalent to the asthenic and close to the athletic type of Kretschmer.

eustress positive stress, a type of stress that has a beneficial effect, e.g., stress that raises the aspiration level. The term was coined by Hans Selye (who also introduced the notion of stress, around 1940).

eutelegenesis = ARTIFICIAL INSEMINATION.

euthanasia the alleviation of pain associated with impending death. More commonly, e. is **mercy killing**, in which the death of an individual suffering from an incurable illness is deliberately brought about by painless means.

euthenics the science concerned with bettering the human condition by improving the environment.

euthymic mood a mood of well-being and tranquillity. Also called **euthymia**.

eutychia a state of general satisfaction.

evaluability-assessment data in evaluation research, information sought to identify problematic areas of program evaluation; a review of expectations for program performance and questions to be answered by evaluation data, followed by a study of program implementation to identify designs, measurements, and analyses that are possible.

evaluation interpretation of test results and experimental data; also, determination of the relative value of phenomena such as therapeutic techniques, hypotheses, and observations. In educational psychology, the term is used for an overall appraisal of a student's progress.
    For the use of the term in e. research, see DISCREPANCY E.; FORMATIVE E.; GOAL MODEL OF E.; IN-HOUSE E.; METAEVALUATION; NETWORK-ANALYSIS E.; OUTCOME E.; PROCESS E.; PROGRAM E.; PROGRAM-IMPACT E.; SECONDARY E.; SUMMATIVE E.; SYSTEMS MODEL OF E.; TRANSACTIONAL E.

evaluation apprehension a worried, uneasy feeling on the part of a subject in an experiment who desires a favorable evaluation by the experimenter.

evaluation contract in evaluation research, a legal contract in which the evaluator is committed to producing a specified product using specified research methodologies. No deviation from the contracted specifications is allowed without the formal authorization of the contracting agency. The term applies also to a contracted commitment by an evaluator to produce a specified product by a specified date.

evaluation dissemination in evaluation research, the distribution of the results of an evaluation project through written reports, oral presentations, or both, to an audience. An audience may include administrators, operating staff, granting agencies, policy-makers, evaluators in related areas, and others, depending upon the nature of the program being evaluated.

evaluation interview an interview conducted as part of a personnel-evaluation program. An e.i. may be a routine or periodic discussion of a subordinate's job performance or may include such psychological incentives as suggesting that the subordinate present at the interview a set of goals to be reviewed by management.

evaluation of training in industrial psychology, a review of training programs with emphasis on motivation, reinforcement, stimulus, orientation, safety, and special skills involved.

evaluation research the application of scientific principles, methods, and theories to identify, describe, conceptualize, measure, predict, change, and control those factors that are important to the development of effective "human-service delivery systems." The experimental approach is generally viewed as the most important, and is generally concerned with discovering the effectiveness of new approaches to a problem as compared with older, more traditional approaches. (E.r. is one of the new divisions of the American Psychological Association.)

evaluation utilization in evaluation research, an effort to act on the findings of an evaluation program. It involves the managing of disparate evaluation outcomes as well as generalizing of solutions for the problems discovered through the evaluation process.

evaluative ratings rank-orderings of judgments of the esthetic value or other qualities of a group of objects. E.r. may be based on hedonic values, such as the relative pleasantness of a series of paintings, or on the relative complexity of a series of problems, or may be expressed as a scale of intelligence quotients.

evaluative reasoning a form of critical thinking that involves appraisal of the effectiveness, validity, meaning, or relevance of any act, idea, feeling, technique, or object.

evaluator an individual whose role is to advise a therapy or sensitivity group about its progress.

evasion a communication disorder in which an idea which is logically next in a chain of thought is replaced by another idea closely related to it. It is a form of paralogical thinking frequently observed in schizophrenia. See PARALOGIA.

event: See INTERBEHAVIORAL PSYCHOLOGY.

eversion theory of aging a concept that aging results from functional deterioration of body tissues due to changes in the structure of the collagen molecule. (Collagen is the major protein of the white fibers of connective tissue, cartilage, and bone.) Also called **cross-linkage theory**. Also see CYBERNETIC THEORY OF AGING.

evil eye: See FASCINUM.

eviration the delusion of a male that he has been emasculated and feminized, or turned into a woman (from Latin *ex-* and *vir*, "male").

evoked potential an electric activity that is observed in a particular part of the brain when a specific sense organ or peripheral-nerve ending is stimulated. E.g., a flash of light will produce an e.p. in the visual cortex while a tone will result in an e.p. in the auditory cortex. An e.p. differs from ordinary brain waves in that the activity occurs at the time of stimulation rather than spontaneously, and also occurs in a sensory area associated with the appropriate nerve tract. The e.p. is predictable and reproducible. Abbrev.: **EP**. Also called **cortical-evoked response (ER)**.

evolution of brain the concept that the human brain has evolved over a period of many millions of years from a set of simple nerve fibers connecting various body areas as in primitive multicellular animals. At a more advanced stage, a neural axis developed to connect the nerve fibers and their cell bodies, becoming a spinal cord. Still later, collections of neurons with control functions developed at the head end of the spinal cord, as in the brains of birds, fish, and reptiles. From those basal conglomerations of brain tissue evolved the highly convoluted cerebral cortex of modern man.

evolution theory the principle that present organisms have developed from preexisting organisms through orderly genetic adaptations to the environment. See DARWIN. Also see CONVERGENT E.

-ex-; -exo-; -exter-; -extra- a combining form meaning outer or outside.

exact replication: See REPLICATION.

exaggeration a defensive reaction in which the individual justifies questionable attitudes or behavior through overstatement, e.g., by exaggerating one's hatred for a parent, or by magnifying the faults of an employer.

exaggeration in wit a term applied to the use of caricature, parody, and exaggeration in order to achieve pleasurable "comical nonsense" (Freud).

exaltation a state of extreme elation and joyous excitement during which the patient may dance, sing, laugh, or declaim in an unrestrained and uninhibited manner. It is a symptom that frequently occurs in acute mania. The term also denotes an abnormal increase in the function of an organ.

exalted paranoia a type of paranoid disorder in which the patient experiences great elation and makes extravagant claims. He may claim, e.g., that he has invented a system that will bring all wars to a halt, or he may appoint himself the head of a new religious sect that has special access to infinity.

examination: See PSYCHIATRIC E.; PSYCHOLOGICAL E.; NEUROLOGICAL E.; MENTAL E.; OBJECTIVE E.

examination anxiety tension and apprehensiveness associated with taking a test. Freud explained e.a. as an unconscious association with childhood punishment for misdeeds.

examination dream a dream that is associated with test or examination anxiety. Also called **matriculation dream**.

Examining for Aphasia a series of tests devised by Jon Eisenson, consisting of identifying objects (agnosia tests) by (a) sight, sound, and touch, (b) answering auditory- and reading comprehension questions, and silent reading comprehension, to identify receptive disturbances, and (c) tests involving action, speech, word-finding, and writing (apraxias, aphasia) to identify predominantly expressive disturbances.

exanthemata an eruption or rash that may appear on the skin as a sign of a fever induced by an infectious agent, particularly a virus. An **exanthematous** reaction also may be caused by an adverse drug effect. Among exanthematous infections are rubeola or measles, rubella or German measles, chicken pox, smallpox, and infectious mononucleosis.

exceptional child a comprehensive term denoting a child who is substantially above or below normal in some significant respect. The term often describes a child who shows marked deviations in intelligence, but it may also be used to indicate the presence of a special talent, or unusual emotional or social difficulty. Also see GIFTEDNESS; MENTAL RETARDATION; SLOW LEARNER.

excitability in child psychology, the intensity of heart rate, cries, and bodily movement in infants. E. varies from child to child. Some infants are easily aroused and extremely sensitive to stimulation while others are even and calm. The relative e. of an infant may affect the mother-child relationship; e.g., a baby who cries often and is not easily pacified is more likely than a tranquil baby to elicit anxiety in the mother.

excitability of neuron the property of a neuron in reacting to irritation, marked by an electric or chemical response. Whereas all living cells display a form of irritability, neurons and some muscle cells show irritability in the form of excitability which is characterized by a sudden, transient increase in their ionic permeability, and change in the electric potential of the neural membrane.

excitant an agent capable of eliciting a response.

excitation the activity elicited in a nerve when it is stimulated.

excitation and conduction a two-stage process in which (a) excitation occurs in a neuron as a response to the irritation of a stimulus, and the potential difference across the membrane becomes an electric sink, causing in turn a flow of current from neighboring areas, and (b) the neighboring areas also become electric sinks and a wave of excitation spreads in a manner known as conduction. See EXCITABILITY OF NEURON.

excitation gradient the principle that the closer the similarity of two stimuli, the greater the probability they will produce the same (though weaker) response. Also called **generalization gradient**.

excitatory agent: See EXCITANT.

excitatory field an area of the brain near the termination of an excited sensory neuron.

excitatory-inhibitory processes according to Pavlov's early theories, antagonistic functions of the nervous system: excitation and inhibition. According to Eysenck, a predominance of the excitatory process predisposes the individual to hysterical neurosis, and a predominance of the inhibitory process is associated with obsessive-compulsive or phobic reactions.

excitatory irradiation the spread of excitation outward from an active neural center.

excitatory-postsynaptic potential the conducted action potential in a postsynaptic fiber which declines rapidly after the forward conduction of a nerve impulse. The rate of depolarization is affected by such factors as the rapidity of repeated transmissions across the synapse, which is susceptible to fatigue. Abbrev.: **EPSP**.

excitatory synapse the firing of a nerve impulse across a synaptic cleft at the end of the axon. Transmitter-chemical changes at the terminal button change the permeability of the receiving neuron that makes possible the e.s.

excitement an emotional state marked by impulsive behavior, tense anticipation, and general arousal.

excitement phase: See SEXUAL-RESPONSE CYCLE.

exclamation theory: See ORIGIN-OF-LANGUAGE THEORIES.

excrement = FECES.

excrement fear = COPROPHOBIA.

executive organ the body organ that plays the major role in responding to a stimulus. When the stimulus is a desire to touch an object, the hand becomes the e.o. Other organs often play subsidiary roles, e.g., the eye that helps direct the e.o. serves as an **auxiliary organ**.

executive stress strain experienced by management personnel who are responsible for major decisions, the effectiveness of subordinates, and the success of the company as a competitive organization.

exercise law: See LAW OF EXERCISE.

exhaustion death − BELL'S MANIA.

exhaustion delirium a delirious state occurring among mountain climbers, long-distance swimmers, explorers, and individuals lost in the wilderness, as well as patients suffering from advanced cancer or other debilitating diseases. E.d. is particularly apt to occur when extreme overexertion is coupled with other forms of stress such as prolonged insomnia, starvation, loneliness, or excessive heat or cold. See DELIRIUM.

exhaustion stage the third and final stage of the general adaptation syndrome, marked by a breakdown of hormone reactions and acquired adaptations to a stressful situation. The e.s. follows the organism's alarm reaction and resistance, the first two stages of the syndrome delineated by Hans Selye in the 1950s. Also called **stage of exhaustion**. See GENERAL ADAPTATION SYNDROME. Also see ALARM REACTION; STAGE OF RESISTANCE.

exhaustive stupor a stupor, sometimes manifested as a coma, that results from a severe infection or toxic condition.

exhibitionism a psychosexual disorder consisting of repeated exposure of the genitals to unsuspecting strangers as a means of achieving sexual excitement, but without any attempt at further sexual activity with the stranger. The act is performed by a male in the presence of female children or adults, and may involve masturbation during the exposure. (DSM-III)

exhibitionistic need a need for attention-getting by arousing, amusing, or shocking others.

existence needs: See EXISTENCE, RELATEDNESS, AND GROWTH THEORY.

Existence, Relatedness, and Growth theory a variation of Maslow's hierarchy of needs as applied in industrial psychology by Alderfer. The categories (of work motivation) include existence needs, related to physical needs of the organism (food, clothing, shelter); relatedness needs that involve interpersonal relations with others on and off the job; and growth needs in the form of personal development and improvement. Abbrev.: **ERG; ERG theory**.

existential analysis a phase in existential psychotherapy in which the individual explores his own being, that is, his values, relationships, and commitments. The object of this analysis, however, is not to accept things as they are, but to develop new and more fulfilling modes of existence. Being, therefore, is not static and fixed; rather, it is the process of becoming. Also called **existential psychoanalysis**.

existential anxiety a general sense of apprehension and Angst associated with the feeling that life is ultimately meaningless and futile, and that we are alienated not only from other people but from ourselves. Also called **existential anguish**. Also see ANGST.

existential crisis according to existentialists, the basic crisis that faces humankind today, that of finding meaning and purpose in life.

existential ego function the activities of the ego in relation to the problem of existence: increased awareness of the self and of the meaning and possibilities of our lives.

existential-humanistic therapy a form of therapy that emphasizes treatment of the entire person, rather than just his biology, behavior, or unconscious features. The therapy requires a concerned and caring orientation of the therapist toward the patient; and emphasis is placed on the patient's subjective experiences, free will, and ability to decide about his own life course. Also called **humanistic-existential therapy**.

existentialism a philosophical and psychological approach which holds that the essential problem of existence is to find oneself, be oneself, and actualize oneself. If this problem is solved, the individual will make his own contribution and think and act creatively because his behavior will draw upon his own experience and the awareness of his own potentialities. E., via Soren Kierkegaard, Maine de Biran, and Blaise Pascal, has its roots in the Stoic philosophers and Socrates. Modern e. derives its emphasis on individual experience and on the quest for identity from the phenomenology of Edmund Husserl and the existential philosophy of Friedrich Nietzsche, Karl Jaspers, Martin Heidegger, and Jean-Paul Sartre. In literature, this quest is reflected by writers like Franz Kafka and Albert Camus, to whom modern man has become alienated from himself. See BEING-IN-THE WORLD; EXISTENTIAL PSYCHOTHERAPY; EXISTENTIAL PHENOMENOLOGY; ZEN THERAPY.

existential living as used by C. Rogers, the capacity to live fully in the present and respond freely and flexibly to new experience without fear. Rogers considers the capacity for e.l. a central feature of the fully functioning person.

existential neurosis = EXISTENTIAL VACUUM.

existential phenomenology the direct, immediate awareness of ourselves and our unique experience, putting aside all preconceptions, hypotheses, and analyses. E.p. means knowing ourselves instead of knowing *about* ourselves. See PHENOMENOLOGY; EXISTENTIALISM

existential psychoanalysis = EXISTENTIAL ANALYSIS.

existential psychotherapy a form of therapy which eschews both the current emphasis on outer adjustment and the standard psychoanalytic approach which focuses on free association, dredging up the past, and unconscious conflicts. Instead, it places the emphasis on an exploration of the individual's present life and values, and development of a more meaningful, integrated, fulfilling existence. To reach these goals, the patient is encouraged to confront his own being, become more aware of his own feelings and relationships, and redefine his own identity.

existential school: See EXISTENTIALISM.

existential vacuum a term introduced by V. Frankl to denote the inability to perceive meaning in life as expressed in feelings of emptiness, alienation, futility, aimlessness. In accord with other existentialists, Frankl considers meaninglessness to be the quintessential symptom or ailment of the modern age. Also called **existential neurosis**. See LOGOTHERAPY. Also see WILL TO MEANING.

exit interview the meeting between student and school counselor before the student leaves to begin high school, college, technical school, a vocational program, or a job. Future plans, future course of study, and the student's degree of preparation are discussed. The term is also applied to the employee's final meeting with his or her supervisor or personnel staff prior to termination.

exocathection Murray's term for a preoccupation with practical, worldly affairs rather than personal matters. Compare ENDOCATHECTION.

exocrine gland any gland that secretes a substance through a duct, e.g., the lacrimal gland.

exogamy /eksog'-/ the practice of marrying outside the tribe, clan, or social unit. Adjective: **exogamous**. Compare ENDOGAMY.

exogenous /eksoj'-/ referring to a mental or physical disorder that is caused primarily by a factor outside the body of the patient, or outside the affected organ system.

exogenous depression = REACTIVE DEPRESSION.

exogenous factors causes of mental disorder originating outside the organism or outside the nervous system or psyche. Examples are traumatic situations, alcohol abuse, or business failure.

exogenous stimulation stimulation that originates in the outer environment, e.g., light and sound waves. Compare ENDOGENOUS STIMULATION.

exogenous stress stress arising from external situations such as natural catastrophes, excessive competition on the job, or climbing a precipitous mountain.

exonerative moral reasoning the process by which an individual consciously formulates moral reasons for an act that would normally be considered immoral or unacceptable. The term refers to a process of self-serving reasoning designed to achieve vindication in the eyes of oneself or others.

exophoria deviation of one eye in an outward direction.

exophthalmic goiter any of the various types of hyperthyroidism in which there are diagnostic signs of exophthalmos, or protruding eyes, and an enlarged thyroid gland. E.g. often is a prominent feature of GRAVES' DISEASE. See this entry.

exophthalmos an abnormal protrusion of the eyeball, a condition commonly associated with hyperthyroidism or toxic goiter. The condition also may be the result of a tumor or infection involving the eye. E. often is characterized by the appearance of a fixed stare by the patient.

exopsychic characterizing mental activity that produces effects on society or the environment, that is, outside the individual. Compare ENDOPSYCHIC.

exorcism the process of driving demons out of the mind by means of certain rites and ceremonies, prayers and incantations. Some individuals believe these evil spirits are the major cause of mental disease or other aberrations.

exosomatic method a technique that uses electrical resistance of the skin in psychogalvanic-response studies. See GALVANIC SKIN RESPONSE.

exotic bias a term used in anthropology to denote the tendency of social scientists to overemphasize those features of a culture that contrast sharply with the investigator's own culture while overlooking those features that are the same or similar.

exotic psychosis a severe mental illness observed in folk cultures or other non-Western societies. The term has been replaced by culture-specific syndrome. See CULTURE-SPECIFIC SYNDROMES.

exotropia the walleye effect caused by the outward deviation of an eye, as in GRIEG'S DISEASE. See this entry.

expanded consciousness a sensory effect of meditation or of the use of mind-altering drugs that cause the individual to feel his mind has been opened to a new kind of awareness or to new concepts.

expansive delusion a generalized delusion of wealth, power, well-being, and importance.

expansive ideas grandiose delusions and extravagant schemes. See DELUSIONS OF GRANDEUR; MEGALOMANIA.

expansive mood a mood that reflects feelings of GRANDIOSITY. See this entry.

expansiveness a personality trait manifested by loquaciousness, overfriendliness, hyperactivity, and lack of restraint.

ex-patient club in psychiatry, an ongoing group organized by a former mental patient or by a hospital as part of its aftercare program. The objective is to provide social and recreational experience, to promote readjustment and rehabilitation, and to maintain improvement through group support and, in some cases, group therapy.

expectancy an attitude of anticipation of a given stimulus or event based upon previous experience with related stimuli or events. In statistics, e. is the probability of an occurrence based on mathematical calculation.

expectancy charts the graphic representation of performance expected on the basis of tests of ability. E.c. may be individual when predicting performance of a single person, or institutional when based on the expectations of a group of individuals who have been tested, such as a group of job applicants.

expectancy theory a purposive-behaviorism theory (Tolman) that cognitive learning involves acquired expectancies and a tendency to react to certain objects as signs of certain further objects previously associated with them.

expectant analysis: See FOCUSED ANALYSIS.

expectation a state of tense, emotional anticipation. See ANTICIPATION.

expected day of confinement: See GESTATION PERIOD.

expected frequency a frequency predicted from a theoretical model, and contrasted with an observed frequency; also, a frequency that would occur on the basis of chance alone.

expediter in psychiatry, an individual who helps the patient obtain the treatment or rehabilitation services he needs by contacting various agencies and facilities. Also see ADVOCATE.

experience an event that is lived through, or undergone, as opposed to one that is imagined or thought about; the present contents of consciousness; also, knowledge or skill resulting from practice or learning.

experiential group a group of persons who come together to share feelings and experiences (e.g., an Alcoholics Anonymous group), as contrasted with a TASK-ORIENTED GROUP. See this entry.

experiential psychotherapy a form of psychological treatment primarily for psychotics, developed by K. A. Whitaker and Th. P. Malone (1953) in which patient and therapist form an "intrapsychic society" in which they penetrate to the id level and share each other's deepest fantasies and experiences. This is accomplished by cutting themselves off from external reality and employing clay, rubber knives, and other materials to stimulate symbolic expression, including dreams. The therapist then indicates that he understands the patient's symbols, fantasies, and immaturities, and encourages him to test out more mature reactions.

experiment a series of observations conducted under controlled conditions to test a hypothesis; a research technique for determining cause-and-effect relationships. An e. may involve the manipulation of an independent variable, the measurement of a dependent variable, and the exposure of subjects to conditions being studied.

experimental analysis of behavior the study of the shaping, maintenance, and extinction of behavior by environmental contingencies. This approach uses experimental manipulation rather than statistical averaging, emphasizes an engineering rather than a theoretical orientation, and analyzes the effects of schedules of reinforcement on rate of response. This field was originated by B. F. Skinner. See BEHAVIOR ANALYSIS.

experimental control the regulation of all extraneous conditions and variables in an experiment so that any change in the dependent variable can be attributed to the independent variable.

experimental design outline or plan of the procedures to be followed in scientific experimentation in order to reach valid conclusions.

experimental error a deviation or false value in experimental data, usually due to a design error.

experimental esthetics the use of experimental-psychology techniques in the study of art forms and qualities. E.e. studies may also involve the use of Gestalt concepts in analyzing emotional effects and preferences for colors and patterns.

experimental group a group of subjects exposed to one or more independent variables or to a set of treatment conditions for purposes of scientific study. Also see CONTROL GROUP.

experimental hypothesis a premise that is the basis for a scientific study and which describes what the researcher hopes to demonstrate if certain experimental conditions are met.

experimental marriage an agreement, written or verbal, between a man and woman to live together as husband and wife for a period of time in order to determine their compatibility and desire to formalize the marriage. Scotland permitted one-year experimental marriages before the Reformation, and seven-year experimental marriages were common in England in the tenth century. Experimental marriages in rural Latin America were permitted in recent years in order to determine the ability of the couple to produce children, an event desired for formal marriage. Also called **trial marriage**.

experimental method a system of scientific investigation, usually based on a design and carried out under controlled conditions with the aim of testing a hypothesis and establishing a causal relationship between independent and dependent variables.

experimental neurosis an artificial neurosis produced in an animal (dog, chimpanzee, pig) during conditioning experiments in which the animal is required to discriminate between sounds, shapes, or other stimuli that differ only slightly. Failure to solve the problem is usually followed by punishment. This situation creates an internal conflict and produces a state of accumulated tension and anxiety that gives rise to such neurotic symptoms as stereotyped behavior, compulsivity, disorganized responses, extreme emotional display, and emotional apathy. Also called **artificial neurosis**.

experimental psychology the scientific study of behavior, motives, or cognition in a laboratory setting, in order to predict, explain, or control behavior. E.p. aims at establishing lawful, quantified relationships and explanatory theory through comparison of responses under various controlled conditions.

experimental realism the attempt to design an experiment, particularly a social-psychological experiment, that is psychologically realistic and elicits valid emotional responses from subjects. Deception may be employed to achieve e.r. Also see MUNDANE REALISM.

experimental series the actual trials in an experiment, as opposed to trial runs and experimental controls.

experimental variable = INDEPENDENT VARIABLE.

experimenter bias systematic experimental error resulting from alteration in the experimenter's behavior due to his special knowledge or motivation. E.b. may result, e.g., from knowledge of the hypothesis being studied, of group membership of the subject, or of a subject's test score.

experimenter effect the distortion in experimental findings caused by mistakes made by the experimenter in handling and interpreting the data, or due to the experimenter's behavior toward the subjects. E.g., a harsh and impersonal experimenter may intimidate subjects so that their responses are unintentionally altered by his attitude.

experimenter-expectancy effect the distortion in experimental findings caused by the impact of an experimenter's expectations on a subject's responses, a type of experimenter effect. The experimenter's body gestures, expressions, and tone of voice have all been found to influence subjects' responses. See EXPERIMENTER EFFECT; EXPERIMENTER BIAS.

expert witness in forensic psychiatry and psychology, a professional individual who is qualified by reason of training and experience to serve as a consultant in legal proceedings, e.g., in bearing witness to the competence or incompetence of an individual.

expiation an action that is performed for the purpose of reducing feelings of guilt.

expiatory punishment Piaget's term for the type of punishment preferred by children up to the age of roughly eight in which the culprit is made to suffer in proportion to the severity of his crime; however, his punishment need not match the crime in content. Compare RECIPROCAL PUNISHMENT.

explicit behavior any overt, observable behavior.

exploitative character = EXPLOITATIVE ORIENTATION.

exploitative-manipulative behavior the use of other people to attain one's ends without regard for their needs or feelings. In industrial or business situations, e.-m.b. means treating workers as commodities rather than persons.

exploitative orientation a term used by Erich Fromm to denote a character pattern marked by the use of stealth, deceit, power, or violence to obtain what one wants. Also called **exploitative character**.

exploration according to E. Ginzberg, the phase of the "realistic period" of adolescence when existing job opportunities are actively explored in light of the adolescent's interests and abilities. The phase of CRYSTALLIZATION follows. See this entry.

exploration drive the motivation that compels an organism to examine areas of its environment, or beyond its immediate environment, because of unsatisfied desires for security, food, sex, or other factors. The e.d. is most highly developed in humans and other higher animals and has been identified as a typical arousal syndrome. Also see CURIOSITY.

exploratory behavior the movements by humans or animals in orienting themselves to new situations.

explosive = PLOSIVE.

explosive disorder: See INTERMITTENT E.D.; ISOLATED E.D.

explosive personality a personality with a pattern of frequent outbursts of uncontrolled anger and hostility, out of proportion to any provocation. See INTERMITTENT EXPLOSIVE DISORDER.

exposition attitude the tendency to explain, demonstrate, lecture, and define relationships (Murray).

ex post facto research research that begins with data that have already been collected, or research conducted after the experimental treatments have already taken place; literally, research after the event, research in retrospect (Latin).

exposure deafness a loss of hearing due to prolonged exposure to loud sounds. The condition may be temporary or permanent, depending upon the loudness, length of exposure, and sound frequencies. A transient form marked by reduced sound-threshold sensitivity for several hours is called **auditory fatigue**.

Expressed Emotions a study by G. W. Brown, J. L. T. Birley, and J. K. Wing, 1972, indicating that a high relapse rate in schizophrenics is associated with the frequency and quality of emotions expressed by the family toward the patient, such as criticism, hostility, and over-involvement, particularly when they spend at least 35 hours a weeks together. Abbrev.: **EE**.

expressionism factor in psychological esthetics, the components of artistic style that emphasize the artist's emotional experience and a reflection of a tense quality. E.f., according to D. E. Berlyne, is based on stylistic ratings that score a high positive loading on the tense-tranquil scale and a high negative on artist's feelings and objective ideas-inner feelings. Also see ABSTRACT EXPRESSIONISM.

expression method the technique of measuring and describing emotions in terms of bodily changes.

expressive amimia: See AMIMIA.

expressive amusia: See AMUSIA.

expressive aphasia a language disorder in which the ability to speak, write, or use gestures is lost or impaired. The condition is often associated with a lesion in Broca's area of the brain. Also called **cortical motor aphasia; expressive dysphasia; verbal aphasia; word dumbness**. Also see RECEPTIVE APHASIA.

expressive language skills the ability to use language effectively for communicating with other individuals. Speaking, writing, or gesturing are forms of expressive language.

expressive movements a subject's body language —particularly posture, gesture, and facial expression—which may be used as a clue to his or her personality.

expressive therapy a form of psychotherapy in which the patient is encouraged to talk out his problems and express his feelings openly and without restraint. Compare SUPPRESSIVE THERAPY.

expressivity in genetics, the degree to which a penetrant gene or genetic complement manifests itself as a phenotype, that is, as an actual trait or disease. See PENETRANCE.

ext. an abbreviation of "external" or "exterior," used, e.g., in prescriptions.

extended care a health-care service provided to patients who have completed a period of hospitalization but require rehabilitation, skilled nursing, or other convalescent care. E.c. may be recommended by an attending physician when it is believed the service will improve the health of the patient.

extended family a family consisting of parents, children, and individuals united by kinship (grandparents, cousins), or by marital ties. Compare NUCLEAR FAMILY.

extended-family therapy group psychotherapy involving not only the nuclear family but other family members as well, such as aunts, grandparents, and cousins. See FAMILY THERAPY.

extended-stay review the review of a continuous hospital stay that equals or exceeds a period defined in the hospital's utilization review plan. Also see CONTINUED-STAY REVIEW.

extension reflex any reflex action that causes a limb or part of a limb to move away from the body. Kinds of e.r. include extensor thrust, stretch or myotatic reflex, and crossed extension reaction.

extensor carpi; extensor digitorum: See EXTENSOR MUSCLE.

extensor motoneurons efferent-nerve cells with fibers that connect with extensor effectors, or muscles that extend a part of the body by contracting. See EXTENSOR MUSCLE.

extensor muscle a muscle that contracts in order to extend a part of the body. An example is the triceps muscle group which extends, or straightens, the arm. Some extensor muscles have names that indicate this function, such as the **extensor carpi** and the **extensor digitorum** muscles, also of the arm. Compare FLEXOR MUSCLE.

extensor rigidity rigid contractions of extensor muscles. The kind of rigidity sometimes indicates the site of the motoneuron lesion associated with the disorder. An injury to the cerebellum produces increased tone of extensor muscles, called **cerebellar rigidity**. Transection of brain tissues below the anterior corpora quadrigemina causes rigid contraction of anti-gravity muscles, maintaining a subject in a standing position.

extensor thrust a reflex extension of the leg caused by applying a stimulus to the sole of the foot. The reflex normally occurs each time a person takes a step in walking or running, signaling a need for body support and providing the thrust for taking the next step. Also see STRETCH REFLEXES.

extent prognosis: See DIRECTION PROGNOSIS.

exteriorization the act of relating one's interior affects and attitudes to external, objective reality; also, outward expression of one's private and personal ideas.

external auditory meatus one of several folds of tissue in the surface of the auricle, or external ear. It is adjacent to the external auditory canal, which, in turn, extends to the tympanic membrane, or eardrum.

external boundary: See EGO BOUNDARIES.

external capsule a thin flat layer of tissue separating the claustrum from the putamen, near the center of the human brain. It consists of white fibers from the anterior white commissure and subthalamic region and is continuous with the internal capsule. Also called **capsula externa**.

external chemical messenger a substance such as an odor that is secreted or released by an organism, and which influences other organisms, e.g., a pheromone. Abbrev: **ECM**.

external ear the part of the ear that extends beyond the surface of the head. It is connected by the auditory canal with the tympanic membrane of the middle ear.

external granular layer: See CELLULAR LAYERS OF CORTEX.

external hair cells of ear minute hairs or cilia arranged in three or four successive rows on the organ of Corti. There are about 12,000 e.h.c.o.e. per cochlea, serving as sensory epithelial cells.

external hydrocephalus a form of hydrocephalus that is associated with a head injury. Symptoms occurring after the injury include intermittent headaches, drowsiness, vomiting, and confusion, followed by mental dullness, apathy, and retardation. The cause is an injury-related blood clot that lodges in the cerebrospinal-fluid pathways and blocks drainage of the fluid.

external inhibition a reduction in a conditioned response that occurs when an external extraneous stimulus accompanies the conditioning stimulus.

externalization the paranoid projection of one's own thoughts into the external world, as in ideas of reference; also, the process of learning to distinguish between the self and the environment during childhood; also, the process by which a drive comes to be aroused by external stimuli instead of internal stimuli—e.g., hunger may be aroused by the sight of tempting food even when we are sated.

externalizing behavior: See EXTERNALIZING/IN-TERNALIZING.

externalizing/internalizing T. M. Achenback's classification of child referrals on the basis of (a) acting out, antisocial behavior, and hostility (externalizing behavior), and (b) anxiety, excessive inhibition, somatization, and depression (internalizing behavior).

external locus of control: See LOCUS OF CONTROL.

external pyramidal-cell layer: See CELLULAR LAYERS OF CORTEX.

external rectus an extrinsic eye muscle that rotates the eyeball outward.

external sense a sense-organ system that depends upon external stimulation, e.g., vision.

external stigmata: See SEGMENTAL INSUFFICIENCY.

external validity representativeness, or the degree to which the results of psychological research or testing can be generalized. Campbell and Stanley originated this usage, and listed a number of threats to e.v., such as the reactive effects of testing. See also INTERNAL VALIDITY.

exteroceptive conditioning conditioning that depends primarily upon external stimuli such as auditory, visual, or somatic cues. Compare IN-TEROCEPTIVE CONDITIONING.

exteroceptor a sense organ that receives stimulation from outside the body.

exteropsychic: See ADULT-EGO STATE.

extinction the gradual diminution in the strength or rate of a conditioned response when the unconditioned stimulus or the reinforcement is withheld. In neurophysiology, e. is a progressive decrease in excitability of a nerve to a previously adequate stimulus until it becomes completely inexcitable. E. for visual and tactile stimuli occurs in occipital-parietal lesions. Verb: **to extinguish**. See E. OF EGO; INATTENTION; SENSORY E.

extinction of ego in psychoanalysis, the impulse to annihilate the ego due to primitive feelings of guilt and repressed hostility toward the self generated by a punitive superego. The obsessive neurotic attempts to protect his loved objects from his hostility by magical rituals, but when these fail, feelings of dejection, apathy, and unworthiness overwhelm him, and this state of mind is equivalent to extinction of the ego.

extinction ratio the proportion of unreinforced responses to reinforced responses emitted by a subject in periodic-reinforcement reconditioning.

extinguish: See EXTINCTION.

extirpation = ABLATION.

-extr-; -extra- a combining form meaning outside or beyond.

extraception an attitude of skepticism, objectivity, and adherence to the facts (Murray).

extradural hemorrhage bleeding that occurs outside the dura mater, the outer layer of membranes that provide a protective covering for the brain surface. E.h. usually involves a ruptured artery resulting from a severe head injury such as a skull fracture. There may be a brief lucid period after the injury, then severe headaches, dizziness, confusion, loss of consciousness, and finally death if the e.h. is not controlled.

extraindividual behavior behavior that is influenced by environmental setting rather than psychological characteristics of the subject. The concept is based on an assumption that, with certain cultural influences considered, an otherwise normal individual will adapt his behavior to his surroundings. Thus, his behavior in a church will be influenced by the church environment, but his behavior will change radically in a gambling casino because of the casino setting. Also see SITUATED IDENTITIES.

extrajection the act of attributing one's own feelings or characteristics to another person.

extramarital sex sexual activity with someone other than one's spouse. Also called **nonmarital sex**.

extrapsychic pertaining to that which originates outside the mind or that which occurs between the mind and the environment.

extrapsychic conflict a conflict arising between

the individual and the environment, as contrasted to internal or intrapsychic conflict. See CONFLICT.

extrapunitive relating to the outward direction of hostility or a tendency to find external factors as the cause of one's frustrations.

extrapyramidal dyskinesia distortions of voluntary movement, such as tremors, spasms, tics, rigidity, gait disturbance, occurring (a) in organic conditions, including PARKINSON'S DISEASE, CHOREA, ATHETOSIS, and HEMIBALLISMUS, and (b) as a side effect of antipsychotic drugs, which produce such conditions as AKATHISIA, ACUTE DYSTONIA, and TARDIVE DYSKINESIA. For details, see these entries.

extrapyramidal effects reactions to drugs such as neuroleptics and tricyclic antidepressants that involve the extrapyramidal system. E.e. also may result from certain drugs administered for the treatment of headaches, such as carbamazepine. Major tranquilizers induce e.e. that include a variety of involuntary movements, such as tremors, rigidity, and dystonia.

extrapyramidal involvement: See EPI.

extrapyramidal motor system a portion of the central nervous system that includes parts of the spinal cord, basal ganglia, and mesencephalon. Its functions are the regulation of muscle tone, body posture, and coordination of opposing sets of skeletal muscles and movement of their associated skeletal parts. Also see PYRAMIDAL SYSTEM.

extrapyramidal syndrome a disorder marked by involuntary movements such as tremors and tics, impaired voluntary movements, and changes in posture and muscle tone. The e.s. also may include violent flinging motions of the limbs. Symptoms of parkinsonism are a part of the e.s.

extrapyramidal tract the part of the central nervous system that is located outside the pyramidal-fiber pathways. The category was established early in the 20th century on the false assumption that pyramidal-tract-nerve fibers were involved in voluntary motor activity while extrapyramidal fibers were not.

extrasensory perception alleged awareness of external events by other means than the known sensory channels. It includes telepathy, clairvoyance, precognition, and, more loosely, psychokinesis. There is considerable difference of opinion as to the existence of these modalities. Abbrev.: **ESP**. Also called **paranormal cognition**.

extra-small-acrocentric-chromosome syndrome: See CAT'S-EYE SYNDROME.

extraspective perspective a methodological approach based on objective, empirical observation of actions and reactions, as contrasted with an introspective, first-person account of experience. The natural-science approach of behaviorism is based on an e.p.

extrauterine pregnancy = ECTOPIC PREGNANCY.

extraversion the tendency to direct one's interests and energies toward the outer world of people and things rather than the inner world of subjective experience; outgoing, outer-directed attitude (from Latin, "turning outward"). Also called **extroversion**. Compare INTROVERSION.

extraverted type a Jungian term for a person who is considered to be habitually extraverted and whose attitudes, values, and interests are directed toward the physical and social environment.

extrinsic asthma a form of bronchial asthma that is precipitated or aggravated by exposure to environmental allergens, e.g., plant pollens, house dust, molds, animal danders. E.a. patients account for about 15 percent of the total number of asthma cases in the United States.

extrinsic cortex the portion of the cortex innervated by fibers that receive impulses from stimuli in the environment, a concept introduced in 1958 by K. H. Pribram. See INTRINSIC CORTEX.

extrinsic eye muscles the muscles attached to the outside of the eyeball that control its movements.

extrinsic motivation any motive or incentive that is external to a specific behavior or activity, especially motivation arising from the expectation of punishment or reward, e.g., studying motivated by the fear of an examination. Compare INTRINSIC MOTIVATION.

extrinsic reward an extraneous reward that is not logically related to the performance or behavior itself.

extrinsic thalamus a part of the thalamus that contains nuclei which relay incoming impulses.

extropunitive a reaction to frustration or distress in which anger or aggression is directed at the person or situation conceived to be the source of the frustration.

extroversion = EXTRAVERSION.

eye: See VISUAL SYSTEM. Also see COMPOUND EYE; LEADING EYE.

eye bank a source of corneal transplants, usually maintained by a local nonprofit charitable organization that obtains donor eyes by bequest. The eyes are stored and supplied to surgeons for use in appropriate cases in which blindness can be treated by removing the damaged cornea of a patient and replacing it with a grafted cornea from the e.b. The donor eyes must be removed immediately after the death of the donor. Also see ORGAN TRANSPLANTS.

eye contact the act of looking at one's interlocutor. Maintaining e.c. is considered essential to communication between therapist and patient during face-to-face interviews. In child therapy, it is often the initial step; and to encourage e.c., the behavior therapist may hold a piece of candy near his eyes, and give it to the child if he looks at him. E.c. is used as a variable in some social-psychological studies to represent the degree of interpersonal intimacy.

eyedness: See LATERALIZATION; EYE DOMINANCE.

eye dominance the preference for the use of one eye over the other. Eye preference is more often right-sided than left-sided, and the main influence of preference is on a differential acuity of the two eyes. There is no valid relationship between e.d. and learning to read. Also called **ocular dominance**.

eyeglasses: See CONTACT LENS.

eye-hand coordination the harmonious functioning of eyes and hands in grasping and exploring objects. By six months, e.-h.c. develops so that most infants can grasp an object within reach, although full use of the thumb develops later, between eight and 12 months.

eyelash sign a reaction of eyelid movement to the stimulus of stroking the eyelashes. The e.s. is part of a diagnostic test for loss of consciousness due to a functional disorder, such as hysteria. If the loss of consciousness is due to an organic CNS disease or injury, the reflex will not occur.

eye movements movements that provide coverage of the fields of vision, as controlled by six muscles: the superior rectus, for looking upward; inferior rectus, for looking downward; medial rectus, for turning the eye toward the nose; lateral rectus, for turning the eye away from the nose; superior oblique, for looking downward and inward; and inferior oblique, for looking upward and inward. The superior and inferior oblique muscles also control rotation movements of the eyeball.

eye phobia = OMMATOPHOBIA.

eye preference: See EYE DOMINANCE.

eye-roll sign an index of susceptibility to hypnosis (Herbert Spiegel): The subject is directed to roll his eyes upward as far as possible and at the same time lower his eye lids slowly. If little or no white space shows under the cornea, he is considered not hypnotizable. These low scorers, on a scale of 0 to 5, tend to be critical and to favor thinking over feeling, while high scorers, who are readily hypnotizable, tend to be uncritical

and suggestible and to favor feeling over thinking.

eye structure the three-layer structure of the eye, consisting of (a) the fibrous outer coating, which forms the cornea in front and continues as the sclera over the rest of the globe, (b) the middle layer called the uveal tract, which includes the iris, and (c) the innermost, or retinal layer, which is composed of nerve tissue. The anterior chamber, between the cornea and lens, is filled with a fluid, the aqueous humor, and the space behind the crystalline lens, a cavity occupying about four-fifths of the globe or eyeball, is filled with the jellylike vitreous humor. The humors serve as refracting media. Also see VISUAL SYSTEM; AQUEOUS HUMOR.

eye-voice span the distance in terms of letters between the word being spoken and the word focused on in oral reading.

Eysenck, Hans Jürgen /ī′zengk/ German-born British psychologist, 1916—. E. has contributed to the factor analysis of personality, and to genetic studies of emotionality and conditioning in rats, intelligence testing, analysis of social attitudes, and the development of behavioral therapy. He is the author of *The Scientific Study of Personality* and founder of the *Journal of Behavior Research and Therapy*. See EYSENCK PERSONALITY INVENTORY; BODY-BUILD INDEX; CONDITIONABILITY; EXCITATORY-INHIBITORY PROCESSES; FACTOR THEORY OF PERSONALITY; INTROVERSION; INTROVERSION-EXTROVERSION; MAUDSLEY PERSONALITY INVENTORY; MESOSOMATIC; NEUROTICISM; PSYCHOTICISM; SYMPTOMATIC TREATMENT.

Eysenck Personality Inventory a self-report personality test of the questionnaire variety, designed to measure two major personality dimensions derived by factor analysis, extroversion-introversion, and neuroticism.

F

fables test a test in which the subject is asked to interpret fables. It is used in intelligence and projective tests.

fabrication: See FABULATION; CONFABULATION.

Fabry, Johannes /fäb′rē/ German physician, 1860–1930. See FABRY'S DISEASE.

Fabry's disease a hereditary disorder involving a sex-linked lipid metabolism abnormality. A complex glycolipid substance accumulates in the tissues, causing skin lesions over the thighs and genitalia and a painful burning sensation in the lower extremities. Hypertension with cerebral complications often is associated with the disorder and a common cause of death. Also called **angiokeratoma corporis diffusum; glycosphingolipid lipidosis**.

fabulation fabrication; a psychological reaction in which falsehoods and fictions are concocted. The term was used by Adolf Meyer. See CONFABULATION.

face: See PERSONA.

face-hand test a test of cerebral dysfunction in which the examiner touches the patient's face and the back of his hand at the same time (double-simultaneous tactile sensation). According to L. Bender, who devised the test, inability to perceive both sensations is indicative of minimal brain damage or schizophrenic tendencies in children, and of diffuse brain damage in adults. Also see DOUBLE-SIMULTANEOUS TACTILE SENSATION.

face-saving behavior an act in which one attempts to redress a social blunder or compensate for a perceived "wrong impression." See IMPRESSION MANAGEMENT.

face-to-face group any group whose members are in personal contact and are thus able to perceive each others' needs and responses, and carry on direct interaction, e.g., a T-group or psychotherapy group. Also called **direct-contact group**.

face validity the degree to which the items or content of a test appear to be appropriately measuring some domain, regardless of whether they are really doing so. A test with f.v. sometimes lacks predictive, empirical, or construct validity.

facial-affect program the relationship or link between a specific emotion and a given pattern of facial-muscular activity.

facial disfigurement any distortion, malformation, or abnormality of the facial features due to injury, disease, or congenital anomaly. Because of the common tendency of people to assign traits to other individuals on the basis of facial features, the patient with f.d. is particularly vulnerable to social, psychological, and economic discrimination and unfavorable stress effects. See DISFIGUREMENT.

facial display facial expressions; a form of nonverbal behavior consisting of facial gestures and position. Darwin advanced the idea that facial expressions are innate reactions that evolved and possess specific survival value; e.g., a baby's smile evokes nurturing responses in parents. Cross-cultural research reveals that certain facial expressions are universally correlated with such primary emotions as surprise, fear, anger, sadness, and pleasure.

facial expression a facial pattern that is indicative of an emotional response or disorder. Many studies have been made of the meaning of various expressions (e.g., baring the teeth when angry) and the identification of various emotions from photographs made during provocative situations. Other observations indicate that physical conditions sometimes produce characteristic facies, such as the masklike countenance in parkinsonism; and it has also been found that the face can be a mirror of emotional disorder as well, as in the anguished look of the depressive or the exalted expression of some paranoid patients.

facial hemiatrophy a progressive wasting of the tissues on one side of the face, starting around puberty, causing an effect of progeria. F.h. is associated with a sympathetic-nerve disturbance. Also called **Parry-Romberg's syndrome**. Also see ROMBERG'S DISEASE.

facial hemiplegia: See HEMIPLEGIA.

facial nerve the seventh cranial nerve, which is the motor nerve of all facial muscles involved in facial expressions. Branches serve parts of the ear and taste sensory organs. The f.n. is more vulnerable to paralysis disorders than any other cranial nerve. The f.n. is referred to as "cranial nerve VII."

facial talk: See CONDITIONED-REFLEX THERAPY.

facial trophoneurosis = ROMBERGS DISEASE.

facial vision: See ECHOLOCATION.

-facient a combining form meaning making or causing.

facies /fā′shē·ēz/ facial expression. It is often a guide to a patient's state of health or emotions (Latin, "form, face, appearance"). Plural: **facies.** See FACIAL EXPRESSION.

facilitation in environmental psychology, a user-benefit criterion of environmental design. Kinds of f. include behavioral f., as measured by how well a design helps a user of space accomplish performance tasks, and social f., as determined by the adequacy of the setting in providing personal space that permits communication with others without the threats of crowding. Also see BEHAVIORAL F.; SOCIAL F.

facilitator a professionally trained or lay group member who fulfills some or all of the functions of a group leader, e.g., a psychotherapist who leads a therapy group.

facioscapulohumeral muscular dystrophy = LANDOUZY-DÉJÉRINE DYSTROPHY.

fact-giver a person who assumes the role of providing information during a group discussion, e.g., on the question of abortion.

factitious disorders a group of disorders that simulate physical or psychological symptoms which are produced by the individual and are under voluntary control, although they serve hidden psychological purposes. In DSM-III, factitious (artificial, sham) disorders include "factitious disorder with psychological symptoms," "chronic factitious disorder with physical symptoms," and "atypical factitious disorder with physical symptoms." These disorders do not include malingering, in which there is voluntary control but no psychological disturbance. (DSM-III)

factitious disorder with psychological symptoms a disorder in which the individual voluntarily produces severe psychological (often psychotic) symptoms that are not explained by any other mental disorder, and are apparently adopted in order to appear like a psychiatric patient. The symptoms are not feigned, as in malingering, but they usually make up a hodgepodge that does not conform to any standard mental disorder. Moreover, the symptoms become aggravated if the individual is aware of being observed, and others may be added if he or she is asked about them. In addition, if the individual is asked simple questions involving calculations or facts, the answers are usually inexact—a symptom known as Vorbeireden, a German word meaning "talking past the point." See GANSER SYNDROME; PSEUDODEMENTIA. (DSM-III)

factor an underlying influence that accounts in part for variations in individual behavior and is relatively independent of other influences.

factor analysis a mathematical procedure for reducing a table of intercorrelations to a small number of descriptive or explanatory concepts.

E.g., a number of tests of mechanical ability might be intercorrelated and then reduced to a few factors such as fine motor coordination, speed, and attention.

factor-comparison method in industrial psychology, a system of comparing key jobs in terms of factors common to all the jobs. The factors include mental requirements, skill requirements, physical requirements, responsibility, and working conditions.

factorial design an experimental design in which two or more independent variables are manipulated, in order to study their joint and separate influences on a dependent variable.

factorial invariance the identity or similarity of factors across different samples.

factoring the process of performing a FACTOR ANALYSIS. See this entry.

factor-loading in factor analysis, a measure of the correlation between an item and a factor. E.g., in a factor analysis of Rorschach scores, the number of Anatomy responses might have a high f.-l. on a neuroticism factor.

factor matrix a table of factor loadings arrayed into several columns of factors.

factor of uniform density: See LAW OF COMMON FATE.

factor I = FIBRINOGEN.

factor reflection a change of the signs of a set of factor-loadings from positive to negative, or vice versa.

factor rotation the movement of mathematical coordinates through an arc relative to a set of data points. F.r. is one of the steps in factor analysis.

factor theories of learning the concept that learning involves two or more processes or factors—particularly, a mechanical, motor process in conditioning and a comprehension factor in other types of learning.

factor theory of personality an approach to the discovery and measurement of personality components through factor analysis. The components are identified primarily through a statistical study of performance on tests covering various aspects of behavior, as contrasted with an intuitive or purely clinical approach. Through exhaustive application of this method, Eysenck arrived at a three-dimensional typology: introversion-extraversion, neuroticism, and psychoticism. R. B. Cattell's studies have resulted in a hierarchy of traits and states, including, among many others, ego strength, harria, surgency, arousal, and zeppia.

fact-seeker a person who takes the role of seeking further information in relation to specific topics, especially during a group discussion.

facts of life: See SEX OFFENDERS.

faculty psychology a theory that mental processes can be divided into separate specialized abilities which can be developed by mental exercises in the same way that muscles can be strengthened by physical exercises. F.p. was formulated in the 18th century by the Scottish philosophers Thomas Reid and Dugold Stewart who held that will, judgment, perception, conception, memory, etc., could be "explained" simply by referring to these "active powers"; that is, we remember because we possess the faculty of memory.

fad a transient interest, custom, or fashion usually of a trivial nature, which sweeps rapidly through a whole population. Examples are the hula hoop, the ultrashort miniskirt, and Rubik's magic cube. Such fads rarely last more than a year (Bogardus, 1942), but while they exist, they are vivid testimony to the power of mass suggestion, conformity, and publicity. Also see FOOD FADDISM.

fading in operant conditioning, a process of shifting one kind of reinforcement or discriminative stimulus to other, different stimuli by "mixing" the new stimuli with the old, and progressively f. the new stimuli in and the old stimuli out.

Fahr, Theodor German neurologist, 1877–1945. See FAHR'S DISEASE.

Fahr's disease a form of cerebral-artery degeneration marked by calcium deposits that are due to parathyroid dysfunction and hypercalcemia. The disorder often is concentrated in deep cortical gray matter, and obstruction of the vessels occurs most frequently in the cerebral capillaries. Pathologic effects include mental retardation and extrapyramidal disorders.

failure fear = FEAR OF FAILURE.

failure through success a Freudian description of the self-injuring trait of the individual who strives to achieve a goal but renounces it when the goal is within grasp because of the influence of conscience (moral veto), which leads to satisfaction from rejecting success. An example is the case of the woman who waits for a married man to divorce his wife, then withdraws from the marriage agreement when the divorce finally makes marriage possible.

failure-to-grow syndrome failure to grow at a normal rate due to inadequate release of growth hormone. It is a childhood condition that appears to be related, in some cases at least, to parental neglect and emotional deprivation. Secretion of the hormone often returns to normal after a period of emotionally supportive hospital care. Also see FAILURE TO THRIVE.

failure to thrive progressive decline in responsiveness, accompanied by loss of weight and retardation in physical and emotional development, among infants who have been neglected, ignored, or institutionalized. See REACTIVE ATTACHMENT DISORDER OF INFANCY. Also see FAILURE-TO-GROW SYNDROME.

fainting a temporary loss of consciousness due to physical or psychological factors. See SYNCOPE.

faith: See RELIGIOUS F.

faith healing the process of alleviating or attempting to alleviate mental or physical illness through belief in divine intervention or the prayers of a professional faith healer. Also called **faith cure**. Also see MAGICAL THINKING;

VOODOO; SUPERSTITIOUS CONTROL; HEADSHRINKING; HEX DOCTORS.

faking in psychological testing, the tendency of some subjects to (a) "fake good" by choosing answers that create a favorable impression, e.g., in applying for a job or admission to an educational institution, or (b) "fake bad" in order to appear so disturbed or incompetent that they will be exempt from military service or exonerated in a criminal trial.

fallacy a reasoning error that leads to a conclusion that appears true but is actually false; also, a mistaken idea (from Latin *fallacia*, "fraud").

fallectomy a sterilization procedure in which the Fallopian tubes are cut or tied off, or both.

falling sickness = EPILEPSY.

Fallopian-tube pregnancy pregnancy that is marked by implantation of a fertilized ovum in the wall of a Fallopian tube rather than in the lining of the uterus. Also called **tubal pregnancy**.

Fallopian tubes slender fleshy tubes that extend from either side of the uterus to the ovary on the same side. During ovulation, an ovum drops into the open end of the tube and migrates toward the uterus. If coitus occurs at the same time, spermatozoa travel through the uterus and F.t. to meet the ovum and attempt to fertilize it.

Fallopio, Gabriello Italian anatomist, 1523–62. See FALLOPIAN-TUBE PREGNANCY; FALLOPIAN TUBES; FALLECTOMY; GRAAFIAN FOLLICLE; HYSTEROSALPINGOGRAPHY; LAPAROSCOPY; OVULATION; PREGNANCY; SALPINGECTOMY; SALPINGITIS; SPERM ANALYSIS; STERILIZATON; TESTICULAR-FEMINIZATION SYNDROME; TUBAL LIGATION; TUBECTOMY.

Fallot, Etienne Louis Arthur /fälô'/ French physician, 1850–1911. See TETRALOGY OF FALLOT; CARDIAC DISORDERS; HEART DISORDER.

Falret, Jean-Pierre /fälre'/ French psychiatrist, 1794–1870. See FALRET'S DISEASE; DOUBTING.

Falret's disease a form of manic-depressive psychosis marked by a range of emotional oscillation from hyperactivity, excitement, and violence to depression with suicidal tendencies in a recurrent pattern. Also called **circular insanity; cyclic insanity; folie circulaire** /fôlē'sērkēler'/.

false association a Stekel term for the identification by a dreamer of several persons who represent the same love object. The association may be partial and misleading.

false conditioning = PSEUDOCONDITIONING.

false memory = PARAMNESIA.

false negative a valid case that is incorrectly excluded from a group by the test used.

false positive a case that is actually unqualified but mistakenly included in a group.

false pregnancy a rare hysterical condition in which a woman shows all the usual signs of pregnancy even though conception has not taken place: "Everything is there except the child," including absence of menstruation, distended abdomen, breast changes, and morning sickness. The disorder usually occurs in immature women who experience intense unconscious conflicts over child-bearing. Also called **hysterical pregnancy; pseudocyesis.** Also see PREGNANCY FANTASY; PREGNANCY.

falsetto the type of thin, high-pitched voice that occurs when only a reduced surface of the vocal cords is activated by the airstream. In the male, this quality of vocal resonance may represent some voice abnormality.

falsifiability the capacity of an assertion, theory, or statement to be promoted as a truth when in fact it cannot withstand the challenge of scientific testing. For a more specific meaning, see FALSIFIABLE HYPOTHESIS.

falsifiable hypothesis a predictive statement whose outcome can be observed, and can therefore be either confirmed or refuted.

familial amaurotic idiocy = TAY-SACHS DISEASE.

familial amyotrophic dystonic paraplegia a disease marked by progressive muscle wasting, dystonia, and spastic limb weakness. The disorder apparently is hereditary, with 12 members of one family afflicted in three generations. Mental retardation is associated with the disease, poor school performance often preceding signs of muscle impairment.

familial dysautonomia an autosomal-recessive disorder characterized by deficient tear production, excessive sweating, drooling, and blotchy skin. Almost all patients observed have been members of families of Ashkenazi Jews. Skin blotches tend to occur in response to excitement and increase rapidly in size and number. Mental impairment may be associated with the disorder, but some patients have normal or superior intelligence. Also called **Riley-Day syndrome.**

familial factors factors in the family that account for a certain disease or trait. The exact nature, or even existence, of these factors is often a matter of conjecture.

familial hormonal disorder a syndrome associated with mental deficiency, deafness, and ataxia, first observed in 1919 by W. Koennicke. Urinary gonadotropins, estrogen, pregnandiol, and 17-ketosteroids are markedly reduced in the patients, who seldom exceed a mental age of five years. Genitalia are impaired, and female patients may never experience menstruation. The disease is believed to be hereditary.

familial microcephaly: See MICROCEPHALY.

familial neurovisceral lipidosis = G_{M1} GANGLIOSIDOSIS.

familial periodic paralysis a hereditary disorder involving a potassium deficiency that leads to periodic attacks of flaccid paralysis lasting from a few hours to a few days. The attacks begin in adolescence with hunger, thirst, or sweating, and loss of deep reflexes. The condition responds to oral doses of potassium salts.

familial Portuguese polyneuritic amyloidosis = ANDRADE'S SYNDROME.

familial psychosis a psychosis that appears to "run in the family" because it occurs in many or all of its members. This occurrence does not necessarily indicate that the condition is hereditary, since members of the family tend to share a common environment and heritage. See SCHIZOPHRENOGENIC MOTHER.

familial retardation any type of retarded or abnormally slow mental or physical development pattern that tends to occur in certain families at a frequency greater than in the general population. The f.r. trait usually is inherited although a genetic link often is difficult to document. Consanguineous marriages tend to increase the rate of f.r. cases.

familial unconscious according to L. Szondi, an area of the mind that contains our genetic tendencies and through which our "repressed ancestors" direct our behavior, choice of friends, occupation, and relationships with the opposite sex. See FATE ANALYSIS.

familianism a tendency to maintain strong intrafamilial relationships which are culturally transmitted and inherited, leading to a state of extreme family solidarity.

familiar a supernatural spirit that supposedly lives in the body of an animal, or one that like the mythical genii of Muslim demonology is thought to be at the service of the individual who controls it.

family: See CHILD-FOCUSED F.; EXTENDED F.; NUCLEAR F.; OCCUPATIONAL F.; PATHOGENIC F. PATTERN; PATRIARCHAL F.; PSEUDOFAMILY.

family care a type of aftercare in which ex-mental patients (also mental retardates, the elderly, and abused or delinquent children) live with foster families on a temporary or permanent basis. The caretakers usually receive instruction about the special needs of the foster person, such as maintenance medication. The chief advantage of this program is to give these individuals an opportunity to live as normal a life as possible, and to keep them out of institutions. Also called **foster-family care; foster placement.** See GHEEL COLONY.

family constellation the number, characteristics, ages, and relationships of members of a family.

family counseling counseling of parents or other family members by psychologists and social workers, who provide information, emotional support, and guidance on problems faced by the family, such as raising a mentally retarded or physically disabled child, adoption, public assistance, family planning, abortion, and mental disorder in the family. Also see GENETIC COUNSELING.

family incubus a family member who because of physical or mental disability creates a burdensome problem or is depressing to the other members.

family-interaction method a study technique for investigating family behavior by observing the interaction of its members in a controlled situation, such as a structured laboratory.

family method in behavior genetics, the study of the frequency of a trait or a form of mental disorder by determining its occurrence in relatives who share the same genetic background.

family neurosis maladaptive patterns that pervade an entire family; also, a family member's neurotic reactions that are interrelated with the psychopathology of other members of the family on an unconscious level.

family pattern a characteristic quality of the relationship between the parents and between the parents and children in a particular family. Family patterns vary widely in emotional tone and in attitudes of the members toward each other. Some families are warm, others cool; some are extremely close and symbiotic, in others the members keep each other at a distance; some are open to friends and relatives, while others are a closed corporation; in some, one or more children are accepted and loved, and in others one or more children are rejected.

family planning controlling the size of the family, and ultimately the size of the population, especially through the use of birth-control measures for determining the number and spacing of children. Also see POPULATION RESEARCH.

family romance in psychoanalysis, a poetic tale (romance) in which a child pictures himself or herself as born of distinguished parents or as saving the life of illustrious persons who represent the parents. Such fantasies are believed to arise out of the child's need for independence and recognition.

family social work a branch of social work that specializes in helping the individual deal effectively with problems involving relationships with his family and community.

family therapy a form of group psychotherapy in which the family is the therapeutic unit. The method was developed largely by Nathan Ackerman, who maintained that since the family is the "matrix" out of which all human interactions develop, it is the logical locus of therapeutic intervention. The object of f.t. is not merely to improve relationships but to modify home influences that contribute to the disorder of one or more family members. In this process, the therapist helps individual members become aware of their distorted reactions and defensive patterns, and encourages them to communicate more meaningfully and handle their difficulties more constructively. Also see CONJOINT THERAPY.

fanaticism a blind, rigid devotion to a set of extreme beliefs, or an overzealous crusade for a cause. F. "often (but not exclusively) occurs in true paranoia or paranoid schizophrenia" (Eidelberg, *Encyclopedia of Psychoanalysis*, 1968).

Fanconi, Guido /fänkō′nē/ Swiss pediatrician, 1892—. See FANCONI'S ANEMIA.

Fanconi's anemia an autosomal-recessive syndrome characterized by microcephaly, genital hypoplasia, broken and otherwise abnormal chromosomes, hyperpigmented skin, and a high risk of death from cancer. Nearly 40 percent of patients studied had neurologic abnormalities

such as mental retardation, defective hearing, or involuntary overextension of the limbs.

fantasm a vivid image of a person or thing perceived as a disembodied spirit.

fantasmic thinking: See FANTASY.

fantasy a figment of the imagination; a mental image, night dream, or daydream in which our conscious or unconscious wishes and impulses are fulfilled. Also spelled **phantasy**. See ANAL FANTASIES; ANAL-RAPE F.; BEATING FANTASIES; CANNIBALISTIC F.; DAYDREAM; FELLATIO F.; FLIGHT INTO F.; FORCED F.; FOSTER-CHILD F.; HETAERAL F.; INCEST F.; KING-SLAVE F.; NIGHT F.; POMPADOUR F.; PREGNANCY F.; PRIMAL FANTASIES; PROCREATIVE F.; REBIRTH F.; RESCUE F.; SPIDER F.; WOMB F.

fantasy cathexis the investment of psychic energy in images or wishes, or in their sources within the unconscious.

fantasy life a form of daydreaming that permits an illusion of wish-fulfillment, as opposed to thinking that is logical and realistic. Some authors believe that fantasies provide a psychic safety-valve for the abreaction of strong affects.

fantasy period according to E. Ginzberg, the period of early adolescence when future occupation or career is envisioned in fantasies that express inner needs. The f.p. is so named because its formulations occur in the absence of realistic judgments of interests, abilities, and opportunities. However, this stage is a necessary forerunner to the "realistic period." Also see CRYSTALLIZATION.

FAR = FETUS AT RISK.

Farber's lipogranulomatosis a lipid metabolic disorder characterized by the development of nodules and pigmentation of the skin. There is involvement of the upper extremities with arthritic swelling and erosion of the bones. Normal body tissues are infiltrated and replaced by foam cells. Respiratory distress and mental retardation appear at a very early age.

far point the farthest, most remote point at which an object can be seen clearly under conditions of relaxed accommodation.

farsightedness: See HYPEROPIA.

FAS = FETAL ALCOHOL SYNDROME.

fasciculi small bundles of muscle or nerve fibers. Singular: **fasciculus**.

fasciculus cuneatus a bundle of nerve fibers that connects the medulla oblongata with an area of white fibers on the dorsal side of the spinal cord. See MEDULLA OBLONGATA.

fasciculus gracilis a bundle of nerve fibers that extends the pathways of the medulla oblongata into the spinal cord.

fasciculus proprius a bundle of nerve fibers in the spinal cord that connects a series of nearby segments. The fibers are believed to represent primitive connecting links between body segments, inherited from a lower form of vertebrate life.

fascinating gaze a term sometimes used to describe the intense gaze of the hypnotist toward his subject.

fascination the enchantment with a person, object, or activity; enraptured attraction. In psychoanalysis, f. is an infant's primitive attempt to master what is perceived (e.g., a light) by identifying with it; also, the attempt of an insecure individual to identify with a heroic personality in order to feel heroic.

fascinum /fas′inəm/ or /fäs′kinōōm/ an "evil eye" (Latin, "evil eye, jinx, charm"). Certain individuals are believed to possess an "evil eye" that can be used to control and injure or destroy others simply by staring at them.

fasciolus gyrus a brain convolution that is a part of the hippocampal system, appearing as a delicate band of tissue that communicates with a thin sheet of gray matter, the indusium griseum, on the surface of the corpus callosum. It is associated with olfactory functions. Also called **gyrus fasciolaris**.

fascism scale = F SCALE.

fashion the style of art, literature, garments, manners, and customs, which may be transient and irrational but often reflects the mood of the period.

fatal illness a disease or other medical disorder that causes death of the patient.

fate analysis a genetic theory of personality developed by L. Szondi, according to which the life of every individual is governed by a hidden plan determined by latent recessive genes. These genes stem from the "familial unconscious," through which our "repressed ancestors" direct our behavior, our choice of friends, our occupation, and the type of diseases to which we are subject. See SZONDI TEST.

fate neurosis = DESTINY NEUROSIS.

father blues: See MATERNITY BLUES.

father-daughter incest sexual relations between father and daughter, the most common form of incest, and the most frequent among men who have been convicted of sexual offenses.

father figure = FATHER SURROGATE.

father fixation an abnormally strong emotional attachment to the father.

father hypnosis a term used by Ferenczi in support of his view that hypnotic submission is derived from blind obedience, a transference of father fixation. F.h. is associated with fear and mother hypnosis with coaxing. See MOTHER HYPNOSIS.

father ideal the father component of the ego ideal, the other component representing the self.

father in 'mothering' role: See MOTHERING.

father surrogate a substitute father; an individual who takes the place of the real father, performing typical paternal functions and serving as an object of identification and attachment. Also called **father figure; surrogate father**.

fatigue a usually transient state of discomfort and loss of efficiency as a normal reaction to emotional strain, physical exertion, boredom, or lack of rest. Abnormal precipitating factors may include emotional stress, improper diet, or a debilitating disease. A sensory system, such as hearing, may experience f. from overexposure to a stimulus. F. may be localized, involving only certain muscles.

fatigue fear = KOPOPHOBIA.

fatigue studies studies of factors that cause both mental and physical fatigue. F.s. by E. S. Robinson in 1928 indicated that some signs of physical fatigue, e.g., by visitors to museums, actually represented mental stress due to attention overload. The investigator found that when persons were shown a series of copies of paintings, they began to lose interest at the same point in the series that other persons showed signs of fatigue by viewing the original paintings, presented in the same order, in a museum. Signs of physical fatigue were alleviated by providing discontinuity in the environment, with a frequent change of pace in the visual stimuli offered.

fatiguing vigil a form of sleep deprivation in which an experimental subject performs mental work while awake.

fat metabolism the physiological processes whereby fat deposits in the body can be converted into the basic fatty acids which in turn can be converted into glucose molecules to be burned as body fuel. By a somewhat reverse process, carbohydrate molecules are converted to fat for future use as a body fuel. Since one gram of fat contains nine calories, compared with four calories per gram of carbohydrate or protein, fat is nature's most efficient method of storing energy sources. F.m. is under the control of the autonomic nervous system, stored fat being converted to free fatty acids in the bloodstream as a reaction to a variety of stimuli ranging from sexual excitement to sports activity.

fatuity stupidity, dullness, a state of feeblemindedness or dementia.

fausse reconnaissance /fōs′rekōnesäNs′/ an alternative term (French, "false recognition") for PARAMNESIA. See this entry.

faute de mieux /fōt·dəmyœ′/ as used in psychiatry, the choice of a homosexual partner when no partner of the opposite sex is available (French, "for lack of something better"). See ACCIDENTAL HOMOSEXUALITY; SITUATIONAL HOMOSEXUALITY.

faxen psychosis = BUFFOONERY PSYCHOSIS.

F body: See AMNIOCENTESIS.

F distribution a mathematical sampling distribution used for testing the significance of variance ratios, that is, one variance divided by another. It is used for comparing between-groups variance and within-groups variance, as well as for assessing variability differences within any two samples. It was named for R. A. Fisher.

fear an intense emotion aroused by a recognized threat, and involving a feeling of unpleasant tension, a strong impulse to escape, and physiological reactions, such as rapid heartbeat, tensing of the muscles, and, in general, mobilization of the organism for flight or fight. F. is aroused not only by direct danger but by situations or objects that represent this danger. See PHOBIA. Also see ANXIETY.

fear appeal an attempt to influence actions and

attitudes by arousing fear, e.g., fear of cancer, body odor, or embarrassment. Studies show that fear appeals frequently backfire by arousing a "defensive avoidance reaction" in which the subjects tune out the message or dismiss it as "only statistics."

fear drive in the Mowrer-Miller theory of avoidance learning, an unpleasant feeling that motivates the subject to avoid a particular situation.

fear-induced aggression: See ANIMAL AGGRESSION.

fear of darkness normal or pathological horror of darkness or night. This fear is neither universal nor inevitable, but when it occurs, it appears to be associated with feelings of helplessness, inability to see what one is doing, and a sense of unfamiliarity because things look different in the dark. The fear first becomes manifest at about three years of age but may develop into a phobia in which darkness has unconscious symbolic significance or is associated with danger and threat. See ACHLUOPHOBIA. Compare PHENGOPHOBIA.

fear of dismemberment a psychiatric disorder in which the patient believes or fears he may lose a part of his body. The symptoms are associated with strong feelings of persecution and occur in cases of schizophrenia and the involutional psychoses. Also called **dismemberment complex**.

fear of eternity a fear related by Fenichel to concern by a patient that his usual means of orientation may be lost. The concept of eternity involves a loss of the usual significance of time and may represent a subconscious fear of the loss of control over sexual and aggressive impulses.

fear of everything = PANPHOBIA.

fear of failure a dread of failing to measure up to standards and goals set by oneself or by others, including anxiety over academic standing, losing a job, sexual inadequacy, or loss of face and self-esteem. The term **kakorrhaphiophobia** has been applied to a pathological f.o.f.

fear of flying a dread of flying in an airplane or other airborne vehicle, considered by some authors to stem from a fear of sexual relations. Also called **aviophobia**.

fear of rejection a dread of being socially excluded or ostracized; also, a fear of sexual rejection, which is sometimes associated with paraphilias such as pedophilia. See REJECTION.

fear response a response to a threatening or unpleasant situation that is covert and not observable but which is assumed to produce changes in overt behavior that are observable.

fear of strangers the fear of unfamiliar people, commonly occurring in children at around eight months of age, and apparently associated with feelings of insecurity and threat. For pathological fear of strangers, see XENOPHOBIA.

feasibility tests in evaluation research, investigations conducted prior to the main evaluation, to establish properties of response measures and to determine the successfulness of evaluation designs. It is used to establish the validity of response measures, to provide early information on the probable level of program implementation, or to try out new methods for gauging differences in the reception of treatments by members of the target sample.

feather fear = PTERONOPHOBIA.

feature indicator design factors of objects that provide visual cues to feature detectors in the visual cortex. Examples of feature indicators include boundaries between dark and light regions, straight or curved edges or surfaces, and connecting features such as crossbars.

-febr- a combining form relating to fever (Latin *febris*). Adjective: **febrile**.

febriphobia a morbid fear of fever. Also called **pyrexeophobia; pyrexiophobia**.

feces /fē'sēz/ waste matter expelled from the bowels. In psychoanalysis, interest in the f. is one of the earliest expressions of curiosity, and withholding the f. is one of the earliest expressions of the drive for aggression and independence. Also called **excrement; fecal matter**. See ANAL-RETENTION STAGE; ANAL SADISM.

feces-child-penis concept in psychoanalysis, the complex of anal-stage factors that have an influence on the oedipal and castration conflicts, e.g., the infantile association between feces as a part of the body that has been lost and the later concern about loss of the penis.

Fechner, Gustav Theodor /fesh'nər/ German physician and philosopher, 1801–87. To advance his philosophical belief that natural events are an aspect of "soul-substance," F. sought to find a relationship between physical and psychological events through experimental investigations on such subjects as sensations, just-noticeable differences, afterimages, and esthetics, thus establishing the psychophysical approach. See FECHNER'S LAW; FECHNER'S PARADOX; PARALLEL LAW.

Fechner's law a psychophysical formula proposing that the sensation experienced is proportional to the logarithm of the stimulus magnitude. Also see WEBER'S LAW; STEVENS' LAW.

Fechner's paradox the apparent increase in brightness of a figure caused by closing one eye after viewing the figure with both eyes open.

fecundation = IMPREGNATION.

fecundity in demography, the biological capacity to have children. If that capacity has been reduced, the term subfecundity is used, and if it is totally lacking, it is termed sterility. In contrast, **fertility** refers to the number of children actually had by an individual or a population. In biology, these concepts are often reversed: Fecundity refers to the number of children, and fertility refers to the capacity to have children. Also see NET FERTILITY.

Federn, Paul /fā'dərn/ Austrian psychoanalyst, 1871–1950. See COMPLETE MOTHER; EGO BOUNDARIES; EGO PSYCHOTHERAPY; EGO STATE; MORTIDO; ORTHRIOGENESIS.

feeble-mindedness an obsolete term for mental retardation and mental deficiency. Also see AFFECTIVE F.-M.

feedback a direct response by an individual or group to another person's behavior, such as the reactions of an audience to a speaker's remarks; also, the process of receiving afferent impulses from the proprioceptors, which enable us to make accurate movements such as reaching for a pencil; also, the reception of appropriate signals by a regulator, such as a thermostat. See PRO-PRIOCEPTION; PROPRIOCEPTOR. Also see AUDITORY F.; INFORMATION F.; PHYSIOLOGICAL F.; POSITIVE F.; NEGATIVE F.; SOCIAL F.; CLOSED-LOOP F. SYSTEM; DEVIATION-AMPLIFYING F.

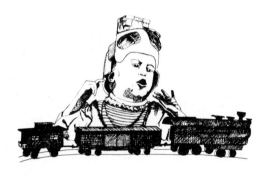

FEEDBACK. Example of use of feedback technique to teach a cerebral-palsy child to hold the head straight; as long as the head is up, the toy train moves.

feedback evaluation = FORMATIVE EVALUATION.

feeding behavior the sequential development of a child's need and skills in taking nourishment, including (a) stimulation and coordination of the sucking and swallowing reflexes in early infancy, (b) adaptation to breast or bottle and to scheduled or self-demand feeding, (c) biting at about the fourth month, (d) anticipatory chewing movements, (e) actual chewing when the teeth are developed, and (f) transferring from finger feeding to the use of various utensils. See SELF-DEMAND SCHEDULE.

feeding problem a behavior disorder among children characterized by refusal to eat at all, by eating an inadequate amount or type of food, or by failure to hold down the food. Problems of this kind are indicative of emotional maladjustment. Also called **feeding disturbance**. See EATING BEHAVIOR.

feeding system a center of the lateral hypothalamus that controls the desire to eat. The urge to eat can be produced by chemical or electrical stimulation of the f.s.

feeding techniques the breast-versus-bottle method of feeding an infant. Various studies (Hernstein, 1963; Taylor, 1969; Newton, 1971) indicate that neither method has an overall advantage for the child, but that the most important factor is an accepting, warm attitude on the part of the mother.

fee-for-service plan a system of charging a patient for each task or procedure authorized with different fees based on the length of time and difficulty of the treatment.

feeling an affective or emotional state, or an intuitive awareness; also, a tactile or temperature sensation.

feeling apperception a Jungian term for an active or passive f.a., the passive undirected form (termed **feeling intuition**) being marked by a content that attracts the feeling while the active form is a directed function, e.g., an act of will.

feelings of unreality: See DEPERSONALIZATION.

feeling-talk: See CONDITIONED-REFLEX THERAPY.

feeling theory of three dimensions: See TRI-DIMENSIONAL THEORY OF FEELING.

feeling tone the affective quality of an experience or object, such as its pleasantness or unpleasantness, or the particular type of emotion it arouses. In consumer psychology, the term applies to the feeling or mood for a particular consumer product created by an advertising appeal. F.t. factors may include color, typography, choice of words, and illustrative matter. Print and broadcast advertising also may modify f.t. through the implied endorsement by a noted personality. At one time, opera singers were portrayed in cigarette-advertising to suggest that tobacco did not harm the throat.

feeling type one of Jung's basic functional types, characterized by a dominance of feeling or affects. The f.t. is included in the rational class of functional types.

Feer, Walther Emil /fār/ Swiss pediatrician, 1864–1955. See FEER'S DISEASE.

Feer's disease a disease affecting mainly infants, who exhibit insomnia, restlessness, anorexia with weight loss, photophobia, pain or paresthesia, loss of teeth, skin discoloration, and sensory loss. The condition has been associated with mercury poisoning from medications, paints, felt, or other products made with mercury. The term is essentially equivalent to ACRODYNIA. See this entry.

Feil, André /fel/ French physician, 1884—. See KLIPPEL-FEIL SYNDROME; BONNEVIE-ULLRICH SYNDROME; NIELSEN'S DISEASE; WILDERVANCK'S SYNDROME.

fellatio the use of the mouth in sexual stimulation of the penis. In psychoanalytic theory, the child's gratification from sucking the nipple (and later the finger) is transferred to the penis. Also called **fellation; penilingus; oral coitus; buccal onanism**. Verb: **to fellate**.

fellatio fantasy the mental image of sexually stimulating the penis with the mouth, or having it stimulated by another person.

fellation = FELLATIO.

fellator a person who performs fellatio. If the person is female, she is preferably called a **fellatrix**.

Fels Parent Behavior Rating Scales scales developed to assess the preschool child's home environment in terms of such factors as child-subordinate versus child-centered, isolation versus close rapport, disapproval versus approval, harmony versus conflict, freedom versus restriction, mild versus severe penalties, uncritical versus critical. Also called **Fels scales of parent behavior**.

female circumcision: See CLITORIDECTOMY.

female ejaculation a lubricating fluid secreted by glands of the vagina during sexual stimulation. The fluid is not a true ejaculate and normally reaches a peak of flow before orgasm, often increasing when preorgasm stimulation is prolonged. The flow also varies with the menstrual cycle, being higher during premenstrual-period coitus.

female genitalia: See GENITALIA.

female-genitals fear = EUROTOPHOBIA.

femaleness the quality of being female in the anatomical or physiological sense; the possession of sexual characteristics derived from the XX (sex) chromosomes. Also see FEMININITY; SUPERFEMALE.

feminine: See FEMININITY.

feminine identification the tendency of the male to adopt feminine characteristics, and in some cases feminine roles. In Adler's view, e.g., feminine traits are softness, tenderness, obedience, and passivity; but such descriptions are culture-bound.

feminine identity an inner sense of affiliation with the female sex.

feminine masochism masochism in male patients who gratify their need to be punished and humiliated by playing the role of a woman in fantasy. In these cases the woman may be pictured as suffering birth pangs or serving as a prostitute against her will.

femininity possession of the secondary sex characteristics of a woman, as contrasted with femaleness, which is determined by the XX chromosomes. The term is also used for a "typically feminine" personality pattern, whether in a female or male. However, there is little agreement today on the description of this pattern, or even whether it exists at all. See MASCULINITY-F. TESTS.

femininity complex in psychoanalysis, the unconscious attempt of the male child to resist castration by the mother by identifying with her and wishing for a vagina and breasts—an expression of "vaginal envy." According to M. Klein (1932), the boy actually dreads the feminine role and may respond to this dread by becoming excessively aggressive. Also see VAGINAL ENVY.

feminism female physiological characteristics in the male such as enlarged breasts due to undersecretion of androgens or oversecretion of estrogens. Also, f. is a pattern of sex-specific female role behavior that is socially oriented rather than related to the female biological functions. F. usually is characterized by activities directed toward political and economic equality with men. See WOMEN'S LIBERATION MOVEMENT.

feminization the process of becoming more feminine, regardless of the gender of the individual.

feminizing-testes syndrome an inherited form of pseudohermaphroditism associated with a defective trait for testosterone response. The typical patient has normal female external genitalia and breasts, a blind vaginal pouch, absence of uterus, and male gonads within the labial folds. The gonads are excised and estrogen therapy is administered to enhance the female appearance. The patient is infertile and does not menstruate.

fenestra ovalis the oval window, or membrane, that separates the middle and inner ears.

fenestra rotunda the round membranous window of the cochlea that equalizes pressures of sounds.

fenestration the surgical procedure in which a substitute window is formed in the bony wall of the middle ear and into the semicircular canal in order to improve hearing in otosclerotic conditions.

Fenichel, Otto Austrian psychoanalyst, 1899–1946. A disciple of Freud, F. accepted his theory of the libido and psychosexual development, but placed special emphasis on disturbing emotional experiences in childhood as the primary causal factor in neuroses (*The Psychoanalytic Theory of Neuroses*, 1945). See BORDERLINE PSYCHOSIS; COPROPHAGIA; FEAR OF ETERNITY; FLIGHT INTO FANTASY; MALIGNANT PSYCHOSIS; MASTERY MOTIVE; PHOBIC CHARACTER; PRECONSCIOUS THINKING; PRIMAL DEPRESSION; SHAMELESSNESS.

feral children children that reportedly have been raised by wild animals and isolated from human contact. For an example, see the WILD BOY OF AVEYRON.

Ferenczi, Sandor /shän'dôr fer'entsē/ Hungarian psychoanalyst, 1873–1933. Starting as an associate and follower of Freud, F. developed a flexible form of psychoanalysis, "active therapy," which was focused on character structure rather than id impulses (instincts). Early in his career he espoused a strict privation philosophy, but it aroused so much hostility in his patients that he switched to a permissive approach that emphasized the healing effect of love and acceptance. See ACTIVE THERAPY; AMBISEXUALITY; FATHER HYPNOSIS; PROTOPSYCHE; PSYCHIC REFLEX ARC; RELAXATION PRINCIPLE; SPHINCTER MORALITY; SUNDAY NEUROSIS.

Féré phenomenon = GALVANIC SKIN RESPONSE.

Fernald method = VAKT.

ferning the development of a fernlike pattern in a specimen of cervical mucus placed on a microscope slide when the hormone estrogen is present in the mucus. The effect usually is observed just before ovulation.

ferric-chloride test one of several laboratory tests used to detect signs of phenylketonuria and other inherited metabolic defects. A piece of filter paper is placed in a baby's diaper to absorb urine. The paper is treated with a ferric-chloride solution which will react with phenylpyruvic acid to turn the paper green if the infant is a possible victim of phenylketonuria. Normally, there is no phenylpyruvic acid in the urine.

Ferry, Erwin Sidney American physicist, 1868–1956. See PORTER'S LAW (also called **Ferry-Porter law**).

fertility: See FECUNDITY.

fertilization = IMPREGNATION.

festinating gait the involuntary gait of the Parkinson patient in which the body leans stiffly forward and the walk becomes a half run (from Latin *festinare*, "to hurry"). Also called **festination**.

Festinger, Leon Amerian psychologist, 1919—. See COGNITIVE DISSONANCE.

fetal activity the activity level of the fetus, which shows low positive correlations with performance on the Gesell maturity tests administered at six months after birth, but inconclusive results on later tests.

fetal alcohol syndrome a group of mental and physical abnormalities, such as microcephaly, mental retardation, hyperactivity, and cardiac and genital anomalies, associated with extreme maternal alcohol intake during pregnancy and occurring in 30 to 50 percent of offspring. Abbrev.: **FAS**.

fetal cephalometry See CEPHALOMETRY.

fetal distress the condition of a fetus whose life or health is threatened by effects of a disease or other disorder originating in the organ systems of the mother. The threat could occur as toxemia of pregnancy, an infectious disease transmitted through the placenta, or an injury that may cause a spontaneous abortion, among various possibilities. Also see FETUS AT RISK.

fetal infection any disease that may affect a fetus as a result of the infectious agent being transmitted from the mother via the placenta. A f.i. usually is caused by a virus, but other agents may include tuberculosis bacteria, the syphilis spirochete, or the toxoplasmosis protozoa. Rubella is a common type of viral f.i., resulting in various kinds of malformations.

fetal-maternal exchange the transfer across the placental barrier of substances required for the maintenance of fetal life and the elimination of its waste products. These include oxygen, water, electrolytes, and urea. Substances of low molecular weight, including thiamine, alcohol, and opiates, cross the placental barrier easily while large molecules do not. Amino acids may cross, but large proteins do not, with the result that a fetus manufactures its own proteins from the mother's amino-acid supply. Some drugs as well as disease organisms such as viruses and syphilis spirochetes may cross the placental barrier to produce congenital defects.

fetal period the final stage of human prenatal development from the eighth or ninth week after conception to the time of birth. The embryonic stage precedes the f.p.

fetal response response of the unborn child to environmental conditions. E.g., there is an increase in the fetal heart rate when the mother smokes, and some investigators claim that there is an increase in activity when the mother is undergoing severe emotional stress. See PRENATAL INFLUENCE.

fetation = PREGNANCY.

fetish a nonsexual object (glove, shoe, handkerchief) or part of the body (foot, lock of hair, ear) that arouses sexual interest or excitement by association or symbolization. Gratification is usually achieved by fondling, kissing, or licking. In anthropology, a f. is an object, such as a talisman or amulet, that embodies a supernatural spirit or exerts magical force. A f. can also be an idea, goal, or mode of behavior that elicits special devotion, e.g., when one makes a f. of success. Also see FETISHISM.

fetishism a psychosexual disorder in which nonliving objects are repeatedly or exclusively used in achieving sexual excitement. Fetishes are most often feminine undergarments, shoes, boots, and occasionally hair or nails, and are frequently associated with a childhood caretaker. See FETISH. Also see PARTIALISM. (DSM-III)

fetishistic cross dressing: See CROSS DRESSING.

fetus: See EMBRYO.

fetus at risk a fetus that has a significant risk of being born with a mental or physical disorder because of known influences observed in the parents or other family members. Examples of parental influences include a mother with diabetes or hypertension. The risk of a mental disease in a child born in a family with no history of mental disease is less than three percent, but the risk may range up to 50 percent in certain cases, e.g., if the defect is a sex-linked recessive trait inherited from the mother's side of the family and the parents are related. Abbrev.: **FAR**. Also see FETAL DISTRESS.

Feuchtersleben, Ernst von /foish′tərsläbən/ Austrian physician, poet, and philosopher, 1806–49. F. was the author of two seminal works on psychiatry (1838 and 1845).

fever fear = FEBRIPHOBIA.

FI = FIXED INTERVAL.

Fiamberti, Adamo Mario /fyämber′tē/ Italian psychiatrist, 1894—. See FIAMBERTI HYPOTHESIS.

Fiamberti hypothesis the theory that schizophrenia results from a nervous-tissue deficiency of acetylcholine, which may be secondary to a toxic or infectious condition.

fiber an elongated threadlike structure which, in a living organism, may be the smallest part of a nerve, muscle, bone, skin, or other organ system.

fibrillary astrogliosis an excess of fibrous neuroglia tissue in the central nervous system. The neuroglia tissue or astroglia is composed of astrocytes.

fibrillary tremor: See TREMOR.

fibrinogen a protein substance in the blood that serves as one of a dozen factors involved in blood clotting. F. is converted to fibrin by an enzyme, thrombin. Fibrin is formed in the first stage of blood clotting and precipitates in the third and fourth stages of a chemical action that requires a total of about five minutes. Also called **factor I**.

fibroma a benign tumor of the connective tissue. Plurals: **fibromas; fibromata**.

fibrositis a rheumatismlike disorder marked by aches, pains, and stiffness in muscles of various body areas. The patients also may show signs of psychologic distress, e.g., tenseness, nervousness, fatigue, and weakness; the condition also seems to be aggravated by excitement or emotional upset.

fiction an Adlerian term for a complex set of lifestyle guidelines that resolve inferiority feelings; also, an imaginary concept that may be accepted for the sake of argument.

fictional finalism Adler's doctrine that human beings are more strongly motivated by the goals and ideals they create for themselves (which he termed fictions), and more influenced by future possibilities, than by past events such as childhood experiences. See INDIVIDUAL PSYCHOLOGY.

fidgetiness a state of increased motor activity associated with anxiety, tics, chorea, or boredom.

fiducial limits = CONFIDENCE LIMITS.

field a complex of personal, physical, and social factors within which a psychological event takes place.

field-cognition mode a combination of perception, memory, and thought that directs the behavior of an individual within his environment.

field defect an abnormality in the normal curvature of a visual field, including tubular vision and total blindness.

field dependence the tendency to respond uncritically to environmental cues, particularly deceptive cues in tasks requiring the performance of simple actions or the identification of familiar elements in unfamiliar contexts. Passivity is associated with f.d., and women tested tend to be more **field dependent** than men. However, in societies where women are more self-reliant, such sex differences diminish sharply; e.g., in Eskimo society no differences were found. See COGNITIVE STYLE. Also see FIELD INDEPENDENCE; FIELD INDEPENDENCE-DEPENDENCE.

field experiment an experiment carried out in a natural "real-world" setting in which subjects are manipulated in some manner and observed for their reactions. Subjects are likely to be unaware of the experiment; e.g., in studies of interpersonal distance, an experimenter may randomly select subjects in a public setting, deliberately jostle or crowd them, and record their reactions.

field force a term used by K. Lewin for a manifestation of drive or energy in relation to the entire psychological field.

field independence the capacity to orient oneself correctly in spite of deceptive environmental cues; the ability to correctly identify familiar elements in unfamiliar contexts. Analytic ability, high achievement motivation, and an active coping style are positively correlated. An individual's degree of f.i. or field dependence is an aspect of his COGNITIVE STYLE. See this entry. Also see FIELD DEPENDENCE; FIELD INDEPENDENCE-DEPENDENCE.

field independence-dependence a cognitive style in which the individual is able to think independently of the environment at one time, and is dependent on environmental stimuli at another. Also see FIELD DEPENDENCE; FIELD INDEPENDENCE.

field of consciousness the total awareness of an individual at a given time.

field of regard the total space and all the objects within that space that can be seen at one time by the moving eye.

field properties the environmental factors that surround and influence a living organism.

field research research conducted outside the laboratory, in a natural social or other setting.

field space: See FIELD THEORY.

field structure the pattern, distribution, or hierarchy of parts of a psychological field, or life space (K. Lewin).

field teacher: See FIELD WORK.

field theory K. Lewin's systematic approach, which describes behavior in terms of patterns of dynamic interrelationships between the individual and the total situation—psychological, social, and physical—in which he is embedded. The situation is termed the field space or life space, and the dynamic interactions are conceived as forces with positive or negative valences, represented diagrammatically as vector lines. The theory attempts to do justice to the totality, or Gestalt, of human experience, and the changing tensions which are constantly occurring in that totality. See CONFLICT; VALENCE; LIFE SPACE.

field work in clinical social-work education, a practicum in which the student supplements and applies classroom theory by taking responsibility for actual cases in psychiatric, medical, or social agencies, under the tutelage of experienced, qualified supervisors, or **field teachers**.

Fiessinger, Noël French physician, 1881–1946. See STEVENS-JOHNSON SYNDROME (also called **Fiessinger-Rendu syndrome**).

fifth cranial nerve = TRIGEMINAL NERVE.

fight-flight reaction according to the physiologist Walter Cannon (1915), a reaction to a stressful situation in which the sympathetic nervous system mobilizes the organism, and puts it on a "war footing," either to fight back or to flee. Also called **fight-or-flight response**.

figural aftereffect a Gestalt-perceptual phenomenon in which a shift of vision from a first figure superimposes its image on a second figure.

figural cohesion a tendency for parts of a figure to

be perceived as a whole figure even if the parts are disjointed (Gestalt psychology). Also see CLOSURE.

figurative knowledge Piaget's term for knowledge acquired by attending to and remembering specific perceptual features, words, or facts, e.g., the ability to recall vocabulary, dates, colors, shapes, impressions, and other details. Piagetians believe that f.k. is overemphasized in schools and intelligence tests. Compare OPERATIVE KNOWLEDGE.

figure-drawing test a test in which the subject draws a human figure. It is used as a measure of intellectual development or as a projective technique. See GOODENOUGH DRAW-A-MAN TEST; MACHOVER DRAW-A-PERSON TEST; ROSENBERG DRAW-A-PERSON TECHNIQUE; LEVY DRAW-AND-TELL-A-STORY TECHNIQUE.

figure-ground the principle that perceptions have two parts: a figure that stands out in good contour and an indistinct, homogeneous ground.

figure-ground distortion the inability to focus on an object without having its setting interfere with its perception. See FIGURE-GROUND PERCEPTION.

figure-ground perception the ability to attend to and discriminate properly between figure and ground in a visual field presentation. An impairment in this perceptual skill can seriously affect a child's ability to learn.

filial-regression law: See LAW OF FILIAL REGRESSION.

film color a filmlike texture-free soft color that lacks localization, as contrasted with the color of a surface.

filth fear = DIRT PHOBIA.

fimbria a part of the hippocampal-system of the brain, consisting of a flattened band of fibers along the surface of the hippocampus. The f. continues as the crura of the fornix passing beneath the corpus callosum.

final common path a motoneuron that serves as a funnel for the routing of a variety of different nerve impulses from many reflex arcs. Motoneurons in general carry impulses from two or more arcs rather than serving one reflex arc exclusively.

finalism: See TELEOLOGY; FICTIONAL F.

final tendency the ultimate objective of a neurosis. According to Stekel and Adler, every neurosis has a central idea around which motives group themselves. It is the objective of the therapist to uncover the f.t. as early as possible.

Finch, Stuart McIntyre American child psychologist, 1919—. See ADOLESCENT PSYCHOTHERAPY.

fine motor activities the selected activities used to develop effective usage of the small muscles needed for eye-hand coordination, speaking, and eye movements.

Fine Motor Composite: See BRUININKS-OSERETSKY TEST OF MOTOR PROFICIENCY.

fine motor skills the ability to coordinate precise movements necessary for such activities as writing, tracing, catching, throwing, cutting, and visual tracking.

fine tremor: See TREMOR.

finger agnosia a type of body-image disorder in which the patient has difficulty in discriminating between different kinds of tactual stimuli applied to the fingers. If the patient's fingers are touched in two places, e.g., the patient may be unable to judge without visual clues whether the sensations come from the same finger or from two different fingers.

finger-biting behavior a form of compulsive self-mutilation observed particularly in children with Lesch-Nyhan syndrome, in which the finger-biting is usually accompanied by **lip-biting**.

finger-nose test a neurological test used to observe a child's facility in alternating movements by having him repeatedly touch a finger to his nose and then to the examiner's finger.

finger painting a type of projective test in which the subject paints on a surface with his fingers; also, a children's play activity which gives them a chance to "mess" and express themselves freely.

finger spelling a form of symbolized language; a manual alphabet used to spell out words for the deaf.

Fink-Green-Bender test: See DOUBLE-SIMULTANEOUS TACTILE SENSATION.

fire phobia = PYROPHOBIA.

fire-setting behavior the tendency to set fires as an expression of aggressiveness, defiance, or revenge by an individual with an antisocial-personality disorder or -conduct disorder, by a schizophrenic responding to delusions or hallucinations, or by an individual with an organic mental disorder who fails to appreciate the consequences of the act. In DSM-III, these forms of fire-setting are distinguished from a persistent compulsion to set fires, termed PYROMANIA. See this entry.

firing the act of initiating a nervous impulse.

first admission a patient admitted for the first time to a hospital for the mentally disturbed or retarded.

first aid emergency medical care that is rendered a victim of an accident or sudden illness until the services of a physician or other health professional can be obtained. The objective is to preserve life signs by preventing heavy loss of blood, and to maintain breathing, prevent further injury, prevent shock, inspire confidence, and do no more than necessary until a physician can take charge.

first cause: See CREATIVE SELF.

first cranial nerve = OLFACTORY NERVE.

first-degree burns: See BURN INJURIES.

first impressions the primacy effect in social relationships; the tendency to regard one's early perceptions of a person as more valid than later information which, when contradicting f.i., may be discounted or rationalized away. See PRIMACY EFFECT.

first negative phase: See SECOND NEGATIVE PHASE.

first phase of repression: See PRIMARY REPRESSION.

first-rank symptoms a system of differential diagnosis of schizophrenia based on the division of symptoms into five categories. The categories include hallucinations, changes in thought process, delusional perceptions, somatic passivity, and other external impositions. The system was introduced by Kurt Schneider and has been tested in nine countries where nearly 60 percent of schizophrenia patients were found to show f.-r.s.

first signaling system a term used by Pavlov to refer to the system of immediate environmental stimuli that are responsible for evoking animal and human behavior. According to Pavlov, the f.s.s. forms the basis of the SECOND SIGNALING SYSTEM. See this entry. Also see SIGNALING SYSTEM. The f.s.s. is also called **sensory-conditioning system; primary signaling system; primary signal system**.

Fisch, L. English physician, fl. 1956. See FISCH-RENWICK SYNDROME.

Fischer, Liselotte American psychologist, fl. 1940. See BOLGAR-FISCHER WORLD TEST.

Fisch-Renwick syndrome a disorder marked by congenital deafness, hypertelorism, a high palatal arch, and a white forelock of hair. The condition may be a variation of the Klein-Waardenburg syndrome.

Fisher, Ronald Aylmer English statistician and geneticist, 1890–1962. See FISHER EXACT TEST; F DISTRIBUTION; ANALYSIS OF VARIANCE.

Fisher exact test a statistical test giving the exact probability of departure from chance for data in a fourfold contingency table.

fish fear = ICHTHYOPHOBIA.

fission the reproduction of a cell or one-celled animal by splitting into two independent parts.

fissure a cleft or indentation in a surface. The cerebral cortex contains numerous fissures which have the effect of increasing the actual surface of the brain. Also called **sulcus**.

fissure of Rolando a prominent fissure that makes a double-S-shaped pattern along the lateral surface of the hemisphere from a point beginning near the top of the medial surface. It marks the border between the frontal and parietal lobes. Also called **central fissure; central sulcus; Rolandic fissure**.

fissure of Sylvius a well-defined fissure that runs along the lateral surface of the cerebral cortex, separating the frontal and parietal areas from the temporal region. It is the most prominent sulcus on the surface of the cortex and isolates much of the temporal lobe. Also called **lateral fissure; lateral sulcus; Sylvian fissure**.

fistula an abnormal passageway between two internal organs or between an internal organ and the outside of the body. A f. may develop as a result of an injury, such as a gunshot wound, as a congenital defect, as an effect of an abcess, or as a result of a surgical procedure. A **craniosinus f.** is marked by loss of cerebrospinal fluid through a sinus into the nose.

fitness for trial competence to stand trial, as determined by the judge on the basis of the defendant's ability to understand the nature of the proceedings if he is being tried, and to cooperate with counsel and plead to the charges. If the question of mental illness is raised, the determination is usually based on a psychiatric examination.

five-day hospital a program of partial hospitalization in which the mental patient is treated on an in-patient basis during the week but returns to his family on weekends. The f.-d.h. is a transitional arrangement designed to bridge the gap between hospital and community life for patients who are not acutely ill.

5-HIAA; five-hydroxyindoleacetic acid = HIAA.

5-hydroxytryptamine = SEROTONIN.

5-hydroxytryptophan: See HYDROXYTRYPTOPHAN.

five-to-seven shift the striking progress in all aspects of children's development between ages five and seven when very significant advances in physical growth, motor coordination, reasoning capacity, linguistic ability, and socioemotional development occur. Among the many observable changes are a decline in egocentrism, the emerging ability to adopt the perspective of others, and a vastly improved competence in communication. According to S. White, the f.-t.-s.s. may represent a basic reorganization in all aspects of the child's life. This view is supported by cross-cultural evidence pointing to a transition process equivalent to the f.-t.-s.s. in children from disparate cultures. (H. Gardner, *Developmental Psychology*, 1978)

fixation in general, obsessive preoccupation with a single idea, impulse or aim, as in an "idée fixe." In psychoanalysis, f. is persistence of an early psychosexual stage, or inappropriate attachment to an early psychosexual object or mode of gratification, such as anal or oral activity. Also, f. is the focusing of both eyes on a single object, or looking quickly and accurately from one object, or word, to another, as in reading; also, the process of strengthening a habit until it becomes "fixed."

fixation hysteria a type of conversion hysteria in which the area or function affected is one that is or has been injured or diseased.

fixation line: See LINE OF FIXATION.

fixation of affect the retention of a feeling or affect after it is no longer appropriate.

fixation pause a period during which the eyes are focused directly on an object.

fixed-action pattern a system of response to stimuli through a neural pathway that involves sensory, cortical, and hypothalamic connections. Because of a presumably preconnected route to be followed by impulses, it is believed a particular stimulus will elicit a predictable response. The term may be applied to instinctive behavior patterns that lack reinforcement.

fixed alternative = CLOSED-ENDED QUESTION.

fixed idea: See IDÉE FIXE.

fixed interval a schedule in which the first response after a set interval has elapsed is reinforced. FI = 3 minutes means that reinforcement is given to the first response occurring at least three minutes after a previous reinforcement. Abbrev.: **FI**.

fixed-interval reinforcement schedule in operant conditioning, a type of interval reinforcement in which the reinforcement or reward is presented at the end of regular, consecutive intervals, e.g., every 30 seconds. See INTERVAL REINFORCEMENT. Compare VARIABLE-INTERVAL REINFORCEMENT SCHEDULE.

fixed model an experimental paradigm used in the analysis of variance, in which the experimenter sets or fixes the independent variables, instead of sampling them at random. Also see RANDOM MODEL; MIXED MODEL.

fixedness: See FUNCTIONAL F.

fixed ratio a schedule in which reinforcement is given after a specified number of responses. FR = 50 means that reinforcement is given after 50 responses have occurred. Abbrev.: **FR**.

fixed-ratio reinforcement schedule in operant conditioning, a type of intermittent-reinforcement schedule in which the reward is consistently presented after the subject makes a fixed number of correct responses; e.g., food might be delivered following every fifth correct response. See RATIO-REINFORCEMENT. Compare VARIABLE-RATIO REINFORCEMENT SCHEDULE.

fl. an abbreviation of "fluid," used, e.g., in prescriptions.

flaccid soft or flabby, usually applied to an absence of muscle tone as in muscular atrophy.

flaccid paralysis a paralysis with loss of tonus and absence of reflexes producing a weak, flabby condition in the affected areas.

flagellantism the practice of whipping or submitting to whippings as a means of sexual arousal and gratification; also, flogging one's self, or being flogged, as a religious discipline. See FLAGELLATION.

flagellation whipping another person or oneself, or submitting to whipping as a religious ritual. F. may be a form of penitence or a means of achieving sexual excitement.

flapping tremor = ASTERIXIS.

flash: See RUSH.

flashback hallucinosis spontaneous recurrence, after a drug-free period, of predominantly visual hallucinations similar to those experienced during an acute toxic episode. Flashbacks are most common after repeated ingestion of LSD, and may occur months after the last use. Popularly called **flashbacks**.

flat affect absence or near absence of emotional response to any situation or event; extreme apathy. F.a. is a common schizophrenic symptom. Also called **emotional flatness; flattening of affect; flatness of affect; flattened affect**.

flatfoot a pedal, or foot, deformity in which one or more of the supporting arches is significantly lower than normal. Kinds of f. include **relaxed f.**, in which the arch is lowered only when weightbearing, **rigid f.**, caused by ankylosis, **transverse f.**, from lowering of the transverse arch, and **spasmodic f.**, caused by a contraction of the peroneal muscle. Also called **pes planus**.

flatness of affect; flattened affect; flattening of affect = FLAT AFFECT.

Flaubert, Gustave /flōber'/ French novelist, 1821 –80. See BOVARISM.

-flav-; -flavo- a combining form meaning yellow (Latin *flavus*).

flavor a sensation produced by a combination of aroma, taste, and texture, involving olfactory, gustatory, and tactile sense organs.

fldxt. an abbreviation used in prescriptions, meaning "fluid extract" (Latin *fluidextractum*).

Fleischer, Richard /flī'shər/ German physician, 1848–1909. See HEPATOLENTICULAR DEGENERATION (there: **Kaiser-Fleischer ring**).

flexibilitas cerea = CATALEPSY.

flexible work hours a work schedule that permits employees to determine the hours worked per day, as long as they work during certain **core hours**, and for a specified number of hours per week. The purpose is to enable them to adjust their schedule to commuting, family, school, or shopping demands. Also called **flextime; flexitime**.

flexion contractures a manifestation of arthrogryposis multiplex congenita, or crooked-joint disorder, in which an infant's arms and legs are fixed in a bent position. The condition may be accompanied by other abnormalities, e.g., mental retardation. In the absence of other physical anomalies, the child often will respond to physical therapy and eventually have normal use of the arms and legs. Also see ARTHROGRYPOSIS MULTIPLEX CONGENITA.

flexion reflex any reflexive response by a limb or part of a limb in which the movement is toward the body. A f.r. often is a reaction to a painful or intense stimulus. Compare EXTENSION REFLEX.

flexion reflex of the leg a deep-reflex response produced by having the patient bend his knee, after which the examiner grasps the tendons of the semimembranosus and semitendinosus muscles with his fingers, and taps the fingers. The muscles contract and flex the leg.

flexitime = FLEXIBLE WORK HOURS.

flexor muscle a muscle that makes a limb bend, such as the biceps muscle of the upper arm. Compare EXTENSOR MUSCLE.

flextime = FLEXIBLE WORK HOURS.

flicker discrimination the ability to perceive a change in brightness of a light source. The ability varies with the frequency of alternating changes in brightness until a point called critical flicker frequency, or fusion frequency, is reached when the observer sees only an apparently steady level of brightness.

flicker fusion an illusion produced by a flickering light source when the rate of flickering is so rapid that the light pulses seem to fuse into a continuous illumination. See CRITICAL FLICKER FREQUENCY.

flicker stimulus a periodically changing visual or auditory stimulus that produces a rapidly alternating sensation.

flight fear = FEAR OF FLYING.

flight from reality withdrawal into inactivity, detachment, or fantasy as an unconscious defense against anxiety; also, a retreat into psychotic behavior as a means of escaping real or fancied problems.

flight into disease = FLIGHT INTO ILLNESS.

flight into fantasy a defensive behavior in which individuals, "fearing their impulses, withdraw and become hypoactive; they feel that as long as they limit themselves to daydreaming, they may be sure that their frightening ideas will not bring about real injury" (Fenichel, *The Psychoanalytic Theory of Neurosis*, 1945).

flight into health in psychoanalysis, an unconscious defense in which a patient gives up his or her symptoms and appears healthy, at least temporarily, in order to avoid further probing and the unpleasant truths it reveals. Also called **transference cure; transference remission**.

flight into illness a tendency to exaggerate minor physical complaints (usually without organic pathology), as an unconscious means of avoiding stressful situations and feelings. Also called **flight into disease; escape into illness**. See HYPOCHONDRIASIS; CONVERSION DISORDER.

flight into reality a defensive reaction in which the individual becomes overinvolved in activity and "busywork" as an unconscious means of avoiding threatening situations or painful thoughts and feelings.

flight of colors an aftersensation of a bright light manifested by a succession of color images.

flight of ideas a disturbance in thinking consisting of a rapid succession of superficially related ideas; a constant series of digressions in the flow of thought observed primarily in acute manic states, and more occasionally in schizophrenia. Also called **topical flight**. See PRESSURE OF SPEECH; PRESSURE OF ACTIVITY.

flippancy in psychiatry, a defensive attitude in which serious problems are avoided or glossed over by taking them lightly.

floaters: See DETACHED RETINA.

floating transference in psychoanalysis, the positive feelings of the patient toward the analyst and analytic situation that occur spontaneously at the beginning of the process. Also called **floating positive**.

floccillation aimless plucking at clothing or bed clothes common in senile dementia, delirium, and high fever (from Latin *floccus*, "little tuft"). Also called **carphology**.

flogging-fear = MASTIGOPHOBIA.

flogging the dead horse a propaganda technique in which the speaker or writer attempts to create an atmosphere of acceptance by starting his message with trite statements designed to elicit enthusiastic agreement.

flood fear = ANTLOPHOBIA.

flooding a behavior-therapy technique in which the individual is exposed directly to a maximum-intensity fear-producing situation without any graduated approach. Also see IMPLOSIVE THERAPY.

floor effect the inability of a test to measure or discriminate below a certain point, usually because its items are too difficult. Compare CEILING EFFECT.

Flourens, Pierre /floŏräNs'/ French physiologist, 1794–1867. In opposition to Franz Joseph Gall's prevailing theory, which localized specific "faculties" in specific parts of the cerebrum, F. performed experiments that appeared to show that the entire cerebrum is involved in thought and volition, and that the reflexes, on the other hand, remain operative if the cerebrum is removed.

flow chart a step-by-step, chronological description of experimental procedures or, in computers, of information-processing; a diagram that presents a visual outline of the orderly progression or sequence of an activity that has been broken down into component features. A f.c. may include possible options and indicate consequences.

flower-spray ending a type of nerve-fiber ending in a muscle spindle in which the fiber spreads into numerous endings among various muscle fibers. Compare ANULOSPIRAL ENDING.

fluctuation of attention sensory clearness that waxes and wanes despite constant stimulation.

fluency the ability to rapidly think of and easily produce words and their associations.

fluid abilities abilities, such as memory span and mental quickness, that are functionally related to physiological condition and maturation. Thus, f.a. improve during childhood and deteriorate in old age. Compare CRYSTALLIZED ABILITIES.

flukes: See SCHISTOSOMIASIS.

fluphenazine; fluphenazine enanthate; fluphenazine hydrochloride: See PHENOTHIAZINES.

flurazepam; flurazepam dihydrochloride: See BENZODIAZEPINES.

flurothyl = HEXAFLUORODIETHYL ETHER.

fly agaric common name for the mushroom Amanita muscaria, so called because it contains a drug that puts flies in a stupor for several hours. Effects on humans range from euphoria through hallucinations to violent behavior. F.a. has been identified as the drug taken by Norse berserkers before battle and as the mushroom eaten by Alice in Wonderland before she experienced macroscopia. The active ingredient of f.a. is muscarine. Also called **soma**.

flying flies: See MOUCHES VOLANTES.

flying saucers: See UFOS.

Flynn-Aird syndrome a hereditary disorder marked by dementia, ataxia, muscle wasting, skin atrophy, and visual problems, as well as bilateral nerve deafness. Blindness, myopia, and bilateral cataracts are among the ocular abnormalities. The condition is believed to be associated with an autosomal-dominant gene, with 15 members of one family afflicted over a span of five generations.

focal-conflict theory a theory developed by Thomas French (1952) which interprets currently experienced personality conflicts in terms of the individual's attempts to solve conflicts that originated very early in life.

focal degeneration the development of a lesion or dysfunction in a specific area of brain tissue. The f.d. may remain limited in focus or degenerate further into neighboring regions, as in cases of Jacksonian seizures. F.d. usually is a causative factor in limited mental disorders, such as a particular form of aphasia or apraxia.

focal dermal hypoplasia = GOLTZ' SYNDROME.

focal epilepsy: See JACKSONIAN EPILEPSY.

focal pathology the study of changes in body tissues and organs involved in a disease at the focal point of the diseased area.

focal psychotherapy brief therapy aimed at the relief of a single symptom, such as homosexual anxiety or feelings of guilt, and not involving a depth approach.

focus the concentration or centering of attention on a stimulus (Latin, "fireplace"). Plurals: **focuses; foci** /fō′sī/ or /fō′kē/.

focused analysis a form of orthodox psychoanalysis in which interpretations are focused on a specific area of the patient's problem, as opposed to **expectant analysis** in which there may be a gradual free-floating unfolding of the patient's psyche. Also called **directed analysis**.

focusing in experiential psychotherapy, a process in which the patient remains silent for a period of time in order to allow himself to experience an entire problem globally, and get in touch with his deeper feelings about it. See EXPERIENTIAL PSYCHOTHERAPY.

focusing mechanism a system of ciliary muscles, lens elasticity, and ocular-fluid pressure that enables the eye to focus an image sharply on the retina. The natural shape of the lens is spherical, but it is partly flattened by the fluid pressure when the ciliary muscles are relaxed to observe distant objects.

Foerster: See FÖRSTER.

fog fear = HOMICHLOPHOBIA.

folie à cinq /fōlē′äseNk′/ a rare paranoid disorder in which five people, usually members of the same family, share the same delusional system. See SHARED PARANOID DISORDER.

folie à deux /fōlē′ädœ′/ a rare psychotic disorder in which two (and occasionally more) intimately related persons simultaneously share identical delusions. The usual pattern reveals a dominant partner who transfers his paranoid delusions to the submissive, suggestible partner. The pair is most commonly comprised of two sisters, a husband and wife, or a mother and child. F.à d. is a psychosis of association. Also called **communicated psychosis; induced psychosis; double insanity**. For the DSM-III description of this disorder, see SHARED PARANOID DISORDER.

folie à double forme /fōlē′ädo͞ob′ləfôrm′/ an obsolete term for bipolar disorders.

folie à trois /fōlē′ätrô·ä′/ a rare psychotic disorder or psychosis of association in which three intimately related persons simultaneously share identical delusions. Also called **triple insanity**. See FOLIE À DEUX.

folie circulaire = FALRET'S DISEASE.

folie des grandeurs /fōlē′degräNdœr′/ a French equivalent of megalomania.

folie des persécutions /fōlē′depersäkēsyôN′/ a French equivalent of paranoid psychosis.

folie du doute = DOUBTING MANIA.

folie du pourquoi /fōlē′dēpo͞orkô·ä′/ a French term, meaning literally a "craze of why" or question-asking insanity, a form of obsessive-compulsive behavior in which a patient has an abnormal urge to ask questions.

folie morale /fōlē′môräl′/ a French equivalent of MORAL INSANITY. See this entry. Also see ACQUIRED F.M.

folklore the traditions, beliefs, myths, legends, customs, tales, and songs that endure in a specific culture because they are transmitted from generation to generation.

folk psychiatry the diagnosis and treatment of behavioral disorders by techniques that are appropriate to a cultural or ethnic group. The techniques may be effective even though they are not based on scientific procedures. However, the efficacy of the system often can be explained in terms of modern psychiatry. In a Puerto Rican centro ritual, e.g., the medium may sing songs, drink special beverages, and blow tobacco smoke toward the patient. But the medium meanwhile seeks the cause of the behavioral problem by asking the patient about the content of his dreams, about any financial difficulties, sex problems, family concerns, and so on, until a diagnosis is possible from the information obtained. The treatment may be a form of exorcism, or the assignment of therapeutic duties or tasks that help restore self-esteem. The term also applies to the study of folklore, including rituals, magic, and fairy tales, as a source of insight into psychopathology observed in literate societies.

folk psychology a branch of psychology that deals with nonliterate or primitive societies, studying their customs, beliefs, legends, religious behavior, folk remedies, and the activities of folk healers.

folk soul a term used to identify a transcendental group mind or collective consciousness that influences the behavior of individuals within the group.

folkways the traditional modes of behavior in a designated culture or society.

follicle-stimulating hormone a hormone secreted by the anterior pituitary portion of the hypothalamus, stimulating the growth of follicles that encase the ova in the ovary. The follicles in turn produce estrogen which, through a physiological feedback mechanism, reduces the secretion of the f.-s.h. The same hormone in the male stimulates the development of spermatozoa in the testis. Abbrev.: **FSH**. See ESTROGEN.

Fölling test a diagnostic test for phenylketonuria devised by Asbjorn Fölling in Oslo, in which the urine turns olive green in response to ten percent ferric chloride. The test has now been replaced by more effective tests, since affected children do not excrete detectable amounts of phenylpyruvic acid until irreversible brain damage has occurred.

following behavior a species-specific trait of certain young animals that run or swim after a parent or surrogate parent. The characteristic is a manifestation of IMPRINTING. See this entry.

follow-through a research technique in which the investigator examines experimental and control subjects in childhood and again at intervals until they reach the age at which outcomes are measured.

follow-up counseling the measures taken by a counselor or clinician in helping the student or client with on-going problems or new manifestations of the original problems. The term also refers to evaluation of the client's progress and the effectiveness of counseling to date.

follow-up history: See CATAMNESIS.

follow-up study a study of discharged patients during an extended period, for such purposes as determining if rehabilitation efforts are continuing, assessing the effectiveness of treatment, gauging the patient's adjustment to the community, and detecting indications of relapse. The term is also used for long-term study of experimental subjects to see if the effects of the experimental conditions are lasting.

fontanelle /-nel'/ a soft, membrane-covered area in the incompletely ossified skull of an infant. Also spelled **fontanel**.

food faddism in psychiatry, strange or inappropriate food patterns and habits resulting from pathological modes of thinking. Individuals exhibiting f.f. are convinced that certain foods are beneficial and others extremely harmful, and give bizarre or complex theories to back up their beliefs.

food fear = SITOPHOBIA.

food-intake regulation a form of behavior observed in some animals that adjust their daily intake of calories according to the temperature of the environment, energy expended at various tasks, and other factors, so that calorie intake and calorie loss are constantly in balance.

food preferences a behavior pattern in which organisms prefer the foods they need for normal body functions. However, experiments usually show that subjects tend to develop habits that override preferences based on bodily require-

ments. An example is the habit of preferring sugar although it is not required by the body in order to function normally. Also see SELF-SELECTION OF DIET.

food-satiation theory the principle that cells in the ventromedial nucleus of the hypothalamus induce an animal to stop eating after a predetermined amount of food has been consumed. Injury to the satiety center is associated with an urge to continue eating beyond the normal point of satiety.

food self-selection: See SELF-SELECTION OF DIET.

food therapy a behavior-therapy technique in which food is used as reinforcement. E.g., a child who fears doctors is given a candy each time he pretends to have a doll stay at a doctor's office. Similarly, if a psychotic patient insists on wearing all his clothing at once, he may be denied access to the dining room until he dresses appropriately.

footcandle one illumination unit; the amount of light falling upon an area of one square foot placed at a distance of one foot from a light of the intensity of one INTERNATIONAL CANDLE. See this entry.

foot-dragging an abnormal-gait pattern of a patient suffering from paretic leg muscles. The patient may walk in a shuffling manner or appear to literally haul or push the defective leg forward while walking.

foot drop a characteristic of certain types of neuromuscular disorders, such as paralysis of the muscles that control movement of the foot or toes. The affected foot may slap against the floor or ground and the patient may depend upon the sound of the foot hitting the walking surface as a signal that the foot is on the ground. The condition also may result from a severed tendon, and from leprosy. The f.d. gait sometimes is called a **steppage gait**.

footedness: See LATERALIZATION.

foot fetishism: See RETIFISM.

foot-in-the-door effect the tendency of a subject who accommodates a minor request to yield to a more sizable request than a subject who is approached with the sizable request from the start. Also see DOOR-IN-THE-FACE EFFECT.

foramen magnum a large opening at the base of the skull through which the spinal cord and the left and right vertebral arteries, as well as other tissues, pass between the neck and the interior of the skull.

foraminotomy a surgical procedure performed to free the nerve roots in patients afflicted by spinal compression. F. involves the removal of a portion of the intervertebral foramen, usually by enlarging the opening above the nerve root. The procedure relieves such disorders as paresthesias, weakness in the lower limbs, pain in the lower back, and in some cases paraplegia. Also see LAMINECTOMY.

Forbes, Gilbert Burnett American pediatrician, 1915—. See CORI'S DISEASE (also called **Cori-Forbes disease**).

forced-choice test = FORCED-RESPONSE TEST.

forced fantasy a fantasy that has been forced to surface by the analyst.

forced-response test an examination that provides the student with fixed responses from which he must choose an answer, e.g., a multiple-choice or matching test. This type of test is sometimes termed **objective test**. Also called **forced-choice test**. Compare FREE-RESPONSE TEST.

forced treatment therapy administered to a patient against his will, particularly unusual or hazardous treatment, specified by the Wyatt v. Stickney decision of 1972 as lobotomy, electroconvulsive therapy, and aversive-reinforcement conditioning. Also called **coercive treatment; enforced treatment**. Also see RIGHT TO REFUSE TREATMENT; CONSUMERISM.

forceps injury a congenital defect, temporary or permanent, induced by the use of forceps to extract a newborn infant from the mother's uterus during labor. F.i. is one of the causes of cerebral palsy, a disorder in which 85 percent of the cases are due to neurologic damage during gestation or delivery.

forceps major = POSTERIOR FORCEPS.

forceps minor = ANTERIOR FORCEPS.

forebrain the part of the brain that includes the cerebral hemispheres plus the basal ganglia, olfactory bulb and olfactory tracts, third ventricle, thalamus, hypothalamus, pituitary bodies, mammillary bodies, optic tracts, and retinas. Collectively, those tissues control virtually all sensation and perception, emotion, motivation, language, learning, and thinking. Also called **prosencephalon**.

foreconscious = PRECONSCIOUS.

foreign accent = BARBARALALIA.

Forel, Auguste-Henri /fôrel'/ Swiss neurologist, 1848–1931. See SUBTHALAMUS (there: **fields of Forel**).

foremilk: See COLOSTRUM.

forensic psychiatry a field of psychiatry concerned with legal issues, hearings, and trials, including insanity pleas, commitment procedures, theories and laws dealing with criminal responsibility, guardianship, conservatorship, confidentiality, competence to stand trial, and legal definition of insanity. Also called **legal psychiatry**. Also see CRIMINAL PSYCHIATRY.

forensic psychology application of psychological principles and techniques in situations involving the law, including (a) the evaluation of testimony, (b) functions of the expert witness in commitment and criminal proceedings, (c) methods of interrogation, (d) guilt detection, (e) legal policies involving human relations, (f) diagnosis and therapy in correctional institutions, and (g) providing assistance in development of laws on such problems as adoption, juvenile delinquency, drug addiction, and intergroup conflicts. Also called **legal psychology**. Also see CORRECTIONAL PSYCHOLOGY; COURTROOM PSYCHOLOGY; CRIMINAL PSYCHIATRY.

foreperiod in reaction-time experiments, the pause between the ready signal and the presentation of the stimulus.

foreplay the first stage of sexual response, marked by psychological as well as physical stimulation. F., which may last from several minutes to several hours, includes kissing, stroking, fantasy, and related activities. F. also is accompanied by such physical effects as erection of the penis and the nipples. Also see FOREPLEASURE.

forepleasure a psychoanalytic term for preliminary sexual play that focuses on any of the erogenous zones and leads to sexual intercourse and end pleasure. Also see FOREPLAY.

Forer, Bertram Robin American psychologist, 1914—. See INTEREST TESTS (there: **Forer Vocational Survey**).

foreshortening the illusion that the length of a line appears shorter when viewed lengthwise.

foreskin a loose fold of skin that normally covers the glans of the penis but may retract during erection or coitus. The f. is a continuation of the skin covering the rest of the penis. The term is usually synonymous with preputium, preputium penis, or prepuce. See PREPUTIUM; PREPUTIUM PENIS.

forest fear = HYLOPHOBIA.

fore-unpleasure a term employed by Anna Freud (from German *Vor-Unlust*) to denote the child's anticipation of punishment and the suffering it will produce (*Ego and Mechanisms of Defense*, 1936).

forgetting: See DECAY THEORY; MOTIVATED F.

formaldehyde: See ALDEHYDES.

formal discipline a concept that certain subjects, e.g., mathematics, should be studied for the primary purpose of exercising and developing the mind.

formal operations a term applied by Piaget to completely developed intellectual functions, such as abstract thinking, logical processes, conceptualization, and judgment. These capacities develop during the **f.o. stage**, which begins at about age 12.

formal parallelism a comparative approach to the concept of development proposed by Heinz Werner, based on relating multiple modes of functioning (that is, different modes of animal life, different kinds of sociocultural organization, or different types of consciousness) to different levels of organization and integration, rather than relating them to a single line of chronological development, as in the law of recapitulation formulated by Haeckel and G. Stanley Hall. Also see RECAPITULATION THEORY.

formal-thought disorder a type of thought disturbance most commonly observed in schizophrenia, in which the patient fails to follow semantic and syntactic rules in spite of adequate education, intelligence, and cultural background.

formants frequency bands of sounds produced by

the vocal cords and other physical features of the head and throat in speaking. A simple sound like the vowel /ä/ may span several kilohertz of frequencies when recorded on a sound spectrogram.

formative evaluation in evaluation research, a process that is concerned with helping the developer of programs or products through the use of empirical research methodology. Ideally, the formative evaluator will work along with the developer from the outset of the work. At the same time as development planning is taking place, problems related to personnel, cost, and procedures of f.e. should also be solved. Also called **feedback evaluation**. Also see SUMMATIVE EVALUATION.

formboard test a performance test in which the subject fits blocks or cutouts of various shapes into depressions in a board.

form discrimination the ability of an individual to use his senses to judge the weight, shape, size, texture, and other features of an object. F.d. tests usually are performed visually but in some instances, as in testing a visually handicapped person, may be done by tactile sensations alone.

formes frustes /fôrm′frēst′/ a French term, meaning literally coarse forms, for indefinite or atypical symptoms or types of a disease.

formication the acutely distressing sensation of ants or other insects crawling on the skin (from Latin *formica,* "ant"). It is a tactile, or haptic, hallucination occurring in cocaine abuse and delirious states associated with acute alcoholic hallucinosis, meningitis, rheumatic fever, scarlet fever, diphtheria, and other infectious disorders. Also see ACAROPHOBIA.

form word = FUNCTION WORD.

fornicate gyrus an arched or horseshoe-shaped prominence on the cerebral cortex between the hippocampal and cingulate gyri. Also called **gyrus fornicatus.**

fornication sexual intercourse involving an unmarried individual. The legal definition varies in different areas and in some instances may be applied to any human sexual intercourse between persons who could not be married within the local laws, as when marriage would be prohibited because of racial or other cultural restrictions. In some states of the United States, an unmarried woman may be charged with f. while an unmarried man would be charged with adultery.

fornix a long tract of nerve fibers that forms an arch between the hippocampus and the hypothalamus. The f. is associated with eating behavior in animals, which develop hyperphagia after lesions of the f. are induced.

Forssman, Hans Axel Swedish physician, 1912—. See BÖRJESON-FORSSMAN-LEHMANN SYNDROME.

Förster, Carl Friedrich Richard /fœrs′tər/ Polish-born German ophthalmologist, 1825–1902. See AUBERT-FÖRSTER PHENOMENON.

48,XXXX = XXXX SYNDROME.
48,XXXY = XXXY SYNDROME.

48,XXYY = XXYY SYNDROME.
45,X = TURNER'S SYNDROME.
45,XX—G = GROUP G MONOSOMY.
49,XXXXX = XXXXX SYNDROME.
49,XXXXY = XXXXY SYNDROME.
47,XX+18 = CHROMOSOME-18 TRISOMY.
47,XX+?G = CAT'S-EYE SYNDROME.
47,XX+13 = CHROMOSOME-13 TRISOMY.
47,XX+21 = TRISOMY 21.
47,XXY: See KLINEFELTER'S SYNDROME.
47,XYY = XYY SYNDROME.
46,XX18q— = CHROMOSOME 18, DELETION OF LONG ARM.
46,XX5p— = CRI DU CHAT SYNDROME.
46,XX4p— = CHROMOSOME 4, DELETION OF SHORT ARM.
46,XX13q— = CHROMOSOME 13, DELETION OF LONG ARM.
46,XX13r: See CHROMOSOME 13, DELETION OF LONG ARM.

forward association the forming of an associative link between one item and an item that succeeds it in a series or sequence. Compare BACKWARD ASSOCIATION.

forward-conduction law: See LAW OF FORWARD CONDUCTION.

fossa any hollow or depressed area of the anatomy. Kinds of f. include the **anterior f., middle f.,** and **posterior f.** in the base of the cranium for the lobes of the brain, the **ethmoid f.** for the olfactory bulb, and the **hypophyseal f.** for the pituitary gland.

fossa navicularis vulvae the depression between the entrance of the vagina and the transverse membrane that connects the hind end of the labia minora.

foster-child fantasy a common childhood belief that the parents actually are foster parents. Also see FAMILY ROMANCE.

foster-family care: See FAMILY CARE.

Foster Grandparents Program an ACTION program developed by the federal government, in which senior citizens are trained to provide care, companionship, and emotional support to developmentally disabled children in residential institutions such as training schools. The foster grandparents may push wheelchairs of nonambulatory children, play board games with the children, and generally provide adult companionship for youngsters who want to sit on a lap or have a special person who will listen to their problems. (ACTION is a merger—1971—of national volunteer organizations, e.g., Peace Corps, Vista, including Foster Grandparents.)

foster home a home in which a mentally or physically handicapped person is placed by a social agency for purposes of family care and sustenance. The family is usually paid by the agency, and the placement may be temporary or permanent. See FAMILY CARE.

foster placement: See FAMILY CARE.

fourchette: See FRENULUM.

four-day week a work schedule that arranges, e.g., a standard 40-hour employment week into four ten-hour days rather than five eight-hour days.

fourfold table a 2×2 contingency table for data presentation.

Fourier, Jean Baptiste Joseph /foored·ā'/ French mathematician, 1768–1830. See FOURIER ANALYSIS; HARMONIC ANALYSIS.

Fourier analysis the analysis of complex sound or light waves into simple sine waves. The principle on which this analysis is based is called **Fourier's law**.

Fournier tests a series of tests for signs of ataxia in a patient who lacks an ataxic gait in normal walking. The patient is commanded to rise quickly from a seated position, walk, stop, turn quickly, or perform other movements.

four phases of medical practice: See REHABILITATION.

fourth cranial nerve = TROCHLEAR NERVE.

fourth-degree burns: See BURN INJURIES.

fourth ventricle: See VENTRICLE.

fovea centralis a small depression in the retina where the lens normally focuses an image most clearly. It is also the portion of the retina in which cone cells are concentrated with the greatest density. Also called **foveal pit**.

Foville, Achille Louis /fōvēl'/ French physician, 1799–1878. See FOVILLE'S SYNDROME.

Foville's syndrome a form of hemiplegia alterans, involving contralateral hemiplegia and homolateral paralysis of the abducens and facial nerves. Two other symptoms are paralysis of outward movement of the eye and paralysis of the conjugate movement as well.

FR = FIXED RATIO.

Fracastoro, Girolamo /fräkästō'rō/ Italian physician and poet, 1483–1553. See SYPHILIS.

fractional analysis a psychoanalytic technique in which therapy is interrupted at various intervals while the patient works through the acquired insights of previous therapy periods.

fractional antedating goal response a reaction that develops earlier and earlier in conditioning a series of responses, and may become a conditioned stimulus for subsequent responses.

fracture a broken bone or part of a bone. A f. may be due to extreme accidental pressure or a powerful muscle spasm, or be caused by indirect means, e.g., a disease that makes the bone weak or brittle. A f. may be identified as **greenstick f.**, if one side is broken and the other side of the bone is merely bent; a f. in which the bone penetrates the skin sometimes is called an **open f.**, or **compound f.**

fractionation a psychophysical procedure to scale the magnitude of sensations. In f. a subject might be asked to adjust a light so that it seems half as bright as a comparison light, that is, to bisect it.

fragile X chromosome a genetic defect that affects mostly male offspring and is associated with mental retardation. The disorder is so named because of the tendency of the long arms of the X-shaped chromosome to break when the defect is present. F.X c. is the second most prevalent cause, after Down's syndrome, of mental retardation among males. Also called **fragile X syndrome**.

fragmentary delusion an unsystematized, undeveloped delusion or series of disconnected delusions. It is especially common in delirium.

fragmentary seizures brief, partial phases of a generalized seizure, such as auras alone or abortive movements and disturbances of consciousness. F.s. may occur in patients under anticonvulsant drugs that have not attained complete control.

fragmentation a psychological disturbance in which thoughts or actions that are normally integrated are split apart, as in loosening of associations, vagueness of ideas, or bizarre actions. Bleuler considered f. to be a primary symptom of schizophrenia (which literally means "splitting of the mind").

fragmentation of thinking an association disturbance that is considered by some authors to be a primary symptom of schizophrenia. The thinking processes become confused to the point that complete actions or ideas are not possible. In a mild form, the patient may give general rather than specific answers to questions.

frame: See PROGRAMED INSTRUCTION; LINEAR PROGRAM.

frame-of-orientation need the term used by Erich Fromm to denote the need to develop or synthesize one's major assumptions, ideas, and values into a coherent world view. Fromm distinguishes between frames of reference based on reason and those based on subjective distortions, superstition, or myth.

frame of reference a standard against which ideas, actions, and results are judged; the set of reality, ethical, and other parameters that form the "cognitive map" of an individual for evaluating and coping with the real world. See COGNITIVE MAP.

Framingham Study a large-scale, long-range survey by the United States National Institutes of Health of possible causes of heart disease. The F.S. selected a population of 5,000 residents of Framingham, Massachusetts, representing a cross section of the country's general population, and followed the daily life-styles of the individuals for a period of more than 20 years. The study found that primary factors associated with heart disease were cigarette-smoking, physical inactivity, high cholesterol levels, and hypertension—as predictors of heart attacks. The F.S. is regarded as one of the most reliable studies of the causative factors of heart disease because its data were compiled from persons who were originally free of heart disease and carefully recorded the dietary and other habits of the subjects before signs of heart disease appeared.

France, Anatole /fräNs/ French writer and Nobel laureate, 1844–1924. See BRAIN WEIGHT.

Franceschetti, Adolphe /fränchesket'ē/ Swiss ophthalmologist, 1896—. See TREACHER COLLINS' SYNDROME (also called **Franceschetti-Zwahlen-Klein syndrome**); DYSOSTOSIS.

Francis of Assisi Italian monk and preacher, saint, ca. 1182–1226. See STIGMATA.

Frank, Jerome David American psychiatrist, 1909—. See GROUP PSYCHOTHERAPY.

Frankl, Victor German-born American psychiatrist, 1905—. F. originated logotherapy, an existential approach based on the will to meaning and the existential neurosis, or inability to see meaning in life. He was a victim of the Nazis and wrote *From Death Camp to Existentialism*, 1959, which was incorporated in *Man's Search for Meaning*, 1963. See EXISTENTIAL VACUUM; FREEDOM OF WILL; LOGOTHERAPY; PARADOXICAL INTENTION; SELF-TRANSCENDENCE; WILL TO MEANING.

Franklin, Benjamin American author, scientist, and statesman, 1706–90. See PUN.

Franz, Shepard Ivory American psychologist and physiologist, 1874–1933. Chiefly noted for his study of brain functions, F. opposed the "new phrenology" which localized psychological activity in specific areas, by showing that extensive damage could occur without permanent loss of function. This led to the development of effective reeducational programs for brain-injured patients.

fraternal twins = DIZYGOTIC TWINS.

free-access environment an environment to which most individuals can easily gain access; an open, unrestricted environment, e.g., a public library or museum.

free association the basic process in psychoanalytic therapy, in which the patient is encouraged to lie on a couch and verbalize whatever comes to mind, no matter how embarrassing or irrelevant it may appear to be. The object is to allow unconscious material, such as traumatic experiences, repressed memories, and threatening impulses, to come to the surface where they can be interpreted. F.a. also helps to discharge some of the feelings that have given this material excessive control over the patient.

free-association test a test in which the subject is offered a stimulus word and is expected to respond as quickly as possible with a word he associates with the stimulus.

free base a highly concentrated and chemically altered form of cocaine that is prepared by treating cocaine with ether. The f.b. is taken by smoking the substance.

freedom of will as used by V. Frankl, conscious volition or the capacity to freely choose an attitude or course of action. In Frankl's logotherapy, f.o.w. is not considered to be significantly compromised by unconscious factors or environmental conditions. See FREE WILL.

free-floating anxiety a diffuse, chronic sense of uneasiness and apprehension not directed to any specific situation or object. It is one of the most characteristic symptoms of anxiety neurosis, but also found in other types of psychoneurosis such as phobic and obsessive-compulsive disorders, as well as some cases of schizophrenia.

free-floating attention in classical psychoanalysis, the analyst's state of mind in which he "focuses his attention on the patient himself and immerses himself in the whole stream of associations, allowing them to flow through his alert, receptive mind without any concentrated effort at intellectual understanding. His is a passive, unguided attention that, in absorbing all the patient's associations, permits the unconscious, intuitive elements of his mind to sense connections among associational fragments, and to see patterns and significant relationships in the seemingly amorphous productions of the patient" (J. C. Nemiah, in *American Handbook of Psychiatry*, 1975).

free-floating fear a generalized sense of fear that is not directed to a particular object or situation.

Freeman, E. A. English physician, fl. 1938. See WHISTLING-FACE SYNDROME (also called **Freeman-Sheldon syndrome**).

free nerve ending a branched afferent neuron ending found in the skin and believed to be a pain or temperature receptor.

free operant avoidance = SIDMAN AVOIDANCE SCHEDULE.

free play play that is not controlled or directed by a group leader, teacher, or play therapist.

free recall a type of memory experiment in which a list of words is presented one by one and subjects attempt to remember them in any order. The first and last words presented are best remembered; proponents of the dual-memory theory attribute this finding to the fact that the last words are still in short-term memory, hence recoverable, while the first words received the most rehearsal and were transferred to long-term memory. Also see DUAL-MEMORY THEORY.

free-response test a type of examination in which the student constructs his answers in his own words, e.g., a short-answer or essay test. This type of test is sometimes termed "subjective." Compare FORCED-RESPONSE TEST.

free will the philosophic concept that we are not entirely ruled by the scientific law of cause and effect, but have the capacity to make our own independent choices and decisions. This concept contrasts with the Freudian view that all our mental processes, including decision-making, are completely determined, and that f.w. is an illusion. See DETERMINISM.

freezing behavior a form of passive avoidance in which the subject remains motionless and makes no effort to run or hide. The behavior is most often observed as a severe reaction to a threatening situation.

Fregoli's phenomenon misidentification of people known to the patient, who may claim they have undergone changes in appearance and intend to persecute him. Also called **illusion of negative doubles**.

French kiss a type of sexual arousal in which the participants kiss with their mouths open so the tongues can touch. Also called **soul kiss; tongue kiss**.

frenulum a small fold of skin or membrane that limits movement of a part of the body. The f. of the prepuce of the penis is a fold of tissue that limits the backward movement of the foreskin. In the female, a f. is formed by the tissues of the labia minora and the clitoris, and a second f., called a **fourchette** (French, "fork"), is formed by a union of the labia minora on the opposite side of the vaginal opening.

frequency a measure of the number of cycles per second of air vibrations perceived or recorded. The range of sound f. that can be detected by the ear varies with the species, age of the individual, and other factors. The range for most humans is between 20 and 20,000 cycles per second.

frequency discrimination the ability to detect variations in sound frequencies. In f.d. testing, the subject may merely be required to differentiate between two frequencies with a reasonably large difference. Occasionally, the test involves gradually narrowing the difference between frequencies until they become so close that differences cannot be perceived.

frequency distribution a plot of the frequency of occurrence of scores of various sizes, arranged from lowest to highest score.

frequency law: See LAW OF FREQUENCY.

frequency polygon a graph depicting a statistical distribution, made up of lines connecting the peaks of adjacent intervals.

frequency theory a generalization that the cochlea functions like a microphone and pitch is determined by the frequency of impulses traveling up the auditory nerve. The theory is supported by studies showing that, e.g., a tone of 500 cycles per second produces 500 evoked responses per second in the auditor nerve.

Freud, Anna /froit/ Austrian-born British psychoanalyst, 1895–1982. The youngest daughter of Sigmund Freud, Anna F. made many contributions to both the theory and practice of psychoanalysis, particularly through her studies of defense mechanisms (*The Ego and Mechanism of Defense*, 1936); through gathering clinical case material on children; and through application of play therapy as a therapeutic and educational tool at the Hampstead Clinic in England. See CHILD ANALYSIS; DEFENSE MECHANISM; FORE-UNPLEASURE; METAPSYCHOLOGIC PROFILE.

Freud, Sigmund /froit/ Austrian neurologist and psychiatrist, born on May 6, 1856, in Freiberg, Moravia, died on September 9, 1939, in London. F. (whose name literally means "joy" or "pleasure") began his professional life as a neurologist, making significant contributions to that field, but turned his full attention to the psychological approach to mental disorders, such as hysteria, after witnessing Charcot's demonstrations of hypnosis in Paris. After discarding hypnosis as a technique limited to removal of symptoms, F. developed the method of free association, which led to recognition of unconscious sexual conflicts and repressions as the major factors in neuroses. These concepts became the cornerstones of the new discipline which he called psychoanalysis, and which focused on such procedures as (a) the interpretation of dreams in terms of hostile or sexual feelings stemming from childhood, (b) analysis of resistances and the relationship between therapist and patient, and (c) a study of the patient's present symptomatology in terms of psychosexual development and early experiences. The goal of this process, which takes many months or years, was not merely to eliminate symptoms, but to restructure the patient's entire life. F., however, did not stop here, but applied his psychoanalytic method to the study of historical figures, such as Leonardo da Vinci, and to the exploration of primitive cultures, drawing a parallel between the childhood of the individual and the childhood of the human race. To disseminate his views, which were regarded as highly controversial at the time, he taught many disciples, was instrumental in establishing the first psychoanalytic association, and published a series of books, including *The Interpretation of Dreams* (1900), *Three Essays on the Theory of Sexuality* (1905), *Totem and Taboo* (1913), *Beyond the Pleasure Principle* (1920), and *The Ego and the Id* (1923). Adjective: **Freudian** /froi'dē·ən/.

See FREUDIAN APPROACH; FREUDIAN SLIP; FREUDIAN THEORY OF PERSONALITY; NEO-FREUDIAN; ABRAHAM; ADLER; BLEULER; BREUER; BRILL; FENICHEL; FERENCZI; HALL; HORNEY; JONES; JUNG; KOHUT; NIETZSCHE; RANK; REICH; STEKEL. This dictionary includes another 205 entries in which F. is mentioned by name, and over 1,000 entries in which Freud's work and ideas are discussed.

Freudian approach a general term sometimes applied to Freud's emphasis on clinical cases and the view that human beings are driven by unconscious, and especially psychosexual, impulses. Also called **Freudianism**. See PSYCHOANALYSIS.

Freudian slip an unconscious error or oversight in writing or speech that Freud attributed to unacceptable impulses breaking through the ego's defenses and exposing the individual's true wishes or feelings, e.g., a slip of the tongue or pen. A F.s. is a symptomatic act.

Freudian theory of personality the general psychoanalytic concept that character and personality are the product of experiences and fixations stemming from the early stages of psychosexual development.

fricative a speech sound made by forcing a stream of air through a narrow opening of the vocal tract. A f. has high-frequency vibrations. It may be voiced, e.g., /v/, /z/, /zh/, /th/, or voiceless, e.g., /f/, /s/, /sh/, /th/. Also see LABIAL.

friction-conformity model the idea that pedestrians' rate of walking is influenced by the number of obstacles met and by conformity to the pace set by adjacent pedestrians.

Friedman, Meyer American physician, 1910—. See TYPE A PERSONALITY; TYPE B PERSONALITY.

Friedmann, Max /frēd′män/ German neurologist, 1858–1925. See POSTTRAUMATIC CONSTITUTION (there: **Friedmann's complex**).

Friedreich, Nikolaus /frēd′rīsh/ German physician, 1826–82. See FRIEDREICH'S ATAXIA; ATAXIA; BIEMOND'S ATAXIA; CHARCOT-MARIE-TOOTH DISEASE; MYOCLONUS; ROUSSY-LÉVY SYNDROME.

Friedreich's ataxia a syndrome of ataxia accompanied by abnormal deep-tendon reflexes in the legs, foot deformity, spine curvature (kyphoscoliosis), and visual and speech defects. The ataxia symptoms begin in childhood, involving the legs first, followed by the arms. Eventually, the patient becomes bedridden. Nystagmus is a common visual problem. Mental retardation has been reported in ten percent of some patient groups but much less in others. Two different types of genetic factors have been established, involving both dominant and recessive genes. Also, because of variations in effects among different patients, it is believed the condition actually may be a complex of several disorders with similar signs and symptoms. Also called **hereditary ataxia**.

fright a fear reaction to an unexpected danger.

frightened to death: See VOODOO DEATH.

frigidity a female sexual disorder consisting of impairment of desire or inability to achieve full gratification. The condition has a wide range, including mild disinterest in sexual relations, sexual interest without orgasm, and active aversion. There are also many possible causes, such as faulty attitudes acquired from parents, conflict or abuse, distasteful early sex experiences, a clumsy or inadequate male partner, and unconscious hostility toward the male sex. Adjective: **frigid**. See VAGINAL HYPOESTHESIA; VAGINISMUS; DYSPAREUNIA; SEXUAL ANESTHESIA.

fringe of consciousness = MARGINAL CONSCIOUSNESS.

frog fear = BATRACHOPHOBIA.

Fröhlich, Alfred /frœ′lish/ Austrian neurologist, 1871–1953. See FRÖHLICH'S SYNDROME.

Fröhlich's syndrome a disorder caused by underfunctioning of the anterior lobe of the pituitary gland (hypopituitarism). Major symptoms are underdeveloped genital organs and secondary sexual characteristics, general sluggishness, obesity, and in some cases polyuria, polydipsia, and mild mental retardation. Also called **adiposogenital dystrophy**.

Frohman, Charles Edward American biochemist, 1921—. See BERGEN'S FRACTION (there: **Frohman factor**).

Froin, Georges /frô·eN′/ French physician, 1874—. See FROIN'S SYNDROME.

Froin's syndrome a condition associated with chronic or syphilitic meningitis, spinal-cord tumors, and polyneuritis in which the cerebrospinal fluid has an excessive protein content, excessive CSF cells, and massive coagulation.

Fromm, Erich German-born American psychoanalyst, 1900–80. F. developed a broad cultural, yet personal, approach focused on (a) the search for meaning, (b) the development of personality and socially productive relationships, and (c) the enrichment of life through character, the need to belong, the development of individuality, and the replacement of the present commercial "marketing orientation" with a "sane society" built around cooperation, caring, and the ability to love. These concepts have been vividly expressed in such books as *Man for Himself* (1947), *The Sane Society* (1955), and *The Art of Loving* (1956). See AUTHORITARIAN CONSCIENCE; BELONGINGNESS; BROTHERLINESS; CULTURALISTS; EXPLOITATIVE ORIENTATION; FRAME-OF-ORIENTATION NEED; HOARDING CHARACTER; HUMANISTIC COMMUNITARIAN SOCIALISM; HUMANISTIC CONSCIENCE; HUMANISTIC THEORY; IDENTITY NEED; INCESTUOUS TIES; IRRATIONALITY; LOVE; MAGIC HELPER; MARKETING ORIENTATION; NEO-FREUDIAN; PERSONALITY TYPES; PRODUCTIVE LOVE; PRODUCTIVE ORIENTATION; PRODUCTIVE THINKING; RECEPTIVE CHARACTER; RECEPTIVE ORIENTATION; ROOTEDNESS NEED; SOCIAL PSYCHOLOGY; SYMBIOTIC RELATEDNESS; TRANSCENDENCE NEED; TRUE SELF; WITHDRAWAL-DESTRUCTIVENESS.

frontal pertaining to the front, or **anterior**, side of the body or an organ such as the brain.

frontal eye-field lesion a lesion, produced surgically or by injury, in a region of the brain anterior to the motor area involved in head and eye movements. Such a lesion may result in unilateral blindness with the effect observed on the side opposite the lesion.

frontalis muscle a muscle layer that covers the scalp immediately beneath the skin of the forehead. Because the f.m. is closely associated with stress reactions of muscles from the cranium to the shoulders, it is utilized in biofeedback training for the treatment of a variety of postural and nervous-tension disorders.

frontal lobe the part of either of the cerebral hemispheres that lies on the frontal, or anterior, side of the central sulcus, or fissure. The f.l. is associated with personality factors in humans, e.g., initiative, foresight, and tact; but intelligence apparently is not affected by f.l. lesions. See BRAIN.

frontal-lobe syndrome an organic mental disorder due to lesions in the frontal lobe, characterized by such symptoms as impairment of purposeful behavior, emotional lability, impaired social judgment and impulse control, and marked apathy. The symptoms vary with the size and location of the lesion. See ORGANIC PERSONALITY SYNDROME.

frontal lobotomy a surgical procedure in which nerve fibers connecting the frontal lobes with the rest of the brain are cut. The procedure has been used as a form of therapy for persons suffering certain forms of chronic psychosis. It also has been used to relieve suffering from pain; the pain may remain as intense as before, but the patient appears better able to tolerate it. Also called **lobotomy**. Also see LEUCOTOMY.

frontal perceptual disorders a condition observed in some patients with tumors or other lesions of the frontal lobes who have difficulty in performing certain problem-solving tasks, such as following a moving target, finding matching numbers, letters, or other symbols, or evaluating thematic pictures.

front-clipping: See CLIPPING.

Frostig, Marianne B. Austrian-born American psychologist, 1906—. See FROSTIG DEVELOPMENTAL TEST OF VISUAL PERCEPTION; FROSTIG MOVEMENT SKILLS TEST BATTERY; FROSTIG-HORNE TRAINING PROGRAM.

Frostig Developmental Test of Visual Perception a group of tests of visual perceptual skills devised by Marianne Frostig as a diagnostic procedure in the rehabilitation of learning-disabled children. The tests include eye-motor coordination, figure ground, form consistency, position in space, and spatial relations. Abbrev.: **DTVP**. See VISUAL-SPATIAL ABILITY.

Frostig-Horne training program a learning program developed to remedy deficiencies in visual perception revealed by the Frostig Developmental Test of Visual Perception.

Frostig Movement Skills Test Battery a series of sensorimotor tests developed by Marianne Frostig and used in evaluating learning problems in children. The sensorimotor skills may include stringing beads and transferring blocks or other objects from one side of the body to the other.

frottage /frôtäzh′/ a sexual disorder, or paraphilia, in which an individual deliberately and persistently seeks sexual excitement by rubbing against other people (French, "rubbing"), possibly because he is unable to face the challenge of mature sexual relations. The person displaying this type of behavior is called a **frotteur** /frôtœr′/ or a **rubber**.

fructosuria a rare familial disorder probably transmitted by a single recessive gene, involving the metabolism of fructose (fruit sugar), and resulting in mental retardation.

frustration the thwarting of impulses or actions by external or internal forces. Typical internal forces are intrapsychic conflicts and inhibitions; typical external forces are the admonitions of parents and the rules of society. According to psychoanalysis, frustration "dams up" psychic energy, which then seeks an outlet in wish-fulfilling fantasies and dreams, or in various neurotic symptoms.

frustration-aggression hypothesis the theory introduced by Dollard and his colleagues in 1939 that frustration nearly always produces aggression and, conversely, that aggression is nearly always an expression of frustration.

frustration-regression hypothesis the theory that frustration does not always lead to aggressive acts (as the frustration-aggression hypothesis is often interpreted), but may lead to regressive behavior, as in children who become infantile dependent, and unable to cope with problems on their own if they are repeatedly thwarted (Barker, Dembo, and Lewin, 1941).

frustration response a reaction to frustration characterized by anger or depression and attempts at control (R. B. Cattell).

frustration tolerance the ability to endure tension; the ability to preserve relative equanimity upon encountering obstacles; also, the ability to delay gratification. The growth of adequate f.t. is a feature of normal ego development. Poor f.t. is a sign of inadequate ego strength.

F scale in the classic study by Adorno and colleagues of the authoritarian personality, a scale designed to measure antidemocratic ideology and authoritarianism. Also called **California F s.; fascism scale**.

FSH = FOLLICLE-STIMULATING HORMONE.

ft. an abbreviation used in prescriptions, meaning "make" (Latin *fac, fiat*, or *fiant*).

FTA-ABS test a highly sensitive and specific test for syphilis based on *f*luorescent *t*reponemal antibody *abs*orption.

ft. pulv. an abbreviation used in prescriptions, meaning "make a powder" (Latin *fiat pulvis*).

fucosidosis a rare metabolic disorder characterized by progressive neurologic deterioration in affected children. The children develop normally for the first few months but begin to show mental development regression at about one year of age. Spasticity and dementia develop in the third and fourth years. All patients show a deficiency of a sugar enzyme, **fucosidase**. Also called **mucopolysaccharidosis F**.

fufuraldehyde: See ALDEHYDES.

fugue /fyo͞og/ an amnesic, dissociated state in which the individual suddenly flees from home, forgets his entire past but not his basic skills, and starts a new life with a new name (French. "flight"). After recovery, the earlier events of his life can be recalled, but not the f. period. Extended f. states can sometimes be traced to an unconscious desire to escape from threatening or distasteful situations, and are usually terminated spontaneously or through hypnotic suggestion or a sodium-Amytal interview. Brief fugues may also occur in epilepsy or states of catatonic excitement. The corresponding DSM-III term is PSYCHOGENIC F. See this entry. Also see PORIOMANIA; AMNESIA.

fulfillment the satisfaction of needs and desires, or attainment of aspirations, sometimes more in fantasy than in reality. See WISH F.

Fullerton-Cattell law a generalization that errors of observation and of just-noticeable differences are proportional to the square root of the magnitude of the stimulus. The F.-C.l. has been proposed as a replacement for Weber's law.

full-thickness burns: See BURN INJURIES.

full word = CONTENT WORD.

fully functioning person the term used by C. Rogers to refer to the healthy personality. According to Rogers, a f.f.p. experiences freedom of choice and action, is creative, and, most important, exhibits the qualities of EXISTENTIAL LIVING. See this entry.

function the typical activity of an organ directed toward a purpose or goal, e.g., secretion of a hormone by a gland, or the control of balance by the cerebellum.

functional = PSYCHOGENIC.

functional activities actions associated with basic daily home and work requirements, e.g., eating, grooming, dressing, and operating simple types of equipment such as typewriters. Skills in f.a. sometimes must be trained or improved upon in persons who have experienced stroke or other neurologic damage or disease.

functional aids devices designed and developed by biomedical engineers to assist disabled persons in basic daily activities, such as eating, grooming, or operating automobiles.

functional ailment a mild, temporary symptom resulting from disturbed physiological functioning, such as a visceral expression of an emotional disturbance.

functional analysis of environments: See REINFORCEMENT ANALYSIS.

functional aphonia the absence of voiced speech due to a psychogenic rather than organic disorder.

functional asymmetry perceptual superiority of the eye or ear on one side of the body for certain kinds of stimuli. Studies show, e.g., that the right ear usually is superior for receiving verbal material or the human voice whereas the left ear has superiority for pitch patterns, melodies, and environmental sounds. In visual asymmetry, the right half-field has superiority for verbal material while the left half-field exhibits superiority for recognition of faces and shapes and for slope of line and depth perception.

functional autonomy the term coined by G. W. Allport for his theory that behavior originally motivated by instinctual forces may develop derivative motives that eventually supersede the primary drives and operate autonomously. E.g., studying first motivated by the need for approval is gradually replaced by love of scholarship, or the gourmet, who started by eating to live, now lives to eat. Also called **autonomy of motives; functional autonomy principle**.

functional bradykinesia: See BRADYKINESIA.

functional conformance in environmental design, the provision of the objects and equipment required to adapt an environment to a given set of functional uses, e.g., providing a study with desk, lights, and comfortable chair.

functional deafness a loss of hearing that is not associated with organic damage or defect to the ear. F.d. may or may not be psychogenic but often is found to be a conversion symptom.

functional disorders = PSYCHOGENIC DISORDERS.

functional distance in environmental psychology, the distance between two residences. In studies of the impact of physical environment on interpersonal behavior, f.d. represents the possibility for interaction between persons in any two residences.

functional dysmenorrhea: See DYSMENORRHEA.

functional dyspareunia a psychosexual disorder in which there is recurrent and persistent genital pain during coitus, in either male or female. The term applies only if the disturbance is not caused exclusively by a physical disorder and is not due to lack of lubrication, functional vaginismus, or another mental disorder. (DSM-III)

functional dysphonia = FUNCTIONAL VOICE DISORDER.

functional encopresis repeated voluntary or involuntary passage of feces in inappropriate settings, occurring at least once a month after age four, and not due to physical disorder. The condition is often associated with lax toilet training and stressful situations, as in entering school or the birth of a sibling, and if clearly deliberate, it may be an antisocial or other pathological act. Also called **encopresis**. (DSM-III)

functional enuresis repeated involuntary voiding of urine during the day or night after the age when continence is expected. The condition is not due to physical disorder, but is often found in near relatives, and is frequently associated with delayed bladder development, lax toilet training, and stressful situations such as hospitalization, entering school, or the birth of a sibling. Also called **aconuresis**. (DSM-III)

functional fixedness in problem-solving, the tendency to cling to set patterns and overlook new approaches. E.g., one may overlook new and different uses to which an object can be put. The opposite of f.f. is CREATIVE THINKING. See this entry.

functional hyperinsulinism: See HYPOGLYCEMIA.

functional invariants in Piaget's theory of cognitive development, the "primary shapers of intellectual growth that are basic modes of interacting with the environment to make behavior appropriate to what has previously been experienced as well as to modify behavior to fit new intellectual challenges. Assimilation and accommodation are the most important f.i." (Philip G. Zimbardo, *Psychology and Life*, 1979)

functionalism a general psychological approach that views behavior in terms of active adaptation to the environment. F. was developed by John Dewey, James R. Angell, Harvey A. Carr, and William James as a revolt against the atomistic point of view of structuralism, which limited psychology to the dissection of states of consciousness and the study of mental contents rather than mental activities. F. emphasized the causes and consequences of human behavior, the union of the physiological with the psychological, the need for objective testing of theories, and the applications of psychological knowledge to the solution of practical problems and the improvement of human life. Compare STRUCTURALISM.

functional leadership the type of behavior of a group member or leader that advances the group's progress toward fulfilling its function or reaching its goal.

functional moneme = FUNCTION WORD.

functional pain pain without an organic cause.

functional plasticity the ability of one of the cerebral hemispheres to adapt to the absence of the other hemisphere by carrying on most of the mental functions of both. The f.p. phenomenon is observed in cases of infantile hemiplegia when it has become necessary to remove by surgery one of the hemispheres in order to control the symptoms of the disorder. See SPLIT BRAIN.

functional psychology: See FUNCTIONALISM.

functional psychosis a psychotic disorder, such as schizophrenia and bipolar conditions, which is believed to originate primarily from psychogenic factors, since no specific organic pathology can be demonstrated. Many investigators, however, believe there may be a hereditary or constitutional predisposition in some cases.

functional skills activities that develop from aptitudes, e.g., mechanical ability, artistic talent, salesmanship, and writing.

functional type a term introduced by Jung in classifying personality types from a functional viewpoint. The four basic functional types are: feeling, thinking, sensational, and intuitive.

functional unity the combination of various parts, traits, or processes working as an integrated unit.

functional vaginismus a psychosexual disorder characterized by a history of recurrent and persistent involuntary spasms of the musculature of the outer third of the vagina, interfering with coitus and not caused exclusively by a physical disorder or due to another mental disorder. (DSM-III)

functional voice disorder abnormality of pitch or melodic patterns, absence of voice, spasticity, or hoarseness associatiated with psychogenic disturbances in the absence of organic factors. Also called **functional dysphonia.**

function engram a memory imprint, or "archaic residue," that constitutes a functional inheritance in Jung's concept of racial memory. The archetypal symbols are function engrams.

function pleasure the performance of a task without anxiety, resulting in a pleasure that encourages a repetition of the act. F.p. accounts for certain activities of children, e.g., playing the same game repeatedly or hearing the same story many times.

function word a word that has no independent lexical meaning and expresses primarily a grammatical relationship or function of other words. Examples are prepositions, conjunctions, articles, and certain pronouns. Also called **empty word; form word; grammatical word; structure word; relational word; functional moneme; functor; closed-class word.** Compare CONTENT WORD.

fundamental attribution error an error of judgment caused by a bias toward dispositional rather than situational factors. An example could be the error of assuming that a person's behavior is due to his attitudes or beliefs while disregarding influences such as financial or social pressures.

fundamental-response processes the several physiological activities believed to produce color vision.

fundamental rule: See ANALYTIC RULES.

fundamental symptoms a term introduced by Bleuler to distinguish primary from secondary symptoms of schizophenias. F.s. would be autism, schizophrenic dementia, ambivalence of emotions, of intellect, or of will, or disturbances of attention, of activity, of behavior, and of associations. Compare SECONDARY SYMPTOMS.

fundamental tone the lowest tone in a complex tone.

funicular myelitis = DANA'S SYNDROME.

Funk, Casimir Polish biochemist, 1884—. F. was the discoverer of vitamins, in 1913. See VITAMIN.

Funkenstein, Daniel Hertz American psychiatrist, 1910—. See ADRENALINE-MECHOLYL TEST (also called **Funkenstein test**).

funnel sequence in surveys and interviews, a method for structuring the order of questions starting with general items and gradually narrowing the focus on more specific items.

furlough psychosis a period of acute schizophrenic behavior, characterized by delusions, suicidal tendencies, and inappropriate feelings that affects some soldiers soon after they begin military leave. The condition, which may subside within a few months, is believed due to the sudden release of a vulnerable individual from military life on which he has become dependent. Also see PRERELEASE ANXIETY STATE.

furor a sudden outburst of rage or excitement during which an irrational act of violence may be committed. The term **f. epilepticus,** or **epileptic f.,** is applied to the rare cases of grand mal or psychomotor epilepsy in which this occurs. See ISOLATED EXPLOSIVE DISORDER.

furthest-neighbor analysis in psychological esthetics, a hierarchical-grouping method for classifying judgments of dissimilarity. The f.-n.a. is used in evaluating how well selected subjects rate differences between works of art when they are given no specific criteria for making judgments.

fusarium moniliform toxin: See MOLDY-CORN POISONING.

fusiform gyrus a long convolution of brain tissue that extends lengthwise along the medial surface of the cerebral hemisphere across the ventral sides of the temporal and occipital lobes.

fusion in psychoanalysis, a merging of different instincts, as in the union of sexual and hostility drives in sadism. Also, f. is the blending of two colors into one (**color f.**), of sounds received by the two ears (**binaural f.**), or of images falling on the two retinas (**binocular f.**). Also see UNITY AND F.

fusion frequency = CRITICAL FLICKER FREQUENCY.

fusion state the experience of merging with a particular person, with all of humankind, or with the whole of reality. It is a state of mind that may be induced by drugs, such as LSD or opiates, but also by religious or mystical experiences.

future shock a term coined by Alvin Toffler to describe the personal confusion and social disorientation that accompany very rapid technological and social change.

futuristics an area of inquiry into expected future patterns of technological, economic, and social organization. F. aims to identify and propose solutions to significant future problems.

G

g = GENERAL FACTOR.

GA = GAMBLERS ANONYMOUS.

GABA an acronym for *gamma-aminobutyric acid*, a substance present in the central nervous system of mammals and believed to be a neurotransmitter. In experiments involving cats, GABA levels were found to be three times as high during the sleeping as during the waking state. GABA stimulates cerebellar Purkinje cells and mimics a cortical inhibitory substance.

GABA shunt a metabolic pathway of GABA and an alternative metabolic route for a substance, alpha-ketoglutarate, which is formed in the Krebs cycle during conversion of carbon chains of sugars, fatty acids, and amino acids to carbon dioxide. The alpha-ketoglutarate is transformed in two steps into GABA. Metabolism of GABA yields succinic acid which feeds back into the Krebs cycle.

GABOB the hydroxyl derivative of gamma-aminobutyric acid, which plays an important role in cerebral metabolism. See GABA.

GAD = GENERALIZED ANXIETY DISORDER.

GAG: See MUCOPOLYSACCHARIDOSES; BETA-GLUCURONIDASE DEFICIENCY.

GAI = GUIDED AFFECTIVE IMAGERY.

gain-loss theory of attraction a theory of interpersonal attraction stating that alterations in the assessment of one person by another have a greater effect than unvarying evaluations on the degree of attraction. That is, persons who are perceived as liking a subject more or less than they used to are liked or disliked more than persons who are perceived to have always liked or disliked the subject.

gait a manner of performing a function, usually applied to the pattern of muscle activity of an individual while walking. Kinds of walking g. include waddling, spastic, tabetic, hemiplegic, and marche à petits pas. G. also may refer to speech mannerisms, e.g., a STUTTERING G. See this entry.

gait apraxia: See APRAXIA OF GAIT.

gait stuttering = STUTTERING GAIT.

-galact-; -galacto- a combining form relating to milk (Greek *gala*).

galactosemia an autosomal-recessive disease marked by cataracts, jaundice, lethargic and hypotonic behavior, and mental retardation in untreated patients. A high infant-death rate occurs among untreated patients, and those that survive are likely to be mentally retarded. Treatment is based on restricted intake of dietary galactose, which accumulates in the blood and urine due to an inability to metabolize the carbohydrate.

Galen (Claudius Galenus) Greek physician and philosopher, ca. 130 to ca. 200 A.D. The most eminent physician of his time, G. wrote 500 treatises summarizing all medical thought to date, and was one of the first to recognize both physical and mental causes of mental illness, citing such factors as head injuries, alcohol excess, shock, economic reverses, and disappointment in love—although his explanations of the specific effects of these factors and his dependence on herbal remedies and opiates were a mixture of science and superstition. See ANIMAL SPIRITS; CHOLERIC TYPE; ORGANIC APPROACH; PHLEGMATIC TYPE; SANGUINE TYPE.

galeanthropy the delusion of being a cat.

galeophobia = AILUROPHOBIA.

Galgenhumor = GALLOWS HUMOR.

Galilean fully scientific, since it explains the individual case, analyzes dynamic causal interaction in the present, and predicts exactly. This meaning of the term—used, e.g., in statistics—was originated by Kurt Lewin. Compare ARISTOTELIAN.

Galileo Galilei /gälēlā′ō/ Italian physicist, astronomer, and inventor, 1564–1642. See GALILEAN; ARISTOTELIAN.

Gall, Franz Josef /gäl/ German physician, 1758–1828. G. abandoned an early interest in brain physiology to develop a popular theory of "phrenology" in which various intellectual and emotional characteristics were correlated with specific areas of the skull; e.g., a protuberance in one area meant conscientiousness, and in another, self-esteem. Though this approach was ridiculed, it served the purpose of challenging its opponents to make studies of LOCALIZATION OF FUNCTION. See this entry. Also see CRANIOLOGY; PHRENOLOGY; FLOURENS; LASHLEY; SPURZHEIM.

gallbladder disease a disorder of the gall bladder, a pear-shaped storage organ located immediately below the liver. The primary type of disorder is the formation of gallstones, or **cholelithiasis**, followed by **cholecystitis**, or inflammation of the gall bladder, which often is due to a bacterial infection.

gallows humor a humorous or comical type of behavior that is inappropriate at a time of death or disaster. G.h. is often observed in cases of organic psychosis and delirium tremens. Also called by its original German name, **Galgenhumor** /gäl′gənho͞omôr′/.

Galton, Francis English scientist, 1822–1911. G. began his professional career by applying the "pedigree method," or study of genealogy, trying to demonstrate that genius is hereditary and the race can be improved through eugenics. To advance this cause, he embarked on the first scientific study of individual differences, in which he carried out experiments on word association, mental imagery, sensory discrimination, and the measurement of vision, hearing, and strength of grip. In the course of these studies he developed tests, apparatus, and statistical methods that had a lasting influence on the field. See GALTON BAR; GALTON WHISTLE; GENIUS; PEDIGREE METHOD; TWIN STUDIES; WORD-ASSOCIATION TEST. Also see CATTELL, J. M.; GODDARD.

Galton bar an instrument for measuring the j.n.d. for visual linear distances.

Galton whistle a high-pitched whistle used to determine the upper threshold for pitch.

Galvani, Luigi /gälvä′nē/ Italian anatomist and physicist, 1737–98. See GALVANIC SKIN RESPONSE; GALVANOTROPISM.

galvanic skin response a response to certain stimuli by a change in electrical resistance of the skin, particularly on the palms or other areas lacking hair. The effect is produced by unconscious activity of the sweat glands and may occur as a reaction to pleasant as well as unpleasant stimuli, to emotional arousal and stress, and even to a novel stimulus or a conditioned neutral stimulus. Abbrev.: **GSR**. Also called **Féré phenomenon; electrodermal response (EDR); psychogalvanic reflex (PGR)**. Also see LIE DETECTOR; PSYCHOGALVANIC SKIN-RESISTANCE AUDIOMETRY.

galvanotropism an orienting response that attracts a body to a source of electrical stimulation.

-gam-; -gamo-; -gamy a combining form relating to marriage or to a union for propagation or reproduction (from Greek *gamos*, "marriage").

Gamblers Anonymous an organization of compulsive gamblers with the objective of controlling the impulse to gamble through mutual understanding, sharing of experiences, and emotional support. G.A. is modeled after Alcoholics Anonymous except for a lack of emphasis on the spiritual. Abbrev.: **GA**. See PATHOLOGICAL GAMBLING.

gambler's fallacy a mistaken belief that one may predict correctly in a completely chance or random situation. E.g., if an unbiased coin comes up head nine times, a gambler might think it was especially likely to come up tails the tenth time, although the true probability of this is still just 0.5.

gambling: See PATHOLOGICAL G.

games in psychotherapy, (a) an interaction, or transaction, in which one individual tries to get the better of others or make his mark in society, or (b) an activity situation set up to elicit emotions or stimulate revealing interactions and interrelationships. In play therapy, g. are often used as a projective or observational technique. In transactional analysis, the term is used to denote recurrent, and often deceitful, ploys adopted by individuals in their dealings with others. In Gestalt therapy, g. are "exercises" or "experiments" designed to increase self-awareness, e.g., acting out frightening situations, or sitting in the "hot seat" next to the therapist, where the participant learns how others view him as well as how he sees himself. Also see RULES OF THE GAME.

games people play: See TRANSACTIONAL ANALYSIS.

gametes: See GERM CELLS.

game theory a model or paradigm for understanding the dynamics of interpersonal conflict. G.t. likens conflict situations to the relationship of two players in a game, such as tennis, that employs offensive and defensive maneuvers. In g.t., each "player" tries to increase his advantage while defending himself from the other "player."

gamma third letter of the Greek alphabet (Γ, γ).

gamma the distance of a stimulus from the threshold.

gamma alcoholism according to E. M. Jellinek, the typical form of alcoholism in countries where hard liquor is consumed. G.a. is characterized by increasing tolerance, physiological adaptation, loss of control, and, if drinking is suspended, a withdrawal or abstinence syndrome consisting of craving for alcohol, convulsions, and delirium tremens. Also called **addictive alcoholism; malignant alcoholism; essential alcoholism; regressive alcoholism**. Also see CHRONIC ALCOHOLISM.

gamma-aminobutyric acid: See GABA.

gammacism a speech pattern, typical of the baby talk of small children, in which dental consonants, e.g., /d/ and /t/, are used to replace velars, such as /g/ and /k/.

gamma-endorphin: See ENDORPHIN.

Gamma hypothesis: See ALPHA, BETA, GAMMA HYPOTHESES.

gamma motoneurons a category of motor neurons usually found in muscle spindles and originally identified as A-gamma fibers because their conduction rate is slower than that of A-alpha and A-beta nerve fibers. Some muscle-spindle motor neurons are large with fast conduction rates and technically are not g.m. Also called **intrafusal motoneurons**.

gamma movement a form of apparent, or illusory,

movement in which an object appears to expand when it is suddenly presented, or to contract when it is withdrawn, and when the intensity of a light is suddenly increased, it appears to grow larger and to approach, and when its intensity is suddenly decreased, it appears to shrink and recede.

gamma waves brain waves with the highest frequency of any recorded on the EEG, reaching 40 to 50 cycles per second at peak amplitude. G.w. are found primarily in the forward part of the cortex and appear to reflect thinking and reasoning.

gamonomania an abnormally strong urge to marry.

gamophobia a morbid fear of marriage.

gang a social group composed of members with a high degree of personal contact who share common interests and standards of behavior, which in some instances are antisocial.

ganglionic blocking agents substances that are antagonists to drugs that stimulate the autonomic ganglia. Hexamethonium is an example of g.b.a. and functions as a double agent that imitates acetylcholine at the junction of nerves and muscles and also antagonizes acetylcholine at the ganglionic synapses, interfering with nerve transmission at both sites.

ganglionic layer: See CELLULAR LAYERS OF CORTEX.

ganglion trigeminale = GASSERIAN GANGLION.

gangliosidosis a lipid-metabolism disease marked by the excessive accumulation of **gangliosides** in the nervous system. Gangliosides are complex chemical agents composed in part of fat and sugar molecules; they normally are present in the nervous system in only trace amounts. G. occurs in a number of different forms, each associated with a specific ganglioside. Tay-Sachs disease is one type of g.

gangrene a pathologic tissue condition in which an area of the body becomes necrotic, usually because of an interruption of a normal blood supply, and putrefying bacteria invade the dead tissue. G. may occur as a result of atherosclerotic occlusion of an artery to one of the extremities, severe frostbite or freezing of a limb, or Buerger's disease aggravated by cigarette-smoking. See BUERGER'S DISEASE.

ganja one of the more potent forms of hashish, or cannabis sativa. G. has been used in experiments to determine if cannabis may increase the incidence of chromosome damage among marijuana smokers. G. smokers reportedly experience respiratory disorders at a rate twice that of the average for cannabis smokers.

Ganser, Sigbert /gän′zər/ German psychiatrist, 1853–1931. See GANSER SYNDROME; AFFECTIVE AMNESIA; AFFECTIVE EUDEMONIA; FACTITIOUS DISORDER WITH PSYCHOLOGICAL SYMPTOMS; PSEUDODEMENTIA; VORBEIREDEN.

Ganser syndrome a relatively rare disorder in which a prisoner awaiting trial or a patient under examination for commitment gives absurd, approximate, or inappropriate answers to simple questions; e.g., a saw may be called a nail, or a horse may be said to have six legs. The condition was first described in 1898 by the German psychiatrist Sigbert Ganser and is probably an unconscious attempt to avoid a distasteful situation rather than a deliberate attempt to malinger. Also called **Ganser's syndrome; syndrome of approximate answers**; and, popularly, **nonsense syndrome**.

Ganzfeld /gänts′felt/ a homogeneous visual field, without any particular point or area of stimulation (German, "entire field"). In an experiment, subjects looked into white spheres, and when colors were introduced, the colors tended to disappear, indicating that the registration of color (and likewise of form) requires stimulus change.

Gardner, Howard American psychologist, fl. 1980. See COGNITIVE STYLE; FIVE-TO-SEVEN SHIFT; LEARNING MODEL; PURE MEANING; SCHEMES; VERBAL THOUGHT.

Gardner-Diamond syndrome a morbid condition of body-surface lesions following a period of emotional distress or trauma. The lesions may occur singly or in clusters, beginning as a stinging, tingling, or burning sensation, and developing into black and blue patches (eccymoses) and painful, red swellings. Also called **psychogenic-purpura-and-painful-bruising syndrome**.

gargalanesthesia the absence of tickle sensitivity.

gargalesthesia sensitivity to tickling.

gargoylism the grotesque facial appearance of patients suffering from mucopolysaccharidosis in Hurler's syndrome. The features include an abnormally long and narrow skull due to premature closure of the sagittal suture, broad nose bridge, an open mouth with a large tongue protruding, thick lips, and clouded corneas. See HURLER'S SYNDROME.

GAS = GENERAL ADAPTATION SYNDROME.

gas chromatography a method of chemical analysis in which an inert gas in injected into a glass tube containing the substance to be tested in order to separate volatile fractions of the substance. G.c. is used to separate and quantify barbiturates, steroid, and fatty acids. Also see CHROMATOGRAPHY.

gasoline intoxication a euphoric reaction induced by gasoline-vapor inhalation. G.i. also results in headache, weakness, CNS depression, confusion, nausea, and respiratory disorders. Inhalation of volatile hydrocarbons is extremely rapid and more toxic than oral ingestion of the same substance. Gasoline inhalation may be more than 100 times as toxic as ingestion of the same amount.

gas poisoning toxic or lethal effects of inhaling a gas. Specific effects vary with the type of substance inhaled. A concentration of five parts per ten million of formaldehyde in the atmosphere will paralyze the cilia of the human respiratory tract. A concentration of 500 parts of carbon monoxide per million for one hour may cause only a slight headache, but twice that concentration for the same period may be fatal.

Gasser, Johann Ludwig /gäs'ər/ Austrian anatomist, 1723–65. See GASSERIAN GANGLION.

Gasserian ganglion a nerve complex at the point in the trigeminal nerve where three branches join. Also called **ganglion trigeminale**. See TRIGEMINAL NERVE; TIC DOULOUREUX.

-gastr-; -gastro- a combining form relating to the stomach (Greek *gaster*).

gastric motility movements of the stomach muscles, particularly those caused by digestive processes. G.m. also may occur in the absence of food in the stomach, as in the reaction of a patient to stress. See STOMACH REACTOR.

gastric neuropathy one of the visceral forms of diabetic neuropathy, marked by delayed emptying of the stomach and irregular food absorption. See DIABETIC ENTEROPATHY; DIABETIC GASTROPATHY.

gastrin: See ZOLLINGER-ELLISON SYNDROME.

gastroduodenal ulceration a peptic ulcer of the alimentary mucosa which is exposed to gastric acid of the stomach. Ulcers on the stomach side of the boundary between the two organ segments tend to develop later in life and are less likely to be associated with increased acid secretion than peptic ulcers on the duodenal side. Since nearly everybody secretes gastric acid but only certain individuals develop ulcers, factors other than acid are assumed to be responsible for the development of peptic ulcers. Stress has been implicated as a causative factor. Also, the g.u. appears, on the basis of some study findings, to occur more frequently in persons with O-type blood, suggesting a possible familial or genetic factor. Also see ULCER; ULCER PERSONALITY.

gastroenteritis an inflammation of the lining of the stomach and intestines. The causes may be food poisoning, infectious diseases, allergic reactions, or psychologic factors, such as fear, anger, or other emotional disturbance. Symptoms may include headache, nausea and vomiting, diarrhea, and gas pain.

gastrointestinal motility the forward motion of contents of the gastrointestinal tract, propelled mainly by the alternate contractions of bands of circular and longitudinal muscle fibers that produce peristalsis.

gastrointestinal problems disorders associated with dysfunctions of the gastrointestinal tract, such as diarrhea, malabsorption syndrome, colitis, flatulence, dysphagia, gastroenteritis, and peptic ulcer.

gastrulation a stage of embryonic development in which the blastula, or clump of undifferentiated cells, begins to evolve into the shape of a primitive organism.

gate-control theory of pain the generalization that the spinal cord regulates the amount of perceived pain reaching the brain by opening or closing "gates" for the flow of pain impulses. See GATING; SPINAL GATE.

gatekeeper a nonprofessional who may have received special training as a liaison worker between a community health center and an area of the community, e.g., a playground, where signs of stress may appear.

Gates, Arthur Irving American psychologist, 1890—. See GATES-MACGINITIE READING TESTS.

Gates-MacGinitie Reading Tests a series of tests (replacing the **Gates Reading Tests**) designed to assess vocabulary, comprehension, reading speed, and reading accuracy at the primary level.

gating the inhibition or blocking of one set of sensory stimuli or one sensory channel when attention is focused on another channel or set of stimuli. That is, while attending to one sensory channel, other channels are either "turned off" or processed at the periphery of awareness. Also called **sensory g.** Also see GATE-CONTROL THEORY OF PAIN; SPINAL GATE.

gating mechanism = SPINAL GATE.

gatophobia = AILUROPHOBIA.

Gaucher, Philippe Charles Ernest /gōshā'/ French physician, 1854–1918. See GAUCHER'S DISEASE; CEREBROSIDE; LIPID-METABOLISM DISORDERS; SPHINGOLIPID; SPHINGOLIPIDOSES.

Gaucher's disease a genetic disorder involving enlarged liver and spleen, associated with large cells that appear to contain fat. A cerebral and noncerebral form of the disease have been described. The cerebral type of G.d. is marked by severe impairment of psychomotor function and, in some cases, progressive dementia. Also called **cerebroside lipidosis.** See LIPID-METABOLISM DISORDERS.

Gauss, Carl Friedrich /gous/ German mathematician, 1777–1855. See NORMAL DISTRIBUTION (also called **Gaussian distribution**).

gay a popular term for homosexual, primarily male homosexual. It is used as noun and adjective.

gay liberation a term used by militant homosexuals seeking recognition of their behavior as normal and to achieve civil rights they feel are denied because of their sexual orientation.

Gegenhalten /gā'gənhäl'tən/ in neurology, involuntary resistance to passive movement of the extremities (German, "holding against, resisting").

Gehrig, Lou: See AMYOTROPHIC LATERAL SCLEROSIS.

Geist Picture Interest Inventory: See INTEREST TESTS.

gelasmus; gelastic epilepsy: See LAUGHTER.

Gelinau, Jean Baptiste Edouard /zhelĕnō'/ French neurologist, 1859—. See GELINAU'S SYNDROME.

Gelineau's syndrome a form of idiopathic narcolepsy.

Gemeinschaftsgefühl: See SOCIAL INTEREST.

-gen-; -genes-; -genet- /-jen-/ a combining form relating to generation or production (from Greek *-genes*, "born, of a certain kind").

gender dysphoria displeasure or unhappiness associated with one's gender role. The state is sometimes associated with the absence of a parent at an early age, as in cases of female-to-male transsexualism that develops in girls who experience maternal deprivation and develop a competitive relationship with the father.

gender identity a sense of maleness or femaleness resulting from a combination of biologic and psychic influences, including environmental effects of family and cultural attitudes. The main biologic factor is the Y-sex-chromosome influence on male-hormone production which appears to affect brain development, resulting in masculine behavior. Female g.i. is the state resulting from absence of the Y-chromosome influence. Also see GENDER ROLE; ROLE CONFUSION; SEXUAL IDENTITY.

gender-identity disorder of childhood a psychosexual disorder consisting of a persistent feeling of discomfort and inappropriateness concerning one's anatomic sex, arising before puberty and involving (a) the desire to be, or insistence that he or she is, of the other sex, and (b) persistent repudiation of the anatomy and activities typical of his or her own sex, going far beyond ordinary "tomboy" or "sissy" behavior. (DSM-III).

gender-identity disorders a group of rare psychosexual disorders characterized by conflict between anatomic sex and sexual identification (male or female). These disorders include TRANSSEXUALISM, GENDER-IDENTITY DISORDER OF CHILDHOOD, and ATYPICAL GENDER-IDENTITY DISORDER. See these entries. (DSM-III).

gender role the pattern of masculine or feminine behavior that characterizes an individual, defining masculine and feminine in terms accepted by the particular culture. The g.r. is largely determined by one's rearing and may or may not conform to the individual's biologically determined sexual identity. Also see GENDER IDENTITY; ROLE CONFUSION.

gene a portion of a chromosome that contains a code for a specific functional product of an organism. The product may be an RNA molecule or a portion of a protein molecule that would be synthesized by the RNA from substances in the environment. A g. carries a particular trait from one generation of the species to the next. The trait may be expressed in the organism if the g. inherited is dominant or if chromosomes inherited from both parents, in the case of higher organisms, are both recessive for that trait. A dominant g. for humans might contain the code for brown eye color while a recessive g. could be the code for producing blue eye color. See DOMINANT G.; RECESSIVE G.

genealogy the study of the ancestry of an individual with emphasis on family history and relationships rather than hereditary traits.

gene mutation a sudden alteration in a genetic trait that results in an individual abnormality and may or may not be transmitted to the individual's offspring. The mutation may or may not be beneficial to the species but could account for evolutionary changes. A g.m. can be caused by radioactive energy, a chemical in the environment, or unknown factors. Most achondroplastic dwarfs are considered examples of spontaneous mutation since they occur about 80 percent of the time in families that have no record of the abnormality. They also represent a type of mutation that can become an inherited trait as the new gene can be transmitted to the offspring of the dwarf. Also see MUTATION.

gene pool the total number of genetic traits distributed within the population of a species. In populations that favor random sexual selection, the genes are distributed along a normal, or bell-shaped, curve. Each gene adds slightly to or subtracts slightly from a given trait. See MULTI-FACTORIAL INHERITANCE.

general ability a measurable ability to handle all types of intellectual tasks. Also see GENERAL FACTOR.

general adaptation syndrome the total mobilization of the organism's resources and defense systems to meet situations of severe stress. According to H. Selye, originator of the concept in 1950, there are three levels of defense, each determined largely by endocrine secretions. In stage one, termed alarm reaction, pituitary-adrenal secretions produce an increase in heart rate, blood sugar, muscle tone, and general alertness. In stage two, termed resistance, secretions from the adrenal cortex (corticoids) help the organism repair damage and sustain continued stress. In stage three, termed exhaustion, the hormone defenses and protective reactions break down, and continued exposure to stress may lead to disintegration, diseases of adaptation (such as hypertension, arthritis, peptic ulcer), and even death. The ability of the individual to survive depends upon the length and severity of the stress condition and the body's ability to cope and endure. Abbrev.: **GAS**. Also called **adaptation syndrome**.

general anesthetics: See ANESTHETICS.

General Anxiety Scale for Children: See ANXIETY SCALES.

general aptitude: See APTITUDE.

General Aptitude Test Battery a group of United States Employment Service tests covering verbal, numerical, and spatial aptitude as well as manual dexterity, form perception, and clerical perception.

general arousal = ORIENTING RESPONSE.

general factor a general ability of intrinsic importance in test results, e.g., intelligence tests. According to C. Spearman, the g.f. represents the capacity to perceive relationships and derive conclusions from them. The g.f. is said to be a basic ability that underlies the performance of different varieties of intellectual tasks in contrast to specific abilities unique to special tasks. As used by L. L. Thurstone in factor analysis, the g.f. is the general ability with which each of the primary factors is correlated. Abbrev.: **g**. Compare SPECIAL FACTOR.

general image an image representing any one of a class of objects.

generalities: See GLITTERING G.

generalizability the accuracy with which results or findings can be generalized or transferred to situations other than those originally studied.

generalization the process of applying a concept, judgment, principle, or theory derived from a limited number of cases to an entire class of objects, events, or people. More simply, g. is the tendency to make the same response to new but similar stimuli, as we often do in stereotyping people. The term is also applied to the process by which stimuli that did not occur in the original conditioning process come to evoke the conditioned response; e.g., a dog conditioned to bark when a particular bell sounds tends to bark to bells of any pitch. See RESPONSE GENERALIZATION PRINCIPLE; STIMULUS GENERALIZATION.

generalization gradient = EXCITATION GRADIENT.

generalized amnesia: See PSYCHOGENIC AMNESIA.

generalized-anxiety disorder an anxiety state, or neurosis, characterized by a generally anxious mood lasting at least a month, and manifested in such symptoms as **motor tension** (jitteriness, muscle aches, fatigue, inability to relax, furrowed brow), **autonomic hyperactivity** (sweating, pounding heart, dry mouth, light-headedness, frequent urination, upset stomach), **apprehensive expectation** (feelings of anxiety and worry, anticipation of catastrophe to self or family), or **vigilance** and scanning (feeling on edge, impatient, and irritable, having difficulty concentrating and sleeping). Abbrev.: **GAD**. (DSM-III)

generalized gangliosidosis = G_{M1} GANGLIOSIDOSIS. Also see LIPID-METABOLISM DISORDERS.

generalized inhibitory potential a conditioned inhibition that results from a stimulus generalization.

generalized reinforcer a rewarding factor that will reinforce a wide range of stimuli and behavior. For humans, money is a g.r.; for laboratory animals, food is a g.r.

general language disability a wide-ranging language disorder in children characterized by delayed speech, prolonged use of infantile speech and grammar, and reading and spelling difficulty. G.l.d. may stem from minimal brain damage.

general paresis the severest form of neurosyphilis, caused by the destructive action of the spirochete on brain tissue. Due to a lengthy incubation period, initial symptoms appear between five and 30 years after the primary infection. Psychological signs are irritability, confusion, fatigue, and forgetfulness, followed by headaches, failure to grasp finer shades of meaning, confabulation, and deterioration in manners, morals, and judgment. If untreated with penicillin, physical signs gradually develop, including sluggish pupils, sagging facial muscles, vacant expression, slurred speech, poor handwriting, unsteady gait, followed by inability to dress, paralyses, convulsions, loss of bladder and bowel control, and gradual deterioration to a vegetative level. For personality types, de-

pending on previous trends, see G.P., DEMENTED OR SIMPLE TYPE; G.P., DEPRESSED TYPE; G.P., EXPANSIVE TYPE; G.P., PARANOID TYPE; ARGYLL-ROBERTSON PUPIL; LOCOMOTER ATAXIA. Also see SYPHILIS; BAYLE'S DISEASE. Also called **general paralysis**. Obsolete terms for g.p. are **general paralysis of the insane; dementia paralytica; paralytic dementia; paretic psychosis**.

general paresis, demented or simple type the most common psychosis occurring in advanced general paresis, characterized by mental deterioration, masklike facies, loss of interest, apathy, and withdrawal.

general paresis, depressed type a psychosis occurring in advanced general paresis, consisting of discouragement due to failing powers, followed by loss of insight, deep despondency, and, in some cases, nihilistic delusions (e.g., "My body is a hollow shell").

general paresis, expansive type a psychosis occurring in advanced general paresis, marked by euphoria, grandiose schemes, and delusions ("I am the richest man in the world"; "I know how we can have an unlimited supply of energy").

general paresis, paranoid type a psychosis occurring in advanced general paresis, in which the most prominent symptom is DELUSION OF PERSECUTION. See this entry.

general-principles transfer: See TRANSFER BY GENERALIZATION.

General Problem Solver a computer program that simulates human problem-solving methods. It sets subgoals and reduces the discrepancies to each following subgoal. Abbrev.: **GPS**.

general psychology the study of the basic principles, problems, and methods underlying the science of psychology, including such areas as the physiological basis of behavior, human growth and development, emotions, motivation, learning, the senses, perception, thinking processes, remembering and forgetting, intelligence, personality theory, psychological testing, behavior disorders, social behavior, and mental health.

General Schedule: See CLASSIFICATION METHOD.

general semantics the science of human responses to signs and symbols, including the meaning of words, signals and gestures, and the psychological and sociological aspects of language in the expression of thought and feeling and in exerting an influence on individuals or groups. See SEMANTIC THERAPY; SEMANTICS.

general-systems theory an attempt to integrate the fragmented approaches and different classes of phenomena studied by contemporary science into an organized whole. Human behavior is viewed as a subsystem of the whole, to be investigated by a holistic approach which draws upon many disciplines and specialties.

general transfer the ability to apply skills and knowledge acquired in one field to problems in another field, e.g., using Jungian theory to analyze a Shakespearian play. Also see SPECIFIC TRANSFER.

generation gap conflict between the young and old; the assumed gulf in contemporary society between the values of adolescents and parents that many social scientists regard as unprecedented owing to extremely rapid technological, social, and moral change. However, other theorists dispute the importance, extent, and novelty of the g.g.

generativity versus self-absorption stage seven of Erikson's eight stages of man. Generativity is the positive goal of adulthood. In contrast to a narrow interest in the self, or self-absorption, generativity is interpreted in terms not only of procreation, but of carrying out one's full parental and social responsibilities toward the next generation. Also called **generativity versus stagnation**. See ERIKSON'S EIGHT STAGES OF MAN.

generator potential a change in the electrical charge of a receptor as a result of a stimulus. G.p. usually is used in visual studies in which the potential may be roughly proportional to the stimulus triggering the effect.

generic skills a term introduced by the Canadian Employment and Immigration Commission to identify work behaviors that are fundamental to the performance of a wide range of occupations. An example of a generic skill is manipulative skill, which involves eye-hand coordination and using the body posture for lifting and carrying. The g.s. are matched in a matrix with jobs requiring one or more g.s.

-genesis a combining form relating to creation, origin, development. Adjective: **genetic**. See -GEN-.

gene-splicing the technique of removing DNA genetic material from one organism and inserting it into another organism, usually of a different species. The purpose is to develop new sources of drugs or similar organic substances from microorganisms or to correct genetic defects in organisms. G.-s. is the basic method of recombinant-DNA efforts. Also see GENETIC ENGINEERING; RECOMBINANT DNA.

genetic code the arrangement of genetic factors in the chain of a chromosome that determines the transmission of hereditary information, such as the sequence of amino acids needed to form the protein of a body tissue.

genetic counseling the presentation of information and guidance that will enable an individual or family to make appropriate, scientifically based decisions involving such areas as analysis of a couple's genetic background, genetic risks, tests administered during the gestation period, abortion, and relevant facts about inherited pathology. Also called **genetic guidance**. See GENE; AMNIOCENTESIS; ABORTION; CONGENITAL DEFECT; FAMILY COUNSELING.

genetic counselor a health professional with special training in genetics who provides counseling and advice to prospective parents in matters of birth defects and inherited diseases. A Princeton University survey found that 91 percent of professional genetic counselors held degrees of M.D. or Ph.D., or both.

genetic defect any physical or mental deformity or abnormality in an offspring that is due to a faulty genetic trait. Generally, a g.d. expresses itself in a failure to synthesize a normally functioning enzyme that is required for a specific step in building a certain body cell or for a vital stage in the metabolism of a food element. In addition to single-gene defects, the term may be applied to chromosomal aberrations, e.g., Klinefelter's syndrome.

genetic drift the chance variation in gene frequency in a population from one generation to the next; e.g., the smaller the population, the greater the random variations.

genetic engineering selective alterations of the genetic contents of living cells or viruses, by methods such as enzymatic transfer of genes between genomes, for purposes such as basic research on genetic mechanisms and bacterial production of medically helpful gene products. Also see GENE-SPLICING; GENETIC MAP.

genetic error a hereditary trait associated with a single-gene defect. The g.e. may be due to a mutation that is spontaneous or caused by an environmental hazard such as radiation that alters the gene's ability to provide the proper instructions for cellular manufacture of an enzyme required to metabolize an important amino acid. A g.e. that becomes hereditary usually is not lethal to the embryo or fetus since the individual is able to survive birth and become a fertile adult and thus able to transmit the g.e. to another generation of individuals. Some genetic errors, however, may result in fetal death or mortality for the individual before maturity. More than 2,000 kinds of genetic errors have been cataloged.

genetic guidance = GENETIC COUNSELING.

geneticism the concept that behavior is inborn, as in Freud's theory of instincts and psychosexual development.

geneticist a health professional who specializes in the study of genetics. A g. may be a member of the staff of a medical-services department of a hospital, medical college, or research institution.

genetic map a plan of a chromosome showing the location of each of the genes. In simple organisms, maps are prepared with the help of mutation-testing techniques. After a region of a chromosome has been identified with a specific function, a mutation is induced at the site and the chromosome is allowed to reproduce. If the function is altered in the next generation, it is assumed that it is the result of manipulation of the gene at the site tested. Human genetic maps are developed retrospectively by analyzing the chromosome patterns in tissue cells of individuals with hereditary abnormalities and comparing the patterns with those from persons considered normal.

genetic material data from the developmental history and previous experiences or relationships of the patient which will throw light on his or her present adaptation, problems, and psycho-dynamics. See CURRENT MATERIAL.

genetic memory a theory that information based on experience or learning may be stored in a DNA or RNA molecule, which might in turn be inherited as part of a chromosome. Also see GENETIC STORAGE.

genetic method the study of behavior in terms of hereditary origins and developmental history.

genetic predisposition a tendency for certain physical or mental traits to be inherited. Schiz-ophrenia, e.g., seems to be a g.p. mental trait which affects less than one percent of the gener-al population, but four percent of distant rela-tives of patients, 12 percent of siblings of pa-tients, and 82 percent of identical twins when one of the pair is schizophrenic. A g.p. in iden-tical twins is found even when the twins have been separated since infancy.

genetic psychology the study of genetic and early environmental factors that influence the de-velopment of a child's personality.

genetics the branch of biology that is concerned with the phenomena of heredity and the laws that determine inherited traits. Also see BE-HAVIOR G.; BIOGENETICS; POLITICAL G.; SOCIOGE-NETICS.

genetic sequences the order in which genetically determined structures or functions develop.

genetic storage a theory that learned informa-tion—e.g., fear of poisonous snakes, or ability to recognize family members—may be stored by the nervous system at the synaptic or meta-bolic level. See GENETIC MEMORY.

genetic technology the study of the biochemical constitution of genes and chromosomes, includ-ing the manipulation of genes of organisms so that they produce substances beyond their natu-ral functions, such as drugs or hormones needed by humans. G.t. also permits the prediction by amniocentesis of the possibility that a fetus may be born with a certain specific congenital defect.

genetic theory the viewpoint that behavior can be explained in hereditary and developmental terms.

genetotropic diseases diseases that are due to an inherited enzyme defect or deficiency, such as the inborn errors of metabolism, of which phenylketonuria is an example.

-genic a combining form meaning (a) produced by, (b) producing. See -GEN-.

geniculate bodies small masses on the surface of the thalamus containing nuclei that relay visual and auditory impulses to the cortex.

genital character the adult stage of psychosexual development which has evolved from the pre-genital levels to serve the interests of genitality.

genital corpuscles = DOGIEL'S CORPUSCLES.

genital eroticism the arousal of sexual excitement by stimulation of the genital organs.

genital-femoral nerve a nerve that receives sen-sory impulses from the genitalia and the leg. It divides into femoral and genital branches. The genital branch innervates the cremaster muscle

and skin of the scrotum in men, and in women the genital branch accompanies one of the liga-ments of the uterus. The femoral branch subdi-vides into other smaller nerves of the leg.

genital herpes a strain of herpes simplex that in-volves the genitals. Although g.h. usually is transmitted by sexual contact, some epi-demiologists believe that because of extreme human susceptibility to the virus it is possible for transmission to occur through other means, e.g., hand-to-hand contact, especially in cities or other sites of high population density. See HERPES.

genitalia the reproductive organs of the male and female of the species. The **male g.** include the penis, testes and related structures, prostate, seminal vesicles, and bulbourethral glands. The **female g.** consist of the vagina, uterus, ovaries, fallopian tubes, and related structures. Singular: **genitalis.** Also called **genitals; privates.** Also see AMBIGUOUS G.

genital intercourse sexual intercourse, usually in a penis-vagina contact as opposed to various other forms of sexual activity.

genitalis: See GENITALIA.

genitality the capacity to experience erotic sensa-tion in the genital organs, starting with child-hood masturbation and culminating in adult sexuality.

genitalization in psychoanalysis, the focusing of the genital libido (pleasure from the sex organs) on nonsexual objects that resemble or symbolize them, such as knives, shoes, or locks of hair. Verb: **to genitalize.** See FETISH.

genital love the love of the genitals during the period of object love; also, in psychoanalysis, sexually mature love of another person.

genital mutilation the destruction or physical modification of the external genitalia. G.m. may be (a) a ritual, (b) self-inflicted as in examples of male schizophrenics who have cut off the penis, or (c) inflicted on others as in war-time reports of castration of enemy soldiers. Krafft-Ebing's *Psychopathia Sexualis* cites cases of g.m. of women's bodies by men. Also see CIRCUMCISION; CLITORIDECTOMY; INFIBULATION; ORCHIECTOMY; SKOPTSY; VULVECTOMY; TRANSSEXUALISM.

genital phase in psychoanalysis, the final stage of psychosexual development, reached in puberty, when erotic interest and activity are focused on a sexual partner. Also called **genital stage.**

genital primacy in psychoanalysis, the final stage of sexual development in which libidinal energy is concentrated on the genital organs and hetero-sexual relations. This stage begins at puberty and is characterized by "subordination of all sexual component instincts under the primacy of the genital zone" (Freud, *A General Introduction to Psycho-Analysis*, 1920). Also called **g.p. stage.**

genitals = GENITALIA.

genital stage = GENITAL PHASE.

genital stimulation a complex set of factors associated with sexual arousal in mammals, in-cluding integration of male and female genital reflexes, odors, hormone secretions, sights, sounds, and tactual and kinesthetic cues. Each factor contributes to g.s., which still may occur in the absence of one or more of the cues.

genital zones the external reproductive organs and adjacent areas which are capable of producing genital sensations. Also see EROTOGENIC ZONE.

genital zones of the nose olfactory receptors that are sensitive to body odors of any kind that cause sexual arousal. Men who find cunnilingus sexually exciting may have olfactory receptors that are particularly sensitive to the odor of the vulva (besides often liking its taste). The active chemical of the vulva odor, a fatty acid, when painted on a female monkey will attract male monkeys who try to copulate even though the female is not in estrus.

genitourinary: See URINARY-TRACT INFECTION.

genius an extreme degree of creative ability, usually demonstrated by exceptional achievement; also, the person who possesses this ability. Francis Galton, the first to investigate g. systematically, mistakenly based his study on the genealogy of eminent individuals (1869). J. M. Cattel favored an environmental explanation. Terman applied the term to children with an IQ of 140 or more, and followed up a large group until they were over 50, but found few geniuses among them. Adler attributed exceptional achievement to overcompensation for feelings of inferiority, while Freud held that geniuses are born with extraordinary ability but are basically conflicted and frustrated individuals who solve their emotional problems by expressing themselves in works of art or science—a theory that has not been widely accepted. Also see TALENT.

Gennari, Francesco /jenär′ē/ Italian anatomist, 1750–95. See STRIPE OF GENNARI; STRIATE CORTEX.

genocopy: See GENOTYPE.

genome /je′-/ a complete set of hereditary factors in the chromosomes. See GENETIC ENGINEERING.

genophobia a morbid fear of anything having to do with sex.

genotrophic disease a disease that tends to be transmitted by a genetic defect, e.g., an inborn error of metabolism.

genotropism a theory proposed by L. Szondi to account for an individual's instinctive choices. The hypothesis argues that the individual acquires through recessive genes the mental traits that determine certain spontaneous actions, such as the choice of male or female companions with a similar genetic background.

genotype the full set of genes of an individual organism. For humans, the g. represents the entire genetic constitution of a person, comprising somewhere between 30,000 and 100,000 traits or trait components acquired through myriad generations of ancestors. An individual whose g. appears to be identical to that of another is called a **genocopy**. A person with a dominant gene for a birth defect may be identified as possessing a **dominant g**. The offspring of a marriage of two individuals with identical domi-

nant genotypes is more likely to suffer a severe form of congenital defect than either of the parents. G. also may refer to alleles present at one or more loci. See PHENOTYPE.

gens an ethnic subgroup whose line of descent follows that of the male members.

genu the knee, or any anatomical structure resembling it (Latin). The term also denotes the anterior portion of the corpus callosum as it bends forward and downward; this portion contains nerve fibers that radiate from the anterior forceps to the frontal lobe on either side.

genuineness: See CONGRUENCE.

genu recurvatum: See BOWING OF BONES.

genu valgum a knee deformity marked by a lateral deviation of the legs from the midline and usually involving both legs. The cause often is a developmental defect and may include a laxity of the ligaments of the knee. Also called **knock-knee**.

genu varum: See BOWING OF BONES.

geophagy /-of′-/ dirt- or earth-eating, a form of pica. G. has been traced to fifth-century China; the "clay holes" of malnourished slaves brought to America; Polynesia and Malaysia, where it is still used to maintain a slender figure and during pregnancy; and parts of Africa, where warriors carried bags of dirt on the mistaken assumption that it would give them strength. Also called **geophagia** /-fā′-/. See PICA.

geotaxis the involuntary movement of an organism that helps it maintain a postural orientation that relates to the force of gravity. Most animals have statocysts, or gravity detectors, as part of their nervous system. The human statocyst is a part of the labyrinth apparatus of the cochlea. See STATOCYST. Also see TAXES.

geotropism the response of an organism to the attraction of gravity.

gephyrophobia /jefī′-/ a morbid fear of crossing a bridge or a body of water (from Greek *gephyra*, "bridge").

-ger-; -gero-; -geront- a combining form relating to old age (Greek *geras*).

geriatric delinquency delinquency among the elderly, from misdemeanors such as shoplifting to serious "crimes of passion." The main motivating factors include neediness and boredom. As a pattern, g.d. was first observed in the 1980s when a higher average-age level began to become a social factor in the United States.

geriatric disorders chronic diseases that occur commonly, but not exclusively, among older persons. Examples of g.d. include tumors, glaucoma, cataracts, heart disease, arthritis and rheumatism, and respiratory diseases.

geriatric psychiatry = GEROPSYCHIATRY

geriatric psychology = GEROPSYCHOLOGY.

geriatric psychopharmacology the branch of pharmacology that deals with diagnosis and treatment of mental disorders associated with the aging process, such as disturbances of sleep patterns, cognitive functioning, mood, and behavior. Because of metabolic changes of aging, drugs may have different biologic activity, and CNS sensitivity to drugs may be increased.

geriatric rehabilitation the restoration of ambulation and independent-living ability to persons afflicted with a geriatric disorder. Gerontologists generally agree that many of the diseases associated with aging are preventable and controllable when the patients seek early treatment, and do not regard infirmities of aging as inevitable.

geriatrics the branch of medicine that deals with old age and the treatment of physical and mental disorders that arise in this period. The term was coined by I. L. Nascher, in 1914. See -GER-.

geriatric screening and evaluation centers agencies that are staffed and equipped to provide physical examinations and care and psychological and financial counseling to older persons. One screening program found that 50 percent of all mental-hospital patients over the age of 65 were actually qualified to be discharged back into their communities.

geriopsychosis a general term for manifestations of brain deterioration and mental disorders associated with aging.

German measles one of the exanthematous viral diseases. It occurs in major epidemics at intervals of six to nine years and produces symptoms similar to measles although it is less highly contagious. Because it is less contagious, more than ten percent of women are not infected during childhood but contract the disease as adults. A woman who develops G.m. during pregnancy has a 25-percent chance of delivering a child with congenital rubella. The rate of malformation in the fetus ranges from a low of six percent during the third month to as high as 50 percent in the first month. The birth defects include malformations of the eyes, ears, and central nervous system. During an epidemic year, about five of every 1,000 live births in the United States are congenital-rubella infants. Also called **rubella**. Also see CONGENITAL-RUBELLA SYNDROME.

germ cells the **gametes**, or reproductive cells, of an organism. In humans, the g.c. are the ova and spermatozoa, which carry the haploid number of chromosomes, as distinguished from the somatic cells.

germ fear = BACILLOPHOBIA.

germinally affected a person who carries a homozygous recessive pair of genes for a disorder that is not expressed in his own body.

germinal period after conception, the first one to two weeks of prenatal life in which the fertilized egg (zygote) travels to the uterus where it is implanted. The embryonic stage follows the g.p.

germ plasm the reproductive tissue from which the male and female gametes develop, as distinguished from the somatoplasm, or tissues that form the rest of the body. Also see SOMATO-PLASM.

germ theory the viewpoint in medicine that infectious diseases are caused by the invasion of the body tissues by microorganisms such as bacteria, viruses, rickettsials, protozoa, or fungi.

gerocomy the medical care of aging patients.

gerontological psychiatry = GEROPSYCHIATRY.

gerontological psychology = GEROPSYCHOLOGY.

gerontology the scientific study of old age and the aging process. Also see SOCIAL G.

gerontophilia = GEROPHILIA.

gerontophobia a morbid fear of growing old or of old age. Also see AGEISM.

gerophilia a love of old people. Also called **gerontophilia**.

geropsychiatry a subspecialty of psychiatry (which is termed g. in the United States and **psychogeriatrics** in Great Britain), concerned with the diagnosis, treatment, and management of mental disorders that first emerge in old age, or first become significant in old age, including those associated with long-term psychiatric hospitalization. In general, these disorders run the gamut from minor maladjustments to major functional or organic syndromes. They contribute to a reduction in adaptive capacity, and may aggravate other illnesses or impairments of the elderly person. The treatment process is generally holistic and multidisciplined, taking into account not only the patient's mental and emotional condition, but also his interests, social and recreational life, living conditions, and, if necessary, placement in an appropriate facility. Also called **geriatric psychiatry; gerontological psychiatry**.

geropsychology the study of old age and the psychological aspects of the aging process. Also called **geriatric psychology; gerontological psychology**.

Gerstmann, Josef /gerst'män/ Austrian neurologist, 1887–1969. See GERSTMANN'S SYNDROME.

Gerstmann's syndrome a set of symptoms of a neurologic disorder marked by dysgraphia, finger agnosia, acalculia, and right-left disorientation. Whether the G.s. is a true set of related conditions due to a defect in the dominant hemisphere or an arbitrary grouping of symptoms has been the cause of considerable controversy among neuropsychologists.

Gesell, Arnold Lucius American psychologist, 1880–1961. A major contributor to the study of child development, G. held that behavior patterns change and mature in a predictable and measurable sequence from the fetal period through adolescence, due primarily to internal forces. This theory was based on observations carried out in controlled situations involving a specially constructed "dome," film recordings, one-way screens, and "co-twin control" studies. See GESELL DEVELOPMENT SCALES; CHILD DEVELOPMENT; FETAL ACTIVITY; INFANT AND PRESCHOOL TESTS.

Gesell Development Scales scales developed at the Yale Clinic of Child Development for assessing the linguistic, motor, adaptive, and social development of infants and preschool children.

Gestalt factor a condition, e.g., proximity, that favors perception of a Gestalt figure.

Gestalt psychology /geshtält′/ a psychological approach that focuses on the dynamic organization of experience into patterns or configurations (German *Gestalt*, "shape, figure, configuration, totality"; plural: *Gestalten*). This viewpoint came into prominence as a revolt against structuralism, which analyzed experience into static, atomistic sensations, and also against the equally atomistic approach of behaviorism, which dissected complex behavior into elementary conditioned reflexes. G.p. holds, instead, that the whole is greater than the sum of its parts, as shown by Max Wertheimer's crucial experiment with successively flashed lights which gave the illusion of motion (1912), and by later experiments that gave rise to principles of perceptual organization (proximity, closure, similarity, Prägnanz) which were then applied to the study of learning, insight memory, social psychology, and art. See KÖHLER; KOFFKA; WERTHEIMER. Also see AUTOCHTHONOUS GESTALT; PRINCIPLE OF PRÄGNANZ; CLOSURE.

Gestaltqualität /geshtält′kvälitāt′/ the form or configuration of a whole, which is dependent on the patterning of the parts (German, "quality of configuration").

Gestalt therapy a form of psychotherapy first proposed by Frederic S. Perls, in which the central focus is on the totality of the patient's "here-and-now" functioning and relationships, as opposed to investigation of past experiences and developmental history. Gestalt techniques, which can be applied in either a group or individual setting, are designed to elicit spontaneous feelings and self-awareness, and promote personality growth. Examples of such techniques are role-playing, placing a group member on a "hot-seat," acting out anger or fright, and reliving traumatic experiences or relationships.

gestation the process of carrying the embryo, later termed the fetus, in the uterus until delivery. See PREGNANCY.

gestational age the age of the fetus calculated from the date of conception. Also see MENSTRUAL AGE.

gestation period the period of pregnancy, or of carrying the offspring in the uterus of the mother. The g.p. ranges from as low as 20 days for the shrew to 550 days for the African rhinoceros and 22 months for the elephant. In human beings, the expected day of confinement (EDC) may be calculated from the beginning of the mother's last menstruation (280 days, 40 weeks, or nine calender months).

gestural automatism: See AUTOMATISM.

gestural communication nonverbal transmission and reception of messages (ideas, feelings, signals) by means of body movements.

gestural-postural language a nonverbal language in which communication is limited to gestures and postures.

getting caught: See ETHICAL-RISK HYPOTHESIS.

geumaphobia a morbid fear of taste or tasting.

-geus-; -geusia /-gōōs-/ a combining form relating to taste or the sense of taste (from Greek *geusis*, "taste").

G$_{M1}$ gangliosidosis a lysosomal enzyme-deficiency disease. **G$_{M1}$ ganglioside deposits** in brain tissue form one clinical feature. Mental retardation and neurologic deterioration develop with tonic-clonic convulsions, skeletal deformities, blindness, deafness, and loss of normal reflexes. Swallowing ability is lost, so that tube feeding becomes necessary. Also called **generalized gangliosidosis; late infantile systemic lipidosis; familial neurovisceral lipidosis.**

G$_{M2}$ gangliosidosis = TAY-SACHS DISEASE.

Gheel colony a group of homes in Gheel, Belgium, in which psychotic patients reside with families. This practice dates from the 13th century and can be traced, in legend at least, to Saint Dymphna, who is said to have dedicated her life to the care of the insane. See FAMILY CARE; SAINT DYMPHNA'S DISEASE.

ghost fear = DAEMONOPHOBIA.

ghost images "apparitions" of disembodied individuals who retain some general bodily characteristics of previously living persons. G.i. are rarely "observed" by more than one individual despite the presence of others and tend to occur in periods of emotional crisis. A ghost image often includes some implausible physical factors; e.g., the ghost wears clothing, rides a horse, or carries an inanimate object such as a heavy chain.

giant-cell arteritis = ARTERITIS.

giant follicular lymphadenopathy: See LYMPHADENOPATHY.

gibberish language that is incoherent and unintelligible and of a type observed in some schizophrenia patients who use a language that appears to be representative of a primitive mentality.

Gibson, James Jerome American psychologist, 1904—. See ECOLOGICAL PERCEPTION.

Gide, André /zhēd/ French writer, diarist, and Nobel laureate, 1869–1951. See NIETZSCHE.

Gierke, Edgar Otto Konrad von /gēr′kə/ German pathologist, 1877–1945. See VON GIERKE'S SYNDROME.

giftedness in children, the possession of outstanding intelligence, ability, or creative talent. G. is frequently calculated as the 0.5 percent of children who score 140 or higher on IQ tests. As a group, the gifted have received less attention and fewer special services than learning-disabled or mentally retarded children.

gigantism an abnormally large body size due to excessive secretion of growth hormone by the pituitary gland. The term sometimes is applied to persons more than 205 cm (81 inches) in height. See CEREBRAL G.; ACROMEGALY.

gigantosomia primordialis a term sometimes used to identify a case of gigantism marked by normal body proportions and normal sex development.

Gilbert, Augustin-Nicholas /zhilber'/ French physician, 1858–1927. See BEHCET'S DISEASE (also called **Gilbert-Behcet syndrome**).

Gilbreth, Frank Bunker American engineer and management scientist, 1868–1924. See THERBLIG; MOTION ECONOMY.

Gilford, Hastings English physician, 1861–1941. See PROGERIA (also called **Hutchinson-Gilbert syndrome**).

Gilles de la Tourette, Georges Edouard Albert Brutus /zhēl'delätoōret'/ French physician, 1857–1904. He was the first to describe, in 1884, the "maladie des tics convulsifs," and in his clinical studies he furthered Charcot's theories on hysteria and hysteroepilepsy. See TOURETTE'S DISORDER (also called **Gilles de la Tourette's syndrome**); ABOIEMENT; BUTYROPHENONES; COPROLALIA; CULTURE-SPECIFIC SYNDROMES; ECHOLALIA; TIC; VARIABLE CHOREA OF BRISSAUD.

gingival = ALVEOLAR.

gingseng root the root of any of the species of plants of the genus Panax, valued for its medicinal properties, particularly in Oriental cultures. It is used as a stimulant, heart tonic, and aphrodisiac.

girl fear = PARTHENOPHOBIA.

give-and-take process: See INTERPERSONAL ACCOMMODATION.

give-up-itis a term referring to the condition in which a prisoner of war or patient with a malignant illness loses hope, relinquishes all interest in survival, and eventually dies.

giving up-given up complex a pattern occurring in depression and bereavement, described by G. Engel (1968) in terms of feelings of helplessness or hopelessness, depreciated self-image, inability to experience gratification from roles and relationships, lack of continuity between past, present, and future, and recurrent memories of previous periods of giving up.

Gjessing, Leiv Rolvsson Norwegian physician, 1918—. See GJESSING'S SYNDROME.

Gjessing's syndrome a nitrogen-metabolism disorder associated with periods of excitement or catatonic stupor in schizophrenics. The metabolic defect leads to nitrogen retention.

glands organs that secrete substances that are needed for some bodily function or that are to be discharged from the body. Kinds of g. include exocrine g., which discharge substances (e.g., tears, sweat) outside the body or into the gastrointestinal tract (e.g., insulin), and endocrine g., which discharge products into the bloodstream. Exocrine g. generally release their product into a duct while endocrine g. are ductless. (The term gland is derived from Latin *glans*, "acorn.")

glandulae preputialis = TYSON'S GLANDS.

glans clitoris a small rounded tubercle at the free extremity of the clitoris.

glans penis the approximately mushroom-shaped cap at the free extremity of the corpus spongiosum. The free extremities of the corpora cavernosa extend into the cavity on the upper side of the cap, and with covering skin and connective tissue the organ part appears to be continuous with the three corpora forming the shaft of the penis.

glare a quality of intense brightness, due either to a reflection from a glass or metallic surface or to any strong and harsh light that hinders visual acuity, e.g., high-beam headlights.

Glaspey, E. American (?) psychologist, fl. 1941. See BRYNGELSON-GLASPEY TEST.

Glasser, William American psychiatrist, 1925—. See REALITY THERAPY.

glass fear = HYELOPHOBIA.

glia = NEUROGLIA.

glial insufficiency a lack of neuroglia cells which provide structural support and aid in the excitation and conduction of nerve impulses in the central nervous system. Some glial cells also serve as a provider of nutrients for the neurons, collecting substances from the blood supply or manufacturing from materials in the blood and storing the nutrients for use as needed by the CNS neurons.

glial RNA a form of RNA presumed to be associated with short-term memory, on the basis of animal experiments that indicated that RNA levels increased in areas associated with learning tasks, following training periods.

glioma /glī·ō′mə/ the most malignant form of brain tumor. A g. can develop from parenchymal cells of the brain, pineal gland, pituitary gland, retina, or other tissues. It usually is a primary tumor and rarely metastasizes beyond the central nervous system. It is the most common kind of brain cancer and accounts for about one-fourth of the spinal-cord tumors.

glissando technique an electroconvulsive-treatment procedure in which the current is slowly stepped up in order to avoid a sudden flow of maximum current and a sudden, extreme convulsion.

glittering generalities vague but catchy phrases and slogans frequently used in propaganda and political campaigns to elicit favorable reactions, e.g., "good, clean government" or "our noble heritage."

global amnesia a type of memory disorder so severe that the patient is incapable of effective thought processes. The condition is associated with severe and diffuse cerebral lesions.

global aphasia = SENSORIMOTOR APHASIA.

global rating a generalized and often ill-defined rating of personality, intelligence, or improvement (such as "improved," or "markedly improved"), as contrasted with more specific ratings based on observations or tests of specific behavior.

globoid-cell leukodystrophy = KRABBE'S DISEASE.

globus hystericus a hysterical (conversion) symptom in which the individual feels he has a lump in the throat, sometimes accompanied by choking sensations. Possible causal factors are frustrations that are "hard to swallow," "distasteful" situations, or difficulty in expressing anger

("My voice gets stuck in my throat"). Also see ESOPHAGEAL NEUROSIS.

glomerular nephritis = GLOMERULONEPHRITIS.

glomeruli a part of the olfactory bulb in which the olfactory nerves terminate; also, a small tuft or cluster of capillaries enclosed in a kidney capsule.

glomerulonephritis an inflammatory kidney disease that involves the glomeruli, or tufts of capillaries, in the kidney-filtration system. The glomeruli usually become enlarged, and there is a proliferation of cellular tissue. Although g. usually occurs after a severe infection, e.g., tonsillitis, the cause of the inflammation generally is an immune reaction rather than a secondary infection. Also called **glomerular nephritis**. Also see KIDNEY DISEASE.

-gloss-; -glosso- a combining form relating to the tongue, and, by way of extension, to speech (from Greek *glossa*, "tongue, speech").

glossodynia a feeling of pain in the tongue, or in the tongue and buccal mucous membranes, without any observable reason. Also called **glossalgia**.

glossolalia unintelligable jargon that simulates coherent speech. It is most commonly found in religious ecstasy ("speaking in tongues"), hypnotic or mediumistic trances, and occasionally in schizophrenia. See NEOLOGISM.

glossopharyngeal nerve the ninth cranial nerve, which supplies the pharynx, soft palate, and posterior third of the tongue including the taste buds of that portion. It is responsible for the swallowing reflex, stimulation of parotid-gland secretions, and reflex control of the heart through innervation of the carotid sinus. The g.n. is referred to as "cranial nerve IX."

glossosynthesis the creation of nonsense words.

glottis the opening between the vocal cords.

glove anesthesia a conversion (hysterical) disorder in which there is a functional loss of sensitivity in the hand and part of the forearm, that is, areas that would be covered by a glove. **Shoe anesthesia** and **stocking anesthesia** are terms applied to similar effects experienced in the foot or leg.

glucagon a polypeptide hormone secreted by alpha cells of the pancreas (the islands of Langerhans) to increase concentrations of glucose in the blood. It is administered in a commercial preparation to relieve symptoms of hypoglycemia, such as the comatose condition resulting from excess levels of insulin in the blood.

glucocorticoids substances produced by the adrenal cortex, or synthetic drugs with similar effects, that increase the concentration of blood sugar or liver glycogen. G. function indirectly by increasing the concentration of amino acids needed to convert fats and proteins into sugar molecules.

glucogenosis = VON GIERKE'S SYNDROME.

glucoreceptors the special cells in the hypothalamus that react to the rate at which glucose passes through them.

glucose-tolerance test a measure of the body's ability to handle carbohydrate metabolism. The patient is required to fast for eight to 12 hours, at the end of which time blood and urine samples are taken for analysis. Then the patient is given a dose of 100 grams of glucose in soda or plain water, and blood and urine samples are taken again 30 minutes afterward. Additional samples of blood and urine are taken every hour for the next five hours to determine how long it takes the body to metabolize the 100 grams of glucose. In certain cases, samples may be taken of cerebrospinal fluids and joint fluids. The g.-t.t. is used primarily to diagnose hypoglycemia and diabetes. Abbrev.: **GTT**.

glucostatic theory the concept that the rate of glucose use by the body is more important in regulation of food intake than actual blood levels of glucose. The rate of use is determined by comparing blood-glucose levels in the arterial and venous parts of the circulatory system, a large difference indicating a high rate of use.

glue-sniffing a form of substance abuse in which the fumes of glue are persistently inhaled as a stimulant that produces a "high." **Toluene** is the usual ingredient in glue that produces psychoactive effects; other hydrocarbons involved in g.-s. may be xylene or benzene.

glutamate a salt or ester of glutamic acid. G. is a neurotransmitter.

glutamic acid $C_5H_9NO_4$—an amino acid that is regarded as nonessential in diets but is important for normal brain function. It is converted by pyridoxine, or vitamin B_6, into GABA. The tuberculosis drug isoniazid blocks the conversion, resulting in a side effect of neuritis for tuberculosis patients unless they also receive large daily doses of pyridoxine. G.a. has been used in dozens of human and animal experiments to determine if it might be supplied in quantities to increase brain-cell function, thereby enhancing learning ability and intelligence. However, results of the studies have been inconclusive. Also called **glutamine**.

glutamic oxalacetic transaminase an enzyme of the human body that may be involved in the cause of muscular dystrophy. Increased blood levels of g.o.t. are a clinical sign of the presence of the disease and also of damage to heart and liver tissues. Abbrev.: **GOT**. When present in blood serum, g.o.t. is usually identified as **serum g.o.t.**, or **SGOT**.

glutethimide: See PIPERIDINEDIONES.

-glyc-; -glyco- /-glīk-/ a combining form relating to sugar.

glycine $C_2H_5NO_2$—an amino acid classified as nonessential for growth and a common component of gelatin. It is converted with the aid of pyridoxine, vitamin B_6, into a constituent of the hemoglobin molecule of red blood cells. It also is used in antacid preparations. Also called **aminoacetic acid**.

glycogen a polysaccharide formed by the liver from glucose molecules and stored in the liver and other body tissues as a primary source of carbohydrate body fuel. It is easily broken down into glucose molecules as needed for energy. Also called **animal starch**.

glycogenosis Type III = CORI'S DISEASE.

glycogenosis Type II = POMPE'S DISEASE.

glycogen-storage disease Type V = MCARDLE'S DISEASE.

glycosaminoglycan: See MUCOPOLYSACCHARI-DOSES; BETA-GLUCURONIDASE DEFICIENCY.

glycosphingolipid lipidosis = FABRY'S DISEASE.

Gmelin, Leopold German chemist and physiologist, 1788–1853. See GMELIN TEST.

Gmelin test a test for the presence of bile in body fluids, particularly urine. If bile is present, the test solution produces zones of colors, according to the varying degrees of oxidation of bile, or bilirubin. Also called **Rosenbach-Gmelin test**.

gnostic function the process of discriminating light touch sensations that stimulate the cutaneous receptors. Also called **gnostic sensation; epicritic sensibility**. Also see PHOTOPATHIC SYSTEM.

goal the objective or end result toward which an organism strives.

goal-attainment model in evaluation research, a process that focuses on the achievement of a particular time-limited goal and measures the degree to which a program has achieved its goals.

goal-directed behavior behavior that appears to be related to an organism's efforts to reach a goal.

goal gradient a principle that an organism works faster with fewer errors as the goal becomes closer.

goal-limited adjustment therapy: See SECTOR THERAPY.

goal-limited therapy brief, or short-term, psychotherapy in which the objective is to treat specific emotional problems and maladjustments in cases where a long-range approach is considered unnecessary, undesirable, or impractical. The focus is usually on the modification of behavior and the removal of symptoms. See SHORT-TERM THERAPY.

goal model of evaluation in evaluation research, a system of assessing organizational effectiveness in terms of meeting the public goals or expectations of the organization rather than assessing the private goals of the organization. It is sometimes considered an inappropriate analysis of a cultural system using a social system as the level of analysis.

goal-setting in industrial psychology, the process of setting goals that provide (a) a basis for motivation, that is, the amount of effort to expend, and (b) guidelines or cues to appropriate behavior if the goal is to be met. G.-s. is effective only if the individual is aware of what is to be accomplished and accepts it for himself or herself.

go-around a group-therapy technique in which each member in turn is requested to react to another member, a discussion theme, or a described or enacted situation.

go berserk: See BERSERK.

goblet figure = RUBIN'S FIGURE.

God complex a term first applied by Ernest Jones to the attitude of some aging psychoanalysts who come to believe that they can accomplish more than is humanly possible, or that their word should be accepted as the final truth. This attitude is not necessarily confined to analysts.

Goddard, Henry American psychologist, 1866–1957. Founder of the Vineland Training School in New Jersey, G. modified the Binet scale for use in detecting different degrees of mental retardation, and showed that individuals in the "moron" category, which he introduced, were capable of holding productive jobs. He later applied Galton's "pedigree method" to the Kallikak family and others, demonstrating to his satisfaction that heredity is the primary factor in mental defect, but ignoring the influence of environment. See KALLIKAK; MORON; PEDIGREE METHOD.

godemiche = DILDO.

God's flesh = TEONANACTL.

Goethe, Johann Wolfgang von /gœ'tə/ German writer, scientist, and statesman. See MIGNON DELUSION; MORPHOLOGY.

goiter: See **exophthalmic g.; Graves' disease; thyrotoxicosis**.

Goldenhar, Maurice Swiss physician, fl. 1952. See GOLDENHAR'S SYNDROME.

Goldenhar's syndrome a congenital disorder that may include small tissue appendages near the ears, tissue growths near the junction of the cornea and inner eyelid, and enlargement of the mouth on one side. There also may be hearing loss and scoliosis. The patients may be mildly retarded. Also called **oculoauriculovertebral dysplasia**.

golden section the esthetic division of a line or area so that the ratio of the smaller to the larger portion is equal to the ratio of the larger portion to the whole line or area. Also called **golden mean**.

Goldflam, Samuel Vulfovich Polish neurologist, 1852–1932. See ERB-GOLDFLAM SYNDROME.

Goldmann, Hans Swiss ophthalmologist, 1899—. See TONOMETRY (there: **Goldmann applanation tonometer**).

Goldstein, Kurt German-born American psychologist, 1878–1965. See GOLDSTEIN-SCHEERER TESTS; WEIGL-GOLDSTEIN-SCHEERER TEST; ABSTRACT ATTITUDE; CATASTROPHIC ANXIETY; CATASTROPHIC BEHAVIOR; CENTERING; CENTRAL APHASIA; CONCEPT-FORMATION TESTS; HOLISM; SELF-REALIZATION.

Goldstein-Scheerer tests a group of tests that require copying color designs, sorting objects into categories (color, form, material), and reproducing designs from memory with sticks. The tests assess ability to abstract and form concepts, and are often used in diagnosing brain damage. See WEIGL-GOLDSTEIN-SCHEERER TEST.

Golgi, Camillo /gōl'jē/ Italian histologist, 1843–1926. See GOLGI APPARATUS; GOLGI STAIN; GOLGI TENDON ORGANS; GOLGI TYPE I NEURON; GOLGI TYPE II NEURON; SOMATIC RECEPTORS.

Golgi apparatus an irregular network of membranes and vesicles within a cell, serving a secretory function.

Golgi corpuscles = GOLGI TENDON ORGANS.

Golgi stain a technique used to enhance the appearance of a neuron or neurons against a background of other cells in a slice of animal tissue. The stain contains silver particles that are absorbed by the nervous tissue. The treated tissue sample is then developed like a piece of photographic film, the nerve tissue appearing as a dark image against a light background of other cells.

Golgi tendon organs receptors in muscle tendons with relatively high firing thresholds. When tension in the tendon becomes high enough to cause damage to bone or other tissues, the organs send inhibitory messages to the motor neurons of the attached muscle. Also called **Golgi corpuscles**.

Golgi Type I neuron a pyramidal neuron with a long axon extending from gray matter to the periphery, carrying impulses from one part of the central nervous system to another.

Golgi Type II neuron a stellate neuron with a short axon found in the retina and cerebral-cerebellar cortices.

Goltz, Robert William American physician, 1923 —. See GOLTZ' SYNDROME.

Goltz' syndrome a congenital disorder marked by eye anomalies, absent or extra digits, and skin lesions, particularly nodules of herniated subcutaneous fat in thin skin areas. Some, but not all, of the patients tested have been found to be mentally retarded. Also called **focal dermal hypoplasia**.

-gon-: See -GONI-.

gonadal cycle the ebb and flow of sexual behavior. Kinds of g.c. include life, seasonal, and estrous, each of which is related in turn to activity of certain sex hormones.

gonadal dysgenesis = TURNER'S SYNDROME.

gonadal hormones the primary male and female sex hormones, including the androgens and estrogens, which generally require the presence of other hormones to perform effectively.

gonadocentric a term relating to a stage of libidinal development, normally reached at puberty, in which the genitals become the central focus of the sex drive with masturbation at the fringe of love object.

gonadotrophic hormones hormones secreted by the anterior pituitary gland to promote the activity of the gonads. See GONADOTROPIN.

gonadotropin an agent that has a stimulating effect upon the gonads. Kinds of g. include the follicle-stimulating, luteinizing, and interstitial-cell-stimulating hormones of the pituitary gland, also **human chorionic g.** (which is used in the treatment of underdeveloped gonads), **human menopausal g.**, and **anterior pituitary g.**

gonads the primary male and female sex organs. They are the testes, which are the source of male spermatozoa, and the ovaries, which produce the female ova.

-goni-; -gonio-; -gon- a combining form relating to an (anatomical) angle or corner (Greek *gonos*).

gonococcal arthritis: See ARTHRITIS.

gonococcal conjunctivitis: See GONORRHEA.

go-no-go test a form of delayed-alternation test, used mainly in animal experiments, in which the subject is trained to respond to cues or signals that are the equivalent of "go" and "no-go," or "stay."

gonorrhea a venereal disease caused by a virulent bacterium that may be transmitted by either sexual or nonsexual contacts. A nonsexual form of the disease is **gonococcal conjunctivitis**, a serious eye infection that can lead to blindness. More common are infections of the genitalia by exposure to g., through sexual contacts.

good-and-evil test a variation of the right-and-wrong test employed in criminal-responsibility evaluations to determine whether the person accused was cognizant of the differences between right and wrong behaviors. See M'NAGHTEN RULES.

good-boy-nice-girl orientation the earlier stage (stage 3) of L. Kohlberg's conventional level of moral reasoning. At this stage, the idea of motive and underlying intention emerge, and moral behavior is that which wins approval. Also called **good-boy-good-girl stage; interpersonal concordance**. See CONVENTIONAL LEVEL.

good breast according to Melanie Klein, the introjection of a part of the mother's breasts as a good object during the first year of life. Compare BAD BREAST.

good continuation the Gestalt principle that a perceived line tends to maintain its direction.

Goodenough, Florence Laura America psychologist, 1886—. See GOODENOUGH DRAW-A-MAN TEST; GOODENOUGH-HARRIS DRAWING TEST; CROSS-CULTURAL TESTING; FIGURE-DRAWING TEST.

Goodenough Draw-a-Man Test an intelligence test in which the subject draws the picture of a man, which is then scored according to age norms for certain features such as eyes, nose, hair, ears, clothing, and facial expression, as well as the basic structure of the figure.

Goodenough-Harris Drawing Test an elaboration of the Goodenough Draw-a-Man Test in which the subject is required to draw a picture of a man, a woman, and himself or herself. An estimate of intelligence is made on the basis of 73 items such as individual body parts, clothing details, proportion, and perspective.

good Gestalt a configuration or Gestalt that is complete, orderly, clear, properly arranged in a pattern or system, as in the spontaneous solution to a problem. Also see GOODNESS OF CONFIGURATION.

good-me according to H. S. Sullivan, the personification of behavior and impulses that meet with the approval of the parents. The g.-m. develops as a part of the socialization process, and serves to protect the child from anxiety about himself. See PERSONIFIED SELF.

goodness of configuration qualities of shapes or forms that emphasize simplicity, regularity, symmetry, and continuity. Wolfgang Köhler speculated that the mind tends to perceive more g.o.c. than may actually exist in a shape. Also see CLOSURE; LAW OF PRÄGNANZ.

goodness of fit the accuracy with which a regression line fits or represents a set of data points; the degree to which empirical data conform to a standard or theoretical value. Also see CHI-SQUARE.

good object a term introduced by Melanie Klein to identify the introjected object that supports the ego in its binding of the death instinct by libido during early infant life.

good sense: See SENSE.

good shape the Gestalt principle that figures are perceived to be as uniform and stable as possible.

goora nut = KOLA NUT.

goose flesh; goose pimples; goose skin = PILOERECTION.

Gordon, Alfred American neurologist, 1874–1953. See GORDON REFLEX.

Gordon Holmes rebound phenomenon = REBOUND PHENOMENON.

Gordon Occupational Check List: See INTEREST TESTS.

Gordon reflex the dorsal extension of the great toe, produced by compression of the calf muscle.

GOT = GLUTAMIC OXALACETIC TRANSAMINASE.

Gottschaldt, Kurt /gôt′shält/ German psychologist, 1902—. See GOTTSCHALDT FIGURES.

Gottschaldt figures simple geometric figures concealed in complex figures for the purpose of testing form perception.

Gough, Harrison Gould American psychologist, 1921—. See MASCULINITY-FEMININITY TESTS (there: **Gough Femininity Scale**); ADJECTIVE CHECK LIST (there: **Gough Adjective Check List**).

gout a hereditary form of arthritis marked by abnormally high blood levels of uric acid and deposits of urate salts in the joints. G. rarely affects women, and generally presents no symptoms during the first three decades of life. Acute g. is characterized by severe pain, inflammation, and swelling about the affected joint. A chronic form of g. can damage the kidneys and the joints. Also called **gouty arthritis**. See ALLOPURINOL; BENEMID; COLCHICINE; ARTHRITIS.

governess psychosis a severe form of schizophrenia reportedly suffered by governesses, although the claim lacks documentation.

GPS = GENERAL PROBLEM SOLVER.

Graaf, Regnier Dutch anatomist and biologist, 1641–73. See GRAAFIAN FOLLICLE.

Graafian follicle a pouchlike cavity in an ovary in which an ovum develops and matures. At ovulation, one of the follicles ruptures and releases a mature ovum which falls into a Fallopian tube to be fertilized.

gracile tubercle an elongated swelling on the upper end of the fasciculus gracilis in the medulla oblongata. The g.t. contains the gracilis nucleus which receives dorsal root fibers from sensory receptors in the leg. Also called **clava**.

gracilis nucleus the nerve cell that is the point of termination of the fasciculus gracilis running from the spinal cord to the medulla. Also called **nucleus gracilis**.

gradation method the psychological technique of measuring change in small equal units.

graded activities a system of grading handicrafts and other occupational-therapy activities according to increments of mental or physical skills.

graded potentials neural potentials that do not fit the traditional all-or-none spike-potential theory. Kinds of g.p. include receptor or generator potentials, postsynaptic potentials, and subthreshold potentials.

grade equivalent a test score expressed in terms of a grade norm. E.g., if a third-grader's score of 99 conforms to fifth-grade norms, his g.e. is expressed as five. See GRADE NORM.

grade norm the standard score or range of scores that represent the average achievement level of a particular school grade. E.g., the mean achievement of all fifth-graders in Wisconsin might be taken to constitute a fifth-grade norm. Also see GRADE EQUIVALENT.

grade scale a standardized scale with scores expressed in terms of grade norms. Also see GRADE EQUIVALENT.

grade-skipping: See EDUCATIONAL ACCELERATION.

grade II astrocytoma = ASTROBLASTOMA.

gradient in the psychology of motivation, a graduated change in the strength of drives in situations involving conflict and ambivalence, that is, the degree to which we feel pulled in different directions. For examples see APPROACH GRADIENT; AVOIDANCE GRADIENT.

gradient of effect the principle that S-R sequences closely preceding or following reinforced sequences are more likely to occur than those that are remote.

gradient of reinforcement the generalization that the closer a response is to the reinforcement, the stronger it will be.

gradient of texture the fact that textures and surface grains of objects appear progressively finer as the viewer moves away from them.

Graduate Record Examination an aptitude-achievement test of verbal and mathematical ability used to select candidates for graduate schools. Abbrev.: **GRE**.

Gräfe, Albrecht Friedrich Wilhelm von /grä′fə/ German ophthalmologist, 1828–70. See GRÄFE'S DISEASE.

Gräfe's disease a gradual paralysis of the eye muscles that is progressive and eventually affects all the extraocular muscles. Also called **chronic progressive ophthalmoplegia**.

graft rejection an immunological phenomenon in which the body's immune-reaction system attacks and destroys transplanted tissue from a donor who is not genetically identical. Among exceptions to the phenomenon are corneal transplants, which do not involve blood vessels, and blood transfusions when the blood groups of the donor and recipient are compatible. G.r. accounts for most failures of whole-organ transplants.

-gram a combining form relating to a record, to tracing something.

grammar the distinctive features and structural principles of a language, especially the construction of words (morphology) and sentences (syntax). See LINGUISTICS; TRANSFORMATIONAL G.

grammatical word = FUNCTION WORD.

Gramophon symptom Mayer-Gross' term for a disorder frequently seen in Pick's disease, in which the patient tells an elaborate anecdote with precise expression and diction from start to finish, ignoring attempts to interrupt the story. After completing the anecdote, the patient may begin the complete story in the same manner and repeat it exactly as before and as if the anecdote had never been told before.

grand crisis an apparently convulsive seizure experienced by Mesmer's patients, which he believed to be a major factor in his "animal magnetism" therapy. Also called **grande crise** /gräNd′krēz′/. The term is essentially equivalent to MESMERIC CRISIS. See this entry.

grande hystérie = HYSTEROEPILEPSY.

grandeur: See DELUSIONS OF G.

grandfather complex in psychoanalysis, the desire of small children to become their parents' parent.

grandiose delusions = DELUSIONS OF GRANDEUR.

grandiose expansiveness a delusional feeling of vast power, importance, or wealth, accompanied by a state of euphoria. Also see DELUSIONS OF GRANDEUR.

grandiose ideas = DELUSIONS OF GRANDEUR.

grandiosity an extreme, totally unrealistic feeling of greatness, importance, or ability, apparently stemming from feelings of inferiority, insecurity, or guilt. Also see DELUSIONS OF GRANDEUR.

grand mal /gräNmäl′/ a major epileptic seizure pattern (French, "great sickness") consisting of a generalized convulsion with tonic and clonic phases, sudden loss of consciousness, often with frothing at the mouth and urinary incontinence, and followed by a period of stertorous (noisy, snoring) breathing, confusion, and deep sleep. Also called **g.m. epilepsy; major epilepsy.** See AURA; EPILEPSY; STATUS EPILEPTICUS; PETIT MAL.

grand mean a mean of a group of means.

grandmother cells a popular term applied to feature-detector cells in the visual cortex that are stimulated by only certain objects in the visual field, such as a moving insect or the outline of a hand. The g.c. refer to hypothetical cells that would be stimulated only by the features of one's grandmother.

Grandry, M. Belgian physician, fl. 1867. See MERKEL'S TACTILE DISK (also called **Grandry-Merkel corpuscles**).

Granit, Ragnar Arthur Finnish neurophysiologist, 1900—. See GRANIT THEORY OF COLOR VISION.

Granit theory of color vision a theory developed by Ragnar Granit in 1959, based on electrical stimulation of extremely small areas of the retina, revealing three types of receptors: scotopic dominators, rods that are most sensitive at 500 millimicrons; photopic dominators, cones that are most sensitive at 560 millimicrons; and photopic modulators, which are other cones that are sensitive to very narrow frequency ranges. Hue is attributed to the activity of the modulators, brightness to the dominators, and color blindness to a defect in particular modulator cells.

Grantham lobotomy = THALECTOMY.

granular cortex the portion of the cerebral cortex that contains granular cells. The granular, or stellate, cells are located in layers II and IV of the brain cytoarchitecture, the areas associated with perception and projection functions.

-graph- a combining form relating to writing or a recording instrument.

grapheme a letter or combination of letters that represents one sound, e.g., the g or the ph in "grapheme"; a minimum distinctive unit of meaning in a writing system. Also see MORPHEME; PHONEME; PHONEME-G. CORRESPONDENCE.

graphic-arts therapy the use of drawing, writing, painting, or printmaking, as a therapeutic tool in the treatment of disturbed children and adults. See ART THERAPY.

graphic rating scale a graph in the form of a line with gradations used to chart degrees of traits or characteristics of subjects.

graphology the analysis of the physical characteristics and patterns of handwriting as a means of identifying the writer, indicating his psychological state at the time of writing, or evaluating his personality characteristics. G. has been called the oldest projective method, since the Chinese used it for character study in the 11th century. Today, psychologists differ as to its value and also as to the techniques of analysis, some stressing specific characteristics such as upward slope or heavy bars on the t's, while others claim that general handwriting patterns can be related to general personality traits. Also called **handwriting analysis**.

graphomania a pathological, inordinate impulse to write, e.g., the tendency of some paranoid patients to write letter after letter to the authorities or to the press as an expression of their persecutory or grandiose delusions.

graphometry a projective test in which a subject draws a figure blindfolded, then describes the drawing while blindfolded and without the blindfold.

graphomotor technique a projective method in which a subject makes a free drawing while blindfolded, after which the clinician attempts to interpret the drawing.

graphophobia a morbid fear of writing.

graphorrhea the writing of long lists of meaningless words, a trait of certain patients (among them, manics) who also may have similar speech habits. See LOGORRHEA.

grasp reflex an involuntary reaction in which the subject automatically grasps whatever touches the palm. In infants this reaction is normal; later, it may be a sign of frontal-lobe lesion. The g.r. is observed mainly in infant humans and monkeys before the cerebral cortex has matured. A similar response occurs when the sole is stimulated. Also called **grasping reflex; grasping and groping reflex**.

gratification the satisfaction of a need or desire, or the pleasant state following such satisfaction. Also see DELAY OF G.

gratification of instincts = SATISFACTION OF INSTINCTS.

Graves, Robert James Irish physician, 1796– 1853. See GRAVES' DISEASE.

Graves, Robert (Ranke) English novelist, poet, and critic, 1895–1975. See MYTHOLOGY.

Graves Design Judgment Test an artistic-aptitude test designed by Maitland Graves to evaluate a subject's concepts of unity, dominance, variety, balance, continuity, symmetry, proportion, and rhythm.

Graves' disease a hyperthyroid disorder affecting mainly adult women between the ages of 30 and 50, and chacterized by an overactive thyroid gland, exophthalmos, reddish nodules on the legs, skeletal-muscle weakness, and other symptoms of thyrotoxicosis. Possible causes include tumors of the pituitary or thyroid glands, medication, or toxic thyroid nodules. Auto-immunity and emotional distress often are associated with G.d. Although scientific data are lacking, many physicians report an apparent emotional trauma linked to the onset of symptoms, e.g., death of a loved one or divorce. Also called **Basedow's disease; Parry's disease; toxic diffuse goiter**.

gravida I: See PRIMIPAROUS.

gravidity = PREGNANCY.

gravity fear = BAROPHOBIA.

Gray, Louis Herbert American comparative philologist, 1875–1955. See ORIGIN-OF-LANGUAGE THEORIES.

Gray, William Scott American educator, 1885– 1960. See GRAY ORAL READING TESTS.

gray commissure an H-shaped portion of the spinal cord that consists of GRAY MATTER. See this entry.

gray market an unauthorized source of drugs, particularly of controlled substances such as anxiolytics. The g.m. sometimes is identified as an **informal source** to differentiate it from an **illegal**, or **black-market, source**. The g.m. may be licensed to sell controlled substances though not properly qualified to diagnose or treat the cause of the symptoms for which the drugs are provided. E.g., a physician who is not a psychiatrist may be authorized to prescribe major tranquilizers.

gray matter cell bodies of neural tissue. G.m.

occurs in masses of cell bodies in the spinal cord, the cerebral cortex, and certain subcortical nuclei.

Gray Oral Reading Tests a graded set of standardized passages administered individually to pupils in grades 1 to 12, to assess oral reading speed, comprehension, and accuracy of pronunciation, and to identify various defects such as word-for-word reading.

gray-out partial loss of consciousness due to deficiency of oxygen in the blood (anoxemia), as in high-altitude flying without an oxygen mask or pressurized cabin, or in mountain-climbing.

gray-out syndrome a psychosis which occasionally occurs in pilots flying in the stratosphere out of sight of the horizon. Major symptoms are a dulling of sensory, motor, and mental capacitives and impairment in judgment, memory, and time sense.

gray rami communicantes gray-matter fibres connecting two nerves of the autonomic system. Some motor fibers pass through g.r.c. after synapsing in the sympathetic ganglia.

gray ramus a collection of unmyelinated axonal fibers of the autonomic system. They are postganglionic fibers which carry impulses back to the spinal nerves from the peripheral branches.

GRE = GRADUATE RECORD EXAMINATION.

great-man theory of leadership the idea that history is determined by "great men" or those who hold commanding positions of influence, power, and authority, in contrast to the idea that history is largely determined by economics, technological development, a broad spectrum of social influences, and Zeitgeist. Also called **great-man theory of history**.

Great Mother: See MAGNA MATER.

Greek love a seldom used term for male homosexuality.

Greenacre, Phyllis American psychoanalyst, 1894 —. See IMPOSTER SYNDROME.

greenstick fracture: See FRACTURE.

greeting behavior a form of attachment behavior that begins to manifest itself clearly at about six months of age. See ATTACHMENT BEHAVIOR.

gregariousness the tendency of animals to congregate in herds or flocks (from Latin *grex*, "herd, group"), and for human beings to associate with others in groups, organizations, and activities, in order to enjoy social life for its own sake. For humans, the drive is probably not instinctual but develops slowly out of the child's helplessness and dependence; g. gives him security, companionship, acceptance, and a sense of belonging. See AFFILIATIVE DRIVE; SOCIAL INSTINCT.

grief a distressing state of sadness in response to a significant loss, usually of a cherished person. It involves a period of mourning in which the bereaved individual may weep, sigh, and become preoccupied with thoughts of the deceased. Where neurotic tendencies or feelings of guilt are minimal or nonexistent, this period is self-limiting. Also see MOURNING; PATHOLOGICAL G. REACTION.

Grieg's disease a form of hypertelorism marked by a flattened bridge of the nose, deformed cranium that presents an appearance of a low forehead, and divergent strabismus (walleye). See FACIAL DISFIGUREMENT.

Griesinger, Wilhelm /grē′zingər/ German psychiatrist, 1817–68. The first systematic organicist in psychiatry, G. attributed all mental illness, from general paresis to hysteria, to brain damage. This one-sided approach was, in part at least, counterbalanced by his conviction that mental disease is treatable, and that mental institutions should be centers for medical research. See ORGANIC APPROACH.

Griffiths, Ruth English psychologist, 1909—. See GRIFFITHS MENTAL DEVELOPMENT SCALE.

Griffiths Mental Development Scale a scale used to determine the level of development of infants up to two years of age in five areas—locomotor, personal-social, hearing-speech, hand and eye development, and performance—and to yield a general quotient derived by dividing the mental age by the chronological age.

grimace a distorted facial expression, sometimes appearing as a facial tic, often observed in catatonic patients and patients with organic neurologic disorders.

Grinker, Roy Richard American psychoanalyst, 1900—. See NARCOSYNTHESIS; TRANSACTION.

Griselda complex the reluctance of the father to allow his daughter to marry because of the father's desire to keep the daughter for himself, a manifestation of an unresolved Oedipus complex.

grooming a basic function of self-care and an important part of the responsibility of rehabilitation of mentally or physically disabled individuals. In addition to the health benefits of g., the function helps build self-esteem in the patient and confidence that he will be accepted by others in the community. In monkeys and other species, g. behavior consists, e.g., in picking parasites or dirt from the fur.

gross motor activities the involvement of the total musculature of the body and the ability to control body movements in relation to such elements as gravity, sidedness, and body midline.

Gross Motor Composite: See BRUININKS-OSERETSKY TEST OF MOTOR PROFICIENCY.

gross motor skills the smooth functioning and effective body movements required for walking, running, hopping, and awareness of one's own body image.

gross stress reaction a transient situational personality disorder in which such symptoms as nightmares, tremors, and anxiety attacks occur as a result of exposure to severe physical demands and extreme emotional stress experienced in military situations or civilian disasters (fire, earthquake, tornados, explosions). The term is a DSM-I category. For examples, see CIVILIAN-CATASTROPHE REACTION; COMBAT REACTIONS; PRISONER-OF-WAR REACTIONS; POSTTRAUMATIC STRESS DISORDER.

ground the relatively homogeneous and indistinct background of figure-ground perceptions.

ground bundles short tracts of the spinal cord that connect different or neighboring levels of the cord. Also called **intersegmental tracts**.

group acceptance the degree to which group members approve of a new, prospective, or potential member as reflected in his actual admission and relative status and role as perceived by the group.

group analysis the study of the pathological behavior of a group; also, analytic group psychotherapy.

group-analytic psychotherapy a term applied by S. H. Foulkes (1948) to a type of group therapy that focuses on the communication and interaction processes taking place in the total group. Interventions make use of group rather than individual forces as the principal therapeutic agent. Also called **therapeutic group analysis**.

group behavior the behavior of a group as a whole or of an individual influenced by a group.

group boundary the rules that govern group membership and activities.

group-centered leader the type of leader who views his function in relation to the desires and potential of the group; a nonauthoritarian leader concerned with the group's needs, abilities, development, independence, and responsibility.

group climate the relative degree of acceptance, tolerance, and freedom of expression that characterizes the relationships within a counseling or therapy group. The work of the group is enhanced to the extent that these qualities exist. Ideally, the status of an individual as full group member is not abridged when he or she engages in disapproved, destructive, or provocative behavior. Rather, a distinction is drawn between such temporary behavior and the individual as a whole while the meaning of the behavior is probed.

group cohesion: See COHESION.

group consciousness an awareness of a member for the group as a whole; also, an awareness of the group that is greater than the sum of members' awarenesses.

group contagion an outmoded term denoting the communication or transmission of emotion through a group or crowd, e.g., the rapid spread of fear. Also see CROWD CONSCIOUSNESS; MASS HYSTERIA.

group counseling a method of providing guidance and support for patients organized as a group, as opposed to individual counseling.

group differences the calculated variations between two or more groups on one or more variables. E.g., the ten-percent variation between men and women in reaction-time studies constitutes a group difference.

group dimension any group trait constituting a variable that can be measured and used to characterize a particular group, e.g., average age, size, or homogeneity of religion.

group dynamics a term applied by K. Lewin to the

study of the interactions and interrelationships that take place within groups as well as between the group and the surrounding social field. It includes investigations of group cohesiveness, the interdependence of group members, collective problem-solving and decision-making, different types of leadership, group conformity, subgroups, and the social climate of different groups. Also called **group process**.

group experience in group counseling, the interactions that afford the client an opportunity to gain insight into his problems by sharing with and learning from other members. Particularly emphasized is the valuable role g.e. plays in helping the client understand others' perceptions of him. When group counseling is an adjunct to individual counseling, the g.e. allows the counselor to directly observe the client's emotional difficulties as manifested in group interactions.

group experiment an experiment in which several subjects are observed or tested either simultaneously or within a given experimental session.

group feeling a desire to be associated with members of a group, and to participate in its activities.

group G monosomy a chromosomal disorder involving the absence of all or part of a G-group chromosome, which includes chromosomes 21 and 22. Patients have mongoloid features, short spadelike hands, and are severely retarded. Because of varied effects, more than one chromosomal defect may be involved. Chromosome 21 often is involved in translocations and aberrations related to Down's syndrome. Monosomy is a rare occurrence among live births but not among aborted fetuses. Also called **45,XX—G**.

group harmony: See GROUPTHINK.

group home a small residence for emotionally disturbed or mentally retarded children or adults, or for the physically disabled, where they can live in a noninstitutional, familylike setting, maintain healthy relationships, and achieve a measure of independence and integration with the community.

group hysteria = MASS HYSTERIA.

group identification the awareness that one is a member of a group; also, the process of sharing, or internalizing, the group's objectives.

grouping in education, the process of assigning pupils to grades, classes, or subgroups. In statistics, g. is the process of arranging scores in categories, intervals, classes, or ranks.

group interview a conference or meeting in which one or more questioners elicit information from two or more respondents in an experimental or real-life situation; a method of obtaining information from a group of individuals who are encouraged to interact with each other in making responses to the interviewer. Group interviews are often employed in motivation research because the participation of a number of people, particularly if they are acquainted with each other as members of a club or similar group, yields deeper responses than are normally possible to obtain through individual interviews.

group marriage a family pattern in which several men and women live together, share the burdens of the household, the rearing of children, and a common sexual life. G.m. has also been practiced among peoples of Brazil, Australia, Siberia, and other parts of the world, often as an insurance against "dying childless." The Oneida community practiced a form of g.m. called stirpiculture (from Latin *stirps*, "stock, offspring"), or selective mating in plural marriages.

group mind an outmoded term for the overall character and behavioral pattern of a group. The concept (a) implies the existence of a group consciousness that exceeds or is qualitatively distinct from individual consciousness and (b) assumes that a group's behavior cannot be understood in terms of individual psychology. See SYNTALITY.

group morale the spirit of the group, marked by confidence and willingness to pursue group goals.

group norms = SOCIAL NORMS.

group pressure psychological pressure exerted by a group to induce individual members to conform to its standards, attitudes, or behavior, e.g., by pointing out the importance of teamwork or majority rule, by threatening expulsion or ostracism, or by rewarding conformity with approval or special benefits. See SOCIAL NORMS.

group problem-solving the collective effort of two or more persons to perform a task or solve a problem. When the nature of the problem is objective, that is, when the problem has a single definite solution, groups generate more and better answers than individuals working alone. However, individuals work faster than groups. When the nature of the problem is subjective, as in questions requiring moral judgment, groups may not be superior to individuals. Also see BRAINSTORMING; GROUPTHINK.

group process = GROUP DYNAMICS.

group psychotherapy collective treatment of psychological problems in which two or more patients interact with each other on both an emotional and a cognitive level in the presence of one or more psychotherapists who serve as catalysts, facilitators, or interpreters. Though group approaches vary, they all appear to be based on the principle that "intimate sharing of feelings, ideas, experiences in an atmosphere of mutual respect and understanding enhances self-respect, deepens self-understanding, and helps a person live with others" (J. D. Frank, *Group Methods in Therapy*, Public Affairs Pamphlet 284, 1959). Also called **group therapy**. For individual types, see ACTIVITY-GROUP THERAPY; ACTIVITY-INTERVIEW G.P.; DIDACTIC G.P.; DIRECTIVE G.P.; FAMILY THERAPY; INSPIRATIONAL GROUP THERAPY; INTERVIEW G.P.; PLAY-G.T.; PSYCHOANALYTIC G.P.; PSYCHODRAMA.

group-relations theory G. W. Allport's view that behavior is influenced not only by one's unique pattern of traits, but by one's need to conform to social demands and expectations. Social determinants become particularly evident in group therapy, since this type of therapy tends to challenge attitudes, such as prejudices, that are based on conformity and restricted thinking.

group residence a homelike setting for a small population of patients or ex-patients who require a certain amount of supervision and care although they no longer need the facilities of a hospital or nursing home. A g.r. may provide shelter and rehabilitation for between ten and 30 patients of the same or both sexes and may be treatment-oriented or work-oriented, according to needs of the patient group.

group rigidity the tendency of a given social group to oppose or thwart structural change; also, its inability to adapt to internal or environmental pressures. Many factors including group size, history, cohesiveness, physical environment, and relationship to other groups may affect g.r.

group risk-taking the willingness of a group to make a decision that involves potential hazards or negative results. In contrast to the traditional belief that groups always tend to make more conservative decisions than individuals, experimental evidence indicates that group decisions tend toward greater extremity or risk than individual decisions.

group roles the behavior patterns carried out by the members of a group. Group members may adopt different roles at different times. Some members may take on multiple roles while other members fill no definable roles.

group sex sexual activity among a heterosexual or homosexual group of people who usually meet with the express purpose of obtaining maximum satisfaction through such means as observing each other, experimenting with different techniques, and exchanging partners.

group solidarity a common bond among a group of people such as a team, combat unit, or therapy group, arising from shared feelings, activities, and objectives. When g.s. is high, the morale of the group is also likely to be high.

group space a "bubble" of personal space that may be established and defended by two or more persons who share the space. Experiments show that members of a group tend to stand or walk closer together when an individual who is not a member of the group approaches. G.s. defense is most aggressive when the group consists of a male-female pair. See GROUP TERRITORIAL BEHAVIOR. Also see PROXEMICS; INTERACTION TERRITORY.

group structure the characteristics of a social group in relation to size, purpose, attitudes, and relationships between individuals, subgroups, leaders, and other members, as well as the relations of the group as a whole to other groups.

group superego the portion of the superego acquired from peer groups as opposed to the part derived from parental influence.

group territorial behavior the tendency for ethnic and other groups to establish and defend areas as separate or shared territories. The behavior is observed in neighborhoods of large cities and in city street gangs. A form of intragroup territorial behavior is seen in family settings where husband and wife regard bedroom areas or dining-table seating patterns as their personal territory.

group test a type of test administered to several students or subjects simultaneously.

group therapy = GROUP PSYCHOTHERAPY.

groupthink a form of thinking or decision-making found in certain relatively small and cohesive groups in which the need to achieve consensus excludes a careful consideration of all the evidence, especially conflicting evidence. Dissenting members tend to voluntarily suppress their doubts, questions, and critical objections in the service of group harmony.

growth center a facility established specifically for the application of group techniques directed to personal change. The common purpose of most of these centers appears to be self-development, or fulfillment of "human potential," in one way or another. For examples, see ENCOUNTER GROUP; SENSORY-AWARENESS GROUPS; BIOENERGETICS; TRANSACTIONAL ANALYSIS; T-GROUP. Also called **human-potential g.c.**

growth curve a graphic representation of the growth rate of an organism or function such as learning.

growth hormone: See PITUITARY GLAND.

growth motivation = METAMOTIVATION.

growth needs: See EXISTENCE, RELATEDNESS, AND GROWTH THEORY.

growth principle Roger's concept that in an atmosphere free of coercion and distortion an individual's creative and integrative forces will lead to fuller adaptation, insight, self-esteem, and realization of potential.

growth spurt the stage of rapid physical development at the onset of adolescence, including the dramatic increase in height and weight as well as development of the reproductive organs and the secondary sex characteristics.

Gruber, Georg Benno Otto /groo'bər/ German pathologist, 1884—. See MECKEL'S SYNDROME (also called **Gruber's syndrome**).

grumbling mania a state of restlessness marked by feelings of dissatisfaction, complaining, and capriciousness.

GSR = GALVANIC SKIN RESPONSE.

gtt. an abbreviation used in prescriptions, meaning "a drop" (Latin *gutta*).

GTT = GLUCOSE-TOLERANCE TEST.

GU: See URINARY-TRACT INFECTION.

guarana paste a chocolate-colored paste made from seeds of a liana plant, Paullinia cupana, that grows in the Amazon basin. The seeds are mixed with water and cassava flour and molded into cylinders. G.p. is shaved from the cylinders as needed and infused as either a hot or cold beverage. The caffeine content of g.p. is about five percent, or about three times that of coffee. Also see YOPO.

guardianship a legal device that places the care of a person and his property in the hands of another. The legal rights of mentally handicapped persons vary in different court jurisdictions. In some areas, the patient loses most legal rights and is considered totally incompetent under a paternalistic guardianship even though the patient may be able to live independently and earn income.

Gubler, Adolphe Marie French physician, 1821–79. See MILLARD-GUBLER SYNDROME (also called **Gubler's hemiplegia**).

guess-who technique a type of personality-rating device used chiefly in school settings. The procedure utilizes short word-pictures of diverse personality types. Students are directed to identify the classmates whose personalities seem to correspond most closely to these descriptions.

guidance the use of personal interviews and tests in providing educational or vocational direction in cooperation with the client.

guidance program the cumulative resources, staff, and techniques used by a school to assist students in resolving a range of scholastic or social problems. A specialized approach will include professionally trained counselors, social workers, and test administrators who each have specified functions within the overall program. In some programs, the use of specialists may be minimized, with teachers and administrators filling guidance functions.

guidance specialist an individual who has been trained in a counselor-education program or who has sufficient credentials and experience to function in one or more guidance capacities.

Guided Affective Imagery the elicitation of emotional fantasies, or waking dreams, in psychotherapy, a technique used primarily in brief psychotherapy and group therapy. Abbrev.: **GAI**.

guide dog a dog that is specially trained to aid in the mobility of a blind person. A g.d. is raised as a normal puppy until the age of three months when it is tested for its role in guiding the blind. In their 13th week, dogs that qualify are placed in private hands and trained only as guide dogs until after they are one year old. About 90 percent of dogs tested initially and selected for training pass the final test after one year's training. Also called **Seeing Eye dog**.

guiding fictions Adler's term for personal principles that serve as guidelines by which an individual can understand and evaluate his experiences and determine his life style.

Guilford, Joy Paul American psychologist, 1897–. See GUILFORD-ZIMMERMAN TEMPERAMENT SURVEY; INTEREST TESTS (there: **Guilford-Zimmerman Interest Inventory**); ARP TESTS; MASCULINITY-FEMININITY TESTS.

Guilford-Zimmerman Temperament Survey a personality inventory for use in grades 9 through 16 and with adults, measuring ten factorially analyzed traits: ascendance, sociability, friendliness, thoughtfulness, personal relations, masculinity, objectivity, general activity, restraint, and emotional stability.

Guillain, Georges /gēyeN'/ French physician, 1876–1951. See GUILLAIN-BARRÉ SYNDROME; ACUTE POLYNEURITIS; INFECTIOUS MONONUCLEOSIS.

Guillain-Barré syndrome an acute progressive type of polyneuropathy with muscular weakness and loss of normal sensation in the extremities at the onset. As the disease progresses, the symptoms spread inwardly. The condition often begins in the feet and ascends toward the head. Since G.-B.s. often develops after an infection, it is believed to result from an immune reaction. Because the symptoms are subtle and the cause is difficult to determine, patients often are misdiagnosed as victims of hysteria or psychosomatic disorders. In severe cases, motor nerves and trunk muscles are involved, leading to respiratory paralysis and death. If the patient survives the acute phase, recovery can be aided by occupational therapy, by orthopedic appliances, and in some cases by surgery to correct effects of muscular deficits. Also called **Guillain-Barré-Strohl syndrome**. Also see ACUTE POLYNEURITIS; LANDRY'S PARALYSIS.

guilt feelings in its normal expression, a feeling of remorse in proportion to actual violations of responsibility or ethical codes. **Pathological guilt** is a highly exaggerated reaction to real or fancied transgressions. In psychoanalysis, this type of guilt feeling is defined as a conflict between the ego and its moral authority, the superego. In most instances, guilt involves loss of self-esteem and a need to make amends. Also see INITIATIVE VERSUS GUILT; NEUROTIC GUILT; SENSE OF GUILT; SURVIVAL GUILT; UNCONSCIOUS GUILT; CRIME FROM SENSE OF GUILT.

guilty fear fear of severe consequences resulting from a forbidden impulse or action.

Guinon, Georges /gēnôN'/ French physician, 1859–1932. See TOURETTE'S DISORDER (also called **tic de Guinon; Guinon's disease**).

gumma: See INTRACRANIAL G.

Gunn, Robert Marcus English ophthalmologist, 1850–1909. See MARCUS GUNN'S SIGN.

Günther, Hans /gin'tər/ German physician, 1884–1929. See GÜNTHER'S DISEASE.

Günther's disease a congenital form of porphyria in which excess porphyrin formation occurs in the bone marrow. Psychic and neurologic changes often accompany pain, nausea, and other effects.

gura nut = KOLA NUT.

guru a Hindu religious leader or spiritual guide; also, colloquially, any spiritual or intellectual leader or counselor. (The term is of Hindi origin.)

guru stage a descriptive term sometimes applied to L. Kohlberg's speculative notion of a stage beyond the highest (postconventional) level of moral reasoning. The g.s. represents an understanding of the basis of one's moral principles, possibly through a philosophical or religious framework. See POSTCONVENTIONAL LEVEL.

gustation the sense of taste, whose receptors are taste buds distributed on the surface of the tongue, palate, and oral cavity, and activated by substances soluble in saliva. Four primary taste qualities—sweet, sour, bitter, and salty— singly or in mixtures, are believed to account for all the tastes we experience. Also see TASTE.

gustatory hallucination a false taste sensation, as in believing that one tastes poison in one's food or acid in one's mouth.

gustatory nerve = LINGUAL NERVE.

gustatory seizure a type of epilepsy attack that is accompanied by distortions of taste and smell sensations, that is, by peculiar tastes and odors.

gustolacrimal reflex = BOGORAD'S SYNDROME.

Guthrie, Edwin Ray American psychologist, 1886 –1959. See GUTHRIE'S CONTIGUOUS CONDITIONING; LEARNING THEORY.

Guthrie's contiguous conditioning a learning concept based on the premise that each response becomes permanently linked with stimuli present at the time; that is, the theory emphasizes contiguity rather than reinforcement or the law of effect.

Guttman, Louis Israeli psychologist, 1916—. See CUMULATIVE SCALE (also called **Guttman scale**).

guttural a general lay term for a **velar** or a **pharyngeal**, speech sound made behind the hard palate, e.g., the /l/ in "all," the /kh/ in Scottish "lo*ch*" or German "Ba*ch*," and the near-/kh/ in French "Pa*r*is" or Spanish "*J*uan."

gutturophonia a form of dysphonia characterized by a throaty voice.

Guyana mass suicide: See COLLECTIVE SUICIDE; MASS MASOCHISM.

-gymn-; -gymno- /-jimn-/ as combining form meaning naked, bare, uncovered (Greek *gymnos*).

gymnemic acid a substance obtained from leaves of a southern Asiatic shrub which is used in taste tests. G.a. abolishes the sense of taste for sweet and bitter but does not affect sensitivity for sour, astringent, or pungent substances.

gymnophobia the fear of naked bodies.

-gyn-; -gyno-; -gynec- a combining form relating to women (from Greek *gyne*, "woman, female").

gynandromorph an organism with both male and female characteristics. In most instances male characteristics occur on one side of the body and female on the other, and in a few cases the head is female and the rest of the body male. Also called **gynander**. Also see ANDROGYNY.

gynecology the branch of medicine that deals with diseases and disorders of women, especially those involving the reproductive organs.

gynecomastia abnormal development of breast tissue in males. In young men, the condition usually occurs on both sides whereas in men after the age of 50, g. ordinarily is unilateral. The cause usually is a hormonal disturbance that may be related to a tumor. Many cases end spontaneously, without treatment. Serious cases of g. can be treated surgically.

gynephobia = GYNOPHOBIA.

gynomonoecism the ability of a person who is genetically a female to produce spermatozoa in the ovaries.

gynophobia a morbid fear of women. Also spelled **gynephobia**. An older term is **horror feminae**.

-gyr-; -gyro- /-jīr-/ a combining form relating to a circle or to rotation.

gyrator treatment a form of alternative psychiatric treatment devised by Benjamin Rush for patients diagnosed as "torpid and melancholic" whose condition he attributed to depletion of blood in the brain. He placed these patients in a revolving cage on the theory that the rotation would drive out the illness by producing vertigo, perspiration, and nausea, and also restore the blood supply to the brain by centrifugal force.

gyrus /jī'rəs/ any of the elevations or convolutions of the surface of the brain caused by folds and clefts of the cortex. Each g. is identified by its location or some other feature, such as the cingulate g., an arch-shaped convolution. Plural: **gyri** /jī'rī/. Also see ANGULAR G.; CINGULATE G.; DENTATE G.; FASCIOLUS G.; FORNICATE G.; FUSIFORM G.; HESCHL'S G.; LATERAL G.; LINGUAL G.; ORBITAL G.; SUBCALLOSAL G.

gyrus cinguli = CINGULATE GYRUS.

gyrus fasciolaris = FASCIOLUS GYRUS.

gyrus fornicatus = FORNICATE GYRUS.

H

h an abbreviation used mainly in prescriptions, meaning "hour" (Latin *hora*).

Haab, Otto /häb/ Swiss ophthalmologist, 1850–1931. See HAAB'S PUPILLARY REFLEX.

Haab's pupillary reflex the normal contraction of both pupils when the eyes focus on a bright object in a darkened room.

habeas corpus /hāb′ē·əs/ in forensic psychiatry, a writ requiring a person to be brought before a judge or court to determine whether confinement in a mental institution has been undertaken with due process of law (Latin, "have the body").

habilitation the process of bringing an individual to a state of fitness through treatment or training. The term (from Latin *habilitare*, "to make fit") usually is applied to cases of disorders that are congenital or acquired during infancy. See REHABILITATION.

habit a persistent pattern of learned behavior which becomes so ingrained that it is almost automatic. We develop habitual ways of thinking, feeling, perceiving, talking, and walking, as well as habitual attitudes, reactions, verbal expressions, gestures, facial expressions, and mannerisms. These patterns help to structure our behavior, but if they become too rigid, they may hinder adaptation to new situations.

habitability the degree to which a specific environment fills the functional and esthetic requirements of its occupants. Also see ENVIRONMENTAL DESIGN.

habit complaint a hypochondriachal tendency in certain children who react to emotional or other problems with health complaints.

habit deterioration a tendency of the patient to regress in social behavior to less integrated patterns as a result of mental or physical illness, particularly schizophrenia.

habit disturbances a DSM-I term for a group of "transient situational personality disorders" in childhood, comprising temper tantrums, persistent thumb-sucking, nail-biting, enuresis, excessive masturbation, and stuttering.

habit family hierarchy Hull's term for alternate routes to goals arranged in a preferential order.

habit formation: See HABIT TRAINING.

habit hierarchy the arrangement of simpler habits into progressively more complex habit patterns.

habit interference the weakening of one or both incompatible responses due to conflict, often leading to the domination of one over the other.

habit reversal a behavior process in which the subject must learn a new correct response to a stimulus and stop responding to a previously learned cue. H.r. is employed in behavioral conditioning, e.g., to control obesity or smoking.

habit spasm a persistent, involuntary mannerism resembling a tic, e.g., repeatedly shrugging the shoulders or nodding the head regardless of the situation. Also called **mimic spasm**. See TIC; SPASM.

habit strength learning strength, which varies with the number of reinforcements, amount of reinforcement, interval between stimulus and response, and between response and reinforcement (Hull).

habit tic a term sometimes applied to a brief, recurrent movement of a psychogenic nature as contrasted with tics of organic origin. Examples are grimacing, blinking, and repeatedly turning the head to one side.

habit training instruction, guidance, and practice aimed at inculcating specific habit patterns in animals or humans, especially the training of children in such functions as eating, dressing, sleeping, and elimination.

habituation in general, the process of growing accustomed to a situation or pattern of behavior; the process of becoming psychologically dependent on the use of a particular drug, such as cocaine, but without the increasing tolerance and physiological dependence that are characteristic of addiction; also, the elimination of side responses that interfere with learning a skill, through repetition and practice.

habitus a susceptibility to certain types of physical disorders associated with particular somatotypes; also, the general appearance of the body. See H. PHTHISICUS; APOPLECTIC TYPE.

habitus apoplecticus = APOPLECTIC TYPE.

habitus phthisicus /tiz′-/ a tendency or susceptibility of a patient to the development of pulmonary tuberculosis. In terms of constitutional disposition, the h.p. person would have a slender, flatchested physique.

HACS an abbreviation of *h*yper*a*ctive-*c*hild *s*yndrome. See HYPERKINETIC-IMPULSE DISORDER; ATTENTION-DEFICIT DISORDER WITH HYPERACTIVITY.

hadephobia = STYGIOPHOBIA.

Haeckel, Ernst Heinrich /hekʹəl/ German biologist, 1834–1919. See FORMAL PARALLELISM.

-haem-; -haemat-; -haemato-: See -HEM-.

hair cells cells in the organ of Corti that initiate response to auditory stimuli. At the bottom of the h.c. are endings of auditory fibers of the eighth cranial nerve. Also see INTERNAL H.C.

hair fear = TRICHOPHOBIA.

hair follicle the protective casing of a root of a hair. The basket-shaped ending about the shaft of hair is surrounded by a flower-spray type of nerve ending, which is one of six basic types of somatosensory receptors. In defense behavior, the follicular nerve ending stimulates muscle fibers that contract and make the hair shaft stand erect.

hair-pulling a compulsion to pull out strands of hair from the head (sometimes from the pubic area). H.-p. is variously interpreted as a substitute for masturbation, an aggressive act, and a denial of castration. The symptom occurs primarily in female children. Also called **trichotillomania**.

Hakim's disease a form of normal-pressure hydrocephalus characterized by enlarged brain ventricles, apraxia of gait, urinary incontinence, and mild dementia, but treatable by shunting procedures.

half-show a form of child therapy in which a psychological problem is presented as a puppet-show drama that is stopped at a crucial moment, and the child is asked to suggest how the story should end.

halfway house a transition facility, such as a group residence, for mental patients who no longer need the full services of a hospital but are not yet ready for completely independent living. See COOPERATIVE URBAN HOUSE; BOARDING HOUSE.

Hall, Granville Stanley American psychologist, 1844–1924. Recipient of what was probably the first Ph.D. in psychology in America (Harvard, 1878), H. went on to open the first official psychological laboratory at Johns Hopkins, in 1883, and to become the first president of the American Psychological Association, in 1892. Concerned primarily with the young, he gathered information on children's interests and attitudes through the use of questionnaires, stimulated interest in child guidance, and published widely-read texts on adolescence, human development, and educational problems. As a side interest, he introduced Freud to the American public by translating his *General Introduction to Psychoanalysis*. See FORMAL PARALLELISM; STORM AND STRESS PERIOD. Also see JAMES.

Hallermann, Wilhelm German physician, 1901—· See HALLERMANN-STREIFF SYNDROME.

Hallermann-Streiff syndrome a congenital disorder marked by craniofacial anomalies, including a small beaked nose, small eyes, and low-set ears. In many patients, the skull sutures are slow to close and may remain open into puberty. Approximately 15 percent of the patients are mentally retarded. Also called **oculomandibulodyscephaly with hypotrichosis**.

Hallervorden, Julius German neurologist, 1882–1965. See HALLERVORDEN-SPATZ DISEASE.

Hallervorden-Spatz disease a progressive neurological disorder marked by muscular rigidity, dementia, and an accumulation of iron pigment in brain tissues. The patients may appear normal until about eight years of age when inward rotation and rigidity of the legs develops. Mental function deteriorates, and speaking ability gradually may be lost. Demyelination and loss of cerebral and cerebellar neurons may occur. Also called **Hallervorden syndrome**.

Hallgren, Bertil Swedish geneticist, fl. 1959. See ALLSTRÖM-HALLGREN SYNDROME.

hallucination a false perception; seeing, hearing, tasting, smelling, touching, or feeling something that is not there. All types are found in paranoid schizophrenia, and specific types occur in infectious diseases, barbiturate or alcoholic intoxication, metallic poisoning, hallucinogen reactions, senile psychosis, epilepsy, brain-tumor disorder, Pick's disease, syphilis, cocaine abuse, and psychosis with cerebral arteriosclerosis. Hallucinations usually occur as visual or auditory images and can be produced experimentally by electrical stimulation of the hippocampus, amygdala, temporal cortex, and other brain areas. Adjective: **hallucinatory**. See AFFECTIVE H.; ANTON'S SYNDROME; AUDITORY H.; BLANK H.; BODY-IMAGE HALLUCINATIONS; ELEMENTARY H.; GUSTATORY H.; HYPNAGOGIC H.; HYPNOPOMPIC H.; INDUCED H.; KINESTHETIC H.; LILLIPUTIAN H.; NEGATIVE H.; NONAFFECTIVE H.; OLFACTORY H.; ORGANIC HALLUCINATIONS; PSEUDOHALLUCINATION; SOMATIC H.; TACTILE H.; TELEOLOGIC H.; TEMPORAL-LOBE ILLUSIONS; VESTIBULAR H.; VISUAL H.

hallucinatory epilepsy a form of focal epilepsy in which the patient experiences transient, paroxysmal hallucinations which seem to repeat during each seizure.

hallucinatory game a childhood game in which fantasy objects are created by the child for his or her amusement, and differ from true hallucinations in that the child is aware the objects do not really exist. Also see IMAGINARY COMPANION.

hallucinatory image a mental image accepted as real.

hallucinatory verbigeration a type of hallucination in which the patient hears the same meaningless sentences echoing through his mind in endless repetition and with few if any changes.

hallucinogen abuse /-lo͞oʹ-/ a disorder whose distinguishing features are (a) pathological use of a hallucinogen for at least one month, that is, inability to reduce or stop use, (b) intoxication throughout the day (with certain hallucinogens), and (c) episodes of hallucinogen-delusional disorder or affective disorder, also (d) impaired functioning, as evidenced by fights, loss of friends, absence from work, loss of job, or repeated legal difficulties. (DSM-III)

hallucinogen-affective disorder a brief-to-long-lasting organic-affective syndrome persisting beyond the period of direct effect of hallucinogen use, and characterized by depression or anxiety, self-reproach, guilt feelings, tension, and concern over brain damage or "going crazy." (DSM-III)

hallucinogen cross dependence: See CROSS DEPENDENCE OF HALLUCINOGENS.

hallucinogen-delusional disorder an organic delusional syndrome, transient or long-lasting, that persists beyond the period of direct effect of a hallucinogen. The user experiences all the perceptual changes that occur in hallucinogen hallucinosis plus the conviction that they correspond to reality. (DSM-III)

hallucinogen hallucinosis a disorder that develops within an hour of oral use of LSD, DMT, or mescaline, consisting of (a) perceptual changes during wakefulness (intense perceptions, depersonalization, derealization, illusions, hallucinations, synesthesias), (b) two or more physical symptoms (dilated pupils, rapid heartbeat, sweating, palpitations, blurred vision, tremors, incoordination), and (c) varied behavioral effects, such as marked anxiety or depression, ideas of reference, fear of losing one's mind, paranoid thoughts, impaired judgment, and disturbed social or occupational functioning. These effects last about six hours for LSD (sometimes with recurrent hallucinations, or "flashbacks") and from an hour to two days for other hallucinogens. (DSM-III)

hallucinogens drugs that produce visual, auditory, or other sensory distortions that may be interpreted as hallucinations. Kinds of h. include mescaline, lysergic acid diethylamide (LSD), psilocybin, bufotenine, and dimethyltryptamine.

hallucinosis a mental disorder in which recurrent hallucinations are experienced. See ACUTE H.; ALCOHOL H.; BROMIDE H.; FLASHBACK H.; HALLUCINOGEN H.; ORGANIC H.; PEDUNCULAR H.; HALLUCINATION.

halo effect the illegitimate extension of an overall impression of a person to judgments of specific attributes. E.g., a person who is seen as "warm" might also be incorrectly judged as intelligent merely because of his warmth. The h.e. can cause errors of judgment by an interviewer or examiner during psychological testing.

haloperidol: See BUTYROPHENONES.

Halstead Impairment Index a measure of biological intelligence devised by W. C. Halstead computed from results of a battery of tests that include time-sense memory, tactual form-board, critical fusion-frequency, auditory flutter-fusion frequency, speech-perception, and rate-of-tapping tests.

Halstead-Reitan Neuropsychological Battery: See CEREBRAL-DYSFUNCTION TESTS.

hamartophobia a morbid fear of committing an error or a sin (from Greek *hamartia*, "sin"). Also see ENOSIOPHOBIA.

hammer = MALLEUS.

hammer toe a foot deformity in which one of the toes, usually the second, is in permanent flexion, giving the foot a clawlike appearance. The condition, which may be disabling, can be corrected by surgery. If a high-arched foot has several toes flexed at the distal joints, the condition is called clawfoot, or PES CAVUS. See this entry.

Hampton Court maze a yew-hedge maze in England whose pattern was copied for the study of animal learning.

Hand, Alfred American pediatrician, 1868–1949. See HAND-CHRISTIAN-SCHÜLLER SYNDROME; XANTHOMATOSIS.

Hand-Christian-Schüller syndrome a rare disturbance of lipoid metabolism marked by the presence of large phagocytic blood cells and an accumulation of cholesterol plus a triad of symptoms: membranous bone defects, diabetes insipidus, and exophthalmos. Growth and mental development are retarded in half the cases. Also called **Schüller-Christian-Hand disease; chronic idiopathic xanthomatosis.**

hand controls special devices for disabled persons that enable them to operate automobiles or other machinery with only the use of the hands. E.g., a car may be equipped with h.c. for the accelerator, brakes, and light-dimming switch, which normally are operated with the feet. See CAR CONTROLS.

handedness a tendency to prefer either the right or left hand for performing certain tasks. The preference usually is related to a dominance effect of the motor cortex on the opposite side of the body. Some investigators have found an association between hemispheric dominance for speech and motor activity. See LATERALITY; CEREBRAL DOMINANCE; MANUAL DOMINANCE; DOMINANCE; LEFT-HANDEDNESS; RIGHT-HANDEDNESS.

handicap a disability that interferes with normal daily-living activities.

handicapped an individual who is unable to participate freely in activities that are normal for the person's age or sex because of a mental or physical abnormality. The term disabled refers to an impairment that may not be a handicap, depending on the degree to which it is overcome and the specific situation with which the person has to cope. Also see EMOTIONAL HANDICAP; DISABILITY.

handicapping strategy: See SELF-H.S.

hand-to-mouth reaction the tendency of infants to bring all objects within reach of the hand to the mouth.

hand-washing obsession a morbid preoccupation with washing the hands, possibly the result of an unconscious feeling of guilt ("Out, damned spot, out, I say!" *Macbeth*, V). See ABLUTOMANIA.

handwriting analysis = GRAPHOLOGY.

Hanfmann, Eugenia Russian-born American

psychologist, 1905—. See HANFMANN-KASANIN CONCEPT FORMATION TEST.

Hanfmann-Kasanin Concept Formation Test a test of conceptual thinking as well as mental impairment, in which the subject classifies blocks of various colors, shapes, heights, and width into four categories: tall-wide, flat-wide, tall-narrow, flat-narrow. Performance is analyzed in terms of interpretation of the task, attempted solutions, discovery of the correct solution, and ability to conceptualize and verbalize. Also see VIGOTSKY TEST.

hanging-arousal: See EROTIZED HANGING.

Hans: See LITTLE H.; CLEVER H.

Hansen, Gerhard Henrik Armauer Norwegian bacteriologist, 1841–1912. See HANSEN'S DISEASE; CLOFAZIMINE; DAPSONE; ERYTHEMA NODOSUM LEPROSUM; LEPROSY; MYCOBACTERIUM LEPRAE.

Hansen's disease an alternative term for leprosy. The eponym was assigned in honor of Gerhard A. Hansen, who identified the causative agent of leprosy in 1873 as Mycobacterium leprae. See LEPROSY.

haphalgesia an extreme sensitivity of cutaneous pain receptors, usually of psychogenic origin as observed by reactions to specific substances. e.g., certain fluids that have special significance, rather than general contact sensitivity. Also called **aphalgesia**.

haphazard sampling in experimental studies, a method of selecting subjects that is inconsistent and unsystematic so that the sample is not representative of the population under study.

haphephobia a morbid fear of being touched. Also called **haptephobia; aphephobia**.

-hapl-; -haplo- a combining form meaning single or simple (Greek *haploos*).

haploid pertaining to cells or similar structures that have a single set of unpaired chromosomes. Also called **monoploid**. Also see DIPLOID.

haploid cells cells that contain half the normal number of chromosomes needed for a complete genetic complement. For humans, the **haploid number** is 23 chromosomes. H.c. are gametes, or the cells of ova or spermatozoa, which, when combined in a fertilized ovum, contain the normal diploid number, or full set of genetic traits.

haploidy the process of meiosis in which the diploid number of chromosomes in a germ cell is reduced by half during a stage of cell division in which each daughter cell receives one, rather than two, of each chromosome in a diploid set.

haplology speech that is so rapid that syllables are omitted. It is common in manic states and schizophrenic disorders in which there is PRESSURE OF SPEECH. See this entry.

happiness a state of joyful well-being and satisfaction.

happy-puppet syndrome a congenital abnormality characterized by playful facial expressions, jerky ataxia, and laughing spells. All of the patients observed have been microcephalic. Their gait is stiff and jerky, they tend to have pro-

truded tongues for long periods, and they are easily provoked to prolonged periods of laughter. None of the patients studied had learned to speak. Also called **Angelman syndrome**.

-hapt-; -hapto- a combining form relating to touch, contact, or combination (from Greek *haptein*, "to fasten").

haptephobia = HAPHEPHOBIA.

haptic pertaining to the sense of touch or contact and the cutaneous sensory system in general.

haptic hallucination = TACTILE HALLUCINATION.

haptic perception the detection of stimuli through tactile-nerve endings in the skin. Also see TOUCH SENSE.

haptometer an instrument that measures tactile sensitivity.

hard determinism: See DETERMINISM.

hard-of-hearing a term used to identify a condition of mild deafness that usually can be corrected with the use of a HEARING AID. See this entry.

Hardy, Godfrey Harold English mathematician, 1877–1947. See HARDY-WEINBERG LAW.

Hardy-Weinberg law a principle of genetic stability in a large population in which random mating occurs. The H.-W.l. states that, with respect to a particular pair of alleles, the frequency of the genes or alleles remains the same, providing there is no mutation, selection, or differential mating.

harelip a cleft in the lip because of failure of the bones of the upper jaw to fuse properly during the embryo stage of intrauterine life. A h. may occur as a single or double cleft, ranging from a notch to a complete interruption of the tissue. The h. in humans is to the left or right of center rather than in the middle where the lip of a hare is divided. Also called **cleft lip**.

Harlow, Harry F. American psychologist, 1905–81. See LEARNING SETS; MOTHERING.

harmaline: See CAAPI.

harm-avoidance need the need to avoid harm, illness, or injury.

harmine a naturally occurring hallucinogen derived from the plant Peganum harmala which grows in the Amazon basin. The bark is stripped and made into a cold-water infusion that is a variation of CAAPI. See this entry.

harmonic an overtone whose frequency is an exact multiple of the lowest, or fundamental, tone.

harmonizer a group member who plays the role of diplomat and facilitates group unity by mediating between opposing points of view and reducing interpersonal tension.

harmony an arrangement of parts such as lines or musical tones into a whole pattern that is balanced and pleasing; also, friendly relations among people.

harmonic analysis the use of Fourier's law or a harmonic analyzer, to resolve complex wave forms into simple sine and cosine components.

harpaxophobia a morbid fear of becoming a victim of robbers.

harp theory = PLACE THEORY.

harria a factor trait marked by assertiveness, decisiveness, and realism in behavior (Cattell).

Harris, Seale American physician, 1870–1957. See HARRIS' SYNDROME.

Harris' syndrome a form of hypoglycemia, or hypcrinsulinism, due to functional or organic disorders of the pancreas and marked by symptoms of jitteriness, mental confusion, and visual disturbances.

Harris Tests of Lateral Dominance tests designed to determine predominance of one side of the body over the other, and, in some cases, crossed dominance. Hand dominance is determined by such activities as hammering and cutting with scissors; eye dominance, by looking through a tube; foot dominance, by kicking or pretending to stamp out a fire.

Harrower, Molly R. American psychologist, 1906—. See PROJECTIVE PSYCHOTHERAPY.

Hartley, David English philosopher and physician, 1705–57. Though H. is credited with extending the associationist doctrine to include all mental and motor processes, his major contribution was his theory that all ideas, sensations, and memories have their physical counterpart in the form of "vibrations"—that is, body and mind are intrinsically related. Despite the crudity of his explanations, he is frequently recognized as a pioneer in physiological psychology. See ASSOCIATIONISM.

Hartmann, Heinz German psychoanalyst, 1894–1970. See ADAPTIVE HYPOTHESIS; SOCIAL COMPLIANCE.

Hartnup disease an amino-acid transport defect, associated with an autosomal-recessive gene. Neurologic signs vary and include mild-to-moderate mental retardation, ataxia, nystagmus, tremor, and psychotic reactions. Most patients also have a skin rash that tends to appear in summer and recede in winter, with exposure to sunlight a precipitating factor. (The disease was named for Edward Hartnup, a hospital patient, around 1950.)

hashish a form of cannabis sativa made from the flowering tops of the marijuana plant. H. generally is several times as potent as marijuana made from the leaves and stems of the same plant. The active ingredient in all forms of cannabis is **delta-9-tetrahydrocannabinol**, which is metabolized in the liver to a related substance that produces intoxicating effects. See PSYCHEDELICS.

Haslam, John British physician, 1764–1844. See PINEL-HASLAM SYNDROME.

hate a hostile emotion combining feelings of detestation, anger, and a desire to retaliate for real or fancied harm. Also called **hatred**.

Hawthorne effect the effect upon behavior of the subject's knowing he or she is in an experiment. The H.e. is named after a Western Electric manufacturing section, in which output increased after experimental changes were made in the working conditions, but apparently as a result of attention rather than due to the specific changes.

Hb = HEMOGLOBIN.

HD: See HUNTINGTON'S CHOREA.

Head, Sir Henry English neurologist, 1861–1940. See EPICRITIC SENSATION.

headache: See CAREBARIA; CLAVUS; CLUSTER HEADACHES; HISTAMINE H.; LEAD-CAP H.; MIGRAINE; NEURASTHENIC HELMET; POSTTRAUMATIC H.; TENSION H.

head-banging the act or habit of repeatedly striking the head on a crib, wall, or floor during a temper tantrum. H.-b. is one of the many expressions of rage in a young child who feels frustrated. Also see HEAD-KNOCKING.

head consciousness overawareness of the head, with a fear that it might suffer injury. It is a posttraumatic symptom that sometimes develops after a severe head injury.

head injury: See HEAD TRAUMA.

head-knocking a habit of bumping the head against a wall, crib side, or other solid object, observed in infants but differentiated from the temper-tantrum type of head-banging.

head-rolling repeated movements of the head from side to side as manifested by some infants prior to going to sleep. The condition has been attributed to inhibition of movement in the crib, lack of stimulating play, and possibly to intrauterine passivity. Also called **jactatio capitis nocturnis**.

head-shrinking the shrinking of severed heads, usually human heads, through the application of heat or herbal liquids, practiced among headhunters and other societies mainly in Asia and South America, who use such heads for mental healing and other ritual purposes. Derived from this practice is the term **headshrinker**, or simply **shrink**, as a slang word for psychiatrist. Also see MAGICAL THINKING; VOODOO DEATH; FAITH HEALING; HEX DOCTOR.

Head Start project a comprehensive child-developmental program designed to give children of disadvantaged backgrounds the services and experiences they need to help them develop as socially competent individuals. It is considered one of the most comprehensive enrichment strategies to date.

head trauma an injury to the head, usually through a severe blow. The h.t. may be a **concussion** (disruption of brain function, with spontaneous recovery), a **contusion** (a diffuse disturbance, with edema and multiple intracerebral hemorrhages), or a **laceration** (severe disturbance due to rupture of brain tissue, with subdural or extradural hemorrhage). Head traumas are of two general types: **acute h.t.**, in which impairment of brain functions is temporary, and **chronic h.t.**, in which impairment is permanent or relatively permanent due to the fact that lasting damage has been done to the brain. Also see BRAIN TRAUMA; CEREBRAL TRAUMA.

health insurance insurance that reimburses the patient for part or all of the cost of physical or psychiatric care, or lost income, resulting from medical disability.

health-maintenance organization a form of multidisciplinary medical care in which physicians, often including psychiatrists, as well as paramedical personnel, provide comprehensive health services to subscribers for a fixed fee. The h.-m.o. then may assume financial responsibility for subsequent hospitalization, if required. The United States Public Health Service Act of 1973 recognized the h.-m.o. program and provided subsidies. Abbrev.: **HMO.**

health professional any individual who has received advanced training that equips him or her to work in the field of physical or mental health. Health professionals include, among others, psychiatrists, psychologists, neurologists, physiatrists, orthopedists, rehabilitation counselors, speech pathologists, physical therapists, occupational therapists, psychiatric social workers, and biomedical engineers.

health psychology as defined by the American Psychological Association Division of Health Psychology, "the aggregate of the specific educational, scientific, and professional contributions of the discipline of psychology to the promotion and maintenance of health, the prevention and treatment of illness, and the identification of the etiology and diagnostic correlates of health, illness, and related dysfunction."

health-related facilities: See PSYCHIATRIC SERVICES.

health visitor a health professional, usually employed by a local agency such as the Visiting Nurses Association, who visits families where health supervision is needed, e.g., to assure that a child does not become a victim of abuse or neglect.

healthy identification modeling one's attitudes or behavior, consciously or unconsciously, on another individual who has sound values, attitudes, and reactions.

hearing the perception of sounds through the auditory sensory mechanism located in the inner ear and brain. The physical stimulus consists of molecules generated by the vibration of physical objects (a whistle, stringed instrument, vocal cords), which vary in frequency, intensity, and complexity. The waves enter the external ear (pinna), vibrate the eardrum (tympanum), and are transmitted by the ossicles to the fluid-filled cochlea in the inner ear, in which the vibrations are transformed into electrical impulses, which are carried by the auditory nerve to the cortex, where they are registered and interpreted. Also called **audition**.

hearing aid an electronic device that amplifies sounds for persons with a hearing deficiency. A h.a. consists of a microphone to collect sounds, a power supply, an amplifier, and an **earphone** that translates electrical impulses from the other components back into audible sound waves. A h.a. may vary somewhat in design for patients with conductive deafness and those with nerve deafness. For patients who have suffered a hearing loss in one ear, a **contralateral h.a.** is available to detect sounds at the deaf ear and transmit the signals around the head to an earphone placed near the good ear, thus producing a normal stereophonic effect that is important in determining sound orientation. The contralateral h.a. usually is concealed in an eyeglass frame.

hearing disorders diseases, injuries, or congenital defects that are the cause of some degree of deafness. Congenital deafness may include persons who may have been born with normal hearing but suffered a loss of that ability before sounds became meaningful. Deafness acquired after sounds became meaningful is called adventitious deafness. The term functional h.d. refers to inability to understand the human voice at certain levels of loudness.

hearing loss the inability to hear a normal range of tone frequencies or a normally perceived level of sound intensity, or both. The degree of loss usually is recorded as a percentage of the normal level.

hearing theories theories of hearing developed to explain the full range of audible pitch (20 to 20,000 cycles per second) and intensity or loudness (about 15 to 160 decibels). The place (or piano or harp) theory of Helmholtz holds that the fibers of the narrow end of the basilar membrane respond to high tones and those at the wide end to low tones, and that nerve fibers attached to the membrane transmit stimuli of different frequencies to the brain. The frequency or telephone theory holds that the basilar membrane is essentially a transmitting instrument which vibrates as a whole at the frequency of the incoming sound, creating an impulse that is transmitted to a portion of the auditory nerve. A third theory, advanced by Wever, holds that fibers respond to the higher frequencies by firing in squads or volleys. See PLACE THEORY; TELEPHONE THEORY; VOLLEY THEORY.

heart attack the common term for a coronary occlusion in which one of the coronary arteries becomes blocked. The condition may or may not result in a myocardial infarction, depending upon the extent of damage to the surrounding heart muscle by the h.a.

heart block: See ARRHYTHMIA.

heart disorder any disease or defect that interferes with normal functioning of the heart. The term may be applied to congenital defects, e.g. tetralogy of Fallot, damage caused by diseases such as rheumatic fever or syphilis, or an atherosclerotic condition, e.g., angina pectoris or coronary occlusion.

heart-lung machine a mechanical device that maintains functions of the heart and lungs for a short period of time during surgery involving those organs. The machine collects blood from the veins before it reaches the heart and circulates it through a plastic chamber where it is freshly oxygenated before being pumped back into the patient's arteries.

heart rate in emotion the effect of strong emotion that can increase the rate of the heartbeat through sympathetic impulses. Parasympathetic reflexes resulting from increased blood pressure during emotion also can have an effect of altering the heart rate. A strong parasympathetic reflex can slow the heart rate to a point at which it may appear on the verge of stopping.

heat = ESTROUS BEHAVIOR.

heat effects changes in mental or physical conditions due to perceived or true ambient temperatures above the normal comfort range. Perceived heat may be affected by humidity or individual cognition factors; high humidity usually makes excessive heat less tolerable. The main physiological h.e. are heat-induced asthenia, marked by fatigue, lethargy, headache, anorexia, insomnia, irritability, and restlessness; heat stroke, characterized by confusion, delirium, staggering, coma, and death; heat exhaustion, marked by vomiting, headache, restlessness, and faintness; and severe circulatory disorders, e.g., heart attacks caused by excessive demands on the cardiovascular system to circulate blood near external surfaces for a cooling effect. Because of variable perceived h.e., studies of psychological effects are less conclusive, although performance enhancement appears to improve with increasing ambient temperatures up to a level of around 90°F (32°C), after which arousal and performance decline. See ACCLIMATIZATION; HEAT-INDUCED ASTHENIA; HEAT EXHAUSTION; HEAT STROKE; OVERHEATING.

heat exhaustion a health disorder marked by circulatory collapse and a comatose condition after exposure to excessive heat. The symptoms result from an inability of the circulatory system to adjust to the dilation of blood vessels in the skin. Excessive sweating, dehydration, alcohol-drinking, or diarrhea can be precipitating factors. The symptoms may resemble those of a drug overdose, but the h.e. patient usually responds rapidly to treatment.

heat hyperpyrexia = HEAT STROKE.

heat-induced asthenia a condition associated with extended exposure to heat and characterized by general physical and mental impairment, fatigue, lethargy, irritability, insomnia, headache, and possible loss of appetite.

heat phobia = THERMOPHOBIA.

heat stress any stress effect on an organism that results from exposure to excessive ambient temperatures, particularly the physiological disorders that include HEAT-INDUCED ASTHENIA, HEAT EXHAUSTION, and HEAT STROKE. See these entries.

heat stroke a physiological heat-stress effect caused by a breakdown of the body's ability to cope with heat by sweating. Symptoms include weakness, headaches, anorexia, nausea, and in some cases cramps and muscle twitches. Since body heat cannot be dispersed by sweating, the skin appears hot and dry. The trapped heat may cause brain damage. Emergency treatment with ice water must be started immediately. Also called **thermic fever; heat hyperpyrexia**.

heavy-particle radiography = PROTON-BEAM RADIOGRAPHY.

Hebb, Donald Olding Canadian psychologist, 1904—. See HEBB'S THEORY OF PERCEPTUAL LEARNING; CELL ASSEMBLY; LEARNING THEORY; PHASE SEQUENCE.

Hebb's theory of perceptual learning a learning theory that assumes that impulses become stored in cell assemblies in the cerebral cortex. Separate assemblies can become coordinated to form a sequence or totality.

hebephrenia a chronic form of schizophrenia characterized by a general disintegration of the personality, involving loss of touch with reality, incoherent speech, silly behavior, bizarre gestures, fragmentary hallucinations and delusions (such as sex change, cosmic identification, and rebirth), and a poor prognosis. The term was coined by the German psychiatrist Ewald Hecker in 1877, from the Greek words *hebe*, "youth, puberty," and *phren*, "mind," in the sense of adolescent insanity. For the DSM-III description of this disorder, see SCHIZOPHRENIC DISORDER, DISORGANIZED TYPE. Also see MANIC H.; DEPRESSIVE H.

Heberden, William, Sr. English physician, 1710–1801. See HEBERDEN'S NODES.

Heberden's nodes small hard nodules that develop on the middle joints and ends of the fingers of some osteoarthritis patients. The nodes may develop suddenly, with or without pain, as soft, tender swellings that gradually change into painless, bonelike knobs. H.n. occur mainly on the hands of women patients and may be a familial or hereditary disorder since most patients have female relatives with the same condition.

hebetude a state of severe emotional dullness or disinterest observed in some schizophrenia patients who not only withdraw from the environment but withdraw from themselves, becoming apathetic and listless.

heboid pertaining to youth, and particularly to puberty (from Greek *hebe*, "youth, puberty"). Also called **hebetic**.

heboidophrenia an obsolete term for the simple form of schizophrenia (coined by Karl Ludwig Kahlbaum).

Hecker, Ewald German psychiatrist, 1843–1909. See HEBEPHRENIA.

-hedon- a combining form relating to pleasure (Greek *hedone*).

hedonic level the level of pleasure, particularly sensual pleasure, as opposed to pain or unpleasantness.

hedonic-tone factor the quality of an experience in terms of its position on a scale ranging from pleasant to unpleasant. The term was proposed by D. E. Berlyne, in 1973, to identify artistic-evaluation variables manifested by verbal expressions of pleasure.

hedonism in philosophy, the doctrine that pleasure

is the prime goal of life; in psychology, the theory that pleasure and the avoidance of pain are the major motivating forces in human behavior.

hedonistic orientation a term sometimes applied to stage 2 of Kohlberg's preconventional level of moral reasoning. See PRECONVENTIONAL LEVEL.

hedonophobia a morbid fear of feeling pleasure.

heel-to-knee test a test for ataxia in which the patient, from a reclining position, must raise his foot, then touch the knee with the opposite heel and move the heel along the shin, with his eyes open or closed.

Heidbreder, Edna American psychologist, 1890—. See HEIDBREDER TEST.

Heidbreder test an alternative term for the Minnesota Mechanical Ability Tests, named for Edna Heidbreder, who helped develop the technique.

Heidegger, Martin /hī′degər/ German philosopher, 1889–1976. H. is often said to be the most eminent critic of metaphysics since Kant. He developed an existential approach which holds that, faced with the inevitability of death, we must find meaning in life, not through outer conformity and adaptation to others, but through self-understanding and self-analysis (Dasein analysis, or analysis of "being there"). By drawing on the uniqueness of our experience and the pattern of our potentialities, we will then develop our own kind of life, our own "being-in-the-world." See DASEIN ANALYSIS; EXISTENTIALISM; UMWELT.

Heidenheim's disease = CREUTZFELDT-JAKOB DISEASE.

height phobia = ACROPHOBIA.

Heinis, Hugo /hī′nis/ Swiss psychologist, 1883—. See HEINIS CONSTANT.

Heinis constant a measure of mental-growth rates by converting mental-age units into theoretically equal mental-growth units and dividing the result by the chronological age. Also called **personal constant**.

Heinroth, Johann Christian /hīn′rōt/ German physician, 1773–1843. H. was the first to claim psychiatry as a separate medical discipline, and eventually occupied the first chair in psychiatry at the University of Leipzig.

Hejna, Robert F. American speech pathologist, fl. 1960. See HEJNA TEST.

Hejna test an instrument used to measure speech articulation by presenting pictures designed to elicit verbal responses which contain specific sounds.

-helc-; -helco- a combining form relating to an ulcer.

helicine artery one of the coiled arteries in the corpora cavernosa of the penis. The artery has a helical shape when the penis is flaccid but assumes a relatively elongated shape when the penis is tumescent. Also called **helicina**.

helicotrema a small opening at the apex of the cochlea where the scala vestibuli and scala tympani communicate.

-helio- a combining form relating to the sun (Greek *helios*).

heliophobia a morbid fear of sunlight. Also see PHENGOPHOBIA.

heliotropism orienting of an organism toward a light source, especially the sun.

hellebore a poisonous plant, Veratrum viride, native to North America and used as an herb by members of Native American nations of New England. It was used by Native Americans as a tobacco substitute and processed for smoking and as a snuff. H. contains more than 20 different alkaloids, including **veratrine**, which produces prolonged muscle contractions. The h. alkaloids have been used to lower blood pressure but generally are avoided because of their potential toxicity.

Hellenic love a seldom used term for male homosexuality.

hellenologomania = HELENOMANIA.

hellenologophobia a morbid fear of Greek terms (such as this one) or, generally, of complex scientific or pseudoscientific terminology.

hellenomania a tendency to use obscure Greek or Latin terms instead of English words in writing. Also called **hellenologomania**.

Hellersberg, Elisabeth F. German-born American psychologist, 1893—. See HORN-HELLERSBERG DRAWING COMPLETION TEST.

hell phobia = STYGIOPHOBIA.

Helmholtz, Hermann von German physiologist and physicist, 1821–94. In support of the mechanistic view, and in opposition to vitalism, H. applied a knowledge of medicine, physiology, anatomy, and physics to experimental studies of the speed of nerve conduction, reaction time, the mechanics of the eye, and the development of theories of color vision and hearing. Many of his findings are widely accepted today. See YOUNG-HELMHOLTZ THEORY OF COLOR VISION; COLOR THEORIES; HEARING THEORIES; PLACE THEORY.

helpful figure a child's make-believe fairylike person, which may be male or female, to which the child can turn for help or sympathy. Also see IMAGINARY COMPANION.

helping behavior a type of prosocial behavior, typically in response to a small request that involves no personal risk.

helping model a broad-based educational orientation that has much in common with humanistic models in its emphasis on the complete individual and the realization of the student's full potential. The h.m. is concerned with the learner's motor development, perceptual skills, cognitive development, emotional maturity, interpersonal skills, expression, creativity, and ethical values.

helping relationship according to C. Rogers, a "relationship in which at least one of the parties has the intent of promoting the growth, development, maturity, improved functioning, improved coping with life of the other. The other . . . may be one individual or a group" (*On Becoming a Person*, 1961).

helplessn ss: See LEARNED H.; PSYCHIC H.

Helson, Harry American psychologist, 1898—. See ADAPTATION-LEVEL THEORY.

-hem-; -hemo-; -hemat-; -hemato- a combining form relating to blood (Greek *haema*).

he-man: See ETHICAL HIGHBROW.

hematophobia morbid fear of blood or, more specifically, the sight of blood. Also called **hemophobia**. Also see ERYTHROPHOBIA.

hemeralopia a form of day blindness in which the person has difficulty seeing in bright light but has good vision in dim light. H. is sometimes used for night blindness. Also called **hemeralopsia**.

hematoxylin stain a stain used in microscopic studies of myelinated-nerve tissues because it is absorbed by the fatty membrane. Also see WEIGERT STAIN.

hematuria the presence of blood in the urine.

hemeraphonia a speech disorder in which the person is unable to vocalize during the day but may be able to speak normally at night, a condition observed in some cases of hysteria.

-hemi- a combining form meaning half (especially when referring to the right or left half of the body).

hemianopia an ocular disorder marked by the loss of vision in half the normal visual field. H. may result from a lesion in the optic chiasma or the optic radiation. Also called **hemianopsia; hemiopia**. Adjectives: **hemianopic; hemianoptic**. For homonymous h., bitemporal h., and binasal h., see HOMONYMOUS H. Also see HETERONYMOUS H.

hemiasomatognosia = ANTON'S SYNDROME.

hemiballismus a type of involuntary movement characterized by flailing of the arms and legs. The condition often is associated with extrapyramidal lesions. Also called **hemiballism**.

hemibulbar syndrome = BABINSKI-NAGEOTTE SYNDROME.

hemicrania cerebellaris = BÁRÁNY'S SYNDROME.

hemidecortication the destruction of motorcortical control of one side of the body, a procedure usually performed surgically in animal experiments. Severing the nerve fibers on the left side of the brain results in paralysis on the right side of the animal, and vice versa. The procedure does not affect retention of a previously learned conditioned response involving the paralyzed side. H. is performed in cases of an expanding brain tumor and for treatment of uncontrolled epilepsy associated with hemiparesis. Despite expectations of mental deterioration following h., the patient actually shows improvement on many tests after removal of the affected portion of the brain. Also called **hemispherectomy**.

hemiopia = HEMIANOPIA.

hemiparesis: See SPASTIC H.

hemiplegia a type of paralysis that affects one side of the body, usually as a result of a stroke. Kinds of h. include **alternate h.**, in which facial muscles are paralyzed on one side and extremities on the other, **facial h.**, marked by paralysis only of the facial muscles on one side, and **ascending h.**, a form of ascending paralysis that affects only one side of the body. Also see WERNICKE-MANN H.; NOCTURNAL H.

hemiplegia alternans a type of contralateral paralysis involving cranial nerves and the limbs on the opposite side of the body. E.g., **h.a. hypoglossica** is a form of hemiplegia due to a lesion of the hypoglossal nerve on the opposite side of the paralyzed area.

hemiplegia cruciata a form of paralysis in which the hemiplegia is crossed so that, e.g., the condition affects the right arm and the left leg.

hemispherectomy = HEMIDECORTICATION.

hemispheres the symmetrical halves of the cerebrum and cerebellum.

hemispherical dominance = LATERAL DOMINANCE.

hemizygote an individual with only one of a possible pair of chromosomes. The condition is normal for males with respect to the X chromosome since they possess only one, the matching chromosome being a Y. Males with the XY complement are **hemizygous** in the matter of X-linked genes. See ZYGOTE.

hemlock: See SORCERY DRUGS.

hemoglobin an iron-rich pigment of red blood cells that has a powerful attraction for oxygen molecules. H. allows the blood to carry 60 times as much oxygen per fluid volume as blood plasma without h. The pigment, when saturated with oxygen, produces the red color of blood. Abbrev.: **Hb**.

hemoglobinopathies disorders associated with genetic defects in the characteristics of hemoglobin. A common effect of h. is anemias, which may be severe in homozygous persons and mild in heterozygous carriers; it is possible for an individual to be affected by more than one of the h. Sickle-cell anemia and Cooley's anemia are examples of h. H. usually are identified by a letter of the alphabet, e.g., Hb C, where Hb is medical shorthand for hemoglobin. Additional variations in hemoglobin molecules are identified by the area in which they were discovered, thus a form of sickle-cell anemia first observed in Memphis, Tennessee, may be designated Hb $S_{Memphis}$.

hemophilia: See BLOOD DISORDER; CHRISTMAS DISEASE.

hemophilia B = CHRISTMAS DISEASE.

hemophobia = HEMATOPHOBIA.

hemothymia a morbid desire to murder, or, almost literally, a lust for blood.

hemorrhage bleeding; any loss of blood from an artery or vein. A h. may be external, internal, or within a tissue, such as the skin; a bruise or hematoma is a sign of bleeding within the skin. A h. from a ruptured artery is bright red in color and erupts in spurts that coincide with heart contractions; it is generally more serious than h. from a vein that shows as a relatively slow, steady flow of dark red blood.

hemorrhage and thirst a theory that loss of blood increases thirst, a concept disputed by some investigators because various animal experiments have produced conflicting evidence regarding an association between blood loss and thirst.

hemosiderosis: See TRANSFUSIONAL H.

hemp plant a common name for cannabis sativa, the source of marijuana, hashish, bhang, charas, and ganja.

henbane a common name (*hen* and *bane*) of Hyoscyamus niger, a source of alkaloids that function as a sedative and mild hallucinogen. One agent, hyoscine, is a drug sometimes associated with "twilight sleep," administered to women in labor. In the Middle Ages, h. was administered to people believed to be possessed by a demon. H. also is identified in Shakespeare's *Hamlet* as the poison poured into the ear of Hamlet's father.

heparitinuria = SANFILIPPO'S SYNDROME.

-hepat-; -hepato- a combining form relating to the liver.

hepatic encephalopathy: See SCHISTOSOMIASIS.

hepatitis an inflammation of the liver marked by diffuse or patchy areas of dead liver cells in all of the lobules. Symptoms range from mild, flulike symptoms to liver-function failure, which could be fatal. Jaundice and bilirubin coloring of the urine are usual signs. The causes include virus Types A and B, alcohol, drugs, mononucleosis, and other infectious agents. Type A virus is associated with contaminated food or water. Type B virus usually is transmitted by blood transfusions, through group use of hypodermic needles, or by sexual contact with an infected person.

hepatolenticular degeneration a somewhat rare familial disease transmitted as an autosomal-recessive trait that occurs most frequently in children of consanguineous marriages. The disease is characterized by copper deposits in the liver, brain, and other organs, including in some cases the cornea which acquires a golden-brown pigment ring (the **Kayser-Fleischer ring**). Other common symptoms are tremors, rigidity, and mental deterioration. Also called **Wilson's disease**.

Heraclitus /-klī'-/ Greek philosopher, of Ephesus, ca. 540 to ca. 480 B.C. See ENANTIODROMIA.

Herbart, Johann Friedrich /her'bärt/ German philosopher and educator, 1776–1841. H. is often considered the founder of educational psychology. He held that ideas are forces that compete for a place in conscious or unconscious mental processes, and that related ideas combine to form an apperceptive mass which forms a background for new ideas acquired in the educational process. See HERBARTIAN PSYCHOLOGY.

Herbartian psychology a 19th-century educational-psychology system built around the idea that a new sense perception, to be recognized, must be related to an apperceptive mass of previously acquired ideas. Also called **Herbartianism**.

Herbst, Ernst Friedrich Gustav German physi-

cian, 1803–93. See PACINIAN CORPUSCLES (there: **Herbst's corpuscle**).

herd instinct a term used by Wilfred Trotter for a universal drive in animals to congregate in flocks and herds, and for human beings to belong to groups and participate in social activities. This drive is no longer considered either universal or instinctual. See GREGARIOUSNESS.

here-and-now approach an emphasis on understanding present feelings and interpersonal reaction as they occur in an ongoing treatment session, with little or no emphasis on past experience or the basic reasons behind the individual's behavior. See ENCOUNTER GROUP; GESTALT THERAPY. Compare THERE-AND-THEN APPROACH.

hereditarian one who maintains that genetic inheritance is the major influence on behavior. Opposed to this view is the belief that environment and learning account for the major differences between people. The question of heredity versus environment or "nature versus nurture" continues to be controversial, e.g., as it applies to intelligence.

hereditarianism the viewpoint that emphasizes the influence of heredity on behavioral traits.

hereditary: See HEREDITY.

hereditary ataxia = FRIEDREICH'S ATAXIA.

hereditary choreoathetosis = LESCH-NYHAN SYNDROME.

hereditary disorder any disease or defect that may be transmitted from one generation to another through genes or chromosomal aberrations. Some geneticists believe nearly all diseases, including bacterial infections, have a h.d. component because of patterns of susceptibility.

hereditary hyperurecemia = LESCH-NYHAN SYNDROME.

hereditary myopathy: See MYOPATHIES.

hereditary predisposition a genetic susceptibility to a disorder whose appearance is determined by environmental factors.

heredity the transmission of genetic characteristics to descendents. The process depends upon the union of sperm and ovum during conception, upon the character of the genes contained in the chromosomes of these cells, and upon the particular genetic code contained in the DNA of which the chromosomes are composed. The term also refers to the transmitted characteristics themselves. Adjective: **hereditary**. See CHROMOSOME; DNA; GENE.

heredity fear = PATRIOPHOBIA.

heredopathia atactica polyneuritiformis = REFSUM'S SYNDROME.

Hering, Heinrich Ewald German physiologist, 1866–1948. See HERING-BREUER REFLEX.

Hering, Karl Ewald Constantin German physiologist, 1834–1918. H. is noted for his demonstration that feelings of warmth and cold are relative to skin temperature, and for his color-vision theory. See HERING'S AFTERIMAGE; HERING GRAYS; HERING THEORY OF COLOR VISION.

Hering-Breuer reflex a nervous mechanism involved in normal breathing, with stimuli from sensory endings in lung tissue limiting inspiration and expiration.

Hering grays a set of 50 gray papers ranging in subjectively equal steps from extreme white to extreme black.

Hering's afterimage a positive aftersensation of the same hue and saturation as the original stimulus.

Hering theory of color vision the opponent-colors theory which assumes that there are three sets of cones, one of which is sensitive to white and black, another to red and green, and the third to yellow and blue. The breaking down, or catabolism, of these substances is supposed to yield one of these pairs (white, red, or yellow), while the building up, or anabolism, of the same substances yields the other (black, green, or blue). Color blindness results from the absence of one or more of the chromatic processes. Also called **opponents theory of color vision**.

heritability the capacity to be inherited; also, an estimate, based on a sample of individuals, of the relative contribution of genetics to a given trait or function.

hermaphrodite an individual possessing both male and female sex organs. The external genitalia may be indistinguishable from those of normal males, and the h. may exhibit elements of both male and female sexual behavior. The true h. may have either male or female sex chromosome combinations or show mosaicism with XX chromosomes in ovarian tissues and XY chromosomes in testicular cells. In an endocrine form, the development of a female fetus may be partially altered by a high level of male sex hormones in the maternal bloodstream during pregnancy. Chromosome abnormalities are not a factor in sexual behavior traits of homosexuals and transvestites. Also see AMBISEXUALITY; AMBIGUOUS GENITALIA; TESTICULAR-FEMINIZATION SYNDROME; BISEXUALITY; INTERSEX; PSEUDO-HERMAPHRODITISM; ANDROGYNY.

hero daydream: See DAYDREAM.

Herodotus /hirod′ətəs/ Greek historian, fl. fifth century B.C. See POLYCRATES COMPLEX.

heroin = DIACETYLMORPHINE.

heroin addiction strong physiological and psychological dependence on heroin characterized by tolerance and, when discontinued, withdrawal syndrome. The preferred term today is dependence rather than addiction. See OPIOID DEPENDENCE; OPIOID WITHDRAWAL.

heroin overdose use of an amount of heroin sufficient to produce opioid intoxication (apathy, psychomotor retardation, drowsiness, slurred speech, impairment of attention or memory) and opioid poisoning (shock, coma, pinpoint pupils, and depressed respiration with the possibility of death from respiratory arrest).

hero worship in psychoanalysis, a need of many people for an authority figure they can admire and submit to as a representative of an idealized father. H.w. helps to explain the willingness of the masses to be dominated by a "great" man.

herpes a category of viruses generally noted for their characteristic effect of producing "creeping" eruptions of the skin and mucous membranes. (The term is derived from the Greek word *herpeton*, "reptile," that is, something that creeps). One strain of herpes simplex is associated with venereal contact and is marked by eruptions of vesicles on the genitalia. See HERPES INFECTION. Also see GENITAL H.

herpes infection a disease produced by one of the strains of herpes virus. A h.i. may be manifested as chicken pox, a cold sore, shingles, eczema, conjunctivitis, encephalitis, stomatitis, or vulvovaginitis. The major types of h.i. are **herpes varicella-zoster**, a strain that causes both chicken pox and shingles, **herpes simplex Type 1**, the cause of fever blisters, and **herpes simplex Type 2**, the cause of genital herpes. See HERPES; PERINATAL HERPES-VIRUS INFECTION; EPSTEIN-BARR VIRUS; INFECTIOUS MONONUCLEOSIS; CYTOMEGALIC DISEASE; ARA-A; CONVENTIONAL VIRUS; HUNT'S SYNDROME; GENITAL HERPES; HERPES SIMPLEX ENCEPHALITIS.

herpes simplex encephalitis a form of encephalitis with symptoms similar to those of other types of viral brain infection. Seizures occur repeatedly early in the course of the disease, and there may be signs of dysfunction indicating focal degeneration in the frontal or parietal lobes. However, the herpes simplex virus rarely invades brain or spinal-cord tissues; and viral encephalitis generally mimics other neurologic disorders, so that a firm diagnosis is difficult.

herpes simplex Type 1: See HERPES INFECTION.

herpes simplex Type 2: See PERINATAL HERPES-VIRUS INFECTION; HERPES INFECTION.

herpes varicella-zoster: See HERPES INFECTION.

hertz /hurts/ a wave frequency of one cycle per second. The unit was named for the German physicist Heinrich Hertz /herts/ (1857–94). Abbrev.: **Hz**.

Heschl, Richard Ladislaus Austrian pathologist, 1824–81. See HESCHL'S GYRUS; AUDITORY RADIATIONS.

Heschl's gyrus one of several transverse temporal convolutions of the cerebral cortex that are associated with the sense of hearing. H.g. is named for the Austrian pathologist Richard Heschl, who first traced the auditory nerve fibers of humans to the convolution.

Hess, Walter Rudolf Swiss physiologist, 1881—. See TROPHOTROPIC PROCESS.

hetaeral fantasy a fantasy in which women play the role of courtesan. In the male version of the fantasy, the man possesses a courtesan. Also called **courtesan fantasy**.

-heter-; -hetero- a combining form meaning other, different.

heterochromic iridocyclitis: See IRIDOCYCLITIS.

heterochrony a speed difference between two processes such as nerve impulses; also, a difference in time of development of an organ as compared with the norm. Also called **heterochronia**.

heteroeroticism an attraction for the opposite sex, or for other love objects outside the self.

heterogamous /-rog'-/ a term applied to the structural and functional differences between female and male gametes of organisms.

heterogeneous grouping the practice of putting students of varying ability or intelligence together. Such groups may be entire classes or smaller groups that work together in a specific area, e.g., art or reading. Compare HOMOGENEOUS GROUPING.

heterohypnosis a state of hypnosis induced in one person by another, as opposed to autohypnosis.

heterolalia the substitution of meaningless or inappropriate words for the intended words in speech or writing. See HETEROPHEMY.

heterologous artificial insemination: See INSEMINATION.

heteronomous stage Piaget's first stage of moral development wherein the young child equates morality with the rules and principles of his parents and other authority figures. In the h.s., discipline is imposed by parents. In the autonomous stage, the child learns to discipline himself. Also called **heteronomous morality**. Also see MORAL REALISM. Compare AUTONOMOUS STAGE.

heteronomous superego an opportunistic type of superego which is controlled by an ego demand to behave in whatever manner is expected at the moment in order to secure the approval of others.

heteronomy the state characteristic of childhood in which a person is emotionally or physically dependent and unable to regulate his behavior. H. may also refer to a child's or a childlike person's dependence on another's ideas or values as in Piaget's heteronomous stage. Compare AUTONOMY.

heteronymous hemianopia a visual field defect in which vision in either the left or right half of both eyes is absent, due to a lesion in the optic chiasma. See HEMIANOPIA.

heteronymous reflex a reflex that begins with stimulation in one muscle of a synergistic group but results in contraction of another muscle in the same group. Compare HOMONYMOUS REFLEX.

heterophemy /het'-/ the unconscious speaking or writing of words other than intended. See HETEROLALIA.

heterophily: See HOMOPHILY.

heterophoria the deviation of an eye because of an extrinsic muscular imbalance.

heteroscedasticity a term indicating that two or more frequency distributions are unequal in variance, that is, one distribution spreads out more than the other. Compare HOMOSCEDASTICITY.

heterosexual anxiety anxiety that is related to heterosexual relationships, e.g., a feeling by the patient that he or she is not sexually attractive in appearance or performance.

heterosexuality normal or morbid sexual attraction to members of the opposite sex; also, the developmental stage in which sexual attraction or actual intercourse with members of the opposite sex occurs.

heterosociality relationships on a social level between members of the opposite sex.

heterosome the X or Y sex chromosome, as distinguished from the autosomes.

heterotopia the congenital development of gray matter in the white-matter area of the spinal cord.

heterotropia = STRABISMUS.

heterozygosity a condition of heterozygosis in which an individual possesses one or more pairs of heterozygous genes as a result of crossbreeding. Also called **heterozygousness**. Also see DOUBLE HETEROZYGOUSNESS.

heterozygote a person with two different alleles for the genetic positions on a pair of matching chromosomes. Compare HOMOZYGOTE.

heterozygous possessing different forms of a genetic trait on each of a pair of otherwise normal chromosomes, e.g., a gene for blue eyes on one chromosome and a gene for brown eyes on the matching chromosome of the pair. If both genes are for blue eyes, the individual is homozygous for that trait.

heterozygousness = HETEROZYGOSITY.

heuristic leading to new discoveries or promoting new conclusions. A theory that leads to new experimentation has h. value.

Hex A = HEXOSAMINIDASE A.

hexafluorodiethyl ether $C_4H_4F_6O$—a CNS stimulant used in psychotherapeutic shock treatments because of its ECT-like convulsant effects. Also called **flurothyl**. Trademark: **Indoklon**.

hexamethonium an ammonium compound used in treating certain types of hypertension by its ganglion-blocking action.

hex doctors medicine men who attempt to alleviate mental or physical conditions by the use of spells, incantations, or charms. See WITCHCRAFT; HEADSHRINKING; FAITH HEALING; SHAMAN.

hexosaminidase A an enzyme involved in the normal metabolism of sphingolipid, a fatty substance that is the cause of Tay-Sachs disease. In the absence of h.A, sphingolipid accumulates in the brain tissues, leading to blindness, seizures, loss of coordination, and mental retardation. Also called **Hex A**. See GANGLIOSIDOSES; TAY-SACHS DISEASE.

Heymans, Corneille Jean François Belgian physiologist, 1892–1968. See HEYMANS' LAW.

Heymans' law a generalization that the threshold level of one stimulus is increased in proportion to the intensity of a second, inhibitory, stimulus.

hey-nonny-nonny theory: See ORIGIN-OF-LANGUAGE THEORIES.

HGPRT = HYPOXANTHINE GUANINE PHOSPHORIBOSYL TRANSFERASE.

HHHO: See PRADER-LABHART-WILLI SYNDROME.

HIAA *h*ydroxy*i*ndole*a*cetic *a*cid, also known as **5-**

HIAA, which is the main metabolite of serotonin. Studies have shown that one group of depressed patients may have a low cerebrospinal-fluid 5-HIAA and a preferential response to chlorimipramine, which blocks serotonin re-uptake, while a second group may be characterized by low secretion of urinary MHPG, the main metabolite of epinephrine, and have a preferential response to imipramine and desipramine, which block norepinephrine re-uptake. See 3-METHOXY-4-HYDROXYPHENYLETHYLENE GLYCOL; UNIPOLAR DEPRESSION.

hibernation a sleeplike period of inactivity accompanied by a significant decrease in body temperature that occurs in certain homoiothermic, or warm-blooded, vertebrates. The h. may occur seasonally or diurnally, and the body temperature may drop to within a few degrees of freezing. Endocrine-gland activity decreases during h., but no single gland has been found to control h. Some species, e.g., bears, consume large quantities of food before h. and maintain bodily functions with energy from fat deposits, but others, e.g., golden hamsters, store food and leave h. periodically to feed. Cold-blooded, or poikilothermic, animals become dormant, like plants, in cold temperatures. See HOMOIO-THERMS; POIKILOTHERMS.

hiccups: See SPASM.

hidden-clue test a test in which the subject must discover a particular feature of the stimulus situation that is the clue to a reward.

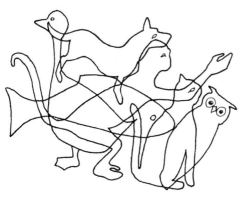

HIDDEN-FIGURES TEST. Name the animals you see in this drawing.

hidden-figures test a test of visual-field defects in which the subject is required to find hidden figures embedded in complex figures of interlocking contours. Poor performance on the test often indicates a lesion or injury in the cerebral cortex.

hidden observer the descriptive term for the dissociated part of consciousness that, under hypnosis, appears to process experience independently of the subject's awareness. Hypnotized subjects can register and later recall auditory, visual, or tactile stimuli to which they were oblivious while in the hypnotic trance.

-hidr-; -hidro- a combining form relating to sweat.

hierarchical theory of instinct a principle that patterns of specific behavioral responses are generated through the hypothalamic, sensory, and cortical systems. In the Tinbergen model, motivational energy accumulates in the neural centers, is released by an appropriate stimulus, and flows through motor-system pathways to produce the behavior most likely to achieve a goal object or reward.

hierarchy of motives; hierarchy-of-needs theory: See NEED-HIERARCHY THEORY.

hierophobia /hīrə-/ a morbid fear of religious or sacred objects (from Greek *hieros*, "powerful, sacred").

HIF an abbreviation of *h*igher *i*ntellectual *f*unctions. See HIGHER MENTAL PROCESSES; HIGHER-ORDER CONSTRUCTS.

high blood pressure a circulatory disorder characterized by persistent arterial blood pressure that exceeds readings higher than an arbitrary standard which usually is 140/90. H.b.p. is a basic sign of hypertension.

highbrow: See ETHICAL H.

higher brain centers the parts of the cerebrum associated with memory, intelligence, and learning.

higher-level skills the work methods and skills that can be applied in many tasks rather than one particular task.

higher mental processes the higher-brain-center functions of intelligence, judgment, imagination, and thinking.

higher-order conditioning a classical-conditioning method utilizing the conditioned stimulus of one series as the unconditioned stimulus of a second.

higher-order constructs the organization of information into coherent constructs that enhance the integration of the information into one's general knowledge.

higher-order interaction in the analysis of variance, the joint effect of three or more independent variables.

higher states of consciousness: See TRANSPERSONAL PSYCHOLOGY.

high Machs: See MACH SCALE.

high-risk approach a research method in which vulnerable, or "high-risk," individuals are studied over a period of time in order to identify factors that differentiate between those who ultimately develop certain disorders and those who do not. For details, see HIGH-RISK STUDIES.

high-risk studies research on individuals or groups who may be predisposed to social, physical, or psychiatric pathology by reason of genetic, constitutional, or environmental factors. The object of h.-r.s. is to identify specific factors and establish the statistical probability of different types of pathology, such as congenital deformity, mental illness, mental retardation, delinquency, or drug abuse.

High School Personality Questionnaire: See CATTELL INVENTORIES.

highway hypnosis a popular term sometimes applied to accident proneness resulting from a state of drowsy inattention experienced during long-distance driving on monotonous roads.

hindbrain the posterior of three bulges that appear in the embryonic brain as it develops beyond the neural tube stage. The bulge eventually becomes the medulla oblongata, pons, and cerebellum in humans. Also called **rhombencephalon**.

Hindu caste system: See SOCIAL IMMOBILITY.

Hinton, William Augustus American physician, 1883–1959. See WASSERMANN TEST (there: **Hinton test**).

hip dislocation: See CONGENITAL HIP SUBLUXATION; HIP DYSPLASIA.

hip dysplasia a form of congenital hip dislocation in which there is asymmetrical joint contact. Like other congenital hip dislocations, the condition usually can be corrected without surgery if treatment is begun in eary infancy. The abnormality can be diagnosed by X-ray and other techniques before the child is old enough to be in a sitting position. Also see CONGENITAL HIP SUBLUXATION.

hippanthropy the belief that one is a horse; a delusion occasionally observed in disorganized (hebephrenic) schizophrenia.

hippie a representative of a subculture starting in the 1960s composed of young people who were in revolt against conventionality in all forms, and developed their own "relaxed," "loose," or "cool" way of dressing, hair style, and living arrangements, such as communes, and frequently used psychedelic or other drugs.

hippocampal commissure: See COMMISSURE.

hippocampus a part of the limbic system associated with emotions. Lesions in the h. have been observed to turn placid animals into ferocious creatures and ferocious creatures into placid animals, depending upon specific areas excised for study. The name derived from the Greek word *hippokampos*, "seahorse"—which it resembles. Adjective: **hippocampal**.

Hippocrates /hipok'rətēz/ Greek physician, ca. 460 to ca. 377 B.C.. Known as the "Father of Medicine," H. sought to divorce the study of both physical and mental illness from religious mysticism. As an example, he held that epilepsy, then known as the divine illness, "appears to me to be in no way more divine or more sacred than other diseases, but has a natural cause from which it originates like other affections." Although his explanations and remedies were in keeping with the times (purgatives, bleeding, herbs), he advanced the knowledge of mental illness by careful observation of causes of depression, phobias, delirium, and other disorders; by giving them names, such as mania and paranoia; and by maintaining that feeling, dreaming, thinking, and other processes are mediated by the brain. See APOPLECTIC TYPE; ATHYMIA; CHOLERIC TYPE; CONSTITUTIONAL TYPE; DEPLETIVE TREATMENT; HUMORAL THEORY; MELANCHOLIC TYPE; ORGANIC APPROACH; PRODROMIC DREAM; SACRED DISEASE; TYPOLOGY; WANDERING UTERUS.

hippophobia = HORSE PHOBIA.

hip replacement a therapeutic measure employed to restore mobility in cases of fractures and arthritic diseases, mainly in older persons. Approximately 100,000 h.r. operations are performed each year in the United States. H.r. surgery is possible also for children although the synthetic joints may have to be replaced periodically to keep pace with changes in body size.

Hirschfeld, Magnus German sexologist, 1868–1935. See SEXUAL NEGATIVISM.

Hiskey, Marshall S. American psychologist, fl. 1980. See HISKEY-NEBRASKA TEST OF LEARNING APTITUDE.

Hiskey-Nebraska Test of Learning Aptitude an individual intelligence test developed and standardized on deaf and hard-of-hearing children, with pantomime and practice exercises to communicate the instructions for the twelve subtests. These include among others bead patterns, paper-folding, picture identification, memory for digits, block patterns, picture analogies, and memory for color.

-hist-; -histio-; -histo- a combining form relating to tissue.

histamine a substance found in all tissues of the body as a metabolic amino-acid product of protein. It is associated in human physiology with headaches, production of gastric juice, dilation of small blood vessels, edema, and inflammation. Injections of h. may cause vomiting, muscle spasms, and diarrhea. See ANTIHISTAMINES.

histamine headache a headache that usually involves only one side of the head and is often associated with common-cold symptoms, due to a release of histamine from body tissues.

histogram = BAR GRAPH.

histologic technician a health professional employed in a clinical laboratory or as an assistant to a pathologist with the responsibility of preparing tissue removed during surgery for microscopic examination. A h.t. becomes qualified by a year of supervised training in a clinical-pathology laboratory. Examination leads to certification as H.T. (ASCP), for h.t., American Society for Clinical Pathologists.

histology the scientific study of the structure and function of tissues at the cellular level.

historical method the technique of studying a client by tracing his personal history.

historical psychoanalysis: See APPLIED PSYCHOANALYSIS.

historical semantics = SEMASIOLOGY.

history-taking in psychiatry and clinical psychology, the process of compiling the history of a mental patient from the patient himself and from other sources such as the family, hospitals or clinics, psychiatrists or psychologists, neurologists, social workers, and others who have been involved in the case. For details, see ANAMNESIS.

histrionic-personality disorder a personality disorder whose essential features are a pattern of long-term, not episodic, self-dramatization in which the patient draws attention to himself or herself, craves activity and excitement, overreacts to minor events, experiences angry outbursts, and impresses others as shallow, only superficially charming, egocentric, inconsiderate, vain and demanding, dependent and helpless, and prone to manipulative suicide threats and gestures. Also called **hysterical-personality disorder**. (DSM-III)

hives a temporary skin inflammation marked by sudden outbreaks of burning and itching swellings. The condition may be caused by psychogenic factors or by an allergy, such as a food allergy. Also called **urticaria**.

HMO = HEALTH-MAINTENANCE ORGANIZATION.

hoarding the carrying and storing of food or other items believed necessary for survival. Various authors have identified h. as instinctive or learned behavior, or both, and as part of a manipulative drive. H. by rodents varies with the environmental temperature, increasing when the temperature declines and decreasing as the temperature rises. For humans, see H. CHARACTER; ANAL CHARACTER.

hoarding character in E. Fromm's theory, a nonproductive personality type who bases his sense of security on what he can save and own. His attitude toward other people is to possess them, and any form of personal intimacy is threatening to him. In addition, he tends to be rigid, stubborn, and obsessively orderly. Also called **hoarding orientation**. Also see ANAL CHARACTER.

Hobbes, Thomas English philosopher, 1588–1679. See ASSOCIATIONISM; ASSOCIATION OF IDEAS; HUMOR.

Hodgkin, Thomas English physician, 1798–1866. See BLOOD DISORDER (there: **Hodgkin's disease**); LYMPHADENOPATHY; LYMPHOMA.

hodometer an instrument invented by R. Bechtel to map the standing and movement patterns of individuals in a museum (from Greek *hodos*, "way"). Pressure-sensitive pads extend over a complete floor space with counters connected to all of the pads, and the counting mechanism records each time an individual moves onto one of the pads.

hodophobia a morbid fear of traveling. Also called **travel phobia**.

Hoefer, Wolfgang /hœ′fər/ Austrian physician, fl. 17th century. See CRETINISM.

Hoffmann, Johann German neurologist, 1857–1919. See HOFFMANN'S SIGN; PROGRESSIVE SPINAL-MUSCULAR ATROPHY (there: **Werdnig-Hoffmann disease**); KOCHER-DEBRÉ-SEMELAIGNE SYNDROME.

Hoffmann's sign a sign of organic brain disease in hemiplegia cases: Snapping the index, middle finger, or ring finger produces a flexion of the thumb. Also called **Hoffmann's reflex; Trömner's sign**.

hog: See PHENCYCLIDINE.

hog-cholera virus a highly contagious RNA myxovirus agent that afflicts swine, producing a wide range of consequences since the virus affects all the cells of the body. Specific lesions occur in the lining of blood vessels, particularly those of the central nervous system. The myxovirus is similar in structure to a cattle virus associated with the birth of calves with CNS abnormalities and the human influenza virus.

-hol-; -holo- a combining form meaning entire, complete.

'hold' functions: See DETERIORATION INDEX.

holergasia a psychosis involving the entire personality (Meyer).

holiday syndrome feelings of dejection and psychic pain that tend to occur during major holiday periods as a result of nostalgic reminiscence and unmet dependency needs. Serious injuries, suicides, and fatal accidents tend to increase significantly during the holiday season. Also see SUNDAY NEUROSIS.

holism a psychological and psychiatric approach developed by Adolf Meyer and Kurt Goldstein, in which human behavior and the human personality are viewed as biological, psychological, and sociocultural totalities which cannot be fully explained in terms of individual parts or characteristics. Adjective: **holistic**.

holistic healing a health-care concept based on the premise that body, mind, and spirit function as a harmonious unit and an adverse effect on one also affects the others, requiring treatment of the whole to restore the harmonious balance.

holistic medicine a branch of medicine that approaches diagnosis and therapy from the viewpoint that an illness may affect the total being, including the mind as well as the body.

holistic psychology an approach to psychology based on the viewpoint that healthy and normal development consists of actualizing oneself and fulfilling one's potentialities, with needs and motives presented in a hierarchical order beginning with primary physiological needs and culminating in an integration of the biological, psychological, and sociocultural aspects of life and the attainment of one's highest and most creative goals.

Holland Vocational Preference Inventory: See INTEREST TESTS.

Holmes, Gordon Morgan English neurologist, 1876–1965. See ADIE'S SYNDROME (also called **Adie-Holmes syndrome**); REBOUND PHENOMENON (also called **rebound phenomenon of Gordon Holmes; Holmes' phenomenon**).

Holmgren, Alarik Frithiof Swedish physiologist, 1831–97. See HOLMGREN TEST.

Holmgren test a color-blindness test devised in the 19th century by A. F. Holmgren, requiring the subject to match skeins of colored yarns with standard skeins.

holography a method of producing three-dimensional images by using light-wave-interference patterns. The technique is used in photography and has been suggested as an explanation for the process whereby images may be formed in the mind.

holophrases the single-word expressions spoken by children, usually by 18 months or earlier, e.g., "Mama," "milk," "no." Some theorists maintain that h. are only name-tags or labels the child attaches to objects; other theorists believe that h. represent more complex intentions, e.g., "milk" for "I want milk." Also see HOLOPHRASTIC; DUOS.

holophrastic referring to the use of a single word to express a complex of ideas. In psychiatry, this tendency is found primarily in schizophrenics. Also see HOLOPHRASES.

holotelencephaly a category of anomalies characterized by a single cerebral ventricle, an absence of sagittal cleavage between the cerebral hemispheres, eye and nose defects, and a variety of other neurologic abnormalities. One type, **h. with cleft lip and hypotelorism**, is a birth-defect complex of anomalies in which the offspring have a small cranium, cleft lip, orbital hypotelorism, absence of a nasal bridge, and, in some cases, absence of olfactory organs; neurologic defects include nystagmus, absence of response to light and sound stimuli, and little evidence of psychomotor development.

home care patient care in the home for physically or mentally disabled persons, including the infirm or senile elderly. H.c. is an alternative to institutionalization, enabling the patient to live in familiar surroundings and preserve family ties. Such services as nursing care, administration of medication, therapeutic baths, physical therapy, and occupational therapy are provided by visiting professionals or paraprofessionals connected with clinics, hospitals, or health agencies. Also called **home-care program**.

home health aide a specially trained person who works with a department of social services or a local visiting-nurses association in providing certain personal-care needs for disabled individuals. E.g., a h.h.a. may be assigned responsibilities for bathing patients or helping them move from a bed to a chair if the patients are unable to perform such tasks alone.

Home Index: See AMERICAN HOME SCALE.

homemaker home health aide a service offered disabled individuals through private or public health agencies to assist disabled persons in homemaking tasks, personal care, and rehabilitation routines. Nearly 2,000 h.h.h.a. programs have been established in North America since the early 1900s. The personnel receive intensive training in the principles and techniques of personal care and rehabilitation after being accepted through a screening process.

homemaker program a service provided for disabled persons who prefer independent living but require assistance in cleaning the home, preparing meals, handling the laundry, and similar tasks.

-homeo-; -homoeo- a combining form meaning similar, like. Also see -HOMO-.

homeopathic principle = ISOPATHIC PRINCIPLE.

homeopathy /hōmē·op′-/ a method of treating disease by administering minute doses of drugs that would produce, in a healthy person, symptoms similar to those of the disease. Compare ALLOPATHY.

homeostasis /-sta′-/ the equilibrium or balance between living cells and their surrounding environment. The h. of a living organism may include such factors as constant temperature, salt-and-water balance, acid-alkali balance, oxygen consumption and carbon-dioxide excretion, and blood-sugar level.

homeostatic model in social psychology, the assumption that all people are motivated by the need to maintain or restore their optimal level of environmental, interpersonal, and psychological stimulation. Insufficient or excessive stimulation automatically causes tension and sets in motion the motive and usually the behavior required to achieve equilibrium.

homeostatic principle in social psychology, the idea that all people tend to seek a comfortable level of environmental stimulation. See HOMEOSTATIC MODEL.

home-service agency a group, which may be a public-health, social-service, or voluntary organization, that provides homemaker or home health aides for mentally or physically disabled persons. The personnel generally are paraprofessionals who are recruited, trained, and supervised by another agency, such as the visiting-nurses association or a hospital with a home-care unit.

homesickness = NOSTALGIA.

home visits visits by hospitalized mental patients to their homes in preparation for discharge; also, visits to patients at home by professional personnel such as psychiatric social workers and psychiatrists, for crisis intervention, aftercare, and assistance in solving personal problems.

homichlophobia a morbid fear of fog.

homicidal behavior attempts to kill other persons, or actual killing. Demographic data indicate that Americans who commit homicide are, typically, 18 to 43 years of age, with a male to female ratio of 5:1. The great majority do not have a classic mental illness, though many are antisocial personalities. However, according to MacDonald (1968), acutely psychotic schizophrenic patients and delirious patients who make homicidal threats should be hospitalized. Among the factors found to be associated with homicidal potential are parental brutality, parental seduction, arson, arrest for assault, and alcoholism.

homicidal monomania an obsolete term for a form of so-called "partial insanity" in which the individual is preoccupied with ideas of killing. Also called **homicidal mania; homicidomania**. Also see MONOMANIA.

homilophobia a morbid fear of sermons; also, the fear that a group of people will criticize one's appearance or manners (from Greek *homilos*, "crowd").

homing the ability of certain animals to return to an original home after traveling or being transported to a point that is a considerable distance from the home and that lacks most visual clues as to its location. In a h. experiment, banded Manx shearwaters transported to North America, 3,050 miles away, were released separately and returned within 13 days to their burrows on an island off the west coast of England. Also see LOCALITY ATTACHMENT.

-homo-; -hom- a combining form with two meanings and two origins: (a) from Greek *homos*, "one and the same," as in "homogenous," meaning of the same kind, uniform, or in "homosexual," meaning of the same sex—also see -HOMEO-; (b) from Latin *homo*, "human being," as in "Homo sapiens," "homage," or "homicide"—also see -HUM-.

homocystinuria a genetic metabolic disorder characterized by a deficiency of an enzyme needed to convert L-homocystine to L-cystathionine. Mental retardation often occurs, along with a shuffling, ducklike gait, and in some cases seizures or hemiplegia. Brain abnormalities often are due to arterial or venous thromboses. Also called **cystathionine synthetase deficiency**.

homoerotism an erotic desire for persons of one's own sex.

homogamy /-mog'-/ in genetics, the interbreeding, in an isolated population group, of members with similar hereditary traits resulting in the reinforcement of such traits in future generations.

homogeneity of variance an assumption underlying some parametric tests of significance that the samples being compared do not differ in variability (spread of scores).

homogeneous grouping /-jēn'-/ the practice of putting students of equal ability together. A homogeneous group may be an entire class or a smaller group formed within a class and based on ability in a specific area, e.g., mathematics. H.g. may also refer to the arrangement of variables in categories. Compare HETEROGENEOUS GROUPING.

homogeneous reinforcement the presentation at the same time of two stimuli that elicit the same or a similar response.

homogenitality an interest in the genitalia of one's own sex.

homographs words that are identical in spelling but different in origin and meaning, whether pronounced the same or not, e.g., "flag" (a piece of cloth) and "flag" (to hang loose), or "tear" /ter/ and "tear" /tir/. If h. have the same pronunciation (that is, if they are also homophones), as "flag" above, they may be called homonyms. See HOMOPHONES; HOMONYMS.

homoiotherms /hōmoi'ə-/ animals such as mammals and birds, the warm-blooded species, which have developed mechanisms for maintaining a fairly constant body temperature that in turn permits their survival over a wide spectrum of environmental conditions (from Greek *homoios*, "same, like," and *therme*, "heat"). Also called **warm-blooded animals**. Adjective: **homoiothermic**. See HIBERNATION. Compare POIKILOTHERMS.

homologous artificial insemination: See INSEMINATION.

homology /-mol'-/ the correspondence or similarity of anatomical structures in different animals, regardless of a relationship in function. An example is the similarity between the arms of humans and the forelegs of lizards. H. suggests evolution of different species from a common remote ancestor. Adjective: **homologous**. Also see ICONICITY.

homo ludens: See PLAY.

homo mollis an obsolete term for a male homosexual (Latin, "soft man").

homonomy drive the motivation to fit into social groups, e.g., the family, the community.

homonymous hemianopia the loss of sight in the same half of the visual field of each eye, e.g., the left half of the visual field of both the left and right eyes. In **bitemporal hemianopia**, half the visual field is lost in both eyes but the affected areas are the left half of the left visual field and the right half of the right visual field. In **binasal hemianopia**, the left visual field of the right eye and the right visual field of the left eye are lost. Also see HEMIANOPIA.

homonymous quadrantic field defect a loss of vision in one quadrant of the visual field of both eyes.

homonymous reflex a reflex in which a stimulus in a muscle produces a contraction of the same muscle. Compare HETERONYMOUS REFLEX.

homonyms words that are both homographs and homophones, that is, words that are spelled and pronounced alike but are different in meaning, e.g., "flag" (a piece of cloth) and "flag" (to hang loose), or "lie" (an untruth) and "lie" (to recline). See HOMOGRAPHS; HOMOPHONES.

homophile a person who loves others of his or her own sex; a homosexual.

homophily /-mof'-/ the principle of communication that interaction between the source of information and the receiver of information is greater when both have similar or shared attitudes, interpretations of language, belief structures, and other similar attributes. The opposite is **heterophily** /-rof'-/.

homophobia fear of, or prejudice against, homosexuals.

homophones words that are identical in pronunciation but different in meaning, whether spelled the same or not, e.g., "flag" (a piece of cloth) and "flag" (to hang loose), or "some" and "sum." If h. have the same spelling (that is, if they are also homographs), as "flag" above, they may be called homonyms. The term h. is also applied to *letters* that have the same pronunciation; e.g., the *c* in "circadian," the *s* in "schizophrenia," and the digraph *ps* in "psychology" are all pronounced /s/. See HOMOGRAPHS; HOMONYMS.

homoscedasticity a term indicating that two or more frequency distributions are equal in variance, that is, neither is significantly more spread out than the other. Compare HETEROSCEDASTICITY.

homosexual behavior in general, sexual impulses, feelings, or relations directed to members of the same sex. H.b., however, may refer only to actual sexual practices such as mutual masturbation, cunnilingus, fellatio, and anal intercourse.

homosexual community a homosexual culture, male or female, which has its own meeting places, customs, social demands, linguistic expressions, organizations, and, in some areas, its own bars, beaches, and shops.

homosexuality sexual relationships between members of the same sex, ranging from sexual fantasies and feelings, through kissing and mutual masturbation, to genital, oral, or anal contact. Also see ABSOLUTE INVERSION; ACCIDENTAL H.; ADOLESCENT H.; CROSS DRESSING; EGO-DYSTONIC H.; EGO-SYNTONIC; FAUTE DE MIEUX; IATROGENIC H.; INVERSION; LATENT H.; LESBIANISM; MALE HOMOSEXUAL PROSTITUTION; MASKED H.; NATURAL HOMOSEXUAL PERIOD; OVERT H.; PEDERASTY; PSEUDOHOMOSEXUALITY; SITUATIONAL H.

homosexual marriage a marital relationship between male or female homosexuals, not legitimized by law. Such "marriages" are usually deeper, more lasting, and more monogamous than other homosexual relationships, but are not necessarily permanent. Participation in such marriages is no longer considered prima facie evidence of psychiatric disorder.

homosexual panic a sudden, acute anxiety attack precipitated by (a) the unconscious fear that one might be homosexual or will act out homosexual impulses, (b) the fear of being sexually attacked by a person of the same sex, or (c) loss, or separation from, a homosexual partner. See KEMPF'S DISEASE.

homosexual rape forcible sexual assault by an individual upon another of the same sex. H.r. usually involves males who are members of a prison population. H.r. is regarded legally as sodomy or buggery.

homosocial peer group a group of individuals, usually children or adolescents, of similar age and the same sex.

homovanillic acid a metabolite of DOPAMINE. See this entry.

homozygote a person with identical alleles at the same genetic positions of each of a matching pair of chromosomes. Adjective: **homozygous**. Compare HETEROZYGOTE.

homunculus a completely formed "minute human" figure thought by some 16th- and 17th-century theorists to exist in the spermatozoon and to simply expand in size in the transition from zygote to embryo to infant to adult. This idea is an illustration of preformism, and is in opposition to the epigenetic principle of cumulative development and successive differentiation. Also see PREFORMISM.

For a different use of the term, see MOTOR-FUNCTION H.; SENSORY H.

honesty in general, truthfulness, uprightness, integrity; in psychotherapy, the ability to express one's true feelings and communicate one's immediate experience, including conflicting, ambivalent, or guilt-ridden attitudes.

honeymoon: See WEDDING NIGHT.

Honi phenomenon the failure of a familiar person (husband, wife) to be perceived as abnormal in size when viewed in the Ames distorted room. See AMES DEMONSTRATIONS.

Hooton, Ernest Albert American anthropologist, 1887–1954. See DEGENERACY THEORY.

Hoover, Charles Franklin American physician, 1865–1927. See HOOVER'S SIGN.

Hoover's sign a diagnostic test for organic hemiplegia, as distinguished from hysterical hemiplegia, by having the patient in a reclining position attempt to raise the paralyzed leg. In organic hemiplegia, the patient unconsciously presses down the heel of the healthy leg during the test.

hopelessness the sense that one's present state—physical, mental, or social—is beyond repair. According to some authorities, about 75 percent of depressed patients believe they will never recover (Cassidy et al., in *Journal of the American Medical Association*, 1957). Feelings of h. are particularly strong in children and adolescents who attempt suicide, as well as in states of alienation and demoralization, and in the grief-stricken.

Hopkins symptoms check list a 58-item self-report inventory designed to identify symptom patterns commonly found in out-patients, such as obsessive-compulsive behavior, anxiety, depressive tendencies, and somatization. Abbrev.: **HSCL**.

hopping reaction a complex series of neuromuscular actions requiring a flexion of the leg followed by a lateral movement, then an extension. Cats, rats, and monkeys may move in hopping patterns but with different cortical-control mechanisms.

horizontal cell a type of association cell found in the retina. H.c. functions include collection of impulses from some receptor cells and carrying the impulses to other retinal cells, much as association cells within the brain relay impulses between cells.

horizontal group a group composed of and restricted to one social class. **Horizontal mobility** refers to a shift of roles within the same social class, e.g., moving from a position on the school board to a position on the chamber of commerce. Also see SOCIAL MOBILITY. Compare VERTICAL GROUP.

horizontal job enlargement: See JOB ENLARGEMENT.

horizontal mobility: See HORIZONTAL GROUP.

horizontal section a theoretical slice of a body or organ, such as the brain, which has been cut at an angle that is perpendicular to the dorsal-ventral axis. See COMPUTERIZED AXIAL TOMOGRAPHY.

horizontal transmission host-to-host transmission of infection as contrasted with **vertical transmission**, or **transplacental transmission**, of infection.

hormephobia a morbid fear of experiencing a shock.

hormic psychology a school of psychology introduced by William McDougall in the 1920s. It emphasizes goal-seeking, striving, and foresight, with human instincts serving as a primary motivation for behavior. H.p. stimulated studies in social psychology. Also called **purposive psychology**. Also see TELEOLOGY.

hormones substances secreted by various glands of the body, serving as chemical messengers to initiate activity in other body tissues. The various hormones are secreted by the anterior and posterior pituitary, adrenal cortex and adrenal medulla, parathyroid, thyroid, pancreas, and testes or ovary glands of internal secretion.

Horn, C. C. American psychologist, fl. 1948. See HORN-HELLERSBERG DRAWING COMPLETION TEST; TOMKINS-HORN PICTURE ARRANGEMENT TEST.

Horner, Johann Friedrich Swiss ophthalmologist, 1831–86. See HORNER'S LAW; BERNARD-HORNER SYNDROME; BABINSKI-NAGEOTTE SYNDROME; SPINAL-CORD DISEASE; WALLENBERG'S SYNDROME.

Horner's law the principle that red-green color blindness is a genetic disorder transmitted indirectly from male to male through a female.

Horney, Karen /hôr′nī/ German-born American psychiatrist, 1885–1952. Trained as a psychoanalyst, H. objected to what she believed to be Freud's overemphasis on the instincts of sex and hostility to the exclusion of social and cultural factors, as well as his structural approach to the mind (id, ego, superego), and his view that unresolved oedipal conflicts are at the root of all neuroses. While retaining the general psychodynamic approach, she advanced her own formulation by interpreting neuroses in terms of maladaptive reactions to basic anxiety originating in disturbed relationships between parents and children, relationships that make the individual feel helpless, isolated, and insecure in a hostile world. Horney's therapy is directed to replacement of the individual's maladaptive reactions, or "strategies," such as extreme competitiveness, or dependence on others, with more constructive approaches to life.

See ADAPTIVE APPROACH; AUXILIARY SOLUTION; BASIC ANXIETY; BASIC CONFLICT; BLOCKAGE; CENTRAL CONFLICT; COMPLIANT CHARACTER; COMPREHENSIVE SOLUTION; CULTURALISTS; DEPENDENCY NEEDS; DEPTH PSYCHOLOGY; DETACHMENT; DISILLUSIONING PROCESS; EMOTIONAL SECURITY; IDEALIZED IMAGE; LONG-TERM PSYCHOTHERAPY; MAJOR SOLUTION; NEO-FREUDIAN; NEUROTIC CONFLICT; NEUROTIC DEFENSE SYSTEM; NEUROTIC NEEDS; NEUROTIC PROCESS; NEUROTIC TREND; OEDIPUS COMPLEX; REAL SELF; RECONSTRUCTIVE

PSYCHOTHERAPY; RESIGNATION; SAFETY DEVICE; SAFETY MOTIVE; SELF; SELF-EFFACEMENT; SELF-EXTINCTION; SOCIAL PSYCHIATRY.

Horn-Hellersberg Drawing Completion Test a projective technique for children in which the subject is required to make complete drawings based on a series of stimulus patterns.

horrific temptation a term applied by Rado to a compulsion by the patient to kill or injure another person, who may be closely related, while at the same time shrinking in horror from the temptation.

horror feminae = GYNOPHOBIA.

horse phobia a morbid fear of horses. Also called **hippophobia**. See LITTLE HANS.

horseshoe crab = LIMULUS.

hor. som. an abbreviation used in prescriptions, meaning "just before sleep" (Latin *hora somni*).

hospital-based home care: See INTENSIVE CARE.

hospital design the basic plan of a hospital building and facilities. While traditional hospitals were designed for the benefit of the staff rather than the patients, newer designs are based on behavior-oriented environmental factors that offer more personal control and privacy for the patients. Studies of traditional h.d. show that as the number of beds per psychiatric ward increases, patient withdrawal symptoms also increase.

hospitalism a term applied by Spitz to a syndrome observed in infants who have been separated from their mothers and institutionalized. According to Bakwin (1949), the outstanding features are "listlessness, emaciation and pallor, relative immobility, quietness, unresponsiveness to stimuli like a smile or coo, indifferent appetite, failure to gain weight." See ANACLITIC DEPRESSION; FAILURE TO THRIVE; MATERNAL DEPRIVATION.

hospitalitis the state of mind of a patient who is so dependent psychologically upon hospital life that his symptoms suddenly recur when he learns he is about to be discharged.

hostile aggression any form of aggression explicitly intended to cause suffering or injury, in contrast to INSTRUMENTAL AGGRESSION. See this entry.

hostility a persistent anger and resentment combined with an intense urge to retaliate. Though hostile impulses may be normal, especially when we are frustrated, deprived, or discriminated against, they may also be a factor in anxiety attacks, obsessive-compulsive behavior, depression, antisocial personality, and paranoid reactions. See ANGER.

hot-line a telephone line maintained by trained personnel for the purpose of providing crisis-intervention service.

hot-seat technique a Gestalt-therapy technique in which a participant sits temporarily in an empty chair next to the therapist and is encouraged to relive distressing experiences and give vent to feelings of guilt or resentment that have been damaging his self-image or relationships for years. The technique is said to generate a new awareness which leads the participant to find his own solutions.

Hottentot apron an overgrowth of the labia minora, so named because it is commonly seen in members of the Hottentots of southern Africa.

Hottentot bustle = STEATOPYGIA.

hottentotism an exaggerated form of stammering or stuttering. The term may have been derived from the Dutch words *hateren*, "to stammer," and *tateren*, "to stutter." Early Dutch settlers of southern Africa are said to have used the same words to derive the name Hottentot for a local tribe whose native speech sounds followed a timing and rhythm that was unfamiliar to Europeans.

housebound housewife's syndrome = HOUSE-WIFE'S SYNDROME.

house fear = DOMATOPHOBIA; OIKOPHOBIA.

House-Tree-Person Technique a projective test developed by J. N. Buck, 1948, to reveal personality dynamics and emotional tone through interpretation of the subject's drawings of a house (representing family relationships and sexual feelings and fantasies), a tree (symbolizing relationship to the environment as well as inner balance), and a person (reflecting the subject's personality, self-image, and sexual role). Abbrev.: **HTP**.

housewife's syndrome a state of frustration and resentment among women who feel trapped and isolated by household chores and child-rearing responsibilities without sufficient outlets for their energies and aspirations. As they grow older, they often become increasingly frigid and suffer from fatigue, backaches, and other somatoform symptoms. The term has also been applied to a "Craig's Wife" compulsion to spend their lives keeping the house spotlessly clean (from the popular play *Craig's Wife*). Also called **housebound h.s.; housewife's neurosis**.

HRF: See PSYCHIATRIC SERVICES.

H.S. an abbreviation used in prescriptions, meaning "just before sleep" (Latin *hora somni*).

HSCL = HOPKINS SYMPTOMS CHECK LIST.

Hsieh-Ping a culture-specific condition observed in Taiwan, characterized by ancestor identification and temporary trancelike states accompanied by tremors, disorientation, delirium, and visual or auditory hallucinations.

H.T. (ASCP): See HISTOLOGIC TECHNICIAN.

HTP = HOUSE-TREE-PERSON TECHNIQUE.

hue color quality, which is determined primarily by wavelength and secondarily by intensity, or amplitude.

huffer's neuropathy peripheral neuropathy, or damage to the peripheral nervous system, resulting from frequently repeated inhalation of organic solvents such as turpentine or naphtha, used as a means of achieving a euphoric reaction, or

high. This inhalation is also called **huffing**. Also see PERIPHERAL NEUROPATHY.

Hughlings Jackson's syndrome = JACKSON'S SYNDROME.

Hugo, Victor /ēgō′/ or /hyo͞og′ō/ French writer, 1802–85. See QUASIMODO COMPLEX.

Hull, Clark Leonard American psychologist, 1884–1952. H. was the originator of the influential theory that all behavior, including conditioning and learning, is initiated by needs and directed to need reduction; and that activities that reduce need reinforce specific responses called habits—e.g., when a hungry rat obtains food by inadvertently pushing a lever, it learns to repeat that response. See HULL'S MATHEMATICO-DEDUCTIVE THEORY OF LEARNING; DRIVE-REDUCTION THEORY; EFFECTIVE-HABIT STRENGTH; HABIT FAMILY HIERARCHY; HABIT STRENGTH; INHIBITORY POTENTIAL; LEARNING THEORY; PURE-STIMULUS ACT; REACTIVE INHIBITION.

Hull's mathematico-deductive theory of learning a complex concept of learning based on classical S-R conditioning with numerous (34) postulates and corollaries to explain various behaviors. Major emphases are on need reduction as a condition of learning, the building up of habit strength by contiguous reinforcement, extinction brought about by nonreinforced repetition of responses, and forgetting as a process of decay with the passage of time.

-hum-; -hom- a combining form from Latin *humus*, "earth, soil." It appears in *homo* and *humanus* or "human," that is, an "earthly being"; but also in "humble" (and "humility," "humiliation"), namely, "on the ground." Also see -HOMO-.

human chorionic gonadotropin: See GONADOTROPIN.

human engineering a branch of psychology concerned with the design of environments and equipment that promote optimum use of human capabilities and optimum efficiency and comfort. Also see ENGINEERING PSYCHOLOGY.

human factors a broad field concerned with the design, maintenance, operation, and improvement of operating systems in which human beings are components, such as industrial equipment, automobiles, health-care systems, transportation systems, recreational facilities, consumer products, and the general living environment.

human-factors psychology a branch of psychology that studies relationships between humans and their work and home environments with the objective of enhancing habitability by redesigning buildings and equipment to fit human abilities and characteristics. New designs are based in turn on user experience with earlier models.

human-growth movement = HUMAN-POTENTIAL MOVEMENT.

humanism any mode of thought or action in which human interests and dignity are valued and which takes an individualistic, critical, and secular perspective (in the tradition of the Humanists of the Renaissance.) Also see HUMANISTIC THEORY.

humanistic communitarian socialism Erich Fromm's term for an ideal society in which humane values would underlie the socioeconomic structure. The goal of h.c.s. is a nonexploitive society in which all members develop to maximum ability, are self-regulating, and contribute fully as individuals and citizens. Fromm believes that social-economic conditions play a major role in determining the character patterns of a given society.

humanistic conscience according to E. Fromm, a feature of the healthy individual in which behavior is regulated by individual standards and not by fear of external authority. See PRODUCTIVE ORIENTATION. Compare AUTHORITARIAN CONSCIENCE.

humanistic-existential therapy = EXISTENTIAL-HUMANISTIC THERAPY.

humanistic perspective the assumption in psychology that people are essentially good and constructive, that the tendency to self-actualize is inherent, and that, given proper environment, human beings will develop to maximum potential. The h.p. has arisen from the contributions of G. Allport, A. Maslow, and C. Rogers. These theorists advocate a personality theory based on the study of healthy as opposed to neurotic or pathological individuals. See HUMANISM; HUMANISTIC PSYCHOLOGY; SELF-ACTUALIZATION. Also see NEED-HIERARCHY THEORY.

humanistic psychology an outgrowth of existentialism and phenomenology that focuses on the individual's capacity to make his own choices, create his own style of life, and actualize himself in his own way. Its approach is holistic, and its emphasis is on spontaneity and the development of the human potential through experiential means rather than analysis of the unconscious or behavior modification. See HUMAN-POTENTIAL MOVEMENT; SENSITIVITY TRAINING; ENCOUNTER GROUP; ENCOUNTER MOVEMENT.

humanistic theory a general approach to human behavior and human life that emphasizes the uniqueness, worth, and dignity of each individual, and the development of personal values and goals that reflect the interplay of physical, psychological, and sociocultural factors. See ERIKSON; FROMM; MASLOW. Also see HUMANISM.

humanistic therapy = THIRD-FORCE THERAPY.

human menopausal gonadotropin: See GONADOTROPIN.

human-motivation theory: See MASLOW'S THEORY OF HUMAN MOTIVATION.

human nature the generally innate but flexible characteristics of humankind as a whole.

human-potential growth center = GROWTH CENTER.

human-potential model a psychological approach in education derived from the basic tenets of humanistic psychology and emphasizing the importance of helping learners achieve maximum individual development of potential in all aspects of their functioning. See HUMANISTIC PSYCHOLOGY. Also see HUMANISTIC PERSPECTIVE.

human-potential movement an approach to psychotherapy and psychology based on the quest for personal growth, development, interpersonal sensitivity, and greater freedom and spontaneity in living. The ideas of F. Perls are an influential force in the h.-p.m. which derives its general perspective from humanistic psychology. Gestalt therapy, sensitivity training, and encounter groups are representative of this approach. Also called **human-growth movement**. Also see GESTALT THERAPY.

human relations relationships and interactions between two or more persons, especially socially and emotionally significant relations. See INTERPERSONAL RELATIONS.

Human Relations Area Files a classification of ethnographic data on a number of primitive tribes, coded in such a way that it is possible to compare the same topic across a number of tribes. H.R.A.F. are useful for cross-cultural research.

human-relations training techniques designed to promote awareness of the feelings and needs of other individuals, and to promote constructive interactions. See SENSITIVITY TRAINING; T-GROUP.

human therapeutic experience a term primarily encountered in educational psychology referring to interactions between teacher and students that foster security, original thinking, and creative expression and help to provide children with a positive model of interpersonal relations.

Hume, David Scottish philosopher, 1711–76. See ASSOCIATIONISM.

humidity effects a principal factor affecting one's experience of ambient temperature. High humidity in hot weather is uncomfortable because it diminishes the "capacity of the air to absorb water vapor from sweat" (P. A. Bell, J. D. Fisher, and R. J. Loomis, *Environmental Psychology*, 1978).

humidity fear = HYGROPHOBIA.

humiliation a feeling of shame due to being embarrassed, disgraced, or deprecated. Some individuals invite h. as punishment for real or fancied wrongdoing; others lose so much self-esteem when they are humiliated that they become depressed. H. of the partner is frequently found in sexual sadism and sexual masochism.

Humm, Doncaster George American psychologist, 1887–1959. See HUMM-WADSWORTH TEMPERAMENT SCALE.

Humm-Wadsworth Temperament Scale a personality inventory designed to assess depressive, paranoid, manic, schizoid, and hysteric tendencies.

humor the semifluid substances (Latin *humor*, "fluid, moisture") that occupy the spaces in the eyeball. The fluid in the anterior chamber, between the lens and the cornea, is known as the aqueous h., and the thicker transparent substance filling the space behind the lens is called the **vitreous h**. See AQUEOUS HUMOR.

In an abstract sense, h. is the capacity to perceive or express the amusing aspects of a situation. There is little agreement about the essence of humor and the reasons we laugh or smile at jokes or anecdotes. Plato (also Thomas Hobbes) claimed that we laugh at people and situations which make us feel superior; Immanuel Kant emphasized surprise and anticlimax: "the sudden transformation of a strained expectation to nothing"; Max Eastman described humor as "playful pain," or taking serious things lightly, and thereby triumphing over them; Freud called attention to the many jokes (especially those having to do with sex and hostility) that enable us to give free expression to forbidden impulses, and explained laughter in terms of release of energy employed in keeping them out of consciousness. The term also denotes a mood or state of mind (good humor, bad humor) and has been used to designate the bodily fluids that were once believed to determine our health and disposition. See HUMORAL THEORY; GALLOWS H.

humoral immunity factors: See IMMUNITY FACTORS.

humoral theory the theory that attributes personality characteristics to the effects of body fluids, or "humors." The h.t. gave rise to the oldest known typology, originated by Hippocrates, who associated a predominance of blood with an sanguine temperament; black bile with a melancholic temperament; yellow bile with a choleric temperament; and phlegm with a phlegmatic temperament. The theory is often considered a forerunner of the modern recognition of the influence of hormones on behavior.

humpback a rounded deformity in the back of an individual due to an abnormal backward curvature, or kyphosis, of the spine. H. is one of the basic orthopedic pathology types of dwarfism. Also called **hunchback**.

Hunermann, Carl German physician, fl. 1937. See CONRADI'S DISEASE (there: **Conradi-Hunermann disease**).

hunger drive a drive or arousal state induced by food deprivation. The h.d. is regulated in large measure by the hypothalamus. Psychological influences play a major role in determining the intensity of an individual's h.d. and in determining individual modes of hunger-related behavior, e.g. types of food preferred or avoided. Also see SPECIFIC HUNGER; NERVOUS HUNGER; SOCIAL HUNGER.

hunger pangs a feeling of emptiness in the stomach, at one time attributed to contractions of the stomach muscles in the absence of food. However, more recent studies found that persons without stomachs also experienced h.p. Also called **hunger pains**.

hunger strike: See NEUROTIC H.S.

Hunt, Howard Francis American psychologist, 1918—. See HUNT-MINNESOTA TEST FOR ORGANIC BRAIN DAMAGE.

Hunt, James Ramsey American neurologist, 1872–1937. See HUNT'S SYNDROME.

Hunter, Charles Canadian (?) physician, 20th century. See HUNTER'S SYNDROME; MUCOPOLYSACCHARIDOSES.

Hunter's syndrome an X-linked recessive mucopolysaccharide disease. As in Hurler's syndrome, there is an excess of mucopolysaccharides in the urine. The child shows normal development until the second year and may learn some words and sentences and achieve toilet training. Hyperkinetic behavior and a clumsy gait develop after age two; physical activity slows down around age five. Mental retardation appears in the second year. Also called **MPS II**.

hunting behavior an instinctive activity of most animals that pursue other animals for food or sport. H.b. may include other forms of behavior such as stalking, running after moving objects, or use of concealment or camouflage.

Huntington, George American neurologist, 1850–1916. See HUNTINGTON'S CHOREA; ABIOTROPHY; ASSAULTIVE BEHAVIOR; AUTOSOMAL ABERRATIONS; BIRTH DEFECT; BRAIN ATROPHY; CHOREA; CONGENITAL DEFECT; DEMENTIA; PHENOTHIAZINES; RAUWOLFIA DERIVATIVES.

Huntington's chorea a hereditary progressive disease marked by involuntary movements and dementia. Two forms, **childhood H.c.** and **adult H.c.**, closely resemble each other in loss of caudate nucleus and putamen neurons. There is a general loss of cerebral-nerve cells. The changes can be observed in pneumoencephalograms. Both childhood and adult forms occur in the same family, but most cases have an average onset age of 35 years. Also called **Huntington's disease (HD)**.

Hunt-Minnesota Test for Organic Brain Damage a three-part organicity test consisting of (a) the vocabulary subtest of the Stanford-Binet Test, which assesses basic verbal ability before impairment occurred, (b) six memory and recall tests which are relatively sensitive to brain damage, and (c) nine tests such as information items, following specific instructions, and counting forward and backward, which indicate whether the subject is too disturbed, uncooperative, or deteriorated to be tested.

Hunt's syndrome a condition resulting from a herpes-zoster infection and characterized by inflammation of the facial nerve, severe otitis media, facial paralysis, and cerebellar ataxia and tremors. Also called **Ramsay Hunt's syndrome; dyssynergia cerebellaris**.

Hunt's tremor: See TREMOR.

Hurler, Gertrud /ho͞or'lər/ Austrian pediatrician, fl. 1919. See HURLER'S SYNDROME; CRANIOFACIAL ANOMALIES; HUNTER'S SYNDROME; MUCOPOLYSACCHARIDOSES.

Hurler's syndrome an autosomal-recessive disease marked by mucopolysaccharide levels in tissues more than ten times normal, plus elevated levels of polysaccharides and a gargoyle appearance. Mental development begins normally but slows after the early months and reaches a plateau around age two. The child may learn a few words, but not sentences, and toilet training is seldom achieved. Also called **Pfaundler-Hurler syndrome; MPS I**. Also see GARGOYLISM.

hurry sickness an obsessive time consciousness, a key trait of the heart-attack-prone TYPE A PERSONALITY. See this entry.

Husserl, Edmund /hŏŏs′erl/ German philosopher, 1859–1938. H. was the founder of the phenomenological school, which studies the mind through the description of immediate experiences, as opposed to the mechanistic approach that focuses on natural causes and bodily functions. To H. the realm of consciousness, not the material world, is the source of all meaning. See EXISTENTIALISM; PHENOMENOLOGY.

Hutchinson, Sir Jonathan English surgeon, 1828–1913. See PROGERIA (also called **Hutchinson Gilford syndrome**).

Huxley, Aldous English novelist and critic, 1894–1963. See PSYCHEDELICS; PHANEROTHYME.

-hyal-; -hyalo- a combining form meaning glassy, transparent.

hyaline membrane a translucent albuminlike substance that forms a glassy surface over the alveoli in the absence of an enzyme that normally would remove the h.m. The enzyme works like a soap or synthetic detergent to break up the h.m. that otherwise blocks the normal flow of oxygen into the alveoli and the release of carbon dioxide carried to the lungs by the pulmonary arteries.

hyaline-membrane disease a disorder of some newborn children who are afflicted by the formation of a hyaline membrane over the alveolar lung surfaces. The membrane causes a **respiratory-distress syndrome** which may worsen progressively until the lungs begin producing a natural surfactant that breaks up the membrane. H.-m.d. almost always occurs in premature babies although infants of diabetic mothers may be afflicted until nearly full term. Also see CONTINUOUS POSITIVE-AIRWAY PRESSURE.

hydantoins a group of drugs developed for the primary purpose of controlling epileptic seizures by hyperpolarizing cortical cells. The h. were introduced in 1938 after careful studies of chemicals capable of suppressing electroshock convulsions without also causing adverse CNS effects. Hydantoin molecules are similar in structure to barbiturates but have the advantage of not altering the threshold for minimal seizures. The prototype of the h., **diphenylhydantoin**—$C_{15}H_{12}N_2O_2$—is prescribed mainly in cases of grand mal and psychomotor epilepsies, but also is administered in some cases of migraine-neuralgia disorders. Other h. include **mephenytoin**—$C_{12}H_{14}N_2O_2$, which is the chemical equivalent of mephobarbital, and **phenylethylhydantoin**—$C_{11}H_{12}N_2O_2$.

Hydergine a trademark for a group of hydrogenated alkaloids employed therapeutically as adrenergic blockers. H. may be prescribed as part of the treatment of organic brain syndrome associated with senile dementia. H. has been found to improve social functioning and mood without significant adverse side effects.

-hydr-; -hydro- a combining form relating to water, waterlike fluid, or sweat.

hydralazine $C_8H_8N_4$—a direct vasodilator drug used in the treatment of essential and malignant hypertension and some cases of peripheral vascular disease. H. often is used with other agents, particularly when the hypertension is complicated by other circulatory disorders, e.g., congestive heart failure.

hydranencephaly a cerebral defect in which the meninges and cranium are intact but the cerebral hemispheres have been almost totally replaced by membranous sacs, which may be filled with fluid. Among infants surviving the neonatal period, most have normal reflexes and responses for several weeks, then show a lack of psychomotor development. Most show no EEG response. One exception was a five-year-old with an IQ of 74 who attended school.

hydration the act or process of accumulating or combining with water. Body cells undergo h. when sodium intake is increased. Compare DEHYDRATION.

hydraulic model an erroneous concept of the nervous system introduced in the early 17th century by the French philosopher René Descartes, who believed that nerves were tubes through which "vital spirits" flowed from the brain to the muscles. Habits were formed, according to the h.m. concept, when repeated use of the nerve tubes caused them to become distended and blocked.

hydrocephalus /-sef′-/ a condition caused by accumulation of cerebrospinal fluid in the ventricles of the brain, resulting in an enlarged cranium and such symptoms as severe mental retardation, epilepsy, and blindness. H. is usually congenital, although it may develop after birth as a result of meningitis, toxic states, head injury, brain tumor, or hemorrhage. The pressure can sometimes be relieved by surgery in which the excess fluid is shunted into the bloodstream. Also called **hydrocephaly**. See NORMAL-PRESSURE H.; LOW-PRESSURE H.; ARNOLD-CHIARI MALFORMATION; HAKIM'S DISEASE; DANDY-WALKER SYNDROME.

hydrocortisone = CORTISOL.

hydrodipsomania a condition of uncontrollable thirst that occurs periodically, especially in epileptic patients.

hydroencephalocele a developmental anomaly of the brain in which a portion protruding through the skull contains a cavity that is linked with the ventricles of the cerebrum.

hydrogen-ion concentration a measure of the degree of **acidity** or **alkalinity** of a substance. When acids and alkaline substances dissociate in water, hydrogen ions, indicated by H+, and hydroxyl ions, indicated by OH−, are released. Acidity or alkalinity is associated with an excess of one or the other ions. The h.-i.c. is indicated by the symbol pH, representing the negative logarithm, p, of the H+ ion. Because it is a negative logarithm, the greater the excess of H+ ions the lower the numerical value. Thus a pH of 0 would represent the largest possible excess of H+ ions, or a "pure" acid. At the other extreme, a pH of 14 would represent the maximum degree of alkalinity in terms of excess OH– ions. Human body fluids have an average pH of about 7.4 or a slightly alkaline pH. If the pH rises about 7.8 or falls below 6.8, enzymes and other biochemical substances in the body malfunction and death may result. See HOMEOSTASIS.

hydromyelia a pathologic accumulation of cerebrospinal fluid in the enlarged central canal of the spinal cord.

hydromyelocele a form of spina bifida in which a protrusion of a portion of the spinal cord is distended with cerebrospinal fluid.

hydrophobia a morbid fear of water; also, a term for rabies, in which water aversion is a major symptom, due to a deglutition reflex irritation that prevents the patient from drinking water regardless of his thirst. See RABIES. Also see WATER PHOBIA.

hydrophobophobia a morbid fear of hydrophobia or of rabies. Also see CYNOPHOBIA.

hydrotherapy in general, the use of water, internally or externally, in the treatment of disease; in psychiatry, the occasional use of wet packs (wet sheets wrapped around the body) or continuous tub baths to calm delirious or agitated patients. The term applies also to the use of hot foot baths for sedation, sprays or douches for stimulation, or swimming and aquatic sports for auxiliary therapy and physical rehabilitation. Also see CONTINUOUS-BATH TREATMENT.

hydroxytryptamine = SEROTONIN.

hydroxytryptophan a naturally occurring substance that is a precursor to serotonin. It is produced from molecules of the essential amino acid tryptophan, which is rapidly transported to the brain for conversion to 5-hydroxytryptophan, and then into 5-hydroxytryptamine, or serotonin.

hydroxyzine: See DIPHENYLMETHANES.

hydroxyzine hydrochloride: See DIPHENYLMETHANES.

hyelophobia a morbid fear of glass. Also called CRYSTALLOPHOBIA.

hygienic inducement a term used to denote those facets of a job, such as salary, working conditions, hours, and benefits, that produce discontent if lacking but do not actually motivate employees to improve their job performance, according to F. Herzberg.

-hygr-; -hygro- a combining form relating to moisture.

hygrophobia a morbid fear of moisture or humidity.

hylephobia a morbid fear of epilepsy.

hylophobia a morbid fear of a forest. Also called **ylophobia**.

hymen a thin membrane that normally covers a part of the opening to the vagina before the first coitus. The h. varies in size among individuals and in some females may be completely absent. It also may remain unruptured after coitus, so the presence or absence of the h. is not a reliable sign of virginity or loss of VIRGINITY. See this entry.

hyoscine = SCOPOLAMINE.

hyoscyamine $C_{17}H_{23}NO_3$—an anticholinergic drug derived as an alkaloid from hyoscyamus, belladonna, and stramonium. It is administered as an antispasmodic, analgesic, and sedative. A sulfate salt of h. is used in the control of symptoms of parkinsonism.

-hyp-: See -HYPO-.

hypacusia a state of partial deafness. Also called **hypoacusia; hypacusis; hypacousia.** Adjective: **hypacusic**.

hypengyophobia a morbid fear of asuming responsibility. Also see PARALIPOPHOBIA.

-hyper- /-hīp-/ a combining form meaning beyond, excessive, abnormal.

hyperactive-child syndrome = HACS.

hyperactivity persistent restless overactivity, particularly among brain-damaged, mentally retarded, or emotionally disturbed children. Such children are constantly on the go, have a short attention span, sleep poorly, and frequently exhibit educational and perceptual deficits. The condition is also observed in adults afflicted with epidemic encephalitis, the manic phase of bipolar disorder, or catatonic excitement. H. should not be confused with the more serious hyperkinetic syndrome. H. behavior is usually purposeful in contrast to the often purposeless hyperkinetic behavior. H. is also called **hyperkinesis**. See MINIMAL BRAIN DYSFUNCTION; HYPERKINETIC SYNDROME; PURPOSELESS H.; DEVELOPMENTAL H.

hyperacusis abnormally acute hearing and a lowered tolerance for loud sounds such as in the presence of COCHLEAR RECRUITMENT. See this entry. Also called **hyperacusia**.

hyperadrenal constitution a body and personality type associated with overactivity of the adrenal gland and characterized by muscular strength and development, hyperglycemia, a tendency toward hypertension, and a personality marked by euphoria, and moral and intellectual energy.

hyperageusia an excessive sensitivity to taste, a condition that may be due to either a neurological or a hysterical disorder.

hyperaggressivity an extreme tendency to express anger and hostility in action, as in assaulting and killing other people. H. is a major symptom of intermittent or isolated explosive disorder, and epileptic furor.

hyperalgesia an abnormal sensitivity to pain. The effect occasionally results from development of new nerve endings in skin areas that have been severely injured. Also called **hyperalgia**.

hyperbolic misidentification: See MISIDENTIFICATION.

hyperbulimia inordinate appetite and excessive intake of food, observed in some schizophrenic patients, in cases of diabetes mellitus, and in patients with hypothalamic lesions. Also see HYPERPHAGIA.

hypercalcemia syndrome = ELFIN FACIES.

hypercarbia a condition of respiratory distress marked by increasing levels of carbon dioxide in the blood. H. may occur in disorders such as emphysema in which the lungs lose their ability to eliminate dissolved carbon dioxide from blood that has been circulated through the tissues. H. effects include impaired mental concentration and attention, irritability, and somnolence. If uncorrected, the condition progresses to coma.

hypercathexis an excess of psychic energy invested in an object (person, activity, goal).

hypercoenesthesia an extreme state of well-being. Also called **hypercenesthesia**. Also see COENESTHESIA.

hypercompensatory type a constitutional type (Lewis) characterized by overdevelopment of blood and lymph vessels, digestive tract, and ductless glands. The hypercompensatory characteristic is expressed in the form of symptoms of paranoid or manic-depressive reactions.

hyperemia: See BLUSHING.

hyperergasia an alternative term for the manic phase of manic-depressive psychosis (Meyer).

hyperesthesia extreme sensitivity to sound, light, heat, cold, and, particularly, tactile stimuli. H. is a common hysterical (conversion) symptom as well as a symptom of some organic conditions such as alcoholic polyneuritis and menopause.

hyperesthetic memory a memory that is abnormally sensitive to past associations, a condition that Freud and Breuer regarded as a causative factor in hysteria cases.

hyperexcitability an extreme tendency to emotional arousal; a tendency to overreact to the slightest stimulus.

hypergargalesthesia an extreme sensitivity to tickling.

hypergenitalism an excessive development of the genital system.

hypergenital type a constitutional type (Pende) characterized by premature and exaggerated development of sexual characteristics, relatively short extremities, and a large chest and skull. The female version also shows extremely sensitive breasts and genitalia, and the female experiences an unusually early menarche.

hyperglycemia an excess of glucose in the blood. In diabetes mellitus, h. is a part of the metabolic syndrome resulting from a relative or absolute lack of insulin needed to remove the excess glucose from the blood. Neuropathic signs range from pain or sensory loss to failure of reflexes and coma.

hypergnosis /hīpərnō'sis/ a perception that is exaggerated to the point of being expanded into a philosophical system or concept, as observed in certain types of paranoid behavior.

hyperhidrosis abnormal production of perspiration by the sweat glands. Although the exact nature of the excessive production is unknown, it commonly occurs in otherwise normal individuals during periods of anxiety or stress. H. usually affects the palms and soles but may occur elsewhere, e.g., the groin or armpits. In severe cases, the skin in the affected areas may become macerated and vulnerable to infections. Also called **hyperidrosis**.

hyperingestion excessive or abnormally high rates of intake of food, fluid, or drugs through the mouth, particularly when intake is greater than the maximum safe level. See BULIMIA.

hyperinsulinism: See HYPOGLYCEMIA.

hyperkalemia: See KIDNEY FAILURE.

hyperkinesis = HYPERACTIVITY.

hyperkinetic encephalopathy extreme restlessness, irritability, impulsivity, and overactivity due to residual brain damage, especially in the hyperkinetic form of epidemic encephalitis.

hyperkinetic-impulse disorder a childhood disorder characterized by extreme impulsiveness, overactivity, restlessness, distractibility, and a short attention span. The syndrome may also include dyslexia, perceptual-motor deficits, defective coordination, and negativism. H.-i.d. is equivalent to the DSM-III category ATTENTION-DEFICIT DISORDER WITH HYPERACTIVITY. See this entry.

hyperkinetic reaction of childhood a DSM-II category which has been replaced in DSM-III by ATTENTION-DEFICIT DISORDER WITH HYPERACTIVITY. See this entry.

hyperkinetic syndrome a childhood or adolescent disorder marked by uncontrolled motor activity, impulsivity, extreme restlessness, perceptual-motor and learning difficulties, a significantly reduced attention span, and possible manic behavior and emotional problems. Psychotherapeutic, pharmacological, and behavior-modification techniques have been used to treat the condition's various manifestations. See ATTENTION-DEFICIT DISORDER WITH HYPERACTIVITY; HYPERACTIVITY.

hyperlipidemia; hyperlipoproteinemia: See LIPID-METABOLISM DISORDERS.

hyperlogia = LOGORRHEA.

hyperlordosis a condition of extreme backward spinal curvature in which the lumbar curve is accentuated. It may develop to compensate or counterbalance another abnormality, e.g., obesity or coxa vara, or result from rickets, or effects of cretinism or dwarfism. A similar posture sometimes is observed in women in an advanced stage of pregnancy.

hypermania an extreme manic state marked by incessant pressure of activity, disorientation, and incoherent speech. Also called **delirium grave; typhomania**. H. is essentially equivalent to COLLAPSE DELIRIUM. See this entry. Also see BELL'S MANIA; DELIRIOUS MANIA.

hypermetamorphosis a form of hyperresponsiveness observed in animals after temporal-lobe ablation. The new behavior is regarded as exploratory or manipulatory. The animal may spend an hour exploring a strange cage whereas a normal subject might devote only a few minutes to this activity.

hypermnesia an extreme degree of retentiveness and recall; unusual clarity of memory images. H. occasionally occurs in normal individuals faced with death and also in mental prodigies, but is most common in cases of hypomania, organic brain syndrome, patients with high fever, hypnosis, and drug intoxication induced by amphetamines and hallucinogens. See CIRCUMSTANTIALITY; PANORAMIC MEMORY.

hypermobile testes testes that move between the scrotum and the abdominal cavity, usually because of an inguinal hernia that has not been corrected. The h.t. may descend into the scrotum when the environment is warm, as when taking a hot tub bath, but retract into the abdominal cavity when the body is exposed to cold temperatures.

hypermotility abnormally increased or excessive activity in a body function, particularly that of the digestive tract. The cholinergic nervous system dominates the upper portion of the gastrointestinal tract while the adrenergic system controls the lower portion. Gastrin and serotonin stimulate digestive-tract motility while secretion and glucagon inhibit contractions. H. is associated with gastric neuropathy, colitis, and irritable bowel syndrome.

hyperobesity a state of extreme overweight, sometimes defined as weighing in excess of 100 pounds above the accepted ideal body weight for one's height, age, and body build.

hyperopia farsightedness. H. is a refractive error due to a defect in the lens of the eye.

hyperorexia = BULIMIA.

hyperosmia an abnormally acute sensitivity to odors.

hyperparathyroidism a disorder caused by overactivity of the parathyroid gland resulting in excessive levels of parathyroid hormone. The cause may be a tumor or overgrowth of one or more of the glands. The disorder is marked by increased calcium but reduced phosphorus levels in the blood and increased excretion of both minerals, with hypertension, weakness, anorexia, and increased urge to urinate. Compare HYPOPARATHYROIDISM.

hyperparesthesia oversensitivity to pressure or touch.

hyperphagia a tendency to overeat, which may be due to a metabolic disorder such as diabetes mellitus or to a brain lesion. Lesions in the amygdala and temporal lobe have been associated with h. Also see HYPERBULIMIA.

hyperphenylalaninemia a severe form of phenylketonuria marked by abnormally high levels of phenylalanine metabolites in the blood of patients even while on a diet that reduces the levels in mild cases. Diagnosis also is made on the basis of liver tests which in h. patients shows a significant level of a phenylalanine hydroxylase that is barely detectable in the milder form of the disease.

hyperphoria deviation of one eye in an upward direction.

hyperphrasia = LOGORRHEA.

hyperphrenia mental activity that is far above normal and in pathologic states may be manifested in the manic phase of manic-depressive psychosis or psychoneurotic preoccupations.

hyperpituitary constitution a body and personality type associated with overactivity of the pituitary gland near or after the end of the normal growth period. The physical characteristics resemble those of Kretschmer's athletic type, with a hypervigilant attitude and a tendency to control emotions through intellectualization.

hyperplasia an abnormal increase in the size of an organ or tissue caused by the growth of an excessive number of new normal cells. H. may be induced by a virus, as in the growth of warts, by a drug such as phenytoin which is prescribed for epilepsy patients, or by bodily changes associated with aging, as in benign prostatic hypertrophy.

hyperpnea = POLYPNEA.

hyperpolarization an increase in the internal charge of a neuron after activation of an inhibitory synapse. The effect is due to an increase in the permeability of the postsynaptic membrane to the degree that potassium ions leave the cell but sodium ions, though smaller, are unable to enter the cell because they are linked to larger water molecules.

hyperpragia excessive mental activity, generally associated with the manic phase of bipolar disorder.

hyperprosexia a compulsion to attend to a stimulus, such as the creaking of a door. Also called **hyperprosessis**.

hyperpyrexia: See HEAT STROKE.

hypersensitivity reactions severe allergylike reactions experienced by individuals after exposure to certain types of drugs. Chlorpromazine neuroleptics, e.g., may produce blood dyscrasias and dermatitis in hypersensitive patients because of an immune response. Also see REVERSE TOLERANCE.

hypersexuality extreme frequency of sexual activity, or an inordinate desire for sexual activity, often stemming from (a) an inability to achieve orgasm, (b) a need to disprove frigidity, impotence, or homosexuality, or (c) a need to achieve recognition or self-esteem through sexual prowess. H. may be associated with temporal-lobe, amygdala, or hippocampus lesions, as demonstrated in animal experiments. See NYMPHOMANIA; SATYRIASIS.

hypersomnia excessive sleepiness or sleep of excessive duration, as in Economo's disease, and, popularly, sleeping sickness. H. may also be a hysterical (conversion) symptom. Also see PSYCHOGENIC H.; ECONOMO'S DISEASE.

hypersomnic encephalitis = ECONOMO'S DISEASE.

hypersthenic in constitutional medicine, pertaining to a conditon of excessive strength and tension associated with hyperactivity of the lymphatic system.

hypertelorism an abnormally great distance between two body organs or areas, as when the eyes of a subject are separated farther from each other than a normal distance. The condition often is associated with mental retardation or other neurologic deficits where cranial anomalies are involved. Also see MEDIAN-CLEFT-FACE SYNDROME; DISFIGUREMENT.

hypertension: See ESSENTIAL H.

hypertensive crisis sudden extreme rise in blood pressure that may result in intracranial hemorrhage, due in some cases to overwhelming emotional stress, and occasionally to certain antidepressant drugs.

hyperthymia an excessive emotional response; also, overactivity that is close to being manic.

hyperthyroid constitution a constitutional type associated with overactivity of the thyroid gland and characterized by youthfulness and well-developed sexual characteristics, hyperemotivity and instability, roughly corresponding to the asthenic type.

hyperthyroidism: See EXOPHTHALMIC GOITER; APATHETIC H.

hypertonic-dyskinetic syndrome = ZAPPERT'S SYNDROME.

hypertonicity a state of increased tension or tonicity. H. in a newborn can be a diagnostic sign of cerebral palsy, particularly if the deep tendon reflexes are exaggerated.

hypertonic type a constitutional type (Pende; Tandler) that corresponds to Kretschmer's athletic type for an individual whose body build is characterized by a high degree of voluntary muscle tone.

hypertransfusion treatment a method of increasing hemoglobin levels in young Cooley's anemia patients by a regimen of intensive blood transfusions, as opposed to occasional or sporadic transfusions. Symptoms of the disease are diminished or postponed, and life expectancy of the patients is increased by as much as 15 years by h.t.

hypertychia a state of elation with excitement and accelerated physical and mental activity.

hyperuricosuria increased urinary secretion of uric acid. H. is one of the major symptoms of the Lesch-Nyhan syndrome. Also called **hyperuricuria**.

hypervegetative type a constitutional type that corresponds roughly to the pyknic type and more closely to the megalosplanchnic and brachymorphic types.

hyperventilation a rapid deep-breathing attack, usually due to anxiety or emotional stress. **Overbreathing**, as it is also called, lowers the carbon dioxide level of the blood and produces such symptoms as light-headedness, palpitation, numbness and tingling in the extremities, perspiration, and in some cases a fainting spell. Also called **h. syndrome**.

hypervigilance a state of heightened alertness, usually with continual scanning of the environment for signs of danger.

hypervitaminoses pathologic conditions caused by excessive intakes of vitamins, with vitamins A and D most often associated with the disorder. Vitamin-A toxicity usually is characterized by drowsiness, irritability, headache, and vomiting, followed by skin peeling and hair loss. Children may suffer from intracranial pressure. Excess vitamin D elevates blood calcium and causes nervousness, weakness, anorexia, nausea, and kidney disorders.

hypervolemia an abnormal increase in the proportion of fluid, or plasma, in the blood. H. can be a hazard of plasma transfusions conducted for the purpose of supplying the missing clotting factors to the blood of hemophilia patients. The incidence of h. among hemophilia patients has been reduced by the development of clotting-factor concentrates. Compare HYPOVOLEMIA.

hypesthesia = HYPOESTHESIA.

hyphedonia a state of diminished pleasure during an experience that normally would produce extreme pleasure.

-hypn-; -hypno- /-hipn-/ a combining form relating to sleep (Greek *hypnos*).

hypnagogic inducing a state of drowsiness or light sleep.

hypnagogic hallucination a hallucination experienced while falling asleep; false perceptions occurring between sleeping and full wakefulness, analogous to hypnagogic imagery. Such hallucinations are ordinarily not considered pathological.

hypnagogic imagery vivid imagery occurring during the drowsy state between wakefulness and full sleep, or while falling asleep.

hypnagogic reverie fantasies occurring between sleeping and waking. Induction of h.r. by hypnosis is sometimes used as a means of encouraging patients to free-associate and bring unconscious material to the surface.

hypnagogic state the drowsy, trancelike period between waking and sleep during which transient, dreamlike fantasies and hallucinations may appear. During a h.s. suggestibility is high and the individual will usually raise his arm or perform some other action on command. Claims have been made that simple material presented during this period will be retained.

hypnalgia literally, dream pain: pain experienced during sleep or in a dream.

hypnoanalysis a modified and shortened form of psychoanalytic treatment in which hypnosis is employed to recover memories and release repressed material, to break through resistances, to help the patient understand and modify faulty attitudes, to enhance the transference process, and to integrate material evoked in the trance with the patient's conscious life.

hypnocatharsis a recapturing and reliving of memories through free association while in a hypnotic state.

hypnodelic therapy the combined use of hypnosis and LSD. It is a controversial form of brief therapy which has not lived up to early claims. See LSD PSYCHOTHERAPY.

hypnodontics the use of hypnotic suggestion in dentistry as a means of relaxing tense patients, relieving anxiety, reinforcing or replacing anesthesia, and correcting such habits as bruxism and nail-biting.

hypnodrama a psychodramatic technique introduced by J. L. Moreno in 1959, in which a hypnotic state is induced and the patient, or "protagonist," is encouraged to act out his relationships and traumatic experiences with the aid of auxiliary egos. The object of the hypnosis is to eliminate the patient's resistance to dramatizing his problems, and to stimulate the revival of past incidents and emotional scenes in their full intensity.

hypnogenic sleep-producing; hypnosis-inducing.

hypnogenic spot a point on the body which when touched may induce hypnosis if the individual is highly susceptible.

hypnograph an instrument used to measure sleep and physiological activities that occur during sleep, e.g., motor activity, pulse, reflexes.

hypnoidization a hypnotic induction technique in which the subject is asked to recline, close his eyes, and attend to a stimulus such as the beat of a metronome, as a means of reaching a hypnagogic state in which he experiences a vivid flow of free associations that frequently evoke memories of early emotional events.

hypnoid state a state of light hypnosis, or a state resembling hypnosis. Also called **hypnoidal state**.

hypnolepsy an obsolete term for narcolepsy.

hypnology the scientific study of sleep and hypnotism.

hypnonarcosis a deep sleep state induced by hypnosis.

hypnophobia a morbid fear of sleeping or falling asleep.

hypnophrenosis a general term applied to any of a variety of sleep disturbances.

hypnoplasty a hypnotic technique in which the subject is put into a light trance and given a claylike substance with which he gives plastic expression to repressed feelings, and he then verbalizes his conflicts with the encouragement of the therapist.

hypnopompic hallucination a false sensory perception occurring in the period between sleeping and full wakefulness.

hypnosigenesis the induction of hypnosis.

hypnosis a superficial or deep trance state resembling sleep, induced by suggestions of relaxation and concentrated attention to a single object. The subject becomes highly suggestible and responsive to the hypnotist's influence, and can be induced to recall forgotten events, become insensitive to pain, control vasomotor changes, and, in the hands of an experienced hypnotherapist, gain relief from tensions, anxieties, and other psychological symptoms. See HYPNOTHERAPY; HYPNOTISM. Also see SELF-H.; HETEROHYPNOSIS; SELF-HYPNORELAXATION; AUTOHYPNOSIS; WAKING H.; MOTHER H.; FATHER H.; PARAHYPNOSIS; HIGHWAY H.; BRAID.

hypnosuggestion the application of direct hypnotic suggestion to such problems as insomnia, intractable pain, uncontrolled hiccuping, functional sterility, severe undernutrition resulting from psychogenic vomiting or anorexia nervosa, and various types of crises including combat situations, panic, and hysterical amnesia.

hypnotherapy the use of hypnosis in psychological treatment, either in short-term therapy directed to removal of symptoms and modification of behavior patterns, or in long-term reconstructive therapy aimed at personality change. A wide variety of conditions can be treated by one or another of the many hypnotic techniques, e.g., obesity, hypertension, asthma, peptic ulcers, insomnia, functional sterility, combat reactions, anorexia nervosa, and bruxism. See the separate entries devoted to each of the major techniques described by M. V. Kline (*Handbook of Clinical Psychology*, 1965): DIRECT SUGGESTION; ABREACTION; AUTOMATIC DRAWING; DREAM SUGGESTION; AGE REGRESSION; HYPNOPLASTY; HYPNOANALYSIS.

hypnotic a drug that helps induce and sustain sleep by increasing drowsiness and reducing motor activity. H. drugs often are employed in smaller doses to produce sedation and may be used in larger doses to produce anesthesia. Barbiturates are among the most widely used hypnotics, but methaqualone, antihistamines, and minor tranquilizers also may be employed for this purpose. As an adjective, the term means pertaining to hypnosis, as in "h. state." Also see SEDATIVE-HYPNOTICS.

hypnotic analgesia a subject's unresponsiveness or substantially reduced sensitivity to pain under hypnotic suggestion.

hypnotic induction the process by which a subject is hypnotized by verbal suggestion, mechanical aids, or drugs. The process depends upon the subject's susceptibility and needs and the hypnotist's skills and experience, but all methods generally involve the subject's fixation of attention and reduction of sensory and motor activities through relaxation.

hypnotic reeducation hypnotic suggestion combined with increased awareness of the emotional basis of the symptom. E.g., a case of torticollis was alleviated by Kraines by (a) relaxation suggestions plus (b) interpreting the symptom as a symbolic representation of the patient's relationship with an overbearing employer whom he could not face "straightforwardly."

hypnotic regression the process whereby an individual under hypnosis is induced to relive an experience from his past. The experience often is repressed or forgotten, but the source of an emotional conflict. The term is often used interchangeably with AGE REGRESSION. See this entry.

hypnotic rigidity a condition of muscular rigidity induced by suggestion during hypnosis.

hypnotic susceptibility hypnotizability, or hypnotic suggestibility or responsiveness. Application of the Stanford Hypnotic Susceptibility Scale indicates that the majority of university students are moderately susceptible, but only five to ten percent exhibit the most advanced phenomena such as posthypnotic visual hallucinations with the eyes open. The latter group tend to have a rich subjective life and to reach out for new experiences, are not afraid to relinquish reality testing for a time, and are not weak or dependent personalities.

hypnotic trance the unconscious dreamlike state of intensified suggestibility elicited in a hypnotized subject.

hypnotism the study of the nature of hypnosis and its diagnostic and therapeutic applications. See BRAID. Also see COLLECTIVE HYPNOTIZATION.

-hypo-; -hyp- /-hīp-/ a combining form meaning under, below, less than normal, deficient.

hypoactivity underactivity, as in the state of psychomotor retardation experienced in depression. Compare HYPERACTIVITY.

hypoacusia = HYPACUSIA.

hypoadrenal constitution a constitutional type associated with underactivity of the adrenal gland. According to Pende, the individual is lean with slender bones, exhibiting developmental deficiency of skeletal and smooth muscles, and a tendency toward melancholia with intelligence that is normal or superior.

hypoaffective type a constitutional body type (Pende) distinguished by an absence of emotional reactivity. The type corresponds roughly to the schizothymic type.

hypoageusia diminished sensitivity to taste, which sometimes occurs in depression or depersonalization states, and as a neurologic disease symptom.

hypoalgesia a reduced sensitivity to pain.

hypobaropathy an alternative term for ACOSTA'S SYNDROME. See this entry.

hypobulia diminished will power; loss of initiative, and impaired ability to make decisions. H. is a common symptom in schizophrenia and depression. Also spelled **hypoboulia**.

hypocalcemia: See MATERNAL DIABETES.

hypocathexis an abnormally low investment of psychic energy.

hypochondriacal delusion a delusion in which a patient insists he is afflicted with an incurable disease which is eating away his stomach, poisoning his brain, or doing some other irreparable harm. For a DSM-III definition, see HYPOCHONDRIASIS.

hypochondriacal neurosis = HYPOCHONDRIASIS.

hypochondriac language = ORGAN LANGUAGE.

hypochondriasis a somatoform disorder characterized by an unrealistic interpretation of physical signs or sensations as abnormal and, as a result, preoccupation with the fear or belief that one has a serious disease. This fear or belief persists and interferes with social and occupational functioning in spite of medical reassurance that no physical disorder exists. Also called **hypochon-**driacal neurosis; nosomania. (DSM-III)

hypodepression a state of simple or mild depression, similar to grief or mourning but with the added factors of self-accusation, self-depreciation, and reduced self-esteem.

hypodermic injection = SUBCUTANEOUS INJECTION.

hypodontia = RIEGER'S SYNDROME.

hypoergasia Meyer's term for the depressive phase of manic-depressive psychosis.

hypoesthesia diminished sensitivity to one or more types of sensory stimuli, such as heat, cold, light, or touch. H. is a common hysterical (conversion) symptom. Also called **hypoesthesis; hypesthesia**.

hypoevolutism an inadequate or deficient development of the morphological, physiological, and psychological aspects of the entire body, or of a body system, body part, or body function.

hypofunction reduced function or activity, especially of an organ, such as a gland.

hypogastric nerve a part of the nervous system that may run as a single large nerve or as several smaller parallel nerves extending into the pelvic region. Postganglionic fibers innervate the bladder, rectum, and genitalia.

hypogenital type a constitutional body type (Pende) in which the lower extremities are abnormally long and the individual shows retarded development of genitalia and other sexual characteristics. A female version of the type has been described, indicating that the characteristics may be inherited. An attenuated form of the h.t. is identified as a **hypogenital temperament**.

hypoglossal nerve the twelfth cranial nerve, which originates in a gray-matter nucleus on the floor of the fourth ventricle and innervates the tongue, lower jaw, and areas of the neck and chest. The h.n. is referred to as "cranial nerve XII."

hypoglycemia a condition involving a low blood-sugar level due to interference with the formation of sugar in the blood or excessive utilization of sugar. In infants the major symptoms are tremors, cyanosis, seizures, apathy, weakness, respiratory problems, and failure to develop intellectually. In adults the major symptoms are debility, profuse sweating, nervousness, and dizziness. The infantile idiopathic form may be due to a single recessive gene, and the adult form may be a psychophysiologic reaction (**functional hyperinsulinism**). Also see HARRIS'S SYNDROME.

hypoglycemic coma: See INSULIN-COMA THERAPY.

hypokinesis a pathological reduction in movement, as in depression and certain organic conditions such as Pick's disease and cerebral arteriosclerosis. Also called **hypokinesia**.

hypokinesthesia a diminished sensitivity to the motion and position of the body, involving reduction in proprioceptive sensation. See PROPRIOCEPTION.

hypolipemia: See LIPID-METABOLISM DISORDERS.

hypologia an abnormal reduction in the capacity to speak, due to mental retardation or a cerebral disorder.

hypomania the mildest degree of mania characterized by a sense of exhilaration, euphoria, and optimism, also by tireless activity, incessant loquacity, effervescence, uninhibited behavior, reckless spending, and preoccupation with unrealistic schemes and solutions to problems. Also called **hypomanic state**. See BIPOLAR DISORDER, MANIC; MANIC EPISODE.

hypomanic personality a DSM-I term for a personality-pattern disturbance marked by a relatively mild degree of exhilaration, overactivity, and loquacity. Such individuals are usually gregarious, exuberant, uninhibited, and overflowing with ideas and unrealistic schemes. Under severe stress they may develop bipolar (manic-depressive) disorder. See HYPOMANIA.

hypomanic state = HYPOMANIA.

hypomenorrhea a condition of diminished menstrual flow or menstruation of abnormally short duration.

hypomotility a reduced or abnormally slow rate of movement.

hypoparathyroid constitution a constitutional type associated with deficient parathyroid gland activity, marked by hyperflexia and hyperkinesis of the skeletal and smooth muscles and a tendency toward rickets or other disorders of calcium metabolism.

hypoparathyroidism a condition of abnormally low secretion of parathyroid hormone due to damage or surgical removal of one or more of the parathyroid glands. Blood levels of calcium are decreased and phosphorus levels increased. **Tetany**, or increased neuromuscular activity due to loss of calcium, is a common symptom. Neurotic behavior and impaired breathing also may result. Compare HYPERPARATHYROIDISM. Also see PSEUDOHYPOPARATHYROIDISM.

hypophagia an abnormally small appetite, as in anorexia nervosa.

hypophoria deviation of one eye in a downward direction.

hypophosphatasia a bone disease that often is associated with shortness of stature, rickets, and osteomalacia. H. is caused by an inborn error of metabolism, a genetic defect that follows an autosomal-recessive pattern of inheritance, and is marked by abnormally low levels of alkaline phosphatase activity. H. usually is involved in cases of rickets that fail to respond to vitamin-D therapy.

hypophrasia a lack of speech or slowness of speech associated with depression. Also called **bradyphrasia**.

hypophrenosis an obsolete term for feeblemindedness.

hypophyseal cachexia a disease caused by total failure of the pituitary gland, resulting in secondary atrophy of the adrenal cortex, thyroid gland, and gonads. Sexual glands and breasts atrophy, teeth and hair fall out, and anorexia, diabetes insipidus, hypoglycemia, and mental changes develop. The disease occurs in two forms, one that affects women after childbirth, called Sheehan's syndrome, and one that affects both sexes and is unrelated to childbirth, called Simmonds' disease. Also called **pituitary cachexia**.

hypophyseal fossa: See FOSSA.

hypophysectomy the surgical removal of the pituitary gland, a procedure rarely of value in treatment of human disorders because of adverse side effects such as the loss of ability to produce vital hormones. H., however, is performed in animal experiments related to motivational studies.

hypophysis; hypophysis cerebri = PITUITARY GLAND.

hypopituitarism: See FRÖHLICH'S SYNDROME.

hypopituitary constitution a constitutional type associated with deficient pituitary-gland activity and corresponding roughly to the Kretschmer hypoplastic type. The infant is characterized by defective growth, small head and hands, short bones, and, in the male, small genitals. The adult male has a large pelvis, feminine distribution of fat and defective sex activity; and the adult female has small breasts and is frigid with a tendency to sterility and masculinism. Both sexes are characterized by low blood pressure, slow pulse, and mental torpor.

hypoplasia an underdeveloped organ, tissue, or organism, usually due to an inadequate number of cells or diminished size of cells forming the structure. When applied to an entire body, h. usually refers to a dwarf of the species.

hypoprosexia an abnormal lack of attentive ability. Also called **hypoprosessis**.

hypopsychosis a state of diminished mental activity.

hyposexuality an abnormally low level of sexual behavior. Hyposexual individuals may show no sex drive or interest in sexual activity. Some cases of h. are associated with epileptic seizures originating in the temporal lobe, the patients showing normal or even hypersexual behavior after surgical treatment of the brain lesion.

hyposomnia a state of reduced total sleep or sleep that occupies shorter-than-usual time periods.

hyposophobia = ACROPHOBIA.

hypospadias a congenital anomaly of the urethra in which it opens below its normal anatomical position. In the male, h. usually is manifested by a urethral opening on the underside of the penis. In the female, the urethra may open into the vagina.

hypotaxia = AFFECTIVE SUGGESTION.

hypotensive: See NORMOTENSIVE INDIVIDUALS.

hypothalamic sulcus a groove in the lateral wall of the third ventricle, on either side, dividing the structure into upper and lower parts, the thalamus and the subthalamus.

hypothalamic theory of Cannon: See CANNON'S THEORY.

hypothalamus a part of the diencephalon which

contains the nuclei with primary control of the autonomic functions of the body. The h. also has responsibility for integrating autonomic activity into appropriate responses to internal and external stimuli. Lesions in metabolic centers of the h. cause increased or decreased appetites, depending upon the h. area affected. Also see LATERAL H.

hypothermesthesia an abnormally diminished sensitivity to heat or heat stimuli. Also called **thermohypesthesia**.

hypothermia a severe loss of body temperature that may be accidental or induced. **Accidental h.** is most likely to affect older persons who are less able to cope with the cooling effect of environmental temperatures in the winter months. H. symptoms include listlessness, drowsiness, apathy, indifference to progressive frostbite, coma, and death. **Induced h.** is employed in surgery and for neurological diseases causing a fever.

hypothesis /hīpoth'-/ a testable proposition about behavior, based on theory, and stating an expected outcome resulting from specific conditions or assumptions.

hypothesis behavior a pattern of behavior by experimental animals in which one particular cue or response is chosen consistently from a number of alternatives. The term was introduced by I. Krechevsky who analyzed patterns followed by rats in running mazes with alternate pathways, according to visual or spatial cues, or both.

hypothetical construct an explanatory concept using terms far removed from observation, or terms with much surplus meaning. Many psychodynamic explanations are hypothetical constructs. Also see INTERVENING VARIABLE.

hypothetical imperative: See CATEGORICAL IMPERATIVE.

hypothetico-deductive reasoning the abstract, logical reasoning that, according to Piaget, emerges in early adolescence and marks the period of formal operations. H.-d.r. is distinguished by the capacity for abstract thinking and hypothesis-testing which frees the adolescent from total reliance on concrete thinking and immediate perception.

hypothymia a subnormal level of emotional tone, as observed in cases of depression.

hypothyroid constitution a constitutional body type associated with a deficiency of thyroid-gland activity. The type corresponds roughly to the pyknic category but with the added features of fatty deposits about the face and neck, short, stubby hands, low basal metabolism, and mental torpor. Also see CONGENITAL HYPOTHYROIDISM.

hypotonia an abnormally severe loss of muscle tone or strength. The muscles tend to assume positions that are influenced by gravity, with overextension and overflexion of the limbs. The muscles are flaccid, and examination may show motoneuron impulses to the affected segments to be subnormal or even absent. Adjective: **hypotonic**.

hypovegetative a term applied to a constitutional type in which the body features correspond to Kretschmer's asthenic type.

hypovigility subnormal awareness or response to external stimuli, as observed in many schizophrenic patients.

hypovolemia a state of reduced extracellular-fluid volume that is associated with the urge to increase water consumption. Compare HYPERVOLEMIA.

hypoxanthine guanine phosphoribosyl transferase an enzyme whose absence in the human body leads to symptoms of the Lesch-Nyhan syndrome. H.g.p.t. was the first enzyme found to be associated with an inherited disorder involving behavioral malfunction and retardation. Abbrev.: **HGPRT**.

hypoxemia a deficiency of oxygen in the blood. In a respiratory disease such as emphysema, the lungs lose their ability to extract oxygen from inhaled air. As a result, blood that leaves the lungs to be pumped into tissues by the left ventricle of the heart lacks sufficient oxygen to maintain normal life functions. H. may be marked by signs of CYANOSIS. See this entry. Also see HYPOXIA.

hypoxia a condition of inadequate oxygen availability to the body tissues. The causes may include anemia or reduced ability of the blood to transport oxygen, a deficiency of oxygen in the environment, disorders of the heart or lungs, or the effect of gas-exchange-blockage disorders such as hyaline-membrane disease. Also see HYPOXEMIA.

hypoxic drive one of the three basic mechanisms that control respiration. It involves the balance between the levels of oxygen and carbon dioxide in the tissues. Normal breathing is stimulated by the presence of carbon dioxide in the blood, and, paradoxically, high levels of oxygen suppress the h.d. by altering the balance between the gases.

hypsarrhythmia an EEG pattern observed in certain infants in the first year of life who exhibit epilepsylike spasms. Also called **major dysrhythmia; myoclonic encephalitis**.

-hyster-; -hystero- a combining form relating to the uterus, the womb. In its concrete sense it occurs, e.g., in "hysterectomy"; but it is also used in an abstract sense, as in "hysteria," literally a "disease of the womb," because hysteria, occurring frequently in women, was ascribed erroneously to the influence of the womb. See WANDERING UTERUS.

hysterectomy the surgical removal of the uterus. H. may be **total h.**, including excision of the cervix, or **subtotal h.**, in which only the uterus above the cervix is removed, or **radical h.**, with excision of a part of the vagina with the uterus and cervix. The h. may be performed through the vagina or through the abdominal wall.

hysteria a neurotic disorder characterized by suggestibility, emotional outbursts, histrionic behavior, repressed anxiety, and transformation of unconscious conflicts into physical symptoms such as paralysis, blindness, and loss of sensation. These symptoms serve to screen out anxiety (primary gains) and at the same time to elicit attention and sympathy (secondary gains). Freud interpreted such symptoms as defenses against guilty sexual impulses (e.g., a paralyzed hand cannot masturbate), but other conflicts are recognized today. He also included dissociative conditions in his concept of h., but these are now regarded as separate disorders. See CONVERSION DISORDER; DISSOCIATIVE DISORDERS; HISTRIONIC-PERSONALITY DISORDER. Also see ANXIETY H.; ARCTIC H.; COMBAT H.; CONVERSION H.; DEFENSE H.; DISSOCIATIVE H.; EPIDEMIC H.; FIXATION H.; GLOBUS HYSTERICUS; MASS H.; RETENTION H.; -HYSTER-.

hysterical amaurosis = HYSTERICAL BLINDNESS.

hysterical amnesia a dissociative reaction characterized by inability to recall anxiety-provoking events, such as experiences associated with guilt, failure, or rejection.

hysterical anesthesia the absence of sensation in certain areas of the body (such as the hands or genital organs) not due to organic pathology or defect. The condition is interpreted as an unconsciously adopted conversion symptom resulting from anxiety, internal conflict, or other emotional disturbance.

hysterical aphonia a sudden loss of voice due to emotional conflicts.

hysterical ataxia = ASTASIA-ABASIA.

hysterical blindness loss of sight, or partial blindness, in eyes that are organically intact. H.b. is a hysterical (conversion) symptom frequently due to an unconscious attempt to screen out a threatening or guilt-laden situation. Despite the "blindness," the pupils continue to react to light and the patient automatically avoids objects that would injure him. Also called **hysterical amaurosis**. Also see ANTON'S SYNDROME; PEEPING TOM.

hysterical character: See HISTRIONIC-PERSONALITY DISORDER.

hysterical convulsions seizures precipitated by psychological rather than organic factors, usually distinguishable from epileptic seizures by the presence of emotional conflict or stress and the fact that the patient does not injure himself, lose his pupillary reflex, or become incontinent during the attack. Also called **conversion seizures**.

hysterical deafness a loss of hearing developed unconsciously usually due to intolerable emotional stress.

hysterical disorder any disorder characterized by involuntary psychogenic dysfunction of the sensory, motor, or visceral activities of the body. An example of a h.d. is the loss of the ability to speak normally after an emotional trauma.

hysterical hiccough a myoclonic spasm of the diaphragm due to emotional causes. Also spelled **hysterical hiccup**.

hysterical hypalgia a decrease in the normal sensitivity to pain in various parts of the body due to psychogenic influences. The h.h. is a defense

against unconscious instinctual demands, e.g., sexual or aggressive sensations or memories that would be painful.

hysterical imitation the imitation by a hysterical individual of symptoms observed in a person with whom the patient identifies. E.g., if one school girl has a fainting spell, other girls also may faint through hysterical identification.

hysterical materialization the symbolic expression of a repressed fantasy in somatic terms; e.g., "an unconscious fellatio fantasy may result in globus hystericus, or an unconscious wish to be pregnant may produce hysterical vomiting" (Eidelberg, *Encyclopedia of Psychoanalysis*, 1968).

hysterical neuroses, dissociative type = DISSOCIATIVE DISORDERS.

hysterical neurosis, conversion type = CONVERSION DISORDER.

hysterical paralysis a conversion symptom affecting one limb (monoplegia), the lower part of the body (paraplegia), or one side of the body (hemiplegia). The condition is functional and psychogenic, and, in contrast to **organic paralysis**, deep reflexes are not lost and there is little or no wasting. Also called **conversion paralysis**.

hysterical paresis a conversion symptom involving muscle weakness, sometimes accompanied by tremors, contractions, tics, spasms, astasia-abasia, or other forms of dyskinesia. See ASTASIA-ABASIA; DYSKINESIA.

hysterical-personality disorder = HISTRIONIC-PERSONALITY DISORDER.

hysterical pregnancy = FALSE PREGNANCY. Also see -HYSTER-.

hysterical pseudodementia a term applied by Wernicke to a conversion syndrome in which the patient of normal intelligence acts as if he had lost the ability to think rationally. He may not be able to answer simple questions, acting as if he were retarded. The disorder is likely to occur in situations where this behavior can be an advantage, as in prisoners at large or awaiting trial, and may be a form of the GANSER SYNDROME. See this entry.

hysterical psychosis an acute psychosis occurring in hysterical personalities and usually lasting three weeks or less without residual symptoms. H.p. is characterized by the sudden onset of hallucinations, delusions, and bizarre and sometimes violent behavior and is most commonly observed in such syndromes as latah, amok, miryachit, windigo, and piblokto.

hysterical puerilism a psychogenic condition in which an adult patient reverts to behavior characteristic of infancy or early childhood. W. McDougall (1926) cites the case of a soldier who, after going through bombardment, regressed to a point where he could not understand language or use utensils, walked with his feet apart, and played with dolls, but still liked to smoke cigarettes and make passes at his nurse. See HYSTERICAL PSEUDODEMENTIA.

hysterical seizure: See HYSTERICAL CONVULSIONS.

hysterical stupor a conversion reaction in which the patient is mute, unresponsive, and immobile. See CONVERSION DISORDER.

hysterical vomiting: See HYSTERICAL MATERIALIZATION.

hysteriform pertaining to a condition characterized by symptoms that resemble those associated with hysteria.

hysteroepilepsy hysterical seizures occasionally occurring in patients with known seizures, and difficult to distinguish from them. Closer study, however, shows that the EEG contains no paroxysmal discharges; the seizure pattern is not a stereotyped tonic-clonic movement sequence; self-injury does not occur; and there is no postictal state of confusion, headache, or drowsiness. Also called **hysteriform epilepsy; grande hystérie; major hysteria**.

hysterogenic zones areas of the body in which stimulation produces a hysterical reaction such as anesthesia, pain, or tenderness, usually in the breasts, spine, head, or ovarian region. Allochiria sometimes occurs in these cases. See ALLOCHIRIA.

hysterosalpingography the study by X-ray or other radiation techniques of the uterus and Fallopian tubes.

hysteroscopy the direct visual examination of the cervix and interior of the uterus with the aid of an endoscope or similar device equipped with lens and light source.

hysterosyntonic a personality type that combines hysterical and syntonic types of personalities. A **syntone** is a normal individual who is in emotional harmony with the environment.

Hz = HERTZ.

I

-iasis /-ī'əsis/ a combining form relating to disease.

-iatr-; -iatro-; -iatrist; -iatry a combining form relating to medical treatment and the physician's role (from Greek *iatreia*, "healing, medical treatment," and *iatros*, "physician").

iatrogenesis the process of producing a iatrogenic (physician-originated) disorder. Also called iatrogeny. See IATROGENIC ILLNESS.

iatrogenic homosexuality homosexual feelings or behavior unconsciously encouraged by the attitude of a doctor or other health professional treating or counseling the patient.

iatrogenic illness a behavior disorder that is induced or aggravated by the physician, especially by incautious comments, overextended examinations, or giving patients too much information. Iatrogenic disorders are particularly common in patients with hysterical or hypochondriacal tendencies, or in suggestible individuals who suspect they have cardiac disorders.

iatrogenic psychosis a functional disorder that develops from attitudes, comments, or other behavior of an attending physician. E.g., an inadvertent remark by an examining physician about an organic abnormality of the subject, even though not serious, may become the basis for a neurosis or psychosis.

iatrogeny = IATROGENESIS.

ibogaine a hallucinogenic agent found in the root of the African forest plant Tabernanthe iboga, used mainly in rituals of members of the Bwiti, or Bouiti, cult of Gabon. Hallucinations reportedly include visitations with specific ancestors and verbalizations related to the history of the people. If death occurs during use of the drug, the event is regarded as divine intervention.

Icarus complex = URETHRAL COMPLEX.

ICD = INTERNATIONAL CLASSIFICATION OF DISEASES.

iceblock theory a concept of behavior change in relation to group dynamics or T-groups or sensitivity training in which existing attitudes and behavior are unfrozen and new attitudes and behavior are first explored and then frozen into new habit patterns (Kurt Lewin).

I-cell disease = INCLUSION-CELL DISEASE.

ichthyophobia a morbid fear of fish; also, a strong dislike for fish (Greek *ichthys*).

ichthyosis-hypogonadism syndrome an X-linked recessive disorder characterized by small genitalia and scaly skin over many areas of the body. Most patients also have anosmia. Mild mental retardation has been noted in some of the patients tested. The hypogonadism may respond to hormone treatments.

icon an image, which may be an aftersensation; a pictorial representation.

iconic content in J. Bruner's theory, the mental images or pictures of particular aspects of reality, e.g., a child's mental representation of a doll. See ICONIC MODE.

iconicity the resemblance between two objects or images despite structural differences, such as the superficial similarity between birds and bats. In psychological esthetics, the term denotes the tendency for visual impressions to remain as short-term images in the mind. I. is associated with whole-word reading methods and subliminal advertising. Also see HOMOLOGY.

iconic mode J. Bruner's term for the representation of reality through mental images based on sensory impressions, e.g., the conversion of one's experience or perceptions of a table into a mental picture based on those perceptions. The i.m. begins to develop in early infancy and is dominant in the preschool years. The other two modes of representation are the ENACTIVE MODE and the SYMBOLIC MODE. See these entries.

iconic representation the representation of stimuli that are stored conceptually according to their perceived image.

iconic stage in Bruner's system of child development, a period between the enactive and symbolic stages when a child develops mental images or perceptual representations of objects and events. See ICONIC MODE.

iconomania a morbid urge to collect and worship images.

iconophobia a morbid fear of images, idols, or works of art, often stemming from religious doctrines.

ICS = INTRACRANIAL STIMULATION.

ICSH = INTERSTITIAL-CELL-STIMULATING HORMONE.

ictal emotions any emotions that suddenly or rapidly occur and disappear, particularly anxiety and depression. I.e. are associated with disorders of the brain, particularly areas in the temporal lobe, and may stem from subclinical epilepsy.

icterus = JAUNDICE.

icterus gravis neonatorum a severe form of jaundice in newborn infants caused by an Rh-factor immune reaction, marked by convulsions, rigidity, and coma, and resulting in retardation or neurologic damage. Also called **erythroleukoblastosis**. See RH BLOOD-GROUP INCOMPATIBILITY; KERNICTERUS.

ictus a sudden epileptic seizure without an aura; also, an apoplectic stroke.

id in psychoanalysis, the collective name (Latin, "it") for the instinctual, biological drives that supply the psyche with its basic energy or libido. Freud conceived of the id as the most primitive component of the personality, and described it as "a cauldron of seething excitement" which resides in the deepest level of the unconscious, has no inner organization, and operates blindly and irrationally in obedience to the pleasure principle. The infant's life is dominated by the desire for immediate, egocentric gratification of instincts (hunger, thirst, elimination, rage, sex) until the conscious ego begins to develop and operate in accordance with the reality principle and the superego. See STRUCTURAL HYPOTHESIS; PRIMARY PROCESS.

id anxiety a Freudian concept of anxiety derived from instinctual drives, and a primary cause of automatic anxieties.

idea a mental image or cognition that may occur without direct reference to perception or sensory processes.

ideal the conception of something in its most perfect form, or the thing or person that embodies such a standard.

idealism: See BODY-MIND PROBLEM.

idealization the conscious or unconscious exaggeration of another person's positive attributes and disregard of his imperfections or failings, thus viewing the other as perfect or nearly perfect. I. is a defense mechanism that protects the subject from conscious feelings of ambivalence toward the idealized object. I., particularly of parents, plays a role in the development of the ego-ideal.

idealized image a term introduced by Horney for a neurotic defense consisting of an exaggerated, unrealistic picture of one's abilities and potentialities, derived from wishful thinking rather than fact.

ideal masochism a Freudian term for psychic or moral masochism, in which the injury is mental rather than physical. Also called **mental masochism**. Also see MORAL MASOCHISM.

idea of influence = DELUSION OF INFLUENCE.

idea of reference = DELUSION OF REFERENCE.

ideation the process of forming ideas and images.

ideational apraxia a condition marked by loss or impairment of the ability to perform a complex series of actions, such as lighting a cigarette, because of failure to conceive the sequence as a whole. The patient may instead perform a part of the sequence of action or a similar but different plan than the one required. The disorder, which may appear as a case of absentmindedness, usually is caused by parietal- and frontal-lobe disease. Also called **ideomotor apraxia; sensory apraxia**.

ideational shield a defense reaction in which an individual who fears the rejection or criticism of others protects himself against anxiety by giving intellectual reasons for not criticizing *them*.

idée fixe /idãfiks'/ an idea that is so rigidly held that every effort to change it is resisted (French, "fixed idea"). Such ideas frequently become obsessions which govern the individual's mental life, and may take the form of delusions maintained despite evidence to the contrary. The term was used by Janet, in 1882, for dissociative ideas that split off from the rest of consciousness and develop an autonomous system or even personality of their own.

id-ego the newborn's psychic matrix from which the id and ego functions develop.

identical-direction law: See LAW OF IDENTICAL DIRECTION.

identical-elements theory the concept that the ability to learn a new task is enhanced if it contains elements of previously mastered tasks.

identical points points on the retinas of the left and right eyes that receive identical images from the same object at a specified distance.

identical twins = MONOZYGOTIC TWINS.

identification the process of associating one's self closely with other persons and assuming their characteristics or views. This process takes many forms: The infant feels he is part of his mother; the child gradually adopts his parents' attitudes, standards, and personality traits; the adolescent takes on the characteristics of the peer group; the adult identifies with a particular profession or political party. I. operates largely on an unconscious or half-conscious level, and may be used as a defense mechanism; that is, allying one's self with others may be a source of security and an antidote to anxiety.

In language development, i. is a two-word extension of a simple pointing response, as in "see kitty."

identification figures the parents, caretakers, or other significant adults who provide role models for a child; the individuals with whom a child consciously and unconsciously identifies. See IDENTIFICATION.

identification test a verbal intelligence test in which the subject identifies objects or parts of objects in a picture.

identification transference a term introduced by S. R. Slavson to distinguish between libidinal and sibling transference in group therapy. I.t. refers to the patient's identification with other members of the group and a desire to emulate them.

identification with the aggressor an unconscious mechanism in which the individual identifies with an opponent he cannot master. This occasionally occurred in concentration camps, and, according to psychoanalysts, occurs on a developmental level when the male child identifies with his rival, the father, toward the end of the oedipal phase. Also see STOCKHOLM SYNDROME.

identity the feeling that we are the same person we were yesterday and last year; a sense of continuity derived from our body sensations (coenesthesia), our body image, and the feeling that our memories, purposes, values, and experiences belong to us; a sense of uniqueness and independence ("I am my own person"). The search for i. is a basic feature of development (Erikson). Also called **personal i**. See EGO I. Also see SENSE OF I.

In cognitive development, the term refers to the awareness that an object remains the same even though it may undergo many transformations; e.g., a piece of clay may be made to assume various forms, but is still the same piece of clay.

identity confusion = ROLE CONFUSION.

identity crisis an acute anxiety state experienced primarily by adolescents who find it difficult to establish a clearly defined personal identity and a consistent role in society. The concept was developed by Erikson. See EGO IDENTITY.

identity diffusion = ROLE CONFUSION.

identity disorder a disorder of late adolescence in which feelings of uncertainty and distress are generated by such identity issues as long-term goals, career choice, sexual orientation and behavior, group loyalty, moral values, and religious identification. (DSM-III)

identity need as used by E. Fromm, the need to achieve a sense of uniqueness, individuality, selfhood. Psychological autonomy or the severing of "incestuous ties" is considered essential for healthy individuality. Unhealthy, spurious individuality is expressed in conformity, a manifestation of the "escape from freedom."

identity versus role confusion the fifth of Erikson's eight stages of man, approximately between the ages of 12 and 18, the years of adolescence. See ERIKSON'S EIGHT STAGES OF MAN.

ideogenetic a term applied to mental processes utilizing images of sense impressions rather than ideas that can be expressed verbally.

ideoglandular pertaining to a glandular function that is initiated by mental processes, e.g., adrenaline secretion.

ideogram a pictograph or figure that symbolizes an object or idea, e.g., hieroglyphics.

ideokinetic apraxia a condition in which a person can perform individual motor responses but is unable to perform a motor-response sequence.

ideology a systematic ordering of ideas with associated doctrines, attitudes, beliefs, and symbols that together form a more or less coherent philosophy or Weltanschauung for a person, group, or sociopolitical movement, e.g., Freudianism or socialism.

ideomotor apraxia = IDEATIONAL APRAXIA.

ideophobia a morbid fear of having or being confronted with ideas.

ideophrenia a form of delirium characterized by ideational disorders.

ideoplasty the process of molding a person's mind by the verbal suggestions of a hypnotist. Also see VERBAL SUGGESTION.

id interpretation in psychoanalytic therapy, an interpretation that penetrates defenses and permits painful thoughts to be released into the consciousness. Also called **impulse interpretation**.

-idio- a combining form relating to an individual's particularity.

idiocy an obsolete term for the lowest level of mental deficiency, characterized by an IQ of less than 20 and a maximum social and intellectual level of a two-year-old. "Idiotic" was replaced by "profoundly retarded." The term i. is something of a misnomer since it is derived from the ancient Greek word for a person in private life as distinguished from a government official, perhaps with the connotation that a private citizen was ignorant or less intelligent than a politician. Also see AMAUROTIC I.; JUVENILE AMAUROTIC I.; KALMUK I.; MORAL I.; TAY-SACHS DISEASE; XERODERMIC I.; IDIOT.

idiodynamics the view that an individual attends to the environmental aspects he considers relevant; that is, the individual plays an essential role in selecting stimuli and organizing responses.

idiogamist /idē·og′-/ a person who is capable of full sexual response only with his or her spouse and is sexually incapable or inadequate with other partners. The term usually refers to a man who is impotent with any partner other than his wife, or other than a very few women (who often resemble his wife).

idioglossia the omission, substitution, and distortion of so many sounds that speech is rendered unintelligible. It is often associated with mental retardation. Also called **idiolalia**.

idiographic pertaining to the description of the individual case, as opposed to the formulation of general laws.

idiographic approach the thorough study of individual cases with emphasis on each subject's characteristic traits (**idiographic traits**) and the uniqueness of the individual's behavior and adjustment, as contrasted with a study of the universal, or nomothetic, aspects of experience. See ALLPORT'S PERSONALITY-TRAIT THEORY. Also see NOMOTHETIC.

idiolalia = IDIOGLOSSIA.

idiom: See PERSONAL I.

idiopathic without known cause; said especially of a disease, such as some forms of epilepsy, whose etiology is obscure.

idiopathic autoscopy: See AUTOSCOPIC SYNDROME.

idiopathic epilepsy epilepsy in which the cause is unknown. Compare SYMPTOMATIC EPILEPSY.

idioretinal light an illusion of shades of gray observed in a dark environment. The effect is caused by chemical changes in the retina or brain cells rather than the wavelength of visible light.

idiosyncracy-credit model the concept that a leader is able to diverge from group standards to the extent that he has built up "credits" or prestige over time by conformity to group norms.

idiosyncratic intoxication = MANIA A POTU.

idiosyncratic reaction an unexpected reaction to a drug resulting in effects that may be contrary to the anticipated results. A barbiturate may have a stimulating rather than a sedative effect, causing a patient to take a larger-than-prescribed dose in an effort to compensate. I.r. is not the same as tolerance, but may be similar to the paradoxical effect of alcoholic beverages which may produce an initial illusion of stimulation.

idiot an obsolete term for an individual with a mental age of less than three years, and an IQ of less than 20. It usually falls in the "profoundly retarded" category. Adjective: **idiotic.** See PROFOUND MENTAL RETARDATION; MENTAL RETARDATION; MONGOLIAN I.; IDIOCY.

idiotism one of Pinel's four categories of insanity, the others being mania, melancholia, and dementia. I. is advanced dementia.

idiotropic egocentric, introspective, introverted (Greek, "turned toward the self").

idiot savant /id′ē·ət savänt′/ a mentally retarded individual who possesses a remarkable, highly developed ability or talent in one area such as rapid calculation, music or feats of memory (French, /idē·ō′sävaN′/, "learned idiot"). Such cases are rare and usually occur in persons who are mildly or moderately retarded. Plural: **idiots savants** /id′ē·ət savänt/ or /-änts′/. See CALENDAR CALCULATION.

idiovariation the phenomenon of genetic mutation in which genotypical structures are undergoing continual mutation and new groups of species are being formed constantly.

idol fear = ICONOPHOBIA.

id omnipotence: See OMNIPOTENCE.

id psychology in psychoanalysis, an approach that focuses on the unorganized, instinctual impulses that seek immediate pleasurable gratification of primitive needs. The id is believed to dominate the life of the infant and possibly the schizophrenic. It is frequently described as blind and irrational until it is disciplined by the other two major components if the personality, the ego and the superego. Also see EGO PSYCHOLOGY; EXPERIENTIAL PSYCHOTHERAPY.

id resistance a type of resistance in psychoanalysis that takes the form of a repetition compulsion; that is, the same material continues to recur regardless of the number or validity of interpretations offered by the analyst. Although the i.r. is difficult to remove, the blind repetition of presentations by the patient becomes a clue in itself. I.r. may precipitate an "analytic stalemate."

id sadism the primitive instinctual destructive urges of the early years of infancy that are associated with omnipotent gratification and security and usually provoked by frustration. Also see INFANTILE SADISM.

id wish the instinctual desires that arise from the repressed, unconscious, infantile, and primitive reaches of the mind. The urges generally are aggressive or erotic.

IEP = INDIVIDUALIZED EDUCATION PROGRAM.

I/E ratio the rate of *i*nspiration divided by the rate of *e*xpiration, sometimes used as an index of emotionality and, if low, as a test of lying.

I-It a relationship in which a person treats himself or another person exclusively as an object. The philosopher Martin Buber, who originated the term, maintained that this type of relationship stands in the way of human warmth, mutuality, trust, and group cohesiveness.

ileostomy: See COLOSTOMY.

iliohypogastric nerve one of the nerves that extend from the spinal cord in the lumbar region, with branches that innervate the skin of the gluteal and lower abdominal regions.

ilioinguinal nerve a nerve that has filaments extending into the genitalia. In the male, the i.n. follows the spermatic cord through the inguinal ring and sends branches into the penis and scrotum. In the female, the i.n. branches extend onto the mons pubis and the labia majora.

illegal source: See GRAY MARKET.

illegitimacy the state of being illegitimate. The term usually is applied when a child is born out of wedlock or the mother is not a legitimate mother with respect to laws governing inheritances. The condition may result if the mother could have married the father at the time of conception, if marriage was not legally possible because of racial or blood-relative relationships, or if the child was conceived by a married woman by a man other than her husband.

Illinois Test of Psycholinguistic Abilities a test designed to measure linguistic abilities considered important in communications and learning disorders, such as the ability to understand spoken words, to manipulate linguistic symbols meaningfully, to express ideas in words, to understand spoken words, to express ideas in movement, to remember auditory stimuli, to reproduce meaningful visual figures, to identify an incompletely presented object, to fill in deletions in an auditory perception, and to synthesize parts of an auditory word to produce a whole word.

illness as self-punishment a form of superego resistance in which guilt feelings and masochistic behavior produce symptoms that are a barrier to their own resolution through psychoanalysis.

illogicality a tendency to draw unwarranted or faulty inferences. It is characteristic of delusional thinking and speech.

illumination conditions the type of illumination, taking into account such factors as intensity and absence of glare, most suitable for performance of different tasks, and for the comfort of the worker.

illumination standards the amounts of illumination recommended for effective performance of certain tasks, as determined by the Illuminating Engineering Society. The i.s., expressed in foot-candles, range from ten for a hotel lobby to 2,500 for a surgical-operating table.

illumination unit the amount of light produced by one FOOTCANDLE. See this entry.

illuminism an exalted hallucinatory state in which the patient carries on conversations with imaginary supernatural beings.

illusion a distorted perception or memory; a misinterpretation of sensory stimuli. Examples are the impression that railroad tracks come together in the distance; that one has been in the same room before, though this is not the case; or that a minute of anxious waiting takes an hour. Illusions occur not only in everyday experience but in delirium, schizophrenia, and reactions to mind-distorting drugs. Also see APPARENT MOVEMENT; ARISTOTLE'S I.; DÉJÀ RACONTÉ; DÉJÀ VU; MEMORY I.; MOVEMENT I.; MÜLLER-LYER I.; OCULO-GYRAL I.; OPTICAL I.; PANUM PHENOMENON; POGGENDORF I.; PROOFREADER'S I.; SIZE-WEIGHT I.; STAIRCASE I.; STROBOSCOPIC I.; WINDMILL I.; ZÖLLNER I.

illusion des sosies; illusion of doubles: See L'ILLUSION DES SOSIES.

illusion of negative doubles = FREGOLI'S PHENOMENON.

illusion of orientation the misidentification of a stimulus because of a clouding of consciousness, as during a febrile or toxic delirium. E.g., a hospitalized patient may appear confused about where he is and about the identity of people in his room.

illusory correlation the lack of a relationship between two variables thought to be related or an exaggeration of the strength of the relationship binding two variables.

illusory movement = APPARENT MOVEMENT.

illustrator a nonverbal body gesture clearly associated with a spoken word or phrase, e.g., pointing to a light switch while saying, "It's in front of your nose." Illustrators are companions of words whereas emblems are substitutes for words. Also see EMBLEM.

image a likeness or copy of an earlier sensory experience recalled without external stimulation.

image agglutinations dream images formed from conglomerations of discrete images influenced by affects and representing day residues. I.a. may be in the form of several objects or faces seen as one. See CONDENSATION.

imageless thought thinking that occurs without the aid of images or sensory content. The Würzburg School upheld the existence of i.t. on the basis of introspective reports, e.g., naming a piece of fruit without picturing it. E. B. Titchener and others in the structural school opposed this view. See KÜLPE.

imagery mental images considered collectively; also, the particular type of i. characteristic of an individual, such as pictorial i. or auditory i.

imagery code the encoding of an object, idea, or

impression in terms of its visual imagery. E.g., if the item "typewriter" is stored in memory via a mental picture of a typewriter, an i.c. is said to have been employed in the memory-storage process. See SEMANTIC CODE.

imagery therapy the use of imagery as a therapeutic technique. E.g., to induce relaxation, a hypnotic subject may be asked to imagine that he is lying on a beach. For another example, see GUIDED AFFECTIVE IMAGERY.

imaginary companion a fictitious person, animal, or object created by a child of two to five years of age. The i.c. is given a name, and the child talks, shares feelings, and pretends to play with it, and may use it as a scapegoat for his misdeeds ("Topo did it, he is *bad*," "Topo made me do it"). Imaginary companions are especially prevalent among lonely or only children, but they are not more common among children with emotional problems than among others. Bright children are more likely to create them and construct elaborate fantasies around them than dull children. Also called **invisible playmate**. Also see SOCIAL OBJECT; HELPFUL FIGURE.

imagination the creation of ideas and images in the absence of direct sensory data, but frequently combining fragments of previous sensory experiences into new syntheses. Also see CREATIVE I.

imaging as used in radioisotopic encephalography, the process of scanning the brain with an isotope-sensitive probe and recording the patterns in graphic form. The i. may be either static or dynamic. See NUCLEAR I.

The term i. is also applied to the use of suggested mental images to control bodily processes, including the easing of pain.

imago in Jung's analytic psychology, the idealized image of a key person in the individual's early life, especially the mother (Latin, "image"). In psychoanalysis, such an image is "preserved indefinitely in the unconscious and often identified with persons other than the original one" (Ernest Jones, *Papers on Psycho-Analysis*, 1938), and has a marked influence on our standards and ideals.

imbecile: See IMBECILITY.

imbecility an obsolete term for a low-to-moderate level of mental deficiency characterized by an IQ between 25 and 50 and a social and intellectual age of a two-to-seven-year-old child. The term was replaced by "severely retarded" and "moderately retarded". See SEVERE MENTAL RETARDATION; MODERATE MENTAL RETARDATION; MENTAL RETARDATION.

imidazole syndrome = BESSMAN-BALDWIN SYNDROME.

imipramine hydrochloride: See TRICYCLIC ANTIDEPRESSANTS.

imitation the process or habit of copying the behavior of another person, group, or object intentionally or unintentionally. It is a basic form of learning which accounts for many of our skills, gestures, interests, attitudes, role behaviors, social customs, and verbal expressions. Though ordinarily normal, i. can take pathological form, as in ECHOLALIA and ECHOPRAXIA. See these entries.

imitative speech the sounds and words that are normally acquired by children between 12 and 18 months of age.

immanent justice Piaget's term for the young child's belief that rules are fixed and immutable and that punishment automatically follows misdeeds regardless of extenuating circumstances. According to Piaget, children up to the age of eight equate the morality of an act only with its consequences and not until later do they develop the capacity to judge motive and subjective considerations. See MORAL REALISM. Compare DISTRIBUTIVE JUSTICE.

immature personality in DSM-I, a personality-trait disturbance characterized by inability to tolerate frustration or stress, lack of emotional control, and, when the individual is opposed or under pressure, reversion to infantile and childish behavior such as sulking, pouting, and temper outbursts. Also called **infantile personality**.

immediacy behavior any action, movement, or physical stance that indicates intimacy or a close relationship between two people, e.g., eye contact or touching.

immediate experience: See CONTEMPORANEITY.

immediate memory a type or stage of the memory process in which a subject recalls information recently acquired, such as a street address or telephone number, although the same information may be forgotten after its immediate use. I.m. is frequently tested in assessing intelligence or cerebral impairment. Also see SHORT-TERM MEMORY.

immissio penis = PENETRATION.

immobility a condition in which an organism shows no signs of motion, as in death-feigning or being "rooted to the spot" by a sudden fright.

immobilization paralysis a functional, sometimes hysterical, type of paralysis in which the patient is unable to move a limb that had been splinted because of injury. The limb is mobile but the patient fails to recognize that it has healed.

immobilizing activity = LIBIDO-BINDING ACTIVITY.

immoral imperative an impulsive subconscious rebellion against moral principles, or a compulsion to act against the rules of society, often seen in compulsive neurotics.

immunity factors the components of humoral and cellular immunity that help protect the body tissues against pathological effects of a foreign substance, such as a disease agent. **Humoral i.f.** include B-lymphocytes that mature in plasma cells and reproduce as clones of "memory" cells that have encountered a specific antigen previously and have acquired means of destroying the substance. They help produce and transport immunoglobin antibodies. **Cellular i.f.** include T-lymphocytes which are thymus-gland-dependent and are mobilized primarily to resist slowly developing bacterial infections, tissues of other individuals such as organ transplants, and

rejection of some of the body's own cells that may have been altered by virus infections or carcinogens. Also see RH FACTOR.

immunization the process of acquiring immunity, as by inoculation or vaccination with an agent that induces the production of natural antibodies by the body's immune system. **Active i.** requires the injection of a specific antigen into the body of the person; in **passive i.** prepared antibodies are introduced into the body. Passive i. occurs commonly during pregnancy when the mother's antibodies pass through the placenta to provide temporary protection for the fetus. The passive-i. effects may last from one to six months, after which active i. may be required.

immunology the branch of medicine that specializes in the study of immunity and immune reactions, e.g., allergies and hypersensitivities.

immunosuppressive drugs drugs that inhibit the formation of antibodies that may develop to resist the antigens of foreign tissues. I.d. are used to prevent rejection by antibodies of transplanted organs or tissues. An unfortunate side effect of i.d. is that they also lower the resistance of the patient to infectious diseases that in many cases prove fatal to the person whose life may have been saved by the transplant operation.

impact analysis in evaluation research, an analytic procedure used to assess the effectiveness of an evaluation program on participant outcomes; a quantitative approach to evaluating the success or failure of a program. Also see PROGRAM-IMPACT EVALUATION.

impairment index a system of measuring impairment of mental functions. An example is the Halstead-Reitan i.i. developed for measuring brain damage in adults and children. It is based on results of a battery of ten tests developed and modified over a period of 30 years in experiments with diagnosed brain-damage patients and normal individuals. The i.i. is regarded as valid for distinguishing true neurologic cases from pseudoneurologic cases.

impasse: See THERAPEUTIC I.

imperative in psychoanalysis, a demand of the superego which represents the commanding voice of parental or social rule, and operates on an unconscious level to direct the behavior of the individual. Also see CATEGORICAL I.; ETHICAL I.; IMMORAL I.

imperative attitude: See ENDOCRATIC POWER.

impersonal projection the process of attributing one's unobjectionable or neutral qualities to another person, as opposed to the projection of objectionable impulses or ideas.

impersonal relationship: See CONTACT BEHAVIOR.

impersonation the deliberate assumption of another person's identity, usually as a means of gaining status or other advantage.

impetus in psychoanalysis, the force or energy behind an instinct or drive.

implantation the attachment of a fertilized ovum to the uterine wall after it has floated freely for several days.

implicit behavior behavior that cannot be observed directly without the aid of instruments.

implicit personality theories the tacit assumptions a person uses in interpreting the personality traits of another and drawing relationships between such traits to form an overall evaluation of the other person.

implicit response a response that is assumed to occur although it cannot be observed directly.

implosion in acoustics, the process of building up air pressure in the air tract just before its explosive release in the production of plosive speech sounds. See PLOSIVE.

implosive therapy a behavior-therapy technique in which the patient is repeatedly encouraged to imagine an anxiety-arousing situation, and to experience anxiety as intensely as possible while doing so. Since there is no actual danger in the situation, the anxiety response is not reinforced and therefore is gradually extinguished. Also see FLOODING; PARADOXICAL INTENTION.

impostor syndrome a personality pattern characterized by pathological lying which takes the form of fabricating an identity or a series of identities (doctor, lawyer, war hero), and playing a role that is designed to bring recognition and status. The dynamics of this pattern are obscure, though P. Greenacre has suggested that the underlying motivation is to steal the limelight from the father, and the pattern of taking different roles may result from failure to develop a full personal identity due to an overpossessive mother who encourages maternal attachment. Also see MUNCHAUSEN SYNDROME.

impotence the inability of the male to complete the sex act due to partial or complete failure to achieve or maintain erection. The condition is usually psychogenic and may also take the form of premature ejaculation, limited interest in sex, orgasm without experiencing pleasure, coitus without ejaculation, and sexual ability only with prostitutes. See INHIBITED SEXUAL EXCITEMENT. Also see ORGASTIC I.; COITUS SINE EJACULATIONE; ANAL I.; PSYCHIC I.; PRIMARY ERECTILE DYSFUNCTION; SECONDARY ERECTILE DYSFUNCTION.

impoverished autism = AUTISME PAUVRE.

impoverished environment: See ENVIRONMENTAL ENRICHMENT.

impoverishment: See INTELLECTUAL I.; POVERTY OF IDEAS. Also see DELUSION OF I.

impregnation the process of initiating pregnancy by the penetration of the secondary oocyte by a spermatozoon and the fusion of the nuclei of the male and female gametes. Also called **fertilization; fecundation; ingravidation**. Also see ORAL I.

impression the neurological effect of stimulation; also, a vague or unanalyzed judgment or reaction.

impressionism factor the designation for an art style characterized by blurred outlines and emphasis on surface qualities and textures. The style was popular with impressionist painters of the 19th century. In D. E. Berlyne's studies of perceptions of art, the i.f. is reflected in evaluation ratings that are highly positive for surface and highly negative for beliefs, imagination, and lines.

impression management in social psychology, a term for the conscious devices and stratagems utilized in a person's effort to portray himself in a desired way so as to control others' impressions of him.

impression method a procedure in which the subject makes an introspective report on a stimulus pattern in terms of his feelings, e.g., pleasant, unpleasant.

impression of universality: See MOB PSYCHOLOGY.

impressive aphasia = RECEPTIVE APHASIA.

imprinting a primitive learning process which occurs during a critical period in the life of some animals. It was first described in 1873 by the English naturalist D. A. Spalding when he observed that newly hatched chicks tended to follow the first moving object, human or animal, that caught their attention. The term itself was coined by the ethologist Konrad Lorenz in 1937. Some investigators believe that such responses (possibly including the smiling response of human infants) are irreversible and instinctual; others regard them as a reversible form of conditioning. Also see CRITICAL PERIOD.

improvement rate the ratio of the number of patients discharged as improved from a hospital or other institution within a given period of time, compared with the total in the original group. The i.r. usually is expressed as a percentage.

improvisation in psychodrama, the spontaneous acting out of problems and situations without prior preparation.

impuberism a state of not having reached puberty because of age or delayed development; also, the continuation of childhood characteristics into adolescence or adulthood. Also called **impuberty**.

impulse a strong, sometimes irresistible, urge; a sudden inclination to act without deliberation. In psychoanalysis, the term denotes the psychological aspect of instinctual drives, such as sex, hostility, hunger, and defecation. It also denotes the wave of electrical energy that passes through a nerve fiber when it discharges. See DISORDERS OF I. CONTROL NOT ELSEWHERE CLASSIFIED; NERVE I. Also see IRRESISTIBLE I.; PRIMORDIAL I.

impulse control the ability to resist an impulse, desire, or temptation, as in restraining an urge to gamble heavily, drink to excess, or give vent to anger.

impulse-control disorder a mental disorder characterized by a tendency to gratify one's immediate desires or express one's immediate impulse to act, without regard to consequences. For individual types, see SUBSTANCE-USE DISORDERS; INTERMITTENT EXPLOSIVE DISORDER; ISOLATED EXPLOSIVE DISORDER; PATHOLOGICAL GAMBLING; KLEPTOMANIA; PYROMANIA. Also see DISORDERS OF IMPULSE CONTROL NOT ELSEWHERE CLASSIFIED.

impulse fear a fear that arises in the absence of a real threat and is usually due to an instinctual factor, e.g., a fear of sudden death in the absence of signs or symptoms of disease.

impulse interpretation = ID INTERPRETATION.

impulse neurosis a term sometimes applied to episodic behavior disorders characterized by precipitous onset, abrupt remission, and a tendency to frequent recurrence. Characteristically, the patient interrupts his typical life-style to act out, or to obey an irresistible impulse, as in choking a sister or brother or marrying an almost unknown person on sudden impulse. For behavior of this kind, which has been termed **episodic dyscontrol**, see INTERMITTENT EXPLOSIVE DISORDER.

impulsion a compelling drive to action in blind obedience to internal drives. It occurs primarily in young children, and in obsessive-compulsive or antisocial adults, who have not developed adequate defenses against their impulses. The term is essentially equivalent to impulsive behavior.

impulsive behavior activity abruptly engaged in without forethought, reflection, or consideration of consequences. Also called **impulsiveness; impulsivity**. See IMPULSION.

impulsive character a personality pattern marked by a tendency to act hastily and without reflection.

impulsiveness = IMPULSIVE BEHAVIOR.

impulsive raptus a seldom used term for a sudden attack of agitation that may occur in cases of catatonic schizophrenia.

impulsivity = IMPULSIVE BEHAVIOR.

impunitive response a reaction to a frustrating experience in which the individual denies or makes light of a problem instead of blaming himself or others. See ROSENZWEIG PICTURE-FRUSTRATION STUDY.

imu a culture-specific syndrome resembling latah, observed among the Ainu women of Japan, and characterized by automatic movements, imitative behavior, and infantile reactions.

Imuran = AZATHIOPRINE.

in absentia in forensic psychology, a term relating to a legal proceeding against an individual that is conducted in his absence. Courts prefer that a person be able to participate meaningfully and personally in his own case and not be tried i.a. because of a mental disorder.

inaccessible unreceptive and unresponsive to external stimuli. In psychiatry, the term refers to the withdrawn state characteristic of autism, schizophrenia, and depression. A patient is i. if he does not react or respond to the therapist in a way that facilitates the development of rapport. Also see WITHDRAWAL REACTION.

inadequate personality a personality disturbance characterized by failure to adapt to the social, emotional, occupational, and intellectual demands of life. Though lacking in effectiveness, stability, judgment, and foresight, these individuals are found to test in the normal range, but frequently become vagrants, ne'er-do-wells, alcoholics, or drug addicts.

inappetence a lack of desire or appetite.

inappropriate affect emotional responses that are not in keeping with the situation, or that are incompatible with expressed thoughts or wishes, e.g., smiling when told about the death of a friend. I.a. is a common schizophrenic symptom.

inattention a state in which there is a lack of concentrated or focused attention, or in which attention drifts back and forth. Also see SELECTIVE I.; SENSORY I.

in-basket test a work-sample test used in management training and selection. The examinee is given an assortment of items (letters, memos, reports) which might be found in an in-basket, and must take action on them as if he or she were on the job.

inborn error of metabolism any biochemical disorder caused by a genetic defect. It often is expressed as a defect or deficiency in the structure or enzymatic function of a protein molecule or in the transport of a vital substance across a cell membrane. Examples of the condition include diabetes mellitus, gout, phenylketonuria, and Tay-Sachs disease. Also called **metabolic anomaly**.

inbreeding the mating of individuals that are closely related, usually for the purpose of preserving certain preferred traits or characteristics while preventing the acquisition of unwanted traits of other genetic stock in the offspring. I. also increases the risk of perpetuating certain genetic defects in the family, as in consanguineous marriages.

incendiarism: See PYROMANIA; FIRE-SETTING BEHAVIOR.

incentive an anticipated reward designed to influence the performance of an individual or group.

incentive systems in industrial psychology, a set of rewards and rules for disbursement, designed to influence future job behavior. Incentives vary in motivating power from group to group and include such items as hospital insurance, pension, increased pay, additional vacation, and shorter work hours.

incentive theory the theory that motivation arousal should be viewed as an interaction or relationship between environmental incentives (stimulus objects) and an organism's psychological and physiological state. Drive-reduction alone is not viewed as an adequate explanation for behavior arousal, although its role in the interaction is not denied. What is emphasized is the role of both positive and negative incentives in arousing the organism and instigating behavior. Also see DRIVE-REDUCTION THEORY.

incest heterosexual activity between persons of closer blood relationship than permitted by law or custom. In some societies sexual intercourse between cousins or between uncles and nieces, aunts and nephews, is prohibited; in others it is permitted. But i. taboos of some kind are found in practically every society. Also see FATHER-DAUGHTER I.; MOTHER-SON I.

incest barrier in psychoanalysis, an ego defense

erected during the latency period against incestuous impulses and fantasies. The barrier is the
result of the introjection of social laws and customs. These internal and external prohibitions
help to free the libido to make an external object
choice.

incest fantasy in psychoanalysis, the young child's
wish to have sexual relations with the parent of
the opposite sex, as expressed in fantasies and
dreams. Incest fantasies directed toward the
mother are particularly prominent among boys
during the act of masturbation, and feed into
castration fears. Incest fantasies toward the
father may be a source of severe conflict in girls.

incest taboo social prohibition against sexual intercourse between persons of closer relationship
than the culture allows. For details, see INCEST.

incestuous desire the desire to engage in sexual
activity with a close relative. The wish is far
more rarely carried out between mother and son
than between father and daughter. In many
cases the father forces the incestuous relationship upon the daughter. Brother-sister sex
play is much more common than a full incestuous relationship, and when incest does occur,
it may be associated with emotional disturbance
or the use of force by the brother. In
psychoanalysis, the emphasis is on i.d. toward
the parent of the opposite sex as an expression
of the Oedipus complex, and its strength is indicated by the fact that an "incest barrier" is
erected, and also by the widespread existence of
incest taboos.

incestuous ties the term used by E. Fromm to denote the condition in which an individual remains psychologically dependent on the mother,
family, or symbolic substitute to the extent that
healthy involvement with others and with society is inhibited or precluded. According to
Fromm, i.t. represent the negative resolution of
the search for rootedness. Also see ROOTEDNESS
NEED. Compare BROTHERLINESS.

incidence the rate of occurrence of new cases of a
given condition in a particular population in a
given period of time. Incidence rates are normally expressed per 100,000 population per
year.

incidental learning learning that is not premedi-
tated, deliberate, or intentional and which is
acquired as a result of some other, possibly unrelated, activity. Some theorists believe that much
learning takes place without motive or any intention to learn; however, others maintain that
no learning occurs in the absence of a motive
and thus there must be a drive at work in i.l.
Latent learning is similar but implies that the
information is subconscious until a specific need
for it arises. Also called **passive learning**.

incidental memory a memory that occurs without
conscious effort or intention, as in remembering
a particular play in a football game.

incidental stimulus an unintentional stimulus that
may occur during an experiment or in another
situation, and which may result in a response.

incipient psychosis = LATENT PSYCHOSIS.

inclusion-body encephalitis = PANENCEPHALITIS.

inclusion-cell disease a rare disorder marked by
the occurrence of large quantities of cytoplasmic
inclusions in the neurons. The inclusions usually
are virus particles from an earlier infection.
Children affected by the disease show severe
psychomotor retardation. Also called **Leroy's
disease; mucolipidosis II; I-cell disease**.

incoherence lack of organization; especially, disjointed or incomprehensible speech.

incommensurable pertaining to two or more characteristics or variables that are not measured in
the same units and thus cannot be compared in
terms of the same scale or standard.

incompatible response a response or action that
conflicts with another when they occur at the
same time, e.g., contracting antagonistic muscles.

incompetence in industrial psychology, the inability
to carry out a task adequately; in legal psychiatry, the lack of the capacity to make sound
judgments regarding transactions, and to assume
legal responsibility for one's life. Also called
incompetency.

incompetency plea the plea, in a court of law, that
the defendant was not legally responsible for the
action in question due to lack of capacity to comprehend its nature or consequences. An i.p. may
be entered on the basis that the defendant,
because of mental disease, defect, or other
reasons, does not understand the nature and object of the proceedings pending against him, or
cannot appreciate or comprehend his own condition in relation to the proceedings, or is unable,
for some other reason, to assist his attorney in
his own defense. Also see COMPETENCY TO STAND
TRIAL.

incomplete-pictures test a test of visual recognition and interpretation in which drawings in
varying degrees of completion are presented,
and the subject attempts to identify the object as
early in the series as possible. Also see PICTURE-
COMPLETION TEST.

incomplete-sentence test = SENTENCE-COMPLETION
TEST.

incongruity the quality of being inconsistent, incompatible, not harmonious, or otherwise in disagreement with an accepted mode or standard.
Perception experiments may include tests of i.,
in which, e.g., a deck of playing cards may contain mismatched colors and suits such as black
hearts or purple spades.

incontinence an inability to control basic body
functions, particularly urination and defecation.
I. is often due to spinal-cord injury, brain damage in the motor region, as in severe cerebral
palsy, or grand mal seizures. The term is also applied to an inability to restrain sexual impulses.

incoordination a lack of harmony or balance in the
action of muscle groups due to a failure to work
together.

incorporation assimilation of the attitudes or attributes of others as part of one's self. In

psychoanalysis, i. is the earliest form of identification and introjection, and the most primitive recognition of external reality. It first occurs in the oral stage when the infant feels, or fantasies, that the mother's breast, and perhaps her total being, are becoming part of himself during the nursing process. It is also considered the earliest expression of sexuality, with the nipple as the object.

incubation in psychology, the stage of creative thinking in which the mind mulls over a problem on an unconscious or semiconscious level in order to give it a chance to ripen (G. Wallas). In medicine, the term applies to growth of cultures in a controlled environment; to maintenance of an artificial environment for a premature or hypoxic infant; and to the asymptomatic stage of development of an infection.

incubation of avoidance the theory that avoidance-learning requires a period of incubation time before it becomes consolidated in the memory. The theory is based on evidence of a delayed appearance of conditioning in experimental animals exposed to electroconvulsive shock.

incubus a medieval term for a demon or evil spirit in male form who is believed to have intercourse with a sleeping woman (from Latin *incubare*, "to lie upon"); also, a nightmare. Also see FAMILY I.

incus one of the tiny bones, or ossicles, located in the middle ear. It is located between the malleus, which is attached to the ear drum, and the stapes, which articulates with the inner ear. Also called **anvil**. See OSSICLES.

in d. an abbreviation used in prescriptions, meaning "in a day" (Latin *in die* /dē'ā/).

indemnity neurosis = COMPENSATION NEUROSIS.

independent events two or more unrelated or noncontingent events. Many statistical tests assume that the observations being compared or added together are i.e.

independent living the ability of an individual to perform all or most of the normal daily functions required in maintaining a home and job, and mobility between home and job, as a self-sufficient person. I.l. is a primary objective of habilitation and rehabilitation, and can be achieved by many disabled individuals with a variety of special devices and equipment designed to compensate for handicaps.

independent-living aids = DAILY LIVING AIDS.

independent variable the stimulus or stimulus situation that is scientifically manipulated by the experimenter while other variables are held constant. Its effects on the dependent variable are then studied. E.g., in studies of high-noise conditions, the i.v. is the level of noise controlled by the experimenter whereas the dependent variable is the subject's reaction. The term i.v. may also be employed to mean the criterion variable used in correlations. Abbrev.: **IV**. Also called **experimental variable**. Compare DEPENDENT VARIABLE.

Inderal $C_{16}H_{22}ClNO_2$—a trademark for propranolol hydrochloride, a beta adrenergic blocking agent. The drug is effective in blocking the actions of most substances that stimulate activity of the heart; exceptions include digitalis and caffeine. The net effect is a slower heart rate and slight decrease in blood pressure. I. may be used in treating abnormalities of heart rhythm.

indeterminism the doctrine that humans are able to act independently of antecedent or current situations, as in making choices.

index adoptees: See CROSS FOSTERING; CONTROL ADOPTEES.

index case = PROBAND.

index number a number used for comparison purposes, such as a percent or an average price over a set period.

Index of Adjustment and Values a personality test based on the subjects' reactions to trait words compiled by Allport, and designed to measure self-concept, self-acceptance, concept of the ideal self, and self-esteem or personal adjustment (Bills, 1951, 1975).

index of body build = BODY-BUILD INDEX.

index of discrimination an index of the sensitivity of a test or test item to differences in subjects tested.

index of forecasting efficiency a measure of the amount of improvement over chance in prediction given by the correlation coefficient. It is equal to $1 - k$, where k is the coefficient of alienation.

index of refraction a number indicating the degree to which a light ray is bent in passing from one transparent medium to another.

index of reliability an estimate of the correlation between actual test scores and the corresponding theoretical true scores.

index variable a variable that is not a determinant or true causal factor but represents or symbolizes the complex process or processes under study. E.g., in developmental studies, age is an i.v. that represents the underlying motor, perceptual, cognitive, or emotional processes.

Indian Health Service an agency of the United States Department of Health and Human Services that provides care for nearly 500,000 Native Americans and Alaskans. The I.H.S. operates 51 hospitals and 83 health centers, some of which, e.g., in Navaho tribal areas, encourage the use of native faith healers for the psychological benefits of the ceremonies.

indifference point the intermediate region between experiential opposites, e.g., on the pleasure-pain dimension, a degree of stimulation that provokes an indifferent or neutral response.

indifferent stimulus a stimulus that has not yet elicited the reaction being studied.

indigenous nonprofessionals: See BLUE-COLLAR THERAPY.

indigenous worker an auxiliary worker in the field of mental health drawn from the same background as low-income clients in order to bridge the gap between these clients and the therapists, who are usually middle class. Indigenous workers also explore the therapeutic needs of residents of a neighborhood served by a community mental-health center, and see that the special characteristics and sociological patterns of an ethnic or cultural group are recognized and utilized in the therapeutic process. See BLUE-COLLAR THERAPY.

indirect associations a symptom of schizophrenic logic in which an association between ideas is not expressed, so that the observer may fail to see the thought connection, and the statement therefore seems bizarre and incoherent.

indirect measurement a measurement that must be transferred or converted to a different scale.

indirect method of therapy a form of client-centered therapy in which the therapist does not attempt to direct the patient's communication or evaluate the patient's remarks, although he may refer back to the patient's remarks or restate them.

indirect vision vision that is possible by stimulation of any part of the retina outside the fovea centralis.

indissociation a Piagetian term for an early child-development stage when perceptions of physical-world phenomena are not clearly distinguished from each other and from the self.

individual difference any trait or other psychological difference by which an individual may be distinguished from other persons.

individualism an approach to life that emphasizes the right to be oneself and to have one's own aims, interests, and idiosyncrasies, as contrasted with conformity to group standards or conventional life-styles.

individualistic motive a type of motivation that influences an individual to advance himself through behavior in which he neither cooperates nor competes with others. Compare COMPETITIVE MOTIVE; COOPERATIVE MOTIVE.

individualistic reward structure a situation in which the success of one person has no bearing on the success of others, e.g., an examination graded on an absolute scale so that all students could potentially receive an A. Compare COMPETITIVE REWARD STRUCTURE; COOPERATIVE REWARD STRUCTURE.

individualization the process whereby an individual is distinguished from one or more others of the same species, sex, or other category.

individualized education program the written statement of objectives and procedures for a handicapped child to be implemented in accordance with the requirements of the federal law. Abbrev.: **IEP**.

individualized instruction an instructional method that permits students to work separately at their own pace. Teachers assist students in identifying skills that need development or knowledge that needs to be acquired. Group projects are incorporated in the program as well.

individualized reading a method of teaching reading that utilizes the child's interests and a variety of books geared to the child's level of skills.

individual man: See PERSONA.

individual program an instructional method in which the student is responsible for developing and carrying out his own program. The i.p. is designed for children who possess a high level of motivation and cognitive development. Compare COMMAND STYLE.

individual psychological motives: See PSYCHOLOGICAL MOTIVE.

individual psychology the psychological theory of Alfred Adler, which is based on the idea that the individual is governed by a conscious drive to develop his own goals and create his own style of life, as opposed to the view that human beings are dominated by "blind," irrational instincts operating on an unconscious level. His concept of self-realization, however, was not purely self-centered, for he held that it must incorporate "social interest," and he optimistically maintained that human beings have a basic, innate urge to cooperate and work for the common good. For other details, see COMPENSATION; FICTIONAL FINALISM; INFERIORITY COMPLEX; OVERCOMPENSATION; STRIVING FOR SUPERIORITY.

individual psychotherapy = INDIVIDUAL THERAPY.

individual test a type of test intended for administration to a single subject only, usually administered by a trained tester, as in the Wechsler and Binet tests.

individual therapy psychotherapy conducted on a one-to-one basis, as contrasted with group therapies, in which there is more than one patient and in some instances more than one therapist. Also called **individual psychotherapy; dyadic therapy**.

individuation a term employed by Jung for the gradual development of a unified, integrated personality which incorporates greater and greater amounts of the unconscious, both personal and collective, and resolves any conflicts that exist, such as those between introversive and extraversive tendencies. Also, i. is a phase of development, occurring between the 18th and 36th month, in which the infant becomes less dependent on the mother and begins to satisfy his own wishes and fend for himself (M. S. Mahler).

indocin: See INDOLE DERIVATIVES.

Indoklon = HEXAFLUORODIETHYL ETHER.

indole an organic molecule that is the basis of many substances involved in CNS activity, such as lysergic aid diethylamide (LSD), serotonin, and tryptophan, and which also contributes to the odor of feces. Also called **2,3,-benzopyrrole**.

indole alkylamines a category of psychedelic drugs that have similar chemical structures and produce similar effects. The group includes lysergic acid diethylamide (LSD), serotonin, and dimethyltryptamine (DMT), psilocin, and psilocybin. See PSYCHEDELICS.

indoleamines compounds formed by an indole

molecule, which is produced as a breakdown metabolite of tryptophan, and an amine group. Serotonin is an example of an indoleamine. See INDOLE DERIVATIVES.

indole derivatives a group of pharmacologically active substances, including natural and synthetic drugs, which have in common an indole molecule and actions that affect CNS functions. One of the i.d. is a nonnarcotic analgesic, **indomethacin (indocin)**—$C_{19}H_{16}ClNO_4$—which has properties similar to those of phenylbutazone. Other i.d. include the INDOLE ALKYLAMINES and INDOLEAMINES. See these entries.

induced abortion deliberate, premature removal of the fetus prior to the stage of viability, by artificial means such as drugs or mechanical devices. Also called **artificial abortion**. Also see THERAPEUTIC ABORTION.

induced color a color change in a visual field that results from stimulation of a neighboring area, rather than from stimulation of the part of the field in which the change appears.

induced hallucination a hallucination that is evoked in one individual by another. It may occur during hypnosis.

induced hypothermia: See HYPOTHERMIA.

induced psychosis: See FOLIE À DEUX.

induced tonus a muscle tonus brought about by a movement of another body part, e.g., holding the head above water while swimming.

induction the formulation of general rules or explanations from specific cases or observations; reasoning from the particular to the general. Compare DEDUCTION.

induction test a series of test items in which the student or subject must derive or formulate a general law, rule, or principle based on several relevant facts or cases.

inductive problem solving a learning situation in which the student is presented with given facts and events from which he must draw relationships and explain the general principles that underlie the relationships.

inductive reasoning the reasoning process whereby inferences and general principles are drawn from specified observations and cases; reasoning from the specific to the general. I.r. is a cornerstone of the scientific method in that it underlies the process of developing hypotheses from particular facts and observations. Compare DEDUCTIVE REASONING.

inductive teaching model an approach in education that strongly emphasizes the role of inductive reasoning in cognitive development. A similarly used term is **inquiry training model**.

indusium griseum a supracallosal gyrus that is formed by a thin layer of gray matter on the dorsal surface of the corpus callosum. The i.g. is a rudimentary component of the hippocampus and is continuous with some of the various tissues of the hippocampal system.

industrial psychiatry the branch of psychiatry concerned with the maintenance of mental health and constructive interpersonal relationships in the work setting. Areas of activity include compensation cases, emergency psychiatric treatment, case-finding, reduction of occupational risks, interpersonal relations among workers or between supervisors and workers, vocational adjustment, accident proneness, absenteeism, executive neurosis, alcoholism, drug abuse, and early detection of mental disorder. Also called **occupational psychiatry**.

industrial psychology the study of the work-related aspects of life, and the application of a knowledge of human behavior to problems that arise in this area, such as personnel selection and training, working conditions, accidents and safety, job analysis, and employee satisfaction.

industrial rehabilitation counselor a rehabilitation counselor who works closely with industry (a) by providing information on available community services such as training opportunities, (b) by offering an alternative recruiting program, (c) by providing assistance in interviewing and placing the disabled in the company, and (d) by providing follow-up services, such as counseling, to the employer and employee, and review of relevant medical and psychological data.

industrial therapy work activities, usually on a paid basis, carried out by mentally ill or physically disabled individuals in a hospital or sheltered workshop for such purposes as morale-building and preparation for outside employment. The work is geared to the individual's interests, personality needs, and level of skill, and is directed by an industrial therapist who usually has a degree in occupational therapy or manual arts.

industry versus inferiority the fourth of Erikson's eight stages of man, covering the Freudian latency period of ages six to 11 years during which the child learns to obey the rules of the game and is interested in how things work and how to make things. If he is not encouraged to be industrious, he will feel inferior. Also called **Robinson Crusoe age**. See ERIKSON'S EIGHT STAGES OF MAN.

inertia a property of the nervous system consisting of a delay between stimulus and response. Also see PSYCHIC I.

ineffability the inexpressible, indescribable character of a state of ecstasy. The individual who undergoes such as state usually maintains that it can be understood only by direct experience. See ECSTASY; EXALTATION.

ineffective stimulus a stimulus that fails to evoke a response, usually because the stimulus is not capable of affecting a receptor.

inertia principle: See PRINCIPLE OF INERTIA.

inf. an abbreviation used in prescriptions, meaning "infusion" (Latin *infusum*).

infancy the earliest period of postnatal life, roughly the first year, during which the child is helpless and dependent upon parental care.

infant and preschool tests individually administered tests designed to assess the development of infants (from birth to 18 months) and preschool children (from 18 to 60 months). The Gesell Developmental Scales determine the level of linguistic, motor, and social behavior on both levels. The California First Year Mental Scale assesses postural adjustment, motor activity, perception, attention, and manipulation. The Merrill-Palmer Scale comprises verbal and performance items standardized for children from 24 to 63 months of age. Other important tests are the Bayley Scales of Infant Development, the Cattell Infant Scale, the Griffiths Mental Development Scale, the McCarthy Scales of Children's Abilities, and the Wechsler Preschool and Primary Scale of Intelligence.

infant at risk a newborn child whose development may be threatened by maternal complications at the time of birth, including conditions that reduce the supply of oxygen to brain tissue. A significant number of children with cerebral palsy, epilepsy, and mental retardation are born prematurely when the mother was experiencing toxemia or bleeding in the uterus. Mechanical injuries resulting from umbilical-cord prolapse, malpresentation, or high-forceps delivery account for some cases of mental retardation.

Infant Behavior Record: See BAYLEY SCALES OF INFANT DEVELOPMENT.

infanticide the killing of an infant or child, as in so-called "mercy killing" when the child is severely defective or incurably diseased, or in the course of extreme child abuse. I. has been practiced in a number of societies, notably Sparta, as a means of eliminating the unfit.

infantile amnesia an inability to remember the first years of life because of repression (Freud).

infantile atrophy = MARASMUS.

infantile autism a severe disorder appearing before 30 months of age, and characterized by (a) a pervasive lack of responsiveness to other people (disinterest, failure to cuddle, lack of eye contact, masklike face, indifference or aversion to affection), (b) impairment in communication development, ranging from total absence of language to immature grammar, echolalia, reversal of "you" and "I," inability to name objects, and idiosyncratic, metaphoric language, and (c) bizarre behavior such as resistance to even minimal changes, extreme attachment to selective objects (a piece of string, a rubber band), and ritualistic acts, such as hand-clapping or staring at spinning objects. Many but not all investigators distinguish this condition from schizophrenia. Also called **Kanner's disease; Kanner's syndrome**. See AUTISM; ECHOLALIA; RITUALS. (DSM-III)

infantile autism, residual state a category comprising individuals who had infantile autism and now show some signs of the illness, such as communication and social peculiarities. (DSM-III)

infantile dynamics psychological forces, such as oral sexuality or the Oedipus complex, that originate in early childhood but continue to exert an unconscious influence on the personality during adulthood.

infantile masturbation self-stimulation during infancy and early childhood, including genital play without discharge, as well as stimulation of other erogenous zones and parts of the body, as in smacking the lips and sucking the fingers.

infantile myxedema = BRISSAUD'S INFANTILISM.

infantile neuroaxonal dystrophy a disease characterized by the swelling of axons in the gray matter of the spinal cord and brainstem. Neurons are lost in the areas of the swellings, or spheroids. Signs of mental deterioration appear in the second or third year after an apparently normal first year of life. The patients gradually lose their sight and ability to speak. Death usually occurs by age 12.

infantile osteopetrosis a rare hereditary disorder marked by poorly formed bone structure, including the skull bones, and sometimes accompanied by retinal degeneration and cranial-nerve palsy. Mental retardation has been reported in more than 20 percent of the patients, with sensory deprivation a possible contributing factor.

infantile paralysis = POLIOMYELITIS.

infantile paresis a congenital form of neurosyphilis that may develop within the first few months of life. It is acquired from an infected mother any time after the first four months of pregnancy.

infantile personality = IMMATURE PERSONALITY.

infantile polycystic disease an inherited kidney disorder that affects newborns and is often fatal. Polycystic renal disorders are marked by the formation of numerous cysts ranging in size from one to ten centimeters in diameter, causing enlargement of the kidney but reducing normal function because of pressure of the cysts. I.p.d. is inherited as an autosomal-recessive trait while adult polycystic disease is an autosomal-dominant trait. Also see POLYCYSTIC KIDNEY DISEASE.

infantile progressive spinal-muscular atrophy: See PROGRESSIVE SPINAL-MUSCULAR ATROPHY.

infantile sadism in psychoanalysis, aggressive and destructive behavior during the early years of life. See ANAL SADISM; ID SADISM; ORAL SADISM.

infantile seduction the use of an immature person, particularly a young child, as a sexual object. I.s. has been associated by some psychoanalysts with an unresolved Oedipus complex that results in the selection of an immature sex partner.

infantile sexuality the psychoanalytic theory that human beings have the capacity for sexual feeling during the first months of life, as manifested in the oral, anal, and early genital stages of development, that is, from sucking the mother's breast, defecating, and masturbatory activities. Also see SEXUAL INFANTILISM.

infantile spasm = WEST'S SYNDROME.

infantile speech speech using the sounds and forms characteristic of very young children (that is, baby talk) beyond the stage where such speech is normal. Immature speech may be encouraged by parents who find it "cute," or it may be an expression of general emotional immaturity. See BABY TALK.

infantilism the regressive behavior of an adult or older child that resembles behavior characteristic of an earlier stage of development.

infantilization the active encouragement of infantile behavior such as extreme dependence on the mother; the process of deliberately keeping the child in an infantile state. Chronically ill or handicapped children are especially likely to be **infantilized** by their parents.

infant learning = INFANT-STIMULATION PROGRAM.

infant narcotic withdrawal a symptom pattern appearing in neonates born to a mother addicted to narcotics, and consisting of vomiting, trembling, hyperactivity, shrill crying, and rapid respiration, which may lead to death if untreated.

infant psychiatry a branch of child psychiatry that focuses on the diagnosis, treatment, and prevention of maladaptive behavior manifested during the period of infancy, that is, during approximately the first year of life.

infant-stimulation program a recently developed program for children born with Down's syndrome or other forms of mental retardation: Under a federal grant the parents receive special instruction in developing their infant's mental and communication capacities through activities involving pictures, sounds, objects, games, and, later, letters and numbers. As a result, many of these children learn to speak fluently, to do simple arithmetic, and to read at slightly-below-grade level. Abbrev.: **infant-stim**. Also called **infant learning**.

infant test a behavior test measuring infantile development, usually through the performance of sensorimotor tasks involving, e.g., coordination and manipulation. Examples are the California First Year Mental Scale, the Gesell Infant Schedule, and the Cattell Infant Intelligence Scale.

infarct: See CEREBRAL I.

infatuation love that usually is short-lived, extravagant, or shallow and based on a superficial reason such as physical attractiveness of the love object.

infavoidance need the need to avoid failure or humiliation, often characterized by not undertaking tasks that are likely to fail.

infection a disease condition caused by the invasion and reproduction of pathogenic microorganisms. e.g., viruses, bacteria, fungi, protozoa, in the body tissues. An i. usually is marked by effects of an immune response, destruction of body cells or conversion of cells as material for producing additional microorganisms, competition with body cells for nutrients, and toxins produced by the microorganisms.

infectious disease any pathological condition caused by the presence of microbes or other organisms in the body. The infectious agents may be bacteria, viruses, plasmodia, yeasts, fungi, rickettsia, or helminths. The mere presence of microorganisms in the body is not a sign of infection as some bacteria live synergistically in the alimentary tract. Also, many individuals carry infectious agents without showing clinical signs of infection.

infectious-exhaustive syndrome a condition of prostration, exhaustion, and in some cases "collapse delirium," associated with a systemic infection such as pneumonia, malaria, typhoid fever, uremia, or scarlet fever.

infectious-exhaustive psychosis an obsolete term for an acute CNS disorder associated with a systemic disease, e.g., a toxic encephalitis.

infectious hepatitis: See HEPATITIS.

infectious mononucleosis an acute infectious disease caused by the Epstein-Barr virus (EBV) and usually transmitted by oral contact. The virus is a member of the herpes line and is found in extracellular fluids of the oral cavity. The disease occurs only in persons with no prior EBV antibodies. Symptoms include malaise, fever, sore throat, chills, and excessive production of lymphatic tissue and lymphocytes. Complications may include CNS involvement, such as meningoencephalitis, Guillain-Barré syndrome, or Bell's palsy. Because the virus is present in fluids of the mouth and throat of recovered persons and is transmitted by oral contact, i.m. sometimes is called the **kissing disease**.

inference statistics = INFERENTIAL STATISTICS.

inference strategies in psychology, the mental processes whereby on the basis of one or more previous judgments the individual reaches still other judgments.

inferential statistics statistics used to draw broad conclusions about the composition or probable behavior of a population. Such inferences are based on statistical measures taken from samples of that population. Also called **inference statistics**. Compare DESCRIPTIVE STATISTICS.

inferior brachium: See BRACHIUM.

inferior colliculi a group of nuclei located behind the aqueduct of Sylvius which serve as relays for auditory nerve impulses.

inferior functions: See SUPERIOR FUNCTIONS.

inferiority: See INDUSTRY VERSUS I.

inferiority complex a basic feeling of inadequacy and insecurity which originates in childhood dependence and helplessness and, according to Adler, "betrays itself throughout life" (1924). Inferiority feelings may be later aggravated by real or fancied deficiencies of a physical, mental, or social nature; but in any case this complex becomes the major driving force of life, impelling normal individuals toward improvement, achievement, and "compensation." On the other hand, those with personality disorders either withdraw from competition or seek to "overcompensate" by becoming excessively competitive and aggressive. Also see ORGAN INFERIORITY.

inferior longitudinal fasciculus a bundle of association fibers that extends from the occipital to the temporal poles of the cerebral hemispheres.

inferior oblique the external eye muscle that rotates the eyeball upward and inward. Also see EYE MOVEMENTS.

inferior rectus: See EYE MOVEMENTS.

inferotemporal cortex a region of the brain immediately beneath the temporal cortex that contains nerve fibers associated with visual perception. Lesions of the i.c. impair visual learning related to either object or form discrimination.

infertility the inability to produce offspring due to a low fertility level on the part of the wife (about 60 percent of cases), the husband (nearly 40 percent of cases), or both. Physical causes predominate, but the condition may be due to psychological factors. In contrast to sterility, many cases can be remedied. Also see STERILITY; FECUNDITY.

infibulation the sewing together of the lips of the vulva or prepuce in order to prevent coitus. If the penile prepuce is stitched over the glans penis, obstructed urine flow and inflammation can result. See SPERMATORRHEA RING.

infinity fear = APEIROPHOBIA.

infinity neurosis an abnormal preoccupation with the concepts of the infinity of space and eternity of time, a condition usually manifested during adolescence or among autistic individuals.

inflammation a localized response of body tissues to injury or invasion by a foreign substance, such as microorganisms. E.g., an immune reaction may produce i. as a defensive measure against the spread of an infection.

inflammatory dysmenorrhea: See DYSMENORRHEA.

influence: See DELUSION OF I.

influencing machine a paranoid delusion in which the patient feels controlled by a machine which serves as an instrument of persecution. In his *Encyclopedia of Psychoanalysis*, 1968, Eidelberg states that the machine is an outwardly projected symbol of the patient's own body, and "the deanimation of the body into a machine is related to the automatizing functions of the preconscious and a sense of the uncanny."

influenza an acute contagious disease caused by a myxovirus infection with symptoms of cough, sore throat, nasal obstruction, upper-chest pain caused by an inflamed trachea, a fever that may reach 41°C (about 106°F), and, occasionally, nosebleeds. I. epidemics have occurred 31 times since 1510. One of the most severe accounted for 20 million deaths in 1918. Encephalitis is a common complication.

informal source: See GRAY MARKET.

informal test a nonstandardized test of a person's abilities that is graded intuitively without norms.

information feedback a response or series of responses that inform an individual about the correctness, physical effect, or social or emotional impact of his behavior. In the field of learning, the concept is similar to the principle behind "knowledge of results," namely, the principle that immediate feedback is beneficial to learning. In interpersonal relations and psychotherapy, i.f. allows an individual insight into others' experience of him. Also see KNOWLEDGE OF RESULTS.

information-input process the CNS mechanism whereby sensory data from the environment are received by the mediation centers of the brain for making judgments or evaluations about appropriate responses.

information-optimization position a conceptual position which states that an organism as an information-processing system has an optimal or preferred level of stimulation. The position further holds that negative affect and avoidance behavior are associated with small and large variations in stimulus while moderate degrees of stimulus variation have a positive affect.

information overload the state that occurs when the amount or intensity of environmental stimuli exceeds the individual's processing capacity, thus leading to an unconscious or subliminal disregarding of some environmental information. According to S. Milgram, the demands of everyday life in large urban centers diminish one's ability to respond to "peripheral" social cues. I.o. is thus said to be a contributing factor to the degeneration of social life in these areas.

information-processing; information science: See INFORMATION THEORY.

Information Test a test that measures the subject's fund of general knowledge in different areas and at different levels of complexity.

information theory a body of principles relating to the communication or transmission of information, which is defined as any message that reduces uncertainty. These principles deal with such concepts as the encoding and decoding of messages, types of communication channels, the capacity of various senses to receive information, application of mathematical principles to the process, and the relative effectiveness of various kinds of feedback. Also called **information science**.

informed consent agreement to an experimental or therapeutic procedure on the basis of the subject's or patient's understanding of its nature and possible risks.

-infra- a combining form meaning below or within.

infradian rhythm a biological rhythm with a cycle longer than one day (from Latin *infra*, "below, within," and *dies*, "day").

infrahuman below human; characterizing all species below the human level. **Infraprimate** refers to behavior, traits, or functions characteristic of animals below the primate level.

infrared spectrophotometer an instrument used in blood analysis and other physiological chemistry studies, using prisms or diffraction gratings to produce a separation of longer-than-visible, or infrared, light wavelengths. In i.s. work, the reflected light is filtered through a medium or potassium or sodium chloride because glass absorbs the wavelengths used. Analysis is based on wavelengths of light absorbed or reflected by various molecules.

infrared-theory of smell a theory that the olfactory sense organ functions at least in part through the absorption of infrared radiation from substances that produce odors. See also RAMAN SHIFT; ULTRAVIOLET ABSORPTION; SMELL MECHANISM.

infundibulum a stalk of tissue that connects the hypophysis, or pituitary gland, to the underside of the brain, just below the third ventricle and above the sphenoid sinus at the base of the skull. The i. is conical and hollow and communicates with the hypothalamus. Ancient anatomists believed the i. was a pathway for mucous secretions to drain from the brain to the nasal cavity.

ingratiation the conscious effort to win the liking and approval of others through conformance, flattery, and other measures designed to create a good impression. I. is an example of impression management.

ingravidation = IMPREGNATION.

in-group an exclusive group characterized by intense bonds of affiliation such that each member feels a sense of kinship and some degree of loyalty to other members by virtue of their common group membership, e.g., an adolescent clique. Also called **we-group**. Compare OUT-GROUP.

inguinal /in'gwinəl/ referring to the region of the groin (Latin *inguen*).

inguinal adenopathy an enlargement of the lymph glands of the groin. I.a. is a diagnostic sign of certain venereal diseases, e.g., TRICHOMONIASIS. See this entry.

INH: See ISONIAZID.

inhalation convulsive treatment method used to prevent death by respiratory failure or anoxia during respiratory-muscle spasms. The basic techniques are administration of oxygen and mouth-to-mouth or resuscitator artificial respiration. Drug-induced convulsions generally involve oxygen deprivation and respiratory depression, regardless of the drug. Anticonvulsant medications are administered in addition to the resuscitation measures.

inhalation of drugs a means of administering a psychotropic substance into the body tissues rapidly when the product is in the form of a gas or aerosol. Anesthetics for major surgery are administered through the lungs, which permits almost instant contact with the bloodstream flowing through the alveoli. I.o.d. also is employed in self-administration of cannabis, nicotine, cocaine, and other volatile substances. Also see VOLATILE-CHEMICAL INHALATION.

inhalation therapy = RESPIRATORY THERAPY.

inheritance psychological or physical traits that have been inherited; also, the process of transmission from parent to offspring. Also see MENDELIAN MODES OF I.; MULTIFACTORIAL I.

inherited disorder: See GENETIC DEFECT: INBORN ERROR OF METABOLISM.

inherited releasing mechanism = INNATE RELEASING MECHANISM.

inhibited female orgasm a psychosexual disorder characterized by recurrent and persistent inhibition of the female orgasm, as manifested by delay in or absence of orgasm following a normal excitement phase during adequate sexual activity. The term only applies if the disturbance is not caused exclusively by physical disorder, medication, or another mental disorder. (DSM-III)

inhibited male orgasm a psychosexual disorder characterized by recurrent and persistent inhibition of the male orgasm, as manifested by a delay in or absence of ejaculation following an adequate phase of sexual excitement. The term only applies if the disturbance is not exclusively caused by physical disorder, medication, or another mental disorder. (DSM-III)

inhibited mania a type of manic state characterized by psychomotor inactivity together with a cheerful and even exultant mood, flight of ideas, and occasionally irritable and even violent behavior (Kraepelin, 1921).

inhibited sexual desire a psychosexual disorder consisting of persistent and pervasive inhibition of sexual desire, taking age, sex, health, and style of life into account. The term only applies if the condition is not due exclusively to such organic factors as medication and physical disorders, or to other mental disorders. (DSM-III)

inhibited sexual excitement a psychosexual disorder characterized by recurrent and persistent inhibition of sexual excitement during sexual activity that is judged to be adequate in focus, intensity, and duration. This disturbance is not due exclusively to medication, physical disorder, or another mental disorder. In males it takes the form of partial or complete failure to attain or maintain erection until completion of the sexual act (impotence); and in females, partial or complete failure to attain or maintain the lubrication-swelling response of sexual excitement until completion of the sex act. (DSM-III)

inhibition the process of restraining one's impulses or behavior, either consciously or unconsciously, due to such factors as lack of confidence, fear of consequences, or moral qualms. In psychoanalysis, it is an unconscious mechanism by which the superego controls instinctual or id impulses that would threaten the ego if allowed conscious expressions; e.g., inhibited sexual desire may result from unconscious feelings of guilt implanted by parents. Also, in the theory of conditioning, i. is the active blocking or delay of a response by the subject, e.g., when a dog is trained to salivate only after the bell has rung for several seconds. Also see PROACTIVE I.; RETROACTIVE I.; RECIPROCAL I.; OCCUPATIONAL I.; REACTIVE I.; SPECIFIC I.; INTERNAL I.

inhibition mechanism a series of biochemical mechanisms within the nervous system that restrict the flow of excitatory impulses. The devices include presynaptic and postsynaptic influences, and depolarization and hyperpolarization of cells. See HYPERPOLARIZATION.

inhibition of delay a reduction in the amount of time that elapses between the onset of a stimulus and a response, or between the onset of a conditioned stimulus and a conditioned response.

inhibitory postsynaptic potential a part of the neural inhibitory mechanism in which hyperpolarization occurs through potassium loss via the postsynaptic membrane, increasing the negative charge of the cell's internal potential. Abbrev.: **IPSP**.

inhibitory potential a hypothesized temporary state in which conditioned inhibition results from a response and reduces the potential of recurrence of that response (Hull).

inhibitory process: See EXCITATORY-I.P.

inhibitory reflex a negative reflex effect that may become established during differential conditioning of an animal. The negative conditioned reflex is not reinforced, does not result in a positive conditioned effect, and hence represents an inhibition of the conditioned reflex.

inhibitory synapse a nerve impulse that does not fire, or fires only with difficulty, across a synaptic cleft because of the failure of an axon terminal to render the membrane of the receiving cell permeable to transmitter substances normally secreted at the terminal button.

in-house evaluation in evaluation research, an organization's internal program assessments, as opposed to evaluation conducted by outside evaluators.

initial cry = EPILEPTIC CRY.

initial insomnia persistent difficulty in falling asleep, usually due to tension, anxiety, or depression. Some anxiety insomniacs become so worried about falling asleep or about the effects of loss of sleep that they are unable to relax sufficiently to induce sleep.

initial interview the first interview with a patient or job applicant. The purpose of the i.i. with a psychiatric patient is to establish a positive relationship, listen to the patient's problem described in his own words, make a tentative diagnosis, and formulate a plan for diagnostic tests, possible treatment, or referral. For the job applicant, see EMPLOYMENT INTERVIEW.

initial spurt the increased productivity or gain in performance frequently noted at the start of a job, task, or series of trials. The i.s. is associated more commonly with new tasks than tasks with which the individual is familiar. Also called **beginning spurt**. Compare END SPURT.

Initial Teaching Alphabet a near-phonemic alphabet of 44 characters, with a single sound for each character. It has been used since the early 1960s in teaching English-speaking children to read—with varying success. The system was devised by Sir James Pitman, and was originally called Augmented Roman. Abbrev.: **ITA**.

initiating structure in social psychology, an important component of the group leader's role consisting in his ability to identify group objectives and create an effective organization aimed at achieving those objectives.

initiation a ritual that represents dedication to a specific goal; in psychoanalytic terms, the redirecting of the infantile libido into mature objectives through ceremonies of i. of an adult into manhood.

initiative versus guilt the third of Erikson's eight stages of man, in the child's fourth and fifth years. Central to this stage is the child's feeling of freedom in planning, launching, initiating all forms of fantasy, play, and other activity. If resolution of the two earlier stages was unsuccessful or if the child is consistently criticized or humiliated, guilt and a feeling of not belonging develop in place of initiative. See ERIKSON'S EIGHT STAGES OF MAN.

initiator a group member who introduces new ideas or helps to launch specific courses of action.

inj. an abbreviation used in prescriptions, meaning "injection" (Latin *injectio*).

injection administration: See ADMINISTRATION.

injury fear = TRAUMATOPHOBIA.

ink-blot test: See RORSCHACH TEST.

innate behavior behavior that appears to be controlled by inborn factors, usually involving motor-nerve responses, rather than learning experiences. An example is the effect observed when limb buds of amphibia are transplanted to opposite sides of the body but function, when developed, according to the way in which they would have moved in their original anatomic sites.

innate releasing mechanism an action pattern in animals that is triggered by specific environmental signals because of an inborn rather than a conditioned response to the stimulus. An example is the zigzag dance performed by male stickleback fish when it sees another fish with a swollen abdomen and apparently assumes it is a pregnant female stickleback even though it has never seen a pregnant female of its own species. Abbrev.: **IRM**. Also called **inherited releasing mechanism**. See also RELEASER.

innate response system the unlearned motor responses with which a child is endowed at birth. An example is turning the head toward a light.

inner boundary: See EGO BOUNDARIES.

inner conflict = INTRAPSYCHIC CONFLICT.

inner controls the inhibitory factors, such as reality and values, that prevent dangerous or undesirable behavior.

inner-directed a term introduced by the sociologist David Riesman to characterize an individual who is self-motivated and not easily influenced by the opinions, values, or pressures of other people. See OTHER-DIRECTED.

inner ear the part of the ear that contains the auditory-nerve endings and organs of equilibrium (utricle, saccule, and semicircular canals).

inner estrangement a term used by Federn to define the unfamiliar and unreal feeling of external objects that may be well perceived, a characteristic of depressive psychoses.

inner language the mental image of words and concepts in terms of visual, auditory, and kinesthetic sensations; speech that is spoken to oneself without any vocalization. According to Vigotsky, i.l. follows egocentric speech and represents the child's recruitment of language in his reasoning efforts. Also called **inner speech**. Also see EGOCENTRIC SPEECH; PURE MEANING; VERBAL THOUGHT; INTERNALIZED SPEECH.

innervation the distribution of nerve fiber endings in muscles, glands, or other tissues. The proportion of muscle fibers to motor-neuron axons is known as the **i. ratio** and may vary from three muscle fibers per axon for small muscles to 150 muscle fibers per motor axon for large muscle bundles of the arms and legs.

-ino- a combining form relating to fibrous tissue and muscle.

in-patient a patient who has been admitted to a hospital for treatment that usually requires an overnight stay, as distinguished from an out-patient or an emergency-room patient.

Inpatient Multidimensional Psychiatric Scale: See ANXIOUS INTROPUNITIVENESS.

in-patient services in psychiatry, diagnostic and treatment services available to hospitalized mental patients and usually unavailable or not completely available in out-patient facilities. Examples are continuous supervision and nursing care and specialized treatment techniques such as electroshock therapy, occupational therapy, and movement therapy, as well as medical treatment, recreation therapy, social-work services, and frequent group therapy.

input the signals fed into a communications channel; also, energy put into a system.

input-output mechanism a function of the human information-processing system that is involved primarily in getting information into and out of the system. The mechanism may be expressed simply as acquiring information needed to accomplish a task, such as studying a diagram in order to assemble a bicycle. Abbrev.: **IO.**

inquiry in Rorschach testing, a period of review and questioning about responses to the ink blots in order to define the nature of the responses.

inquiry training model: See INDUCTIVE TEACHING MODEL.

insane asylum: See ASYLUM.

insanity the legal, nonpsychiatric term for a severe mental illness that renders the individual incapable of managing his or her own affairs in a competent manner. In the United States the definition and legal aspects of i. vary from state to state and may involve such concepts as guardianship, lack of responsibility for contracts or crimes, inability to distinguish between right and wrong, and necessity for commitment. See PSYCHOSIS. See also CONSTITUTIONAL I.; CRIMINALLY INSANE.

insanity defense the criminal-law defense plea that an individual lacks criminal responsibility by reason of insanity.

insanity fear = LYSSOPHOBIA.

insanity of negation a psychosis characterized by delusions of nihilism. See COTARD'S SYNDROME.

insect fear = ENTOMOPHOBIA. Also see ACAROPHOBIA.

insecurity a feeling of inadequacy, lack of self-confidence, and inability to cope, as well as general uncertainty and anxiety about one's goals, abilities, or relationships to others.

insemination the deposit of seminal fluid within the vagina, usually during coitus. If the semen is introduced by means other than coitus, the process may be termed artificial i. **Homologous artificial i.** involves introduction of the husband's semen; and **heterologous artificial i.** is the term used to identify i. with the semen of a donor other than the husband. Also called **semination**. Also see ARTIFICIAL I.

inside density the number of persons per room within a residence; also, the number of rooms per residence. A significant relationship has been found in the United States between persons-per-room density and various kinds of social pathology, including crimes of homicide and rape. This relationship may be culture-bound. Compare OUTSIDE DENSITY.

insight a grasp or understanding of relationships that illuminate experience or help to solve a problem—sometimes called the "aha experience." In psychotherapy, i. is the awareness of underlying, often unconscious, sources of emotional difficulty, and is usually considered essential to the therapeutic process. Also, the term applies to a patient's recognition that his symptoms, such as fears or obsessions, are abnormal, in contradistinction to delusions or other psychotic symptoms that are not recognized as abnormal. Also see AHA EXPERIENCE.

insight therapy a general type of psychotherapy based on the theory that deep and lasting personality changes cannot be brought about unless the patient understands the origin of his or her distorted attitudes and defensive measures. This approach contrasts with therapies directed toward removal of symptoms or behavior modification.

insomnia temporary sleeplessness usually caused by transient physical or emotional conditions; or chronic sleeplessness resulting from persistent physical disorders or deep-seated psychological disturbances. Also called **agrypnia; ahypnia; ahypnosia; aypnia**. See DYSSOMNIA; INITIAL I.; INTERMITTENT I.; MIDDLE I.; PSEUDOINSOMNIA; TERMINAL I.; SLEEP CHARACTERISTICS.

insomnium dream a type of dream that reflects the current state of an individual's psyche and body (according to Artemidorus, who lived in the second century A.D. and wrote the most important work on dreams in ancient times, *The Oneirocritica*). Insomnium dreams differ from **somnium dreams**, which arise from deeper, more obscure sources—a distinction that was made by Jung.

inspectionalism = VOYEURISM.

inspiration the act of inhaling, or drawing air into the lungs; also, the sudden grasp of a creative idea.

inspirational group therapy a therapeutic approach in which a dynamic leader uses a wide variety of supportive measures to arouse and encourage a group. Among them are testimonials, acceptance by the group, esprit de corps, group identification, the realization that others are in the same boat, sharing of experiences, reassurance, and, in the case of Alcoholics Anonymous, recognition of a higher spiritual power.

inspiration-expiration: See I/E RATIO.

instability a tendency toward lack of self-control, erratic behavior, and rapidly changing or excessive emotions. See EMOTIONALLY UNSTABLE PERSONALITY.

instigation therapy behavior therapy in which the therapist provides a positive model and reinforces the patient's progress toward self-regulation and self-evaluation.

instinct an inborn behavior pattern that appears in every member of a species at a given point in its development, e.g., nest-building in ants, and the mating behavior of rats. Such patterns are more readily found in animals than in human beings. Even the human sex and maternal drives, two of the most likely candidates, have been called in question because they vary greatly in intensity and expression. In psychoanalysis, the term is applied to basic biological drives (hunger, thirst, sex, elimination, aggression) which must be fulfilled in order to maintain physical or psychological equilibrium. Also called **instinctual drive; instinctual impulse.** Also see ACQUISITIVENESS; COMPLEMENTARY I.; COMPONENT I.; DEATH I.; DESTRUCTIVE DRIVE; DESTRUDO; DRIVE; EROS; EROTIC I.; HERD I.; HIERARCHICAL THEORY OF I.; LIBIDO; MASTERY MOTIVE; MCDOUGALL; SATISFACTION OF INSTINCTS; SELF-PRESERVATION I.; SEXUAL INSTINCTS; SOCIAL I.

instinctive behavior innate behavior patterns that develop through maturation and are released by specific types of stimulation. I.b. generally is species-specific and thus characteristic of a particular species. Various authors cite migration, hibernation, hunger, sex, or other activities as types of instinctive behavior, but there is lack of agreement regarding what should be included. See INSTINCT.

instinctive monomania an obsolete, 19th-century term for what is now called obsessive-compulsive disorder.

instinctoid needs the universal human needs that must be met if we are to develop to maximum potential. A. Maslow uses the term to emphasize what he considers the innate aim of striving toward self-actualization.

instinctual aim in psychoanalysis, the gratification of an instinct through an activity that discharges it and restores the organism to a state of equilib-

rium. E.g., eating food fulfills the aim of the hunger instinct. See AIM INHIBITION.

instinctual anxiety a Freudian term for anxiety based on an unknown or instinctual danger, as opposed to a **true anxiety** caused by a known and real danger from an external source.

instinctual drive = INSTINCT.

instinctual dyscontrol a form of primary dyscontrol in which the individual makes an explosive response to a situation in order to gratify an impulse, whim, or sudden urge: "I just did it, I don't know why."

instinctual fusion in psychoanalysis, a balanced union of life and death instincts.

instinctual impulse = INSTINCT.

instinctualization of smell the capacity of smell to play a part in coprophilia, anal fixations, and, as a "component instinct," in sexual foreplay. However, there are wide differences from culture to culture: In some societies genital odors are a potent sexual stimulant; in the United States body odors of all kinds are taboo, as indicated by the wide use of perfumes and deodorants. See COMPONENT INSTINCT; COPROPHILIA; SMELL.

instinctual renunciation in psychoanalysis, a refusal of the ego to satisfy a demand of the id. Reasons for i.r. include the concern that satisfying the instincts would result in a threat to the ego from the outside world and would require disobedience to the superego.

institutional care any type of psychiatric, medical, nursing, or other care or treatment received by a patient in a mental hospital, training school, or other residential institution.

institutionalism = SOCIAL-BREAKDOWN SYNDROME.

institutionalization placement of an individual in an institution for therapeutic or correctional purposes; also, the individual's gradual adaptation to institutional life.

institutional neurosis = SOCIAL-BREAKDOWN SYNDROME.

institutional peonage the practice of using patients of mental hospitals as indentured labor for the maintenance of the institution. Under i.p., the patients may operate the hospital laundry, the patients may operate the hospital laundry and kitchen, clean the building and grounds, pensation and without benefits ordinarily required by an employer to grant workers. The patients also are deprived of the therapeutic value of financial incentives. Also see RIGHTS OF DISABLED.

institutional review board a group named by an agency or institution to review research proposals originating within the agency for scientific and ethical acceptability. Abbrev.: **IRB.**

institutional transference emotional dependence upon an institution, such as a hospital, rather than upon a health professional on the staff of the institution. The trait is observed in latent schizophrenics.

instrument any tool or device used in measuring, recording, testing, or similar functions; in general, an implement used in performing specific operations, such as cutting or writing.

instrumental act any activity that is directed toward a specific objective or toward meeting certain needs.

instrumental aggression hostile action directed at acquiring or retrieving an object, territory, or privilege. Also see HOSTILE AGGRESSION.

instrumental conditioning any form of conditioning in which the subject's response is instrumental in reaching a goal, as when a rat is trained to run a maze or push a lever to obtain food. Also called **instrumental learning; Type II conditioning; Type R conditioning**. See OPERANT CONDITIONING.

instrumental dependence the tendency to depend on others for accomplishing a task or while engaging in activities.

instrumentalism John Dewey's view that advocated the translation of theory into practice, the solution of problems by a scientific application of intelligence and critical inquiry, and the evaluation of ideas by testing them in actual situations. In social psychology, i. is a tendency to exploit other persons for pleasure or profit.

instrumentality theory the concept that the subject's attitude about an event depends on his perception of its function as an instrument in bringing about desirable or undesirable consequences.

instrumental learning = INSTRUMENTAL CONDITIONING.

instrumental-relativist orientation a term sometimes applied to the second stage of L. Kohlberg's preconventional level of moral reasoning, when unselfish acts are undertaken only if they benefit the actor in the long run. See PRECONVENTIONAL LEVEL.

instrumental response any response that achieves a goal or contributes to its achievement; a response that is effective in gaining a reward or avoiding pain, e.g., the rat's bar-pressing to obtain food.

insulin a hormone secreted by the beta cells in the islands of Langerhans, with a basic function of facilitating the transfer of glucose molecules through cell membranes. In the absence of i., glucose accumulates in the blood and is excreted. Normal levels of i. increase the rate of glucose transfer by as much as 500 percent compared with the metabolic activity without i. I. also is involved in fat metabolism.

insulin abnormalities any of several metabolic disorders involving the hormone insulin which is produced by cells in the islands of Langerhans in the pancreas. Insulin is a simple protein molecule that affects the metabolism of proteins and fats as well as carbohydrates. When there is an absence or deficiency of insulin in the body, the carbohydrate glucose is not converted to glycogen, or body starch, the form in which it is stored in the liver, and the glucose accumulates in the blood, spilling into the urine, and producing the symptoms of diabetes mellitus. Biochemical complications of insulin deficiency include also fluid and electrolyte disturbances, acidosis, ketosis, coma, and death. Fat metabolism is accelerated so that end products of fat oxidation accumulate in the blood. An excess of insulin in the blood produces a form of shock with unconsciousness.

insulin-coma therapy a treatment for severe mental disorder (especially schizophrenia) developed in 1933 by Manfred Sakel, consisting of prolonged **hypoglycemic coma**, with or without convulsions, induced by intramuscular administration of insulin. Though still used as a last resort in some hospitals, the technique has been almost completely replaced by electroshock therapy and psychoactive drugs, which involve less danger and produce greater and more lasting improvement. Also called **insulin-shock therapy**.

insulin lipodystrophy: See LIPODYSTROPHY.

insulin-shock therapy = INSULIN-COMA THERAPY.

int. an abbreviation of "internal" or "interior," used, e.g., in prescriptions.

intake the initial interview between a patient (or, if the patient is a child, a member of the family) and the therapist or member of the psychiatric team, upon admission to a psychiatric clinic, mental hospital, or psychiatric department of a general hospital.

integrated model in evaluation research, one possible administrative relationship used in formative evaluations between the program director and two production units. Writers, designers, and evaluators are all members of both production units and are involved in program development as well as program evaluation. Members of these units do not necessarily share equal importance or equal access to the program director. Also called **dependent model**. See SEGREGATED MODEL.

integration in general, the unification of parts into a totality. In psychiatry, i. is the developmental process in which separate drives, experiences, abilities, values, and personality characteristics are gradually brought together into an organized whole. See PRIMARY I.; SECONDARY I. Also see PERSONALITY I.

integrative learning the process of learning tasks that involve simultaneous or successive functioning of several modalities, as in reading and writing.

integrative properties the tendency of living organisms to maintain their functional integrity.

integrity the quality of moral consistency, honesty, and truthfulness with oneself and others. Also see EGO I. VERSUS DESPAIR.

intellect the cognitive function of the mind, including reasoning, conceiving, judging, and relating.

intellectual detachment: See DETACHMENT.

intellectual functions mental functions involving

the acquisition, development, and application of ideas, hypotheses, and theories to the solution of problems. I.f. include such processes as cognition, memory, judgment, evaluation, and creative thinking. Also called **intellectual operations**.

intellectual impoverishment depletion of intellectual resources, such as the power to think and solve problems and to maintain an adequate information level and an interest in ideas and events. I.i. occurs in many chronic schizophrenics, senile and depressive individuals, and persons living in a deprived, unstimulating environment. The term is sometimes used interchangeably with poverty of ideas.

intellectual inadequacy: See MENTAL RETARDATION.

intellectual insight in psychotherapy, an objective, rational awareness of experiences or relationships, which by itself does not advance the therapeutic process and may even impede it because little or no feeling is involved.

intellectualism the doctrine that all mental processes, including emotions, can be explained in terms of cognitive functions.

intellectualization a defense mechanism in which emotional problems are attacked abstractly, or concealed by excessive intellectual activity. E.g., a diffident person may avoid the hazards of social intercourse by "keeping his head in books."

intellectual maturity the young-adulthood or fully adult stage of intellectual development; generally, a high level of good judgment, often combined with wisdom.

intellectual monomania an obsolete, 19th-century term for a type of so-called partial insanity which appears to be equivalent to paranoia.

intellectual operations = INTELLECTUAL FUNCTIONS.

intellectual rigidity a tendency to be inflexible in responding to a stimulus. I.r. may be manifested in various ways, depending upon the individual and the stimulus. E.g., an aging person may display i.r. when confronted by new appliances such as a computer, or the necessity to move to a nursing home. Also see CATASTROPHIC REACTION; EINSTELLUNG.

intellectual subaverage functioning a term denoting an IQ more than two standard deviations below the test mean obtained on an intelligence test.

intelligence general mental ability, especially the ability to make flexible use of memory, reasoning, judgment, and information in learning and dealing with new situations and problems. There is widespread agreement that intelligence is a multifaceted concept, and there is no consensus on its specific components, including those just cited. Many psychologists have abandoned the attempt to arrive at a final definition, and frequently conceive i. broadly as the ability to learn and apply learning, or describe it simply as "what i. tests measure." See I. TEST. Also see MARGINAL I.; MECHANICAL I.; MULTIMODAL THEORY OF I.; NONVERBAL I.; SUPERIOR I.; VERBAL I.; ARTIFICIAL I.; BIOLOGICAL I.; CONCRETE I.

intelligence quotient = IQ.

intelligence test a test composed of mental tasks of graded difficulty that have been standardized by use on a representative sample of the population. Examples of an i.t. include the Stanford-Binet test and the Wechsler Adult Intelligence Scale (WAIS). An i.t. is sometimes called an **intelligence scale**. See IQ.

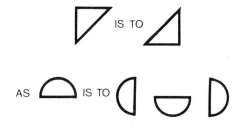

INTELLIGENCE TEST. Example of relationship problem.

intensity the quantitative value of a stimulus or sensation; also, the strength of any behavior, such as an impulse or emotion.

intensive care a hospital service for severely ill or injured patients who require a considerable amount of personal nursing care and supervision. The degree of severity of the illness is equivalent to that of a heart attack. I.c. is the highest priority of a hospital-services program of progressive patient care. At the lowest level of priorities is hospital-based home care.

intensive-care syndrome a type of psychotic behavior observed in certain intensive-care patients who are immobilized in an isolated, unfamiliar environment that may have the effect of sensory deprivation. Variable factors may include the mental and constitutional condition of the patient previous to the need for intensive care, age of the patient, medical-surgical complications, and behavioral effects of drugs administered.

intention a resolve to act in a certain way, or an impulse for purposeful action.

intentional accident = PURPOSIVE ACCIDENT.

intentional behavior goal-oriented behavior emerging between eight and 12 months, that is, behavior in which the child employs strategies to achieve various ends or effects. According to Piaget, i.b. in an infant or young child may be identified when a goal is pursued willingly and in spite of delays or obstacles.

intentional forgetting forgetting that is due to repression or to an unconscious wish to forget.

intentionality a characteristic of psychic acts, which always refer to, or intend, something outside themselves. I. is a key term in Brentano's ACT PSYCHOLOGY. See this entry.

intention tremor a tremor that is associated with voluntary movement, as when the hand trembles while performing a delicate task.

interaction a relationship between two or more systems, persons, or groups that results in mutual or reciprocal influence.

interactional synchrony: See SYNCHRONY.

interaction effect in the analysis of variance, a term that indicates the joint effect of two or more independent variables upon a dependent variable, and contrasted with the MAIN EFFECT. See this entry.

interactionism: See BODY-MIND PROBLEM.

interaction-process analysis a technique developed by F. Bales for the study of the emotional and intellectual interactions that take place in the group-therapy process.

interaction territory in social psychology, a space around two people or a small group of persons while they converse. It is recognized by outsiders that the i.t. should not be invaded as long as the interaction is in progress. Also see GROUP SPACE; PROXEMICS.

interactive measurement a measurement of energy flow of activity between a person and the environment.

interaural rivalry the competition within the auditory system to comprehend conflicting inputs received simultaneously in both ears. I.r. may be employed diagnostically in the study of temporal-lobe lesions or surgical effects since patients recall less of the information heard in the left ear if a lesion is on the right side, and vice versa.

interbehavioral psychology a system of psychology that deals with interactions between the organism and the environment. The focus is on the "event" (learning, perceiving, etc.) which is studied in terms of interbehavior of the organism with other organisms and objects.

interbrain: See DIENCEPHALON.

intercalation the automatic, illogical, and irrelevant insertion of spoken words or sounds between words or phrases.

intercerebral fibers = COMMISSURAL FIBERS.

intercorrelation the correlation between each variable and every other variable in a group of variables.

intercourse = COITUS.

interdental sigmatism the substitution of /th/ for /s/ and /z/, a form of lisping. Also called **sigmation**. See LISPING.

interdisciplinary approach a procedure for treatment or rehabilitation of a disabled person that utilizes the talents and experiences of therapists from a number of appropriate medical and psychological specialties. Also called **multidisciplinary approach**.

interdisciplinary environmental design the design of buildings, houses, and other facilities with contributions from representatives of many areas of environmental expertise, e.g., architecture, psychology, ecology, and social sciences.

interego a Stekel term for Freud's superego, based on the viewpoint that the part of the ego associated with moral standards serves as a mediator or compromiser rather than as a vigilant authority.

interest an attitude characterized by a need to give selective attention to something that is significant to the individual, such as an activity, goal, research area, or social theory.

interest factors the vocational interests of individuals that are matched with personality factors by industrial psychologists in determining probable success in an employment assignment. The i.f. also may include hobbies, recreation, leisure-time activities, and previous jobs.

interestingness a psychological-esthetics term applied in evaluation of a subject's reaction to a work of art and associated with factors of complexity and uncertainty, as opposed to hedonic effects. On a scale of uninteresting-interesting, judged i. tends to increase with levels of complexity and uncertainty.

interest inventories: See INTEREST TESTS.

interest tests self-report inventories in which the subject expresses likes or dislikes for activities and attitudes, especially as associated with different types of work. These are compared with the interest patterns of successful members of different occupations. Important examples are the Kuder Preference Record and the Strong-Campbell Interest Inventory. Other i.t. include the Brainerd Occupational Preference Inventory, the Minnesota Vocational Interest Inventory, the Gordon Occupational Check List, the Thurstone Interest Schedule, the Forer Vocational Survey, the Geist Picture Interest Inventory, the Holland Vocational Preference Inventory, and the Guilford-Zimmerman Interest Inventory.

interface the point at which two or more components of a system meet and interconnect. The term is used as a noun, verb, or adjective.

interference effects effects of brain stimulation that may interfere with a learning task by producing an overloading of neural activity in the brain. The effects can be demonstrated experimentally by introducing electrical stimulation of certain brain centers in animals during training in visual discrimination, bar-pressing, or similar activities.

interference theory a theory of forgetting based on the idea that information is lost or forgotten when new, incoming information conflicts or interferes with it.

intergroup-contact hypothesis the belief that prejudice between two hostile groups can be diminished and positive attitudes fostered by mere social contact.

interhemispheric transfer the transfer of memory traces or learning experiences from one cerebral hemisphere to the other. I.t. can be demonstrated with experiments using laboratory animals and can be observed in humans who transfer handedness from the right to the left hand, or vice versa, following an injury or loss of a hand.

interindividual differences the variations between persons in one or more traits, e.g., variations in intelligence. Also see INTRAINDIVIDUAL DIFFERENCES.

interiorized imitation a term applied by Piaget to the child's ability to form a mental image during the period of sensorimotor intelligence. This period starts during the second year of life when the child begins to manipulate representations as contrasted with direct, objective action. From there on, images can be combined and organized, and even imitated on their own, as in make-believe play.

interjectional theory: See ORIGIN-OF-LANGUAGE THEORIES.

interlocking reinforcement an intermittent-reinforcement schedule involving a decreasing ratio of required responses per reinforcement.

intermale aggression: See ANIMAL AGGRESSION.

intermarriage a marriage between two individuals belonging to different racial, ethnic, or religious groups; also, a marriage between two closely related persons, as in a consanguineous marriage.

intermediate-acting barbiturates: See SHORT-TO-INTERMEDIATE-ACTING BARBITURATES.

intermediate-care facilities hospital-care services for moderately ill patients. The patient may be incapable of fully independent living and usually requires routine medication and nursing care. Intermediate care generally is second to intensive care in a hospital's progressive patient-care priorities.

intermediate gene a dominant gene that is modified by a recessive gene so that the offspring resembles a blend of the parental traits. E.g., genetic traits for red and white flowers may blend into an i.g. for pink flowers.

intermediate precentral area one of three general areas of the frontal lobes, lying anterior to the precentral motor area. The i.p.a. is also involved in motor functions. Also called **premotor area; Brodmann's area 6.**

intermission in psychiatry, the interval between attacks of a mental disorder, when the symptoms temporarily subside or disappear, as frequently occurs between episodes of manic-depressive, or bipolar, disorder.

intermittent explosive disorder a disorder of impulse control consisting of several episodes in which aggressive impulses are suddenly released and expressed in serious assault or destruction of property. The behavior is often called an attack or spell by the individual, and is grossly out of proportion to any precipitating stress. There are no signs of generalized impulsive or aggressive behavior between episodes, nor is the condition caused by any other mental disorder such as schizophrenia or antisocial-personality disorder. (DSM-III)

intermittent insomnia periods of insomnia occurring several times a night, followed by difficulty in falling asleep. The condition occurs primarily in middle-aged and elderly individuals suffering from such disorders as hypertension and precordial stress.

intermittent-positive-pressure breathing machine a respirator or mechanical ventilator used to aid the breathing of a patient with a respiratory disorder. It is intermittent in function, applying pressure only when the patient inhales. An i.-p.-p. b.m. frequently is used to provide an aerosol mist deep in the pulmonary system for the relief of bronchospasms.

intermittent processing = SERIAL PROCESSING.

intermittent psychosis a term applied primarily in Europe to manic-depressive (bipolar) psychosis to indicate that the attacks are recurrent.

intermittent reinforcement in operant conditioning, any pattern of reinforcement that is not continuous; periodic reinforcement. See PARTIAL REINFORCEMENT.

internal boundary: See EGO BOUNDARIES.

internal capsule a large tract of nerve fibers found in the corpus striatum. It contains afferent and efferent fibers from all parts of the cerebral cortex as they converge near the brainstem.

internal carotid artery one of the main arteries supplying blood to the neck and head areas. It begins as a bifurcation of the common carotid artery at about the level of the thyroid cartilage in the neck, on either side of the body, and enters the skull at about the level of the eye. Inside the skull, the i.c.a. breaks up into the anterior cerebral artery branches.

internal conflict = INTRAPSYCHIC CONFLICT.

internal consistency the degree to which all of the items on a test measure the same thing.

internal environment the metabolic, hormonal, homeostasis, and other chemical, thermal, or other influences that affect the normal functioning of the body organs, and excluding factors that are external to the body.

internal feedback = PHYSIOLOGICAL FEEDBACK.

internal granular layer: See CELLULAR LAYERS OF CORTEX.

internal hair cells one of the two types of hair cells in the organ of Corti. The i.h.c. form a single row of auditory hairs, separated from the four rows of **outer hair cells** by other tissue structures. See HAIR CELLS.

internal inhibition any neural inhibitory process that reduces a conditioned-response magnitude despite the use of reinforcement.

internalization in psychoanalysis, the incorporation of attitudes, standards, and opinions of others, and particularly of the parents, into one's personality. I. is the major process involved in the formation of the superego.

internalizing behavior: See EXTERNALIZING/INTERNALIZING.

internalized sentences: See RATIONAL PSYCHO-
THERAPY.

internalized speech silent speech in which we
argue with ourselves over a course of action, rehearse what we are going to do, or reassure
ourselves when we feel threatened. Piaget has
found that children frequently reflect parental
injunctions in talking to themselves ("Kim, if
you touch that, you'll get spanked"), and Albert
Ellis claims that one of the sources of self-
defeating behavior is "self-talk" in which we repeatedly reinforce faulty beliefs (e.g., "You
have to be highly successful in every situation").
Also see SELF-TALK; INNER LANGUAGE.

internal locus of control: See LOCUS OF CONTROL.

internal rectus the external eye muscle that rotates
the eyeball inward.

internal rhythm = BIOLOGICAL RHYTHM.

internal senses the interoceptive and proprioceptive systems within the body. See INTEROCEPTOR;
PROPRIOCEPTOR.

internal-state ratings in psychological esthetics,
one of several methods of evaluating a subject's
reactions to a work of art. I.-s. r. are based on a
subject's mood while exposed to a pattern.
Other types of rating scales include descriptive
ratings and evaluative ratings. See STYLISTIC RAT-
INGS.

internal validity accuracy in establishing an experimental effect, without reference to the issue
of generalizability or representativeness (external validity); the validity of experimental results
that is assured by manipulation of the independent variable by techniques such as using a control group.

international candle an arbitrary amount of light
intensity equivalent to the total light emitted by
an ordinary candle having a flame one inch in
height. See FOOTCANDLE.

International Classification of Diseases a system
of categories of disease conditions developed by
the World Health Organization and based on
principles similar to the system of classifications
used in biology. Basic disease categories are
assigned a three-digit code number with optional
additional digits and other codes for specific disease entities. In the I.C.o.D. system, hemiplegia
is assigned the three-digit code 342; flaccid
hemiplegia is designated 342.0, utilizing the
fourth digit; spastic hemiplegia is identified as
342.1, and so on. Related disorders, e.g., multiple sclerosis (340), other demyelinating diseases
(341), and infantile cerebral palsy (343) precede
and follow 342 in numerical order. The system
was initiated in 1946 and is revised periodically.
Abbrev.: **ICD.** Also see DSM-III.

International Pilot Study of Schizophrenia: See
PRESENT STATE EXAMINATION.

interneurons = INTERNUNCIAL NEURONS.

interneurosensory learning a process of learning
that occurs when two or more systems function
together, such as the auditory and visual modalities.

internuncial neurons neurons that connect sen-

sory and motor neurons within the central nervous system. Also called **interneurons; connector neurons; connectors**.

interoceptive conditioning conditioning that employs techniques requiring direct access to internal organs, through fistulas, balloons inserted
into the digestive tract, or implanted electrical
devices. Compare EXTEROCEPTIVE CONDITIONING.

interoceptive sense = SYSTEMIC SENSE.

interoceptor any receptor consisting of sensory-
nerve cells that respond to changes within the
body, such as blood acidity or the stretching of
muscles.

interocular distance the distance between the
pupils of the left and right eyes when the eyes
are in normal fixation.

interosystem a part of the autonomic nervous system that functions wholly within the body, e.g.,
the cardiac system.

interpersonal accommodation the "give-and-
take" process that is involved in developing
satisfactory interpersonal relationships.

interpersonal concordance = GOOD-BOY-NICE-
GIRL ORIENTATION.

interpersonal conflict a conflict that takes place
between persons who differ with respect to
goals, values, or attitudes. See EXTRAPSYCHIC
CONFLICT.

interpersonal distance the distance that individuals choose to separate their "bubble" of personal space from one or more other individuals.
Studies show that most individuals maintain a
smaller i.d. for friends than for strangers. A
Comfortable Interpersonal Distance Scale
(CIDS) was developed in 1972 by M. P. Duke
and S. A. Nowicki for measuring the i.d. preferred by individuals. Also see PROXEMICS.

interpersonal morality a term proposed to
emphasize the interpersonal aspect of moral
reasoning in contrast to the cognitive, abstract
qualities of moral judgment emphasized in most
major theories. According to Haan, moral judgment occurs within a social context as a process
of discussion, dialogue, compromise, and negotiation.

interpersonal process in psychoanalysis, the
transference and countertransference between
patient and therapist, with the additional exchange of overt feelings of like or dislike for
each other.

interpersonal psychiatry the treatment technique
formulated by H. S. Sullivan, based on the study
of the interpersonal relationships of the patient,
both in and out of the therapeutic situation. The
therapist functions as a "participant observer"
who identifies with the patient's anxiety, anger,
or delusions in order to discover and modify the
faulty "security operations" and "parataxic distortions" which he is attempting to screen out by
"selective inattention," or dissociation. See
PARATAXIC DISTORTION.

interpersonal relations interactions among individuals; the pattern of our dealings with other
people, which H. S. Sullivan regarded as the

most crucial aspect of our personality and the basic source of our emotional security or insecurity.

interpersonal skill an aptitude to carry on effective relationships with others, such as cooperating, communicating thought and feeling, assuming appropriate social responsibilities, and exhibiting adequate flexibility.

interpersonal theory H. S. Sullivan's theory of personality, which is based on "the relatively enduring pattern of recurrent interpersonal situations which characterize human life." Our interactions with other people, particularly "significant others," determine not only our sense of security and our sense of self, but also the "dynamisms" that motivate our behavior. For Sullivan, personality is not "set" at an early age, nor is it primarily an expression of biological, psychosexual drives, as in Freud. Rather, it is the product of a long series of stages in which the individual gradually develops "good feeling" toward others and a sense of a "good-me" toward himself (particularly if he has had a "good mother"). The individual also learns how to ward off anxiety and correct distorted perceptions of other people ("parataxic distortions"); learns to verify his ideas through "consensual validation"; and above all seeks to achieve effective interpersonal relationships on a mature level.

interpersonal therapy a term used by J. L. Moreno for a type of psychotherapy in which there is emphasis on the interpersonal relationships of the various persons involved, such as husband, wife, and one or more other parties. The i.t. may be conducted on a cyclic basis, with alternating sessions for each of the individuals involved.

interpersonal trust in social psychology, an individual's basic assumption about the reliability of other people or groups, specifically the degree to which one can depend on others to do what they say they will do. In this usage, the key factor is not the intrinsic honesty of the other person, but his predictability.

interpolated reinforcement the temporary insertion of one reinforcement schedule into another.

interposition a monocular cue to depth perception occurring when two objects are in the same line of vision and the closer object, which is fully in view, partly conceals the farther object. Also called **relative position**.

interpretation in general, elucidation of the meaning of a play, musical composition, work of art, or other material that is not easy to understand. In psychoanalysis, it is the attempt to explain the inner significance of the patient's attitudes, impulses, dreams, memories, and characteristic behavior.

interpretive therapy a form of active, directive psychotherapy in which the therapist elicits the patient's conflicts, repressions, dreams, and resistances, which he interprets and teaches the patient to interpret in the light of the patient's experience. Also called **interpretative psychiatry.**

interquartile range the middle 50 percent of a frequency distribution, from the 26th to the 75th percentile. The i.r. is a measure of dispersion or spread of scores.

interrater agreement the correlation between several ratings by independent evaluators of a subject's performance, that is, the extent of agreement among the evaluators. See RELIABLE.

interrole conflict: See ROLE CONFLICT.

interruption tone a beat or tone heard when a constant-pitch tone is interrupted. If an interruption is slow, a beat is heard; if fast, a tone.

intersegmental arc reflex a reflex arc formed by sensory neuron or interneuron fibers that travel up or down the spinal cord to communicate with motoneurons. In some instances, the pathways may cross from one side of the spinal cord to the other, creating a crossed i.a.r.

intersegmental tracts = GROUND BUNDLES.

intersensory disorders a condition associated with damage to brain tissues involved in association or integration functions. The areas can be in the temporal, parietal, or occipital lobes and are usually in the dominant hemisphere. I.d. are characterized by difficulty in performing cross-modal matching tasks, such as tactual-visual or auditory-visual tests.

intersensory perception = CROSS-MODAL PERCEPTION.

intersex an individual who exhibits sexual characteristics of both male and female. A true i. individual is the hermaphrodite who possesses one or more contradictory sex features and has both male and female gonadal tissue. See HERMAPHRODITE; BISEXUALITY.

intersexuality the possession of the sexual characteristics of both sexes, particularly secondary characteristics and in some cases partial development of the internal or external sex organs. Also called **intersexualism**.

interstimulation the modification of behavior by the presence of others, e.g., peer-group members, resulting in either increases or decreases in interest, activity, or anxiety.

interstitial cells cells that are in spaces or between parts of a tissue. In the testis, i.c. produce the male hormone testosterone. Also called **Leydig's cells**.

interstitial-cell-stimulating hormone a hormone that stimulates the interstitial cells, or Leydig's cells, of the testes. It is the same as the luteinizing hormone that stimulates activity in the ovaries. Abbrev.: **ICSH**.

interstitial nephritis a form of kidney inflammation that involves mainly the interstitial tissue, between the functioning units. The causes include (a) excessive use of medications containing phenacetin, e.g., APC drugs, (b) systemic diseases, such as gout, and (c) exposure to heavy metals, e.g., mercury; and i.n. may be (d) a complication of a disorder involving functioning units, such as the glomeruli. I.n. often is a chronic progressive disorder leading to kidney atrophy.

interstitial neurosyphilis = CEREBRAL SYPHILIS.

interthalamic adhesions a mass of gray matter that sometimes extends across the midline of the third ventricle from the medial surfaces of the thalamic nuclei masses. Although the tissue band sometimes is identified as the **commissura cinera**, the i.a. have no particular commissural function. Also called **massa intermedia**.

intertrial interval in a series of trials, the amount of time that intervenes between each initial presentation of the stimulus.

interval: See CLASS I.

interval estimate an estimate of a parameter placing it somewhere between upper and lower limits. Also see POINT ESTIMATE.

interval reinforcement reinforcement delivered on the basis of a predetermined time schedule regardless of the number of responses per interval, in contrast to ratio reinforcement which is contingent on the number of responses. I.r. may be delivered at uniform, consecutive intervals or at variable intervals. Also see FIXED-I.R. SCHEDULE; VARIABLE-I.R. SCHEDULE; RATIO REINFORCEMENT.

interval scale a scale based on equal intervals, e.g., a temperature scale or any scale that increases and decreases in equal magnitudes. The zero point is arbitrary on the i.s. Also see NOMINAL SCALE; ORDINAL SCALE; RATIO SCALE.

intervening variable an unseen process inferred to occur within the organism between the stimulus event and the time of response; a process or event that links stimulus and response, e.g., a neural response or a psychological expectation that influences the eventual response. E. C. Tolman spoke of cognitions as intervening variables. Also called **mediating variable**. Also see HYPOTHETICAL CONSTRUCT.

intervention services provided by mental-health practitioners and others such as the clergy, workers in social-welfare agencies, and specially trained police, during a period of community disaster or personal crisis. I. includes such approaches as short-term psychotherapy, psychological first aid, and telephone crisis (hotline) service. Studies have shown that a small number of interviews, in some cases even one, conducted during a time of crisis, can have profound effects. In psychiatry, more specifically, the term applies to active efforts to ameliorate a mental patient's condition as through prescribing drugs, manipulating the environment, interpreting his behavior, or committing him to an institution.

intervention research activities designed to measure how much better a situation is often a systematic modification is imposed between two points in time, or how much better a situation is after one type of intervention program than after an alternative program. The term is used in evaluation research.

interventricular foramen of Monro an opening that connects the third ventricle of the brain with the lateral ventricle. There is an i.f.o.M. in each of the cerebral hemispheres to facilitate the flow of cerebrospinal fluid through the normal spaces in the brain tissue.

interview a face-to-face dialogue for the purpose of obtaining information, establishing a diagnosis, assessing interpersonal behavior and personality characteristics, or counseling the individual. See PSYCHIATRIC I.

interview contrast effect: See CONTRAST EFFECTS IN INTERVIEWING.

interviewer effects influence of an interviewer's attributes and behavior on a respondent's answers and on the subsequent interpretation of collected data. Included in the various i.e. are the attitudes, preconceptions, training, age, sex, and race of the interviewer. The term **interviewer bias** refers more definitely to interviewer expectations, beliefs, and prejudices as they influence the interview process.

interviewer training the instructional methods employed in training individuals to be effective interviewers. The various techniques include the use of videotapes of interviews and group discussions in addition to instructions in basic principles of interviewing.

interviewer stereotype in industrial psychology, the interviewer's concept of an "ideal" job candidate, which becomes the standard for actual job applicants.

interview group psychotherapy a type of group therapy developed by S. R. Slavson for adolescents and adults in which a therapeutically balanced group is selected on the basis of common problems and general intelligence level, and a therapeutic atmosphere is created in which the participants are encouraged to reveal their attitudes, symptoms, and feelings. For details, see ANALYTIC GROUP PSYCHOTHERAPY.

interview therapy a general term for a therapeutic dialogue in which the object is to discover the roots of a patient's problem, and help him resolve his conflicts and achieve a better emotional adjustment.

intestinal lipodystrophy: See LIPODYSTROPHY.

intestinal sepsis: See SEPSIS.

intimacy principle in Gestalt psychology, the concept that configurations are interdependent wholes with parts that cannot be changed without altering the whole.

intimacy versus isolation the sixth of Erikson's eight stages of man. The period extends from adolescence through courtship and early family life to early middle age. During this period, the individual must learn to share and care without losing himself; if he fails, he will feel alone and isolated. See ERIKSON'S EIGHT STAGES OF MAN.

intimate zone in social psychology, the area of physical distance adopted by persons in very close relationships such as that of mother and infant. The i.z. is defined as an area of no more than ½ m (1½ ft.). See PROXEMICS.

intimidation the act or habit of threatening and inspiring fear in other people. According to some psychoanalysts, especially R. P. Knight, this behavior may be used as a defense against anxiety associated with unconscious passive homosexual impulses.

intonation the sound pattern, melody, accent, and pauses of a language or an individual speaker.

intoxication an organic mental disorder characterized by maladaptive behavior (impaired judgment, belligerence, poor job performance, irresponsibility) due to the recent use of a specific substance, such as alcohol, amphetamines, or cannabis (marijuana). The clinical picture involves disturbances in attention, perception, and emotional control, but not delirium or clouding of consciousness, as in the organic brain syndromes. (DSM-III)

intraception an outlook that is warm, humanistic, and dominated by aspirations and feelings (Murray).

intraceptive signaling impulses generated and transmitted internally as stimuli for imaginative thinking. The concept was introduced by H. A. Murray.

intracerebral hemorrhage a type of stroke that tends to affect younger persons, occurring during activity and particularly during periods of stress. The symptoms and signs often include headaches, vomiting, and hypertension. I.h. differs from a typical stroke of the type that affects older people in that lost blood tends to spread throughout the brain areas instead of affecting mainly the area of the cerebrovascular accident. This is easily identified on the CAT scan.

intraconscious personality a phenomenon of multiple personalities in which one personality is aware of the thoughts and outer world of another personality.

intracranial gumma a rare form of cerebral syphilis marked by delirium, emotional lability, and some memory loss for recent events. Some cases may exhibit stupor and loss of sphincter control. The **gumma** or **syphiloma** is a granulomatous nodular growth.

intracranial hemorrhage bleeding in the brain tissues, usually as a result of a rupture of small cerebral blood vessels that have been damaged by hypertension. An i.h. almost always occurs in the putamen, thalamus, pons, or cerebellum, in that order of frequency. I.h. in the frontal, temporal, or occipital lobes usually is the result of injury or of the use of anticoagulant drugs. I.h. generally is further identified by its site, e.g., **pontine hemorrhage**.

intracranial stimulation stimulation of the brain cells of a human or other animal by direct application of an electric current or other stimulus. **Electrical i.s.** has been used for research and diagnostic purposes since the 1930s. Other types of i.s. include the use of chemicals, such as hormones and neurotransmitter substances. Abbrev.: **ICS**.

intrafusal fibers muscle cells that are located within muscle spindles and have a specialized function of sensitivity to stretching.

intrafusal motoneurons = GAMMA MOTONEURONS.

intragroup territorial behavior: See GROUP TERRITORIAL BEHAVIOR.

intraindividual differences the variations between two or more traits of a single person. E.g., certain aptitude tests measure a subject's strengths in mathematical, verbal, and analytic abilities. The three separate scores represent i.d. Also see INTERINDIVIDUAL DIFFERENCES.

intralaminar nuclei nuclei located in the internal medullary laminae (layer of fibers) of the thalamus. The nuclei are believed to have an inhibitory function since stimulation of the cells can cause moving laboratory animals literally to freeze in their tracks.

intralaminar system a diffuse system of thalamic nerve cells associated with sleep and wakefulness and believed to be a part of the reticular activating system. Also called **recruiting system**.

intramuscular injection the injection of a substance into a muscle with a hypodermic needle. The i.i. usually is made into the muscle of the upper arm, the thigh, or the buttock. The choice of muscle area is important in order to avoid damage to a nerve or blood vessel. A needle one and a half inches long is used, and it is inserted at a 90-degree angle, if possible. Also see ADMINISTRATION.

intraneurosensory learning a process of learning via one single system. Most likely, learning is never purely an intraneurosensory function. See INTERNEUROSENSORY LEARNING.

intraocular pressure: See TONOMETRY.

intrapartal eclamptic symptoms: See ECLAMPTIC SYMPTOMS.

intrapersonal conflict = INTRAPSYCHIC CONFLICT.

intrapsychic pertaining to impulses, ideas, conflicts, or other psychological phenomena that arise or occur within the psyche or mind.

intrapsychic ataxia in psychiatry, lack of coordination between feelings, thoughts and volition. I.a. is a common symptom of schizophrenia. An example is laughing while depressed. Also called **mental ataxia**. See INAPPROPRIATE AFFECT.

intrapsychic conflict the clash of opposing forces within the self, such as conflicting drives, wishes, or goals. Also called **inner conflict; intrapersonal conflict; internal conflict**.

intrapsychic society: See EXPERIENTIAL PSYCHOTHERAPY.

intrarole conflict: See ROLE CONFLICT.

intraserial learning learning of the relationships among items within a series or sequence as opposed to learning relationships between material in separate sequences.

intrasubject replication design = SINGLE-CASE EXPERIMENTAL DESIGN.

intrauterine device a device made of plastic or other material, such as copper or rubber, that is inserted into the cervix as a contraceptive device. The i.d. usually has a coil design or the shape of a T, Y, or other configuration and interferes with implantation of an embryo in the wall of the uterus. Abbrev.: **IUD**.

intravenous injection the injection by hypodermic needle of a substance into a vein. I.i. is used when rapid absorption of a drug is needed, when the substance would be irritating to the skin or muscle tissue, and when it cannot be administered through the digestive tract. I.i. also is used for blood transfusions, for feeding of parenteral nutrients, or for introducing a dye for X-ray examination of an organ or body area. Also see ADMINISTRATION.

intrinsic behavior a type of behavior expressed through a specific organ, e.g., smiling.

intrinsic cortex an area of the cerebral cortex that receives impulses from non-sensory thalamic neurons. The term was introduced by K. H. Pribram in 1958. Also called **association area**. See EXTRINSIC CORTEX.

intrinsic eye muscles muscles that are located within the eyeball, and control the size of the pupil, such as the iris and ciliary muscles. See EXTRINSIC EYE MUSCLES.

intrinsic motivation any motive or incentive that is inherent in a specific behavior or activity, e.g., studying that is motivated by genuine interest or pleasure in the subject rather than the need for course credit. Compare EXTRINSIC MOTIVATION.

intrinsic reward a reward that is implicit in an activity, e.g., the pleasure or satisfaction of developing a special skill.

introitus /intrō′itəs/ an opening or entrance, such as the i. of the vagina.

introjection the process of incorporating another person's or group's standards and values into one's own personality. E.g., a child adopts his parents' attitudes, or an adolescent adopts the behavior of the peer group. This process may also be used as a defense mehanism in situations that arouse anxiety ("If you can't beat 'em, join 'em"). See IDENTIFICATION; INCORPORATION.

intromission the act of sending or putting in something. The term is generally used to describe the insertion of the penis into the vagina.

intropunitive response a reaction to a frustrating experience in which the individual takes the blame upon himself and apologizes for his behavior ("It was my fault. I did a stupid thing"). The tendency of an individual to demean himself or direct anger against himself may be a personality characteristic or a symptom of depression. See ROSENZWEIG PICTURE-FRUSTRATION STUDY; SELF-ACCUSATION.

intropunitiveness = SELF-ACCUSATION.

introspection the examination of one's own thoughts and feelings, sometimes for the purpose of reporting on them in the introspective method of study.

introspectionism the doctrine that the basic method of psychological investigation is introspection.

introspective method a study approach in which subjects describe their conscious experiences.

introversion preoccupation with one's self and one's inner thoughts, feelings, and fantasies rather than with the outer world of people and things (Latin, "a turning inward"). Jung considered this orientation to be the basis of a distinct personality type which he characterized as contemplative, reserved, sensitive, and somewhat aloof. Eysenck has found that anxiety states, obsessive reactions, and depressive disorders tend to be associated with this pattern. Also see PASSIVE I.

introversion-extroversion a term originally introduced by Jung to describe the range of self-orientation from introversion, or preoccupation with one's own thoughts, to extroversion, characterized by outward-directed concerns. H. J. Eysenck has applied the bipolar i.-e. concept to show a conditioning relationship, with extroverts acquiring conditioned responses slower and losing them faster than introverts.

introversion-extroversion continuum the concept that most normal individuals are neither true introverts or extraverts but possess traits of both types.

introverted type a Jungian term for a person whose attitudes and feelings are habitually introverted.

intrusive treatment the imposition of a treatment or therapeutic procedure against the will of the patient.

intuition immediate insight or perception as contrasted with reasoning or reflection. Intuitions appear to be products of feeling, minimal sense impressions, or unconscious forces rather than deliberate judgment. They often have a mystical or paranormal (ESP) flavor. Jungians claim this type of awareness taps the accumulated wisdom of mankind stored in the racial, or collective, unconscious.

intuitive sociogram: See SOCIOGRAM.

intuitive type one of Jung's four functional personality types, characterized by an ability to adapt "by means of unconscious indications" and "a fine and sharpened perception and interpretation of faintly conscious stimuli." It is also one of Jung's TWO IRRATIONAL TYPES. See this entry.

inundation fear = ANTLOPHOBIA.

in utero /yōō′tərō/ inside the uterus; while in the uterus; unborn (Latin).

invalidism the acceptance of the role of a chronic invalid as expressed by preoccupation with one's state of health or refusal to recognize the fact that one's illness or disabling condition has been remedied. The motivation, usually unconscious but sometimes conscious, is to enjoy the benefits and "secondary gains" of illness such as attention and concern, being excused from responsibilities, or achieving power over others. See HYPOCHONDRIASIS.

invariance the quality of remaining constant although the surrounding conditions may change; also, the tendency of an image or after-image to retain its size despite variations in the distance of the surface upon which it is projected.

inventory a list of items, often in question form,

used in diagnosing behavior, interests, and attitudes.

inventory test the type of achievement test that contains questions in the major areas of instruction so that an overview or profile of the individual's achievement may be obtained. In addition, the term inventory is commonly applied to tests of interest and personality designed to provide a broad overview of personality patterns in a variety of areas.

inverse derivation = BACK-FORMATION.

inverse relationship a negative relationship, meaning that as one variable increases, the other variable decreases.

inverse-square law a law of physics that states that energy decreases in proportion to the square of the distance from its source. The law applies to sound, light, heat, and odors.

inversion in psychology, a term variously used for homosexuality and assumption of the role of the opposite sex. The term also applies to the reversed images on the retina. Also see OCCASIONAL I.

inversion of affect = REVERSAL.

inversion relationship a change in the usual roles of members of a family or group, e.g., when a boy replaces the father as the family breadwinner.

invert an infrequently used term for a homosexual.

inverted factor analysis a factor-analysis technique for investigation among persons and their traits by correlating their scores on a series of tests. Also called **Q technique**.

inverted Oedipus complex = NEGATIVE OEDIPUS COMPLEX.

inverted-U function the term for a correlation between arousal level and level of performance that indicates that an intensification of arousal up to a moderate level improves efficiency but that beyond the moderate range the performance declines. That is, a moderate arousal level is associated with maximum performance.

investment = CATHEXIS.

inveterate drinking = DELTA ALCOHOLISM.

inviolacy motive the need to defend one's name and prevent self-depreciation (Murray).

invisible playmate = IMAGINARY COMPANION.

in vitro /vē′trō/ referring to biological conditions or processes that occur or are made to occur outside the living body, usually in a test tube (Latin, "in glass").

in vivo /vē′vō/ referring to biological conditions or processes that occur or are observed within the living organism (Latin, "inside something alive").

invocational psychosis a psychotic reaction to religious rituals, such as prayers or incantations in revivalist meetings or voodoo ceremonies.

involuntary hospitalization commitment of a patient with a mental illness to a mental hospital. The trend is toward encouraging voluntary hospitalization wherever possible, and limiting i.h. to patients who are considered dangerous to themselves or others, who are seriously ill but fail to recognize their need for treatment, or who cannot meet their own needs in the community or survive without medical attention. The problem is complex and knotty; e.g., some authorities advocate involuntary confinement of dangerous patients in correctional facilities which provide psychiatric care if they have already been convicted of overt offenses.

involuntary movements movements occurring without intention or volition, such as tics and mannerisms; also, movements carried out in spite of an effort to suppress them, as in athetosis.

involuntary muscles = SMOOTH MUSCLES.

involuntary response a response that is not under conscious control; an automatic, unlearned response or reflex, e.g., the contraction of the pupils.

involution a retrograde change in development, marked by physical and psychological deterioration.

involutional occurring in the years of menopause; menopausal.

involutional paraphrenia an obsolete term for a paranoid state occurring during the involutional period. See INVOLUTIONAL PSYCHOTIC REACTION.

involutional paranoid state a psychosis occurring in the climacteric period characterized by delusions of sin, guilt, poverty, nihilism, or persecution in addition to depressive symptoms. This DSM-II term was replaced in DSM-III by ATYPICAL PARANOID DISORDER. See this entry. Also see INVOLUTIONAL PSYCHOTIC REACTION.

involutional psychotic reaction a mental disorder occurring in late middle life or during the menopausal period, characterized by severe depression, and less often by paranoid thinking. The depressed type was long known as involutional melancholia, but that term has been abandoned by the American Psychiatric Association. Salient symptoms of the depressed type are agitation, apprehensiveness, feelings of despair and worthlessness, persistent insomnia, chronic fatigue, and loss of appetite. The paranoid patient also suffers from agitated depression and anxiety, and in addition manifests persecutory delusions or, in some cases, self-condemnatory, hypochondriacal, or nihilistic delusions. These symptoms are believed to be psychological reactions to physical changes and external stresses. The treatment of choice is electroshock therapy, though psychoactive drugs may also be useful. Also called **climacteric psychosis**. See MELANCHOLIA; MAJOR DEPRESSION.

inward picture an internally perceived image such as the images in dreams and fantasies. Jung, who introduced the term, emphasized that the i.p. not only occurs inwardly but is a picture of the inner, true self.

IO = INPUT-OUTPUT MECHANISM.

iodopsin a photosensitive chemical pigment found in the cone cells of the retina. See RHODOPSIN.

ionizing radiation the radiation of ionizing energy

or particles, as in the emission of X-rays, or alpha or beta particles that are capable of altering the atomic structure of elements within living tissues.

ion pump an ion-transport system through a cell membrane. The i.p. regulates the flow of ions or molecules through tiny holes in the membrane according to their size and the internal metabolic needs of the cell.

iontophoresis in orthopedic therapy, the use of a low-voltage electric current with a vasodilating drug or analgesic ointments to raise superficial and deep-skin-layer temperatures for a longer period than alternative techniques of applying external heat. I. also is used to introduce electrolytes into body tissues.

IOP: See TONOMETRY.

iophobia = TOXIPHOBIA.

iota /ī·ōt′ə/ ninth letter of the Greek Alphabet (I, ι).

Iowa Silent Reading Tests: See DIAGNOSTIC EDUCATIONAL TESTS.

Iowa Stuttering Scale a series of 39 recorded samples of stuttering ranked according to the equal-appearing-intervals method. The object is to assign a scale value to the subject's speech.

Iowa Tests of Basic Skills an achievement battery providing tests for reading, vocabulary, language, arithmetic, and work-study skills for each grade from 3 to 9, with norms for the beginning, middle, and end of each year.

I-persona a term introduced by Burrows to represent a synthesis of the individual's cortical, social, and symbolic functions in the personality.

iproniazid $C_9H_{13}N_3O$—a monoamine oxidase inhibitor developed in the 1950s for the treatment of tuberculosis and later found to have therapeutic value in the treatment of affective disorders. I. was found to elevate the mood of tuberculosis patients, and clinical trials led to its use as a "psychic energizer" to treat depression. However, it has been replaced in recent years by other antidepressant drugs. Also see MONOAMINE OXIDASE INHIBITORS.

ipsation a seldom used term for autoerotism.

ipsative scale a scale in which the individual's characteristic behavior is used as the standard. See IPSATIVE SCORE.

ipsative score a person's score relative to his own baseline, rather than compared with other individuals. Thus an individual with generally low ability will still have relative strength in certain areas, and an i.s. will emphasize this. Also see NORMATIVE SCORE.

ipsilateral existing on the same side, said, e.g., of an abnormality that occurs on the same side of the body. Also called **ipsolateral**. Compare CONTRALATERAL.

ipsilateral deficit a loss of ability to perform a learned task on one side of the body following an injury or induced lesion to a cortical area on the same side of the body. A cortical lesion usually results in a contralateral deficit, or loss of a normal function on the opposite side of the body.

ipsolateral = IPSILATERAL.

IPSP = INHIBITORY POSTSYNAPTIC POTENTIAL.

IPSS: See PRESENT STATE EXAMINATION.

IQ *i*ntelligence *q*uotient; a rating of intelligence based on psychological tests, calculated by dividing the mental age (MA) by the chronological age (CA), and multiplying by 100 to eliminate decimals. Also see CONSTANCY OF THE IQ; DEVIATION IQ.

There are critics who consider the concept of IQ (and other intelligence scales) deeply flawed, mainly in reflecting a biological determinism that often serves racist purposes; they point out that the IQ test is largely a measure of prior learning of skills and knowledge and not simply a measure of some underlying native ability (and that many testees may just not have the middle-class habit of sitting still and following orders, while functioning well "in the real world"); and they refer to cases of misrepresentation of facts in the history of IQ research. (Binet himself was dismayed at seeing the tool that he had devised to identify learning-disabled children applied to normal individuals.) Also see CULTURE-FAIR TESTS; CULTURE-FREE TESTS; SIX-HOUR RETARDED CHILD.

IRB = INSTITUTIONAL REVIEW BOARD.

-irid-; -irido- a combining form relating to the iris.

iridocyclitis an inflammation of the iris and ciliary body of the eye. **Heterochromic i.** is a form of the disorder that results in a loss of pigment in the iris.

iris a muscular disk that surrounds the pupil of the eye and controls the amount of light entering the eye by contracting or relaxing. The i. contains a pigment that gives the eye its coloration, which is determined by hereditary factors.

iris coloboma a congenital defect of the iris which shows as a cleft or fissure (coloboma) extending outward from the edge of the pupil. A coloboma usually occurs in the lower portion of the iris. The defect may be one of several signs of a chromosomal anomaly.

iris dysgenesis = RIEGER'S SYNDROME.

iritic reflex the action of the iris in adjusting the diameter of the pupil as the intensity of the light in the environment changes.

IRM = INNATE RELEASING MECHANISM.

ironed-out facies a flattened facial expression observed in general-paresis patients, due to atonicity of the facial muscles.

iron lung the common name for a ventilator or respirator that provides artificial respiration by alternating positive and negative pressure of the patient's chest. The i.l. was developed originally as a large metal tank that enclosed the body of the patient, except for the exposed head, and used to sustain life in poliomyelitis patients who had suffered paralysis of the respiratory muscles.

iron overloading the accumulation of dangerous levels of iron in the body tissues, a pathologic effect of Cooley's anemia. The iron is needed for the patient's hemoglobin molecules, but because of an inborn error of metabolism it cannot be utilized in the hemoglobin but is deposited as a toxic substance in the heart, liver, and other organs. Therapies for Cooley's anemia are directed toward compensation for i.o.

irradiation an outward diffusion of energy, e.g., nerve impulses, light, or diffusion of conditioned responses.

irradiation effects a factor in the occurrence of ionizing radiation, based on evidence of congenital-malformation rates in geographic areas where natural background radiation is high. Examples include anencephaly, microcephaly, mongolism, cerebral atrophy, and mental retardation. I.e. on cells of the testes appear as abnormal cell divisions within two hours after exposure to radioactivity.

irradiation theory of learning a concept that learning involves selective reinforcement of one of many responses within a response hierarchy.

irrationality as used by E. Fromm, a distorted perception of reality; a highly subjective world view or "frame of orientation."

irrational types the category of functional types established by Jung for individuals whose functions seem to be determined by the intensity of perceptions rather than reasoned judgment. The category includes the intuitive and sensational types.

irreality level a part of a person's life space that is dominated by fantasy, desire, prejudices, and needs (Kurt Lewin).

irrelevant language a language composed of sounds, phrases, or words that are understood only by the speaker, as observed in cases of schizophrenia and autistic children.

irresistible apprehension Kraepelin's term for obsessive-compulsive disorder.

irresistible impulse in forensic psychiatry, an uncontrollable urge, particularly the urge to perform a criminal act. The **i.i. test** is a supplement, in some states, to the M'Naghten rules, to the effect that a prisoner is exempt from criminal responsibility if at the time of the crime he was acting under an impulse which he was powerless to resist by reason of mental disease. Also see M'NAGHTEN RULES.

irresponsibility a legal term used in claiming a person is not responsible for his conduct because of mental impairment.

irritability a state of excessive, easily provoked anger, annoyance, or impatience; also, the capacity of living matter, and particularly nervous tissue, to respond to stimulation.

irritability of cell a loss of equilibrium in a cell because of a mechanical, chemical, electrical, or other stimulus that alters the status of ions or ion charges on or near the cell membrane. I.o.c. usually causes an expression of cell activity, such as transmission of a nerve impulse.

irritable heart of soldiers a Civil War term for what is now known as combat reaction or battle fatigue. According to some authorities, it corresponds most closely to Da Costa's syndrome, an anxiety reaction experienced by soldiers in active combat.

irritable mood: See IRRITABILITY.

Isakower, Otto /ēˈzäkōvər/ Austrian psychoanalyst, 1899–1972. See ISAKOWER PHENOMENON.

Isakower phenomenon strange sensations in the mouth, skin, hands, and the border region around the body, including vaguely perceived advancing or receding objects. The phenomenon occurs primarily while one falls asleep, but may also occur in high fever and stress situations. Isakower compared these sensations to déjà vu and the epileptic aura, and attributed them to a revival of traumatic experiences involving oral deprivation very early in life ("A Contribution to the Psychopathology Associated with Falling Asleep," *International Journal of Psychoanalysis*, 1938). See ABSTRACT PERCEPTIONS; BLANK HALLUCINATION; DREAM SCREEN.

-ischi-; -ischio- /-iskē-/ a combining form relating to the hip, the **ischium**.

ischophonia /iskō-/ an alternative term for stuttering or stammering (from Greek *ischein*, "to keep back, stop"). Also called **ischnophonia**. See STUTTERING.

Ishihara, Shinobu Japanese ophthalmologist, 1879–1963. See ISHIHARA TEST.

Ishihara test a test for color blindness utilizing a series of plates in which numbers or letters are formed by dots of a given color against a background of dots in varying degrees of brightness and saturation. The test, developed by the ophthalmologist Shinobu Ishihara, is used to diagnose specific types of color blindness.

island deafness: See TONAL GAP; TONAL ISLAND.

island of Reil a feature of the cerebral cortex of primate brains consisting of a cleft or division (invagination) near the lower end of the fissure of Sylvius.

islands of Langerhans clusters of cells within the pancreas that secrete two hormones, insulin and glucagon. Cells that secrete glucagon are called **alpha cells**, those that secrete insulin are called **beta cells**.

-iso- a combining form meaning same, equal, alike.

isocarboxazid: See MONOAMINE OXIDASE INHIBITORS.

isocortex = NEOCORTEX.

isohippocampal rhythm a theta-wave electrical rhythm that is detected in the hippocampal region of the limbic system in response to arousal stimuli. It is demonstrated in laboratory animals during performance of learning tasks.

isolate on a sociometric test, the individual chosen often or not at all; also, the group member who is psychologically isolated. More generally, an i. is any person who maintains no, very few, or exceedingly shallow personal relationships. Also called **outsider; social island**. Also see SOCIOMETRY. Compare STAR.

isolated brain: See ENCÉPHALE ISOLÉ; CERVEAU INSOLÉ.

isolated environment: See ENVIRONMENTAL ENRICHMENT.

isolated explosive disorder a disorder of impulse

control characterized by a single discrete episode in which the individual commits a violent, catastrophic act, such as shooting total strangers and then himself during a sudden fit of rage. The episode is out of all proportion to any precipitating stress, and there are no signs of generalized impulsive or aggressive behavior, or any other mental disorder such as schizophrenia or antisocial personality disorder. Also called **catathymic crisis**. Also see CROCODILE MAN. (DSM-III)

isolate monkey: See SOCIAL-ISOLATION SYNDROME; MONKEY THERAPIST.

isolation an unconscious defense mechanism in which the individual screens out painful anxiety-provoking feelings by such methods as recalling traumatic events without experiencing emotion, or adopting a stoical attitude. Pathological forms are found in obsessional preoccupation with repetitive thoughts and actions; dissociative reactions, such as amnesic episodes; and the schizophrenic's loss of contact with reality. Also called **i. of affect**. Also see COMPARTMENTALIZATION; SOCIAL-I. SYNDROME; SENSORY I.; INTIMACY VERSUS I.

isolation amentia a type of mental deficiency due to extreme childhood isolation from social stimuli.

isolation effect a learning technique in which an item is isolated in a list by a distinctive color or type.

isolation experiments the removal of a subject from social or other contact with other members of its group in order to observe behavioral or other effects. Rats reared in isolation show brain-cell deficits ranging from 11 percent in the medulla to 59 percent in the neocortex, when compared with littermates raised together.

isolation of affect: See ISOLATION.

isometric contraction a type of muscle contraction in which tension develops although the muscle does not shorten, as when a weightlifter grasps a set of bar bells. Compare ISOTONIC CONTRACTION.

isomorphism a one-to-one relationship. The term is applied in various ways, e.g., in the relationship between a perceived stimulus and the resulting verbal process, such as pronunciation of a printed word, and in the concept that the excitatory fields of the brain increase with the size of the perceived stimulus. In Gestalt psychology, i. is a relationship in size between a stimulus and the area of the brain responding to the stimulus. In genetics, i. is the production of similar gametes by polypoid organisms even though homologous chromosomes may contain genes in different combinations.

isoniazid a drug of choice for the treatment of tuberculosis because of the sensitivity of tuberculosis mycobacteria to the chemical. Use of the drug can cause a form of neuritis by blocking the function of pyridoxine, or vitamin B_6, in metabolizing glutamic acid in the GABA shunt. I. is a precursor of the monoamine oxidase inhibitor iproniazid, and has some antidepressant activity. Also called **isonicotinic-acid hydrazide (INH)**.

isopathic principle a generalization that a symptom can be relieved by the simple expression of the emotion that has been repressed; e.g., guilt caused by hate can be relieved by an exhibition of hate. The term was introduced by E. Jones. Also called **homeopathic principle**.

isophilia a term coined by H. S. Sullivan for feelings of affection or affectionate behavior toward members of one's own sex, but without the genital component characteristic of homosexuality.

isopropanol C_3H_8O—an isomer of propyl alcohol used as an ingredient in cosmetics, e.g., hand lotions, and medications for external use. It also may be used as an antiseptic. Taken internally, as a drug of abuse, i. is extremely toxic after initial effects similar to those of ethyl alcohol. Also called **isopropyl alcohol**.

isoproterenol $C_{11}H_{17}NO_3$—an adrenergic drug administered as a bronchodilator in respiratory disorders and as a heart stimulant in cardiac block. It is one of the most active of the sympathomimetic amines that affect beta receptors. It is similar to epinephrine in excitation of the central nervous system and resembles epinephrine in most other actions, e.g., vasodilation.

isotonic contraction a type of muscle contraction in which the muscle bundle shortens and thickens, as when a person flexes the biceps muscle of the upper arm. Compare ISOMETRIC CONTRACTION.

ITA = INITIAL TEACHING ALPHABET.

Itard, Jean /zhäN ētär'/ French otologist, 1774–1838. See WILD BOY OF AVEYRON.

itch a cutaneous sensory experience related to pain. The nerve endings associated with i. are the same as those sensitive to the prick-pain sensation produced by a needle or electric stimulus. A rapidly repeated prick-pain sensation produces the i. reaction.

item analysis a statistical comparison of the items in a test against some particular criterion, usually in order to select the items that are most valid.

item difficulty the difficulty of a test item for a particular group as determined by the proportion of individuals who pass or fail the item.

item scaling the assignment of a test item to a scale position according to its difficulty.

item selection the selection of a test item on the basis of factors such as validity, reliability, and freedom from ambiguity.

item validity the degree to which the structure and form of a test item conveys the intention or main point of the item's designer; also, the degree to which a test item actually expresses a question's meaning or a problem's essence.

item weighting assigning a numerical value to a test item that expresses a percentage of the sum total of the test's score. E.g., an essay question may be assigned a value of 40, representing 40 out of 100 possible points.

I-Thou a term used by the philosopher Martin Buber for the relationship of mutual trust, partnership, and recognition of each other's uniqueness which he believed to be essential to the development of individual identity as well as a constructive group process.

itinerant teacher an educationally trained individual who travels to several schools providing specialized instruction to children in many classrooms.

-itis /-īt'is/ a combining form relating to an inflammation.

IUD = INTRAUTERINE DEVICE.

IV = INDEPENDENT VARIABLE.

J

Jackson, John Hughlings English neurologist, 1835–1911. Though primarily known for his studies of focalized seizures (which he attributed to sudden explosive discharges in the motor area of the cortex), J. also described the evolution of the nervous system from the primitive reflexes of the old brain and spinal cord to the middle level which controls motor activities, and to the frontal lobe which controls abstract thought. See JACKSONIAN EPILEPSY; JACKSON'S LAW; JACKSON'S SYNDROME; CONVULSIVE DISORDERS; FOCAL DEGENERATION.

Jacksonian epilepsy a type of epilepsy characterized by recurrent focal seizures which usually start with muscle twitching, localized tonic contractions or clonic movements in one region or side of the body, which then increase in severity and spread to the other side of the body, often terminating in a generalized convulsion with loss of consciousness.

Jackson's law the principle that when mental deterioration results from brain disease, the higher and more recently developed functions are lost first.

Jackson's syndrome a set of symptoms including paralysis of the soft palate, tongue, pharynx, and larynx plus paralysis of shoulder muscles on the same side of the body due to a medulla disorder involving the hypoglossal, vagus, and spinal accessory nerves. Also called **Hughlings Jackson's syndrome; MacKenzie's syndrome.**

Jacobson, Edmund American physician, 1888— See PROGRESSIVE RELAXATION.

jactatio capitis nocturnis = HEAD-ROLLING.

jactation extreme restlessness marked by convulsive movements and tossing about. Also called **jactitation.**

Jakob, Alfons /yä′kôp/ German psychiatrist, 1884–1931. See CREUTZFELDT-JAKOB DISEASE; SLOW VIRUS; UNCONVENTIONAL VIRUS.

jamais phenomenon /zhämä′/ a defense mechanism in which the individual wards off painful feelings or events by insisting that "I have never experienced anything like that before" (French *jamais,* "never"). The reaction varies in intensity and appears to be related to a form of denial. Also called **jamais.**

jamais vu /zhämävē′/ a falsification of memory, or paramnesia, in which a situation that has actually been experienced appears to be completely unfamiliar (French, "never seen").

James, William American psychologist and philosopher, 1842–1910. J., the most influential psychologist of his time, served as professor of physiology, philosophy, and psychology at Harvard University, teaching many students who contributed to the development of American psychology (Hall, Woodworth, Thorndike, and others); introduced the functional approach as well as theories of emotion, habit, and consciousness to students through his monumental text, *Principles of Psychology* (1890); and made lasting contributions to the psychology of religion (*Varieties of Religious Experience,* 1902) and to psychical research as a means of uncovering unconscious factors in mental life. See JAMES-LANGE THEORY; FUNCTIONALISM; PRAGMATISM; SELF; STREAM OF ACTION; STREAM OF CONSCIOUSNESS; TENDER-MINDED; TOUGH-MINDED.

James-Lange theory a combination of viewpoints of William James, who believed that emotions consist of experiences of muscular and visceral reactions to provoking stimuli, and Carl Georg Lange, who contended that emotions coincide with vascular changes. James argued that we do not run because we are afraid but are afraid because we run, and that "a disembodied emotion is a sheer nonentity."

Janet, Pierre Marie Félix /zhäne′/ French psychologist, 1859–1947. After studying at the University of Paris, J. was appointed director of the psychological clinic at Salpêtrière Hospital by Charcot. Focusing his attention on neuroses, he used hypnosis as a therapeutic technique, and was the first to make a clear distinction between neurasthenia and psychasthenia. But he attributed these and other psychiatric disorders, such as hysteria and multiple personality, to physical disability and stress rather than unconscious factors. See JANET'S DISEASE; JANET'S TEST; APHORIA; CANALIZATION; IDÉE FIXE; LA BELLE INDIFFÉRENCE; LIQUIDATION OF ATTACHMENT; MANIA OF RECOMMENCEMENT; PSYCHASTHENIA.

Janet's disease psychasthenia, characterized by stages of pathologic fear or anxiety, obsessions, fixed ideas, feelings of inadequacy, self-accusation, and feelings of strangeness and depersonalization.

Janet's test a tactile-sensibility test in which the subject simply answers in the affirmative or negative when asked if he feels the touch of the examiner's fingers.

Janimine $C_{19}H_{25}ClN_2$—a trademark for imipramine hydrochloride, an antidepressant drug of the tricyclic class used for both psychotic and psychoneurotic depression.

Jansky, Jan Czechoslovakian physician, 1873–1921. See NEURONAL LIPIDOSIS (there: **Bielschowsky-Jansky disease**); SPHINGOLIPIDOSES.

Janusian thinking an alternative term for oppositional thinking, or the capacity to conceive contradictory ideas or images. The term is derived from the name of a Roman god, Janus, who was able to face in opposite directions simultaneously.

Japanese B encephalitis a viral infection of the brain that is transmitted by mosquitoes, usually in warm-weather epidemics. The infection spreads through the brainstem, basal ganglia, and white matter of the cerebrum, causing a mortality rate that averages above 50 percent. Children who survive may experience paralysis, mental retardation, or personality changes.

jargon aphasia = WORD SALAD.

Jaspers, Karl /yäs′pərs/ German philosopher and psychiatrist, 1883–1969. See EXISTENTIALISM.

jaundice a condition associated with a variety of disorders of the liver, gallbladder, and blood and marked by the deposition of bile pigments in the skin, eye surfaces, and excrement. The pigment, which usually is first observed in discoloration of the normally white areas of the eyes, is produced as bilirubin, a breakdown product of the hemoglobin of red blood cells. J. is associated with liver infections but also may be caused by a drug reaction, and is a causative factor in neurologic birth defects. Also called **icterus**. Also see BILIRUBIN; ICTERUS GRAVIS NEONATORUM.

jaw-grinding an unconscious habit of grinding or gnashing the teeth that often is associated with intense mental or physical effort. The term is essentially equivalent to BRUXISM. See this entry.

jaw jerk a reflex test used in the diagnosis of corticospinal-tract lesions: The examiner strikes a downward blow on the lower jaw while it hangs passively open; if the lesion is present, the jaw closes reflexively.

jaw-winking sign = MARCUS GUNN'S SIGN.

JDI = JOB DESCRIPTION INDEX.

jealousy a common but complex emotion composed of feelings of psychic pain, loss of self-esteem, envy, hostility towards a rival, and self-blame. It frequently makes its first appearance at the age of two or three in the form of hostility when a new baby arrives. In adults it may lead to "crimes or passion," or take the form of a paranoid delusion in which the patient maintains his conviction of infidelity despite evidence to the contrary. Also see DELUSIONAL J.; ALCOHOLIC J.; PROJECTED J.

jejunal-bypass operation a surgical procedure for treating obesity. The operation involves removing a portion of the **jejunum**, an eight-foot-long section of the small intestine from which much of the digested food is absorbed. The digestive tract is then reconnected so that it bypasses the jejunal portion.

Jellenik, Elvin Morton American physiologist, 1890–1963. See ALPHA ALCOHOLISM; BETA ALCOHOLISM; GAMMA ALCOHOLISM; DELTA ALCOHOLISM; EPSILON ALCOHOLISM.

Jendrassik, Ernö Hungarian physician, 1858–1921. See JENDRASSIK REINFORCEMENT.

Jendrassik reinforcement a technique of reinforcing the patellar reflex response by having the subject grasp his hands and pull on them while the reflex is tested.

Jespersen, Otto Danish philologist, 1860–1943. See ORIGIN-OF-LANGUAGE THEORIES.

jet-lag phenomenon a maladjustment of circadian rhythms that results from being transported through several global time zones within a short span of time. Rest-work, eating, body temperature, and adrenocortical-secretion cycles may require several days in extreme cases to adjust to local time, which may be several hours earlier or later than the time for which the body originally was adjusted.

jimmy-legs syndrome = EKBOM'S SYNDROME.

jimson weed common name of Datura stramonium, which grows wild in eastern North America and contains an intoxicating agent. The agent is a mixture of hyoscyamine, scopolamine, and atropine, which produces hallucinations, loss of motor coordination, and amnesia for the period of intoxication. The name is a corruption of "James-Town weed," the identity given the plant by early settlers of Virginia.

j.n.d.: See DIFFERENCE THRESHOLD.

job analysis in industrial psychology, the collection of information on a specific job from supervisors or incumbents, or through questionnaires, films, and recordings. The information includes work descriptions, worker behavior, tools, working conditions, and skills involved in the job.

job-characteristics model the basic parameters of a job that affect the psychological state of the employee. They include skill variety, task identity, task significance, autonomy, and feedback.

job-component method a job-evaluation technique based on the assumption that similarities in job content impose similar job demands on the employees and should therefore warrant corresponding pay scales. The j.-c.m. may be applied through a statistical analysis of data obtained from a Position Analysis Questionnaire that covers 194 different job components.

Job Description Index a system of measuring employee attitudes in areas of work, supervision, pay, promotions, and coworkers by allowing the employee to indirectly describe the job from his viewpoint. Abbrev.: **JDI**.

job design in industrial psychology, systematic efforts to improve work methods, equipment, and the working environment through such approaches as (a) methods analysis, or industrial engineering, focused on the development of efficient work methods, (b) human factors, an approach that is primarily concerned with the design of physical equipment and facilities as well as the environment in which people work, and (c) job enlargement or enrichment aimed at expanding the complexity and responsibility of jobs. See JOB ENLARGEMENT; HUMAN ENGINEERING; HUMAN-FACTORS PSYCHOLOGY; ENGINEERING PSYCHOLOGY.

job dimensions the basic features of jobs, such as operating machines or equipment, performing clerical or related activities, or having decision or communicating responsibilities, as well as the work schedules and environment.

job enlargement in industrial psychology, the expansion of responsibilities associated with a particular job, either "horizontally," by increasing the number of subtasks involving the same level of complexity, and by performing different duties at different times, or "vertically," by requiring the employee to perform more complex tasks and undertake increased responsibility and autonomy.

job enrichment the enhancement of interest and attitude by employees toward work tasks by improving the "quality of life" on the job. J.e. methods include reducing boredom by giving employees a variety of different tasks during a work schedule and allowing employees freedom to design their own ways of doing work if it improves their effectiveness on the job.

job evaluation in industrial psychology, determination of the rate of pay for jobs by such methods as (a) comparison with other jobs and with the going rate, (b) assigning jobs to specific classifications on the basis of overall worth, (c) assigning point values to jobs according to such factors as education, experience, and the initiative or effort needed, (d) comparison with rankings and ratings of key jobs according to skill and responsibility requirements; and (e) weighting of the various components of the job.

job information the data relating to jobs and workers used in job-analysis studies. The data may include work activities, such as weaving or welding, human behaviors required, such as communicating or making decisions, personnel requirements, and types of materials processed and equipment used.

job interview = EMPLOYMENT INTERVIEW.

job inventory = TASK INVENTORY.

job performance a criterion of job-related behavior that usually is measured in terms of quantity or quality of output, or both.

job placement the assignment of employment on the basis of the person's abilities and interests, and job availability.

job-placement stage a level of rehabilitation training and work conditioning from which the disabled person is presumed to be ready to move into the competitive job market. The sheltered-workshop personnel also help the patient advance from the j.-p.s. by training him to fill out job applications and preparing him to cope with the job interview.

job requirements the personnel requirements that are reasonably necessary for performing a work task safely and effectively. J.r. may include good eyesight, ability to drive a truck, or ability to perform mathematical calculations quickly.

job-sample experiences vocational rehabilitation for individuals with disabilities. The program enables the clients to obtain training in a sheltered environment for jobs in the community workforce. J.-s.e. are also useful to the nondisabled.

job satisfaction the attitude of a worker toward his job, sometimes expressed as a hedonic response of liking or disliking the work itself, the rewards (pay, promotions, recognition), or the context (working conditions, benefits).

job specifications = PERSONNEL SPECIFICATIONS.

job-specific test a test of the particular abilities required for a particular job, such as typing or welding. It is used primarily in personnel selection and placement and in measuring performance in a training program.

job tenure: See TURNOVER.

Jocasta complex an abnormal attachment of a mother for her son, a disorder named for Jocasta, the mother and wife of Oedipus.

Johnson, Frank Chambliss American pediatrician, 1894–1934. See STEVENS-JOHNSON SYNDROME.

Johnson, Virginia American psychologist, 1925 —. See BIOPHYSICAL SYSTEM; DUAL-SEX THERAPY; PSYCHOSOCIAL SYSTEM; SENSATE-FOCUS-ORIENTED THERAPY; SPECTATOR ROLE.

Johnston, Christopher American physician, died 1891. See JOHNSTON'S ORGAN.

Johnston's organ a sense organ that is part of the antenna of flies. J.o. is vital for **anemotaxis**, or orientation in air currents, and aids the fly in making the necessary postural changes to compensate for variations in air flow.

John the Baptist saint, first century A.D. See CHOREA (also called **Saint John's disease**).

joint alignment the natural symmetry of adjoining bones of the skeleton when appropriate standing or sitting posture is maintained. Many of the movable parts of the body form geometric patterns when j.a. is normal. E.g., the bony prominences of the upper arm form an equilateral triangle when the elbow is flexed; any distortion of the triangle is a sign of faulty or damaged alignment.

joke a witty story which provokes laughter by pointedly and succinctly making fun of the high and mighty, by releasing sexual repressions, or by taking serious things lightly and thereby helping us to get them in perspective. See HUMOR; WIT; PUN.

joking mania: See WITZELSUCHT.

Jones, (Alfred) Ernest British psychoanalyst, 1879–1958. An early disciple of Freud and founder of the British Psychoanalytic Society, J.

wrote the definitive biography of Freud, as well as numerous essays in which art, literature, and folklore were interpreted in the light of psychoanalytic concepts. See ROSS-JONES TEST; APHANISIS; DEUTEROPHALLIC PHASE; GOD COMPLEX; IMAGO; ISOPATHIC PRINCIPLE; MAMMALINGUS; PROTOPHALLIC PHASE; TALKING CURE; TRUE SYMBOLISM; VERBAL SUGGESTION.

Jones, Henry Bence: See BENCE JONES.

Jonestown mass suicide: See COLLECTIVE SUICIDE.

Jost, Adolf /yŏst/ German psychologist, 1874—. See JOST'S LAW.

Jost's law the principle that of two associations of equal strength but unequal age, practice is of greater benefit to the older.

judgment in psychiatry, the capacity to recognize relationships, draw conclusions from evidence, and make critical evaluations of events and people. In psychophysics, j. is the ability to determine the presence or relative magnitude of stimuli.

Juke the pseudonym for an American family studied by psychologists in the early 1900s because most members were retarded or social misfits.

Jumping Frenchmen of Maine syndrome a culture-specific syndrome occurring among members of a religious sect which originated in Wales, the United Society of Believers in the Second Appearing of Christ. Their rites involve jumping, rolling on the ground, and uttering barking sounds until a state of ecstasy is achieved. This state usually subsides at the end of the ceremony, but some members remain affected and begin to jump and shake any time a sharp command is directed at them, or even if a finger is pointed toward them.

junction: See PARAPATHETIC PROVISO.

Jung, Carl Gustav /yo͝ong/ Swiss psychiatrist and philosopher, 1875–1961. A wide-ranging student of medicine, archeology, mysticism, and philosophy, J. associated himself with the psychoanalytic school because it recognized the influence of the unconscious, but after five years he broke with Freud over Freud's theories of infantile sexuality, his emphasis on instinctual impulses, and his limitation of mental contents to personal experiences. In contrast, J. held that we are molded by our "racial" as well as personal history, and motivated by moral and spiritual values more than by psychosexual drives. On this basis he constructed a theory of "analytic psychology," in which the key concepts are (a) the ego, a developing entity in which conscious and unconscious forces are integrated and individualized, (b) the personal unconscious, consisting of half-forgotten memories and experiences which in some cases become fragmented into complexes, due to traumatic experiences or internal conflicts, (c) the collective unconscious, a dynamic store of ancestral images, or "archetypes," which constitute the inherited foundation of our intellectual life and personality, (d) personality dynamics, viewed in terms of opposing forces, such as conscious versus uncon-

scious values, introversive versus extraversive tendencies, and rational versus irrational processes, and (e) personality development, in which the basic psychic energy, which he termed the libido, is constructively utilized in resolving these conflicts and achieving a new integration. If, on the other hand, the conflicts persist and generate emotional disturbances, J. advocated a form of therapy aimed at facing and overcoming difficulties by eliciting unconscious forces that will help the individual solve his problems and realize his potential. This process usually involves the study of dreams and drawings, and exploration of new activities that will express the individual's personality, but does not utilize the Freudian couch or the method of free association. Adjective: **Jungian**.

See JUNG ASSOCIATION TEST; ACTIVE-DAYDREAM TECHNIQUE; AFFECT-FANTASY; ANAGOGIC INTERPRETATION; ANALYSIS IN DEPTH; ANALYST; ANALYTIC PSYCHOLOGY; ANAMNESTIC ANALYSIS; ANIMA; ANIMUS; ANTHROPOS; ARCHAIC INHERITANCE; ARCHAIC RESIDUE; ARCHAISM; ARCHETYPE; ASSIMILATION; ASSOCIATIONISM; ATTITUDE TYPE; AUTOHYPNOTIC AMNESIA; BEHAVIOR TYPE; CENTRAL FORCE; COLLECTIVE UNCONSCIOUS; COMPLEX; CONCRETISM; CONFESSION; CONTRASEXUAL; DEPTH PSYCHOLOGY; DREAM EGO; DREAM FUNCTION; EDUCATION STAGE; EGO COMPLEX; ELUCIDATION; ENANTIODROMIA; EUPHORIC APATHY; EXTRAVERTED TYPE; FEELING APPERCEPTION; FEELING TYPE; FUNCTIONAL TYPE; FUNCTION ENGRAM; GENERAL TRANSFER; IMAGO; INDIVIDUATION; INSOMNIUM DREAMS; INTROVERSION; INTROVERSION-EXTROVERSION; INTROVERTED TYPE; INTUITION; INTUITIVE TYPE; INWARD PICTURE; IRRATIONAL TYPES;
LAND OF CHILDHOOD; LIBIDO; LIBIDO ANALOG; MAGNA MATER; MANDALA; MENTAL LEVELS; MOTHER ARCHETYPE; MYTHOLOGICAL THEMES; MYTHOLOGY; PALEOPSYCHOLOGY; PARALLEL DREAM; PERSONA; PERSONAL IMAGE; PERSONALITY TYPES; PERSONAL UNCONSCIOUS; PHYLOGENY; POWER COMPLEX; PRIMORDIAL IMAGE; PRIMORDIAL IMAGE OF HERO BIRTH; PRODROMIC DREAM; PROPHETIC DREAMS; PSYCHIC ENERGY; PSYCHIC INERTIA; PSYCHIC ISOLATION; PSYCHOLOGICAL RAPPORT; PSYCHOSYNTHESIS; PUER AETERNUS; QUATERNITY; RACIAL MEMORY; RACIAL UNCONSCIOUS; RATIONAL TYPE; RECONSTRUCTIVE PSYCHOTHERAPY; RECURRENT DREAMS; REDUCTIVE INTERPRETATION; SELF; SENSATION TYPE; SHADOW; SOUL IMAGE; SUPERIOR FUNCTION; SYMBOLISM; SYNTHESIS; TELEOLOGY; THINKING TYPE; TOPOGRAPHICAL PSYCHOLOGY; UFOS; UNCONSCIOUS FACTORS; WORD-ASSOCIATION TEST; ZURICH SCHOOL. Also see BLEULER.

Jung association test a word-association test designed to reveal complexes by observing or eliciting strong emotional reactions to specific words.

juramentado a culture-specific syndrome (Spanish, "cursed person") limited to Muslim men that are ethnically related to the Malays and Moros. Victims are suddenly overwhelmed by frenzy, rush about stabbing everyone they encounter, after which they lapse into a stuporous sleep from which they awaken with a complete amnesia for the episode. Though the causes are none too clear, the seizures are often preceded by exciting religious rites or by a devastating emotional experience such as the death of a loved one.

jurisprudential teaching model a teaching model that emphasizes the role of social interaction and uses the model of law and the system of laws as an information-processing model and paradigm for evaluating social issues.

jus primae noctis the "law of the first night" (Latin) which, according to some sources, permitted feudal lords, as a symbol of authority, to take to bed the bride of a serf—specifically, to deflower her. J.p.n. also reflected the medieval European attitude that regarded women as sexual property. Also called **right of the first night; droit du seigneur** /drô·ä′dēsenyœr′/ (French, "right of the lord"); **virginal tribute.**

Justitia pectoralis stenophylla the botanical name for an herb that grows wild in Brazil and Venezuela and is a source of a hallucinogenic snuff used by local populations. The drug contained in the plant leaves, **bolek-hena,** contains tryptamines.

just-noticeable difference = DIFFERENCE THRESHOLD.

just-noticeable-differences method a psychophysical technique in which a standard stimulus is presented along with a variable stimulus whose magnitude is increased in some trials and decreased in others until a just-perceptible difference is reported. The average of the two series is taken, and the threshold is calculated at the point where the difference can be recognized 50 percent of the time.

just-world phenomenon the belief that what happens to a person is justifiable and logical; the notion that people get what they deserve. The j.-w.p. is attributed to a wide-spread need to believe that events proceed rationally and not by chance. As a response, it is especially noteworthy in the case of clearly innocent victims of violent crime. Also called **just-world hypothesis.**

juvenile amaurotic idiocy a neuronal-lipidosis type of metabolic disorder in which the brain shows no accumulation of sphingomyelin, a type of fatty material found in egg yolk, CNS tissues, and kidneys. The brain is atrophied, the cortex is thinned, and the neurons are reduced in number. Cerebellar ataxia occurs, and dementia begins in childhood.

juvenile delinquency illegal behavior by a minor including behavior that would be considered criminal in an adult. Examples are vandalism, truancy, petty thievery, auto theft, forceable rape, arson, drug abuse, and aggravated assault. Major causes of j.d. appear to be home environment (broken home, low standards, sociopathic father) and community influences (gangs, criminal subculture, drug subculture), among both the privileged and underprivileged.

juvenile general paralysis an obsolete term for juvenile paresis.

juvenile paresis congenital syphilis in which the spirochete infection is transmitted from mother to fetus after the fifth month of pregnancy. Due to a lengthy incubation period, onset of symptoms usually occurs between the ages of ten and 12, starting with confusion and restlessness, and progressing to visual disturbances, motor incoordination, impairment of memory and judgment, and gradual deterioration in all areas if the condition is not arrested by penicillin while it is still manageable. Also called **juvenile general paresis.** Also see JUVENILE TABES.

juvenile period the time span extending from the start of puberty to the end of adolescence.

juvenile progressive spinal-muscular atrophy: See PROGRESSIVE SPINAL-MUSCULAR ATROPHY.

juvenile tabes a type of tabes that occurs in children who have acquired syphilis either in very early childhood or congenitally. The symptoms usually appear after the age of ten and often include optic atrophy, mental deterioration, and general nerve atrophy with paralysis. The patient may show a negative Wassermann-test result. Also see JUVENILE PARESIS.

-juxta- a combining form meaning near, beside (Latin *juxta*).

K

Kafka, Franz /käf'kä/ Austrian writer, 1883–1924. His novels and stories dealt profoundly with the dilemma of modern man. See EXISTENTIALISM.

Kahlbaum, Karl Ludwig /käl'boum/ German physician, 1828–99. See PRESBYOPHRENIA (also called **Kahlbaum-Wernicke syndrome**); HEBOIDOPHRENIA; PARANOID; SCHNAUZKRAMPF.

Kahn, Eugen German psychologist, 1887—. See KAHN TEST OF SYMBOL ARRANGEMENT.

Kahn, Reuben American bacteriologist, 1887—. See WASSERMANN TEST (there: **Kahn test**).

Kahn Test of Symbol Arrangement a standardized diagnostic test in which the subject, child or adult, arranges 16 plastic objects (heart, anchor, etc.) as a means of identifying his cultural-symbolic thinking, and comparing the typical patterns of normal and clinical groups, including schizophrenic, neurotic, and brain-damaged subjects.

kainophobia; kainotophobia = NEOPHOBIA.

kakorrhaphiophobia: See FEAR OF FAILURE.

Kalinowsky, Lothar B. German-born American neuropsychiatrist, 1899—. K. is known as a specialist in somatic treatments who brought electroshock treatment to America and demonstrated its effectiveness in depressive and other mental disorders.

Kallikak the pseudonym for a large American family that included one line of continuing distinguished citizens and one of social misfits, mental defectives, alcoholics, criminals, and mentally disturbed individuals. Henry Goddard, who studied the case, concluded that his "pedigree method" established heredity as the prime factor in mental defect, since the "eminent branch" derived from a normal and the "degenerate branch" derived from a retarded girl. He ignored the fact that offspring by this girl were raised in squalid conditions. (The pseudonym is derived from the Greek words *kalos*, "beautiful, good," and *kakos*, "bad.") See GODDARD.

Kallmann, Franz Josef German-born American geneticist and psychologist, 1897–1965. K. applied twin-study and family-study methods to investigations of the role of heredity in schizophrenia, manic-depressive disorder, involutional psychoses, homosexuality, and aging. See KALLMANN'S SYNDROME; TWIN-STUDIES.

Kallmann's syndrome a hereditary disorder characterized by hypogonadism, sometimes in the form of eunuchoidism, mental retardation, color blindness, anosmia, and synkinesia. K.s. is transmitted as an X-linked dominant trait.

Kalmuk idiocy an alternative but seldom used term for Down's syndrome. The term is derived from the name of the nomadic Mongol tribe.

kamikaze: See ALTRUISTIC SUICIDE.

Kandinsky, Victor Chrisanfovic Russian psychiatrist, 1825–90 (?). See CLÉRAMBAULT-KANDINSKY COMPLEX.

Kanner, Leo Austrian-born American child psychiatrist, 1894—. Author of *Child Psychiatry* (1935), the first textbook on the subject in English, K. is best known for his studies of early infantile autism, which he differentiated from childhood schizophrenia. See INFANTILE AUTISM (also called **Kanner's disease; Kanner's syndrome**); AUTOAGGRESSIVE ACTIVITIES; CHILD PSYCHIATRY; EARLY INFANTILE AUTISM; REFRIGERATOR PARENTS.

Kant, Immanuel /känt/ German philosopher, 1724–1804. See CATEGORICAL IMPERATIVE; COMIC; HUMOR. Also see HEIDEGGER.

kappa /kap'ə/ tenth letter of the Greek alphabet (K,κ).

kappa waves brain waves with a frequency similar to that of alpha waves (ten cycles per second) but with a much weaker amplitude. They normally occur while one is reading, thinking, or dreaming.

Kardiner, Abram American psychoanalyst, 1891–1981. K. was a student of Freud, and a co-founder of the first American psychoanalytical school in New York in 1930. See ACTION SYSTEM; BASIC PERSONALITY.

karezza = CAREZZA.

-kary-; -karyo- a combining form relating to a cell nucleus (from Greek *karyon*, "nut, nucleus").

karyotype /kar'-/ the chromosomal constitution of a cell; the chromosomal structure of an individual or a species. Also see TRIPLOID K.

Kasanin, Jacob Sergi American psychologist,

1897–1946. See HANFMANN-KASANIN CONCEPT FORMATION TEST.

kat = KHAT.

-kat-; -kata-; -kato-; -kath- a combining form meaning (a) downward, going down, beneath, (b) against.

katagogic tendency the psychic impulses that tend to prevent an individual from achieving a positive and constructive life goal. The k.t. is the opposite of the **anagogic tendency**, which represents the upward-leading, constructive impulses (Stekel).

katasexuality a sexual preference for dead persons or humans with animal-like characteristics. See NECROPHILIA.

katatonia = CATATONIC STATE.

kathisophobia a morbid fear of sitting down. Also see THAASSOPHOBIA.

kation = CATION.

kava an aromatic resin derived from a shrub, Piper methysticum, that grows on islands of the Pacific Ocean. The active ingredients of the plant, alkaloids that produce sedation without clouding of consciousness, are released from the root and lower stem cells by chewing them. Human saliva causes the necessary chemical changes in the plant substances which are spit into a bowl, diluted with water, and strained before being ingested. Also called **kavakava; ava; keu.**

Kayser, Bernhard /kī'zər/ German ophthalmologist, 1869–1954. See HEPATOLENTICULAR DEGENERATION (there: **Kayser-Fleischer ring**).

K complex a generalized cortical response elicited by an auditory stimulus during sleep and recorded in EEG changes.

Keeler, Leonard American criminologist, 1903–49. See KEELER POLYGRAPH.

Keeler polygraph the original lie detector developed by Leonard Keeler, an apparatus for simultaneous recording of pulse, respiration, blood pressure, and the electrodermal response as the subject is asked questions. See LIE DETECTOR.

keep-awake pills a popular name for stimulant pills that contain caffeine as the active ingredient and can be obtained without a doctor's prescription. A keep-awake pill usually contains approximately 100 milligrams of caffeine, the equivalent of the amount of caffeine in one cup of regular coffee or two cups of strong tea.

Kegel exercises exercises developed by A. H. Kegel in 1952 to help females control the pubococcygeus muscle. Control of the muscle during coitus enables women to enhance their (and the male's) sexual pleasure. The muscle increases abdominal pressure by contracting, drawing the anus toward the pubis as when an individual tightens control of the urinary sphincter. See PUBOCOCCYGEUS.

Keller, Helen American writer, 1880–1968. Deaf and blind from the age of 19 months as the result of an attack of scarlet fever, K. became the most prominent example of motivation and success in overcoming a handicap. See MULTIHANDICAPPED.

Kempf, Edward J. American psychiatrist, 1885–1971. See KEMPF'S DISEASE; HOMOSEXUAL PANIC.

Kempf's disease an acute anxiety episode based on fear that the subject will be attacked by a homosexual or that other people may believe he is a homosexual. The disorder was first described by Kempf in 1920. The term is essentially equivalent to HOMOSEXUAL PANIC. See this entry.

Kendall, Maurice George English statistician, 1907—. See KENDALL'S TAU; COEFFICIENT OF CONCORDANCE (also called **Kendall coefficient of concordance**).

Kendall's tau a nonparametric measure of correlation.

kenophobia a morbid fear of the void or of wide empty spaces. Also called **cenophobia**.

Kent, Grace Helen American psychologist, 1875—. See KENT-ROSANOFF TEST; KENT SERIES OF ENERGY SKILLS; WORD-ASSOCIATION TEST.

Kent EGY = KENT SERIES OF EMERGENCY SKILLS.

Kent-Rosanoff Test a 100-word free-association test, with tables of relative frequency of responses which can be used in determining whether the subject's associations tend to be common and normal, unusual and eccentric, or somewhere in between.

Kent Series of Emergency Skills a series of individual tests designed to yield a preliminary estimate of the general intelligence of children at various ages. Also called **Kent EGY; EGY test**.

-kerat-; -kerato- a combining form relating to the cornea.

keratitis: See COGAN'S SYNDROME.

keratosis a horny tumorlike growth, such as a callus or wart. An **actinic k.** or **senile k.**, which sometimes forms on the skin of an older person who has been exposed to the sun for many years, often evolves into a cancer. A **pharyngeal k.** is a growth on the wall of the pharynx that can cause speech disorders and may also develop into a cancer.

keraunoneurosis a type of traumatic neurosis associated with the experience of fear of lightning or other forms of intense electric shock.

keraunophobia: See ASTRAPHOBIA.

kernel an elementary sentence composed of a noun phrase and a verb phrase. Kernels are the foundation for longer and more intricate constructions. Also called **k. sentence**.

kernicterus a congenital disorder associated with excessive levels of bilirubin in the newborn infant. It is characterized by severe jaundice and has the potential of causing severe CNS damage. K. often is a complication of Rh-factor incompatibility. See BILIRUBIN; BILIRUBIN ENCEPHALOPATHY; ICTERUS GRAVIS NEONATORUM.

Kernig, Vladimir Michailovich Russian physician, 1840–1917. See KERNIG'S SIGN.

Kernig's sign a reflex action that is a diagnostic sign for meningitis. The test is positive if flexing the thigh at the hip while extending the leg at the knee results in resistance and pain.

Ketalar; ketamine: See ARYLCYCLOHEXYLAMINE COMPOUNDS.

ketones chemical compounds formed in the body tissues by the inadequate metabolism of lipids, or fats, in the diet. Fat metabolism requires the presence of an adequate amount of carbohydrates; when carbohydrate intake is restricted, fats are incompletely burned and excreted as k. If k. are not excreted normally, as in cases of uncontrolled diabetes mellitus, a condition called **ketosis** develops, resulting in turn in an acid-base imbalance known as ACIDOSIS. See this entry.

keu = KAVA.

key a set of symbols or concepts used in coding or decoding; a set of answers used in scoring a test.

key question a question designed to reveal the patient's purpose in being ill and his or her personal feelings associated with the symptoms (Adler).

key-word method a technique used in learning foreign-language vocabulary: If the native language is English, the key word would consist of an English word associated with the sound of a foreign word and linked to the foreign word's meaning in a mental image; e.g., the French word *livre* ("book") may remind us of the sound of "leaf"; the key word "leaf" can be connected to "book" in a mental image—visualizing a leaf in a book as a bookmark. The k.-w.m. is essentially a mnemonic strategy.

khat a mild hallucinogen and stimulant derived from the leaves, buds, and twigs of a perennial shrub, Catha edulis, that grows in tropical Africa. Active ingredients include ephedrine- and amphetamine-type drugs. K. herbs have been exported from Africa throughout Arabia for centuries and were the source of a tea used in the Arab world before the development of coffee beverage. Also called **quat; chat; cafta; kat.**

kibbutz a voluntary Israeli settlement with a collective form of economic and social life and communal provisions for rearing children. The children reside in their own infant house at first, and later in shared quarters apart from the parental residence. The mothers breast-feed their infants and play with their growing children at arranged times, but while they are at work, the nurses, or "metapelets," act as mother surrogates. See MULTIPLE MOTHERING.

kidney disease any of the disorders marked by inflammation, infection, structural defects, tumors, or stone formation in the kidneys. Inflammation of the renal pelvis of the kidney is identified as **pyelitis;** in deeper kidney areas the condition may be called pyelonephritis; and inflammation of the glomeruli usually is termed glomerulonephritis. A form of kidney damage caused by hypertension is known as **nephrosclerosis.** Also called **renal disorder.** Also see GLOMERULONEPHRITIS; PYELONEPHRITIS; POLYCYSTIC K.D.; END-STAGE RENAL DISEASE; UREMIA.

kidney failure an inability of the kidney to perform the normal functions of excreting metabolites at normal blood-fluid levels or to retain an appropriate proportion of electrolytes. If uncorrected, k.f. leads to uremia, diminished urine production with accumulation of fluid in the body tissues, and hyperkalemia, or excess potassium in the blood causing muscular weakness and cardiac arrest. Treatment can be obtained through dialysis, used by nearly 50,000 patients in the United States alone to remove excess potassium and uremic products.

kidney transplant the surgical removal of a diseased kidney and its replacement with a kidney donated by bequest of a deceased person or by a living individual, usually a relative with two healthy kidneys. The first k.t. was performed in 1954 and involved identical twins. About 20,000 kidney transplants have been performed with an average survival rate of more than 80 percent. Most failures involve immune-response rejection of the grafts. Also see ORGAN TRANSPLANTS.

Kierkegaard, Soren Aaby /kir'kəgôr/ Danish philosopher and theologian, 1813–55. See EXISTENTIALISM.

kilobytophobia: See COMPUTER ILLITERACY.

kimilue a culture-specific syndrome found among the Native American Diegueno of lower California. Characteristically, the patient loses all interest in daily life, is generally apathetic, suffers a loss of appetite, and experiences vivid sexual dreams.

Kindler, Werner /kin'dlər/ German otorhinolaryngologist, 1895—. See ZANGE-KINDLER SYNDROME.

-kine-; -kinesis a combining form relating to movement.

kinephantom an illusion of movement, often seen as a shadow of wheels moving in an opposite direction.

kinesic behavior a form of behavior in which individuals communicate by the use of body motions rather than formal language. Winking, shrugging, blushing, and eye movements are examples of k.b.

kinesics the study of movement, particularly as it is involved in communication through gestures, posture, and facial expressions.

kinesiology the study of the relationship of anatomical characteristics and physiological functions to body movement.

kinesophobia a morbid fear of motion. Also see ERGASIOPHOBIA.

kinesthesis = KINESTHETIC SENSE.

kinesthetic hallucination a false perception of body movement. E.g., a schizophrenic patient may feel that his head is enlarging, an individual under hallucenogenic drugs may feel that his arms or legs are lengthening, or an amputee may feel movement in the missing limb. See PHANTOM LIMB.

kinesthetic method a therapeutic technique for speech and writing disorders in which attention is focused on the muscle sensations involved in correct and incorrect performance.

kinesthetic sense the sense that provides information through receptors in the muscles, tendons, and joints, which enables us to control and coordinate our movements, including walking, talking, facial expression, gestures, and posture. Also called **kinesthesis; movement sense**. See PROPRIOCEPTION.

kinetic pertaining to movement, as in the term hyperkinetic.

kinetic information the observed gestures, postures, and other body-language clues used in making an evaluation of a patient.

king-slave fantasy a fantasy in which the individual plays a role of king or slave or, alternating between the roles, plays both parts.

kinky-hair disease a familial disorder affecting the normal absorption of copper from the intestines, characterized by sparse, kinky hair. Infants suffer cerebral degeneration, retarded growth, and early death. Early diagnosis and administration of copper may prevent irreversible damage. Also called **Menkes' disease**. Also see HEPATOLENTICULAR DEGENERATION.

Kinsey, Alfred American zoologist, 1894–1956. K. was director of the Institute for Sex Research, Bloomington, IN, which conducted a 15-year study of all phases of sexual behavior, known as the *Kinsey Report*, the first comprehensive empirical study on sexology.

kinship network the system of blood relationships recognized by a given culture or society. Also called **kinship system**.

Kirkbride, Thomas American physician, 1809–83. While serving as physician in chief of the Pennsylvania Hospital for the Insane from 1840 to 1880, K. played an active part in what has been called "the Renaissance of American psychiatry" by opposing such procedures as blood-letting, emetics, and restraint, and by instituting a "moral-treatment" approach based on caring for patients with courtesy and understanding, and engaging them in occupational therapy and religious, educational, and social activities. As one of the founders, and later president, of the Association of Medical Superintendents of American Institutions for the Insane, he collaborated on a series of tenets which held that insanity is a curable disease and is most successfully treated in well-organized institutions designed especially for this purpose. He himself presented a design, **Kirkbride Plan**, for airy, well-equipped buildings which, though a vast improvement over the almshouses and penal institutions in which the mentally ill were usually incarcerated, encouraged construction of huge complexes in isolated locations. See DECENTRALIZATION; MORAL TREATMENT. Also see RAY.

kissing behavior the activity of making contact with the lips, usually as a sign of friendship or affection. The kiss may involve lip contact with any part of the body and with varying degrees of pressure. Mouth-to-mouth k.b. may include extension of the tongues of the parties. K.b. probably is related to licking behavior as manifested by domestic animals. It is not observed in all cultures. Also see FRENCH KISS; CUNNILINGUS.

kissing disease = INFECTIOUS MONONUCLEOSIS.

Kjersted, Conrad Ludwig American psychologist, 1883—. See KJERSTED-ROBINSON LAW.

Kjersted-Robinson law the principle that the amount of material learned in a given time is relatively constant and does not depend on the length of the material.

Klauder, Joseph Victor American dermatologist, 1888–1962. See STEVENS-JOHNSON SYNDROME (also called **Klauder's syndrome**).

Klebedenken /klā′bədengkən/ a schizophrenic association disturbance in which thinking is sticky or adhesive and perseverative (German, "sticky thinking").

Kleeblattschädel syndrome /klā′blätshedəl/ a type of birth defect characterized by a three-lobed skull (from German *Kleeblatt*, "cloverleaf," and *Schädel*, "skull") caused by upward and lateral bulging of the brain through skull sutures. The patients also have hydrocephalus, severe mental retardation, and abnormally short limbs. Also called **cloverleaf skull**.

Klein, David /klīn/ Swiss geneticist, 1908—. See TREACHER COLLINS' SYNDROME (also called **Franceschetti-Zwahlen-Klein syndrome**).

Klein, Melanie /klīn/ Austrian psychoanalyst 1882–1960. K. was the first therapist to use play as an analytic and treatment technique, and also theorized that the Oedipus complex, paranoid attitudes, and the superego originate in very early infancy. See BAD BREAST; CHILD ANALYSIS; DEPRESSIVE POSITION; EGO NUCLEI; EGO-SPLITTING; FEMININITY COMPLEX; FISCH-RENWICK SYNDROME; GOOD BREAST; GOOD OBJECT; PARANOID-SCHIZOID POSITION.

Kleine, Willi /klī′nə/ German psychiatrist, fl. 1925. See KLEINE-LEVIN SYNDROME; EATING BEHAVIOR.

Kleine-Levin syndrome a brain disorder (possibly due to a malfunction of the frontal lobe or hypothalamus) characterized by episodes of clouded consciousness, bulimia, hypersomnia resembling narcolepsy, partial amnesia, and psychomotor retardation.

-klepto- a combining form meaning stealing.

kleptolagnia a morbid urge to steal, usually associated with sexual excitement.

kleptomania a disorder of impulse control characterized by (a) a repeated failure to resist impulses to steal objects not for immediate use or monetary value, and which are either given away, returned surreptitiously, or hidden away, (b) feelings of increased tension before committing the act, and (c) either pleasure or relief while committing it. Stealing of this kind is not due to a conduct disorder or antisocial personality disorder, and is not carried out after long-time planning or with the assistance or collaboration of others. (DSM-III)

kleptophobia a morbid fear of becoming a thief or of stealing.

Kline, Nathan Schellenberg American research psychiatrist, 1916–83. See PSYCHIC ENERGIZER.

Klineberg, Otto American social psychologist, 1899—. K. is noted for his pioneering studies of race differences, ethnic groups, and the cultural aspects of personality and mental health. See RACE DIFFERENCES.

Klinefelter, Harry Fitch American physician, 1912—. See KLINEFELTER'S SYNDROME; GENETIC DEFECT; MICROORCHIDISM; SEX-CHROMOSOME ABERRATIONS.

Klinefelter's syndrome a chromosomal disorder affecting males born with a karyotype of 47,XXY, resulting in small testes, absence of sperm, enlarged breasts, and excretion of follicle-stimulating hormone. Mental retardation is uncommon, but behavioral problems are indicated by a high rate of unemployment, divorce, and alcoholism. The rate of confinement in mental institutions for 47,XXY males is three times that of normal males. Also called **XXY syndrome**.

Klinger, Friedrich Maximilian von German dramatist and novelist, 1752–1831. See STORM AND STRESS.

klinotaxis: See TAXES.

Klippel, Maurice /klipel'/ French neurologist, 1858–1942. See KLIPPEL-FEIL SYNDROME; BONNEVIE-ULLRICH SYNDROME; NIELSEN'S DISEASE; WILDERVANCK'S SYNDROME.

Klippel-Feil syndrome a congenital defect characterized by shortened neck, low hairline, and a reduced number of vertebrae, some of which may be fused into a single mass. The condition often is accompanied by deafness and mental retardation. Also see NIELSEN'S DISEASE.

klismaphilia a psychosexual disorder characterized by dependence on the use of enemas to obtain sexual stimulation. See PARAPHILIAS.

Klumpke's paralysis = DÉJÉRINE-KLUMPKE'S SYNDROME.

Klüver, Heinrich German-born American neurologist, 1898–1979. See KLÜVER-BUCY SYNDROME; EATING BEHAVIOR.

Klüver-Bucy syndrome a condition resulting from temporal lobectomy or certain atrophic changes in the cerebral cortex, and marked by a tendency to examine all objects by touch or by placing them in the mouth. Other effects include increased sexual activity of all kinds, lack of concentration, and development of a special appetite for meat. The syndrome is observed in both humans and laboratory animals following temporal lobectomy.

knee-jerk reflex an involuntary contraction of the quadriceps muscle of the leg following a sharp tap on the patellar ligament. The k.-j.r. provides a test of the integrity of the nervous system as the tap on the tendon stretches the muscle and causes a volley of impulses from the spindle receptors to travel to the spinal cord. This in turn triggers a motoneuron response that travels back to the muscle, causing its contraction. Also see PENDULAR KNEE JERK.

knock-knee = GENU VALGUM.

knockout drops a popular name for chloral-hydrate drugs that are added to alcohol to produce a sudden loss of consciousness. The efficacy of the combination of k.d. and alcohol has been disputed by findings that in controlled experiments the dramatic effects anticipated were not observed. Theoretically, alcohol and k.d. should have a synergistic effect when coadministered. Also called **Mickey Finn**.

Knoll's pins threaded pins that are inserted in the headcap of the femur, or thigh bone, to correct a childhood orthopedic disorder called slipped epiphysis. The cartilaginous portion at the top of the femur slips off the bony surface, causing the child to suffer a painful limp.

knowledge of results a principle of learning that states the learner profits from immediate information about his progress, e.g., about the accuracy of his responses on a test or quiz. According to this principle, prompt feedback is more effective than delayed feedback in reinforcing correct responses and helping the learner to focus on problem areas.

Knox, Howard Andrew American psychiatrist, 1885—. See KNOX TUBE TEST.

Knox Cube Test a performance test in which the subject taps a series of four cubes in various sequences determined by the examiner.

Koch, Robert /kôkh/ German physician and bacteriologist, Nobel laureate, 1843–1910. See CONSTITUTIONAL PSYCHOPATHIC INFERIOR.

Kocher, Emil Theodor /kôkh'ər/ Swiss surgeon, 1841–1917. See KOCHER-DEBRÉ-SEMELAIGNE SYNDROME.

Kocher-Debré-Semelaigne syndrome a disorder of infants and children marked by muscular weakness and hypertrophy along with cretinism and mental retardation in some cases. The condition is similar to that of Hoffmann's syndrome except that K.-D.-S.s. lacks the symptoms of pseudomyotonia and painful spasms. Also called **Debré-Semelaigne syndrome**.

Koenig, Karl Rudolph German-born French physicist, 1832–1901. See KOENIG CYLINDERS.

Koenig cylinders a set of cylinders tuned to emit high-pitch tones for use in determining the upper absolute threshold of hearing.

Koffka, Kurt /kôf'kä/ German-American psychologist, 1886–1941. After obtaining his Ph.D. at the University of Berlin, K. worked with Wolfgang Köhler and Max Wertheimer on studies that led to the Gestalt theory. He later became its chief spokesman through articles and books that explained the theory and its applications—most notably *Principles of Gestalt Psychology*, which he published in 1935 while serving as professor at Smith College. See GESTALT PSYCHOLOGY. Also see KÖHLER; WERTHEIMER.

Kohlberg, Lawrence American educator and psychologist, 1927—. See CONVENTIONAL LEVEL; DEVELOPMENTAL TEACHING MODEL; GOOD-BOY-NICE-GIRL ORIENTATION; GURU STAGE; HEDONISTIC ORIENTATION; INSTRUMENTAL-RELATIVIST ORIENTATION; LAW-AND-ORDER ORIENTATION;

LEGALISTIC ORIENTATION; MORAL JUDGMENT; NAIVE EGOTISTIC ORIENTATION; POSTCONVENTIONAL LEVEL; PRECONVENTIONAL LEVEL; PREMORAL STAGE; PRINCIPLED STAGE.

Köhler, Wolfgang German-American psychologist, 1887–1967. K. opposed the atomistic theories of his time, and joined Max Wertheimer and Kurt Koffka in developing the Gestalt approach. He is also known for his studies of insight, showing that even chimpanzees can "get an idea" such as piling up boxes or putting sticks together to reach a piece of fruit. See GESTALT PSYCHOLOGY; DYNAMIC THEORY; GOODNESS OF CONFIGURATION. Also see KOFFKA; WERTHEIMER.

Kohnstamm, Oskar /kōn'shtäm/ German physician, 1871–1917. See KOHNSTAMM TEST.

Kohnstamm test a demonstration frequently used in preparing a subject for hypnosis: He is asked to stand next to a wall and press an arm tightly against it for two minutes; when he steps away, the arm spontaneously rises—which shows him how it feels to yield automatically to an external force, as in hypnosis. Also called **Kohnstamm maneuver; Kohnstamm's phenomenon.**

Kohs, Samuel Calmin American psychologist, 1890—. See KOHS BLOCK DESIGN TEST.

Kohs Block Design Test a performance test of intelligence included in the Arthur Performance Scale, consisting of a set of colored cubes which the subject must arrange into designs presented on 17 test cards.

Kohut, Heinz Austrian-born American psychoanalyst, 1913–81. K. developed a "self" theory which challenged Freud's. See DISORDERS OF THE SELF; MIRROR TRANSFERENCE.

kola nut the seed of a tree, Cola acuminata or Cola nitida, that is a native of tropical Africa and is cultivated in South America and the West Indies. The active ingredient is caffeine, which comprises about one and one-half percent of the dry weight of the k.n. The nut was discovered in 1667 by a Congo missionary, Father Carli, who observed that local tribesmen chewed the k.n. before meals. Also called **cola nut; goora nut; gura nut; colla; kolla.**

Kolmogorov, Andrey Nikolaevich Russian mathematician, 1903—. See KOLMOGOROV-SMIRNOV TEST.

Kolmogorov-Smirnov test a nonparametric significance test for comparing an observed frequency distribution with a theoretical distribution.

kopophobia a morbid fear of fatigue.

-kopr-; -kopro-: See -COPR-.

koprolagnia = COPROLAGNIA.

koprolalia = COPROLALIA.

koprophagia = COPROPHAGIA.

koprophemia = COPROPHEMIA.

koprophilia = COPROPHILIA.

koprophobia = COPROPHOBIA.

koro an acute phobic reaction in which the patient suddenly fears that his penis is shrinking, will disappear into his abdomen, and bring on death; it is observed in Southern China and the Malay Archipelago. A female form of the disorder, in which the patient feels that her breasts are shrinking and her labia are being sucked inward, has been found in Borneo. Male patients may tie a ribbon around the penis or use other devices to maintain physical control over its presence. The disorder generally is associated with guilt feelings about masturbation or sexual promiscuity. Cases of k. have been observed in North America and other areas in connection with drug abuse, brain tumors, or other disorders. Also called **suk-yeong; shook yong.**

Kornzweig, Abraham Leon American physician, 1900—. See BASSEN-KORNZWEIG TEST.

Korsakoff, Sergei Sergeivich Russian neurologist, 1854–1900. See KORSAKOFF'S PSYCHOSIS; WERNICKE-KORSAKOFF SYNDROME; ALCOHOL-AMNESTIC DISORDER (also called **Korsakoff's disease**); AMNESIC SYNDROME (also called **Korsakoff amnesia**); ALCOHOL DEMENTIA; ALCOHOLIC PSYCHOSES; AMNESIC CONFABULATION; AMNESIC-CONFABULATORY SYNDROME; CONFABULATION; DEMENTIA; MEMORY DEFECT; MEMORY DISORDER; MEMORY FALSIFICATION; ORGANIC DEMENTIA; POLYVITAMIN THERAPY; REGISTRATION; SEMANTIC PARAPHASIA; THIAMINE DEFICIENCY; WERNICKE'S ENCEPHALOPATHY.

Korsakoff's psychosis an organic syndrome occurring primarily in chronic alcoholics and occasionally in patients with severe head trauma, prolonged infections, metallic poisoning, pellagra, or brain tumor. It was first described in 1887 by the Russian neurologist Sergei Korsakoff. Major symptoms include anterograde amnesia with confabulation (invented stories), confusion, disorientation, and in some cases polyneuritis. Also called **Korsakoff's syndrome.** For other details see AMNESTIC SYNDROME; ALCOHOL-AMNESTIC DISORDER.

Korte's laws a group of laws for the perception of apparent movement when two stationary visual stimuli are given in succession. The laws cover conditions of constant time, constant distance, and constant intensity.

Korzybski, Alfred Habdank Polish-born American scientist and writer, 1879–1950. K. is known for his research and writings in semantics. See SEMANTIC THERAPY.

Krabbe, Knud H. Danish neurologist, 1885–1961. See KRABBE'S DISEASE; PROGRESSIVE DEGENERATIVE SUBCORTICAL ENCEPHALOPATHY.

Krabbe's disease an autosomal-recessive disorder characterized by rapidly progressive neurologic deterioration in the first months of life. The brain atrophies due to a loss of white matter, and myelin may be almost totally absent. Death usually occurs within two years. Early symptoms include fretfulness and apathy, rigidity, vomiting, convulsions, and loss of vision and hearing. The cause is a profound deficiency of the enzyme galactocerebroside beta-galactosidase. Also called **globoid-cell leukodystrophy.**

Kraepelin, Emil German psychiatrist, 1856–1926.

K. performed pioneer experiments on the effect of bromides, ether, and other drugs on mental processes, as well as on fatigue and work pauses; but he is best known for his classification of mental illnesses based upon thousands of case studies. He fully accepted the somatic viewpoint, attributing his first major category, dementia, to organic brain changes arising within the organism, and resulting in irreversible deterioration. His second major category, manic-depressive psychosis, was attributed to external factors and did not lead to incurable deterioration. Personality factors, on the other hand, were regarded as by-products of a diseased brain or faulty metabolism. These organic interpretations held sway until challenged by the psychodynamic approach. See KRAEPELIN'S DISEASE; BIOGENIC PSYCHOSIS; BY-IDEA; CONSTITUTIONAL PSYCHOPATHIC INFERIOR; DELUSIONAL MANIA; DEMENTIA PARANOIDES; DEMENTIA PRAECOX; DEPRESSIVE MANIA; DESCRIPTIVE PSYCHIATRY; ECHO PHENOMENON; INHIBITED MANIA; IRRESISTIBLE APPREHENSION; NOSOLOGIC APPROACH; ORGANIC APPROACH; PARABULIA; PARANOID; PARAPHRENIA; PARAPHRENIA SYSTEMATICA; PARERGASIA; SIMPLE SCHIZOPHRENIA; WORD-ASSOCIATION TEST. Also see BLEULER.

Kraepelin's disease a form of atypical depressive psychosis, a residual category of persons whose symptoms do not satisfy the criteria for a major affective disorder. The patients often respond favorably to administration of tricyclic antidepressant or monoamine oxidase inhibitor drugs.

Krafft-Ebing, Baron Richard von /kräft'ä'bing/ German neurologist, 1840–1902. Though his early contributions were in the field of forensic psychiatry, Krafft-Ebing's name is primarily associated with *Psychopathia Sexualis*, a revolutionary work on a subject that was almost completely ignored in the puritanical Victorian age. His clinical descriptions of sexual pathology vividly illustrated the many forms the sexual drive can take, and opened the way to further scientific investigation, including his own studies of general paralysis (paresis), which stimulated research directed toward curing syphilitic infections. See GENITAL MUTILATION; PSYCHOPATHIA SEXUALIS; RELIGIOUS DELUSIONS; WHIPPING.

Krämer, Heinrich /krā'mər/ German inquisitor, fl. 15th century. See WITCHCRAFT.

Krause, Wilhelm /krou'zə/ German anatomist, 1833–1910. See KRAUSE END BULB; CORPUSCLE; DOGIEL'S CORPUSCLES; NERVE ENDING; SOMATIC RECEPTORS.

Krause end bulb a specialized sensory nerve ending enclosed in a capsule. It is associated with temperature sensations.

Krebs, Sir Hans Adolf German-born British biochemist, 1900—. See KREBS CYCLE; GABA SHUNT.

Krebs cycle a metabolic mechanism in which carbohydrates, fatty acids, and amino acids from ingested foods are oxidized to yield carbon dioxide, water, and high-energy phosphate compounds. This mechanism is the principal source of energy for mammals. Also called **citric-acid cycle**. See GABA SHUNT.

Krech, David Russian-born American psychologist, 1909—. See PREJUDICE.

Kretschmer, Ernst German psychiatrist, 1888–1964. Though he performed basic research in psychotherapy and criminal behavior, Kretschmer's name is primarily associated with his work *Physique and Character*, 1921, which presented a constitutional typology in which schizophrenia was linked to the thin, leptosome-asthenic type, and manic-depressive psychosis to the rotund pyknic type. He also suggested that many normal individuals manifest similar characteristics in milder form, terming them schizothymic and cyclothymic. See KRETSCHMER TYPOLOGY; CONSTITUTIONAL TYPE; ACUTE AFFECTIVE REFLEX; APOPLECTIC TYPE; ASTHENIC TYPE; ATHLETIC TYPE; DIGESTIVE TYPE; DYSPLASTIC TYPE; EURYPLASTIC; EUSTHENIC; HYPERPITUITARY CONSTITUTION; HYPERTONIC TYPE; HYPOPITUITARY CONSTITUTION; HYPOVEGETATIVE; LINEAR TYPE; LONGILINEAL; MACROSKELIC; MUSCULAR TYPE; NORMOSPLANCHNIC TYPE; PHTHINOID; PSYCHOBIOGRAM; PYKNIC TYPE; STHENIC TYPE.

Kretschmer typology a controversial classification of individuals based on a "clear biological affinity" between specific physiques and specific personality tendencies, advanced by the German psychiatrist Ernst Kretschmer in the 1920s. He held that a short, stocky "pyknic" tends to be jovial and subject to mood swings (that is, cycloid, and in extreme cases manic-depressive); the frail "asthenic" or "leptosome" is likely to be introversive and sensitive (schizoid, and in extreme cases schizophrenic); the muscular "athletic" type is usually energetic and aggressive; and the disproportioned "'dysplastic" presents a combination of traits but tends toward the asthenic. These tendencies were attributed to endocrine secretions.

Kruskal, William Henry American mathematical statistician, 1919—. See KRUSKAL-WALLIS TEST.

Kruskal-Wallis test a nonparametric method for determining statistical significance with ranked data. It is analogous to one-way analysis of variance.

Kuder, G. Frederic American psychologist, fl. 1934, 1975. See KUDER PREFERENCE RECORD; KUDER-RICHARDSON FORMULAS; INTEREST TESTS.

Kuder Preference Record an interest inventory based on a series of activities to be marked most and least liked, and yielding percentile scores in ten vocational areas: clerical, computational, art, music, social service, outdoor, science, persuasive, literary, and mechanical.

Kuder-Richardson formulas equations for estimating the reliability of a test. Also called **Kuder-Richardson coefficients of equivalence**.

Kufs, H. /kōōfs/ German psychiatrist, 1871–1955. See KUFS' DISEASE; CEREBROMACULAR DEGENERATION; NEURONAL LIPIDOSIS; SPHINGOLIPIDOSES.

Kufs' disease a late juvenile or adult form of amaurotic family idiocy. It differs in signs and symptoms from other forms, such as Tay-Sachs disease, in that the incidence is not related to an ethnic group and there is an absence of ocular lesions. The onset is between the ages of 15 and 26, and the effects are associated with cerebellar or basal-ganglia disorders.

Kugelberg, Eric Klas Henrik Swedish neurologist, 1913—. See PROGRESSIVE SPINAL-MUSCULAR ATROPHY (there: **Wohlfart-Kugelberg-Welander disease**).

Kuhlmann, Frederick American psychologist, 1876–1941. See KUHLMANN-ANDERSON TESTS.

Kuhlmann-Anderson Tests a series of tests of general intelligence ranging from kindergarten to adulthood.

Külpe, Oswald /kil'pə/ German psychologist, 1862–1915. As director of the influential laboratory in Würzburg, K. showed the importance of the "conscious attitude" in thinking, demonstrated that most of thought is imageless, and showed that higher thought processes, such as judging, abstracting, and remembering, could be investigated through systematic experimental introspection. See WÜRZBURG SCHOOL; IMAGE-LESS THOUGHT.

Kundt, August /ko͝ont/ German physicist, 1839–94. See KUNDT'S RULES.

Kundt's rules the principles that distances divided by graduated lines appear larger than undivided distances, and that when bisecting a horizontal line using one eye, the subject tends to place the midpoint too near the nasal side of the eye.

kurtosis a descriptive statistic which describes the degree of peakedness in a set of data. The normal curve is MESOKURTIC. See this entry.

kuru a culture-specific CNS disease that afflicts some natives of the New Guinea highlands and is associated with cannibalism. Symptoms include ataxia, tremors, difficulty in walking, and strabismus. It is believed to be transmitted by eating the brains of persons previously infected with a k. virus.

Kussmaul, Adolf /ko͞os'moul/ German physician, 1822–1902. See LANDRY'S PARALYSIS (also called **Kussmaul-Landry paralysis**).

kwashiorkor a protein-deficiency disease observed in infants and small children who are deprived of essential amino acids they obtained during breast feeding. The symptoms include fluid accumulation in the tissues, liver disorders, impaired growth, distention of the abdomen, and pigment changes in the skin and hair. Normal cerebral development also may be impaired. The condition is found mainly in Third World countries.

kymograph a rotating drum used for recording temporal data in psychology or physiology studies.

kyphoscoliosis: See FRIEDREICH'S ATAXIA.

kyphosis a forward curvature of the spine, producing a hunchback effect. Variations of k. include dowager's hump, when senile osteoporosis is involved, and ankylosing spondylitis, when bones of the spinal column tend to fuse in the curved posture. K. can cause respiratory disorders by compressing the chest area. Also see LORDOSIS; HUMPBACK.

L

L an abbreviation of *l*anguage score. See ACE TEST.

Labananalysis an objective analysis of movement as an expression of the individual, together with a system of graphic representation known as **Labanotation**. L. was developed by the choreographer Rudolf Laban. Also see EFFORT-SHAPE TECHNIQUE.

labeling the act of classifying a patient according to a certain diagnostic category. Patient l. may be misleading since not all cases conform to the sharply defined characteristics of the standard diagnostic categories and some patients may display the traits associated with normal individuals.

labeling theory the view that a label may have a significant effect on behavior. E.g., describing an individual as deviant tends to become an automatic, self-fulfilling prophecy that may result in mental disorder or delinquency. Also called **societal-reaction theory**.

la belle indifférence /läbel′eNdifäräNs′/ a term originally used by Janet to characterize the air of unconcern (French, "nice indifference") manifested by many hysteric patients toward their physical symptoms, possibly due to the fact that the symptoms help to relieve anxiety and bring secondary gains in the form of sympathy and attention. See SECONDARY GAINS.

Labhart, A. /läb′härt/ Swiss physician, fl. 1956. See PRADER-LABHART-WILLI SYNDROME.

-labi-; -labio- a combining form relating to the lips.

labial a speech sound made with the lips, e.g., /b/, /p/, /m/, /w/, /f/, or /v/. If the sound is made with both lips, it is called a bilabial, or labiolabial; if the sound is made with the lower lip and the upper teeth, it is called a labiodental, or dentolabial. See BILABIAL; LABIODENTAL; PLOSIVE; FRICATIVE.

labia majora two folds of tissue that extend downward and backward from the mons pubis to the frenulum pudendi of the female genitalia. The l.m. enclose the labia minora, vagina, urethra, and clitoris. The l.m. develop from the same primordial structures as the male scrotum. Singular: **labium majus**.

labia minora two small folds of tissue between the labia majora, extending backward from the clitoris around the vaginal orifice. The l.m. develop from the urethral folds of embryonic tissue which, under the influence of the androgenic hormone, become the penile urethra of the male. Singular: **labium minus**.

labile affect unstable, changeable, uncontrolled expression of feelings and emotions. It is common in histrionic individuals and in early schizophrenia and organic brain syndromes.

lability-stability: See STABILITY-LABILITY.

labiodental a speech sound made with the lower lip touching or near the upper teeth, e.g., /f/ or /v/. Also called **dentolabial**. Also see BILABIAL; FRICATIVE.

labiolabial = BILABIAL.

labium majus: See LABIA MAJORA.

labium minus: See LABIA MINORA.

laboratory-method model an educational approach in which the role of social interaction is emphasized. The development of personal awareness and interpersonal skills is a major area of concern.

laboratory training a training process directed to the improvement of interpersonal relations, group functioning, and organizational behavior through free expression and experimentation under the general guidance of a trained leader. See GROUP DYNAMICS; SENSITIVITY TRAINING; T-GROUP.

labyrinth the fluid-filled, bony chamber of the inner ear containing the receptors for the sense of hearing and the sense of balance. See COCHLEA; SEMICIRCULAR CANALS.

labyrinthine characterizing speech that is hard or impossible to follow because it wanders from topic to topic with no apparent associative connections, observed primarily in schizophrenia.

labyrinthine sense = SENSE OF EQUILIBRIUM.

laceration: See HEAD TRAUMA; ACUTE TRAUMATIC DISORDER.

lacing agents chemicals used as fillers or substitutes for portions of the active ingredients in drug products, particularly illicit drugs. Strychnine is used as a l.a. for black-market marijuana. Oregano also is commonly mixed with marijuana as a l.a. Caffeine may be used as a l.a. for cocaine.

laconic speech excessively brief, unelaborated speech; also, speech lacking spontaneity (from Greek *Lakon*, "Spartan"). L.s. is frequently found in major depression, schizophrenia, and organic brain syndromes. Also called **poverty of speech.**

lacrimation tearing, mainly excessive tearing; crying. Adjective: **lacrimal.**

-lact-; -lacti-; -lacto- a combining form relating to milk (Latin *lactis*).

lactation the production of milk by the mammary glands of mammals.

lactic dehydrogenase an enzyme that is widely distributed in body tissues where it catalyzes the conversion of lactic acid and pyruvic-acid salts, waste products of carbohydrate metabolism. Like creatine phosphokinase (CPK) and glutamic oxaloacetic transaminase (GOT), l.d. blood levels increase as a diagnostic sign of heart- or skeletal-muscle damage, as in a heart attack or muscular dystrophy. Abbrev.: **LDH.**

lactogenic hormone = PROLACTIN.

lacuna a gap or break, e.g., a gap in memory. Plural: **lacunae.**

lacunar amnesia = LOCALIZED AMNESIA.

LAD = LANGUAGE-ACQUISITION DEVICE.

ladder fear = CLIMACOPHOBIA.

Ladd-Franklin, Christine American psychologist and logician, 1847–1930. See LADD-FRANKLIN THEORY; COLOR THEORIES.

Ladd-Franklin theory an explanation of color vision introduced by Christine Ladd-Franklin based on gradual evolution of color-sensitive visual receptors from a normal state of color-blindness in primitive animals. The theory proposes that yellow and blue receptors evolved first, then red and green receptors developed out of yellow-sensitive cones. Regression to a more primitive stage would account for absence of certain receptors in color-blind humans.

-laevo-: See -LEVO-.

Laffer, W. B. American physician, fl. 1909. See ASCHER'S SYNDROME (also called **Laffer-Ascher syndrome**).

lagophthalmos a disorder marked by the inability to close the eyelids completely (from Greek *lagos*, "hare," and *ophthalmos*, "eye"). The condition occurs in cases of leprosy. Also spelled **lagophthalmus.** See LEPROSY.

laissez-faire group in social psychology, a group with passive leadership and a minimum of control.

laissez-faire leader /les′āfer′/ the type of leader who provides minimal or no structure for group activities. Goals and procedures are entirely determined by members. In studies by Lewin, Lippitt, and White, laissez-faire leaders were passive, providing information or guidance only if directly asked; their groups showed low productivity, low cohesiveness, and apathy. See DEMOCRATIC LEADER. Compare AUTHORITARIAN LEADER.

Lake v. Cameron: See LEAST-RESTRICTIVE ALTERNATIVE.

-lal-; -lalia a combining form relating to speech.

laliophobia = LALOPHOBIA.

lalling an infantile form of speech which persists beyond the age at which precise speech sounds should have been acquired. It is characterized by sound omission, or substitutions, e.g., tep/step, lellow/yellow, wed/red. Also called **lallation.**

lalopathy any form of speech disorder.

lalophobia a morbid fear of speaking. Also called **laliophobia.**

laloplegia inability to speak due to paralysis of the speech muscles, not including the muscles of the tongue.

lalorrhea = LOGORRHEA.

la main étrangère = STRANGE-HAND SIGN.

Lamarck, Jean-Baptiste Pierre Antoine de Monet de /lämärk′/ French naturalist, 1744–1829. Adjective: **Lamarckian.** See LAMARCKISM.

Lamarckism the theory advanced by Lamarck that changes acquired by an organism through use or disuse can become hereditary. Also called **Lamarckianism.**

Lamaze, Fernand /lämäz′/ French obstetrician, 1890–1957. See LAMAZE METHOD.

Lamaze method a variation of the natural-childbirth technique, developed in the 1950s by the French physician Ferdinand Lamaze. The L.m., which is relatively painless, evolved from the psychoprophylaxis method used in Russia, based in turn on work by Pavlov. The woman learns about childbirth anatomy and physiology and is active during labor, guided by her husband, or by family and friends. Emphasis is put on the husband's sharing in the birth experience. See NATURAL CHILDBIRTH.

lambda /lam′də/ 11th letter of the Greek alphabet (Λ, λ).

lambert a measure of luminance; the amount of light reflected from a perfectly diffusing and reflecting surface emitting one lumen per square centimeter (named for J. H. Lambert). See LUMEN; LUMINANCE.

Lambert, Edward Howard American physiologist, 1915—. See EATON-LAMBERT SYNDROME.

Lambert, Johann Heinrich German mathematician, astronomer, and philosopher, 1728–77. See LAMBERT; MILLILAMBERT; LAMBERT'S LAW.

Lambert-Eaton syndrome = EATON-LAMBERT SYNDROME.

Lambert's law the principle that the incidence, emission, and reflection of light vary directly as the cosine of the angle of the rays perpendicular to the surface.

laminectomy a surgical procedure used to relieve symptoms caused by a ruptured intervertebral disk, or slipped disk. A l. involves the excision of the posterior arch of the vertebra to relieve pressure; or when several vertebrae are associated with the disorder, they may be fused to stabilize the position of the spinal column in the area affected. Also see FORAMINOTOMY.

lamineria: See ABORTIFACIENT.

Lamy, Maurice Émile Joseph /lämē′/ French physician, 1895—. See MAROTEAUX-LAMY SYNDROME; MUCOPOLYSACCHARIDOSES.

Land, Edwin Herbert American inventor, 1909
—. See LAND THEORY OF COLOR VISION.

Landau reflex a normal reaction observed in infants between the ages of three and 12 months when the child is supported horizontally in the prone position; the head raises and the back arches. An absence of the reflex is a sign of a neurologic disorder such as cerebral palsy or motor-neuron disease.

land of childhood a Jungian term for the period in which the rational consciousness has not yet separated from the collective unconscious, and mythological images and associations predominate.

Landolt, Edmund French ophthalmologist, 1846–1926. See LANDOLDT CIRCLES.

Landolt circles a set of circles with gaps of varying size used to test visual acuity.

Landouzy, Louis Théophil Joseph /läNdōōzē′/ French physician, 1845–1917. See LANDOUZY-DÉJÉRINE DYSTROPHY.

Landouzy-Déjérine dystrophy a form of muscular dystrophy that involves mainly the muscles of the face, shoulders, and upper arms. It may begin at any time from childhood to early adulthood, usually as a gradual weakening of the facial muscles or difficulty in raising the arms above the head. Some patients are only slightly affected by the L.-D.d. form of the disease, and it is rarely life-shortening. Also called **facioscapulohumeral muscular dystrophy.**

Landry, Jean Baptiste Octave /läNdrē/ French physician, 1826–1865. See LANDRY'S PARALYSIS.

Landry's paralysis an acute ascending paralysis which begins in the lower limbs and spreads upward to involve the bulbar and respiratory muscles. The cause may be an infection, an autoimmune reaction, or of toxic origin. About half the patients die within two weeks of the onset of symptoms; survivors usually recover within three months. Also called **Kussmaul-Landry paralysis**.

Landsteiner, Karl Austrian-born American pathologist, 1868–1943. See ABO BLOOD-GROUP INCOMPATIBILITY.

Land theory of color vision a theory suggested by E. H. Land (inventor of the Polaroid camera), based on the idea that color registration is carried out in the brain. Experiments involving color separation through filters have indicated that various wavelengths register on the color-sensitive components of the retina as a large number of color-separated "photos," and the visual mechanism in the brain then acts as a computer, averaging together and comparing long-wave photos with the average of the shorter-wave photos, and assigning different colors to them according to the ratios between them.

Langdon Down's disease = DOWN'S SYNDROME.

Lange, Carl /läng′ə/ German physician, 1883—. See LANGE'S COLLOIDAL GOLD REACTION; PARETIC CURVE; TABETIC CURVE.

Lange, Carl Georg Danish psychologist, 1834–1900. See JAMES-LANGE THEORY.

Lange, Cornelia Catharina de Dutch physician, 1871–1950. See DE LANGE'S SYNDROME; OLIGODACTYLY.

Langerhans, Paul /läng′ərhuns/ German pathological anatomist, 1847–88. See ISLANDS OF LANGERHANS; GLUCAGON; INSULIN; INSULIN ABNORMALITIES.

Lange's colloidal gold reaction a diagnostic procedure in which varying amounts of cerebrospinal fluid are added to ten test tubes containing gold solution. Also called **Lange's test**. See PARETIC CURVE.

language any means, vocal or other, of expressing or communicating thought or feeling.

language-acquisition device the innate mechanism of children in developing a language structure using linguistic data from parents. Abbrev.: **LAD**.

language arts the part of the school curriculum that incorporates the language skills of listening, speaking, reading, writing, spelling, and handwriting.

language centers the areas of the cerebral cortex, such as Broca's area, involved in spoken or written language functions as well as music.

language deficit a delay, or deviance, in the normal speech and language development of a child due to some neurological dysfunction.

language development: See ORIGIN-OF-LANGUAGE THEORIES.

language disability: See LANGUAGE DISORDER; GENERAL L.D.

language disorder a disturbance of speech or writing characterized by failure to follow the rules that govern meaning (semantics) or structure (syntax). Also called **language dysfunction**. For examples, see AGRAMMATISM; APHASIA; CLANG ASSOCIATION; INCOHERENCE; NEOLOGISM; WORD APPROXIMATION; WORD SALAD.

language-experience approach to reading a method of teaching language skills based on children's experiences. Experience-based materials may be dictated by the child to the teacher, then used as material for teaching reading.

language localization areas of the brain in which various functions of written and spoken words and music are centered. Although Broca's original discovery found l.l. near the third frontal convolution of the left hemisphere, later research has identified numerous cortical centers associated with visual and auditory language processing as well as neural pathways linking the areas. Also see SPEECH LOCALIZATION.

language origin: See ORIGIN-OF-LANGUAGE THEORIES.

language pathology the study of the causes and treatment of disorders of symbolic behavior.

language retardation developmental lag in cerebral maturation resulting in delayed language skills manifested by lisping, lalling, baby talk, congenital auditory agnosia, and word deafness. However, the term l.r. is not applied to cases of language difficulty associated with mental retardation, impaired hearing, or structural abnormalities in the speech organs.

language score: See ACE TEST.

language theories: See ORIGIN-OF-L.T.

Lansing (II) virus: See LEON (III) VIRUS.

lanugo the fine hair that appears in the later months of fetal development. It may still be visible on parts of a newborn's body before disappearing within a few weeks. Also called **l. hair**.

-laparo- a combining form relating to the loins or the abdomen.

laparoscopy the examination of the peritoneal cavity by means of an endoscope equipped with a lens and light source. The procedure permits the study of ovaries, Fallopian tubes, and related organs through a small incision in the abdominal wall.

lapsus calami /cal′əmē/ a "slip of the pen" (Latin) dictated by unconscious feelings or impulses. See PARAPRAXIS; SYMPTOMATIC ACT; FREUDIAN SLIP.

lapsus linguae /lin′gwī/ a "slip of the tongue" (Latin); an unconscious, unintentional error that alters the surface meaning of what one is saying while revealing an unconscious association, motivation, or wish. See SYMPTOMATIC ACT; FREUDIAN SLIP.

lapsus memoriae /memôr′ē·ī/ a "memory lapse" (Latin); a temporary inaccuracy in memory or a temporary inability to remember a common fact, especially when the lapse has unconscious significance, as in forgetting the name of a person we dislike. See SYMPTOMATIC ACT.

large-numbers law: See LAW OF LARGE NUMBERS.

large-object fear = MEGALOPHOBIA.

Larsson, Tage Konrad Leopold Swedish scientist, 1905—. See SJÖGREN-LARSSON SYNDROME.

larval sadism a type of sadism that is masked or concealed.

larval schizophrenia latent or incipient schizophrenia, that is, schizophrenia that is assumed to be present but has not advanced to the level of psychosis.

-laryng-; -laryngo- a combining form relating to the larynx.

laryngeal cancer a malignant growth of the upper respiratory tract that affects mainly men over the age of 40 and accounts for about 3,000 deaths each year in the United States. The risk of l.c. increases with cigarette-smoking, drinking alcoholic beverages, and living in urban areas; the incidence among cigarette smokers is approximately seven times that of the general population. Early symptoms include hoarseness or a feeling of soreness or a "lump" in the throat. As the l.c. progresses, it interferes with breathing and swallowing. Treatment usually includes surgery or radiation, or both, the appropriate procedure depending upon the cancer site and the extent of its growth. If it is possible to correct the problem by excising only one vocal cord, the patient is trained to speak with the remaining vocal cord. If it is necessary to remove the entire voice box, or larynx, the patient is trained to speak with the aid of an electronic de-

vice or by a technique of swallowing air into the esophagus and forcing it out again while the lips and teeth are manipulated to form speech sounds. However, the vocabulary of words that can be produced in this manner is limited. See LARYNGECTOMY.

laryngeal reflex the reaction to laryngeal irritation manifested by coughing.

laryngectomy the surgical removal of all or a part of the larynx, commonly because of laryngeal cancer. A l. usually is accompanied by severe psychological trauma because of the patient's anxiety about being unable to communicate in the usual manner. There also is fear, partly justified, that the patient may suffocate after surgery because of an inability to alert the doctors and nurses if the trachea becomes blocked during the recovery period. See LARYNGEAL CANCER.

laryngopharynx the lower portion of the pharynx situated between the larynx and oropharynx.

larynx the muscular and cartilaginous structure at the top of the trachea and below the tongue roots; the organ of voice consisting of nine cartilages connected by ligaments, and containing the vocal cords.

Lasègue, Ernest Charles /läzāg′/ French physician, 1816–83. See LASÈGUE'S SIGN.

Lasègue's sign a diagnostic sign of sciatic-nerve disorder consisting of painful flexion of the hip when the knee is extended but not when it is flexed.

Lashley, Karl Spencer American psychologist, 1890–1958. L. experimented on localization of brain function, demonstrating that undamaged areas can take over some of the functions of damaged areas (the principle of equipotentiality), and that learning and retention depend more on the amount of intact cortex than on the location, since extensive areas work together in these processes (the principle of mass action). See ENGRAM; LAW OF EQUIPOTENTIALITY; LAW OF MASS ACTION.

Lasswell, Harold Dwight American educator, 1902—. See CONTENT ANALYSIS.

latah a culture-specific syndrome first discovered in Malaya, but also found in Thailand, Siberia, the Congo, and the Philippines. The condition develops mainly in dull, submissive women who have been subjected to a sudden fright. Its major symptoms, besides fearfulness, are mimicking behavior (echolalia, echopraxia) and a compulsion to utter profanities and obscenities (coprolalia). These reactions are believed to stem from an inability to cope with the threatening, anxiety-provoking situation.

latch-key children children who come home from school to an empty home because both parents work.

late infantile systemic lipidosis = G_{M1} GANGLIOSIDOSIS.

latency in psychoanalysis, the stage of psychosexual development when overt sexual interest is repressed and sublimated, and the child's attention is focused on skills and peer activities with members of his or her own sex. This stage lasts roughly from the resolution of the oedipal phase (fourth or fifth year) to the onset of puberty (11th or 12th year). Also called **latency stage**.

latency of response the amount of time intervening between the onset of a stimulus and the onset of the response. L.o.r. may be used as a criterion of the strength of conditioning. Also called **latency of reply; response latency**. See RESPONSE TIME.

latency stage = LATENCY.

latent addition period a brief time span when a second stimulus may add to the effects of a first stimulus. The l.a.p. varies with the size of the nerve and synaptic factors but lasts approximately one-half millisecond.

latent content in psychoanalysis, the concealed or disguised impulses and ideas that lie beneath the symbolic images, or manifest content, of a dream or fantasy. According to Freud, unconscious wishes and impulses seeking expression in dreams encounter "censorship" and are distorted into symbolic representations, that is, the manifest content or dream as experienced. Through free association and interpretation, the l.c. is uncovered. See DREAMWORK. Compare MANIFEST CONTENT.

latent goals in evaluation research, objectives of a program or organization that are not publicly stated; or program objectives known to the staff that are unacceptable for public statement; also, functions that result from the attempt to obtain manifest goals that are not obvious, apparent, or planned by the program director.

latent homosexuality homosexual tendencies that have never been expressed overtly and are usually unrecognized by the individual. The latter condition is also called **unconscious homosexuality**.

latent learning learning acquired unintentionally and remaining subconscious or latent until a specific need for it arises. E.g., a student writing an exam may be able to accurately cite a quotation subconsciously memorized without any previous effort to do so. L.l. is a form of INCIDENTAL LEARNING. See this entry.

latent psychosis an underlying psychotic disorder, such a schizophrenia, which has not reached the full-blown, or florid, stage. Also called **prepsychotic psychosis; incipient psychosis**.

lateral bundle a bundle of nerve fibers in the spinal cord that carry impulses from pain- and temperature-sensory end organs.

lateral cervical nucleus a part of the lemniscal system, appearing as a small mass of gray matter beneath the medulla. Axons of the l.c.n. communicate with the medial lemniscus.

lateral confusion = MIXED LATERALITY.

lateral corticospinal tract one of the two primary motoneuron pathways in the spinal cord, consisting of crossed fibers running between the spinal motor mechanisms and the direct sensory fibers.

lateral dominance the tendency for one hemisphere to be dominant over the other for most functions, leading to preferential use of one side of the body. Also called **hemispherical dominance**. See LATERALITY; HARRIS TESTS OF LATERAL DOMINANCE.

lateral fissure = FISSURE OF SYLVIUS.

lateral geniculate body an oval elevation on the side and to the rear of the thalamus and connected to the superior colliculus through the superior brachium. Most of the fibers of the optic nerve end in the l.g.b. and are relayed to the visual cortex.

lateral geniculate nucleus a nerve cell located on the lateral surface of the thalamus and serving as a relay neuron for visual impulses being transmitted to the cortex. Abbrev.: **LGN**.

lateral gyrus a convolution in the surface of the brain located in the area of the cingulate gyrus above the corpus callosum.

lateral horns the lateral portion of gray matter located between the dorsal and ventral horns of the spinal cord. The l.h. contain the autonomic-motor fibers that innervate the smooth muscles, heart, and glands.

lateral hypothalamic syndrome a pattern of recovery from lateral hypothalamic lesions, marked by aphagia and adipsia, during which an experimental animal is kept alive by tube feeding, followed by a period of adipsia-anorexia when only wet, palatable foods are accepted. In the third stage, the animal will eat hydrated dry food but continue to avoid water intake and may suffer dehydration. Recovery is the fourth stage.

lateral hypothalamus the portion of the hypothalamus that regulates eating. Lesions of the l.h. in animal experiments result in a loss of interest in food. Stimulation of that part of the brain increases the animal's appetite. Abbrev.: **LH**.

lateral inhibition a theory that discrimination between various sensory inputs, such as taste sensations, involves a feedback mechanism of second-order cells and collaterals relaying impulses into an inhibitory network which in turn raises the threshold for the sensation.

laterality the preferential use of one side of the body for certain functions such as eating, writing, sighting, and kicking. The trait is associated with CEREBRAL DOMINANCE. See this entry. Also see HANDEDNESS; LATERALIZATION; MIXED L.; RIGHT-LEFT DISORIENTATION; SPEECH LATERALIZATION; LANGUAGE LOCALIZATION; SPLIT BRAIN; FUNCTIONAL PLASTICITY; DIRECTIONAL CONFUSION.

lateralization the relationship between handedness, eyedness, footedness, and cerebral dominance as manifested by learning tasks and also signs of localized brain damage. Right-left confusion and dyslexia are among disorders diagnosed through l. tests. L. is observed more frequently in humans than in primates. Also see SPEECH L.

lateral lemniscus a bundle of nerve fibers running longitudinally upward through the pons, terminating in the medial geniculate body and inferior colliculus. The l.l. carries auditory-nerve fibers from one side of the body to the other. Also see LEMNISCAL SYSTEM.

lateral olfactory tract a bundle of axons of mitral cells which forms the primary communication between the olfactory system and portions of the brain. Also see OLFACTORY TRACT.

lateral orbital gyrus: See ORBITAL GYRI.

lateral rectus: See EYE MOVEMENTS.

lateral section the portion of a body or organ that is located on or toward a side and away from the medial, or middle, section. See CONTRALATERAL; IPSILATERAL.

lateral specialization the development of special abilities in the right or left hemisphere. Examples include the general tendency for speech, writing, calculation, and language to be controlled by the left hemisphere and nonverbal ideation and spatial construction to be controlled by the right hemisphere. See LATERALITY.

lateral spinothalamic tract one of the long sensory-nerve bundles that runs through the lateral, or outer, areas of the spinal cord. It contains second-order neurons and fibers that ascend all the way to the thalamus without synapses. Also see SPINOTHALAMIC TRACT.

lateral sulcus = FISSURE OF SYLVIUS.

lateral thalamic nucleus a large mass of cell bodies on the lateral side of the thalamus which relay incoming sensory impulses.

lateral ventricle a reservoir of cerebrospinal fluid found in each of the cerebral hemispheres. The lateral ventricles on each side communicate with each other and with the third ventricle at a point near the thalamus.

lateropulsion a symptom of certain CNS disorders, e.g., parkinsonism, in which the patient makes rapid, short steps sidewise.

lateroventral nucleus of hypothalamus one of a group of relay nuclei located in the thalamus where it transmits impulses from the cerebellum to the frontal lobe. Its function is related to coordination of muscular movements.

Latin square an experimental design in which treatments are administered in orders that are systematically varied and denoted by Latin letters. E.g. one group might receive treatments A, B, and then C, while a second group receives them in order B, C, A, and a third group in order C, A, B.

laudanum a mixture of alcohol and opium once commonly used as an analgesic and anesthetic. Historical records indicate the mixture was introduced around 1530 by Paracelsus and was used as an intoxicating beverage in 18th-century England.

laughter pleasurable convulsive sounds which serve to release tension built up when we listen to an amusing story or watch an amusing event. Eidelberg states that "a joke permits us a temporary return from the reality of the adult to the simple pleasure realm of the child," and points out that "laughter may also be used as a defense against crying and against embarrassment"

(*Encyclopedia of Psychoanalysis*, 1968). In psychiatry, l. means unrestrained or paroxysmal **laughing spells.** Such spells have been found (a) to precipitate cataplectic attacks, (b) to be a common manifestation in manias, and a symptom of the **Angelman,** or "**happy-puppet,**" **syndrome,** and (c) to be an occasional symptom of psychomotor seizure among children (termed **gelastic epilepsy**). Spasmodic l., called **gelasmus,** is also found in schizophrenia, hysteria, and organic (especially bulbar) and pseudobulbar diseases of the brain, as well as in dancing mania. Also see COMPULSIVE L.

Laurence, John Zacharias English physician, 1830–74. See LAURENCE-MOON-BIEDLE SYNDROME.

Laurence-Moon-Biedl syndrome an autosomal-recessive disorder which may be characterized by some degree of obesity, polydactylism, subnormal intelligence, and ocular abnormalities, particularly of the retina. A common finding is progressive cone-rod degeneration and night-blindness. Hypogonadism and hearing difficulty often are associated with the disorder. More than 75 percent of the patients tested have been mentally retarded. Also called **Laurence-Moon-Biedl-Bardet syndrome; retinodiencephalic degeneration.**

Lavater, Johann Kaspar /lävä′tər/ Swiss poet and theologian, 1741–1801. See PHYSIOGNOMY.

law in science, a theory that is widely accepted as correct, and one that has no significant rivals in accounting for the facts within its domain.

law-and-order orientation a term applied to the stage of Kohlberg's conventional level of moral reasoning in which the emphasis is on authority, established rules, doing one's duty, and maintaining the social order. See CONVENTIONAL LEVEL.

law of advantage the principle that of two or more incompatible or inconsistent responses one has the advantage of being more reliable and occurring more frequently.

law of assimilation the principle that organisms respond to new situations in a manner similar to their reactions to familiar situations.

law of avalanche the spreading of neural impulses from a stimulus receptor to a number of other neurons, resulting in an effect that is disproportionate to the initial stimulus, as in an epileptic seizure.

Law of Bichat an early concept (18th century) that the vegetative body system provides for assimilation and augmentation of mass while the animal body system provides for the transformation of energy, the two systems being in inverse ratio in the development of ontogenetic evolution.

law of cohesion the principle that acts occurring close to each other in time and space tend to become integrated into more complex acts.

law of combination the principle that simultaneous stimuli or stimuli in close proximity may produce a combined response, or will occur together when a stimulus eliciting either response is presented.

law of common fate the Gestalt principle that objects functioning or moving in the same way appear to belong together. Wertheimer called this principle the **factor of uniform density**.

law of constancy the Freudian principle that all mental processes tend toward a state of equilibrium and the stability of the inorganic state. Also called **principle of constancy**. See DEATH INSTINCT; NIRVANA PRINCIPLE.

law of contiguity the principle that learning depends upon the proximity of stimulus and response in space or time. The l.o.c. is a principle of associationism. Also see CONTIGUITY OF ASSOCIATIONS.

law of contrast a principle of association which states that thinking about any special quality tends to remind one of its opposite. In later associationist doctrine, this principle was considered a special case of contiguity.

law of diminishing returns the principle that each practice session produces a smaller gain.

law of effect the principle that subjects tend to learn satisfying behavior more easily than habits leading to an unpleasant state.

law of equality a Gestalt principle that parts of a figure perceived as equal tend to form a whole.

law of equipotentiality the principle introduced in 1929 by K. S. Lashley that, due to the complexity of the nervous system, intact areas of the cortex can take over some functions of areas that have been destroyed. The theory was based on studies of rats with cortical lesions running a maze. Other investigators have challenged the validity of the l.o.e. because of difficulty in reproducing the findings in different species. Also called **principle of equipotentiality; equipotentiality law**. See LAW OF MASS ACTION.

law of exercise the principle that the learning rate increases as the degree of practice increases.

law of filial regression the principle that inherited traits tend to revert toward the mean for the species. E.g., very tall fathers tend to have shorter sons, and very short fathers tend to have taller sons.

law of forward conduction the rule that nerve impulses always travel in the same direction, which is from the terminal knob of the axon to the postsynaptic membrane of the dendrites. The l.o.f.c. prevails in nature, but the direction can be reversed under experimental laboratory conditions.

law of frequency the principle that the rate of learning increases with the rate of practice. Also called **law of repetition; law of use**.

law of identical direction the physiological principle that in normal binocular vision the images focused on the retinas of the left and right eyes become fused to appear as a single image focused onto the median plane of the head.

law of initial values the principle that the initial level of a physiological response is a major determinant of a later response in that system.

Thus, if an individual's pulse rate is high, his cardiovascular response to an emotion-provoking stimulus will be smaller than if the initial pulse rate had been low. Also called **Wilder's l.o.i.v.**

law of large numbers a mathematical principle indicating that as the sample size increases the theoretical expectations of its statistical properties will be more and more closely realized. In a purely chance series there may be apparent deviations from randomness in the short run, but in the long run chance will be more and more closely approximated, as predicted by the l.o.l.n.

law of least action = LEAST-EFFORT PRINCIPLE.

law of mass action the theory that large areas of the cortex function together in the learning process, and that if cortical lesions occur, their size is more important than their location. The concept evolved from 1929 experiments by K. S. Lashley on the effects of different amounts of destruction on the ability of rats to escape from a problem box. The theory developed into the LAW OF EQUIPOTENTIALITY. See this entry. L.o.m.a. is also called **principle of mass action**.

law of parsimony = OCCAM'S RAZOR.

law of Prägnanz = PRINCIPLE OF PRÄGNANZ.

law of precision a Gestalt principle that all percepts tend to become organized into regular, symmetrical forms with precise contours. See PRINCIPLE OF PRÄGNANZ.

law of primacy = PRIMACY EFFECT.

law of prior entry the principle that of two simultaneous stimuli, one attended to and the other not, the attended stimulus will be perceived as having been introduced sooner than the other.

law of progression the principle that successive increments of sensation increase in arithmetic progression while stimulus increments increase in geometric progression.

law of proximity = PROXIMITY PRINCIPLE.

law of readiness a learning theory postulate that when a conduction unit (that is, neural mechanism) is ready to conduct, conduction by it is satisfying (Thorndike).

law of recency = RECENCY EFFECT.

law of repetition; law of use = LAW OF FREQUENCY.

laws of color preference an order of preferred colors based on results of more than 50 studies of choices made by adults. The order for nearly all humans of both sexes, regardless of ethnic or cultural background, has been found to be blue, red, green, violet, orange, and yellow. Infants appear to prefer yellow but shift toward blue and red in later childhood. Exceptions to the rule have been found among Native Americans and Filipinos, whose first choice is red.

laws of learning principles that state the conditions under which learning occurs. For the major l.o.l., see LAW OF CONTIGUITY; LAW OF DIMINISHING RETURNS; LAW OF EFFECT; LAW OF EXERCISE; LAW OF FREQUENCY; PRIMACY EFFECT; RECENCY EFFECT. For other principles and practices that enhance learning, see PROGRESSIVE EDUCATION;

SPACED PRACTICE; MEANINGFUL LEARNING; ROTE LEARNING; OVERLEARNING; ASSOCIATIVE LEARNING.

laxative addiction a dependence upon the use of laxatives to induce bowel movements. L.a. evolves as a vicious cycle in which the laxative use itself gradually reduces normal bowel activity so that laxatives or enemas become increasingly necessary to prevent constipation problems. See ENEMA ADDICTION; KLISMAPHILIA.

lay analysis psychoanalysis performed by a non-medical practitioner, or **lay analyst**, who has been trained in psychoanalytic theory and practice.

layman a man or woman who has not received formal training or enough formal training to qualify for membership in a profession, or who, generally, is not a member of one's own profession or does not have one's special knowledge or skills. A priest may consider a physician a l., and vice versa.

LCU = LIFE-CHANGE UNITS.

LD = LEARNING DISABILITIES.

L-data an abbreviation for *l*ife-record data, compiled as the subject reacts to life situations (Cattell).

LDH = LACTIC DEHYDROGENASE.

L-dopa: See DOPAMINERGICS.

lead-cap headache a headache that has the sensation of a heavy weight or a severe constriction about the head, sometimes described as **skull-lifting headache** or **splitting headache**.

lead encephalitis an acute inflammation of the brain due to lead intoxication. It usually is marked by suddenly increased intracranial pressure that is relieved by infusions of a urea solution repeated as necessary or by craniotomy. The mortality rate is very high, and among those who survive there may be permanent blindness, paralysis, and mental retardation..

lead encephalopathy a brain disorder most commonly found in children who eat paint that contains lead. Symptoms include convulsions, cortical blindness, mania, delirium, and coma. Increased intracranial pressure may result in projectile vomiting and a bulging of the fontanelles in very young children. L.e. occurs in adults who inhale tetraethyl lead in gasoline fumes.

leader: See AUTHORITARIAN L.; BUREAUCRATIC L.; CONTINGENCY THEORY OF LEADERSHIP; DEMOCRATIC L.; DISCUSSION L.; FUNCTIONAL LEADERSHIP; GREAT-MAN THEORY OF LEADERSHIP; GROUP-CENTERED L.; LAISSEZ-FAIRE L.

leaderless group a special or experimental group in which subjects discuss or work together on a problem without a leader. The subject's behavior may be observed and rated in order to evaluate specific skills related to leadership ability, e.g., ease in verbal communication, problem-solving, and social situations. The l.g. technique may be used to screen candidates for positions in business, social work, teaching, and the military.

leaderless-group therapy a form of group psychotherapy in which leaderless meetings are held either (a) on an occasional or regularly scheduled basis as an adjunct to the traditional therapist-led process, or (b) on an entirely self-directed basis, in which a group meets for its entire life span without a designated leader. (The pros and cons of the alternatives are presented by Irvin D. Yalom in *The Theory and Practice of Group Psychotherapy*, 1975.)

leader match a concept of leadership training in which it is assumed that leader style tends to resist change but that leaders can be trained to diagnose a situation and alter it to fit their own style.

leadership the capacity to influence the actions and attitudes of individuals or groups through such means as organizational skill, superior knowledge and expertise, the power of personality, and, in general, the ability to evoke the cooperation and commitment of others.

leadership role the specific functions and activities of an individual who heads a group, serving, e.g., as director, guide, catalyst, or mobilizer. Some leaders play an authoritarian, others a democratic or a laissez-faire role.

leadership theories competing theories advanced to explain leader effectiveness, particularly, (a) trait theories, which focus on such characteristics as supervisory ability, intelligence, self-assurance, and decisiveness, (b) behavior theories, which focus on a combination of employee-centered supervision (characterized by friendliness, treating others as equals, eliciting suggestions) with production-centered supervision (assigning tasks, scheduling the work), and (c) situational-moderator theories, which attempt to describe what works best in different situations, since no single leader or leadership style is equally effective in all settings.

leading eye the eye that is the first to turn toward a visual stimulus.

lead-pipe rigidity a plastic type of muscle hypertonus involving opposing muscle groups. The condition occurs in some cases of parkinsonism and cerebral palsy.

lead poisoning: See LEAD ENCEPHALOPATHY; LEAD ENCEPHALITIS.

leaping ague a type of dancing mania sometimes called CHOREOMANIA. See this entry.

learned autonomic control the individual's capacity to learn to regulate visceral functions such as blood pressure and temperature, which are ordinarily under the control of the autonomic nervous system. The learning is accomplished primarily by the use of biofeedback techniques, and in some cases by the use of hypnosis. Also called **visceral learning**. See BIOFEEDBACK; HYPNOTHERAPY.

learned helplessness a term applied by Maier and Seligman (1976) to a sense of helplessness and lack of motivation generated by exposure to aversive events over which the individual has no control. Animals exposed to inescapable electric shocks failed to learn to escape shocks in situations where escape was possible, and human beings subjected to continual stresses and deprivations frequently become depressed and fatalistic, and feel they can do nothing about their problems. Also see BEHAVIOR-CONSTRAINT THEORY.

learning the process of acquiring new and relatively enduring information, behavior patterns, or abilities; modification of behavior as a result of practice, study, or experience.

learning by doing: See PROGRESSIVE EDUCATION.

learning curve a graph that records the course of learning. A measure of performance (e.g., gains, errors) is represented along the vertical axis. The horizontal axis plots trials or time. The learning of a group or individual may be represented by the curve.

learning disabilities disorders in one or more of the basic psychological processes involved in understanding or using spoken or written language. The term includes perceptual handicaps, brain injury, minimal brain dysfunction, dyslexia, and developmental aphasia. Excluded are visual or hearing handicaps, mental retardation, or emotional disturbance as the primary handicapping conditions. Abbrev.: **LD**.

learning-disabilities specialist an individual trained to identify and remedy the problems associated with learning disabilities. He or she often acts as the school's team coordinator in an interdisciplinary approach to the child.

learning model an orientation to the study of human development and behavior that stresses the critical influence of environmental conditions on the physical, cognitive, interpersonal, and emotional functioning of the individual. The l.m. primarily regards the child as passively absorbing the relevant features of the environment in a continuous line of development in contrast to the cognitivist emphasis on development as an active construction of knowledge in several specific stages characterized by distinct modes of organization and expression. (Howard Gardner, *Developmental Psychology*, 1978) Also called **environmental-learning theory**. Also see COGNITIVE STRUCTURE.

learning paradigm in abnormal psychology, a theory that abnormal behavior is learned through the same processes as other forms of behavior.

learning session: See PRACTICE PERIOD.

learning sets a form of discriminative learning in which the subject is given a number of different problems and each problem is offered for a fixed number of trials. The number of trials is repeated for each problem regardless of whether it is solved the first or second time. The purpose is to improve the learning ability of the subject. The "learn-to-learn" concept was introduced in 1949 by H. F. Harlow.

learning theory a body of concepts and principles rather than a single theory, which seeks to explain the learning process. For the major approaches, see CONDITIONING; GUTHRIE'S CONTIGUOUS CONDITIONING; HABIT; HEBB'S THEORY OF PERCEPTUAL LEARNING; HULL'S MATHEMATICODEDUCTIVE THEORY OF LEARNING; INSIGHT; LAWS OF LEARNING; OPERANT CONDITIONING; THORNDIKE'S TRIAL-AND-ERROR-LEARNING; TOLMAN'S PURPOSIVE BEHAVIORISM.

learn-to-learn concept: See LEARNING SETS.

least-effort principle the hypothesis that an organism tends to choose the means or course of action that appears to entail the smallest amount of effort or the least resistance. Also called **law of least action**.

least-noticeable difference = DIFFERENCE THRESHOLD.

Least-Preferred Coworker Test a measure of leadership style based on the extent of the leader's esteem for his least-preferred coworker, or **LPC**, that is, the one with whom it has been most difficult to cooperate. The leader is then asked to rate this worker from 1 to 8 on a set of bipolar dimensions (friendly-unfriendly, supportive-hostile, unproductive-productive, etc.). The ratings have been used to distinguish between task-oriented and relationship-oriented leaders.

least resistance: See LEAST-EFFORT PRINCIPLE.

least-resistance site: See LOCUS MINORIS RESISTENTIAE.

least-restrictive alternative the concept that less treatment rather than more is the most desirable objective, with the minimum level of restrictions on the patient's freedom. This position was emphasized in two decisions of Judge D. Bazelon in 1966: **Rouse v. Cameron**, and **Lake v. Cameron**.

least-squares criterion a term referring to the success of fitting a regression line to a set of data points. The more closely the line fits, the smaller the sum of squares of the differences between the line and each data point.

leaving the field reacting to frustration or conflict by removing oneself from the situation or escaping into psychogenic illness.

Lebenslüge = LIFE LIE.

Leber, Theodor /lā′bər/ German ophthalmologist, 1840–1917. See LEBER'S DISEASE; AMAUROSIS.

Leber's disease a hereditary visual disorder characterized by slowly progressive optic atrophy with normal peripheral vision but blind areas of the retina toward the center. The symptoms begin around the third decade of life. The genetic defect is transmitted by the female but males are most often affected.

Le Bon, Gustave /ləbôN′/ French physician and social psychologist, 1841–1931. See CROWD CONSCIOUSNESS.

Leboyer technique a psychological approach to childbirth devised by the French obstetrician Frédéric Leboyer. The L.t. focuses on the feelings and sensations of the baby, and advocates peace and quiet, dim lights, delay in severing the umbilical cord, body contact between the newborn and the parents, and an immediate warm bath that approximates the conditions within the womb.

lecanomancy a system of divination in which a medium looks into a basin of water and sees visions. L. has been used in psychoanalytic studies to show relationships between the medium's supposed visions and his dreams and complexes. (The term is derived from the Greek words *lekane*, "dish, pan," and *manteia*, "oracle, divination.")

lécheur /lāshœr'/ a man or woman who touches genitals with his or her mouth, that is, performs cunnilingus or fellatio (French, "licker"). If the person doing this is female, she is more properly called a **lécheuse** /lāshœs'/. Also see OROGENITAL ACTIVITY.

lecture method a personnel-training procedure used primarily to present new material to large groups, especially when classroom time is limited. It is also used to introduce other instructional methods, such as films, or to summarize material developed by other instructional methods.

left-handedness preferential use of the left hand for major activities, such as eating, writing, and throwing. It is a component of SINISTRALITY. See this entry. Also see LATERALITY; CEREBRAL DOMINANCE; HANDEDNESS; DEXTRALITY-SINISTRALITY.

left-sided apraxia a disorder marked by the inability of a right-handed individual to carry out actions with his left hand that he is able to carry out with his right hand. The condition is due to a lesion in the anterior portion of the corpus callosum that prevents information from the right motor region from reaching the left motor-association area.

left-side fear = LEVOPHOBIA.

left temporal lobectomy: See TEMPORAL LOBECTOMY.

legal capacity the mental capacity to manage one's legal affairs, that is, to make and understand a contract, to make a will, and to stand trial and understand the nature of the proceedings.

legalistic orientation a term applied to the lower stage of L. Kohlberg's postconventional or principled level of moral development, in which the emphasis is on rights and standards that have been agreed upon by the whole society. See POSTCONVENTIONAL LEVEL.

legal psychiatry = FORENSIC PSYCHIATRY.

legal psychology = FORENSIC PSYCHOLOGY.

legasthenia a condition that appears to be both congenital and hereditary, characterized by difficulty in visual and auditory synthesis of individual letters into a total word pattern, or difficulty in analyzing a given word into its component letters despite apparently adequate intellectual and perceptual ability (from Latin *legere*, "to read," and Greek *astheneia*, "weakness"). Also called **dyslexia with dysorthographia**.

Legg, Arthur Thornton American surgeon, 1874–1939. See LEGG-CALVÉ-PERTHES DISEASE.

Legg-Calvé-Perthes disease a bone disorder of the upper portion of the femur due to faulty circulation, resulting in necrosis, or death, of the cartilage cells near the top of the upper leg bone. L.-C.-P.d. affects mainly children between the ages of four and 12 and is treated by surgery to replace the deformed natural joint with an artificial one that in many instances will allow the patient to participate in certain sports. Also called **Waldenström's syndrome.**

legitimacy knowledge in social psychology, the role played by an individual's major group identifications in contributing to self-image and estimate of personal value. L.k. derives from the individual's perceptions of the culture's relative acceptance of his racial, sexual, ethnic, or religious group. Competence knowledge refers to that component of self-image that derives from individual gifts and accomplishments.

Lehrmann, Orla J.O.L. Swedish physician, fl. 1961. See BÖRJESON-FORSSMAN-LEHRMANN SYNDROME.

Leibniz, Gottfried Wilhelm von /lĭp'nĭts/ German philosopher and mathematician, 1646–1716. See PREESTABLISHED HARMONY.

-leio- a combining form meaning smooth.

Leiter, Russell Graydon American psychologist, 1901—. See LEITER INTERNATIONAL PERFORMANCE TEST.

Leiter International Performance Test a non-verbal intelligence test primarily for cross-cultural administration, and consisting of such materials as number series, concealed figures, picture-completion tasks, and matching wooden blocks according to colors, forms, and pictures.

Lemli, Luc American pediatrician, fl. 1964. See SMITH-LEMLI-OPITZ SYNDROME.

lemniscal system a part of the somatosensory network of nerve fibers, composed mainly of large-diameter myelinated A fibers. It includes the dorsal columns, the tract of Morin, and the neospinothalamic tract of nerve fibers, extending from the spinal cord to the thalamus and cortex. Also see LATERAL LEMNISCUS.

length of stay: See LOS.

lens of eye a transparent, biconvex structure enclosed in an elastic membrane capsule. It is composed of tiny hexagonal prism fibers fitted together in concentric layers. The fetal lens is nearly spherical, not perfectly transparent. In adulthood, the lens is convex, clear, and transparent. In old age, it becomes flattened, slightly opaque, and amber-tinted.

lenticular-fasciculus stimulation the self-stimulation that occurs in a rat when an electrode is inserted in a subthalamic pathway near the lenticular nucleus of the brain and wired to a lever that the animal can press. When the level is pressed, a mild electric current flows to the electrode. Because the rat tends to press the lever repeatedly when wired to the electrode, it is assumed that l.-f.s. has a pleasurable effect.

lenticular nucleus a lens-shaped portion of the corpus striatum and the outermost of the large nuclei located near the thalamus, as a result of pressure from the developing fore-brain about midway through a human pregnancy. It consists of a wedge of gray matter with fibers associated in motor-neuron activity. Also called **lentiform nucleus**.

Leonardo da Vinci /lä·ōnär′dō dä vin′chē/Italian artist, scientist, and philosopher, 1452–1519. See APPLIED PSYCHOANALYSIS; FREUD.

Leon (III) virus one of three enterovirus strains known to cause poliomyelitis in humans. The others are identified as **Brunhilde (I)** and **Lansing (II)** strains. Some primates and rodents also can be infected with at least one of the three strains.

leprechaunism a familial disorder characterized by a large head with small, emaciated body, large, wide-set eyes, long, low-set ears, and an abundance of hair at birth. The patients have poor psychomotor development and muscular hypotonia. The syndrome is believed to be due to an autosomal-recessive gene which becomes manifested through consanguinity. Also called **Donohue's syndrome**.

leprostatic medication: See DAPSONE.

leprosy an infectious disease caused by the bacterium Mycobacterium leprae. The first sign is usually a spot, or macule, with loss of sensation at the center. This may be followed by damage to the peripheral nerves, leading to many types of deformity such as drop foot, claw hand, and facial paralysis. Anesthesia of the body surface then develops, and burns, ulcers, and cuts become infected, destroying many parts of the body since there is no pain signal. Today treatment with Dapsone or other drugs can arrest the disease if given in time, but many victims are still socially isolated and suffer the psychological stigma of "spoiled identity." Also see HANSEN'S DISEASE; LAGOPHTHALMOS.

-lept-; -lepto- a combining form meaning thin, slender, slight, small, delicate (Greek *leptos*, literally, "peeled").

Leptazol = PENTYLENTETRAZOL.

leptokurtic a frequency distribution that is more peaked than a comparison distribution, such as the normal curve. Also see PLATYKURTIC; MESOKURTIC.

leptomorph: See BODY-BUILD INDEX.

leptosome type = ASTHENIC TYPE.

Leroy's disease = INCLUSION-CELL DISEASE.

LES = LOCAL EXCITATORY STATE.

Lesbianism female homosexuality. The term is based on the name of an Aegean Island, Lesbos, where the poetess Sappho (ca. 600 B.C.) wrote glowing accounts of erotic activities between women. Also called **Sapphism**. Also see IATROGENIC HOMOSEXUALITY.

Lesch, Michael American pediatrician, 1939—. See LESCH-NYHAN SYNDROME; AUTOAGGRESSIVE ACTIVITIES; FINGER-BITING BEHAVIOR; HYPERURICOSURIA; HYPOXANTHINE GUANINE PHOSPHORIBOSYL TRANSFERASE; SELF-MUTILATION.

Lesch-Nyhan syndrome an X-linked recessive disease associated with a hypoxanthine-guanine

enzyme deficiency, overproduction of uric acid, and a tendency to self-mutilation by biting the lips and fingers. All reported patients are mentally retarded, with IQs below 50. Motor development deteriorates after the first six to eight months of life, marked by spasticity, chorea, and athetosis. Also called **hereditary choreoathetosis; hereditary hyperuricemia**.

lesion any change in the structure or function of an organ or part of an organ due to injury, disease, or surgical procedure that results in a discontinuity of the normal condition of the tissue. Generally, a l. may be a wound, ulcer, tumor, cataract, or any other pathological change in tissue.

lethal catatonia = BELL'S MANIA.

lethality scale a set of criteria used to predict the probability that an individual is likely to attempt or commit suicide. The l.s. is based on ten factors, including sex, age, prior suicidal behavior, medical status, degree of stress, and symptoms such as alcoholism, depression, or sleep disturbances.

lethargy a listless, drowsy, apathetic state usually accompanied by a low energy level and lack of motivation. It can be observed in various degrees in depressive disorders, and in an extreme degree in lethargic encephalitis (sleeping sickness).

lethologica temporary inability to recall a proper noun or name.

letting off steam: See TALKING IT OUT.

-leuc-; -leuco-; -leuk-; -leuko- a combining form meaning white or lack of color.

leucocyte an alternative spelling of leukocyte. See LEUKEMIA.

leucoencephalitis = LEUKOENCEPHALITIS.

leucoencephalomalacia = LEUKOENCEPHALOMALACIA.

leucotomy a type of psychosurgery in which an incision is made in the white matter of the brain, as sometimes distinguished from frontal lobotomy in which an incision is made in a lobe of the brain. In l. the prefrontal lobes of the brain are separated from the rest of the brain by cutting the connecting nerve fibers; the purpose is to sever the brain areas associated with emotion in an effort to reduce anxiety or violent behavior. L. treatment has been replaced to a large extent in recent years as a result of the development of tranquilizing medications. Also called **prefrontal lobotomy; leukotomy**. Also see FRONTAL LOBOTOMY; TRANSORBITAL LOBOTOMY; LOBECTOMY.

leu-enkephalin: See ENKEPHALIN.

-leuk-; -leuko-: See -LEUC-.

leukemia a severe progressive disease of the blood-forming tissues, characterized by a proliferation of **leukocytes** (white blood cells) and diminished production of normal red blood cells and blood platelets. L. results in anemia and increased susceptibility to infection and hemorrhage, joint pain, fever, and enlarged liver, spleen, and lymph nodes. Kinds of l. include **acute lymphoblastic l., acute myeloblastic l., chronic lympho-**

cytic l., and **chronic granulocytic l**. L. may be due to an autosomal aberration such as the Philadelphia chromosome disorder in which a portion of chromosome number 22 is deleted and translocated to other chromosomes, such as chromosome number 9, a common occurrence in chronic l. The incidence of acute l. is about 15 times higher in cases of Down's syndrome than in the general population. Also see BONE-MARROW DISEASES.

leukocytic sarcoma: See SARCOMA.

leukoencephalitis an inflammation of the white matter of the brain. It may be caused by an infection that usually does not involve the central nervous system, as a complication of a disease in another body system, or as a reaction to an immunization. The acute hemorrhagic form of l. is marked by death of cerebral venules resulting in multiple hemorrhages in the white matter, which is fatal. Also spelled **leucoencephalitis**.

leukoencephalomalacia a softening of the tissue of the white matter of the brain. The condition usually is the result of a circulatory disturbance that causes a reduced blood flow to the affected area and infarction. A form of l. observed in fowl can be induced by a deficiency of vitamin E; it is known as **crazy-chick disease**. L. is also spelled **leucoencephalomalacia**.

leukotomy = LEUCOTOMY.

-lev-; -levo-; -laevo- a combining form relating to the left side (from Latin *laevus*, "left").

levadopa: See SINEMET.

levallorphan: See NARCOTIC ANTAGONISTS.

levee effect /lev′ē/ a type of reaction to disaster or threat of disaster characterized by the acquisition of devices that are believed to protect the individual or group. The term is derived from the belief that a home or workplace in a flood plain is safe from floods if a levee or dike forms a boundary between the people and the water. The levee may not protect against the next flood, but its presence provides a sense of security against floods.

leveling a family-therapy technique in which verbal aggression is encouraged on the assumption that it will reduce tensions that would otherwise lead to physical aggression.

leveling effect the tendency for repeated measurements to cluster about the mean due to practice effects.

leveling-sharpening the tendency to perceive and remember any object or event in a way that minimizes or omits small features, details, and irregularities (leveling) while emphasizing or exaggerating the highlights (sharpening). Leveling and sharpening occur simultaneously; e.g., as a rumor is retold, the insignificant details are dropped but the outstanding aspects are heightened.

level of aspiration = ASPIRATION LEVEL.

Levin, Max Russian-born American neurologist, 1901—. See KLEINE-LEVIN SYNDROME; EATING BEHAVIOR.

levirate: See SORORATE.

Lévi-Strauss, Claude /lāvē′ strôs′/ Belgian social anthropologist, 1908—. See ORIGIN-OF-LANGUAGE THEORIES.

levitation the illusion of ascending into the air without support, that is, in the absence of any known cause. The term is mainly used in relation to dreams and parapsychological phenomena.

levodopa: See DOPAMINERGICS.

levophobia a morbid fear of anything situated to the left. Compare DEXTROPHOBIA.

levorphanol $C_{17}H_{23}NO$—a narcotic analgesic with a molecular structure and withdrawal symptoms like those of morphine. L. is more potent than morphine, a dose of two to three milligrams producing effects equivalent to a ten-milligram dose of morphine. However, abuse liability and some adverse effects are increased proportionally. Also see SYNTHETIC NARCOTICS.

Levy, David Mordecai American psychiatrist, 1892–1977. See RELEASE THERAPY.

Lévy, Gabrielle /lāvē′/ French neurologist, 1886–1935. See ROUSSY-LÉVY SYNDROME.

Levy Draw-and-Tell-a-Story Technique a projective test in which the subject draws two figures of his own sex and one of the opposite sex, and tells a story about them. The technique frequently reveals oedipal and sibling-rivalry reactions. (S. Levy, 1950)

Lewin, Kurt /lōō′in/ German-born American psychologist, 1890–1947. Though schooled in Gestalt psychology, L. developed a distinct and influential approach of his own, as expressed in such concepts as LIFE SPACE, FIELD THEORY, VECTOR ANALYSIS, and ASPIRATION LEVEL. See these entries. Also see ARISTOTELIAN; AUTHORITARIAN LEADER; DEMOCRATIC ATMOSPHERE; DEMOCRATIC LEADER; DREAM SCREEN; ENCOUNTER GROUP; FIELD FORCE; FIELD STRUCTURE; FRUSTRATION-REGRESSION HYPOTHESIS; GALILEAN; GROUP THEORY; ICEBLOCK THEORY; IRREALITY LEVEL; LAISSEZ-FAIRE LEADER; LOCOMOTION; MOTORIC REGION; ORAL TRIAD; PSYCHOLOGICAL FIELD; SENSITIVITY TRAINING; TOPOLOGICAL PSYCHOLOGY; TOPOLOGY; T-GROUP.

Lewin, Louis /lā′vēn/ German toxicologist, 1850–1929. See PHANTASTICUM.

Lewis, W. Lee American chemist, 1878–1943. See BRITISH ANTI-LEWISITE.

Lewisite: See BRITISH ANTI-L.

lexical word = CONTENT WORD.

lexicology the study of the meaning of words and their idiomatic combinations. Applied l. is called **lexicography**, the science and art of compiling dictionaries.

Leyden, Ernst Viktor von /lī′dən/ German physician, 1832–1910. See WESTPHAL-LEYDEN SYNDROME.

Leyden's ataxia = WESTPHAL-LEYDEN SYNDROME.

Leydig, Franz von /lī′dik/ German zoologist, 1821–1908. See INTERSTITIAL CELLS (also called **Leydig's cells**); INTERSTITIAL-CELL-STIMULATING HORMONE.

L-5-hydroxytryptophane a naturally occurring

substance that is used in the treatment of certain forms of myoclonus. The chemical functions by crossing the blood-brain barrier to serve as a precursor for the synthesis of serotonin, a neurotransmitter. Abbrev.: **L-5-HTP**.

LGN = LATERAL GENICULATE NUCLEUS.

LH = LATERAL HYPOTHALAMUS.

LH = LUTEINIZING HORMONE.

liability: See MULTIFACTORIAL MODEL.

liaison psychiatry: See CONSULTANT; CONSULTATION-L.P.

libidinal development = PSYCHOSEXUAL DEVELOPMENT.

libidinal phases in psychoanalysis, the four stages in the development and expression of the sexual instinct, each of which is focused on a single erotogenic zone: the mouth (sucking the breast), anus (defecating), phallus (urinating and playing with the penis or clitoris), and genitals (discharge of semen or vaginal secretions). See PSYCHOSEXUAL DEVELOPMENT.

libidinal transference the transference of the patient's libidinal drives from his parents to his therapist.

libidinal types a personality classification devised by Freud and based on a three-fold distribution of libidinal (sexual) energy in the psyche. In the **erotic type**, the libido remains largely in the id, the main interest is in loving and being loved, and if decompensation occurs, a hysterical disorder will develop. In the **obsessional type**, the libido is largely invested in the superego, and the individual is dominated by conscience and may develop an obsessive-compulsive neurosis. In the **narcissistic type**, the libido is primarily invested in the ego, and the main interest is in self-preservation, with little concern for others or for the dictates of the superego; and if decompensation takes place, mental illness takes the form of psychosis or antisocial disorder.

libidinization = EROTIZATION.

libido in psychoanalysis, the energy of the sexual instinct in all its manifestations (Latin, "desire, lust"). In his first formulation (1905) Freud conceived of this energy as narrowly sexual. However, he gradually broadened the concept to include all expressions of love and pleasure; and toward the end of his life, he included in l. both the life and death instincts (Eros and Thanatos). Jung expanded Freud's original concept to apply the term to the general life force which provides energy for all types of activities: biological, sexual, social, cultural, and creative. Also see L. THEORY.

libido analog an object that substitutes for the libidinal object. As examples, Jung cites fetishes, figures of the gods, and churingas (sacred objects of wood or stone in Australia).

libido-binding activity a term used by S. R. Slavson for an activity in which members of a group concentrate libidinal energies on a specific interest or occupation, as contrasted to activities that stimulate the libido. Also called **immobilizing activity**.

libido organization in psychoanalysis, the hierarchical system in which weaker or residual erotogenic areas are subordinate to the dominating or primacy zone, that is, oral, anal, phallic, or genital zone.

libido theory in psychoanalysis, the hypothesis that the impetus for psychosexual development and expression stems from a single instinctual energy source, the libido. In 1920, when Freud promulgated his dual-instinct theory, the l.t. was broadened to include the energy of the death or aggressive drive as well as the sex drive. Also see LIBIDO.

library design the conceptual planning of a library to provide optimum environmental space for the persons who usually use libraries. E.g., studies of library use have revealed that many people utilize libraries as quiet, comfortable areas for reading or study and are not particularly concerned about methods of displaying books and periodicals that may be of primary interest to librarians. See ENVIRONMENTAL DESIGN.

licensed practical nurse a health professional who has completed a special eight-to-15-month training course in practical nursing in an approved school and has been licensed by a state nursing board. L.p.n. training programs in local vocational or technical schools, or community colleges or hospitals, were authorized under the 1917 Vocational Educational Act. Abbrev.: **LPN**. In some states a l.p.n. is called **licensed vocational nurse (LVN)**.

Lichtheim, Ludwig /lisht′hīm/ German physician, 1845–1928. See LICHTHEIM'S TEST.

Lichtheim's test an inner-language test for persons with serious speech disturbances or expressive aphasia. The test requires the patient to indicate the number of syllables in words he cannot pronounce.

licking behavior the act of an animal licking itself or another animal, particularly an offspring. L.b. appears to be part of the maternal instinct of many mammals; the pregnant female licks itself before giving birth, then licks the offspring, thereby establishing a means of identifying her own young. Some mothers lick their young before licking themselves; others lick themselves first.

lidocaine $C_{14}H_{22}N_2O$—a topical anesthetic and antiarrhythmic drug. L. is used mainly to control abnormal heart rhythms but may cause convulsions and respiratory arrest in some patients. CNS effects include drowsiness, paresthesias, and temporary loss of auditory acuity. Some patients become agitated by these side effects.

lie: See LYING.

Liebeault, Ambroise August /lēbō′/ French psychiatrist, 1823–1904. L. was a pioneer in the use of hypnosis for treatment of hysterical patients, and leader of the Nancy School, which he founded with H. Bernheim. See BERNHEIM; NANCY SCHOOL; CHARCOT.

lie detector a device that presumably determines the truthfulness of a person by detecting gal-

423

vanic skin responses, changes in heart rates, respiration, or other physiological signs of anxiety or similar emotions associated with stress. Although results are considered accurate in roughly 80 percent of cases, the technique is not reliable when applied to hardened criminals, psychopaths, and the mentally retarded, among others. See KEELER POLYGRAPH.

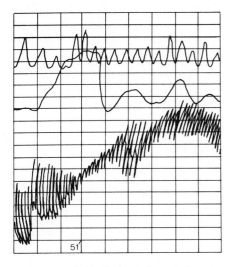

LIE DETECTOR. Sudden fluctuation in respiration rate (top line), galvanic skin response (center line), and pulse and blood pressure (lower line) seem to indicate that the subject lied in answering a particular question.

-lien-; -lieno- a combining form relating to the spleen.

Liéou, Young Choen /lē·ā·ōō′/ French physician, fl. 1928, 1942. See BARRÉ-LIÉOU SYNDROME.

life age = CHRONOLOGICAL AGE.

life-change rating scale a scale used in measuring the relative impact of diverse stress-producing life experiences, changes, and crises. Also see LIFE CRISIS; LIFE-CHANGE UNITS.

life-change units the units of measurement on the life-change rating scale on which diverse life experiences are assigned numerical values in accordance with their stress-generating potential; e.g., divorce is high on the scale while moving to a new house would be relatively low. A study in this area indicates that individuals with a high cumulative life-change-unit score (high potential-stress score) show more health changes than other subjects. Abbrev.: **LCU**. Also see LIFE-CHANGE RATING SCALE; LIFE CRISIS.

life crisis a serious or significant life experience that produces stress and necessitates major adjustment, e.g., divorce, marriage, career change, and death of a close family member. In one study relating health to life crises, subjects who had recently had major stress-producing experiences were more apt than other subjects to show significant alterations in health status. Also see LIFE-CHANGE RATING SCALE; LIFE-CHANGE UNITS.

life cycle the progression from birth to maturity to death which characterizes a particular species, group, institution, or culture. Also, l.c. is the average time this process takes, that is, its life span or life expectancy.

life energy a term applied by Wilhelm Reich to the "orgone," or cosmic energy, which he believed to be emitted by energy vesicles called bions. See ORGONE.

life expectancy the number of years that a person born in a certain calendar year can, on the average, expect to live. The l.e. of an average person may be influenced by such factors as the region of birth and early childhood and the development of new medical techniques, e.g., drugs or surgical procedures, that may extend the l.e.

life fear a term used by Otto Rank for a pervasive feeling of terror experienced during the birth process, which generates a lasting urge to return to the safety of the womb and live a dependent life.

life goal an Adlerian term for the secret strivings of the individual based on his concept of what he could attain in life and how he might compensate for real or imagined inferiority.

life history a systematic account of a person's development from birth to the present. As a counseling term, l.h. refers to the meaningful aspects of an individual's emotional, social, and intellectual development as recorded in autobiographical and biographical material. The l.h. is a more structured and formal document than the autobiography. Emphasis is less on external circumstances and more on an understanding of the individual's life goals and values.

life instinct = EROS.

life lie a term coined by Adler (German *Lebenslüge*) to denote the false conviction of some neurotics that their life plan is bound to fail due to other people or circumstances beyond their control. He interpreted this conviction as a method of freeing themselves from personal responsibility. The term was also used for a false belief around which the individual's life is built.

life plan an Adlerian term for an individual's style of life and guiding fiction as he strives to reach his life goal.

life rhythm = BIOLOGICAL RHYTHM.

life script a term applied by Eric Berne to the scenario which the individual uses in "performing" his roles and playing his interpersonal games throughout life. The l.s. is viewed as an unconscious plan based largely on fantasies derived from early experience. See SCRIPT ANALYSIS.

life space the fundamental concept of K. Lewin's field theory comprising the "totality of possible events" for one person at a particular time or, in other words, a person's possible options together with the environment that contains them. The l.s. is a representation of the environmental, biological, social, and psychological influences that define one person's unique reality at a given moment in time. Contained within the l.s. are positive and negative valences, that is, forces or pressures on the individual to approach a goal or move away from a perceived danger.

life-space interviewing a technique originated by Fritz Redl in which children in residential treatment are interviewed by staff members during moments of stress, e.g., immediately after receiving an upsetting letter or after being attacked by another child. Efforts are made to convert these everyday events into therapeutic experiences by such means as restoring the child's belief in himself and strengthening his ego.

life span the precise length of an individual's life or the typical duration in the life of a species. The l.s. is not derived from statistical calculations. Also see LIFE EXPECTANCY.

life stress events or experiences that produce severe strain, such as failure on the job, marital separation, or loss of a love object.

life-style the general behavior pattern of an individual as expressed by his motives, his manner of coping, attitudes, and other factors. In many cases, the l.-s. characteristics of a person are so well defined that his reactions to certain situations are fairly predictable.

lifetime personality the pattern of behavior that dominates a person's life-style between birth and death (Murray).

Lifton, Robert Jay American psychologist, 1926 —. See SURVIVOR SYNDROME.

ligated tubes: See TUBAL LIGATION.

light adaptation a decline in the sensitivity of cone cells in the retina during exposure to light so that more light is required to obtain the same degree of visual acuity. In general, the amount of time required to be able to achieve dark adaptation varies inversely with the amount of light exposure during a previous l.a.

light reflex = PUPILLARY REFLEX.

light-sensitivity: See PHOTOPHOBIA.

light trance: See TRANCE.

Likert, Renses American social scientist, 1903—. See LIKERT SCALE.

Likert scale a scale made up of items with gradations of response along a single dimension. E.g., "strongly agree, agree, undecided, disagree, strongly disagree" (with a given statement) would form a five-point L.s. Also called **Likert procedure**. Also see ATTITUDE SCALE; THURSTONE ATTITUDE SCALES.

Lilliputian hallucination a visual hallucination (more properly, an illusion) of objects, animals, or people greatly reduced in size. The most vivid examples are found in delirium tremens (alcohol withdrawal delirium) in which tiny animals dart around the room and terrify the patient. Also called **diminutive visual hallucination; microptic hallucination**. See MICROPSIA. Also see ACAROPHOBIA.

l'illusion des sosies /lilēzyôN'desōzē'/ literally, "the illusion of doubles" (French). See CAPGRAS' SYNDROME.

limbic cortex the portions of the brain that are associated with the limbic system, a part of the brain that is relatively old in terms of evolution.

The cortical portion of the limbic system is the cingulate gyrus, which, with other limbic structures such as the amygdala, is involved primarily in emotion, activation, and motivation functions. (The term is derived from Latin *limbus*, "fringe, border.")

limbic lobe a part of the brain that includes the hippocampal formation and the cingulate, dentate, parahippocampal, and subcallosal gyri. The l.l. forms a ring of neural tissue about the brainstem and is a part of the limbic system. It is associated with emotional function. Also called **Brodmann's area 24**.

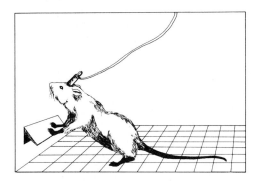

LIMBIC SYSTEM. With an electrode implanted in the septal area of the brain, a rat presses a bar to give himself a mild electric shock up to 5,000 times an hour, until exhausted. The shock is assumed to stimulate a "pleasure center" in the limbic system.

limbic system the parts of the brain that include portions of the cerebral cortex, the thalamus, and certain subcortical structures such as the amygdala, hippocampus, and septal area. It is involved in most involuntary aspects of behavior and called limbic because it represents a part of the primitive cerebral cortex that is considered borderline, in terms of cerebral evolution. See SELF-STIMULATING MECHANISM. Also see CROCODILE MAN.

limen = THRESHOLD.

liminal pertaining to the threshold; or, at the THRESHOLD. See this entry.

liminal stimulus a threshold-level stimulus that elicits a response half the time.

limited-capacity retrieval the assumption that short-term memory is of finite capacity and can store relatively few impressions or facts at one time. Assuming it is true that short-term memory has a significant role in thought processes, its limited capacity would appear to restrict the number of ideas, feelings, or cognitive functions that can be considered or carried out at one time.

limited responsibility a forensic term applied to cases of so-called partial insanity, which means "a mental impairment which is not so complete as to render the victim irresponsible for his criminal acts". H. Weihofen (*Insanity as a Defense in Criminal Law*, 1933) cites (a) cases where mental disorder is probably a contributing cause but not of a type to render the person irresponsible, and (b) cases of mental disorder of which the person "is not capable of deliberation, premeditation, malice or other mental state usually made a requisite for first degree offenses, and in which, therefore, a lesser offense than that charged was in fact committed." Also see PARTIAL INSANITY.

limophoitas a psychotic episode induced by starvation.

limophthisis the physical and mental signs of emaciation caused by severe undernourishment.

limulus a species of Arachnida merostomata used in certain animal vision experiments. Also called **horseshoe crab**.

lin. an abbreviation used in prescriptions, meaning "liniment" (Latin *linimentum*).

Lincoln, Robert Stanley American psychologist, 1923—. See LINCOLN-OSERETSKY MOTOR DEVELOPMENT SCALE.

Lincoln-Oseretsky Motor Development Scale a test designed to assess general motor ability of children between six and 14 years of age through their performance on 36 sensorimotor items.

Lindzey, Gardner Edmond American psychologist, 1920—. See ALLPORT-VERNON-LINDZEY STUDY OF VALUES.

linear correlation a measure of relationship between two variables that assumes the underlying data points fall along a straight line.

linear perspective the principle that the size of an object's visual image is a function of its distance from the eye. Thus, the same object looks smaller when removed to a distance. Two objects appear closer together at a distance, e.g., the tracks of a railroad appear to converge on the horizon.

linear program a form of programed learning in which information is presented in small, discrete, step-by-step **frames** that usually are progressively more complex. Correct answers are given after each frame, thus eliminating error practicing and providing immediate feedback and continuous reinforcement. See PROGRAMED INSTRUCTION; BRANCHING PROGRAM.

linear regression a regression analysis that assumes that the predictor variable is related to the predicted variable along a straight line.

linear system a system in which the units of input summate in a straight line, or in which the response to a complex stimulus is a simple summation of individual responses.

linear type a term occasionally applied to Kretschmer's asthenic body type, characterized by a slender, narrow-chested, long-necked, long-nosed physique.

line of fixation a straight line between the object of visual focus and the retinal fovea.

line of regard a straight line between an object being viewed and the center of rotation of the eye.

lingam = DILDO.

linguadental a speech sound made with the tongue placed against the teeth, e.g., /th/.

lingual pertaining to the tongue or, by way of extension, to speech.

lingual frenum the tissue that attaches the front of the tongue to the floor of the mouth.

lingual gyrus a relatively short convolution of the brain, running horizontally from the occipital to temporal lobes immediately above the fusiform gyrus.

lingual nerve a branch of the fifth cranial nerve that supplies fibers to the anterior two-thirds of the tongue, including the taste-bud papillae and mucous membrane. Also called **gustatory nerve**.

lingual papilla any of the four types of papillae (nipplelike projections on the surface of the tongue): circumvallate (in back), filiform (largely tactile), foliate (taste buds on back and edges), and fungiform (taste buds in front).

linguistic approach a method of teaching reading which assumes that children have mastery of oral language. Letters and sound equivalents taught in reading are embedded in meaningful words with regular spelling patterns.

linguistic-kinesic method the objective study of disordered behavior in terms of language and movement involved in interactions between individuals.

linguistics the study of speech habits; the study of languages and their structure and origins. L. includes phonology, grammar (morphology, syntax), lexicology, and, in a wider sense, phonetics and semantics. See PSYCHOLOGICAL L.; PSYCHOLINGUISTICS.

linkage a tendency for two or more genetic traits to be inherited together, so that an offspring may show the combination of traits or none of them.

linkage worker: See ADVOCATE.

Link trainer a trademark for a ground-based mockup of an airplane cockpit capable of simulating actual flying conditions and used to train pilots.

linonophobia a morbid fear of string. Also called **string phobia**.

-lip-; -lipo- a combining form relating to fat (Greek *lipos*).

lip-biting: See FINGER-BITING BEHAVIOR.

lip eroticism the use of the lips to obtain sexual arousal or satisfaction.

lipid-metabolism disorders a group of metabolic anomalies characterized by abnormal levels of fatty substances in the blood or other tissues, resulting from genetic, endocrine, organ-failure, or external factors. Kinds of l.-m.d. include hyperlipoproteinemia or hyperlipidemia, hypolipemia, Tangier disease, Gaucher's disease, Niemann-Pick disease, and generalized gangliosidosis. See LIPODYSTROPHY.

lipodystrophy any disorder of lipid metabolism. Kinds of l. include **intestinal l.**, in which a malabsorption of fats from the digestive tract may be associated with CNS lesions, as in Whipple's disease, and **progressive l.**, marked by a symmetrical loss of subcutaneous fat deposits and fat-deposit abnormalities around the kidney, heart, and abdominal cavity. No consistent neurologic abnormalities are associated with the latter form of l., but nearly 20 percent of the patients in one study showed signs of mental retardation. The cause of progressive l. is unknown. L. also is associated with diabetes mellitus in a form marked by loss of subcutaneous fat in areas injected with insulin. It also is known as **lipotrophic diabetes mellitus**, or **insulin l**. Also see LIPID-METABOLISM DISORDERS; PARTIAL L.; TOTAL L.

lipoid pertaining to any of a variety of organic substances that are fatty, oily, or waxlike. L. substances often are an integral part of a plant or animal cell.

lipotrophic diabetes mellitus: See LIPODYS-TROPHY.

Lippitt, Ronald, American psychologist, 1920 —. See AUTHORITARIAN LEADER; DEMOCRATIC LEADER; LAISSEZ-FAIRE LEADER.

lip-reading the use of visual clues in determining what a speaker says. The newer term **speech-reading** is preferred because visual clues come from watching the entire speaker speak rather than the lips alone.

liq. an abbreviation used in prescriptions, meaning "solution" (Latin *liquor*).

liquidation of attachment a term used by Janet for freeing the patient from a painful situation by unraveling the attachments in which he is embedded.

lisping the defective production of sibilant sounds caused by improper tongue placement or abnormalities of the speech mechanism. Also called **sigmatism**. Also see INTERDENTAL SIGMATISM.

Lissauer, Heinrich /lis′ou·ər/ German neurologist, 1861–91. See LISSAUER'S TRACT; LISSAUER TYPE PARESIS.

Lissauer's tract an area near the tip of the dorsal horn of the spinal cord where C fibers and some A fibers enter the cord.

Lissauer type paresis an uncommon form of general paresis in which the patient may experience severe focal symptoms, e.g., hemiplegia and aphasia, but retain most intellectual functions. Also called **Lissauer's dementia paralytica**.

lissencephaly = AGYRIA.

lissencephaly syndrome a congenital disorder characterized by microcephaly, ferretlike features, and lissencephaly brains, which have smooth surfaces (from Greek *lissos*, "smooth"). The patients show little response to light or sound stimuli, are hypotonic, and die within the first year. The condition is believed to be due to an autosomal-recessive gene defect. See AGYRIA.

lissophobia = LYSSOPHOBIA.

listening attitude a behavior set in which a person prepares himself to receive a message. Arieti claims that a schizophrenia patient who habitually prepares himself to experience a hallucination may learn to avoid it.

listening with the third ear a form of empathy in which the analyst or another therapist develops a special sensitivity to the unspoken thoughts and feelings behind the patient's spoken words. The term was originally used by Nietzsche, and adopted by Theodore Reik as the title of a book published in 1948.

literacy the ability to read and write.

literacy test any test that examines the ability to read and write.

literal alexia a form of alexia in which individual letters or numerals are not recognized and letters like *d* and *b* are confused. Also called **literal dyslexia**. See ALEXIA.

literalism: See OBJECTIVE ORIENTATION.

literal paraphasia a type of aphasia in which phonemes are substituted in speech, making it difficult to comprehend what the individual is trying to say, e.g., "lar" for "car." See PARAPHASIA.

literary psychoanalysis: See APPLIED PSYCHOANALYSIS.

-lith-; -litho- a combining form relating to stone (Greek *lithos*).

lithic diathesis an inherited disorder of the urinary system marked by a tendency to form kidney stones, or urinary calculi.

lithium a chemical element with antimanic effects. Because l. can partially replace the sodium in body tissues, it appears to control mood swings associated with shifts in sodium levels in the body, and to alter the permeability of neural membranes. L. also affects serotonin metabolism in brain cells. The prototype drug is **l. carbonate**—CLi_2O_3.

lithium therapy the use of lithium, usually in the form of lithium carbonate, as a therapeutic agent in manic states and in preventing the recurrence of both manic and depressive episodes in bipolar disorder. Dosage must be carefully regulated and blood-level tests must be regularly administered because of possible toxicity.

litigiousness a personality characteristic consisting of contentiousness, quarrelsomeness, and readiness to threaten a lawsuit.

litigious paranoia a type of paranoid reaction in which the individual is constantly quarreling, claiming persecution, and insisting that his rights have been breached. He usually threatens to go to court, and frequently does, to seek redress for exaggerated or fancied wrongs. Also called **paranoia querulans; paranoid litigious state**.

littering the strewing of trash, garbage, or other waste materials over the surface of an area. L. contributes to urban blight and rural unsightliness, and is a form of environmental pollution. (Litter is derived from the Latin word *lectus*, "a place to lie down," an area frequently prepared by scattering a layer of straw or similar material on the ground or floor.)

Little, William John English surgeon, 1810–94. See LITTLE'S DISEASE.

Little Hans /huns/ a landmark case of Freud's in which a child's phobia for horses was traced by the father, with Freud's help, to castration anxiety stemming from masturbation, to repressed death wishes toward the father due to rivalry with the mother, and to fear of retaliation, with displacement of that fear onto horses. The case was reported in "Analysis of a Phobia in a Five-Year-Old Boy" (1909).

Little's disease a disorder of newborn infants who show muscular weakness, convulsions, spasticity, mental retardation, and various visual difficulties including cataracts and optic atrophy. The condition is associated with neonatal asphyxia, maternal illness during pregnancy, and birth injuries. The patients often are born prematurely. Also called SPASTIC DIPLEGIA.

Littré, Alexis /liträ'/ French anatomist, 1658–1726. See LITTRÉ'S GLANDS.

Littré's glands small oil glands on the corona of the penis and the inner surface of the foreskin that secrete smegma, which resembles melted soap in appearance. The term also applies to small mucous glands in the lining of the male urethra.

Lloyd Morgan's canon a principle that an action of an animal cannot be interpreted as an exercise of a higher psychical faculty if it can instead be interpreted in terms of a faculty that stands lower in the psychological scale. L.M.c., proposed in 1894 by Lloyd Morgan, helped eliminate the older concept of anthropomorphism, or the endowment of animals with human traits. Also called **Morgan's canon; Morgan's principle**.

loading the weight or relative significance given to a statistic; also, the degree to which a test is correlated with a factor.

load theory: See ENVIRONMENTAL-L. T.

lobar divisions the major topographic regions of the cerebral hemisphere separated generally by principal sulci of the cerebrum. The l.d. include the frontal, parietal, temporal, and occipital lobes. There also may be subdivisions, e.g., the inferior, middle, and superior temporal lobes.

lobectomy a psychosurgical technique in which the prefrontal region of the frontal lobes is surgically removed as a means of alleviating chronic, severe psychoses. The operation is rarely performed today, and is a last-resort procedure. Also see LEUCOTOMY.

lobotomy = FRONTAL L. Also see LEUCOTOMY; LOBECTOMY; THALECTOMY; TRANSORBITAL L.

local excitatory state the localized increase in negative potential on the surface of a neuron as an initial response to a stimulus. Abbrev.: **LES.** Also called **local excitatory potential**.

locality attachment the ability of an organism to detect its position in space with reference to other points, such as the home or nest of the individual animal. L.a. may be associated with the ability of domestic animals to return to their place of birth or a former home after being removed to another locality many miles away. Also see HOMING.

localization the assignment of mental functions to nervous-system tissues involved in specific activities. Visual functions, e.g., are associated with specific nerve tracts, projection and association neurons of the cortex, receptor neurons, and

other cells that mark l. of the function. Also see L. OF FUNCTION; VICARIOUS FUNCTION.

localization of function the assignment of different mental functions, such as vision and speech, to specific areas of the cortex. Also called **cortical l.o.f.** See PHRENOLOGY.

localization of symptoms a term used by Freud for the unconscious selection of a particular bodily function or part of the body to express a neurotic impulse. E.g., a man might develop hysterical constipation as a defense against his wish to engage in anal intercourse. Also see SYMPTOM CHOICE.

localized amnesia a memory loss restricted to specific or isolated experiences. Also called **lacunar amnesia; circumscribed anmesia**.

localized functions: See LOCALIZATION OF FUNCTION.

local potential the phase of a graded or generator potential that precedes the spike potential, if the localized stimulation is above threshold level. Also called **local response**.

local sign a theory advanced in the 19th century by Rudolph Lotze to explain how the nervous system is able to localize a stimulus, visual or tactual, by an association between experience and one or more cortical cells. A l.s. helps the body determine, e.g., the specific area of the skin that has been stimulated and the type of stimulation. Sight and sound inputs also carry a l.s. indicating the source in space and its modality.

local theory of thirst a concept introduced in 1932 by W. Cannon to explain the association between thirst and dryness of the mouth. The l.t.o.t. asserted that the dryness of the mouth represented the general state of body-tissue hydration. Later studies found hormonal, neural, and other factors of greater significance in the control of water intake.

location in early language development, the stage in which such words as "here" and "there" are first used in identifying the location of objects.

location constancy the tendency for a resting object and its setting to appear to have the same position even if the relationship between setting and observer is altered as the observer shifts position. Also see OBJECT CONSTANCY.

loci: See LOCUS.

loci method: See METHOD OF L.

Locke, John English philosopher, 1632–1704. See ASSOCIATIONISM; ASSOCIATION OF IDEAS; EMPIRICISM; TABULA RASA CONCEPT.

locked ward a hospital unit in which mentally disturbed patients are kept under lock and key. The present trend is toward elimination of the l.w., since the patient feels he is being incarcerated and punished for being ill. Other factors responsible for eliminating locked rooms and units are the concept of the mental hospital as a treatment rather than custodial institution, the effectiveness of psychoactive drugs, increase in the staff-patient ratio, and the concepts of the open hospital and therapeutic community.

lockjaw: See TETANUS.

locomotion movement of an organism from one place to another. K. Lewin used the term for psychological movement in one's life space due to a change in the valence of a region or regions. See LIFE SPACE.

locomotor activity a form of general bodily activity involving movement from one area to another, as when an animal explores or chases. Also see RESTLESSNESS.

locomotor arrest the inhibition of movement, an effect that can be produced in experimental animals by electrical stimulation of the hippocampus.

locomotor ataxia muscular incoordination in walking, producing an unsteady gait. It is due to **tabes dorsalis**, a progressive syphilitic disease involving degeneration of the posterior columns of the spinal cord. See GENERAL PARESIS.

locomotor maze a maze that requires bodily movement to reach a goal. Also see STYLUS MAZE; MAZE.

loco plants any of a number of species of Astragalus or Oxytropis that grow wild in western North America, particularly in the Rocky Mountain region. *Loco* is the Spanish word for "crazy" and identifies the effects the plant alkaloids have on humans and animals that ingest them. The loco toxin produces irreversible changes in the central nervous system, including brain lesions and eventual paralysis. Also called **loco weed**.

locus the place or position (Latin, "place") of an anatomical entity, e.g., a hemorrhage in the brain, a butterfly rash on the skin, or a gene on a chromosome. Plural: **loci** /lō'sī/ or /lō'kē/.

locus caeruleus bluish-tinted nuclei found on the floor of the fourth ventricle (from Latin *caeruleus*, "blue"). The area cells contain large amounts of catecholamines, primarily norepinephrine. Lesions of the l.c. in experimental animals have resulted in disturbances in normal sleep patterns.

locus minoris resistentiae a site or area of the body or an organ that offers the "least resistance" to an invasion by pathogenic microorganisms or the toxins produced by the organisms. A wound or break in the skin becomes a l.m.r. for tetanus, syphilis, rabies, or other disease agents that might otherwise be less of a threat of infection.

locus of control The center of responsibility for the control of behavior. **Internal l.o.c.** refers to the conviction that one can use one's behavior to achieve desired goals; **external l.o.c.** refers to the belief that real power resides outside the individual, and that forces other than oneself determine one's life.

Loeffler, Wilhelm /lœf'lər/ Swiss physician, 1887 —. See LOEFFLER'S SYNDROME.

Loeffler's syndrome a simple form of eosinophilic pneumonia, with low-grade fever, mild respiratory symptoms, and generally rapid recovery. A characteristic feature is a filling of the alveolar spaces of the lungs with eosinophils, usually as a hypersensitivity reaction to metal compounds, parasites such as fungi, or psychotropic and psychedelic drugs.

-log-; -logo- a combining form relating to speech or words (from Greek *logos*, "word, speech").

logagnosia; logamnesia = RECEPTIVE APHASIA.

logic the branch of philosophy that deals with correct and fallacious reasoning procedures, including use of syllogisms, and inductive and deductive thinking processes.

logical positivism the viewpoint that verifiable, factual, experiential knowledge and intersubjective scientific language must be employed in philosophy and psychology, rather than metaphysical concepts and theories. Also see PHYSICALISM.

logicogrammatical disorders a manifestation of semantic aphasia, which affects patients with lesions of the dominant parietal region. The patient uses the correct words, but they are arranged in a sequence that gives a different meaning, e.g., "the plate is on the table" versus "the table is on the plate."

logic-tight compartments a term sometimes used to describe a manner of intellectualization in which contradictory ideas or motives are segregated in separate regions of the person's consciousness.

logistic curve an S-shaped curve showing the growth of a population dependent upon fixed resources. Growth is initially slow because of the small number of individuals, then picks up speed, then slows again at a saturation point as the limited resources become constraining.

log-log coordinate paper graph paper in which both ordinate and abscissa are in logarithmic form, used especially for plotting psychophysical data.

Logo a trademark for a computer-programing language designed to encourage the development of problem-solving skills. L. is based on Piaget's research in the development of thinking in children. (The term is not an acronym but derived from the Greek word *logos*, "word, reason.")

logoclonia a speech characteristic in which parts of words are repeated in a manner similar to that of stuttering. L. often is a symptom of senile or presenile disorders, e.g., Alzheimer's disease.

logodiarrhea; logomania = LOGORRHEA.

logopathy a general term for a speech disorder of any kind.

logopedics the study and treatment of speech disorders.

logorrhea /-rē'ə/ a rush of rapid, uncontrollable, and incoherent talking typically observed in the manic phase of bipolar (manic-depressive) disorder. Also called **hyperlogia; hyperphrasia; lallorhea; logodiarrhea; logomania; polylogia; polyphrasia; tachylalia; tachylogia; tachyphrasia; verbomania**. See PRESSURE OF SPEECH; TACHYPHEMIA.

logospasm a speech disorder marked by explosive utterances or stuttering, similar to logoclonia.

logotherapy an approach developed by Frankl in the 1950s and 1960s, which focuses on the "human predicament," and helping the patient to overcome what he terms "existential neurosis," the inability to see meaning in life. The therapeutic process consists of examining three types of values: creative (work, achievement); experiential (art, science, philosophy, understanding, loving); and attitudinal (courageously facing pain and suffering). Each patient is encouraged to arrive at his own solution, which Frankl believes should incorporate social responsibility and constructive relationships. See EXISTENTIALISM.

-logy; -ology a combining form relating to a field of study. See -LOG-.

Lombroso, Cesare Italian criminologist and alienist, 1836–1909. L. is chiefly noted for two controversial theories, (a) that genius is closely akin to insanity and (b) that criminals can be identified by hereditary "stigmata of degeneracy," such as low foreheads, close-set eyes, and small, pointed ears. See DEGENERACY THEORY; PHYSIOGNOMY; STIGMATA OF DEGENERACY.

loneliness fear = AUTOPHOBIA.

long-acting barbiturates derivatives of barbituric acid that are metabolized and excreted at a slow rate. L.-a.b. include phenobarbital, mephobarbital, and barbital. L.-a.b. are among the drugs of choice for epilepsy because of the chronic nature of the disease.

long-circuiting a term used by Cattell for the renunciation of immediate satisfactions in favor of attaining remote, long-term goals.

long-hot-summer effect the supposition that incessant heat conditions can cause or contribute to increased aggression and outbreaks of violence.

longilineal denoting a constitutional type of body that is long rather than broad and roughly equivalent to Kretschmer's asthenic type. Also see BRACHYMORPH.

longitudinal study the study of a variable or group of variables in the same cases or subjects over a long period of time, e.g., a comparative study of the same group of children in an urban and a suburban school over several years for the purpose of recording their cognitive development in depth. Also called **longitudinal method**. Compare CROSS-SECTIONAL STUDY.

longitudinal sulcus a fissure that runs along the top of the cerebral cortex and marks the division between the left and right hemispheres of the brain. The fissure is quite prominent at the frontal and occipital poles. At the bottom of the l.s. the hemispheres are connected by the corpus callosum.

long-term care facilities extended-care institutions, such as nursing homes, that provide medical and personal services for patients who are unable to live independently but do not require the in-patient services of a hospital. Patients utilizing l.-t.c.f. are generally over the age of 65 and suffer from disorders such as Alzheimer's disease, parkinsonism, and stroke. However, about 12 percent of the more than 1,000,000 l.-t.c.f. patients in the United States are young adults.

long-term memory memory that endures for long periods of time; the ability to practice a skill, recall events, or reproduce names and numbers long after they were originally learned, due to a slow rate of decay. Abbrev.: **LTM**. Also called **remake memory**. Also see SHORT-TERM MEMORY.

long-term psychotherapy psychotherapy requiring a number of sessions per week over a period of many months. The most extended technique, psychoanalysis, takes on the average two to three years since it seeks to evoke unconscious material stemming from the patient's earliest experiences and is directed toward the reorganization of his entire emotional life. Somewhat less extended are the client-centered, existential, Horney, Sullivan, and Adler approaches.

looking-glass self the concept of the self as a reflection of other people's reactions and opinions.

looming a type of space perception in which the retinal image of an object is magnified as it approaches. Reactions to l. vary: Chicks run away, kittens avert their heads, monkeys leap backward and make alarm cries, while human infants attempt to withdraw their heads at two weeks and blink at three weeks.

loop colostomy: See COLOSTOMY.

loosening of associations a schizophrenic disturbance in which thought and speech processes are disconnected and fragmented, and the patient jumps from one idea to a totally unrelated and irrelevant idea instead of following the usual lines of association. Also called **loose association**. Also see COGNITIVE SLIPPAGE.

lorazepam: See BENZODIAZEPINES.

lordosis an abnormal curvature of the spine which, when viewed from the side, shows a concavity in the lumbar and cervical portions. A l. effect may be observed in a woman in an advanced stage of pregnancy who adopts the posture in order to maintain balance. With that exception, the l. patient displays a posture that sometimes is termed **swayback** or **saddle-back**. Also see KYPHOSIS; HYPERLORDOSIS.

Lorenz, Konrad Austrian naturalist and ethologist, 1903—. See CRITICAL PERIOD; IMPRINTING; OVERPOPULATION.

Lorr Scale = MULTIDIMENSIONAL SCALE FOR RATING PSYCHIATRIC PATIENTS.

LOS length of stay. LOS is an aspect of the medical review procedure involving continued-stay review, which consists in part of a comparison of the case under review with regional norms usually expressed as the average LOS for each diagnosis.

loss of affect an inability to respond emotionally; apathy, emotional flatness. L.o.a. is a common symptom of schizophrenia, but is also found in presenile and senile brain disorders.

loss of personal identity a failure to recall one's identity and past life. It is a major symptom in disassociative, or psychogenic, amnesia.

lost in thought: See PREOCCUPATION.

lot. an abbreviation used in prescriptions, meaning "lotion" (Latin *lotio*).

Lotze, Rudolph Hermann /lôt′sə/ German physician, philosopher, and psychologist, 1817–81. See LOCAL SIGN.

loudness a partly subjective measure of the amplitude of sound waves, the perception of intensity varying with the individual listener. L. also varies with the wavelength of the sound, with human sensitivity being greatest for sounds in the middle range of sound-wave lengths. L. is measured in decibels. Also see PITCH; TIMBRE; MOST COMFORTABLE L.

Lou Gehrig's disease = AMYOTROPHIC LATERAL SCLEROSIS.

Louis-Bar, Denise European physician, fl. 1941. See LOUIS-BAR'S SYNDROME.

Louis-Bar's syndrome a familial disorder marked by cerebellar ataxia and progressive mental deterioration accompanied by frequent respiratory infections. A common sign of the disorder is the dilation of blood vessels in the skin and eyes, giving the eyes a "bloodshot" appearance, beginning around the age of five years. Ataxia symptoms appear when the child begins to walk. The syndrome, named for Denise Louis-Bar, is believed to be an autosomal-recessive trait. Also called **ataxia-telangiectasia**.

love a complex yet basically integrated emotion comprising strong affection, feelings of tenderness, pleasurable sensations in the presence of the love object, and devotion to his or her well-being. It is an emotion that takes many forms: concern for one's fellow humans (brotherly love); responsibility for the welfare of a child (parental love); sexual attraction and excitement (erotic love); self-esteem and self-acceptance (self-love); and identification with the totality of being (love of God) (Erich Fromm, *The Art of Loving*, 1956). See BEING L.; DORIAN L.; GENITAL L.; HELLENIC L.; MONKEY L.; MOTHER L.; OBJECT L.; PHALLIC L.; PLATONIC L.; POSTAMBIVALENT PHASE; PREGENITAL L.; PRODUCTIVE L.; PUPPY L.; SELF-L.; TRANSFERENCE-L.

love needs the next level in A. Maslow's hierarchy of needs beyond physiological and safety needs, characterized by the striving for affiliation and acceptance. Also called **belongingness and l.n.** See NEED-HIERARCHY THEORY.

love object the person in whom the individual invests the emotions of affection, devotion, and, usually, sexual interest.

Lowe, Charles Upton American pediatrician, 1921—. See OCULOCEREBRAL SYNDROME (also called **Lowe's disease; Lowe's syndrome**).

low Machs: See MACH SCALE.

low-pressure hydrocephalus a type of hydrocephalus that occurs in some men after middle age because of midbrain tumors or a previous attack of meningitis or encephalitis. The cerebrospinal-fluid pressure is near normal, but the ventricles of the brain are large and dilated. The symptoms of l.-p.h. include dementia and a shuffling gait.

LPC: See LEAST-PREFERRED COWORKER TEST.

LPN = LICENSED PRACTICAL NURSE.

LSD: See PSYCHEDELICS; LSD PSYCHOTHERAPY.

LSD psychotherapy an experimental technique in which LSD was administered to chronic alcoholics and patients with character disorders during the 1960s as a means of facilitating the process of uncovering and reliving repressed memories, and increasing the patient's ability to communicate his thoughts and feelings. According to some reports, the method was moderately successful, but has been abandoned due to the risks involved, particularly the risk of releasing latent psychotic tendencies. See PSYCHEDELICS. Also see PSYCHOLYTIC THERAPY.

LTM = LONG-TERM MEMORY.

lucidity a mental state or interval in which a person may not have complete ability to reason or comprehend complex matters but has adequate mental powers to be legally responsible for his actions.

ludes: See METHAQUALONE.

ludic activity = PLAY.

luding out: See METHAQUALONE.

ludotherapy = PLAY THERAPY.

lues /lōō′əs/ a synonym for syphilis. The term (Latin, "infection, plague") may be combined with an anatomical or other term, e.g., **l. nervosa**, for syphilis of the nervous system. Adjective: **luetic** /lōō·et′ik/.

luetic curve = TABETIC CURVE.

Luft, Rolf Swedish endocrinologist, 1914—. See LUFT'S DISEASE.

Luft's disease a metabolic disorder marked by an abnormally high rate of basal metabolism, profuse perspiration and polydipsia without polyuria, polyphagia without weight gain but accompanied by muscular wasting and weakness. The causative factor is a mitochondrial-enzyme defect that affects the ability of the nervous system to control respiration rate.

-lumb-; -lumbo- a combining form relating to the loin, the **lumbar** region.

lumbar nephrectomy: See NEPHRECTOMY.

lumbar nerves: See SPINAL NERVES.

lumbar puncture a procedure used to obtain a cerebrospinal-fluid sample for laboratory diagnostic studies by inserting a hypodermic needle into the spinal cord at a point between two lumbar vertebrae.

lumen /lōōm′ən/ the amount of illumination (Latin, "light") shed by a light of one candlepower over an area of one square meter.

luminance the amount of light reflected from an object as measured in millilamberts.

luminosity the relative brightness of a light source as measured in terms of reflectance of surfaces in the environment and other factors that may influence the perceived light intensity. E.g., a light of a given intensity will appear brighter in a room with white walls than the same light in a room with dark walls.

luminosity curve the brightness values of visible wave lengths as plotted with the wave length on the abscissa and luminosity on the ordinate.

lumpectomy: See MASTECTOMY.

lump in the throat: See GLOBUS HYSTERICUS.

lunacy; lunatic; lunatismus: See MOON-PHASE STUDIES; ASYLUM LUNACY.

lunacy commission an ad hoc group of psychiatrists appointed by judicial order to evaluate the mental state of an individual whose case is being considered by the court.

lupus erythematosus a collagen (or connective-tissue) disease of unknown origin occurring primarily in young women. Common signs are fatigue, fever, migratory joint pains, l.e. cells in the blood, often a butterfly rash on the nose and cheeks, and scaly red patches on the skin. Psychiatric symptoms are common, starting with anxiety and exaggeration of previous personality tendencies, and frequently progressing to depressive and paranoid reactions. Abbrev.: **LE.** If the effects are disseminated throughout the body, the condition is known as **systemic l.e. (SLE).**

Luria, Alexander Romanovich Russian psychologist, 1902—. See LURIA TECHNIQUE; CEREBRAL-DYSFUNCTION TESTS (there: **Luria-Nebraska Neuropsychological Battery**).

Luria technique a method of measuring emotional tension, in which a subject holds his fingers on a tremor recorder during a free-association test.

lust a very intense desire, usually associated with erotic excitement or arousal.

lust dynamism a term used by H. S. Sullivan for overtly expressed sexual desires and abilities.

lust murder a term occasionally applied to an extreme form of sexual sadism in which a rapist murders his victim and then mutilates the body.

-lut-; -luteo- a combining form meaning yellow or yellowish.

luteal phase the stage of the menstrual cycle beginning immediately after ovulation, when the ruptured follicle becomes the corpus luteum, a temporary endocrine gland that secretes the hormone progesterone. If fertilization of the ovum does not occur, the l.p. ends with menstruation.

luteinizing hormone a gonadotrophic hormone secreted by the pituitary gland that causes the rapid growth of a follicle in the ovary until it ruptures and releases an ovum. The same hormone is secreted by the pituitary in males, where it is called the interstitial cell-stimulating hormone. Abbrev.: **LH.**

luteotrophic hormone = PROLACTIN.

lux a measure of illuminance on a surface of one square meter receiving a uniformly distributed flux of one lumen from a light source (Latin, "light").

LVN: See LICENSED PRACTICAL NURSE.

lycanthropy the belief that the individual can change himself or others into a wolf or other animal (from Greek *lykos*, "wolf"). The delusion reached epidemic proportions in Europe during the 16th century; one judge sentenced 600 **lycanthropes** to death, since many "werewolves" were accused of violent crimes. L. is still occasionally reported, as in the mountainous villages of Italy. Also called **lycomania; zoanthropy.**

lygophilia an abnormal desire to be in dark or gloomy places (from Greek *lyge*, "twilight").

lying making false statements with conscious intent to deceive. Nonpathological l. is often found in children or adults seeking to avoid punishment or to save others from distress ("white lies"). Pathological lying is a major characteristic of the antisocial personality, and may be a symptom of brain disorder resulting from severe head injury, alcoholism, congenital syphilis, or encephalitis. See CONFABULATION; MALINGERING; PATHOLOGICAL L.

lymph a yellowish, relatively clear fluid found in the lymphatic vessels and derived from tissue fluids. Nutrients and oxygen are delivered to body cells dissolved in water, and the l. (containing occasional red blood cells, fat globules, and waste products) represents the excess fluid that is drained back into the blood-circulation system, via the lymphatic vessels.

lymphadenopathy any of several diseases involving the lymph nodes. Kinds of l. include **dermatopathic l.**, marked by regional lymph-node enlargement with skin disorders, **giant follicular l.**, in which the normal structure of the nodes is disrupted by a proliferation of follicular nodules, and effects of Hodgkin's disease, leukemia, and second-stage syphilis.

lymphoma any neoplastic disorder of the lymphatic system. Kinds of l. include **Burkitt's l.**, which usually is manifested as a cancerous growth in the jaw or abdomen; **Hodgkin's disease**, which usually begins as enlarged lymph nodes; and **lymphocytoma**, which is composed primarily of lymphocyte cells.

lymphosarcoma: See SARCOMA.

lynching: See CROWD BEHAVIOR; COLLECTIVE BEHAVIOR.

Lyon, Mary Frances English geneticist, 1925—. See X-LINKED ABNORMALITIES (there: **Lyon hypothesis**).

lypemania a now-obsolete term used by Esquirol for melancholia, one of his five classes of mental disorders (the others being monomania, mania, dementia, and imbecility).

-lys-; -lysi-; -lyso-; -lytic a combining form relating to dissolution. Lysis (Greek, "loosening") is used to refer to subsidence of symptoms and is sometimes contrasted with crisis.

lysergic acid amide; lysergic acid diethylamide: See PSYCHEDELICS.

lysinuria the presence of **lysine** in the urine, an effect of an amino-acid metabolism enzyme deficiency. It is an inherited condition associated with muscle weakness and mental retardation.

lysis: See -LYS-.

lyssophobia a morbid fear of becoming insane, or of dealing with insanity. Also called **maniaphobia; lissophobia.**

-lytic: See -LYS-.

lytic cocktail a mixture of antipsychotic (neuroleptic) drugs, such as chlorpromazine, promethazine, and Hydergine used in treating acute or impending delirium.

M

m. an abbreviation used in prescriptions, meaning "minim" (Latin *minimum*).

M = MEMORY. Also see PRIMARY ABILITIES.

M. an abbreviation used in prescriptions, meaning "mix" (Latin *misce*).

MA = MENTAL AGE.

mace an aromatic spice made from the fibrous seed coat of the nutmeg. M. has been associated with the euphoric effects produced by nutmeg intoxication although the active ingredients that are related chemically to hallucinogenic drugs are concentrated primarily in the oil of the NUTMEG itself. See this entry.

MacGinitie, Walter Harold American psychologist, 1928—. See GATES-MACGINITIE READING TESTS.

Mach, Ernst /mäkh/ Austrian physicist and philosopher, 1838–1916. See MACH BANDS.

Mach bands an illusion produced during the ramp-stimulus-visual test when a dark line is observed at the dark transition zone and a bright line at the light end of the ramp.

Machiavelli, Niccolò /mäkē·ävel′ē/ Florentine statesman and author, 1469–1527. See MACHIAVELLIANISM; MACH SCALE.

Machiavellianism a personality trait characterized by expediency and a belief that ends justify means. A **Machiavellian** is one who views other people more or less as objects to be manipulated and, he hopes, dominated through deception and dishonesty if needed to achieve his goals.

machina docilis: See AUTOMATON.

machine: See INFLUENCING M.

machine fear = MECHANOPHOBIA.

Machover, Karen Alper American psychologist, 1902—. See MACHOVER DRAW-A-PERSON TEST; FIGURE-DRAWING TEST.

Machover Draw-a-Person Test a projective technique based on the interpretation of drawings of human figures of both sexes (K. Machover, 1951). The examiner notes the sequence of the drawings, the subject's verbalizations and attitudes, self-image, and evidence of such reactions as hyperactivity, anxiety, sexual conflicts, aggressiveness, impulsivity, mood swings, and bizarre tendencies. The interpretation of the specific signs is usually based on the examiner's individual clinical experience. Abbrev.: **DAP**

test. Analogous to this test is the **Machover Draw-a-House Test (DAH test)**.

Mach scale /mäk/ a measurement of the degree to which individuals condone, tolerate, or condemn the use of manipulation and deceit in pursuit of material or other aims (abbreviation of "Machiavelli"). Low Machs affirm absolute ethical standards; high Machs reveal relative, shifting standards of behavior. See MACHIAVELLIANISM.

MacKenzie, Sir Stephen English physician, 1844–1909. See JACKSON'S SYNDROME (also called **MacKenzie's syndrome**).

MacQuarrie, Thomas William American psychologist, fl. 1927. See MACQUARRIE TEST FOR MECHANICAL ABILITY.

MacQuarrie Test for Mechanical Ability a paper-and-pencil test focusing primarily on spatial relations and eye-hand coordination. The items include tracing a twisting line through other lines, tapping, block analysis and counting, and pursuit.

-macr-; -macro- a combining form meaning large, long, enlarged.

macrobiotic diets a series of diets based on ratios of foods that are considered "Yin" or "Yang," according to their originator, George Ohsawa. Meals are prepared so that they contain five parts of yin foods to one part of yang foods. Fruits generally are yin, although some are considered too heavily yin, while meats are too heavily yang for most meals. The macrobiotic dieter progresses through a series of six very restrictive yin and yang diets, each more severe than the preceding diet, ultimately reaching a "perfect diet" of brown rice and tea. The m.d. are claimed to cure epilepsy and various other disorders. Although promoted as an ancient Zen Buddhist health regimen, m.d. are not ancient, not Buddhist, and not healthy, according to nutrition scientists who have evaluated the diets.

macrocephaly a rare congenital defect involving gross enlargement of the head due to abnormal growth of the supporting tissue of the brain, resulting in moderate-to-severe mental retardation, frequently with impaired vision and seizures. Also called **megalocephaly**.

macrocosm: See MICROCOSM.

macroglossia an abnormally large-size tongue, affecting production of lingual sounds in speech.

macrogyria = PACHYGYRIA.

macromastia abnormally large female breasts.

macrophage a scavenger cell (a phagocyte, or a cell able to digest bacteria, cell debris, etc.) found in connective tissue and major organs and tissues.

macropsia a false perception that objects are larger than they actually are, due to disease of the retina or hysterical (conversion) disorder. Also called **megalopsia**. Compare MICROPSIA.

macroskelic a constitutional type of body build in which the most prominent characteristic is abnormally long legs. The m. individual would be classified as asthenic in Kretschmer's system.

macrosomatic animals animals whose body sizes are statistically larger than the mean for the species. The mean of the general body size for humans is calculated as the product of the standard score for body height multiplied by the standard score for transverse chest measurement. Sizes one or more standard deviation larger are classified as macrosomatic. Compare MICROSOMATIC ANIMALS.

macrosomatognosia: See SOMATOGNOSIA.

macrosplanchnic build a body type in which the trunk is disproportionately large compared with the limbs.

macula lutea = RETINAL MACULA.

made shaunda a Hindu term for nutmeg. It is translated as "intoxicating fruit."

Maddox, Ernest Edmund English ophthalmologist, 1860–1933. See MADDOX ROD TEST.

Maddox rod test a test of eye-muscle balance: The patient views a candle flame through glass rods which convert it into a line of light; the differential images perceived by the two eyes indicate the degree of heterophoria.

madness: See RAVING M.

MAF = MINIMAL AUDIBLE FIELD.

Magendie, François /mäzhäNdē'/ French physiologist, 1783–1855. See BELL-MAGENDIE LAW.

magic the illusory possession of supernatural or paranormal powers, as in tricks involving sleight of hand; the attempt to control natural events through incantations, dances, or gestures; or the effort of the obsessive-compulsive neurotic to allay anxiety by invoking certain numbers, performing certain rituals, or repeating long lists of feared persons or objects. Also see COMMUNICATION M.; COMPULSIVE M.; CURSING M.

magical communion = COMMUNION.

magical thinking a primitive cognitive process based on the illusion that thought can influence events, fulfill wishes, or ward off evil. Thinking of this kind originates in early childhood and is manifested in superstitions, dreams, fantasies, obsessive thoughts, ritual acts, as well as the belief found in some schizophrenics that they can "think" an enemy to death or right the world's wrongs through the power of thought. See OMNIPOTENCE OF THOUGHT; PALEOLOGIC THINKING; PRELOGICAL THINKING; PRIMARY PROCESS; VOODOO DEATH; CURSING MAGIC; FAITH HEALING.

magic bone: See VOODOO DEATH.

magic helper a term applied by Fromm to a person on whom a neurotic individual has bestowed a sort of magical omnipotence to solve all the patient's problems. The m.h. also may be influenced by the relationship and assume a position of irrational authority, or a neurotic need for power.

magic mushroom = TEONANACTL.

magic omnipotence: See COSMIC IDENTIFICATION.

magic phase a stage of thinking in which the mere thought of an event or object is the equivalent of reality in a world created by the subject. In Freudian terms, the m.p. is defined as omnipotence of thought, and is characteristically observed in young children and schizophrenics.

Magna Mater a term meaning literally "great mother" (Latin), representing Jung's archetype of the primordial mother image and the **Great Mother** of the Roman Gods, Cybele. Also see MOTHER ARCHETYPE.

magnesium deprivation the lack of magnesium in the diet. Rats deprived of magnesium experimentally develop an aversion to the mineral when it is returned to their diet, whereas deprivation of other minerals results in a preference for the chemical after it becomes available again. The effect is believed to be due to adverse health conditions such as gastric distress experienced when magnesium is first restored to the diet.

magnetic crisis; magnetic pass: See MESMERIC CRISIS.

magnetic sense an ability of an organism to orient itself according to the lines of force of a magnet or the magnetic fields of the earth. The roots of certain plants have been found to align themselves with magnetic fields, and it has been postulated that migrating birds tend to follow magnetic fields of the earth with the aid of sensory apparatus that detects the force of magnetism.

magnet reflex a response of some animals to the sensation of touch on the plantar surface (sole) of the foot. Rather than withdraw the foot, the animal extends its foot toward the source of the sensation as it normally would extend the foot in making contact with the ground.

magnitude estimation judgment of the size of a stimulus by assigning it a numerical value along a scale. Also see METHOD OF LIMITS; METHOD OF CONSTANT STIMULI.

magnitude of response: See RESPONSE AMPLITUDE.

Magnus-de Kleyn postural reflexes a series of leg movements associated with head movements. E.g., when the head of a cat is turned to one side, legs on the side toward which the head points become extended while those on the other side are flexed; if the head turns downward, the front legs flex and the hind legs extend; upward movement of the head produces the opposite effect, with front legs extended and hind legs flexed.

Mahler, Margaret Schoenberger Hungarian-born American psychoanalyst, 1897—. See AUTISTIC PHASE; AUTISTIC PSYCHOSIS; END-STATE; INDIVIDUATION; RAPPROCHEMENT; SEPARATION-INDIVIDUATION; SYMBIOTIC PSYCHOSIS.

maiden fear = PARTHENOPHOBIA.

maieusiophobia /mā·ōōsē·ō-/ a morbid fear of childbirth (from Greek *maieuesthai*, "to act as a midwife").

Main, Thomas Forrest English psychiatrist, fl. 1937, 1972. See MAIN'S SYNDROME.

Maine de Biran, François Pierre Gauthier /men'dəbiräN'/ French philosopher, 1766–1824. See EXISTENTIALISM.

main effect in the analysis of variance, a term that estimates the effect of an independent variable acting alone, and contrasted with the INTERACTION EFFECT. See this entry.

main en griffe = CLAWHAND.

main étrangère: See STRANGE-HAND SIGN.

mainliner a street term for a drug abuser who takes illicit drugs by intravenous injection—who is **mainlining**. Also see SKIN-POPPING.

main sensory trigeminal nucleus: See TRIGEMINAL NUCLEUS.

Main's syndrome a condition in which a female psychotic patient who has been a health professional, e.g., a nurse, exploits her background to obtain therapeutic privileges and special sympathy from doctors, nurses, and attendants.

mainstreaming education of physically disabled, mildly retarded, and learning-disabled children within regular schools, but with special assistance where needed. M. is also the return of recovered mental patients or deinstitutionalized chronic patients to the community, where they receive rehabilitative assistance directed toward helping them achieve as full and normal a life as possible.

maintaining cause an influence in a person's environment that tends to maintain and reinforce his maladaptive behavior. An example is the required participation at cocktail parties of a professional person who suffers from alcoholism.

maintenance drugs medications that are prescribed regularly for a long period of supportive therapy (e.g., **methadone maintenance**), rather than for immediate control of a disorder. After an acute psychotic episode subsides, a patient may receive a daily dose of m.d. for six months or more, followed by a period of gradual withdrawal if that step is warranted.

maintenance functions the functions that keep the organism's physiological activities in homeostasis.

maintenance level the stage of maturity when physiological development has progressed as far as it can, and size and weight remain at a constant level.

maintenance minimum the minimum number of persons needed to maintain a behavior setting.

In a hospital or clinic, the m.m. would be the smallest number of staff members, professionals and nonprofessionals, required to provide adequate service for the patients accepted.

maintenance strivings the needs and motives that are directed toward maintaining a biological and psychological steady state. M.s. may include such basic needs as food, water, sleep, sexual gratification, psychological stimulation, and physical and mental activity.

major affective disorders (DSM-III): See BIPOLAR DISORDER, MIXED; BIPOLAR DISORDER, MANIC; BIPOLAR DISORDER, DEPRESSED; MAJOR DEPRESSION; MAJOR DEPRESSIVE EPISODE.

major asynergia of Babinski: See ASYNERGIA.

major depression an affective disorder in which the individual has experienced one or more major depressive episodes (subtyped **m.d., single episode**, and **m.d., recurrent**), but has never experienced a manic episode. Also see MAJOR DEPRESSIVE EPISODE. (DSM-III)

major depressive episode an affective disorder characterized by (a) a relatively persistent unhappy (dysphoric) mood, with loss of interest or pleasure in practically all activities, (b) feelings of sadness,, hopelessness, and irritability, and (c) the occurrence of several of the following symptoms every day for at least two weeks: poor appetite with significant weight loss, or increased appetite with significant weight gain; insomnia or excessive sleep; psychomotor agitation or retardation; decrease in sexual drive; loss of energy with fatigue; feelings of worthlessness, self-reproach, or excessive, possibly delusional, feelings of guilt; reduced ability to think, concentrate, or make decisions; and recurrent thoughts of death, the wish to die, or suicide attempt. (DSM-III)

major dysrhythmia = HYPSARRHYTHMIA.

major epilepsy = GRAND MAL.

major hysteria = HYSTEROEPILEPSY.

major-role therapy vocational counseling focused on the selection of occupational goals and vocational retraining, to enable an individual in need of rehabilitation to work at maximal capacity and satisfaction as a useful member of society.

major solution a Horney term for a neurotic tendency to repress or deny trends that may conflict with the idealized self. The m.s. also may be one of withdrawal into resignation as a means of reducing anxiety.

major tranquilizers drugs that calm agitated or psychotic patients and induce a lowered state of reaction to emotional stimuli with little overall effect on consciousness, as compared with sedative-hypnotic drugs. M.t. are used mainly in the treatment of schizophrenias and natural or drug-caused manic states. They include the phenothiazines, thioxanthenes, and some opiates. For other examples, see NEUROLEPTICS.

Make a Picture Story a projective test for children or adults in which the subject tells stories about cardboard figures which he selects and places against a background. The subject is then questioned about the feelings and attitudes of the characters, the title of the story, and the situation depicted. The stories are analyzed qualitatively to reveal personality dynamics, as in the TAT, and also scored objectively as to choice and placement of figures and other details. (E. S. Shneidman, 1947) Abbrev.: **MAPS**.

make-believe a form of dramatic play in which the child pretends to be another person, real or imaginary, and imitates activities involved in such situations as preparing a dinner or putting a baby to bed. Piaget describes such activities as "symbolic play." Also see IMAGINARY COMPANION.

-mal- a combining form meaning bad, wrong, ill, diseased, abnormal (Latin *malus*).

maladaptation the failure of an organism to acquire biological traits needed to interact effectively with an environment.

maladaptive in psychology, pertaining to a behavior pattern that is ineffective or counterproductive when used as a means of coping with the problems and stresses of life.

maladaptive behavior behavior that is detrimental to a person, group, or society; ineffective or self-defeating coping behavior. The term is often preferred by social-learning theorists as a substitute for mental illness, particularly when emphasizing the fact that detrimental patterns represent learned behavior and are thus modifiable.

maladaptive mechanisms patterns of behavior that interfere with the individual's capacity to adjust to the demands of life; e.g., overmobilization under stress, a "workaholic" pattern, self-defeating behavior, retreat from reality, and use of certain defense mechanisms such as denial.

maladie des tics = TOURETTE'S DISORDER.

maladie du doute = DOUBTING MANIA.

maladjustment the inability to maintain effective relationships and meet the demands of life satisfactorily. Also, m. is a catchall term for any emotional disturbance of a relatively minor nature.

malaise a slight feeling of illness, a vague feeling of discomfort and uneasiness (French).

malaria a febrile disease caused by a plasmodium, or protozoal parasite, that attacks the red blood cells. The agent is transmitted through the bite of a mosquito that previously has sucked blood from a m. victim, which may be a human or primate. The symptoms, paroxysms of chills and fever, differ somewhat according to the species of plasmodium. See MIASMA THEORY.

mal de pelea = PUERTO RICAN SYNDROME.

maldevelopment the defective development of an individual because of genetic, dietary, or external factors that interfere with the normal rate of growth of tissues and bodily functions. A protein deficiency of children weaned prematurely, in particular in Third World countries, may result in forms of m. known as marasmus and kwashiorkor which are marked by retarded physical and mental growth.

male climacteric the so-called **male menopause** which occasionally occurs in men, about ten years later than in women. Unlike the true menopause, it appears to be the result of psychological reactions to glandular changes more than the changes themselves, as well as anxiety over diminished potency. Symptoms, when they do occur, include nocturnal urinary frequency, fatigue, flushes, decreased sexual desire, and fear of being "put on the shelf." Also called **male climacterium**.

male continence = EJACULATIO RETARDATA.

male ejaculation: See EJACULATION.

male genitalia: See GENITALIA.

male homosexual prostitution sexual contact by one male with another for financial gain, or other personal gain, such as favors and protection in prison. Studies indicate that a social hierarchy exists, as in female prostitution. Lowest in status are the "street hustlers" who are usually teenage boys and not necessarily homosexuals themselves; next are the "bar hustlers"; and highest in prestige are the "call boys," who do not solicit in public.

male member = PENIS.

male menopause: See MALE CLIMACTERIC.

maleness the male anatomical structures and physiological functions associated with the male sexual and reproductive role. Also see SUPERMALE.

malergy a term used by Cattell for a condition of subnormal or inefficient functioning.

malevolent transformation a term coined by H. S. Sullivan for the feeling that one lives among enemies and can trust no one. This attitude is usually based on harsh or unfair treatment during childhood, and may be the basis for social withdrawal and, in some cases, mental disorder of a paranoid nature.

malfunction the failure of an organ or mechanical process to function properly.

malignant: See BENIGN.

malignant alcoholism = GAMMA ALCOHOLISM.

malignant neoplasm: See NEOPLASM.

malignant neurosis a type of progressive neurosis in which the symptoms become increasingly severe until the individual withdraws into a room or his bed, fails to perform any activity, and may become literally paralyzed by doubts and indecision. Such cases may be diagnosed as pseudoneurotic schizophrenia.

malignant psychosis a term introduced by Fenichel to identify a form of progressive schizophrenia that terminates in permanent dementia. M.p. is approximately equivalent to process psychosis and nuclear schizophrenia.

malignant stupor a psychogenic stupor from which there is little or no chance of recovery.

malingering a deliberate feigning of an illness or disability for financial gain or to escape responsibility. Examples are faking mental illness as a defense in a trial, faking physical illness to win compensation, or faking mental defect to avoid military service.

Malin syndrome a symptom pattern occasionally occurring as a side effect of major tranquilizers, in which the outstanding symptoms are dehydration, hyperhidrosis, hypersalivation, hyperthermia, and mental confusion.

malleation a spasmodic activity of the hands that resembles the movements of hitting or hammering; a tic that usually involves striking the thighs.

malleus the largest of the three ossicles in the middle ear and the bone closest to the tympanic membrane, or eardrum (Latin, "hammer"). It transmits vibrations of the eardrum to the incus. Also called **hammer; mallet**. See OSSICLES.

Malleus Maleficarum: See WITCHCRAFT.

malnutrition a state of health characterized by an improper balance of carbohydrates, fats, proteins, vitamins, and minerals in the diet with respect to energy needs as reflected in physical activity. M. may be due to excessive intakes of food categories as well as inadequate levels, as in examples of obesity or hypervitaminoses. Dietary deficiencies are associated with many physical and psychological disorders, such as pellagra which is marked by depression and other mental disturbances as a result of inadequate levels of niacin in the diet, thiamine deficiency which is manifested by sensory and motor disorders, and familial periodic paralysis, which is caused by a potassium deficiency.

malonic acid $C_3H_4O_4$—one of the components of **barbituric acid**, which is the basic substance used in the manufacture of two dozen different kinds of sedative-hypnotic drugs. The m.a. is combined with urea to yield **malonyl urea**—$C_4H_4N_2O_3$, a chemical name for barbituric acid. See BARBITURATES.

malpractice unethical or negligent behavior on the part of a professional person (e.g., a therapist) which may lead to legal action.

malvaria: See MAUVE FACTOR.

mammalingus the act of suckling the breast during intercourse, particularly in terms of the Ernest Jones concept that the act represents a type of fellatio when it involves the mother and father.

mammary gland the gland of the female breast that secretes milk.

mammillary bodies a pair of small spherical masses located on the underside and forming a part of the hypothalamus. Also called **corpus mamillare; bulla of fornix**.

mammography a technique for studying the human breast for cancer or other disorders by X-ray. Simple m. is done without injection of an opaque medium into the ducts of the breast, but use of a contrast medium is an alternative procedure.

mammotrophic hormone = PROLACTIN.

management by objectives the use of specific programs developed and implemented by organizations which may incorporate one or more of a set of general procedures, including job design, incentive systems, participatory decision-making, and goal-setting. Abbrev.: **MBO**.

managerial grid an alternative term for **two-dimensional leader-behavior space** in which the dimensions are concern for people and concern for production.

mandala /mun'-/ a circular oriental figure (Sanskrit, "circle") believed to represent the cosmos, which Jung used as an archetypal symbol of the union of conflicting conscious and unconscious forces in the self. Also see UFOS.

mand function an utterance that makes a de*mand* on the listener (e.g., "Listen here!"), rewarding the speaker in the form of listener compliance (Skinner).

mandibulofacial dysostosis = TREACHER COLLINS' SYNDROME.

mandrake an herb made from the roots, leaves, bark, or berries of a plant, Mandragora officinarum, used for millenia as an anesthetic, aphrodisiac, hallucinogen, and folk remedy. One of the active ingredients is hyoscyamine, a form of atropine. Another, **mandragora**, is a traditional analgesic employed by practitioners of herbal medicine.

mania a pathological state of excitement, overactivity, and agitation, as in the manic phase of bipolar disorders; a violent, frenzied, deranged state of mind, as in the popular concept of a maniac; also, morbid preoccupation with an activity or idea, or an uncontrollable impulse to perform a certain kind of act, as in collecting m. or kleptomania. See MANIC EPISODE.

Also see ABLUTOMANIA; ABSORBED M.; ACROMANIA; ACUTE M.; AFFECTIVE MONOMANIA; AGROMANIA; AKINETIC M.; ALCOHOLOPHILIA; AMENOMANIA; AMURAKH; ANDROPHONOMANIA; ANTIMANICS; ARITHMOMANIA; APHRODISIOMANIA; ASOTICAMANIA; BELL'S M., BITING M.; CHOREOMANIA; CHRONIC M.; COLLECTING M.; CONSTITUTIONAL MANIC DISPOSITION; COPING M.; DELIRIOUS M.; DELUSIONAL M.; DEPRESSIVE M.; DIPSOMANIA; DOUBTING M.; DROMOMANIA; ECDOMOMANIA; ECOMANIA; EGOMANIA; EMETOMANIA; EROTOGRAPHOMANIA; EROTOMANIA; GAMONOMANIA; GRAPHOMANIA; GRUMBLING M.; HAIR-PULLING; HELLENOMANIA; HYDRODIPSOMANIA; HYPERMANIA; HYPOCHONDRIASIS; HYPOMANIA; HYPOMANIC PERSONALITY; ICONOMANIA; INHIBITED M.; INSTINCTIVE MONOMANIA; INTELLECTUAL MONOMANIA;

LOGORRHEA; LYPEMANIA; MEGALOMANIA; METROMANIA; MICROMANIA; MONOMANIA; MONOMANIE BOULIMIQUE; MONOMANIE DU VOL; MONOMANIE ÉROTIQUE; MONOMANIE INCENDIÈRE; MYTHOMANIA; NARCOMANIA; NAUTOMANIA; NECROMANIA; NYMPHOMANIA; OIKIOMANIA; OINOMANIA; ONOMANIA; ONOMATOMANIA; OPIOMANIA; PARATERESIOMANIA; PHAGOMANIA; PHANEROMANIA; PHARMACOMANIA; PHONOMANIA; PHOTOMANIA; PLUTOMANIA; POLYTOXICOMANICS; PORIOMANIA; PORNOGRAPHOMANIA; PSEUDOMANIA; PSEUDONOMANIA; PYROMANIA; REACTIVE M.; RELIGIOUS M.; SCHIZOID-MANIC STATE; THANATOMANIA; TOMOMANIA; TOXICOMANIA; TRICHORRHEXOMANIA; TUBERCULOMANIA; UNIPOLAR MANIC-DEPRESSIVE PSYCHOSIS; UTEROMANIA; WITZELSUCHT.

mania a potu an acute psychotic state precipitated in most cases by a moderate amount of alcohol

(Latin, "drinking mania"), and characterized by confusion, disorientation, hallucinations, and impulsive violence with complete amnesia for the episode. Some authorities believe the condition is actually psychomotor epilepsy released by alcohol, although in normal persons it may occur after a period of prolonged stress. Also called **pathological intoxication; idiosyncratic intoxication**. See FUROR.

maniac popular term for a seriously disturbed person who is, in the public mind, totally deranged and likely to be dangerous to others.

maniacal exaltation: See MANIA TRANSITORIA.

mania of recommencement a form of obsessive-compulsive behavior in which the patient feels compelled to repeat simple operations, e.g., locking a door, many times before he feels the task has been performed properly (Janet).

mania phantastica infantilis a rare childhood mental condition characterized by exaltation, fugues, confabulations, fantasies, and retardation. The symptoms may be an autochthonous reaction or occur during a delirious state following a febrile disease.

maniaphobia = LYSSOPHOBIA.

mania transitoria an obsolete term for an acute, transient form of "maniacal exaltation," which develops suddenly and is characterized by "incoherence, partial or complete unconsciousness of familiar surroundings, and sleeplessness" (T. S. Clouston, *Clinical Lectures on Mental Diseases*, 1904). Also called EPHEMERAL MANIA.

manic a term applied to a person suffering from the m. phase of bipolar disorder. It is also a lay term for a mentally disturbed person, especially one who tends to be overactive or violent.

manic-depressive illness a severe affective disorder characterized by a predominant mood of elation or depression, and in some cases an alternation between the two states. Also called **manic-depressive psychosis**. For details, see BIPOLAR DISORDER, DEPRESSED; BIPOLAR DISORDER, MANIC; BIPOLAR DISORDER, MIXED; MAJOR DEPRESSIVE EPISODE; MANIC EPISODE. Also see UNIPOLAR MANIC-DEPRESSIVE PSYCHOSIS.

manic-depressive reaction a DSM I term for the category "bipolar disorder" in DSM-III. See BIPOLAR DISORDER, DEPRESSED; BIPOLAR DISORDER, MANIC; BIPOLAR DISORDER, MIXED.

manic episode an affective disorder characterized by (a) one or more periods of elevated, expansive or irritable mood, (b) a duration of at least a week, with three of the following symptoms: increase in activity or restlessness; talkativeness or pressure of speech; flight of ideas or racing thoughts; inflated self-esteem with grandiosity; decreased need for sleep; extreme distractibility; and involvement in activities with painful but unrecognized consequences, such as buying sprees, foolish investments, sexual indiscretions, or reckless driving. Episodes of this kind generally begin abruptly, escalate quickly, and are briefer than major depressive episodes. See MANIA. (DSM-III)

manic excitement a state of elation with hyperactivity occurring in manic episodes.

manic hebephrenia a manic phase similar to that of manic-depressive psychosis that occurs in some hebephrenic- (disorganized-) schizophrenia patients.

manic mood: See CONSTITUTIONAL MANIC DISPOSITION.

manic state a mental state characterized pressure of activity and speech, flight of ideas, and elation, ranging from relatively mild hypomania to the extreme of delirious mania.

manic stupor a mixture of manic and depressive reactions, in which the patient is elated but inactive, unresponsive, and unproductive of ideas. This state is occasionally found in bipolar (manic-depressive) disorder, and has been cited as one of the "mixed" types (in DSM-I). Also called **stuporous mania; unproductive mania**.

manifest anxiety an anxiety with overt symptoms that indicate an emotional confict.

Manifest Anxiety Scale: See ANXIETY SCALES.

manifest content the images and events of a nightdream or daydream as experienced and recalled by the dreamer. Compare LATENT CONTENT.

manifest goals in evaluation research, openly stated, objectively defined goals or objectives of an organization or program; goals specified by indicators of success and assessed in an evaluation program.

manikin test a performance test item in which wooden pieces must be fitted together to form a man. The test is an item on the Pintner-Paterson and other performance scales.

manipulanda the characteristics of an object such as solidity or plasticity that can be changed by an organism's motor activity, or which facilitate motor activity.

manipulation behavior designed to exploit or control others, e.g., weeping, throwing a tantrum, threatening suicide, and lying or scheming to gain special consideration or advantage. Also called **manipulative behavior**.

manipulation check in an experiment, the question or questions designed to help the experimenter evaluate the efficacy of the experimental manipulation. The m.c. is intended to verify that subjects perceive the manipulation as the experimeter intends.

manipulative behavior = MANIPULATION.

manipulative drive = MANIPULATORY DRIVE.

manipulative techniques various devices used particularly in brief psychotherapy, such as exhortation, suggestion, advice, prescription of drugs, and environmental modification or manipulation.

manipulatory drive motivations that have no direct relationship to food or other survival needs and may be by-products of other neural development. A m.d. may be directed toward a learning experience that exposes the subject to new stimuli which may in turn contribute to survival. E.g., a primate may perform tasks merely for the reward of watching a mechanical toy move. Also called **manipulative drive**.

Mann, Henry Berthold Austrian-born American mathematician, 1905—. See MANN-WHITNEY U TEST.

Mann, Ludwig /mun/ German neurologist, 1866–1936. See WERNICKE-MANN HEMIPLEGIA.

mannerism a gesture, facial expression, or verbal habit peculiar to the individual. Behavior of this kind may have hidden significance that must be worked through in psychoanalytic treatment.

mannitol $C_6H_{14}O_6$—a sugar alcohol obtained from seaweed, fungi, and other plant sources and used as a diuretic and diagnostic aid in the study of kidney function and cardiac disorders.

mannosidosis a rare disorder involving a possible deficiency of an enzyme needed to metabolize mannose molecules. Clinical case reports indicate the patient may have slow motor development, mental retardation, and hypotonic muscles. Laboratory tests may find brain and liver levels of mannose (a form of sugar) eight to ten times normal.

Mann-Whitney U test a nonparametric statistical test of ranked data for two independent samples.

manoptoscope an instrument for measuring eye dominance. It is a hollow cone through which the subjects sights.

Manouvrier, Léonce Pierre /mänōōvrē·ā'/ French anthropologist, 1850–1927. See MESO-SKELIC.

mantle layer the middle layer of the embryonic neural plate that develops into cerebral gray matter.

man-to-man rating scale a rating scale that compares dimensions or traits of the ratee with a selected group of persons who illustrate varying degrees of the traits in question. The rater selects the person in the comparison group with whom the ratee is most closely matched on a given trait.

mantra in transcendental meditation, a word or phrase (often in Sanskrit) repeated over and over to block out extraneous thoughts and induce a state of relaxation which enables the individual to reach a deeper level of consciousness. The m. is assigned by a teacher and is kept secret by the devotee. See TRANSCENDENTAL MEDITATION.

manual-arts therapist a health professional who assists in the rehabilitation process by training mentally or physically disabled patients in creative projects that require the use of the limbs, e.g., woodworking, metalworking, animal care, gardening, and printing. The purpose is to build self-esteem, confidence, and a sense of achievement while also preparing the patient for outside employment.

manual dominance the tendency to favor one hand over the other and to use it more frequently in acts that require only one hand. Also see LATERAL DOMINANCE; HANDEDNESS.

manualism a method of instruction for the deaf consisting of communication by means of finger spelling and sign language. Also called **manual method**.

MAOI; MAO inhibitors = MONOAMINE OXIDASE INHIBITORS.

maple-sugar urine disease an amino-acid metabolism disorder involving a deficiency of enzymes required for processing of leucine, isoleucine, valine, and alloisoleucine amino acids. A symptom is a distinctive maple-syrup odor of the patient's urine and perspiration. Other symptoms are mental retardation, hypertonicity, altered reflexes, and convulsions. Diet, dialysis, and transfusions are among therapeutic measures needed in m.-s.u.d. Abbrev.: **MSUD**. Also called **maple-syrup urine disease**.

mapping of genes: See GENETIC MAP.

map-reading test a test of the ability of a subject to orient in space. The test may require that the subject use a map to follow a path while holding the map in a position other than in the direction of movement. Thus, the direction of the path on the map would be different from that of the subject following the path.

MAPS = MAKE A PICTURE STORY.

marasmus in infancy, a condition characterized by apathy, withdrawal, and emaciation resulting from extreme emotional deprivation and leading, in some cases, to death (Greek *marasmos*, "consumption"). M. may occur in institutionalized infants who do not receive warmth and emotional security, or the marasmic state may be induced by an exceptionally anxiety-ridden mother. Also called **infantile atrophy**.

marathon group an encounter group that meets in seclusion for a period varying from eight hours to a week. These groups are based on the theory that a single extended session will elicit more intense interactions, foster a greater sense of intimacy and sharing, and encourage a freer expression of feelings than a series of shorter, interrupted sessions. See TIME-EXTENDED THERAPY.

marche à petits pas /mär'shäptēpä'/ a shuffling, mincing gait with short steps with loss of related body movements. The gait occurs in some cases of parkinsonism and in patients with brain damage due to multiple small CVA infarcts.

Marchi stain a stain used in the study of myelinated nerve fibers. M.s. contains osmium which stains the myelin residue black.

Marcus Gunn's sign a phenomenon in which the closed upper eyelid raises when the mouth opens and the jaw moves to the opposite side. It is a sign of facial-nerve or muscle paralysis, usually congenital. Also called **Gunn's syndrome; jaw-winking sign**. Also see MARIN AMAT'S SYNDROME.

Marfan, Antoine Bernard Jean /märfäN'/ French pediatrician, 1858–1942. See PECTUS CARINATUM (there: **Marfan's syndrome**); SKELE-TAL-SYSTEM DEFORMITY.

marginal characterizing an individual or group that has not been assimilated into the culture and therefore remains on the periphery of a particular society. The term is also applied to individuals whose intelligence level is borderline or whose emotional adjustment is tenuous.

marginal branch of the cingulate sulcus = MARGINAL SULCUS.

marginal consciousness those contents of consciousness that, while above the threshold of awareness, are not the center or direct focus of attention. Marginal stimuli are not equivalent to subliminal stimuli. Also called **fringe of consciousness**.

marginal group in a relatively homogeneous country or community, a distinct group that is not absorbed into the social mainstream because it differs in one or more significant dimensions, e.g., a specific religious, national, or racial group.

marginal individuals persons who live on the fringe of their own sociocultural group, or who are in a state of transition between two social worlds and not fully accepted in either. Marginal status of immigrants, Mexican-Americans, and other national or ethnic groups frequently generates role conflicts and feelings of alienation.

marginal intelligence an intelligence level between normal and mentally deficient.

marginals the row and column totals in a bivariate frequency distribution. Also called **marginal numbers**.

marginal sulcus a branch of the cingulate sulcus that turns upward between the paracentral lobule and superior frontal gyrus. Also called **marginal branch of the cingulate sulcus**.

Marie, Pierre French physician, 1853–1940. See MARIE'S ATAXIA; CHARCOT-MARIE-TOOTH DISEASE; ANKYLOSING SPONDYLITIS; BRAIN ATROPHY; PROGRESSIVE SPINAL-MUSCULAR ATROPHY; TOE DROP.

Marie's ataxia a form of ataxia, or failure of muscular coordination, that affects mainly adults. M.a. is usually a hereditary disorder caused by a lesion in the cerebellum and first identified by the French Physician Pierre Marie. The condition is progressive and disabling, involving not only gait disturbances but tremors, slurred speech, and difficulty in swallowing.

Marie-Strümpell disease: See ANKYLOSING SPONDYLITIS.

marihuana: marijuana: See PSYCHEDELICS; HASHISH.

Marin Amat, Manual Spanish ophthalmologist, 1879—. See MARIN AMAT'S SYNDROME.

Marin Amat's syndrome a pathologic condition in which the eyelid closes when the jaws move, as in chewing or opening the mouth. The condition is due to a spasm or paralysis of the ipsilateral facial nerve. Also see MARCUS GUNN'S SYNDROME.

Marinesco, Georges Rumanian pathologist, 1863–1938. See MARINESCO-SJÖGREN SYNDROME.

Marinesco-Sjögren syndrome an autosomal recessive hereditary disorder marked by cataracts, short stature, cerebellar ataxia, and mental retardation. All patients studied had bilateral cataracts; some were microcephalic. Cerebellar ataxia is present at infancy, and the patients are mildly to moderately retarded. Patients may live well past middle age but often lose their ability to walk because of progressive muscle weakness.

marital adjustment an ability to meet the demands and opportunities of marriage, especially (a) the sharing of experiences, interests and values, (b) respect for the partner's individual needs, aims, and temperament, (c) maintenance of open lines of communication and expression of feeling, (d) clarifying of roles and responsibilities, (e) cooperation in decision-making, problem-solving, and rearing of children, and (f) attainment of mutual sexual gratification.

marital conflict open or latent conflict between marriage partners. The nature and intensity of conflicts varies greatly, but studies indicate that the prime sources are often sexual disagreement, child-rearing differences, temperamental differences (particularly the tendency of one partner to dominate), and, to a lesser extent, religious differences, differences in values and interests, and disagreements over money management.

marital schism a condition of open discord between husband and wife, which puts a strain on the marriage and may lead to separation or divorce. Studies by Rosenbaum and others indicate that m.s. may be a causative factor in schizophrenia among the children.

marital skew a defective family pattern in which the pathological behavior of the dominant partner is accepted by the other partner. The condition may be pathogenic and is sometimes cited as a possible factor in schizophrenia.

marital therapy = MARRIAGE THERAPY.

markedness hypothesis the hypothesis that oppositional terms or antonym pairs are learned by children piecemeal. According to the m.h., children first concentrate on the more obvious or salient term; e.g., a child will learn to use the word "big" before learning to use "little" and will, in the early stages, employ "big" to designate small as well as large objects.

marker a term used in social psychology for any item or article used to indicate territorial possession in a public setting, e.g., a coat or briefcase left on a seat in a waiting room.

marketing orientation the term used by E. Fromm to denote a prevalent contemporary character pattern in which the individual regards people as commodities and evaluates personal worth in terms of salability. Attributes perceived as leading to business or social success are valued more than knowledge, creativity, integrity, or dedication. According to Fromm, the m.o. contributes to shallow relationships and alienation from self and society.

market research = CONSUMER RESEARCH.

Markoff, Andrei Andreevich Russian mathematician, 1856–1922. Also spelled **Markov**. See MARKOFF CHAIN; MARKOFF CHAINING.

Markoff chain in statistics, a sequence consisting

of a number of steps or events, with probability governing the transition between each pair of steps. Also spelled **Markov chain**.

Markoff chaining the theory that central motor mechanisms involve a chain reaction in which each movement depends upon a preceding movement which sends a feedback signal. The theory has been challenged on several points, including the fact that a chain of movements may not be repeated in exactly the same manner each time a task is performed. Also spelled **Markov chaining**.

Maroteaux, Pierre /märōtō'/ French physician, 1926—. See MAROTEAUX-LAMY SYNDROME; MUCO-POLYSACCHARIDOSES.

Maroteaux-Lamy syndrome an inherited disorder of connective tissue and skeletal development marked by dwarfism of the trunk and extremities and in some cases delayed closure of the cranial sutures and maldevelopment of the facial bones. One type of the disorder is classed as **systemic mucopolysaccharidosis**. Mental retardation and deafness often accompany the condition.

marriage: See CLUSTER M.; EXPERIMENTAL M.; GROUP M.; HOMOSEXUAL M.; INTERMARRIAGE; OPEN M.; SYMBIOTIC M.; SYNERGIC M.; TRADITIONAL M.; TRIAL M.

marriage fear = GAMOPHOBIA.

marriage therapy psychotherapy directed to improving a disturbed marital relationship, and "centered on the effort to alter the psychodynamics and behavior" of the partners (Sager, 1966). The sessions are usually conjoint, but a combination of individual and joint sessions is often more productive. They may be conducted on a problem-solving level in which grievances are aired and clashes worked through, or on a more analytic level focusing on dreams, unspoken communications, and the sources of defensive or aggressive attitudes. Also called **marital therapy; couples therapy**. Also see CONJOINT THERAPY.

Martinotti, Giovanni Italian physician, 1857–1928. See MARTINOTTI CELLS.

Martinotti cells spindle-shaped cells in the inner stellate (bottom) layer of the cortex, with axons that extend to the surface and communicate with the pyramidal cells of the cortex.

masculine attitude a term introduced by Adler to identify the masculine protest against feminine sensations in the female neurotic and manifested by unconscious tendencies to play a masculine role.

masculine identity a well-developed sense of affiliation with males, or identification with what are conceived to be masculine attitudes and values.

masculine protest a term applied by Adler to an urge to rebel against characteristics associated with femininity, such as submissiveness and inferior status, and to adopt characteristics associated with masculinity, such as assertiveness and competitiveness. This "protest" occurs primarily in women but may also be found in men who have identified with the so-called feminine role. In either case Adler interpreted it in terms of overcompensation for feelings of inferiority and believed that it sets up a "fictive" neurotic goal which may be substituted for healthy motives such as friendship, love, and social interest.

masculinity social-role behaviors, as distinguished from reproductive functions, that identify an individual as a boy or man. See MALENESS; SEX ROLES; VIRILITY.

masculinity-femininity tests tests designed to measure the degree of masculinity or femininity in individual subjects. The earliest was the Terman-Miles Attitude-Interest Analysis Test (1938); others, usually in inventory form, are the MMPI, the Guilford-Zimmerman Temperament Survey, and the Gough Femininity Scale. The recently developed Bem Sex-Role Inventory (1974, 1981) consists of 60 personality characteristics on which subjects rate themselves, yielding androgyny (high feminine, high masculine), feminine (high feminine, low masculine), masculine (high masculine, low feminine), and undifferentiated scores. The Bem inventory is one of the few that includes androgyny.

masculinization = VIRILISM.

Mashburn, Neely Cornelius American physician, 1886—. See MASHBURN COMPLEX COORDINATOR.

Mashburn Complex Coordinator an instrument for measuring eye-hand and eye-foot coordination by lining up rows of red and green lights with a stick and rudder bar.

mask a Stekel term for a character disguise. E.g., love of children may be a m. for homosexuality. Also see PERSONA.

masked affection expressions of love and tenderness toward another that actually mask a feeling of hatred for the person.

masked depression a condition in which psychosomatic symptoms occur episodically and in association with some degree of depressed mood.

masked deprivation = AFFECTIVE SEPARATION.

masked disorder an emotional disturbance concealed by a form of abnormal behavior that appears to be unrelated to the cause of the disturbance. The m.d. often represents an unconscious effort to treat a real problem as if it did not exist.

masked epilepsy: See EPILEPTIC EQUIVALENT.

masked homosexuality an unconscious form of homosexuality in which a person seeks in heterosexual activities the pleasures usually obtained in homosexual acts, e.g., anal intercourse.

masked obsession an obsession that manifests itself in the form of a physical symptom, e.g., pain. The organic symptom may represent a pleasurable but tabooed memory and can defy both physical diagnosis and relief through medication.

masking the partial or complete obscuring of one sensation by another. E.g., noises frequently screen out speech; smoking dulls the sense of taste; and body odors are masked by soap containing carbolic acid. Screen memories are also a form of m. See SCREEN MEMORY.

Maslow, Abraham Harold American psychologist, 1908–70. M. originated the concept of a hierarchy of needs that motivate all individuals: basic physiological needs, and needs for safety, belonging, love, esteem, understanding, and self-actualization. His emphasis on self-fulfillment made him a leader in the human-potential movement. See MASLOW'S MOTIVATIONAL HIERARCHY; MASLOW'S THEORY OF HUMAN MOTIVATION; BEING COGNITION; BEING LOVE; DEFICIENCY LOVE; DEFICIENCY MOTIVATION; ESTEEM NEEDS; EXISTENCE, RELATEDNESS, AND GROWTH THEORY; HUMANISTIC PERSPECTIVE; HUMANISTIC THEORY; INSTINCTOID NEEDS; LOVE NEEDS; META-MOTIVATION; METANEEDS; METAPATHOLOGY; MOTIVATION; NEED-HIERARCHY THEORY; PEAK EXPERIENCES; PERSONALITY STRUCTURE; PHYSIOLOGICAL NEEDS; SAFETY NEEDS; SELF-ACTUALIZATION; SELF-REALIZATION.

Maslow's motivational hierarchy the hierarchy of human motives, or needs, described by Maslow: physiological needs at the base, followed by safety and security; then love, affection, and gregariousness; then prestige, competence, and power; and, at the highest level, esthetic needs, the need for knowing, and self-actualization. Also see MASLOW'S THEORY OF HUMAN MOTIVATION.

Maslow's theory of human motivation the humanistic view that advocates an emphasis on the higher human motives for understanding, esthetic values, self-realization, and peak experiences. These Maslow called abundancy needs, which contrast with the usual emphasis on deficiency needs which stem from physical needs, insecurity, and alienation. See PEAK EXPERIENCES; MASLOW'S MOTIVATIONAL HIERARCHY.

Masoch: See SACHER-M.

masochism a disorder in which the individual derives pleasure from pain inflicted by others or, in some cases, by himself. The term is based upon the name of Leopold V. Sacher-Masoch, whose stories frequently included scenes of sexual gratification associated with being whipped, choked or bitten, or other forms of cruelty. However, the term is also applied to experiences that do not involve sex (or in which it may exist in disguised form), such as martyrdom, humiliation, religious flagellation, or asceticism. In psychoanalysis, m. is interpreted as aggression turned inward when outward expression is laden with guilt and anxiety. For kinds of m., see SACHER-MASOCH.

masochistic character an individual who persistently and characteristically obtains gratification or freedom from guilt feelings as a consequence of humiliation, self-derogation, self-sacrifice, wallowing in misery, and, in some instances, submitting to physically sadistic acts.

masochistic fantasies fantasies of being whipped, choked, or otherwise abused as an expression of masochistic tendencies, particularly as a means of achieving sexual excitement.

masochistic sabotage patient behavior that tends unconsciously to provoke punishment, scorn, or other adverse reactions from persons or objects in his environment. Self-defeating behavior may also be manifested by the patient's uncooperative attitude or insulting remarks in therapy.

masochistic wish-dream a dream in which injury is inflicted upon the dreamer.

mass action the concept that although the brain has specific sensory- and motor-function centers, the cortex is relatively nonspecific in learning and the general mass of the cortex is involved in that function. See LAW OF M.A.

massage the systematic stroking or kneading of a body area by hand or a mechanical or electrical device, e.g., a vibrator. Manual m. usually is administered for therapeutic and rehabilitative purposes because the hands can detect abnormalities, such as swellings or muscle spasms. M. may be performed in a fluid environment, as in a whirlpool bath.

massa intermedia = INTERTHALAMIC ADHESIONS.

mass contagion = MASS HYSTERIA.

massed practice a learning procedure in which material is studied either in a single lengthy session or in sessions separated by very short time intervals. In many learning situations, m.p. is found less effective than distributed or spaced practice. Compare DISTRIBUTED PRACTICE; SPACED PRACTICE.

mass hysteria an epidemic of extreme suggestibility and irrational behavior among an entire group of people, such as the dancing manias, werewolf delusions, and biting manias that swept through Europe between the 13th and 16th centuries, tulipmania in 17th-century Holland, the Florida real-estate boom of the 1920s, bank runs during the Depression, and mass reactions to the Orson Welles broadcast based on H. G. Wells' *War of the Worlds*, in 1938. Also called **epidemic hysteria; collective hysteria; mass contagion**. See COLLECTIVE PSYCHOSIS.

mass masochism a term used by Theodore Reik to describe the willingness of a population to endure sacrifices and suffering as demanded by a dictatorial leader to whom people have surrendered their own power. An example is the mass suicide of Jim Jones cult members in Guyana in 1978.

mass methods experimental, testing, or measurement procedures that are administered simultaneously to a large number of subjects, as in giving reading tests to all school children in a certain city.

mass movement a concerted effort by a large number of people to bring about social changes.

mass observation a survey technique in which a large number of people are interviewed, as in a public-opinion poll.

Masson, W. scientist, fl. 1845. See MASSON DISK.

Masson disk a device for measuring the threshold of brightness vision by observing a rotating disk with concentric rings of diminishing grayness.

mass polarization the focusing of attention of an entire population on a single message or propaganda theme.

mass psychology the study of the characteristic actions and reactions of crowds, mobs, gangs, audiences, or the public at large, including such phenomena as mass hysteria, fads, rioting, lynching, group revelry, group conformity, political movements, and relationships to leaders. Also see MOB PSYCHOLOGY.

mass reflex an indiscriminate response of many body effectors to a single stimulus, as in "freezing" with fear.

mass-to-specific development in fetal and infantile development, progression from gross, random movements involving the whole body to more refined movements of body parts.

-mast-; -masto- a combining form relating to the breast (Greek *mastos*).

mastectomy the surgical removal of the breast or breast tissue. M. usually is performed to remove breast tissue invaded by malignant breast tumors and to prevent metastasis of tumor cells to other body areas. But m. is performed occasionally to remove a benign tumor or to correct a condition of chronic cystic mastitis. A m. that is limited to the area of the neoplasm may be called a **lumpectomy**; a **simple m.** results in excision only of the breast; a **modified radical m.** removes the breast and the lymph nodes in the armpit; a **radical m.** removes the breast, the lymph nodes in the armpit, and the underlying muscle tissue.

Masters, William Howell American physician, 1915—. See BIOPHYSICAL SYSTEM; DUAL-SEX THERAPY; PSYCHOSOCIAL SYSTEM; SENSATE-FOCUS-ORIENTED THERAPY; SPECTATOR ROLE.

mastery motive the impetus to master or control outer demands and inner drives; also, the drive to achieve and be successful. Some authors (e.g., Fenichel) call it **mastery instinct**.

mastery training experimental or "real-world" training that prepares subjects for aversive situations or conflict by teaching methods of assertion and constructive control over environmental conditions.

mastigophobia a morbid fear of receiving a flogging, also of witnessing a flogging.

Mast syndrome an inherited type of presenile dementia, with symptoms that begin before the age of 20, followed by progressive deterioration to complete incapacity before middle age. Symptoms include mental deterioration, spasticity, dysarthria, difficulty in walking, and a blank facial appearance dominated by an unblinking stare. (The syndrome is named for an American Amish family in which the disease was first found, in the middle of the 20th century.)

masturbation manipulation of the sex organs, especially the penis and clitoris, for purposes of sexual gratification. The act is usually accompanied by sexual fantasies. Some investigators also include in m. the use of mechanical devices such as vibrators, self-stimulation of other organs such as the anus or nipples, as well as nail-biting, hair-plucking or -twisting, and inserting a finger in the nose, mouth, or ear. (The word m. is derived from the Latin *masturbari*, "to masturbate," which probably comes from *manu stuprare*, "to defile oneself with the hand.") See AUTOEROTISM; ONANISM; ANAL M.; COMPULSIVE M.; INFANTILE M.; MUTUAL M.; PSYCHIC M.; SYMBOLIC M.

masturbation equivalents activities that have been identified as psychological substitutes for masturbation, e.g., gambling, nail-biting, pulling on one's earlobe, twisting strands of one's hair. Also see PREPHALLIC M.E.

matatabi = METATABI.

matched dependent behavior: See IMITATION.

matched-group design an experimental design in which experimental and control groups are equated or matched on a background variable before being exposed to the experimental procedure. Compare RANDOMIZED-GROUP DESIGN.

matched sample a sample that is equal to another sample with respect to the relevant variables. E.g., for a study in which weight and blood pressure are considered, matched samples will show an equivalent range and mean for the two factors.

matching a research technique for assuring comparability of subjects by equating them on background variables. E.g., the individuals in a control group and in an experimental group might be matched on years of education, income, and marital status.

matching hypothesis the finding that people tend to be attracted to and interact with individuals who roughly equal them in physical beauty. This equation appears to be true for both opposite-sex and same-sex relationships.

matching test a test based on selection of items from one list and matching them with the appropriate items on another list.

matching to sample a procedure for studying learning, in which an animal is shown a stimulus, and is then required to pick out an example of it from an array of several alternatives.

maté = PARAGUAY TEA.

materialism: See BODY-MIND PROBLEM.

materialization in parapsychology, the alleged production of a body or its parts by supernormal or spiritualistic methods.

maternal aggression: See ANIMAL AGGRESSION.

maternal attitudes attitudes of the mother toward her children, particularly those attitudes that play an important role in character formation, emotional adjustment, and self-image. Negative examples are permissive, indulgent, overprotective, rigidly disciplinary, neglectful, and abusive attitudes. Positive examples are caring, accepting, and recognition of the child's need for independence and self-esteem.

maternal behavior the behavior associated with caring for offspring by the mother or, in some cases, caring for the young of other mothers.

Some forms of m.b. in animals are impaired by medial-cortex lesions, and males of some species exhibit m.b. after receiving injections of prolactin, the lactogenic hormone.

maternal deprivation a lack of adequate affection, care, and stimulation from the mother or mother substitute, particularly during infancy. It is a situation that occurs in disturbed families and institutions, and which may have an effect on all aspects of the child's personality—emotional reactions, intellectual development, self-concept, interpersonal relations, and physical well-being. In some cases this type of deprivation may lay the basis for severe mental disorder. See FAILURE TO THRIVE; MARASMUS.

maternal diabetes a common cause of congenital anomalies and fetal death *in utero*. Congenital anomalies are about five times more frequent among offspring of diabetic mothers. Fetal mortality rates in cases of m.d. range from ten to 30 percent. The newborn may suffer from hypoglycemia and hypocalcemia, the latter condition being marked by tremors and convulsive movements.

maternal drive the female parental drive to feed and otherwise care for the offspring.

maternity blues a popular expression for transient feelings of "let-down" and dejection that frequently occur after giving birth to a child, in contrast to the more severe and lasting depression that occasionally occurs. Also called **postpartum blues**. See POSTPARTUM PSYCHOSIS; POSTPARTUM EMOTIONAL DISTURBANCES.

Recent studies indicate that the new father may experience a similar reaction, especially if he is unprepared for the change in routine and the complete attention needed by the infant (**paternity blues; new-father blues**).

mathematical biology a branch of biology that deals with the development of mathematical models of biological phenomena, such as conditioning and nerve conduction.

mathematical model the representation of a psychological or physiological function in the form of a mathematical formula or equation, as in Weber's law.

mathematico-deductive method the use of postulates and corollaries in mathematical form to develop a system or theory.

Mathematics Usage Test: See ACT ASSESSMENT.

Mathews, Chester Ora American psychologist, 1895—. See WOODWORTH-MATHEWS PERSONAL DATA SHEET.

Mathurin, Saint French priest, fl. fourth century. M. was the patron saint of idiots and fools. See SAINT MATHURIN'S DISEASE.

mating behavior behavior related to the selection of sexual partners for reproduction of their species. M.b. varies with the species and, with the exception of birds, is generally polygamous, the female being attracted to the male who appears to have the greatest resources for parenting the offspring through size, strength, amount of territory controlled, or other, similar factors demonstrated during courtship.

matriarchy a society in which lineage is **matrilineal**, that is, traced through the female; also, a society ruled by women, who are either symbols of power or of love and motherhood. Many investigators believe the **matriarchal** society preceded the patriarchal because the first relationship of infants of both sexes is to the mother. Others believe the patriarchal came first because of the superior strength of the male.

matriculation dream = EXAMINATION DREAM.

matrilineal: See MATRIARCHY.

maturation the process of "unfolding from within" as contrasted with development through learning and contact with the environment. M. includes (a) biological development, such as growth and differentiation of cells and the development of sensory and motor functions, and (b) personality development from infancy through childhood, adolescence, and adulthood. Biological development is governed primarily, though not wholly, by heredity; and personality development is a product of both inborn, constitutional tendencies (that is, maturational factors) and environmental influences.

maturational crisis a crisis, characterized by a period of acute disorganization of behavior or affect precipitated by a transition from one developmental phase to another, such as entering kindergarten, becoming engaged, getting married, becoming a parent, and retiring. Also called **developmental crisis; normative crisis**. See ACCIDENTAL CRISIS.

maturational lag a slowness, or delay, in some aspects of neurological development which affects learning but does not involve specific brain damage.

maturation-degeneration hypothesis the principle that functions and abilities between birth and death can be plotted as a trajectory curve that reaches a peak in the early years and then gradually declines.

maturation hypothesis a generalization that some behaviors are solely hereditary but do not appear until appropriate organs and neural systems have matured.

maturity: See DEVELOPMENTAL LEVELS.

maturity-onset diabetes a form of diabetes mellitus that usually does not present symptoms until after the age of 40. It is generally less severe and slower in development than the juvenile form of the disease. Obesity often is associated with m.-o.d. and may be controlled simply with oral hypoglycemic pills or by weight-control diet, or both.

maturity rating an evaluation of adult behavior on a particular trait as compared with a peer-group norm.

matutinal insomnia = TERMINAL INSOMNIA.

maudlin drunkenness a silly, blissful, unpleasantly sentimental type of behavior frequently observed in intoxicated persons.

Maudsley Personality Inventory a personality test developed by E. J. Eysenck, containing 24 items characteristic of neuroticism (N) and extraversion (E). The validation of the M.P.I. has been established by significant discriminations between normal health groups and clinical groups, as well as correlations with other tests of the same dimensions.

mauve factor a purplish spot found in chromatographic tests of urine samples of many schizophrenics. Because the m.f. also is found in urine tests of mental patients who are not schizophrenic and of persons considered normal, it has not been accepted as a basis for diagnosis. Abram Hoffer and Humphry Osmond termed the condition **malvaria** (from Latin *malva*, "mallow"); most investigators attribute it to phenothiazines.

maximum-security unit a section of an institution for the mentally ill reserved for patients who are dangerous to themselves or others.

Maxwell, James Clerk Scottish physicist, 1831–79. See MAXWELL DISKS.

Maxwell disks a series of slotted color disks on a rotating spindle used to produce mixed hues.

May, Rollo American psychoanalyst, 1909—. M. is known as a spokesman for the existential movement, particularly concerned with combatting feelings of emptiness, cynicism, and despair by emphasizing basic human values, such as love, free will, and self-awareness. See ANGST.

maze a patterned device of correct and incorrect pathways (including many blind alleys) that must be followed from an entrance to an exit. Various types of mazes are used in learning experiments for animals and humans. A common human m. device is a printed paper pattern on which the subject traces the correct pathway with a pencil. Also see STYLUS M.; T-MAZE; LOCOMOTOR M.; TEMPORAL M.; ELITHORN MAZE; PORTEUS MAZE.

maze behavior a manifestation of ability to perform intelligent planning. There is evidence that mental rehearsal or planning for intelligent acts is impaired by frontal-lobe lesions because some patients perform poorly on m.b. tests after the lesions have occurred.

maze learning learning to reach a certain objective by starting from a designated point and following a circuitous pathway that has more or less randomly placed blind alleys. The m.l. process usually involves multiple trials and is regarded as successful when the subject can reach the goal in the most direct way and without errors on two successive trials.

MB: See CREATINE PHOSPHOKINASE.

MBD = MINIMAL BRAIN DYSFUNCTION.

MBO = MANAGEMENT BY OBJECTIVES.

McArdle, Brian English neurologist, fl. 1936, 1972. See MCARDLE'S DISEASE; MYOGLOBINURIA; TARUI'S DISEASE.

McArdle's disease a disorder characterized by an abnormal accumulation of glycogen in skeletal muscle tissue. M.d. is an autosomal-recessive disease that can be marked by muscle pain, contractures, myoglobinuria, and some degree of exercise intolerance. The precise causative factor is a deficiency of an enzyme, myophosphory-lase B. Also called **Type V glycogen-storage disease; McArdle's syndrome**.

McCarthy, Dorothea American psychologist, 1906–74. See MCCARTHY SCALES OF CHILDREN'S ABILITIES; EGOCENTRIC SPEECH.

McCarthy Scales of Children's Abilities a comprehensive instrument for children between two and one-half and eight and one-half years of age, consisting of six overlapping scales: Verbal, Perceptual-Performance, Quantitative, General Cognitive, Memory, and Motor. It is suitable for children from different socioeconomic groups, and for identifying learning disabilities.

McClelland, David C. American psychologist, 1917—. See ACHIEVEMENT DRIVE; ACHIEVEMENT MOTIVATION; AFFECTIVE-AROUSAL THEORY; NEED FOR ACHIEVEMENT.

MCD = METAPHYSIAL CHONDROPLASIA.

McDougall, William American psychologist, 1871–1938. In opposition to the stimulus-response approach of behaviorism, this independent thinker held that all activity is motivated by instincts and purposive striving; in opposition to the prevailing environmentalist view, he supported eugenics as the road to human improvement; and in opposition to the then current emphasis on observable phenomena, he took a position at Duke University and sponsored the ESP investigations of J. B. Rhine. See HORMIC PSYCHOLOGY; HYSTERICAL PUERILISM; INSTINCT; NEURIN; RHINE.

MCE = MEDICAL CARE EVALUATION.

McGregor, Douglas M. American psychologist, 1906–64. See NEED-HIERARCHY THEORY.

MCL = MOST COMFORTABLE LOUDNESS.

McNaughton rules = M'NAGHTEN RULES.

McNemar, Quinn American psychologist and statistician, 1900—. See TERMAN-MCNEMAR TEST OF MENTAL ABILITIES.

MD = MUSCULAR DYSTROPHY.

m. dict. an abbreviation used in prescriptions, meaning "as directed" (Latin *modo dictu*).

Mead, Margaret American anthropologist, 1901–78. See COFIGURATIVE CULTURE; POSTFIGURATIVE CULTURE; PREFIGURATIVE CULTURE.

mean the arithmetic average, the most widely used statistic for describing central tendency; also, the arithmetic m. Symbol: M or $\bar{X} = \Sigma X/N$.

mean deviation = AVERAGE DEVIATION.

mean-gradation method = EQUAL-APPEARING-INTERVALS METHOD.

meaning the cognitive or emotional significance of a word, theory, signal, or symbolic act. Also see CONTEXT THEORY OF M.; WILL TO M.

meaningful learning acquisition of material that relates to the learner's experience or enriches his life in an interesting or challenging way—as contrasted with material that has little or no relevance and can only be learned by rote. Also see READINESS.

meaninglessness the absence of meaning, particularly when associated with a pervasive feeling that one's life, life in general, or the entire world lacks significance, purpose, or direction. The perception or feeling of m. poses the major problem which the existential approach attempts to solve, or to live with. See EXISTENTIALISM. Also see WILL TO MEANING.

means any object, process, or activity utilized by an organism in its movement toward a goal or toward solution of a problem.

means-end capacity according to E. C. Tolman, the ability to perceive and respond to the linkages between means objects and goals, e.g., the ability to judge cues to distance, depth, and direction on the way to a goal.

means-end relations according to E. C. Tolman, all the objects and factors, such as time and distance, that are interposed between the means and a given end or final goal and must be perceived by the organism.

means-ends readiness E. C. Tolman's term for the state of selective responsiveness of organisms to means-object stimuli in the environment. Essentially, m.-e.r. constitutes a predisposition, established through the contributions of experience and inheritance, to judge stimuli in a certain way or to prefer one behavior over another potentially effective behavior in pursuit of a specific goal. Also called **means-ends expectation**.

means object any object, response, event, or condition that contributes to an organism's progress toward a goal. The term refers not only to objects as such but to environmental cues that alert the organism to the correct route or response. Also called **means situation**.

mean square in the analysis of variance, the sum of squares divided by its degrees of freedom. The m.s. between groups divided by the m.s. within groups yield an F ratio. The m.s. is a variance estimate.

means situation = MEANS OBJECT.

measure of central tendency a value near the center of a distribution of scores that is used to represent the total distribution; an average or typical value. The mean, median, and mode are all measures of central tendency. Also called **central-tendency measure**. Also see MEASURE OF VARIATION.

measure of variation a statistical measure that reveals the degree to which scores in a frequency distribution are dispersed or concentrated around the center values. A typical distribution shows most values clustering around the middle while the number of values that deviate from midpoint or midscore diminish in proportion to their degree of deviation. The standard deviation and the range are frequently used measures of variation. Also called **measure of dispersion; measure of variability**. Also see AVERAGE DEVIATION; RANGE; STANDARD DEVIATION; MEASURE OF CENTRAL TENDENCY.

mechanical aptitude an ability to comprehend and deal with machines or mechanisms.

mechanical-aptitude tests tests designed to measure various abilities related to mechanical work, such as mechanical information, mechanical reasoning, spatial relations, perceptual skills, understanding of mechanical principles, mechanical assembly, and manual dexterity.

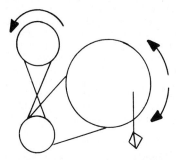

MECHANICAL-APTITUDE TESTS. Example of mechanical reasoning: If the left upper pulley turns left, is the weight (at right) lowered or raised?

mechanical intelligence the mental ability to understand concrete objects and mechanical relationships.

mechanical-man concept the view that human beings and life itself can be understood as forms of machinery subject only to physical processes and not subject to nonphysical phenomena such as consciousness: "Every Detail of the Past and Future History of Mankind would be the same if consciousness were completely nonexistent, just so long as the physical laws of nature were kept unchanged" (D. E. Wooldridge, *Mechanical Man, The Physical Basis of Intelligent Life*, 1968).

mechanism in psychiatry, a general term applied to a large number of psychological functions that help us meet environmental demands, protect our ego, satisfy our inner needs, and alleviate internal and external conflicts and tensions. Among them are language, which enables us to retain and express our thoughts; memory, which stores the information we need in solving problems; perception, which involves recognition and interpretation of events; and the thought processes involved in overcoming difficulties. In addition, there are various defense mechanisms such as rationalization and compensation, with which we protect ourselves from anxiety and loss of self-esteem. Also called **mental m.**

mechanistic approach the assumption that complex psychological processes can ultimately be understood as the outcome of underlying physiological processes; e.g., perception is explained by recourse to the scientific principles (especially chemical and electrical) that govern the nervous system. The m.a. forms the basic outlook of physiological psychology. See MECHANISM. Also see DESCARTES; REDUCTIONISM.

mechanophobia a morbid fear of machinery.

mechanoreceptors receptors that are sensitive to mechanical forms of stimuli. Examples of m. are receptors in the ear that translate sound waves into nerve impulses and receptors in the joints and muscles. See CHEMORECEPTORS.

Mecholyl: See ADRENALINE-M. TEST.

Meckel's syndrome a congenital disorder marked by microcephaly, eye, ear, and olfactory abnormalities, and varying degrees of brain-tissue anomalies. Some of the children afflicted with the disorder show premature closure of skull sutures. The patients either are stillborn or die in early infancy. Also called **dysencephalia splanchnocystia; Gruber's syndrome.**

Medea complex the compulsion of a mother to kill her children as revenge against the father, named for the Medea of Greek myths who killed her children fathered by Jason after he deserted her in favor of a younger woman.

medial pertaining to the middle or center of a body area or organ.

medial bundle a group of sensory fibers located between the dorsal ganglion and the spinal cord and composed mainly of large myelinated nerves including pressure-receptor fibers. The m.b. fibers communicate with the dorsal column of white matter.

medial geniculate body an enlargement on the surface of the thalamus that contains nerve-cell nuclei. It functions as a relay point for auditory impulses between the inferior brachium and the auditory cortex.

medial lemnisci sensory tracts from the spinal cord that communicate with the thalamus. Singular: **medial lemniscus.**

medial olfactory stria a nerve tract that connects the olfactory bulbs through the anterior commissure.

medial orbital gyrus: See ORBITAL GYRI.

medial rectus: See EYE MOVEMENTS.

medial saggital: See SAGGITAL.

median a description of the central tendency in a set of data. It is the point below which 50 percent of the cases fall. It is the preferred measure of central tendency in a markedly skewed distribution, since it is less sensitive to a few extreme cases than the mean is.

median class = MEDIAN INTERVAL.

median-cleft-face syndrome a congenital disorder characterized by defective fusion of structures in the midline of the face. The cleft may involve the eyes, the tip of the nose, the palate, and the premaxilla. The lower-lip area is rarely affected. Visual acuity may be normal, but strabismus is common. About 20 percent of the patients tested had some degree of mental retardation. Also called **ocular hypertelorism.**

median gray a gray halfway between pure white and pure black.

median interval the class or class interval of a frequency distribution in which the median is found. Also called **median class; median group; midinterval.**

mediate association a connection between two ideas that is formed indirectly by means of an intermediate, or intervening, idea, as in remembering a chemical formula by making a word out of the symbols.

mediated generalization a type of conditioning in which a generalized response follows a stimulus that is dissimilar to the original stimulus, e.g., responding the same way to toy as to the original stimulus, ball.

mediating variable = INTERVENING VARIABLE.

mediational learning a concept of learning that assumes the presence of mediators to bridge the association between two or more events that are not directly contiguous in space or time. The mediators are events or processes that serve as cue-producing responses.

mediation processes the processes involved in decision-making, including retrieval of stored information, judgments and evaluations, computations, reasoning, and other mental operations.

mediation theory the hypothesis that stimuli affect behavior indirectly through an intervening process.

mediator a process or system that exists between a stimulus and a response, or between the source and destination of a neural impulse, or between the transmitter and receiver of communications.

medical audit a system of evaluation of the effectiveness of diagnostic and therapeutic procedures. A m.a. may take the form of analyses of individual cases or of a patient population. Kinds of m.a. include **retrospective m.a.,** based on a review of patients' charts after they have been discharged, and **concurrent m.a.,** which is conducted while the patient is still under treatment.

Medical Care Evaluation a medical audit in which an assessment of the quality of care and its utilization is made, including investigation of suspected problems, analysis of the problems identified, and a plan for corrective action. Abbrev.: **MCE.**

medical history in psychiatry, the portion of the developmental history, or anamnesis, that focuses on the patient's health throughout life, including illnesses and disorders, congenital or acquired. The object is to uncover, where possible, etiological clues to his or her present condition.

medical-laboratory technician a specially trained health professional who works in a hospital clinical laboratory or similar environment. In the United States a registered m.-l.t. is required to have at least three years of college plus one year of training in an approved clinical-laboratory school, and successful completion of an examination by the American Society for Clinical Pathologists.

medical model a systems-analysis approach to evaluation, that is, an approach dealing empirically with the interrelatedness of all the factors that may affect performance, and monitoring possible side effects of the treatment. The m.m. is in contrast to the **engineering model,** which is a simple comparison of gains for different groups, some of which have been exposed to the program of interest. Both terms are used in evaluation research.

medical model of disease a theoretical pattern or conceptualization of a disorder, which may be idealized or modified as needed to represent signs and symptoms, diagnosis, therapy, and prognosis. The m.m.o.d. may be presented in mathematical form or as a computer program. A m.m.o.d. can represent a behavioral or other psychological disorder.

medical psychology an area of applied psychology devoted to psychological questions arising in the practice of medicine, such as emotional reactions to illness, attitudes toward terminal illness and impending death, psychological means of relieving pain (e.g., through hypnotic suggestion), reactions to disability, studies of iatrogenic factors, development of techniques for testing drug side effects on psychological functions ("behavioral toxicity"), and application of personality tests to patients with migraine, ulcers, and other stress-related disorders.

medical psychotherapy psychotherapy that utilizes medicines and medical techniques in the treatment of mental illness.

medical social worker a health professional who receives special training and education in helping individuals and families with problems associated with disabling diseases and injuries. The areas of expertise of the m.s.w. include social life, employment, finances, living arrangements, marriage, child care, and emotional reactions. A m.s.w. generally is required to have at least one graduate degree in appropriate studies, and a doctoral degree is needed for administrative posts.

medicine fear = PHARMACOPHOBIA.

meditation contemplation; reflection; thinking quietly but deeply about one's aims and relationships, or the meaning of life. Also see TRANSCENDENTAL M.

medium any agency through which something is achieved, including the air or a wire through which messages are transmitted. In parapsychology, a m. is the person who functions as the instrument of alleged communication between the living and the dead.

mediumistic hypothesis the theory that a schizophrenic patient is close to the collective unconscious and therefore in a position to see the trend of events and signs of his own disintegration.

medium trance: See TRANCE.

medulla oblongata the portion of the spinal cord that becomes enlarged at the base of the brain. It contains many nerve tracts that conduct impulses between the spinal cord and higher brain centers. The m.o., or "bulb," also contains autonomic nuclei involved in the control of breathing, heartbeat, and blood pressure. It is one of the three structures of the hindbrain, the most primitive part of the brain, the others being the pons and cerebellum. Also called **myelencephalon.**

medullary cystic disease a kidney disorder characterized by the formation of cysts in the medulla, or area of the organ in which the filtering function occurs. See KIDNEY DISEASE; KIDNEY FAILURE.

medullary sheath a fatty insulating sheath that covers peripheral sensory and motor neurons.

medullary tegmental paralysis = BABINSKI-NAGEOTTE SYNDROME.

Meduna, Ladislas J. von Hungarian-born American psychiatrist, 1896–1964. See ATYPICAL PSYCHOSIS; CARBON-DIOXIDE THERAPY; METRAZOL SHOCK TREATMENT; ONEIROPHRENIA.

Meehl, Paul Everett American psychologist, 1920 —. See COGNITIVE SLIPPAGE.

-mega- a combining form meaning large, enlarged.

megadoses pharmacotherapy the use of massive doses of pharmacologic agents in the treatment of certain disorders, e.g., the administration of megadoses of nicotinic acid to control schizophrenia. Various vitamins, minerals, and hormones are employed in the therapies of orthomolecular psychiatrists. See ORTHOMOLECULAR PSYCHIATRY; OSMOND.

megalocephaly = MACROCEPHALY.

megalomania a highly inflated conception of one's importance, power, or capabilities, bordering on DELUSIONS OF GRANDEUR. See this entry.

megalophobia a morbid fear of anything large.

megalopsia = MACROPSIA.

-megaly a combining form relating to an abnormal enlargement.

megavitamin therapy: See ORTHOMOLECULAR PSYCHIATRY.

Meier, Norman Charles American psychologist, 1893–1967. See MEIER ART JUDGMENT TEST.

Meier Art Judgment Test a test to determine artistic abilities of subjects by asking them to express a preference for one of two copies of a masterpiece, one of which has been rendered esthetically inferior by subtle changes. The complete test, designed by N. C. Meier, includes 100 sets of pictures.

Meige, Henry /māzh/ French physician, 1866–1940. See BRISSAUD'S INFANTILISM (also called **Brissaud-Meige syndrome**).

meiosis a stage in the production of ova and spermatozoa in which each daughter cell is haploid, or contains only one of each pair of chromosomes from the original diploid set in the parental gonads. During the process of fertilization, the ova and spermatozoa undergo a fusion that restores the double set of chromosomes within the nucleus of the zygote thus formed.

Meissner, Georg /mīs'nər/ German physiologist and anatomist, 1829–1905. See MEISSNER'S CORPUSCLES; ENCAPSULATED END ORGANS; NERVE ENDINGS; SOMATIC RECEPTORS.

Meissner's corpuscles small oval sensory nerve receptors that are sensitive to touch. They are located in the skin and mucous membranes of the mammary papilla, the lips, and the tip of the tongue.

mel a unit of pitch measurement in which a tone of 1,000 cycles per second is equivalent to 1,000 mels. (The term is an abbreviation of *mel*ody.)

-melan-; -melano- a combining form meaning black (Greek *melas*).

melancholia a pathological state of depression characterized by feelings of dejection, loss of interest and initiative, inability to feel pleasure, low self-esteem, and preoccupation with self-reproaches and regrets. See ABDOMINAL M.; CLIMACTERIC M.; IDIOTISM; PARANOID M.

melancholia agitata a 19th-century term for the excited phase of catatonic schizophrenia. It is occasionally used today for agitated depression, especially when it is associated with senile psychosis.

melancholic mood: See CONSTITUTIONAL DEPRESSIVE DISPOSITION.

melancholic personality a DSM-I term for a personality-pattern disturbance characterized by a subdued emotional tone, persistent mild depression, inability to enjoy life, self-depreciation, insecurity and fear of disapproval, and a tendency to develop a severe depressive disorder under stress.

melancholic type the morose personality type which Hippocrates attributed to an excess of black bile. See CONSTITUTIONAL TYPE.

melanocyte-stimulating hormone: See PITUITARY GLAND.

melanomas: See SKIN CANCER.

melatonin: See PINEAL GLAND.

melioristic having a tendency to make things better.

melissophobia a morbid fear of bees (from Greek *melissa*, "bee," literally "honey fly"). Also called **apiphobia**.

Melkersson, Ernst Gustav Swedish physician, 1899–1932. See MELKERSSON-ROSENTHAL SYNDROME.

Melkersson-Rosenthal syndrome a hereditary disorder often precipitated by stress, and characterized by chronic noninflammatory swelling of the lips, folds in tongue, peripheral facial palsy, and a variety of visual symptoms, including opaque corneas, swollen eyelids, and lagophthalmos. Also called **Miescher's cheilitis**.

Mellaril: See ELECTROCARDIOGRAPHIC EFFECT.

member = PENIS.

membership character a Gestalt relationship in which a change in a member influences the whole and a change in the whole influences the members; also, the character of an element derived from the totality.

membership group any social group to which an individual belongs as a genuine member. Also see REFERENCE GROUPS.

membrane growth the development of a neuron, which presumably releases a substance that enhances the building of membrane tissue from available protein and lipoid molecules under genetic control. The membrane gradually advances toward a target organ or a synaptic communication with another neuron. Each neuron has its own m.g. pattern and is not influenced by neighboring neurons growing in opposite directions to other targets.

membranous dysmenorrhea: See DYSMENORRHEA.

membrum virile = PENIS.

memorandum as a whole: See OBJECTIVE PSYCHOTHERAPY.

memory the ability to revive past experience, based on the mental processes of learning or registration, retention, recall or retrieval, and recognition; the total body of remembered experience; also, a specific past experience that is recalled. Abbrev.: **M**. See RECALL; RECOGNITION; RELEARNING METHOD; REPRODUCTION; RETENTION; PRIMARY ABILITIES; REMEMBERING; VON RESTORFF EFFECT; ASSOCIATIVE M.; AUDITORY M. SPAN; AUTOMATIC M.; CONSTRUCTIVE M.; DUAL-M. THEORY; EIDETIC IMAGE; GENETIC M.; GENETIC STORAGE; HYPERESTHETIC M.; IMMEDIATE M.; INCIDENTAL M.; LONG-TERM M.; MINUTE M.; MOTOR M.; PANORAMIC M.; PARAMNESIA.; PHOTOGRAPHIC M.; PHYSIOLOGICAL M.; PRODUCTIVE M.; PSEUDOMEMORY; RACIAL M.; REDUPLICATIVE M. DECEPTION; REMOTE M.; REPLACEMENT M.; SERIAL-M. SEARCH; SHORT-TERM M.; TWO-STEP-M. THEORY; UNCONSCIOUS M.; VERBAL M.; VISUAL M.; VISUAL SEQUENTIAL M.

memory afterimage a clear and strikingly intense memory of an experience shortly after it has occurred. E.g., after hearing the closing notes of Beethoven's Ninth Symphony, one may "hear" them again distinctly and vividly in memory. (M.a. is not equivalent to the term afterimage.)

memory aids: See MNEMONIC STRATEGY.

memory color any object's color as modified in memory. The term emphasizes the fact that the quality of remembered color often differs substantially from the actual hue. Color perception is considered a compromise between m.c. and present sensory input.

memory cramp the constant recurrence in an individual's mind of certain melodies or lines of poetry or similar usually irrelevant material.

memory curve = RETENTION CURVE.

memory defect an impairment of the ability to recall, due to the effect of an organic condition on brain functioning, as in stroke, cerebral arteriosclerosis, senile brain disease, or Korsakoff's syndrome. Some investigators also include psychogenic memory distortions among memory defects. See MEMORY DISTORTION.

memory disorders a general term for both organic and psychogenic disorders of memory, including amnesia (anterograde, retrograde, dissociative), hypermnesia, long-term and short-term memory defects, and pseudoreminiscence. A m.d. may be partial or total, mild or severe, permanent or transitory, anterograde or retrograde. The cause may be injury, a disease that is marked by faulty cerebral-blood circulation, a lesion, psychological trauma, fugue states, intrapsychic conflicts, or, in the case of Korsakoff's amnesic syndrome, a result of malnutrition. See AMNESIA; GLOBAL AMNESIA.

memory distortion inaccurate or illusory recall or recognition. See PARAMNESIA; DÉJÀ VU; DÉJÀ

VÉCU; DÉJÀ RACONTÉ; JAMAIS VU; CONFABULATION; RETROSPECTIVE FALSIFICATION.

memory drum a drum that turns at a given speed while presenting a list of items to be remembered singly or in pairs.

memory falsification a symptom of Korsakoff's psychosis in which the patient fills in memory gaps with detailed fabrications. The term is essentially equivalent to CONFABULATION. See this entry.

Memory-for-Designs Test a perceptual-motor test for brain damage in which 15 geometric figures are presented for five seconds each, then removed and drawn from memory.

memory illusion the act of describing another person's experiences as if they were one's own. The person often believes implicitly that he actually experienced the event and may be able to "recall" the details quite accurately.

memory image the mental reconstruction of an object or event with an awareness that it originated in the past.

memory impairment: See MEMORY DEFECT.

memory retention: See CONSERVATION.

memory span the number of items that can be recalled immediately after one presentation. Usually, the items consist of letters, words, numbers, or syllables that the subject must reproduce in order. The distinction may be drawn between **visual m.s.** and auditory m.s. depending on the nature of the presentation. See AUDITORY M.S.

memory storage the retention of memories in the organism. Explanations of this process are theoretical, including, e.g., the continuous operation, or "reverberation," of loops of neurons; growth of new nerve endings grouped in "synaptic knobs"; the recording of messages similar to the operation of a digital computer; and encoding of information in complex molecules such as RNA.

memory trace = ENGRAM.

memory transfer the transfer of acquired information from one individual to another by transplantation of brain cells. Experiments attempting to demonstrate that memory traces in RNA molecules might be transferred among flatworms and mice have produced conflicting results.

ménage à trois /mānäzh′ätrô·ä′/ a relationship involving three persons who are members of the same household, e.g., a married couple and the mistress of the husband sharing an apartment.

menarche /mənär′kē/ the first menstruation, usually occurring between the 11th and 17th year, marking the onset of puberty in the female.

Mencken, Henry Louis American editor and satirist, 1880–1956. See ECDYSIASM.

mendacity in psychiatry, PATHOLOGICAL LYING. See this entry.

Mendel, Gregor Johann /men′dəl/ Austrian monk, 1822–84. Adjective: **Mendelian** /-dēl′-/. See MENDELIAN MODES OF INHERITANCE; MENDELIAN RATIO; MENDELISM; COUPLING; REPULSION.

Mendel, Kurt /men′dəl/ German neurologist, 1874–1946. See BEKHTEREV-MENDEL REFLEX.

Mendelian modes of inheritance the principles of genetics as developed around 1865 by the Austrian monk Gregor Mendel. They are the **principle of independent segregation**, or **Mendel's first law**, which states that recessive traits are neither modified nor lost in future generations as both dominant and recessive genes are independently transmitted and so are able to segregate independently during the formation of sex cells. **Mendel's second law**, the **principle of independent assortment**, states that there is no tendency for genes of one parent to stay together in future offspring. As a result, the average distribution of two traits in the F_2 generation, representing grandchildren of the original mating, will show a ratio of 9:3:3:1, with nine of 16 grandchildren expressing the dominant genes of both traits, three expressing one dominant and one recessive gene for each of the traits, and one expressing only the recessive traits. Not all genes express only a dominant or recessive trait, as can be demonstrated in human skin colors in which the genes are expressed as a trait that is intermediate between the dominant and the recessive.

Mendelian ratio the ratio in which dominant and recessive heredity traits are likely to occur in the offspring of a specific type of mating. See MENDELIAN MODES OF INHERITANCE.

Mendelism the doctrine of genetic principles of heredity as established by Gregor Mendel in the 19th century. See MENDELIAN MODES OF INHERITANCE.

Mendel's first law; Mendel's second law: See MENDELIAN MODES OF INHERITANCE.

menerik a culture-specific syndrome, mainly among Eskimos of both sexes, manifested in paroxysms of wild screaming and dancing, often culminating in epileptiform seizures.

Ménière, Prosper /mānēyer′/ French physician, ca. 1801–1862. See ADULT SENSORINEURAL LESIONS (there: **Ménière's disease**); BULBOCAPNINE; TINNITUS; VERTIGO.

meningeal syphilis a form of tertiary syphilis in which the leptomeninges, the pia-arachnoid layers, are involved.

meninges the three layers of membranes that provide a protective cover for the surfaces of the brain and spinal cord. They consist of a tough outer layer, the dura mater, the arachnoid tissues that also serve as a reservoir of cerebrospinal fluid, and a thin pia-mater layer that fits over the various contours and fissures of the cerebral cortex. The m. vary somewhat in structure from the cortical areas to the end of the spinal cord.

meningioma a tumor that develops in the arachnoid-tissue layer of the meninges. Between 15 and 25 percent of tumors of the brain and spinal cord are meningiomas. The typical m. grows slowly and causes damage mainly by pressure of its growth against delicate neural tissues. Patients may complain of headaches or seizures as first symptom. The tumor is benign.

meningismus psychosis: See TYPHOID FEVER.

meningitis an inflammation of the meninges, the three-layered membrane that covers the the brain and spinal cord. Kinds of m. include meningococcal m. and tuberculous m., caused by bacteria; viral m., caused by mumps, poliomyelitis, or herpes viruses; and aseptic m., which is caused by ECHO viruses and affects mainly young children during the summer months. Complications of m. are blindness, deafness, paralysis, and mental retardation. Also see PNEUMOCOCCAL M.; TUBERCULOUS M.; BACTERIAL M.

meningitophobia a morbid fear of brain disease.

meningocele a herniation of meninges through an abnormal opening in the skull with seepage of cerebrospinal fluid into the protrusion. The disorder sometimes is associated with hydrocephalus or other neurologic defects, which reduce the chances of a favorable prognosis. If the herniation contains neural tissue, the condition is identified as an encephalocele. Also see CRANIUM BIFIDUM WITH ENCEPHALOCELE.

meningococcal meningitis: See BACTERIAL MENINGITIS.

meningoencephalitis a form of encephalitis that involves the meninges covering the brain. A common cause is swimming, diving, or water skiing in lakes that contain large populations of free-living amebae, which may be forced by water pressure through the cribiform plate of the olfactory system and into the cerebrospinal fluid. M. also is a complication of **Chagas' disease** and rubella, or German measles.

meningomyelocele a hernia of the spinal cord and meninges through a defect in the spinal column of vertebrae. The defect may, as in a case of spina bifida, be due to a failure of a pair of vertebral arches to form a perfect union at the midline. M. may be visible or concealed beneath the skin and detectable only by radiological examination. See MYELOMENINGOCELE.

meningovascular syphilis = CEREBRAL SYPHILIS.

Menkes, John H. Austrian-born American pediatric neurologist, 1928—. See KINKY-HAIR DISEASE (also called **Menkes' disease**).

menopausal depression a state of despondency occurring during the feminine climacteric, or menopause, particularly among women who have had a prior tendency to depression or feelings of inadequacy and dissatisfaction with life. See INVOLUTIONAL PSYCHOTIC REACTION; MIDLIFE CRISIS.

menopausal myopathy a form of polymyositis that occurs in some menopausal women, characterized by atrophy of proximal muscle tissue.

menopause the period during which menstruation ceases; the end of the reproductive cycle in women. See CLIMACTERIC.

menorrhagia excessive bleeding during menstruation. Also called **epimenorrhagia**.

menses = MENSTRUATION.

mens rea a Latin term literally translated as "guilty mind," and employed in legal records to contend that a person has guilty intent or the mental ability for such intent.

menstrual age the age of the fetus calculated from the beginning of the mother's last menstruation. Also see GESTATIONAL AGE.

menstrual cycle the period of time, averaging approximately 28 days in the human female, during which the endometrial lining of the uterus proliferates and sheds. The m.c. is repeated more or less continuously, except for periods of pregnancy, between puberty and menopause. Ovulation normally occurs about midway in the m.c.

menstrual disorders in psychiatry, psychophysiologic conditions associated with menstruation, including premenstrual tension, dysmenorrhea (painful menstruation), menorrhagia (profuse and persistent bleeding), and oligomenorrhea (scanty menstruation). While these conditions may have organic causes, at least in part, they may also be due to emotional factors such as hidden conflicts, feelings of guilt, or negative attitudes toward sex implanted by the patient's parents.

menstruation a cyclic discharge of blood and uterine cells that occurs in fertile females. Also called **menses; monthly period; period; catamenia**. See MENSTRUAL CYCLE.

mental aberration a pathological deviation from normal thinking. It is a general term for mental or emotional disorder of any kind; it is also applied to individual symptoms such as a delusion of persecution or hysterical paralysis.

mental abilities abilities as measured by tests of an individual in areas of spatial visualization, perceptual speed, number facility, verbal comprehension, word fluency, memory, and inductive reasoning.

mental age a numerical scale unit derived by dividing an individual's intelligence-test results by the average score for other persons of the same age. Thus, a four-year-old child who scored 150 on an I.Q. test would have a mental age of six. The m.a. measure of performance is not effective beyond the age of 14. Abbrev.: **MA**.

mental apparatus = PSYCHIC APPARATUS.

mental asthenia an apparent lack of energy or motivation for mental tasks, often expressed as **concentration difficulty**.

mental asymmetry an unbalanced relationship between opposite mental processes, often manifested by the patient as a concern about his physical symmetry, e.g., one arm larger than the other. Comparisons are also made with others in the family.

mental ataxia = INTRAPSYCHIC ATAXIA.

mental blind spot = BLIND SPOT.

mental chemistry the viewpoint that mental activity obeys the physical laws of chemistry, synthesizing elements into new compounds.

mental claudication a type of temporary interruption of blood flow to a portion of the brain that results in brief episodes of mental confusion.

mental confusion = CONFUSION.

mental defective a person who is mentally retarded or intellectually subnormal.

mental deficiency an alternative term for mental retardation, which is the term used in DSM-III.

mental development the progressive changes in mental processes due to maturation, learning, and experience.

mental discipline the idea that specific areas or subjects of study strengthen mental ability in such a way as to generalize or transfer to all other subjects and intellectual pursuits and to enhance learning in those areas; e.g., the study of mathematics, Greek, Latin, and classic literature was once thought to promote such improvement.

mental disease a general term for a serious mental problem of an organic or psychogenic nature. Mental disorder is the preferred term today since the term disease is primarily associated with organic conditions.

mental disorder a disorder defined by the American Psychiatric Association as "an illness with psychologic or behavioral manifestations and/or impairment in functioning due to a social, psychologic, genetic, physical/chemical, or biologic disturbance" (*A Psychiatric Glossary*, 1980). Also called **psychiatric disorder; mental illness; psychiatric illness**.

mental dynamism: See DYNAMISM.

mental eclipse a delusion, common in schizophrenia, that somebody is stealing the patient's ideas.

mental energy = PSYCHIC ENERGY.

mental evolution the increase in the complexity of brain structure and function that follows the phylogenetic pattern of evolution.

mental examination a comprehensive evaluation of an individual's behavior, attitudes, and intellectual abilities for the purpose of establishing or ruling out pathology.

mental faculties: See FACULTY PSYCHOLOGY.

mental fog: See CLOUDING OF CONSCIOUSNESS.

mental function a mental process or activity such as thinking, sensing, and reasoning.

mental growth the gradual increment in a mental function with increasing age, usually applied to intelligence.

mental healing an alternative term for FAITH HEALING. See this entry.

mental health a state of mind characterized by emotional well-being, relative freedom from anxiety and disabling symptoms, and a capacity to establish constructive relationships and cope with the ordinary demands and stresses of life.

mental-health clinic an out-patient facility for the diagnosis and treatment of mental disorders. It is usually operated by a mental hospital, but is sometimes free-standing and operated by a group of psychiatrists, clinical psychologists, or psychiatric social workers.

mental-health counselor: See ADVOCATE.

mental-health worker a staff member who assists core mental-health professionals in handling the social and psychological problems of patients. The m.-h.w. has special training either in supportive therapy or as an expediter-ombudsman. Also see ADVOCATE.

mental hospital a public or private institution providing a wide range of diagnostic techniques and treatment modalities to disturbed individuals on an in-patient basis. The treatment modalities include, among others, psychotherapy (group and individual), pharmacotherapy, occupational therapy, sociotherapy, and recreational therapy. Also called **psychiatric hospital**. See PRIVATE M.H.; PUBLIC M.H.; MILIEU THERAPY; THERAPEUTIC COMMUNITY.

mental hygiene a general approach aimed at maintaining mental health and preventing mental disorder through such means as educational programs, promotion of a stable emotional and family life, prophylactic and early treatment services, and public-health measures. The term itself is falling into disuse; one indication of this is that the International Committee for Mental Hygiene, which Clifford Beers helped to found, is now known as the National Association for Mental Health.

mental-hygiene clinic a center devoted to the promotion of mental health and prevention of mental illness through such means as public education, diagnosis, counseling, and treatment of conditions not requiring hospitalization. The term has been replaced in most instances by MENTAL-HEALTH CLINIC and COMMUNITY MENTAL-HEALTH CENTER. See these entries.

mental illness = MENTAL DISORDER.

mental imagery mental pictures, fantasies, hallucinations, or representations of objects, people, or events.

mental institution a treatment-oriented facility in which mentally retarded or disturbed patients are provided supervised general care and therapy by trained psychiatric professionals and an auxiliary staff. The m.i. patients generally are those who are unable to function independently as out-patients when supported by psychoactive drugs. A m.i. is required by most, but not all states, to be licensed by a government agency. The National Center for Health Statistics in one recent year listed approximately 434,000 patients in mental institutions in addition to 202,000 in residential facilities for the mentally handicapped.

mentalism the theory that mental phenomena cannot be reduced to physical or physiological phenomena. The term is also used as a synonym for animism.

mentality mind, or mental capacity. The term is used to denote intellectual powers, as in rating mental ability superior, inferior, or average.

mental levels a system of Jung for organizing mental activity in categories of consciousness, personal unconscious, and collective unconscious.

The term refers also to the psychoanalytic division into conscious, preconscious, and unconscious.

mentally defective: See DEFECTIVE CHILDREN.

mentally handicapped the condition of being unable to function independently in the community because of arrested or incomplete development of the mind or any severe and disabling mental disorder.

mentally retarded persons' rights: See RIGHTS OF THE MENTALLY RETARDED.

mental masochism = IDEAL MASOCHISM.

mental maturity the achievement of an adult level of intelligence and behavior.

mental measurement the use of quantitative scales and methods in measuring psychological processes. Also called **mental testing**. See PSYCHOMETRY.

mental mechanism = MECHANISM.

mental metabolism the rate of energy exchange between the individual and the environment as a result of mental processes. Certain individuals, e.g., manics, are said to have a higher rate of m.m. than others.

mental-patient organization a club or other organization established to provide social and recreational activities to former mental patients, to help them maintain their morale, and to readjust to community life. Many mental-patient organizations are independent, but others are affiliated with clinics, hospitals, and mental-health associations or centers.

mental process a psychological process; any activity of an organism that involves the mind.

mental retardation a disorder characterized by significantly subaverage general intellectual function, an IQ of 70 or below, with impairment in adaptive behavior (including thinking, learning, and social and occupational adjustments), and manifested during the developmental period (below age 18). Abbrev.: **MR**. See MILD M.R.; MODERATE M.R.; SEVERE M.R.; PROFOUND M.R.; UNSPECIFIED M.R. (DSM-III)

Mental Scale: See BAYLEY SCALES OF INFANT DEVELOPMENT.

mental set readiness to make a particular response or to perform a psychological function such as solving a problem in a particular way that is usually determined by instructions. See SET.

mental status in psychiatry, the psychological state of a patient as revealed by a mental examination which covers such factors as general health, appearance, mood, speech, sociability, cooperativeness, facial expression, motor activity, mental activity, emotional state, trend of thought, sensory awareness, orientation, memory, information level, general intelligence level, abstraction and interpretation ability, and judgment. See PSYCHIATRIC EXAMINATION.

Mental Status Examination Report a component part of the Multi-State Information System consisting of an optical scan form made up of structured, multiple-choice items covering the usual mental-status categories. Also included is a **Periodic Evaluation Record (PER)** which is administered at frequent intervals to provide a running narrative of the patient's progress. Abbrev.: **MSER**.

mental structure the stable organization of the mind, or the personality, composed of complex but interrelated traits.

mental tension a term used to describe the level of psychic activity in an individual as a relative state of emotional charge. E.g., the manic phase of manic-depressive psychosis represents a state of high m.t.

mental test any test that measures one or more of an individual's psychological traits. The term is sometimes used as a synonym for intelligence test.

mental testing = MENTAL MEASUREMENT.

mental topography = TOPOGRAPHICAL PSYCHOLOGY.

menticide the deliberate and systematic effort to brainwash or otherwise alter an individual's allegiances, beliefs, standards, or values in favor of a different set of attitudes and ideas.

meperidine hydrochloride: See SYNTHETIC NARCOTICS.

mephenesin: See PROPANEDIOLS.

mephenytoin: See HYDANTOINS.

mephobarbital: See BARBITURATES.

meprobamate: See PROPANEDIOLS.

meralgia paresthetica a rare neuritis of the lateral femoral cutaneous nerve, with pain, numbness, burning, tingling, and hypersensitivity of the thigh due to pressure from obesity or corsets, and relieved by a nerve block with a local anesthetic.

mercury encephalopathy a form of brain damage that can occur from exposure to mercury in various forms. Mercury generally disrupts normal motor functions but also can produce a type of dementia that is irreversible. An antidote is dimercaprol. In the Minamata incident, an entire community was contaminated by a mercury-based pesticide. Also see MINAMATA DISEASE.

mercy killing: See EUTHANASIA.

merergasia a term introduced by Adolf Meyer to identify a condition of partial personality disorganization, as in cases of psychoneurosis in which the patient also has partial ability to work or function (from Greek *meros*, "part, lot," and *ergasia*, "work").

mere-exposure effect the hypothesis that repeated exposure to the same stimulus object (e.g., name or face) increases the attraction for that stimulus object. There is considerable evidence for this hypothesis, but it has been questioned by some investigators.

merger state a state of consciousness characterized by a feeling of fusion with an idealized object, with reality as a whole, or with other people. Merger states are sometimes sought through drug use as a means of overcoming feelings of alienation and emptiness. See FUSION STATE.

merit ranking the arrangement of people, data, or

objects in order of size, value, or other characteristics. Also called **order of merit**.

merit rating an evaluation of an individual's performance at a particular task.

Merkel, Friedrich Siegmund German anatomist, 1845–1919. See MERKEL'S TACTILE DISK; SOMATIC RECEPTORS.

Merkel, Julius German psychologist, fl. 1885. See MERKEL'S LAW.

Merkel's corpuscles = MERKEL'S TACTILE DISK.

Merkel's law the principle that equal suprathreshold sense differences correlate with equal stimulus differences.

Merkel's tactile disk a sensory-nerve ending in the mucous membranes of the mouth and tongue. Also called **Merkel's corpuscles; Grandry-Merkel corpuscles**.

merogony a type of reproduction in which an enucleated egg of one species is fertilized with the sperm of another, producing an embryo with the characteristics of the species from which the sperm was obtained. M. is generally an experimental procedure used to demonstrate the dominance of the genetic contents of the nucleus in determining the traits of the embryo.

Merrill, Maud Amanda American psychologist, 1888—. See MERRILL-PALMER SCALE; INFANT AND PRESCHOOL TESTS; STANFORD-BINET INTELLIGENCE SCALE.

Merrill-Palmer Scale a series of 93 verbal and performance items designed to measure the intellectual ability of children between 24 and 63 months of age.

merycism the voluntary regurgitation of food from the stomach to the mouth, where it is masticated and tasted a second time. It is frequently found in severely retarded individuals, although some think the retarded development may be due, in part at least, to the disorder. (The term is derived from Greek *merykismos*, "chewing the cud".)

Merzbacher, Ludwig /merts′bäkhər/ German neurologist, 1875—. See PELIZAEUS-MERZBACHER DISEASE.

-mes-; -meso- a combining form meaning middle or medium.

mescal buttons: See PEYOTE.

mescaline: See PSYCHEDELICS; PHENYLETHYLAMINE DERIVATIVES; PEYOTE; PHENYL ALKYLAMINES.

mesencephalic nucleus one of the three nuclei of the trigeminal nerve. The m.n. extends through the pons into the lower part of the mesencephalon. Its fibers innervate the muscles and joints of the head.

mesencephalic tegmentum a region of the midbrain behind the substantia nigra with neural connections between the cerebrum, spinal cord, thalamus, and subthalamus, forming an indirect corticospinal tract. Lesions in the tegmentum affect the eating habits of laboratory animals, producing in some cases subjects that feed voraciously and indiscriminately.

mesencephalon a relatively small mass of neural tissue lying between the forebrain and hindbrain. It contains the inferior and superior colliculi, a portion of the reticular formation, sensory tracts, and motor tracts and reflex centers. Also called **midbrain**.

Mesmer, Franz Anton German physician, 1733–1815. After writing his doctoral thesis on the magnetic effects of the planets on the human body, M. sought to capture "celestial forces" with iron rods and magnetized water, and to focus them on ailing patients, who experienced a "grand crisis," or seizure. His showmanlike manner and extravagant claims of a "final cure" led to an official investigation in which he was declared to be a fraud—but his methods nevertheless stimulated interest in the power of suggestion. Verb: **to mesmerize**. Adjective: **mesmeric** /-mer′-/. See MESMERIC CRISIS; ANIMAL MAGNETISM; BAQUET; GRAND CRISIS. Also see PARACELSUS.

mesmeric crisis a therapeutic reaction produced by the "magnetist" Anton Mesmer. One of his techniques was the so-called "magnetic pass" in which he clasped the patient's knees between his own and repeatedly drew his hands down the patient's body until the patient lost consciousness and experienced a hysterical seizure which frequently eliminated or alleviated his symptoms. Also called **magnetic crisis**. Also see GRAND CRISIS.

Mesmerism an archaic name for HYPNOTISM. See this entry. Also see MESMERIC CRISIS.

mesmerize: See MESMER.

mesocephalic a moderate relationship between the length and width of the head.

mesoderm the middle of the three primary germ layers of the developing embryo (literally, "middle skin"). The m. cells evolve into cartilage and bone, connective tissue, muscle, blood vessels and blood cells, the lymphatic system, notochord, gonads, kidneys, and pleural membranes. Adjective: **mesodermal**. See EMBRYONIC PERIOD.

mesokurtic moderately peaked; describing a statistical distribution that is neither flatter nor more peaked than a comparison, such as the normal distribution. Also see PLATYKURTIC; LEPTOKURTIC.

mesomorph literally, middle structure, one of W. H. Sheldon's constitutional types, or somatotypes, characterized by a muscular, athletic physique he found to be highly correlated with a **somatotonic temperament** (tendencies toward energetic activity, assertiveness, physical courage, and love of power). Also called **mesomorphic body type**.

mesontomorph a constitutional body type characterized by a broad, stocky body and roughly the equivalent of a mesomorph.

mesopic luminosity the brightness of a color of a designated wavelength at an intermediate level of adaptation of both rods and cones.

mesopic vision vision that is in between photopic (daylight) and scotopic (twilight), representing a joint function of rods and cones.

mesoskelic a constitutional body type that in the Manouvrier system is intermediate between brachyskelic and macroskelic and roughly equivalent to the athletic type.

mesosomatic denoting an individual whose body build is within one standard deviation of the mean after scores for height and chest measurements have been multiplied (Eysenck).

message any symbolic or other communication between individuals or groups; the output of a transmitter that is fed into a receiver.

messenger RNA *ribo*nucleic *a*cid molecules that carry genetic-code instructions from the inherited gene to the subcellular mechanisms responsible for building protein or other molecules from chemicals present in the cell's cytoplasm.

Mestinon: See PYRIDOSTIGMINE.

-met-; -meta- a combining form meaning beyond, behind, or implying change (from Greek *meta*, "among, between, with, beyond").

metabolic anomaly = INBORN ERROR OF METABOLISM.

metabolic defect any deficiency in the structure or enzymatic function of protein molecules or in the transport of substances across cell membranes due to inborn errors or derangements caused by toxic agents or dietary excesses, e.g., alcoholism or cholesterol-rich foods. A m.d. may manifest its effects in the kidney functions as well as in the gastrointestinal system.

metabolic dysperception a term for schizophrenia suggested by Bella Kowalson (1967) to emphasize the variety of perceptual changes in schizophrenic patients as well as the probable metabolic origin for these changes.

metabolic encephalitis encephalitis that is associated with the metabolism of chemical components of foods or drugs. Certain dyes, antibiotics, and heavy metals are presumed causes of encephalitis symptoms.

metabolic-nutritional model a system of study of mental disorders in which the emphasis in on long-term assessments of influences of such factors as toxins and deprivations in populations.

metabolic screening examination procedures used in predicting or diagnosing possible inborn errors of metabolism, such as phenylketonuria. The m.s. procedures include routine ferricchloride diaper tests for newborns, examining liver and eyes for signs of galactosemia, genetic counseling of parents with known familial metabolic deficiencies, and amniocentesis.

metabolism the biochemical processes by which chemical substances in the environment are ingested as sources of energy and structural materials. The breaking down of large complex molecules in food is the catabolic phase of m. The synthesis of new molecules from the process of catabolism is anabolism. The human body can synthesize most substances required for normal functioning from basic molecules in a variety of common foods. But a few fatty acids and amino acids, as well as vitamins and minerals, cannot be synthesized by the body's chemical factories and must be present in the foods ingested. Also see BASAL M.; INBORN ERROR OF M.; CARBOHYDRATE M.; FAT M.; ANABOLISM; MENTAL M.

metachromatic leukodystrophy an autosomal-recessive disorder characterized by a loss of myelin in the central and peripheral nervous system with a concurrent accumulation of metachromatic lipids within macrophages, glial cells, and Schwann cells. Loss of motor function and mental ability tends to develop after the first year of life. Laboratory studies show a five- to 100-fold excess of sulfatides in nerve tissue.

metacommunication auxiliary or covert messages, usually in the form of subtle gestures, movements, and facial expressions.

metaerg a motivational trait that is affected by environmental rather than constitutional influences (Cattell).

metaevaluation in evaluation research, an attempt to make judgments on the merit of evaluation work; systematic evaluation of evaluation activities; focus on assessing methodological rigor, utility, cost, relevance, scope, importance, credibility, timeliness, and pervasiveness of dissemination as criteria for merit in evaluation studies.

metalanguage a language or set of symbols that is used to describe another language or set of symbols. Examples are English words used in teaching a foreign language; the English instructions that accompany a computer program; also, in a language dictionary, any passage whose part of speech is different from that of the headword, e.g., "(garment)" in "SEE-THROUGH *adj.* (garment) of transparent material." M. is sometimes developed for a specific purpose, and may be esoteric or meaningless to the outsider. Also called **second-order language**. Also see SOURCE LANGUAGE; TARGET LANGUAGE.

metallophobia a morbid fear of metals.

metamorphopsia a visual disorder in which objects appear to be distorted. It is seen in migraine and temporal-lobe epilepsy as a symptom and characterized by the illusion that the relative size of parts of objects is deformed. It is frequently observed in parietal-lobe lesions and in mescaline intoxication. The condition may also be due to displacement of the retina. M. is sometimes called **Alice in Wonderland effect**. Also see MACROPSIA; MICROPSIA.

metamorphosis: See BEHAVIORAL M.; DELIRIUM OF M.

metamorphosis sexualis paranoica a rarely used term for a relatively common delusion in paranoid patients who believe their sex has been changed.

metamotivation according to A. Maslow, motives that impel an individual to "character growth, character expression, maturation, and development"; the motivation that operates on the level of self-actualization and transcendence in the hierarchy of needs, the metaneeds. In Maslow's view, m. is distinct from the motivation operating on the lower-level needs characterized by a striving to counteract a physical or psychological deficiency. The metaneeds emerge after the lower-level needs are satisfied. Also called **Being motivation; B motivation; growth motivation**. Also see METANEEDS; NEED-HIERARCHY THEORY. Compare DEFICIENCY MOTIVATION.

metaneeds according to A. Maslow, the highest level of needs that come into play primarily after the lower-level needs have been met. M. constitute the goals of self-actualizers; they include the need for knowledge and various creative pursuits. In Maslow's view, the inability to fulfill the m. results in metapathology. Also called **Being values; B-values**. See METAPATHOLOGY. Also see NEED-HIERARCHY THEORY.

metapathology the term used by A. Maslow to describe the state of vague frustration or discontent experienced by individuals who are unable to satisfy their higher-level needs, or metaneeds, e.g., specific creative, intellectual, or esthetic needs. According to Maslow, this state appears in persons who have sufficiently fulfilled the lower-level needs. See METANEEDS.

metapelet /metäpel'ət/ a surrogate mother. The term is derived from the name of the substitute mothers who care for the children in an Israeli kibbutz.

metaphase the second stage of mitotic cell division characterized by the flow of nuclear material through the cytoplasm to a hypothetical line in the center, called the equatorial plane. There, the chromosomes form a line in pairs but begin to separate into matched sets of individual chromosomes about to be divided.

metaphoric language in psychoanalysis, the use of metaphors and allegories to express feelings and experiences that apparently occurred very early in life, particularly in the pregenital stage. Examples might be "straining at the leash," to indicate tension or pent-up energy, or a bow-and-arrow image to express a fear of "letting go." Language of this kind is considered primary-process thinking, and is found mainly in psychotics, but also in dreams and in temporary neurotic regression. See PRIMARY PROCESS.

metaphoric paralogia = BY-IDEA.

metaphoric symbolism = CRYPTOPHORIC SYMBOLISM.

metaphrenia a condition marked by libidinal withdrawal from the family or group while psychic energy is directed toward material gains.

metaphysical chondroplasia a progressive bone disorder characterized by a gradual bowing of the long bones, particularly in the legs. The condition leads to a misalignment of the limbs that makes walking difficult. The disorder can be corrected by surgery in most cases. Abbrev.: **MCD**.

metapsychological profile a systematic classification of signs and symptoms of patients developed by Anna Freud. The m.p. relates to the patient's unconscious and is used therapeutically to help protect the psychotic from threats by his inner mental life.

metapsychiatry an area of psychiatry that deals with phenomena and issues beyond the scope of standard psychiatric practice, e.g., altered states of consciousness, parapsychology, or mystical experiences.

metapsychology a speculative, theoretical approach to philosophical problems relating to human behavior (literally, "beyond psychology"), e.g., the relation between mind and body and the place of mind in the universe. Such issues lie "beyond" the facts and principles of scientific psychology. Freud, on the other hand, applied the term to a comprehensive system that involves six different approaches to mental processes: the dynamic (instincts, drives), structural (id, ego, superego), topographic (conscious, preconscious, unconscious), economic (distribution of mental energy), genetic (origin and development of mental processes and symptoms), and adaptive (adjustment to the environment).

metastasis /mətas'-/ the spread of a disease from one part of the body to another through blood vessels or lymph ducts. The term usually is applied to the movement of cancer cells from one organ or site to another but also may be used to describe the transfer of pathogenic organisms, e.g., tuberculosis, from the original disease site to another. The original area of disease usually is identified as primary and the tissues involved by m. as secondary, e.g., primary cancer and secondary cancer. Verb: **to metastasize**.

metatabi an agent produced by an Oriental vine, Actinidia polygama, that has a euphoric and sedating effect. The leaves and twigs of the plant are used to make a substance called **cat powder** that is employed as a veterinary tranquilizer. Actinidia polygama and a related species, Actinidia collosa, are cultivated in Japan and parts of China for their green berries. Also called **matababi**.

metathalamus a term sometimes applied to the medial and lateral geniculate bodies, the thalamic nuclei bodies associated with the senses of hearing and vision respectively. The m. is located immediately below the posterior extremity of the thalamus.

metempirical pertaining to phenomena that lie beyond empirical investigation and are considered speculatively.

metempsychosis the belief in transmigration of a soul to another human or animal body following death, often carrying its memories with it—as, e.g., in Hindu religions.

metencephalon the portion of the brain that includes the pons and cerebellum. With the medulla oblongata, the m. forms the hindbrain. Also called **epencephalon**.

met-enkephalin: See ENKEPHALIN.

meteorophobia a morbid fear of meteors.

meth = METHEDRINE.

methacholine infusion test a diagnostic procedure for detecting evidence of familial dysautonomia in newborns. The corneas of dysautonomia patients generally are insensitive to **methacho-**

line, a powerful form of acetylcholine used in the treatment of glaucoma. Thus, methacholine-chloride infusion of the eye of a dysautonomia patient fails to produce a reaction, including lacrimation, observed when the drug is applied to the cornea of a normal individual.

methadone /meth′-/ $C_{21}H_{27}NO$—a narcotic drug used, in the form of its hydrochloride, for relieving pain and treating heroin addiction (from *meth-* + *a*mino + *d*iphenyl + *-one*). Also see SYNTHETIC NARCOTICS.

methadone center a drug-rehabilitation facility that may be a part of a hospital, clinic, or storefront community-health office where previously addicted heroin patients can obtain a daily oral dose of methadone to blunt a craving for opiate drugs. A m.c. also may provide medical treatment for addiction complications, psychotherapy, legal aid, family counseling, and welfare assistance, depending upon local funding and laws.

methadone hydrochloride: See SYNTHETIC NARCOTICS.

methadone maintenance: See MAINTENANCE DRUGS.

methamphetamine: See AMPHETAMINES.

methapyrilene: See ANTIHISTAMINES.

methaqualone $C_{16}H_{14}N_2O$—a synthetic drug that has sedative and hypnotic effects although it is not related chemically to other drugs producing such effects. The potency of m. is approximately that of pentobarbital, and it is employed in therapies of patients who are unable to tolerate barbiturate drugs. M. depresses the sensory cortex in small doses, and in larger doses affects the spinal reflexes. It causes more deaths from overdose than drugs such as phencyclidine ("angel dust") or heroin. M. was discovered about 1950 in a search for antimalarial drugs. (The term is a contraction of *meth-* + *-a-* + *qu*inazolone.) A common abbreviation for m. tablets is **ludes**, from the trademark **Quaalude**; and **luding out** is a street term for m. abuse.

Methedrine a trademark for methamphetamine chloride. (The term is a contraction of *meth*amphetamine and eph*edrine*.) Street terms are **meth** and SPEED. See this entry. Also see AMPHETAMINES.

methocarbamol a member of a group of chemicals used to produce relaxation of skeletal muscles. M. acts through the central nervous system to relieve tremors of alcoholism and parkinsonism. It also may be administered in the treatment of convulsions marked by acute muscle spasms, and to control electroshock seizures.

method of approximations = METHOD OF SUCCESSIVE APPROXIMATIONS.

method of constant stimuli a psychophysical procedure for determining the sensory threshold by repeatedly presenting several constant stimuli known to be close to the threshold. Also see METHOD OF LIMITS; MAGNITUDE ESTIMATION.

method of limits a psychophysical procedure for determining the sensory threshold by gradually increasing or decreasing the magnitude of the stimulus presented. Also see METHOD OF CONSTANT STIMULI; MAGNITUDE ESTIMATION.

method of loci /lō′sī/ or /lō′kē/ a mnemonic strategy (memory aid) in which the items to be remembered are converted into mental images and associated with specific positions or locations. E.g., to remember the name of each person sitting around a table, one might envision the table as a clock and associate the face of each person with an hour position. Also see MNEMONIC STRATEGY.

method of successive approximations the technique of reinforcing each operant response that approximates a response desired by the experimenter. At first, all responses that roughly approximate the desired behavior are reinforced. Later, only responses that more closely approximate the desired behavior are reinforced. The rewarding of these successive responses gradually leads to the desired behavior. The process as a whole is often referred to as shaping. Also called **approximation method; method of approximations; successive-approximations method**. Also see SHAPING.

methodology the analysis and systematic application of procedures used in scientific investigation or in a particular research project.

methods analysis the development of improved ways of performing a job, through analysis of the particular operation, process charts, micro-motion studies, and application of the principles of MOTION ECONOMY. See this entry.

methoxamine one of more than 25 chemically related sympathomimetic amine drugs with physiological effects similar to epinephrine and norepinephrine. The hydrochloride salt of m. may be used in the control of tachycardia, or pathologically rapid heart rhythm, as a blood-vessel constrictor in cases of hypotension, and as a nasal decongestant.

methsuximide: See SUCCINIMIDES.

methyergol carbamide maleate: See SEROTONIN INHIBITORS.

methyldimethoxyamphetamine: See PSYCHEDELICS; PHENYLETHYLAMINE DERIVATIVES; AMPHETAMINES.

methyl dopa an adrenergic blocking agent used in the treatment of hypertension. M.d. acts as an enzyme inhibitor, preventing the natural synthesis of catecholamines that would in turn elevate blood pressure. Side effects of m.d. use may include sedation, psychic depression, and stimulation of lactation.

methylene blue stain a synthetic organic compound that can be used to stain nerve fibers in the skin and cornea of living animals, for experimental and pathological studies. Other tissue stains cannot be used on living organisms because of their toxic effects.

methylenedioxy-5-methoxyphenylisopropyla-mine: See PSYCHEDELICS.

methylphenidate: See ANALEPTICS.

methylxanthines a group of plant alkaloids that

have in common similar molecular structures and pharmacologic activities, including CNS stimulation, although the actions vary in intensity. The prototype of the group is CAFFEINE (see this entry). Other m. include THEOBROMINE (see this entry) and **theophylline**—$C_7H_8N_4O_2$, a stimulant present in tea. The three m. vary in structure as to the number and position of methyl groups, which can be manipulated so that, e.g., caffeine for medications can be manufactured from theobromine by adding a CH_2 radical. Also see CAFFEINE EFFECTS; ASPIRIN COMBINATIONS.

methyprylon: See PIPERIDINEDIONES.

methysergide $C_{21}H_{27}N_3O_2$—a serotonin antagonist used in the treatment of migraine headaches. It reduces the frequency and intensity of migraine attacks in most patients although the mode of action is uncertain. M. is closely related to lysergic acid diethylamide (LSD) and has similar effects at some tissue sites. Neurologic side effects of m. include light-headedness, euphoria, insomnia, unsteadiness, and nervousness. Also see SEROTONIN INHIBITORS.

metonymic distortion a cognitive disturbance found in schizophrenics, in which the patient uses related but inappropriate verbal expressions in place of the proper expression; e.g., he may say that he had three menus instead of three meals a day. See METONYMY.

metonymy /mǝton'-/ a figure of speech in which not the literal word but one associated with it is used, as "the sword" for "war." In speech pathology, m. is a disturbance, most commonly seen in schizophrenia, in which imprecise or inappropriate words and expressions are used.

metopon: See OPIUM ALKALOIDS.

Metrazol = PENTYLENETETRAZOL.

Metrazol shock treatment a form of shock therapy introduced by the Hungarian psychiatrist Ladislas von Meduna in 1934, based on his observation that the psychotic symptoms of schizophrenic patients who were also epileptics tended to disappear following a seizure. The intravenous injections of Metrazol, however, produced intense feelings of dread, and the incidence of fatality was high. The technique is rarely used today. Also called **Metrazol therapy; Metrazol treatment.**

metric methods psychological methods that involve numbers or quantities, or quantitative methods in general, especially those using the metric system.

metric ophthalmoscopy: See OPHTHALMOSCOPY.

metromania a compulsion to write continuously in verse form.

metronoscope a device that exposes printed material at a given rate for use in measuring and increasing reading speed.

Metropolitan Achievement Tests five batteries of tests for grades 1 to 2, 3 to 4, 5 to 6, and 7 to 9, consisting of items that measure vocabulary, reading, arithmetic skills, and language usage at the elementary levels, and social studies, science, and study skills at the higher levels.

Meyer, Adolf Swiss-born American psychiatrist, 1866–1950. Practicing at Johns Hopkins for most of his professional life, M. earned the title of Dean of American Psychiatry by contributing to every phase of the field: to individual therapy by focusing on the reeducation of faulty patterns of adjustment and the environmental forces that helped produce the disorder; to hospital treatment, by enlisting the family of the patient in the treatment and recovery program; and to public education, by encouraging Clifford Beers to crusade for reform, and by collaborating with him in forming the International Committee for Mental Hygiene. In view of this many-sided approach, he is considered the originator of holism and the theory of psychobiology. See ANALYST; ANAMNESIS; ANERGASIA; CHILD PSYCHIATRY; CONSTITUTIONAL PSYCHOPATHIC INFERIOR; DISTRIBUTIVE ANALYSIS AND SYNTHESIS; DYSERGASIA; ERGASIA; ERGASIATRY; ERGASIOLOGY; EUERGASIA; FABULATION; HOLERGASIA; HOLISM; HYPERERGASIA; HYPOERGASIA; MERERGASIA; OBSESSIVE-RUMINATIVE TENSION STATE; OLIGERGASIA; ORTHERGASIA; PARERGASIA; PATHERGASIA; PLURALISM; PSYCHOBIOLOGICAL FACTORS; PSYCHOBIOLOGY; SCHIZOID-MANIC STATE; SYNTROPY; THYMERGASIA.

MF = MULTIFACTORIAL MODEL.

MHPG = 3-METHOXY-4-HYDROXYPHENYLETHYLENE GLYCOL.

miasma theory /mī·az'mǝ/ a theory of disease prevalent in the 18th and early 19th century, which explained typhoid fever, tuberculosis, cholera, malaria ("bad air") and other diseases in terms of putrescent organic matter, especially sewage, that produced noxious odors, or miasmas. The public-health movement began with the attempt to prevent these by attacking pollution.

Mickey Finn = KNOCKOUT DROPS.

-micr-; -micro- a combining form meaning small or enlarging what is small.

microangiopathy any disease or disorder involving small blood vessels, such as capillaries and arterioles. E.g., a thrombus in a capillary may be identified as thrombotic m. The condition is frequently associated with diabetic retinopathy and secondary glaucoma caused by degeneration of the capillaries and hemorrhages in the retina.

microbiophobia = MICROPHOBIA.

microcephalia vera = PURE MICROCEPHALY.

microcephaly a head that is small in relation to the rest of the individual's body. There are numerous causes and manifestations, such as **familial m.** which is an autosomal-recessive trait marked by a small head with sloping forehead and with ears and nose that are relatively large. Mental retardation ranging from moderate to profound often accompanies the condition of m. Also see PRIMARY M.; PURE M.

microcosm a term sometimes used to represent the inner world of the individual, as opposed to the **macrocosm,** or environment.

microelectrode an electrode with a tip that may be

less than one micron in diameter. Some microelectrodes are slightly larger but with tips no larger than a few microns in diameter. They are used to record electrical activity or stimulate activity within a single cell, such as a neuron.

microelectrode technique the use of microelectrodes in the study and diagnosis of nervous-system disorders. Intracellular microelectrodes with tips less than one micron in diameter are able to record activity within a single nerve cell; several working together can be used to study behavior patterns. M.t. in therapy may be used to locate specific foci of brain damage associated with parkinsonism, epilepsy, or other disorders.

microgeny the series of small steps that lead up to a patient's symptoms, or to an individual's specific behavior or mental processes. The term is used in the psychodynamic approach.

microglossia an abnormally small-sized tongue, resulting in a disturbance in the speech production of lingual sounds.

micrognathia a form of facial disfigurement characterized by an abnormally small jaw, or jaws. M. usually involves the lower jaw, a condition that can be corrected by surgical implantation of an artificial chin.

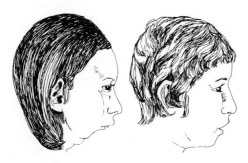

MICROGNATHIA. Before and after corrective surgery.

micromania a psychiatric state in which the patient believes his body has diminished to the size of a dwarf or small child. The condition occurs most frequently in organic depressions and may include a small-penis complex.

micromastia abnormally small female breasts.

micromelia a developmental defect marked by abnormal shortness or smallness of the limbs, a condition sometimes associated with retarded mental development.

micron /mīk'-/ one thousandth of a millimeter (1/1,000 mm).

microorchidism an abnormal smallness of a testicle or the testicles, as in Klinefelter's syndrome. Also called **microrchidia**.

microphobia a morbid fear of anything small. Also called **microbiophobia**.

microphonia a very weak or barely audible voice.

microphthalmos-corneal   opacity-spasticity syndrome a presumably hereditary disorder of children born with microcephaly, small eyes with opaque corneas, spastic diplegia, and mental retardation. Scissoring, or crossing, of the legs is a common sign in such patients.

micropsia a visual disorder in which objects appear to be much smaller than they actually are. The condition may be due to retinal defect or disease, but is more often a conversion symptom or hallucination, and possibly an unconscious attempt to shrink the world to less threatening size. See LILLIPUTIAN HALLUCINATION. Compare MACROPSIA.

micropsychophysiology the study of psychological processes, such as the formation of a delusion or obsession, in minute detail, paralleling the microscopic investigations conducted by physiologists.

micropsychosis: See PSEUDONEUROTIC SCHIZOPHRENIA.

microptic hallucination = LILLIPUTIAN HALLUCINATION.

microscopic level a psychological approach that focuses on the smallest recognizable units of analysis, e.g., cellular components and reactions. The term is usually associated with physiological psychology.

microsleeps brief intervals of dozing or sleeping that occur during periods when a subject presumably is awake. M. may be an effect of sleep deprivation, which also may result in a shift of some desynchronized sleep signs, as normally observed on EEG tracings, to appear during slow-wave sleep, when they usually are absent.

microsocial engineering a descriptive term applied to behavioral contracting, or contract therapy, in which a technique of conflict resolution among family members is established through a specific schedule of responsibilities, privileges, sanctions for violations, and bonuses for compliance. See CONTRACT.

microsomatic animals animals that are abnormally small, as calculated in terms of general body size. Sizes one or more standard deviation smaller are classified as microsomatic. Compare MACROSOMATIC ANIMALS.

microsomatognosia: See SOMATOGNOSIA.

microsplanchnic type a constitutional type characterized by a small abdomen and an elongated body, according to the Viola classification.

micturition reflexes a series of nerve signals that are organized along the spinal cord by the autonomic nervous system as the need arises to empty the urinary bladder. The response begins with pressure-sensitive receptors in the wall of the urinary bladder which stimulate motoneurons that contract the bladder muscles, thereby increasing the pressure further. At the same time, other neurons in the complex relax the sphincter and assist in adjusting the body posture for urination. Through training, cerebral control of the reflexes is developed, as in toilet-training a child or house-breaking a dog. Humans who lose cerebral control through spinal-cord injuries sometimes are able to learn techniques for emptying the bladder by stimulating the m.r. as a response to autonomic skin receptors in the pelvic region.

Midas punishment a term applied to some forms of compulsive masturbation when the behavior is interpreted as a type of self-punishment, similar to the punishment of king Midas in Greek mythology who was ruined through the fulfillment of his wishes.

midbrain = MESENCEPHALON.

midchildhood: See DEVELOPMENTAL LEVELS.

middle cerebral artery the largest branch of the internal carotid artery, running first through the Sylvian fissure, then upward on the surface of the insula where it divides into several branches that spread over the lateral surface of the cerebral hemispheres, including the anterior choroidal branch.

middle class a general social class, which, according to H. Waitzken (1978) consists of an upper-m.c. of professionals (14 percent of the population) and of middle-level executives (six percent), and a lower-middle class of shopkeepers, artisans, and craftsmen (seven percent) and of clerical and sales workers (23 percent). Also see INDIGENOUS WORKER; CULTURE-FAIR TESTS; SIX-HOUR RETARDED CHILD; IQ.

middle commissure: See COMMISSURE.

middle ear a membrane-lined cavity in the bone of the skull, adjacent to the mastoid cells. It is filled with air and communicates with the nasopharynx through the Eustachian tube. The space is occupied by the ossicles—malleus, incus, and stapes—which transmit sound vibrations from the tympanic membrane to the oval window of the inner ear. Also called **tympanic cavity.** See EAR.

middle fossa: See FOSSA.

middle insomnia a period of sleeplessness occurring after falling asleep normally, with difficulty in falling asleep again.

midget: See DWARF.

midinterval = MEDIAN INTERVAL.

midlife crisis a psychological crisis occurring during the middle years, roughly from 45 to 60. Frequently mentioned trauma-producing events for women are the menopause and the departure of the children from the home; and for men, health problems, sexual concerns, and the threat of younger workers on the job. These events, however, do not inevitably assume crisis proportions, depending, in women, on attitudes toward menopausal discomforts and the "empty nest," and the development of satisfying activities to replace dependence on the children. Similarly, the effects on men have often been exaggerated by writers in the field; they "may produce new stresses for the individual, but they also bring occasions to demonstrate an enriched sense of self and new capacities for coping with complexity" (B. L. Neugarten and Nancy

Datum, in *American Handbook of Psychiatry*, 1974). See MENOPAUSAL DEPRESSION.

midparent a term pertaining to an average measure of both parents with regard to height, intelligence, or other characteristics.

midpoint the point or value halfway between the highest and lowest values in a frequency distribution or class interval.

midpontine wakefulness an effect of a lesion in the brainstem at the level of the middle of the pons marked by loss of signals associated with drowsiness or sleep. Animals subjected to midpontine sectioning remain permanently awake.

midrange value a rough measure of central tendency gained by averaging the highest and lowest scores in a frequency distribution.

midscore the median.

Midtown Manhattan Study an interview study of the Yorkville area of New York City entitled "Mental Health in the Metropolis," conducted by L. Srole and colleagues in 1962. The Study resulted in revealing psychiatric findings, e.g., that nine percent of the upper class, 18 percent of the middle class, and 28 percent of the lower class were afflicted with severe mental and emotional disturbances; that even though nearly three percent were actually incapacitated by mental illness, less than half of them had any psychiatric contact; and that of the total group impaired by mental illness, less than one-third had any psychiatric contact. These findings indicate that those who come to the attention of psychiatric facilities do not constitute the majority of those who need help, and may be a nonrepresentative sample of the mentally ill.

Miescher, Guido /mē′shər/ Swiss dermatologist. See MELKERSSON-ROSENTHAL SYNDROME (also called **Miescher's cheilitis**).

Mignon delusion a variation of the family-romance fantasy in which the child believes his parents actually are foster parents and his real family is one of distinguished lineage. The M.d. sometimes is an unconscious defense against aggressive sexual factors of the oedipal period, and is observed most frequently in the schizophrenias. (The term is derived from the child character in Goethe's novel *Wilhelm Meister's Apprenticeship*, 1796.)

migraine a headache that usually is severe, recurrent, often limited to one side of the head, and likely to be accompanied by nausea, vomiting, and diarrhea or constipation. A m. headache also may be associated with an aura of flickering or flashing light, blacking out of part of the visual field, or illusions of colors or patterns. A commonly observed sawtooth pattern may be so vivid that the patient can trace the outline on a piece of paper. In most cases there is evidence of hereditary predisposition, but the precipitating cause is usually psychological stress or fatigue. Remedies include drugs that constrict the cerebral arteries. Also called **sick headache.** Also see BÄRTSCHI-ROCHAIX'S SYNDROME; CLUSTER HEADACHES.

migraine-neuralgia analgesics drugs that relieve the pain and related symptoms of migraine headaches. The m.-n.a. include ergot-derived vasoconstrictors, antihistamines, and serotonin antagonists. Diphenylhydantoin, which has been found effective in the treatment of some types of headaches, also may be employed. See ASPIRIN COMBINATIONS; ERGOT DERIVATIVES; SEROTONIN INHIBITORS; HYDANTOINS; ANTIHISTAMINES; CYPROHEPTADINE; ADRENERGIC BLOCKING AGENTS.

migraine personality a personality pattern found in many migraine victims, who tend to be perfectionistic, overambitious, highly competitive, and overcritical. When disappointed or frustrated, they "hold everything in," and may nurse resentments for long periods, thus keeping themselves under constant emotional tension.

migration adaptation adjustment to a new community or area; an ability to withstand the stresses involved in geographic mobility: the strain involved in making the decision, in separation from familiar surroundings, in the process of moving, and in contact with unfamiliar surroundings and customs. Though stressful, such factors have not been proved to be a common source of mental illness. Also see UPROOTING NEUROSIS.

migration behavior a form of instinctive behavior marked by travel over hundreds or thousands of miles to or from breeding areas. The behavior is observed in birds, fish, and newts. The m.b. of some species is seasonal; in others, particularly the salmon, it is observed only once in the lifetime of an individual. Factors influencing m.b. include sensitivity to chemical cues, pituitary or other hormones, daylight, and temperature.

mild depression the lowest degree of depression, characterized by dejection, loss of interest and enthusiasm, inertia, and vague aches and pains without organic basis. Patients with m.d. sit by themselves, ruminate about their failures or unworthiness, find it next to impossible to talk, work, or think, but are not disoriented and do not show any impairment of memory. Also called **simple depression**.

mild mental retardation a diagnostic category applying to persons with IQs of 50 to 70, comprising 80 percent of the retarded population. Classified as "educable," these individuals usually develop good communication skills, reach the sixth grade in their late teens, and do not go beyond the social level of adolescents, but are usually capable of learning simple vocational skills adequate for minimum self-support. (DSM-III)

Miles, Catherine Cox American psychologist, 1890—. See MASCULINITY-FEMININITY TESTS (there: **Terman-Miles Attitude-Interest Analysis Test**).

milestones: See MOTOR M.

Milgram, Stanley American psychologist, 1933—. See DESTRUCTIVE OBEDIENCE; INFORMATION OVERLOAD; OBEDIENCE; STIMULUS OVERLOAD.

milieu the environment in general; in psychiatry and psychology, the particular climate of the home and character of the neighborhood as they affect the personality and adjustment of the individual.

milieu therapy psychiatric treatment based on modification or manipulation of the patient's life circumstances or immediate environment; also, the concept of a hospital as a therapeutic community. This form of therapy is an attempt to organize the social and physical setting in which the patient lives or is being treated in such a way as to promote recovery. The term is essentially equivalent to environmental therapy. Also see THERAPEUTIC COMMUNITY.

military psychiatry the treatment of psychiatric illness at induction points, training centers, and in combat situations. **Military psychiatrists** are responsible for psychiatric treatment units within military medical facilities, crisis intervention, and development of emergency-treatment techniques to be used on the battlefield or immediately behind the lines.

military psychology the branch of applied psychology concerned with evaluation, selection, assignment, and training of military personnel, as well as the design of equipment and application of clinical and counseling techniques to the maintenance of morale and mental health.

Mill, James Stuart English philosopher (father of John Stuart Mill), 1773–1836. See ASSOCIATIONISM.

Mill, John Stuart English philosopher and economist (son of James Stuart Mill), 1806–73. See ASSOCIATIONISM.

Millard, Auguste /milär'/ French internist, 1830–1915. See MILLARD-GUBLER SYNDROME.

Millard-Gubler syndrome a type of crossed paralysis involving the limbs on one side of the body and the face on the opposite side, including paralysis of the external rectus muscle of the eyeball on the affected facial side. It is caused by a lesion of the pons involving the sixth and seventh cranial nerves and the corticospinal tract. Also called **Gubler's hemiplegia**.

Miller, Wilford Stanton American psychologist, 1883—. See MILLER ANALOGIES TEST.

Miller Analogies Test a test designed to predict scholastic ability on the graduate-school level, consisting of 100 verbal analogies drawn from a variety of fields.

Milligan annihilation method a type of electroshock therapy in which three treatments are administered the first day, followed by two treatments daily until the desired level of regression is achieved.

millilambert 1/1,000 of a lambert; the amount of light reflected from a perfectly diffusing and reflecting surface area of one square foot and illuminated by a light equivalent to 0.93 footcandle.

millimicron a unit of length commonly used to measure wavelengths of light, being one billionth (1/1,000,000,000) of a meter. The wavelength of yellow light is approximately 560 millimicrons, or 5,600 Ångstrom units. Also called **nanometer (nm)**.

milling crowd: See CROWD BEHAVIOR.

Miltown: See PROPANEDIOLS.

mimesis imitation; also, a process of instinctively copying the behavior of another member of the species in the absence of teaching or previous learning.

mimetic pertaining to imitation, e.g., a young chimpanzee's imitation of its mother's actions. The term is often applied to species-specific behavior, that is, behavior that appears spontaneously and in identical or nearly the same form in all members of a species. A **m. response** is a copying or imitative response.

mimic spasm = HABIT SPASM.

min. an abbreviation used in prescriptions, meaning "minim" (Latin *minimum*).

Minamata disease a term for mercury poisoning derived from an epidemic in Minamata, Japan, in which seafood contaminated with mercury was consumed locally, resulting in severe CNS disorders, with brain damage, birth defects, and death. Hydrocarbon compounds of mercury cross the placental barrier, causing mental retardation and cerebral palsy in the offspring. Also see MERCURY ENCEPHALOPATHY.

mind the organized totality of mental and psychic processes of an organism, and the structural and functional components on which they depend; also, psyche, intellect, and characteristic modes of thinking of a group, such as "the primitive m."

mind-altering drugs substances such as mescaline or LSD that produce altered states of consciousness through pharmacological activity. The state of mind may become hallucinogenic, euphoric, excited, depressed, anxious, or a combination of such responses. Also see MOOD-ALTERING DRUGS; PSYCHEDELICS.

mind-body problem: See BODY-MIND PROBLEM.

mind control the control of physical activities of the body, particularly autonomic functions, by mental processes. See AUTOGENIC TRAINING; BIOFEEDBACK; MEDITATION; YOGA.

mind-reading a form of purported paranormal perception in which it is alleged an individual has access to the thoughts in the mind of another person by extrasensory means.

mind stuff a term introduced by W. K. Clifford to denote the elemental material which constitutes reality, consisting internally of the constituent substance of mind, and appearing externally in the form of matter.

mineral regulation a relationship between mineral metabolism and behavior. Loss of parathyroid glands in animals, e.g., disrupts calcium-phosphate balance and results in convulsions. Animals may show food preferences for items rich in calcium, sodium, or potassium when such minerals are lacking in their diets.

miniature end-plate potentials very small variations in postsynaptic end-plate potential due to random release of tiny amounts of acetylcholine at axonal end-plates.

miniature mind the mind possessed by a psychoinfantile person; a mentality that is equally retarded in all aspects. See PSYCHOINFANTILISM.

miniature system the organized knowledge, including facts and assumptions, relating to a restricted area of psychological study, e.g., theories of perception.

minimal audible field an auditory threshold test in which the subject faces the sound source while the intensity is measured at the midpoint of his head. Abbrev.: **MAF**.

minimal audible pressure an auditory-threshold measuring technique in which the pressure on the subject's eardrum is measured.

minimal brain damage the presumption of a mild degree of organicity based upon equivocal "soft signs" which vary from individual to individual, including overactivity, restlessness, learning problems, short attention span, perceptual deficit, and poor coordination. The term is usually avoided today because in most cases the condition cannot be attributed to known organic factors such as rubella, anoxia, or birth injury.

minimal brain dysfunction a relatively mild impairment of brain function which subtly affects perception, behavior, and academic ability. The term has been applied by Health Education and Welfare Task Force to "children of near average, average, or above average general intelligence with certain learning or behavioral disabilities, ranging from mild to severe, which are associated with deviations in function of the central nervous system. These deviations may manifest themselves by various combinations of impairment in perception, conceptualization, language, memory, and control of attention, impulse, or motor function." The effects of the condition are extremely varied, including such symptoms as faulty body image, clumsiness, confusing foreground with background, hyperactivity, emotional lability, untidiness, short attention span, and speech disorders. Abbrev.: **MBD**.

minimal-change method an experimental technique in which a variable stimulus is presented in very small ascending and descending steps.

minimal cue the smallest measurable stimulus that will evoke response. The subject usually is not aware of the stimulus; emotional responses can often be detected by slight changes in expression or posture. Also see REDUCED CUE; CUE REDUCTION.

minimization a cognitive style consisting of a habitual tendency to play down the significance of bodily changes or illnesses.

minimum-change therapy a descriptive term sometimes applied to personal counseling when emphasizing that the aim is limited change or adjustment, in contrast to those approaches in psychiatry and clinical psychology that stress reconstruction, that is, basic alteration of underlying personality patterns. M.-c.t. provides reassurance and support, focusing on helping the individual make the most of available resources. It is not usually associated with exploration of unconscious, deep-seated conflict.

minimum separable method: See VISUAL ACUITY.

Minnesota Clerical Aptitude Test a test designed to measure perception of detail, accuracy, and speed by requiring the subject to compare pairs of names and numbers, and determine which are identical and which nonidentical.

Minnesota Mechanical Assembly Test an individual mechanical-aptitude test in which the subject is given a time limit of 30 minutes within which to put together ten common objects such as a bicycle bell and a mousetrap.

Minnesota Multiphasic Personality Inventory a widely used self-report test designed by Hathaway and McKinley (1942) to measure nine significant phases of personality: hypochondria, depression, hysteria, psychopathic deviate, masculine-feminine interest, paranoia, psychasthenia, schizophrenia, and hypomania. The subject indicates agreement or disagreement with 550 statements (e.g., "I wish I could be as happy as others seem to be," or "It takes a lot of argument to convince some people of the truth"), and the results are scored by the examiner or by computer to determine the subject's personality profile as well as any tendency to lie or to fake good or bad. Abbrev.: **MMPI.**

Minnesota Paper Formboard Test a mechanical-aptitude test requiring the subject to select printed parts of geometric figures which, when correctly assembled, will make one of five figures shown.

Minnesota Rate of Manipulation Test a test of manual dexterity and aptitude in which multicolored disks are fitted into a pegboard in a prescribed order, first with one hand and then with the other after turning them over.

Minnesota Spatial Relations Test a mechanical-aptitude test measuring speed and accuracy in fitting 58 cutouts of different shapes and sizes into the proper spaces on four boards.

Minnesota Vocational Interest Inventory: See INTEREST TESTS.

minor: See EMANCIPATED M.

minor analysis a type of psychoanalysis that is of short duration and limited to the important aspects of a patient's problem, as opposed to a deeper, more exhaustive orthodox analysis.

minor asynergia of Babinski: See ASYNERGIA.

minor epilepsy = PETIT MAL.

minor hemisphere the cerebral hemisphere that is nondominant for an individual or a particular function. The m.h. usually has a complementary or supporting role, which can be demonstrated in many visual tests that involve embedded figures, depth perception, or other visual-spatial functions.

minority group a population subgroup with unique social, religious, or other interests that differ from those of the majority of the population.

minority-group psychiatry the study and treatment of mental disturbances in minority groups, and the relation between these disturbances and such factors as economic deprivation, oppression, racial discrimination, family disorganization, alienation from the rest of society, and inner-city conditions. Also, the term is used for the study of the incidence and types of specific disorders such as schizophrenia, drug abuse, and mental retardation among different minority groups.

minor tranquilizers drugs of the anxiolytic category that resemble barbiturates in their mild sedative action and are prescribed mainly for patients experiencing anxiety and tension. M.t. also may be employed in the treatment of petit mal epilepsy, but they are not recommended for use in the therapy of psychoses. The term is essentially equivalent to ANXIOLYTICS. See this entry.

minute memory a term sometimes used for short-term memory, or immediate recall.

-mio- a combining form relating to (a) a reduction or a diminution, (b) a rudimentary state.

miosis = MYOSIS.

mirror drawing a motor-skill test in which a subject traces an image while looking into a mirror that shows only the image and the pencil. The object is to test ability to alter a manual-habit pattern.

mirror fear = EISOPTROPHOBIA.

mirror focus a secondary focus or tissue-malfunction site that is observed in patients with epilepsy and in animals with certain types of cortical lesions. The secondary focus is symmetrically located in the opposite hemisphere due to impulses traveling through the corpus callosum.

mirror-imaging a type of reversed asymmetry of characteristics often found in sets of twins, particularly monozygotic twins. Examples include handedness, fingerprints, hair whorls, and certain inherited pathological traits.

mirroring = MIRROR TECHNIQUE.

mirror reading reading in a pattern that is the reverse of the pattern generally followed. See PALINLEXIA.

mirror sign a symptom of autistic withdrawal observed in schizophrenic patients who tend to stand in front of a mirror or other reflecting surface for a long period. Advanced Alzheimer's patients may not only look at their image but talk to it, not realizing it is their own.

mirror technique a psychodrama technique in which an auxiliary imitates the individual's behavior patterns if he is unable to participate in the action. The object is to show him how other people perceive and react to him. Also called **mirroring.**

mirror transference a term used by H. Kohut in the treatment of narcissistic-personality disorders: The patient's grandiose self is reactivated in the transference as a replica of the early phase in his life when his mother established his sense of perfection by her admiration of his exhibitionistic behavior. This reactivation process helps to restore the patient's self-esteem.

mirror writing the mirrorlike inversion of letters and words often noted in children with severe reading disability. Also called **palingraphia**. M.w. is related to strephosymbolia, a perception reversal of left and right. See STREPHOSYMBOLIA.

miryachit a culture-specific syndrome marked by indiscriminate, apparently uncontrolled, imitation of the actions of other people encountered by the patient. (The term is derived from a Russian expression meaning to play the fool.)

-mis-; -miso- a combining form relating to hatred (Greek *misos*; unrelated to Old English *mis-*, "bad, wrong").

misala: See TROPENKOLLER.

misanthropy a hatred, aversion, or distrust of all human beings.

miscarriage the spontaneous abortion of a fetus before it is able to survive outside the womb, usually before the 28th week of pregnancy. Also see SPONTANEOUS ABORTION.

miscegenation the marriage or cohabitation of two individuals of different "races" of mankind (Latin *miscere*, "to mix," and *genus*, "race"). Historically, m. has been a common result of slavery and wars, e.g., the conquest of Spain by the Moors in the eighth century. American laws against m. were first enacted in the period of European colonization to discourage cohabitation between slave and master.

miserliness = STINGINESS.

misidentification a failure to identify individuals correctly due to impaired memory or a confused state, as in alcoholic intoxication (**amnesic m.**), failure to recognize people or objects due to a delusion that they have been transformed (delusional m.), or calling a person by someone else's name in a flippant manner (**hyperbolic m.**, occasionally observed in manic patients). Also see DELUSIONAL M.

misocainia = MISONEISM.

misogamy /-sog'-/ a hatred of marriage. In some cases, m. is based on an unresolved Oedipus complex; in schizophrenics, m. may be a defense against a concept that marriage is a form of incest.

misogyny /-soj'-/ a hatred of women. In psychoanalysis, this may be due, in part at least, to such factors in the male as the trauma of weaning, castration threats by the mother, homosexual conflicts, or a frustrated desire to become a woman. The condition may also occur in women who wish to be men, in some cases because their fathers were disappointed when their mother gave birth to a girl.

misologia an aversion to speaking or arguing, which in catatonic schizophrenics may be related to a fear that speaking may have destructive effects. Also called **misology**.

misoneism an extreme resistance to change; intolerance of anything new. It is a common symptom in presenile patients. Also called **misocainia**.

misopedia a hatred of children, which in some cases may be associated with a morbid compulsion to kill them since they represent incest.

missile fear = BALLISTOPHOBIA.

missing fifth-digit nails: See SYNDROME OF M.F.-D.N.

missing-parts test a test in which the subject is required to point out what is missing in a picture. It is frequently used as an observation test in IQ scales such as the Wechsler.

mist. an abbreviation used in prescriptions, meaning "mixture" (Latin *mistura*).

mistrust: See BASIC M.; TRUST VERSUS M.

Mitchell, Silas Weir American physician and poet, 1829–1914. Although he made many contributions to neurology, M. is recognized primarily as the chief proponent of the "rest-cure" approach to nervous disorders, which he attributed to such factors as the hectic pace of the "Railroad Age," women attending college, and combat exhaustion. In addition to rest, his therapeutic regimen included good nutrition, physical therapy, massage, and a change of scene. See REST-CURE TECHNIQUE.

mitochondria small organelles within cells that produce adenosine triphosphate molecules from substances in fats and sugars. Because the product is important as a source of cellular energy, m. usually tend to concentrate in areas of a cell where metabolic activity is at a high level. Adjective: **mitochondrial**.

mitochondrial disease a relatively rare inherited form of muscular dystrophy, marked by a failure in function of the mitochondria, the primary source of energy within muscle cells. Mitochondria, subunits of body cells, contain the enzymes necessary for the metabolism of amino acids and fatty acids; their normal function in turn depends upon the availability of oxygen and nutrients delivered by the bloodstream. M.d. may involve a breakdown of any component of the system.

mitosis the process by which a body cell reproduces by dividing into two daughter cells, each having the same number and kinds of chromosomes. **Mitotic** cell division usually requires that a cell possess enough DNA to permit doubling of its chromosomal material. Compare MEIOSIS.

mitral cell any of the pyramidal cells that form a layer of the olfactory bulb. Each m.c. may receive signals from hundreds of olfactory filaments embedded in the nasal epithelium.

mitral stenosis a narrowing of the opening through the mitral valve that separates the left atrium from the left ventricle of the heart. The disorder can be congenital or a result of a disease, e.g., rheumatic fever, that produces inflammation of the cusps of the valve so that they tend to stick together. The result in either case is a restricted blood flow into the left ventricle, which pumps blood to tissues throughout the body.

Mittelschmerz /mit'əlshmerts/ a pain experienced

by some females about midway in the menstrual cycle, or at the time of ovulation (German, "midpain"). The pain is observed in the region of the ovary and is caused by the rupture of the ovarian follicle and bleeding into the peritoneum. Also see OVULATION.

mitten pattern an unusual slow spike-and-wave EEG pattern that resembles the thumb and hand outline of a mitten. The m.p. occurs mainly in EEGs of adult schizophrenics and epileptic patients with psychosis, and is also found in EEGs of some criminals.

Mitwelt /mit′velt/ an existentialistic term for man's interpersonal relationships and encounters with his fellow men (German, "shared world"). Also see EIGENWELT; UMWELT.

mixed cerebral dominance a condition in which neither cerebral hemisphere is clearly dominant in motor control, causing speech disorders or conflicts in handedness.

mixed deafness: See DEAFNESS.

mixed design an experimental study method in which subjects who can be divided into two or more discrete and typically overlapping population groups are assigned to different experimental conditions, such as two different types of therapies. The experiment is intended to reveal the relative effectiveness of the therapies.

mixed laterality the tendency to shift from right to left side for some activities, or perform some acts with a preference for the right side and others with a preference for the left. Also called **lateral confusion**.

mixed model an experimental paradigm used in the analysis of variance, in which the experimenter fixes one or more variables and samples one or more additional variables. Also see RANDOM MODEL; FIXED MODEL.

mixed-motive game a situation that contains elements of both a cooperative reward structure and a competitive reward structure such that the individual must choose between cooperating and competing. See COMPETITIVE REWARD STRUCTURE; COOPERATIVE REWARD STRUCTURE.

mixed neurosis an early Freudian term for a condition in which the patient showed symptoms of two or more neuroses. Many of the cases once diagnosed as m.n. would be classified today as a type of schizophrenia, especially pseudoneurotic schizophrenia.

mixed reinforcement an intermittent reinforcement in which the reinforcement pattern changes randomly, or by design, e.g., from intervals of four minutes to 40 responses.

mixed sampling = DOUBLE SAMPLING.

mixed schizophrenia a form of schizophrenia that is manifested by symptoms of two or more of the basic categories of schizophrenia: simple, paranoid, catatonic, and hebephrenic (disorganized).

mixed specific developmental disorder a diagnostic category that applies when no single developmental disorder predominates but all the child's reading, arithmetic, and language skills are impaired to relatively the same degree. (DSM-III)

mixoscopia a form of voyeurism in which an orgasm is achieved by observing sexual intercourse between one's love object and another person.

mixoscopia bestialis a type of sexual deviation in which a person achieves excitement by watching another individual have coitus with an animal.

mixovariation in genetics, the combination of multiple hereditary factors over several generations, due to the union of individuals with unlike hereditary equipment (hybridization). Also called **combination**.

MM: See CREATINE PHOSPHOKINASE.

MMECT *m*ulti*m*onitored *e*lectro*c*onvulsive *t*reatment, in which an attempt is made to shorten the time for treatment by inducing four to five seizures in each session and monitoring the patient by means of an EEG and an EKG.

MMPI: See MINNESOTA MULTIPHASIC PERSONALITY INVENTORY.

M'Naghten rules in forensic psychiatry, a set of rules established by the Judges of England in 1843 stating that to plead insanity as a defense, the accused must be "laboring under such a defect of reason, from disease of the mind, as not to know the nature and quality of the act he was doing, or if he did know it, he did not know that what he was doing was wrong." The rules resulted from the case of Daniel M'Naghten, who suffered from delusions of persecution involving Sir Robert Peel, but who mistakenly shot his private secretary. (He died in 1865. His name has no firm spelling.) Also called **McNaughten rules; McNaughton rules; M'Naughten test**. See AMERICAN LAW INSTITUTE GUIDELINES; COMPETENCY TO STAND TRIAL; CRIMINAL RESPONSIBILITY; GOOD-AND-EVIL TEST; IRRESISTIBLE IMPULSE; PARTIAL INSANITY.

mneme = ENGRAM.

mnemonic strategy /nimon′ik/ any device or technique employed to assist memory, usually by forging a link or association between the new information to be remembered and information previously encoded. E.g., one might remember the numbers to a combination lock by associating them with familiar birth dates, addresses, phone numbers, or room numbers. Also called **mnemonic system**. Also see METHOD OF LOCI; MEDIATE ASSOCIATION.

mnemonic trace = ENGRAM.

mob a disorderly, unruly crowd of people characterized by (a) unanimity of feeling, thought, and action, (b) heightened emotional response and irrationality, and (c) a sense of anonymity (or deindividuation) and loss of a sense of responsibility among its members. Mobs frequently lead to aggressive behavior which the individual members would not engage in on their own. Also see CROWD BEHAVIOR; CROWD CONSCIOUSNESS; MOB PSYCHOLOGY.

mobbing behavior a form of behavior often

observed among birds which join together to drive away a predator such as a cat or a hawk.

mobile clinic a group of medical specialists representing various phases of diagnosis and therapy whose members travel as a team to small communities that are unable to support a full-time facility with an equivalent amount of talent and experience. The m.c. members work with local physicians in each of the communities visited.

mobility the state or quality of movability, a term usually applied to the ability of an individual to transport himself between home and work or community facilities. For an infant, m. is the ability to creep, crawl, or walk; for a disabled adult, m. may be the capability of driving a car or traveling by public transportation if blind or partially paralyzed. Also see MOTILITY.

mobility of libido in psychoanalysis, the transfer of libidinal energy from one subject to another, that is, from one part of the body, or one person, to another.

mobilization reaction a reaction to acute or prolonged stress in which the individual becomes emotionally aroused, tense, and alert, and calls upon all available psychological and physical resources to meet the threat. See GENERAL ADAPTATION SYNDROME.

Möbius, Paul Julius /mœ′byōos/ German neurologist, 1853–1907. See MÖBIUS' SYNDROME.

Möbius' syndrome a familial disorder marked by absence of facial expression when crying, failure to close the eyes when sleeping, and various other cranial-nerve abnormalities and muscle defects. About one-third of the patients have skeletal or muscular anomalies such as syndactyly or clubfoot. About ten percent have intellectual or behavioral defects. Also called **congenital facial diplegia**.

mob psychology the tendency of individuals to be swept into action by crowd emotions, as in lynchings, bombings, and demonstrations. The members of the mob lose their inhibitions and give free vent to their feelings when they have the support of a group. Various psychological reasons have been given for the fact that ordinarily law-abiding citizens commit violent acts: the anonymity of the crowd, the "impression of universality" (everybody's doing it), and the tendency to release feelings of frustration stemming from other areas in their lives. Also see MOB; MASS PSYCHOLOGY; CROWD BEHAVIOR; COLLECTIVE BEHAVIOR; CROWD CONSCIOUSNESS; MASS HYSTERIA.

modality a type of sensation, e.g., vision, or a kind of therapeutic technique or process. See SENSE MODALITY.

mode a statistic describing the central tendency of a set of data. It is the highest point or peak in a bar graph or frequency polygon, since it is the most frequently occurring score. Also see MEAN; MEDIAN; UNIMODAL; BIMODAL DISTRIBUTION.

model a graphic or other type of representation of a type of disorder that can be used to show cause-and-effect relationships, differential diagnostic techniques, epidemiological patterns, or similar biomedical study methods. The m. may be an analog-computer program.

modeling a behavior-therapy technique in which learning occurs vicariously through observation alone, without comment or reinforcement by the therapist. The client simply watches someone else perform a particular action such as answering the telephone or responding to a complaint on the job. Models are often parents or other adults and children; they may also be symbolic, e.g., a book or television character. M. is a form of social learning and is often called OBSERVATIONAL LEARNING. See this entry. Also see SOCIAL-LEARNING THEORY; BEHAVIORAL M.

model psychosis a psychosis deliberately produced, usually by a psychotomimetic drug such as LSD, for purposes of research.

moderate depression a depression marked by (a) persistent feelings of anguish, or "psychic pain," (b) despondent ruminations, (c) periods of silence, (d) a dispirited manner, (e) constant complaints about being unwanted and unappreciated, (f) difficulties in thinking and concentrating, and (g) various somatic disturbances such as fatigue, insomnia, loss of appetite, and constipation.

moderate mental retardation a diagnostic category applying to persons with IQs of 35 to 49, comprising about 12 percent of the retarded population. Classified as "trainable," these individuals rarely go beyond the second grade in academic subjects, but though often poorly coordinated, they can be trained to take care of themselves and to develop sufficient social and occupational skills to be able to perform unskilled or semiskilled work under supervision in sheltered workshops. (DSM-III)

moderator variable a variable that is unrelated to a criterion variable, but is still retained in a regression equation because of its significant relationship to other predictor variables. In consumer psychology, a m.v. is an influence by an individual factor, e.g., a personality trait, that may alter, or moderate, a prediction of product choice. Several studies have found that personality variables in consumer groups may account for 20 to 30 percent of brand-choice decisions; an example of a m.v. is self-confidence of the purchaser.

modified replication: See REPLICATION.

modified simple mastectomy: See MASTECTOMY.

modifier in genetics, a gene that appears to have an effect of modifying other hereditary factors and which has no significant effect when the main factor is absent. Some investigators believe a m.-gene plays a role in constitutional medical conditions, including manifestation of psychoses.

modulator in retina a set of ganglion cells that responds to narrow ranges of light wavelengths with peaks corresponding to different colors. See DOMINATORS.

modus operandi a specific form of behavior pattern that may be typical of a particular individual. A criminal may follow a m.o. that is unique in many details so that it can be used to identify the culprit.

Moebius: See MÖBIUS.

mogigraphia = WRITER'S CRAMP.

mogilalia a difficulty or hesitance in speaking (including stuttering) that is frequently associated with resistance to psychotherapy. Also called **molilalia**.

moisture fear = HYGROPHOBIA.

molar pertaining to a level of analysis focusing on a few large components or divisions, without reduction to a number of small elements. Compare MOLECULAR.

molar approach any theory or method that stresses comprehensive concepts and problems, e.g., the cognitivist approach to learning, or humanistic psychology. It avoids highly structured, detailed prescriptions for achievement of stated goals. Compare MOLECULAR APPROACH.

molar behavior a large but unified segment, or holistic unit, of a person's total behavior, as in playing chess. Compare MOLECULAR BEHAVIOR.

moldy-corn poisoning toxic effects resulting from the ingestion of corn or other cereal products contaminated by one of several molds. **Fusarium moniliform toxin** produces massive necrotic lesions in the white matter of the cerebral hemispheres. **Aspergillus flavus** can produce a tremorgenic toxin that causes sustained trembling and convulsions. Several **Patulin fungal toxins** cause neurologic disorders.

molecular pertaining to a level of analysis focusing on reduction to many small components or elements. Compare MOLAR.

molecular approach any theory or method that stressses the particular elements of a problem, focusing on systematically detailed procedures for the achievement of specifically defined goals, as in operant conditioning. Compare MOLAR APPROACH.

molecular behavior behavior that can be analyzed into small units such as reflexes, as opposed to molar behavior. Compare MOLAR BEHAVIOR.

molecularism = ATOMISM.

molestation the act of making sexual advances despite the protests of the individual subjected to the act. Although local laws vary, m. generally implies sexual fondling or touching an individual "without lawful consent." When the victim of m. is a child or a person of impaired mentality, it may be assumed the victim does not have the capacity to give lawful consent. Also see SEX OFFENSES.

molilalia = MOGILALIA.

molimina the unpleasant symptoms experienced by some women during the premenstrual or menstrual periods. Singular: **molimen**.

molysophobia a morbid fear of contamination. Also see MYSOPHOBIA.

momism a popular term for excessive dependence on maternal care; acceptance of maternal dominance, resulting in lack of independence and maturity. (The term was popularized by the novelist Philip Wylie.)

-mon-; -mono- a combining form meaning one, single, alone (Greek *monos*).

monamines = MONOAMINES.

monestrous: See ESTRUS.

money in psychoanalysis, a concept with various dynamic interpretations: (a) as an unconscious representation of the feces, (b) as a gratification of anal impulses to hold back (hoard), evacuate (spend), or play with the feces (handle coins), or (c) as an opportunity to exert power over others.

money phobia = CHREMATOPHOBIA.

Mongolian idiot a term suggested about 1865 by Langdon Down who observed what he believed to be ethnological features in various forms of congenital defects. Although original categories included Caucasian, Ethiopian, and Malayan, as well as Mongolian, only the M.i. classification continued in the medical literature, but is now rarely used. See DOWN'S SYNDROME.

mongolism: See DOWN'S SYNDROME.

moniliasis a disease caused by a systemic fungus infection of the genus Candida, most commonly Candida albicans. The infection can be a source of septicemia, endocarditis, meningitis, or osteomyelitis. The meningitis form of the disease is similar to **chronic cryptococcal meningitis**, another fungal infection of the nervous system that may be characterized by infarcts, nervous-tissue destruction, and increases in neuroglia cells, although the m. invasion of the nervous system rarely is fatal. Also called **candidiasis**. Also see ANAL ITCHING.

monism the philosophical concept that mind and matter are the same, and that there is only one kind of reality. Also see NATURAL M.

monitoring watching patients or experimental subjects (or machines), and checking at intervals to see how they are functioning.

monkey love a form of immoderate maternal love in which the mother attempts to satisfy every whim of the child (from German *Affenliebe* /äf'ənlēbə/, "monkey love, ape love").

monkey therapist a type of monkey used in animal-behavior studies who plays the role of companion for an isolate monkey, one that has been raised in total isolation. In time the isolate monkey's behavioral deficits of huddling and self-clasping tend to disappear and he becomes more sociable. Also called **monkey psychiatrist**.

monoamine oxidase inhibitors a group of antidepressant drugs that function by inhibiting the activity of **monoamine oxidase** in the presynaptic bulb. By interfering with the action of the enzyme monoamine oxidase, which is responsible for the degradation of monoamines, the level of transmitter amines is increased at the synapses. The prototype of the group is IPRONIAZID (see this entry), which has been replaced generally by other m.o.i. because of its high incidence of toxic side effects. Other m.o.i. are **isocarboxazid**— $C_{12}H_{13}N_3O_2$, **nialamide**—$C_{16}H_{18}N_4O_2$, **phenel-**

zine—$C_8H_{12}N_2$, tranylcypromine—$C_9H_{11}N$, tranylcypromine sulfate — $C_{18}H_{24}N_2O_4S$. Abbrev.: **MAO inhibitors; MAOI**. Also called **thymeretics**.

monoamines amines that contain only one amine group, formed from ammonia by the replacement of one or more hydrogen atoms by a hydrocarbon radical. Also called **monamines**.

monochorionic twins a set of twins that shared the same chorionic membrane as embryos.

monochromatism = ACHROMATISM.

monocular cues the cues to the perception of distance and depth that may involve only one eye. The m.c. are linear perspective, relative position, relative movement, chiaroscuro or light and shadow, accommodation, and atmospheric perspective. Also see BINOCULAR CUES.

monocular suppression the tendency of one eye to be dominant while the other is suppressed, resulting in a failure of binocular vision.

monocular vision the use of only one eye.

monoideic somnambulism a term for ideational content related to a single idea that occurs in a state of somnambulism. When more than one idea is involved, the appropriate term is **polyideic somnambulism**.

monoideism an obsessive preoccupation with a single idea, and inability to think of anything else. The condition is found in its most extreme form in schizophrenic and senile patients.

monomania an obsolete term for "partial insanity," in which the patient is preoccupied with one topic and is believed to be pathological only with reference to that topic. Examples of other archaic terms for monomanias are homicidal monomania, affective monomania (corresponding to hypomania), monomanie boulimique (bulimia), monomanie du vol (kleptomania), monomanie érotique (erotomania), and monomanie incendière (pyromania).

monomanie boulimique an obsolete term for bulimia. See MONOMANIA; BULIMIA.

monomanie du vol /dēvol'/ an obsolete term for kleptomania. See MONOMANIA; KLEPTOMANIA.

monomanie érotique an obsolete term for erotomania. See MONOMANIA; EROTOMANIA.

monomanie incendiaire /eNsäNdyer'/ an obsolete term for pyromania. See MONOMANIA; PYROMANIA.

monomatric having one mother. The term pertains to a family or household in which all or most of the child-rearing responsibilities are fulfilled by one person. Compare POLYMATRIC.

monopathophobia a morbid fear of a particular disease. Also see NOSOPHOBIA.

monophasic sleep rhythm the form of sleep pattern in which sleeping occurs in one long period once a day. The m.s.r. is associated with canaries, snakes, and human adults. Also see SLEEP-WAKE CYCLE. Compare POLYPHASIC SLEEP RHYTHM.

monophobia = AUTOPHOBIA.

monoplegia the paralysis of a single part of the body, e.g., one arm, one leg, or one digit.

monopolar depression an affective disorder consisting of one or more depressive episodes with no manic episodes.

monorchid a male with only one testis in the scrotum. The second testis may be undescended. Also see CRYPTORCHID; ECTOPIC TESTIS.

monosomy: See GROUP G M.

monosymptomatic denoting a disorder that is characterized by a single marked symptom.

monosymptomatic circumscription a mental disorder characterized by a single symptom.

monosymptomatic neurosis a neurosis in which the patient exhibits a single symptom of the disorder, such as an obsessive thought.

monosymptomatic psychosis a term sometimes applied to a type of dysmorphophobia in which an obsession or delusion of deformity is the patient's single symptom or complaint.

monosynaptic arc a simple synaptic communication between two neurons, such as a synapse between a sensory fiber and a motoneuron in the spinal cord.

monotonic describing a variable that progressively either increases or decreases, but does not change its direction. E.g., a monotonically increasing variable is one that rises.

monozygotic twins twins that develop from a single ovum fertilized by a single sperm. Approximately 25 percent of human twins are m.t., and the incidence of m.t. is about the same throughout the world. M.t. are identical in genetic composition, having inherited the same sets of genes from both parents. A single-ovum may go through double twinning to produce identical quadruplets, or triplets if one dies *in utero*. Also called **enzygotic twins; identical twins; monovular twins; uniovular twins**. See DIZYGOTIC TWINS; TWIN STUDIES.

Monro, Alexander Secundus Scottish anatomist, 1733–1817. See INTERVENTRICULAR FORAMEN OF MONRO.

monster a term sometimes applied to an individual with a congenital defect or acquired injury that has severely disfigured his appearance. Also see TERATOGENIC.

monster fear = TERATOPHOBIA.

Montagu, Ashley British anthropologist and social biologist, 1905—. See NEOTONY.

Monte Carlo method a method of mathematical simulation in which random variables are calculated.

Montessori, Maria Italian physician and educator, 1870–1952. See MONTESSORI METHOD.

Montessori method an educational system developed by Maria Montessori in Italy early this century, with the first American school established in 1913. Her system focuses on self-education of preschool children through the development of initiative by means of freedom of action; sense-perception training with objects of different shapes and colors; and development of coordination through games and exercises.

monthly period = MENSTRUATION.

mood a mild, usually transient, feeling tone such as euphoria or irritability.

mood-altering drugs substances that change the affective state of the patient through pharmacological action, usually without clouding of consciousness. M.-a.d. include certain tranquilizing, sedating, and antidepressant agents. Also see MIND-ALTERING DRUGS.

mood-congruent psychotic features delusions or hallucinations that consistently reflect a depressed mood (themes of personal inadequacy, guilt, disease, death, punishment) or a manic mood (inflated worth, power, knowledge, or special relationship to a deity or famous person). (DSM-III)

mood-cyclic disorders a category of Rado's adaptational psychodynamics in which the patient may show any of a variety of cycles of depression and/or elation.

mood-incongruent psychotic features delusions or hallucinations whose content does not involve the characteristic themes cited among mood-congruent psychotic features. Examples of m.-i.p.f. are persecutory delusions, thought broadcasting, delusions of being controlled, and the catatonic symptoms of stupor, mutism, negativism, and posturing which sometimes occur in manic episodes.

moodiness an affective state characterized by ill humor, sullenness, and sulking. M. is usually a response to disappointment or frustration, and generally subsides if the individual gets what he wants.

mood swings periodic alternation between feelings of well-being and dejection. If mild and occasional, these changes are normal; but if they are more severe, they may be a neurotic reaction; and if they are intense and persistent, they may be symptomatic of manic-depressive disorder.

Moon, Robert C. American ophthalmologist, 1844–1914. See LAURENCE-MOON-BIEDLE SYNDROME.

Mooney, Ross L. American (?) psychologist, fl. 1950. See MOONEY PROBLEM CHECK LIST.

Mooney Problem Check List a personality inventory containing statements of problems compiled from students, case records, and counseling interviews, and presented in several forms: Junior High School, High School, College, and adult levels. The subject identifies problems relevant to himself or herself, and the results are used in finding individuals with problems and in facilitating interviews and counseling.

moon-phase studies research on the possible relationship between the phases of the moon and epiodes of violence or mental disorder. The relationship has long been expressed in folklore, folk medicine, and language itself ("lunacy," "lunatic"). D. H. Tuke cites the archaic term **lunatismus,** applied to somnambulists who walk in their sleep only when the moon shines. Observational studies indicate that many institutionalized mental patients become restless or agitated during a full moon, and Lieber and Sherin found that the murder rate in Florida began to rise about 24 hours before full moon and reached a peak when this occurred (Arnold L. Lieber and C. R. Sherin, in *American Journal of Psychiatry*, 1972; Arnold L. Lieber and Jerome B. Agel, *The Lunar Effect. Biological Tides and Human Emotions*, 1978).

moral characterizing a person or group whose conduct is ethical or proper.

moral anxiety in psychoanalysis, the anxiety experienced by the ego in terms of guilt or shame, usually as an expression of fear of punishment by the superego for a failure to maintain proper standards of conduct.

moral code a set of rules of conduct accepted by a society or group as binding on all members.

moral conduct behavior that conforms to the accepted set of values, customs, or rules of a given society or religious group.

moral consistency a stable, predictable pattern of moral attitudes and character throughout the years. According to a longitudinal study of children observed by Peck and Havighurst (1960) from age ten through 17, the children tended to maintain a consistent pattern characterized by either (a) expediency (b) conformity, (c) an irrational-conscientious attitude "with an internal standard of right and wrong regardless of the situation or consequences"; or, in a few cases, (d) a rational-altruistic attitude appearing during adolescence and marked by a stable set of moral principles applied with an eye toward both the young person's own good and the good of others.

moral development the gradual development of an individual's concepts of right and wrong, conscience, ethical and religious values, social attitudes, and behavior.

moral idiocy Bleuler's now obsolete term for a total incapacity to feel sympathy or "be concerned with the welfare and woes" of other people, though capable of other emotions.

moral imbecility Bleuler's now obsolete term referring to individuals who are intellectually and emotionally sound but ethically defective and lacking in appreciation for the feelings and rights of others.

moral independence Piaget's term for the older child's recognition that an act's morality may be substantially determined by its motive and other subjective considerations. M.i. is a principle of the autonomous stage. Also see MORAL RELATIVISM. Compare MORAL REALISM.

moral insanity a term coined by Prichard in 1835 for an intellectually normal individual in whom "the moral and active principles of the mind are strongly perverted and depraved," making him "incapable . . . of conducting himself with decency and propriety in the business of life." The term is obsolete. See ANTISOCIAL-PERSONALITY DISORDER.

morality a system of beliefs and a set of values relating to right conduct, against which behavior is judged to be acceptable or unacceptable.

morality of constraint as used by Piaget, the young child's attitude toward morality which consists of an unquestioning, unchallenging obedience to the rules laid down by parents. Obedience is based on fear and on the perception that rules established by parents are fixed, eternal, and sure to be valid. M.o.c. is characteristic of children until roughly age ten. See RULES OF THE GAME. Compare MORALITY OF COOPERATION.

morality of cooperation as used by Piaget, the ten-to-11-year-old child's attitude toward morality characterized by the perception that rules are social conventions that can be challenged and modified when concerned parties agree. M.o.c. means the child willingly accept rules and adheres to them on the basis of reason and not on the basis of fear and not in the spirit of unquestioning obedience. See RULES OF THE GAME. Compare MORALITY OF CONSTRAINT.

moral judgment the beliefs an individual applies in discriminating between right and wrong; the attitudes that comprise a person's moral orientation whether or not they govern behavior in each situation. Some of the major theorists in the area of moral development are Freud, Piaget, Erikson, and Kohlberg.

moral masochism in psychoanalysis, an unconscious need for punishment by authority figures representing the father. Freud believed this need arises out of the childhood desire for passive intercourse with the father, which has been distorted into the desire to be beaten by him.

moral pride: See PRIDE.

moral realism Piaget's term for the type of thinking characteristic of younger children who equate good behavior with obedience just as they equate the morality of an act only with its consequences; e.g., 15 cups broken accidentally is far worse than one cup broken mischievously because more cups are broken. M.r. marks the child's thinking until the age of roughly eight when the concepts of intention, motive, and extenuating circumstances begin to modify the child's early absolutism.

moral relativism as used by Piagetians, the developed ability to consider the intention behind an act along with possible extenuating circumstances when judging its rightness or wrongness. Piaget observed that young children focus strictly on the objective consequences of an act and only later develop m.r. The term is similar to moral independence, and is analogous to the concept of **situation ethics** as used by modern theologians.

moral treatment humane treatment of mental patients, in which mechanical restraint, bloodletting, and unkempt conditions were gradually replaced by a comfortable, healthy environment, occupational and social activities, and reassuring talks with physicians and attendants. This type of approach originated in the family-care program established in Gheel, Belgium, during the 13th century, but came to fruition in the 19th century through the efforts of Philippe Pinel and Jean Esquirol in France, William Tuke in England, and Benjamin Rush, Isaac Ray, and Thomas Kirkbride in America. The therapeutic community of today has its roots in this movement.

moratorium Erikson's term for the experimental stage in adolescence when youths try out alternative roles before making permanent commitments. However, an extended m. is not a universal feature of adolescence; it is more likely to occur in nontraditional societies and in economically advantaged classes. See IDENTITY CRISIS. Also see ERIKSON'S EIGHT STAGES OF MAN.

morbid dependency: See DEPENDENCY NEEDS.

morbidity a disease (pathological) condition, either organic or functional.

morbidity risk a term employed in epidemiology studies to indicate the statistical chance that an individual will develop a certain disease or disorder. The probability often is expressed in terms of risk factors, using 1.0 as a base; the larger the number, the greater the m.r.

morbid perplexity a schizophrenic symptom associated with loss of ego boundaries, and characterized by profound confusion about personal identity and the meaning of existence.

Morel, Ferdinand Swiss psychiatrist, 1888–1957. See STEWART-MOREL SYNDROME.

Morel's syndrome = STEWART-MOREL SYNDROME.

Moreno, Jacob L. Austrian-American psychiatrist, 1890–1974. M. is responsible for widening the armamentarium of the psychotherapist to include psychodrama, in which relationships are acted out; the method of sociometry, which diagrams group relationships; and group psychotherapy and encounter groups, both of which he named and helped to develop. See ENCOUNTER GROUP; HYPNODRAMA; INTERPERSONAL THERAPY; NETWORK; PSYCHODRAMA; PSYCHODRAMA FORMS; PSYCHOLOGICAL GEOGRAPHY; SOCIOGRAM; SOCIOMETRY; SPONTANEITY TEST; SPONTANEITY TRAINING; TELE; THEATER OF SPONTANEITY.

mores the social customs that are accepted by members of a culture or population even though the behavioral standards may lack legal sanction.

Morgan, Conway Lloyd English zoologist and psychologist, 1852–1936. See LLOYD MORGAN'S CANON.

Morgan's canon; Morgan's principle = LLOYD MORGAN'S CANON.

moria an obsessive or morbid desire to joke, particularly when the humor is inappropriate, as in cases of dementia. See GALLOWS HUMOR.

Morita, Shoma Japanese psychiatrist, fl. early 20th century. See MORITA THERAPY.

Morita therapy a therapy for hypochondriasis introduced in the early 20th century by Shoma Morita in Japan. The treatment consists of a period of absolute bed rest, during which the patient is allowed only to sleep and suffer, followed by a period of increasingly difficult and tiring work in a communal setting, with the objective of teaching the patient to accept his life as it is at the moment, a process called **arugamama**.

morning-after pill a popular name for a formulation of *di*ethyl*s*tilbesterol (**DES**) that when administered no later than 72 hours after intercourse will cause the uterus to expel any fertilized ovum. The DES medication is very powerful, requires five days of supervised treatment, and can have serious side effects including failure to expel the embryo while causing it to develop instead as a deformed infant. The drug is used mainly to prevent pregnancy by rape.

morning-glory seeds: See PSYCHEDELICS.

morning sickness attacks of nausea and vomiting experienced by some women during the first months of pregnancy or throughout the entire pregnancy. Although m.s. usually occurs soon after arising in the morning, some women have the symptoms throughout the day. For a small proportion of patients, the symptoms are severe enough to require hospitalization. At the other extreme are women who do not experience m.s. Also called **nausea gravidarum**.

Moro, Ernst Austrian pediatrician, 1874–1951. See MORO REFLEX; ACOUSTIC REFLEX.

Moro reflex the reflex in which the newborn infant, when startled, throws out his arms, extends fingers, and often quickly brings the arms back together as if clutching or embracing. In normal, healthy babies, the M.r. disappears in the course of the first year. Also called **Moro response**. See STARTLE REACTION.

moron a term introduced by Henry Goddard, who applied it to individuals with mild retardation (IQ 50 to 70), who are usually capable of performing simple tasks under supervision in spite of limited academic ability (from Greek *moros*, "foolish").

-morph-; -morphous a combining form relating to (a) a specified form or structure (Greek *morphe*), (b) sleep (from *Morpheus*, the Greek god of sleep, literally, "maker of shapes").

morpheme /môr′fēm/ a minimum distinctive unit of grammar. E.g., in "cats," *s* is a m. (indicating the plural) and *cat* is a m. (because it cannot be divided into its parts *c*, *a*, and *t* without losing its meaning). Any word is composed of one or several morphemes. Also see PHONEME; GRAPHEME.

morphine: See OPIUM ALKALOIDS.

morphine dependence a condition that develops in the body tissues as a result of continued use of morphine so that increasingly larger doses are required to relieve a given degree of pain. M.d. can be rapid, developing in a normal individual in three weeks as a result of a daily therapeutic dose. As tolerance develops, the drug produces excitatory rather than CNS depression effects.

morphine withdrawal interruption of a supply of morphine to a person who has developed dependence on the narcotic. M.w. symptoms begin

with restlessness and yawning, followed by complaints of feeling cold and difficult, jerky breathing. After prolonged sleep, the patient's symptoms intensify, accompanied by abdominal cramps, vomiting, diarrhea, excessive sweating, and muscle twitching. The symptoms begin to subside after about ten days.

morphogenesis the development of the form and structure of an organism.

morphological index the index or relationship among body proportions that describes a particular body build.

morphologic inferiority a term introduced by Adler to describe a subgroup of organ inferiority, characterized by a deficiency in the shape, size, or strength of an organ or a part of it.

morphology the science that deals with anatomy or the body's forms and structures (coined by Goethe, in 1817—German *Morphologie*). In grammar, m. is the study of the inflection, derivation, and composition of words, as distinct from syntax.

Morquio, Luis Urugayan physician, 1867–1935. See MORQUIO'S SYNDROME; MUCOPOLYSACCHARIDOSES; PECTUS CARINATUM.

Morquio's syndrome a congenital disorder due to an enzyme deficiency. It is characterized by bone dystrophy with flaccid muscles. The patient usually is barrel-chested or pigeon-breasted, or both, knock-kneed, and short of stature. However, the autosomal-recessive trait is not accompanied by mental retardation as are many of the similar mucopolysaccharidoses. Also called **MPS IV; Brailsford-Morquio syndrome; chondroosteodystrophy**.

morsicatio buccarum literally, cheek-biting (Latin), a form of compulsive self-mutilation. Also see FINGER-BITING BEHAVIOR.

morsicatio labiorum literally, lip-biting (Latin), a form of compulsive self-mutilation. See FINGER-BITING BEHAVIOR.

mortality = ATTRITION.

mort douce /môrdōōs′/ literally, sweet death (French). The term is used to describe the mutual bliss at the end of sexual orgasm. It is also a synonym for euthanasia.

mortido the death instinct. The term was coined by P. Federn as the counterpart of Freud's libido, or life instinct.

morula /môr′-/ an early stage of embryology, extending from the first cleavage of the zygote until the blastula is formed by further divisions of daughter cells.

Morvan, Augustin Marie /môrväN′/ French physician, 1819–97. See MORVAN'S DISEASE.

Morvan's disease a form of syringomyelia accompanied by painless ulceration of the fingertips and analgesic paralysis and atrophy of the hands and forearms.

mosaicism a condition of genetic abnormality in which an individual's chromosomes represent two or more different cell lines although derived from a single zygote. In a typical case, an individual may have one normal cell line and another with an extra chromosome, such as 45,X/46,XX. The cell lines may differ within tissues and organs of the same person. M. is associated with Down's syndrome and Turner's syndrome. Such individuals or body areas are called **mosaic**.

mosaic test a projective test in which the subject, usually a child, is asked to "make anything you like" out of about 400 pieces of different colors and shapes. Mosaic materials are also used in some intelligence tests.

mosaic theory of perception the concept that each nerve fiber of a peripheral organ, such as the ear, communicates directly with a specific neuron in the brain, complex sensations being produced by combinations of sensory-fiber impulses.

Moschowitz, Eli American physician, 1879–1964. See MOSCHOWITZ'S DISEASE.

Moschowitz's disease a type of hemolytic anemia in which ischemia of the central nervous system is a complication. Autopsy usually shows disseminated thrombi in the brain and other organs. Symptoms include retinal hemorrhages, paresthesia, paralysis, confusion, and headaches. Jaundice, hematuria, and fever are additional diagnostic clues.

most comfortable loudness the level of hearing at which speech is most comfortable for the person. This has important educational implications for a hearing-impaired child. Abbrev.: **MCL**.

mote-beam mechanism a term used to identify a personality characteristic in an individual who expresses concern about an undesirable trait in members of a minority group but ignores the presence of the same trait in himself.

mother complex a strong emotional attachment to the mother, usually accompanied by sexual desire.

mother archetype the primordial image of the mother figure that occurs repeatedly in various cultural concepts and myths since ancient times (Jung). See MAGNA MATER.

mother figure = MOTHER SURROGATE.

mother fixation an abnormally strong emotional attachment to the mother.

mother hypnosis a type of hypnotic submission that is traced to a transference of mother fixation and an obedient response to the coaxing of the mother. See FATHER HYPNOSIS.

mothering a relationship in which the mother or mother surrogate provides the infant and child with adequate emotional warmth, personal care, and sensory stimulation, all of which are believed to be essential to the development of a sense of security, feelings of self-worth, and the capacity to deal with the environment. Today it is widely recognized that the child should be "mothered" by the father as well as the mother. Also see MULTIPLE M.; SCHIZOPHRENOGENIC MOTHER; COMPLETE MOTHER.

A classic study of mothering has been conducted by Harry F. Harlow and associates on monkeys taken away from their mothers shortly after birth and placed in cages that contain two types of **artificial** "**mothers**," one made of wire and the other of sponge rubber and terrycloth attached to a wire frame. In one experiment they were given a choice of the two surrogates, and most of them clung to the cloth mother, suggesting that softness and "cuddliness" have a significant effect. Another experiment indicated that the monkeys preferred to feed as well as cuddle with the soft mother, and still another showed that when the monkeys were placed in a strange room with the wire mother, they cowered in a corner, but when the cloth mother was available, they clung to it and gained enough confidence and security to explore their new surroundings, just as human infants do.

mothering one the term used by H. S. Sullivan for the person who has chief responsibility for the feeding, loving, nurturance, protection, and overall care of an infant or small child.

mother instinct the mother's "instinct" to protect and care for offspring, usually but not always her own. This behavior pattern appears to be unlearned and instinctive in animals, but its instinctual character is less clear among humans.

mother love the natural protective and possessive affection a mother displays toward her child. The feeling, sometimes called instinctive, usually is reinforced by pressures of the social group which expects the mother to show tender feelings toward her offspring.

mother-son incest sexual activity between mother and son, believed to be considerably rarer than father-daughter incest, and associated with such factors as absence of the father, an ethically defective home, disturbed marital relations, alcoholism, and psychosis or other emotional disturbance on the part of one or both partners. Also see PHAEDRA COMPLEX.

mother substitute = MOTHER SURROGATE.

Mother Superior complex the tendency of some therapists to play a maternal role in relations with patients, often to the detriment of the therapy.

mother surrogate a mother substitute (sister, father, friend, teacher, foster mother) who assumes the basic functions of the real mother. In psychoanalysis, a m.s. is a person on whom the patient unconsciously projects acceptable or unacceptable feelings and attitudes which he or she had toward the real mother. Also called **mother substitute; surrogate mother; mother figure**.

motility the capacity to move either voluntarily or involuntarily (as in sleepwalking); also, the style and speed of movement. M. may be inhibited for physical reasons or for psychological reasons, as in hysterical paralysis. Also see MOBILITY.

motility disorder any abnormality of posture, gesture, or other motion or movement, especially as observed in catatonia and childhood schizophrenia.

motion detection the ability of the eye to observe motion even under conditions of cortical blindness. In animal experiments, retinal cells are found to respond to the image of either a moving object or the movement of the eye across an area marked by a light-dark contrast point.

motion economy a set of principles developed by Gilbreth and others for the efficient performance of industrial operations. M.e. recommends, e.g., simultaneous use of both hands moving in opposite directions; arrangement of work to permit an easy, natural rhythm; fixed, convenient location of tools; bins with materials close to the point of use; adequate illumination and workplace height; and the use of jigs and fixtures to relieve hands of unnecessary work.

motion fear = KINESOPHOBIA. Also see ERGASIO-PHOBIA.

motion sickness a type of discomfort marked by nausea, dizziness, headache, pallor, cold sweats, and in some cases vomiting and prostration. The cause is irregular or abnormal motion that disturbs the normal sense of balance maintained by the semicircular canals of the inner ear. The condition may be aggravated or initiated by an emotional disturbance such as anxiety or grief.

motion study: See TIME-M.S.

motivated error a mistake or miscue that reveals a hidden motive, e.g., a "Freudian slip."

motivated forgetting a memory lapse motivated by a desire to avoid a disagreeable recollection.

motivation the process of initiating, sustaining, and directing psychological or physical activities; also, any internal force (impulse, drive, desire) that is involved in this process. Motives may operate on a conscious or unconscious level, and are frequently divided into (a) physiological, primary, or organic (such as hunger and elimination), and (b) personal and social, or secondary (affiliation, competition, and individual interests and goals). See MASLOW; MURRAY.

motivational factors any factor—conscious or unconscious, physiological or psychological—that stimulates, maintains, and directs behavior. Among these factors are basic or immediate needs, interests, incentives and rewards, social drives, and personal drives for security, self-esteem, or superiority.

motivational hierarchy: See MASLOW'S M.H.

motivational selectivity a term used to indicate the influence of individual motives on cognitive processes as an explanation for the differences in ways that an event or object may be perceived by different persons.

motivation research in consumer psychology, research that is designed to reveal the true motives behind the decisions of individuals in such matters as purchases of food, clothing, automobiles, and other products. M.r. also is employed to determine why consumers may refuse to buy a certain product. M.r. utilizes approaches that are clinical, intensive, and qualitative, but are conducted with great accuracy because of the tremendous advertising budgets that may be affected by the results.

motive a conscious or unconscious reason for behavior that directs a person's energies toward a goal. The term has various loose as well as specific meanings, especially as used by theorists of MOTIVATION. See this entry.

motives hierarchy: See NEED-HIERARCHY THEORY.

motokinesthetic method a technique for developing or improving speech whereby the speech pathologist manually manipulates the speech muscles of the patient, or touches specific areas to suggest movement at that point. He may help the patient position the articulators, e.g., jaws, lips, tongue, and soft palate, so that a desired sound is produced. The therapist simultaneously emits the correct sound. Also called **motor-kinesthetic method**.

motone a motor-muscular action pattern (Murray).

motoneuron pool a collection of motor neurons that may be scattered over several segments of the spinal cord although all members of a m.p. terminate in a single muscle.

motoneurons = MOTOR NEURONS.

motor a term characterizing muscular or glandular body functions.

motor amimia: See AMIMIA.

motor amusia a loss of the ability to reproduce melodies, resulting from cortical lesion. The individual may be able to recognize melodies but can no longer sing or play correctly, even though he or she has studied music for years. Also see AMUSIA.

motor aphasia an inability to perform specific muscular movements involved in speaking due to brain damage.

motor apraxia a disorder marked by the loss of ability to perform certain skilled motor tasks involving the arm and hand on one side of the body. The tasks may include typing or such simple movements as manipulating buttons on clothing or safety pins. The condition is associated with a lesion of the precentral gyrus on the side of the body opposite that of the affected limb.

motor area one of three areas of the frontal lobes which, when stimulated, produces movements of skeletal muscles in various parts of the body. Also called **Brodmann's area 4; precentral area**.

motor behavior a general term for any activity resulting from stimulation of muscles or glands. The term is essentially equivalent to MOTOR FUNCTION. See this entry.

motor compliance a type of motor response observed in many schizophrenic children with motility disturbances. The patient will change positions or turn toward the examiner as an automatic reaction to light palm contact.

motor conversion symptoms: See CONVERSION SYMPTOMS.

motor coordination the cooperative action of reflexive or involuntary and voluntary movements of the body, requiring accuracy, timing, and manipulation of cortical and subcortical controls in order to carry out complex activities.

motor development the development of muscular coordination and control required for physical activities and skills. M.d. follows predictable maturational patterns associated with the development of muscles, nerves, and skeleton, as well as the cerebellum for balance and the cerebrum for motor learning and fine muscle coordination. More specifically, the sequence (with varying dates) is: eye control, smiling, head control, trunk control, sitting, bowel control, bladder control, arm and hand movements and reflexes, leg and foot movements, and hand skills. For attainment ages, see MOTOR MILESTONES.

motor disorder the loss of ability to perform simple or complex acts or skills because of temporary or permanent damage to tissues in the motor or premotor areas of the central nervous system. The cause of damage may be a congenital or inherited defect, injury or surgical excision, or a psychochemical factor.

motor disturbance a disturbance of motor behavior, such as hyperactivity, retarded activity, automatism, repetitive movements, rigid posture, grimacing, and tics.

motor end plate a junction between the terminal of a motor neuron and a group of muscle fibers.

motor equivalence a muscle-feedback mechanism that permits higher animals to perform an act, e.g., eating a meal, repeatedly without using the same combinations of nerve and muscle fibers in exactly the same way each time. The feedback function permits other nerve and muscle fibers in the same body area to perform equivalent body movements.

motor function any activity that results from stimulation of motor neurons, including glandular activity as well as reflexes and voluntary and involuntary muscle contractions.

motor-function homunculus an atlas of the brain that displays the motoneuron areas of humans or other mammals in proportion to bodily function. Motoneurons associated with hand functions, e.g., occupy a larger proportion of brain area than those required for the trunk or legs.

motor habit a habit described in terms of movement responses.

motoric region Lewin's term for the experience aspect of personality that is manifested in terms of motor responses and outward appearance.

motoric reproduction processes a term referring to the processes involved in the motor reproduction of modeled behavior. M.r.p. include the constituent capacities, skills, and functions that permit an individual to translate what is learned through observation into actual behavior, e.g., the ability to physically reproduce the motions comprising a tennis serve following a teaching demonstration.

motor impersistence an effect observed in some patients with a lesion in the left cerebral hemisphere and characterized by difficulty in holding the tongue in a protruded position while the eyes are closed. The patient is able to initiate the activity but presumably because of a motor dysfunction cannot maintain persistent control of the act.

motor inhibition: See PSYCHOMOTOR RETARDATION.

motorium the brain areas that control the voluntary or skeletal muscles; the motor cortex.

motor-kinesthetic method = MOTOKINESTHETIC METHOD.

motor learning a type of learning in which muscular and glandular functions are emphasized, as in acquiring new skills and habit patterns.

motor memory the capacity to remember previously learned movements or series of movements, e.g., the sequential elements of an exercise or dance. Also see VERBAL MEMORY; VISUAL MEMORY.

motor milestones the significant achievements in motor development during an infant's first two years. Although individual children vary, norms show that on the average an infant will support his head while prone at three months; support his head in other positions at four months; sit with props at five months; sit supported by his hands and reach with one hand at six months; pick up small items, using thumb opposition, and stand if holding onto a crib railing at eight months; creep, pull to standing position and take side steps while holding on at ten months; walk alone, throw a ball, and walk backwards, sideways, upstairs, and downstairs with assistance at 16 months; and run and walk up and down steps easily or with minimal assistance at 24 months. Also see MOTOR DEVELOPMENT; DEVELOPMENTAL SEQUENCE.

motor nerve an efferent nerve that terminates in a muscle or gland.

motor-neuron disease any disease that involves neurons of the motor functions of the nervous system. However, the term often is applied specifically to AMYOTROPHIC LATERAL SCLEROSIS. See this entry.

motor-neuron lesion any damage to a motor nerve, particularly if the disease or injury involves the cell body.

motor neurons spinal neurons with a cell body in the ventral horn of the spinal cord and numerous synaptic connections with fibers communicating to the cerebral cortex and peripheral body areas. Also called **motoneurons**.

motor neurosis a neurosis in which a primary symptom is an abnormality of motor function, e.g., tremors, tics, or hyperactivity.

motor-primacy theory the concept that body mechanisms associated with motor-nerve functions develop before sensory-nerve mechanisms.

motor-reaction type the type of person whose attention is focused on the motor response rather than the stimulus in a situation (such as a reaction-time experiment or the start of a race) that calls for rapid action.

Motor Scale: See BAYLEY SCALES OF INFANT DEVELOPMENT.

motor set preparatory adjustments or readiness to make a certain response or begin an activity, as in "Ready, Set, Go!" at the start of a foot race.

motor system the complex of skeletal muscles, neural connections with muscle tissues, and the CNS structures associated with motor functions. Also called **neuromuscular system**.

motor tension: See GENERALIZED-ANXIETY DISORDER.

motor tests tests designed to measure manipulative skills such as finger dexterity or the use of hand tools.

motor theory of thought a concept popularized by behaviorists in the 1920s that motor-system responses are controlled by conditioned-reflex links between the motor-cortex and sensory-cortex areas. The theory has been challenged by investigators who note a lack of physiological and anatomical evidence to support it. Also called **motor theory of consciousness**.

motor unit a group of muscle fibers that respond collectively and simultaneously because they are innervated by nerve endings from a single motoneuron.

mouches volantes /mo̅o̅sh′voläNt′/ a French term ("flying flies") used to describe particles or specks sometimes observed floating in one's own eyeball.

mountain-climber's syndrome; mountain sickness: See ACOSTA'S SYNDROME.

mourning grief reactions due to loss of a loved one, involving feelings of dejection, loss of interest in the outside world, and diminution in activity and initiative. These reactions are similar to depression and melancholia, but are less persistent and are not considered pathological. Also see GRIEF; ANTICIPATORY M.; WIDOWHOOD CRISIS.

mourning work a stage of mourning during which, according to Freud, the mourner can separate himself from the identity of the deceased person while recalling memories of the deceased. M.w. follows the period of introjection in which the mourner identifies with the deceased.

mouse fear = MUSOPHOBIA.

movement education a technique designed to help students or patients develop motor skills, creative expression, and self-awareness through physical movement. Also see MOVEMENT THERAPY.

movement illusion an illusion that a part or all of the body is in motion when it is not.

movement learning = RESPONSE LEARNING.

movement perspective a visual illusion produced by the relative distance of moving objects. E.g., a nearby bird flying at 30 miles an hour may appear to be traveling faster than a jet airliner in the distant sky moving at nearly 600 miles an hour.

movement sense = KINESTHETIC SENSE.

movement-sensitive retinal cells cells in the retina of lower animals that respond to various specific movements across the visual field. Examples include the bug-detector cells of amphibia that respond best to small dark spots that move, and newness cells that adapt quickly to objects moving in a particular direction. M.-

s.r.c. seem to be absent in higher animals with binocular vision.

movement therapy a therapeutic modality in which mental patients and disabled individuals are encouraged to express emotion, work off tensions, develop an improved body image, and achieve greater body awareness and social interaction through rhythmic exercises and responses to music. M.t. is carried out under the supervision of a trained movement or dance therapist. See DANCE THERAPY.

movigenic theory a motor-based curriculum developed by Barsch (1967) for the learning-disabled.

Mowrer, Orval Hobart American psychologist, 1907–82. See FEAR DRIVE (there: **Mowrer-Miller theory of avoidance learning**); TWO-FACTOR THEORY.

MPS: See MUCOPOLYSACCHARIDOSES.

MPS V = SCHEIE'S SYNDROME.

MPS IV = MORQUIO'S SYNDROME.

MPS I = HURLER'S SYNDROME.

MPS III = SANFILIPPO'S SYNDROME.

MPS II = HUNTER'S SYNDROME.

MR = MENTAL RETARDATION.

MS = MULTIPLE SCLEROSIS.

MSER = MENTAL STATUS EXAMINATION REPORT.

MSIS = MULTI-STATE INFORMATION SYSTEM.

MSRPP = MULTIDIMENSIONAL SCALE FOR RATING PSYCHIATRIC PATIENTS.

MSUD = MAPLE-SUGAR URINE DISEASE.

M.T. (ASCP) B.B.: See BLOOD-BANK TECHNOLOGIST.

mu /mo̅o̅/ or /myo̅o̅/ 12th letter of the Greek alphabet (M, μ).

-muc-; -muco-; -myx-; -myxo- a combining form relating to mucus (Greek *myxa*).

mucin: See MUCUS.

mucinous carcinoma: See CARCINOMA.

mucolipidosis II = INCLUSION-CELL DISEASE.

mucopolysaccharidoses a group of six metabolic disorders that have in common an excess of mucopolysaccharide (a mucus component) in the tissues. Biochemists have proposed the term **glycosaminoglycan (GAG)** for the diseases. Three of the six forms of the disease are associated with mental retardation. A common abbreviation of mucopolysaccharidosis is **MPS**. See HUNTER'S SYNDROME; HURLER'S SYNDROME; MORQUIO'S SYNDROME; SANFILIPPO'S SYNDROME; SCHEIE'S SYNDROME; MAROTEAUX-LAMY SYNDROME; GARGOYLISM; FUCOSIDOSIS; BETA-GLUCURONIDASE DEFICIENCY.

mucopolysaccharidosis F = FUCOSIDOSIS.

mucous: See MUCUS.

mucous colitis: See COLITIS.

mucous ophthalmia: See OPHTHALMIA.

mucoviscidosis a pathologic condition associated with cystic fibrosis and characterized by a thick accumulation of mucus from exocrine glands in the pancreas. M. can result in blockage of the ducts of the pancreas so that digestive enzymes are unable to flow into the small intestine. The interrupted flow of digestive enzymes in turn prevents the complete digestion of food.

mucus the slimelike secretion of mucous-membrane glands. It may contain discarded tissue cells, leukocytes, water, mineral salts, and mucin, a mixture of glycoprotein molecules. M. is produced in mucous glands and secreted by mucous cells. Adjective: **mucous**.

Müller, Georg Elias /mil′ər/ German psychologist, 1850–1934. As head of the Göttingen laboratory, M. advanced experimental psychology through basic research on Weber's law of psychophysics, color vision, space perception, and memory, which he studied from both an objective and an introspective point of view. See MÜLLER-SCHUMANN LAW; MÜLLER-URBAN WEIGHTS.

Müller, Heinrich /mil′ər/ German histologist, 1866–98. See MÜLLER'S FIBERS.

Müller, Johannes Peter /mil′ər/ German physiologist, 1801–58. M. developed the doctrine of specific energy of nerves, proving that each nerve has its own special sensory or motor function. In his renowned *Handbook of Human Physiology*, 1834–40, he also described the reflex arc, which he had studied in frogs. See SPECIFIC-ENERGY DOCTRINE.

Müller, Max /mil′ər/ German philologist, 1823–1900. See ORIGIN-OF-LANGUAGE THEORIES.

Müller-Lyer, Franz Karl /mil′ər lē′ər/ German psychiatrist and sociologist, 1857–1916. See MÜLLER-LYER ILLUSION; ILLUSION; PERCEPTUAL DISTORTION.

Müller-Lyer illusion /mil′ər lē′ər/ a perceived difference in the length of a line depending upon whether arrowheads at either end are pointing toward each other or away from each other.

Müller-Schumann law a principle that when two items have been closely associated it is difficult to form an association between one of the items and a third item. Also called **paradigm of associative inhibition**.

Müller's fibers a type of glial cell that is elongated and traverses and supports all of the layers of the retina except the rods and cones. Also called **sustenacular fibers**.

Müller-Urban weights a psychophysical procedure for determining the best value of *h*, the measure of precision, by fitting observations to the normal curve. Also called **Müller-Urban weighting; Urban's weights**.

multa loca tenens principle a rule which states that if a drug can substitute for or mimic an action of a natural physiologic agent, it may be able to simulate other natural functions as well. Because of such multiple effects, the administered drug may compete for receptors, enzymes, and other physiological targets.

multiattribute-utility analysis in evaluation research, a method of trying to use the ratings of involved judges to quantify the social utility of a given program. Dimensions relevant to program outcomes are weighted in terms of their compar-

ative social importance; each program is scored on all social-value dimensions. This analysis allows comparison of different social programs.

multiaxial classification a system of classifying mental disorders according to several categories of factors, e.g., social and cultural influences plus etiology and clinical symptoms. See DSM-III.

multidetermination the interaction of several different factors in the etiology of a neurosis.

multidetermined behavior the concept that human behavior is determined by multiple influences, past and present, that interact and interact to produce its current state. The major influences are, in general, genetic, environmental, physiological, and psychological.

multidimensional composed of many dimensions and therefore not a pure reflection of any one. Compare UNIDIMENSIONAL.

Multidimensional Scale for Rating Psychiatric Patients a grouping of psychiatric symptoms into ten representative manifestations, comprising perceptual distortion, conceptual disorganization, motor disturbance, paranoid projection, disorientation, excitement, hostile belligerence, anxious intropunitiveness, retardation and apathy, and grandiose expansiveness. Also called **Lorr Scale**. Abbrev.: **MSRPP**.

multidimensional variable an object of study that represents complex behavior which necessitates (a) analysis of its several dimensions and (b) investigation of the ways in which those dimensions fuse and interrelate. E.g., the study of creative processes represents study of a m.v.

multidisciplinary approach = INTERDISCIPLINARY APPROACH.

multifactorial inheritance the inheritance of a trait, or traits, governed by a myriad of genetic factors from a large population gene pool. Each of the thousands of possible genes in the total pool may act independently but cumulatively to form an individual phenotype. See MULTIFACTORIAL MODEL.

multifactorial model a mode of inheritance that posits that the genetic and environmental causes of a trait constitute a single continuous variable, the **liability**, and if that liability is exceeded, the trait will manifest itself. Also, genetic defects are believed to be due to the adverse effect of many genes, and environmental effects are exerted through many minor events that also have an additive effect. Abbrev.: **MF**. Also see MULTIFACTORIAL INHERITANCE.

multihandicapped the condition of having more than one mental or physical disability. E.g., a patient who suffers from epileptic seizures also may be afflicted with end-stage renal disease, or, as in the classic case of Helen Keller, may be both deaf and blind.

multiinfarct dementia a syndrome whose essential feature is a step-wise patchy deterioration of intellectual functions, due to cerebrovascular disease, with onset earlier than in primary degenerative dementia. This DSM-III category replaces the DSM-II category of "psychosis with cerebral arteriosclerosis," because of evidence of the occurrence of repeated infarcts (small strokes). (DSM-III)

multimodal behavior therapy an approach to psychotherapy initiated by Arnold Lazarus, based on the premise that to produce lasting therapeutic results, it is necessary for the therapist to assess and manipulate where appropriate seven basic modalities of functioning: *b*ehavior, *a*ffect, *s*ensation, *i*magery, and *c*ognition, within the context of *i*nterpersonal relationships and under the influence of *d*rugs or internal chemical reactions. The first letters (in italic type) spell out the acronym BASIC ID. The first five fall within the context of the last two, and the therapist constructs a multimodal profile that assesses the patient's condition, and suggests specific treatment for each problem.

multimodal distribution a distribution curve that has more than one mode.

multimodal theory of intelligence a theory that intelligence is a composite of many abilities.

multimonitored electroconvulsive treatment: See MMECT.

multiparous /-tip'-/ pertaining to a mother (a **multipara**) who has had two or more pregnancies resulting in live births. The pregnancies may be successive or concurrent, as in the case of a birth of twins.

multiple-aptitude test a battery of separate tests designed to measure a wide range of relatively independent functions, and to yield a profile of the subject's abilities in different areas, as contrasted with a single global IQ. Different batteries measure different patterns of abilities; an example is the **Differential Aptitude Test (DAT)**, primarily for use in educational and vocational counseling, and yielding scores on verbal reasoning, numerical ability, abstract reasoning, space relations, mechanical reasoning, clerical speed and accuracy, spelling, and sentence usage.

multiple-base-line design an experimental design in which several items of behavior are assessed before and after an experimental manipulation.

multiple-choice experiment an experiment in which a subject decides which of several possible choices is correct, usually on the basis of a specific cue which must be learned.

multiple-choice test any test in which the subject must make a choice between several answers, of which one is correct or close to being correct.

multiple correlation a correlation estimating the degree of relationship between a target variable and two or more predictors, e.g., the correlation between the amount of anxiety, depression, and stress taken together and used to predict the number of psychosomatic symptoms. Symbol: R.

multiple delusions concurrent delusions, not necessarily interconnected.

multiple-factor pertaining to the concept that in a process being studied more than one variable may be responsible for the observed result.

multiple-factor inheritance the transmission of a genetic trait determined by the combined action of several pairs of genes.

multiple family therapy a form of group psychotherapy in which a family unit meets with two or more therapists at once. See MULTIPLE THERAPY.

multiple identification a manifestation of hysterical seizures in which a patient identifies with two or more persons and acts out their roles as if in a drama. M.i. also occurs in cases of multiple personality.

multiple mothering the use of several warm and caring mother surrogates in a facility for infants, such as a university center for training in home management. Studies indicate that these infants, when tested after adoption, did not differ materially from home-reared children in school achievement, personal and social development and anxiety level, and response to frustration. See KIBBUTZ; MATERNAL DEPRIVATION.

multiple myeloma a progressive and eventually fatal form of cancer involving overproduction of an immunoglobulin protein molecule (**Bence Jones proteins**), bone-marrow blood-cell tumors, and erosion of bones in a punched-out pattern of holes. The round holes frequently develop in the skull and spinal column, leading to pressure on the spinal cord and nerve roots. A further neurologic complication is infiltration of peripheral nerves by amyloid deposits.

multiple myositis: See MYOSITIS.

multiple personality a dissociative disorder in which two or more distinct personalities exist within the individual, each of which is dominant at a particular time. The original personality is unaware of the subpersonalities which are usually of a contrasting character and have their own unique identity, names, and relationships. The transition from one personality to another is sudden and frequently occurs during a period of stress. (DSM-III)

multiple regression a statistical technique for estimating a score from a combination of two or more predictor variables. Stepwise m.r. systematically selects the best predictor, followed by the next best, and so on. Also see REGRESSION ANALYSIS.

multiple reinforcement a reinforcement program using multiple schedules which are changed at random.

multiple-role playing a management, or executive, development technique in which a large group is broken up into smaller groups by having every three persons in alternate rows meet with the three persons directly behind them. Each six-person group is then given the same problem, and the members are assigned roles in a decision-making discussion. The solutions arrived at by each group are then reported to the entire body.

multiple sclerosis a progressive disease of the central nervous system in which patches of myelin are eroded from white matter. Most often affected are the lateral and posterior columns in early stages. As the disease progresses, axons and cell bodies are destroyed, gray matter is invaded, along with optic nerves, cerebrum, pons, midbrain, and cerebellum. Weakness, clumsiness, and visual disturbances are among the first symptoms. Apathy, inattention, and faulty judgment may occur, along with depression or euphoria. The onset of m.s. usually is between the ages of 20 and 40, and, with periods of remission, the disease may continue for as long as 25 years or more. A rapid progression to death from m.s. is rare. The cause is unknown. Abbrev.: **MS**.

multiple-spike recording the recording and analyzing of potentials from rapidly firing neurons using microelectrodes connected to high-speed electromechanical oscillographs, spectral analysis filters, and analog-to-digital computer equipment. Such devices may be used for studies in which spike inputs are recorded at rates in excess of 100 per second.

multiple therapy individual or group psychotherapy in which more than one therapist participates at the same time. Also called **cotherapy; cooperative therapy; dual-leadership therapy; role-divided therapy; three-cornered therapy**.

multiple tics with coprolalia = TOURETTE'S DISORDER.

multiplexing in speech the process of vocal communication whereby several information channels may be functioning independently and simultaneously, utilizing various resonant cavities which are rapidly tuned as needed by neuromuscular control of the tongue, lips, cheeks, and so on. See FORMANTS.

multiplication of personality a schizophrenic phenomenon in which individual psychic functions of the patient's personality become autonomous and are identified as different people within his body. Also see MULTIPLE PERSONALITY.

multiplicity-versus-unity dimension a system of evaluating a work of art in terms of its effects on the viewer, including the degree to which he experiences heightened arousal by complexity or multiplicity factors and lowered arousal by elements of harmony, or unity. Multiplicity in art is believed to be associated with historical periods of political or economic insecurity when tensions are reflected in deformation of art styles.

multipolarity S. R. Slavson's term for the transference in group psychotherapy toward other patients as well as the therapist.

multisensory method an approach to teaching reading and spelling which incorporates the *v*isual, *a*uditory, *k*inesthetic, and *t*actile modalities, often abbreviated as VAKT. See this entry.

Multi-State Information System an automated record-keeping system developed and applied in New York and other states, designed to provide comparative statistics for evaluation of programs and treatment procedures in mental hospitals and community mental-health facilities. Abbrev.:

MSIS. See MENTAL STATUS EXAMINATION REPORT.

multisynaptic arc a neural pathway that involves the routing of an impulse through several synapses. Also called **polysynaptic arc**.

multivariate consisting of many variables, especially in experimental design or correlational analysis.

multivariate analysis a statistical method for testing the effects of a number of variables acting simultaneously.

mummy attitude a term used to describe the immobilized state of a patient in a catatonic stupor.

Munchausen syndrome /muntshou′zən/ a condition characterized by repeated fabrication of clinically convincing symptoms and a false medical and social history. The syndrome was named by R. Asher (1951) after Baron Karl Friedrich Hieronymus von Münchhausen (1720–97), a German soldier-adventurer famous for his tall tales. In DSM-III, the corresponding term is CHRONIC FACTITIOUS DISORDER WITH PHYSICAL SYMPTOMS. See this entry. Also see IMPOSTOR SYNDROME; MALINGERING; PATHOMIMICRY; TOMOMANIA.

mundane realism in experimental psychology, the attempt to design an experiment that corresponds as closely as possible to ordinary "real-world" events. A related term, experimental realism, refers to designing experiments that elicit valid emotional responses even if the events of the experiment do not resemble ordinary occurrences. Also see EXPERIMENTAL REALISM.

Munich Cooperative Model hospital group therapy in which typical intrafamilial conflicts are reproduced. The ward staff observes the sessions and applies its observations and interpretations to patient-personnel interactions, while the patients form autonomous groups for emotional support.

Munsell, Albert Henry American painter, 1858–1918. See MUNSELL COLOR SYSTEM; CHROMA.

Munsell color system a method of color notation devised by Albert H. Munsell for use mainly in science, industry, and technology. The M.c.s. was introduced in 1905 with numerical designations for hues, tint, and shades of color for accurate identification and specification. It has been revised several times.

murder: See HOMICIDAL BEHAVIOR; LUST M.

Murphy, Gardner American psychologist, 1895–1979. See BIOSOCIAL THEORY; CANALIZATION.

Murray, Henry Alexander American psychologist, 1893—. Murray's major contributions were in the fields of personality theory, testing, and diagnosis. Especially important was his theory of "personology," which drew heavily on Freud, but recognized a large number of needs (28 in all) to explain the complex dynamics of behavior; and the Thematic Apperception Test, which is designed to explore individual feelings and reactions related to these needs. SEE ACHIEVEMENT MOTIVATION; AFFILIATIVE NEED;

COGNIZANCE NEED; CONSTRUCTION NEED; COUNTERACTION NEED; DEFENDANCE; DEFERENCE; DOMINANCE NEED; DURANCE; EDWARDS PERSONAL PREFERENCE SCHEDULE; ENDOCATHECTION; ENVIRONMENTAL PRESS; ESTABLISHMENT; EXOCATHECTION; EXPOSITION ATTITUDE; EXTRACEPTION; INTRACEPTIVE SIGNALING; INVIOLATE MOTIVE; LIFETIME PERSONALITY; MOTIVATION; MOTONE; NEED-PRESS THEORY; PERSONOLOGY; PRESS; PRESS-NEED PATTERN; REGNANCY; SECLUSION NEED; SENTIENCE NEED; SUCCORANCE NEED; THEMA; THEMATIC APPERCEPTION TEST; URETHRAL COMPLEX; VERBONE; VISCEROGENIC NEEDS.

muscarine: See PSYCHEDELICS.

muscle contraction the effect of the pull of muscle fibers on the tissues to which they are attached. The pull is due to an electrochemical action in which alternating filaments of actin and myosin, which form muscle fibers, slide in opposite directions, producing an effect of a myriad of muscle fibers that are shorter but thicker. See ISOMETRIC CONTRACTION; ISOTONIC CONTRACTION; MUSCLE FIBER.

muscle fiber a microscopic strand of muscle tissue composed in turn of millions of longitudinally aligned filaments of actin and myosin protein molecules. The actin filaments are attached at intervals to membranes called Z lines. The myosin filaments are arranged in alternate layers with the actin filaments. Also see MUSCLE CONTRACTION.

muscle-reading the technique of interpreting slight involuntary muscle actions by light physical contact with the subject's hands, to detect, e.g., the location of a hidden object.

muscle relaxants agents that act on the central nervous system or its associated structures to reduce muscle tone and spontaneous activity. Although the precise mode of action varies with the drug, m.r. generally act by depressing spinal polysynaptic reflexes, without loss of consciousness. Mephenesin and methocarbamol are commonly prescribed m.r. Meprobamate blocks circuits between the cortex and thalamus without affecting sensory feedback. Benzodiazepines depress limbic-system activity as a means of enhancing skeletal-muscle relaxation. Most skeletal-m.r. also function as minor tranquilizers. Also see RELAXATION THERAPY.

muscle sensation a kinesthetic awareness of movements and tensions in muscles, tendons, and joints.

muscle spindle a collection of muscle fibers enclosed in a fluid-filled capsule of connective tissue which also contains various nerve endings, receptors, and associated tissues.

muscle-tension gradient a measure of the rate of change of muscle tension during performance of a task such as taking a test. The m.-t.g. is measured on an electromyograph.

muscle tonus: See TONUS.

muscular dystrophy a group of genetic diseases marked by painless degeneration of the muscles which gradually weaken and atrophy. Kinds of m.d. include the Duchenne type or progressive m.d., pseudohypertrophic m.d., limb-girdle m.d., facioscapulohumeral m.d. or Landouzy-Déjerine m.d., distal m.d., and ocular m.d. Sometimes two or more forms affect a patient at the same time. Not all forms are totally disabling, but there is no specific cure for m.d. Abbrev.: **MD**.

muscular type a constitutional type characterized by dominance of the muscular and locomotor systems over other body systems. The m.t. corresponds to Kretschmer's athletic type.

musculoskeletal system the combined organ systems of skeletal bones and skeletal muscles, which generally function as a single system in that muscle contractions are required to produce movements of the bones and their associated body tissues.

musical therapy = MUSIC THERAPY.

musician's cramp a symptom of occupational neurosis in which a musician experiences a painful cramp, usually in the arm or hand, which prevents him from performing. The condition is psychogenic and may be a hysterical (conversion) reaction.

musicogenic epilepsy epileptic seizures precipitated by music. See REFLEX EPILEPSY.

music therapy the use of music as an adjunct to psychiatric treatment and rehabilitation. A hospital m.t. program, under the direction of a specially trained therapist, provides a variety of listening and participating experiences adapted to the needs of individual patients, such as an opportunity for nonverbal communication, shared experience, emotional expression, relaxation, and nonthreatening enjoyment. Also called **musical therapy**.

musophobia a morbid fear of mice (from Latin *mus*, "mouse," which is also the root of the word "muscle"; also see -MY-).

mussitation unintelligible muttering, or lip movements without producing speech.

mutagenic having the power to alter the genetic structure of cells, resulting in the production of new forms. See MUTATION.

mutation any change in the genetic material of a species that is permanent and transmissible to future generations. A m. may be produced experimentally or accidentally by exposure to external influences (**mutagens**) such as chemicals or radiation. A m. also may occur spontaneously for no observable cause, as in achondroplastic dwarfism. Also see GENE M.

mutative interpretation an interpretation that penetrates the neurotic vicious circle as the therapist allows some of the id energy to be released through the consciousness as an aggressive impulse directed at the therapist. As the patient gains insight into the problem, more of the infantile material can be recovered through the breach, resulting in a m.i. that produces genuine change.

mutilation: See SELF-M.; GENITAL M.

mutism inability to speak due to physical defect, as

in congenital deafness and impaired speech organs; or voluntary refusal to speak, as in certain religious orders, or as an expression of anger, particularly in children; or involuntary (psychogenic) inhibition of speech as a hysterical symptom which usually expresses hostility or withdrawal from a threatening world, or a symptom of catatonic schizophrenia. Also see AKINETIC M.; ELECTIVE M.

Mutt and Jeff approach an interrogation strategy in which an apparently gentle, friendly inspector (Jeff) is paired with a harsh, ruthless inspector (Mutt) in order to increase the suspect's confidence in the kindly inspector to whom it is hoped he will confess.

muttering delirium a type of delirium in which the patient's speech is marked by slurring, iteration, dysarthria, and perseveration. The patient's movements are dominated by tossing and trembling.

mutuality according to E. Erikson, the capacity to affirm and strengthen oneself and others. M. is a hallmark of maturity. Erikson also uses the term to mean "mutuality of [genital] orgasm with a loved partner . . . with whom one is able and willing to share a mutual trust . . ." (*Childhood and Society*, 1963).

mutually exclusive events two or more events that have no common elements; disjoint events. See DISJOINT SETS.

mutual masturbation masturbation activity in which two or more individuals stimulate each other's genitals at the same time for the purpose of sexual gratification. If it involves two individuals, m.m. is also called **dual masturbation**.

-my-; -myo- a combining form relating to muscle (Greek *mys*, literally "mouse").

myasthenia muscular weakness or fatigability observed in certain diseases such as **m. gravis** but also in depressed or schizophrenic patients. Also see MYOPATHIES.

myasthenic syndrome of Lambert-Eaton = EATON-LAMBERT SYNDROME.

-myc-; -myco-; -mycet- a combining form relating to fungus (Greek *mykes*).

Mycobacterium leprae the disease organism that causes leprosy, or Hansen's disease. The bacterium is a rod-shaped microorganism that is generally prevalent in tropical and subtropical regions throughout the world, including California and the Gulf Coast states of North America. Five subgroups of M.l. have been identified according to immunologic features and types of lesions produced.

mycoplasmas: See T-MYCOPLASMA.

mydriasis an excessive dilatation of the pupil of the eye caused by such drugs as atropine, scopolamine, epinephrine, and cocaine, or the use of phenothiazines or antiparkinsonian medications (**mydriatic drugs**). Also see PARASYMPATHOLYTIC.

mydriatic = PARASYMPATHOLYTIC.

-myel-; -myelo- a combining form relating to the spinal cord or bone marrow (Greek *myelos*).

myelencephalon = MEDULLA OBLONGATA.

myelin a lipid, or fatty, substance that forms a **myelin sheath** around certain nerve fibers, mainly those of the cranial and spinal nerves. M. accounts for the whitish coloration of white matter of the brain, as distinguished from gray matter. Transmission of nerve impulses is generally more rapid in fibers sheathed in m., which is believed to function primarily as an electrical insulator.

myelinated axon a nerve fiber that is covered by a fatty membrane sheath. The fatty membrane contributes to the coloration of neural tissue sometimes identified as white matter.

myelinization the production of myelin around a nerve fiber, a process generally confined to axons of nerves. It develops through a spiral infolding of the surface membrane, or neurilemma, which proliferates outward along the path of the axons after they have become established.

myelin sheath: See MYELIN.

myelitis an inflammation of the spinal cord.

myeloarchitecture the study of the development and distribution of the fiber processes of the nerve cells of the brain, with special emphasis on the myelinated fibers. The development of various areas of the cortex is linked to the stage of life when the myelin sheaths form on the fibers. M. is the counterpart of cytoarchitecture, which deals mainly with the functional distribution of various types of neural cell bodies in the cortex.

myelodysplasia: See OCCULT M.

myelomeningocele a sac containing the spinal cord and the meninges that protrudes from the vertebral area of a patient with spina bifida cystica. The sac usually is closed before birth but postnatally fills with cerebrospinal fluid to protrude from the lumbar, low thoracic, or sacral region of the spine. See MENINGOMYELOCELE.

myelon an alternative name for the spinal cord.

Myers-Briggs Type Indicator a test designed to classify individuals according to their expressed choices between contrasting alternatives in certain categories of traits. The categories include judgment-perception, thinking-feeling, extraversion-introversion, and sensing-intuition. The subject is assigned a type according to the pattern of choices made. Also called **Briggs-Myers Type Indicator**.

myoclonic pertaining to the involuntary movement of voluntary muscles, as observed in the uncontrolled jerking of limbs of persons experiencing an attack of epilepsy.

myoclonic dementia a condition of dementia that is accompanied by sudden, brief, jerking contractions of the muscles. The effects may involve almost any muscles or groups of muscles in nearly any part of the body, including the diaphragm which produces hiccups as a result of myoclonus. M.d. often is associated with Alzheimer-type senile dementia.

myoclonic encephalitis = HYPSARRHYTHMIA.

myoclonic epilepsy = MYOCLONIC SEIZURE.

myoclonic movements spasmodic involuntary muscle contractions that may involve almost any part of the body, depending upon the location of involved neurons. Lesions in the area of the red nucleus are associated with m.m. of the eyes, tongue, palate, larynx, face, and neck muscles. When neck muscles are affected, m.m. cause involuntary nodding of the head. M.m. of the limbs may be caused by a disease of the cerebellum.

myoclonic seizure a severe petit mal seizure characterized by spasmodic muscular contractions on both sides of the body, usually appearing several years after a series of generalized epileptiform attacks in childhood. Also called **myoclonic epilepsy**.

myoclonus rapid, involuntary spasms of skeletal muscles. Myoclonic activity may be normal as when a limb or other part of the body suddenly jerks while falling asleep, but it may also occur on a wider scale in an epileptic attack. The condition may be limited to a group of muscle fibers. In Friedreich's disease, a multiplex form of m. occurs, with muscle spasms or twitchings happening simultaneously or consecutively in unrelated muscle groups. Also see NOCTURNAL M.

myoclonus epilepsy a familial type of grand mal epilepsy that begins in childhood and may affect siblings of the patient. The initial attacks occur as nighttime loss of consciousness, but, after several years, myoclonic contractions of face, trunk, and limb muscles develop with strength enough to throw the patient to the ground. Progressive dementia, dysarthria, and dysphagia replace the attacks in a third stage.

myoelectric arm /mī·ō·ilek′-/ an artificial arm, or prosthesis, that can be manipulated by voluntary nerve impulses. The nerve impulses are received by an electronic transducer which converts them into appropriate movements of the prosthesis through tiny electric motors.

myoesthesis the muscle sense.

myofascia fibrous tissue that surrounds and ensheathes units of muscle tissue. M. helps separate neighboring muscles and reduces friction produced by muscles rubbing against adjacent tissues as the muscles contract and relax.

myoglobinuria the presence of myoglobin in the urine. **Myoglobin** is a substance similar to hemoglobin of the red blood cells and is present in muscle tissue as a physiological means of storing oxygen. Occasionally after physical exertion, normal individuals may excrete myoglobin, which generally is not present in the urine. In patients with disorders such as McArdle's disease, m. may be a common occurrence after physical activity.

myography a diagnostic technique that utilizes an electrical apparatus to record the effects of muscle activity. The principle is similar to that of EEG or EKG recording in that contractile action of the muscle fibers generates a small but measurable electrical discharge. The term also may be applied to a procedure in which a muscle is studied by radiography after the injection of a contrast medium to produce radiopaque images.

myokinetic-psychodiagnosis test a test devised by Mira in which the subject makes drawings of patterns using alternately both the left and right hands. The drawings made by the left hand are presumed to reveal information about the genotype, and the right-hand drawings represent phenotype reactions. The left- and right-hand drawings are compared for diagnostic purposes. The test is administered to both children and adults.

myoneural junction the point of contact between a motor nerve and a muscle. Also called **neuromuscular junction**.

myopathies muscular disorders in which the cause is a deficiency of the muscle-fiber function. The specific cause may be hereditary, metabolic, endocrinal, or infectious. An example is myasthenia gravis, which involves a defect at the junction of the nerve fiber and the muscle fibers. A similar condition may be induced by certain drugs and chemicals used as pesticides. The term usually is employed with another that specifies the type of myopathy or its cause. E.g., **alcoholic myopathy** and **hereditary myopathy** suggest a cause while **ocular myopathy** defines the affected area as the muscles that control eye movements. Also see NEMALINE MYOPATHY; ACUTE ALCOHOLIC MYOPATHY; THYROTOXIC MYOPATHY; MYASTHENIA.

myopia nearsightedness, or closesightedness. M. may be combined with another term to define a specific kind of nearsightedness, e.g., **chromic m.**, for defective color perception of distant objects, **progressive m.**, to denote a gradual loss of accommodation for distant vision associated with aging, and **prodromal m.**, for accommodation changes that permit a return of normal sightedness after a period of m.

myosin: See ACTIN.

myosis an extreme contraction of the pupil, usually due to drugs or disease. Also spelled **miosis**.

myositis a muscle inflammation, particularly involving a voluntary muscle. Kinds of m. include **multiple m. (or polymyositis)**, **m. a frigore**, a muscle inflammation due to exposure to cold temperatures, **m. fibrosa**, an inflammation complicated by formation of fibrous tissue within the muscle, and **m. ossificans**, a condition marked by ossification of the muscle tissue.

myotatic reflexes = STRETCH REFLEXES.

myotenotomy a surgical procedure involving dissection of the tendon of a muscle, usually performed to correct a deformity. M. may be employed to relieve a torticollis condition.

myotonia congenita = THOMSEN'S DISEASE.

myotonic disorders muscular diseases, generally inherited, marked by voluntary muscles that have increased powers of contractility but relax slowly and with great difficulty. The condition often affects the muscles of the hands, as in myotonic dystrophy, or is manifested by general muscle stiffness, e.g., in Thomsen's disease. Dementia or mental retardation often accompany the m.d.

myotonic dystrophy a disorder of myotonia and muscle wasting, usually beginning in the upper part of the body, often accompanied by hypogonadism, cataracts, and heart disease. Males lose their potency and females have no menses or abnormal menses. Age at onset may range from early childhood to adulthood. Some patients are mentally deficient or have personality disorders. Young patients have expressionless faces, an open mouth, and are likely to drool. Also called **dystrophia myotonica; Steinert's disease**.

myotonic pupillary reaction = ADIE'S SYNDROME.

myotypical response the tendency of transplanted muscle tissue to respond as it would in its normal location in the body. Thus, when a salamander leg bud is transplanted to the opposite side of the body, it continues to move in the same patterns as in the original body connection.

myringotomy a surgical incision in the ear drum to enhance drainage following a severe infection, and thus prevent rupture and excessive scar tissue which can impede hearing.

myristic acid: See PSYCHEDELICS.

mysophilia a pathological interest in dirt or filth, often with a desire to be unclean or in contact with dirty objects (from Greek *mysos*, "dirtiness" of body or mind). M. may be expressed as a paraphilia in which the person is aroused sexually by a dirty partner.

mysophobia a morbid fear of contamination by germs or dirt, usually accompanied by compulsive hand-washing, cleaning, or constantly wearing gloves. Also see DIRT PHOBIA.

mysticism a belief in spiritual sources of knowledge and inspiration, and that truth can be reached through intuition and contemplation, and not merely through sense experience.

mystic union the feeling of spiritual identification with God, nature, or the universe as a whole.

M.u. may be a religious experience or, in some cases, a schizophrenic symptom. Also called **unio mystica**. See COSMIC CONSCIOUSNESS; OCEANIC FEELING; COSMIC IDENTIFICATION; COSMIC SENSITIVITY; UNITY AND FUSION; BUDDHISM; ZEN THERAPY; TRANSCENDENTAL MEDITATION; COMMUNION.

Mytelase a trademark for **ambenomium**, an anticholinesterase drug that can be taken orally to relieve the symptoms of myasthenia gravis.

mythological themes a term applied by Jung to the contents of the collective unconscious. Jung believed the whole of mythology could be taken as a projection of the collective unconscious. Also see UFOS.

mythology the study of myths; or the body of myths themselves. In Jung, they represent basic ideas, or archetypes, which are stored in the collective unconscious. Freud compared myths to dreams, which contain hidden meanings, and believed they throw unique light on the cultures from which they stem, and in some instances, as in the Oedipus story, on human nature in general. To use an example from R. Graves, *Adam's Rib*, 1955: The power of the male in Greece is revealed by the legend that Athene was born from the head of Zeus.

mythomania an abnormal interest in myths, and a tendency to fabricate imaginary experiences and incredible stories.

mythophobia a morbid fear of hearing myths or stories.

-myx-; -myxo-: See -MUC-.

myxedema a metabolic disorder that develops in adulthood due to a deficiency of thyroid hormone. The condition is characterized by subnormal heart rate, circulation, and body temperature, and subnormality in most other metabolic activities. The patient tends to be fatigued, listless, and overweight, but may respond to administration of thyroid extract. See CRETINISM.

N

N: See PRIMARY ABILITIES.

n-Ach = NEED FOR ACHIEVEMENT.

Nageotte, Jean /näzhôt'/ French histologist, 1866 —. See BABINSKI-NAGEOTTE SYNDROME.

nail-biting the compulsive habit of chewing on one's fingernails, usually interpreted as a means of discharging inner tension and, in some cases, feelings of hostility. If it is persistent, some observers regard it as a neurotic symptom, a substitute for masturbation, or a fixation at the oral stage of development. Also called **onychophagia; onychophagy.**

naive egotistic orientation a descriptive term sometimes applied to stage 2 of L. Kohlberg's preconventional level of moral reasoning. See PRECONVENTIONAL LEVEL.

naive observer: See PHENOMENAL ABSOLUTISM.

naive realism the act of identifying or equating one's perceptions with reality. Piagetian psychology stresses the child's progress away from n.r. and toward conceptualization and logical reasoning. As conceptualization and reasoning develop, n.r. is irrevocably diminished.

naive subjects: See CONFEDERATES.

Najjar, Victor Assad Lebanese-born American pediatrician, 1914—. See CRIGLER-NAJJAR SYNDROME.

nakedness fear = GYMNOPHOBIA.

Nalline test the use of an injection of Nalline to determine abstinence from opiates, since it precipitates withdrawal symptoms if opiates have recently been used.

nalorphine; naloxone: See NARCOTIC ANTAGONISTS.

name fear = ONOMATOPHOBIA.

naming a type of association disturbance observed in schizophrenia in which the patient relates to the external world solely by naming objects and actions, e.g., naming furniture or other objects in an examining room.

naming area: See SPEECH AREAS.

-nan-; -nano- a combining form meaning (a) extremely small, (b) specifically, 10^{-9}, one thousand-millionth part (from Greek *nanos*, "dwarf").

Nancy School /näNsē'/ a turn-of-the-century group of therapists led by H. Bernheim who believed hypnosis to be a normal phenomenon induced by suggestion, and effective in treating hysterical disorders. See BERNHEIM; LIEBEAULT.

nanism an alternative term for dwarfism, sometimes used to denote dwarfism of glandular origin characterized by an underdeveloped skeleton and an overgrown skull.

nanocephalic dwarfism = SECKEL'S BIRD-HEADED DWARFISM.

nanometer = MILLIMICRON.

nanosomia body type: See PYGMYISM.

Napalkov, A. V. Russian neurophysiologist, fl. 1957, 1962. See NAPALKOV PHENOMENON.

Napalkov phenomenon an unusual conditioned-reflex response observed in phobic patients exposed to a fear stimulus. Instead of exhibiting an immediate fear reaction followed by extinction when unreinforced, the fear increases over a period of time.

naphtha: See PSYCHEDELICS.

narcissism excessive self-love; egocentricity. N. is a common pattern in immature and neurotic individuals, and in some forms of schizophrenia. In psychoanalytic theory, n. stems from an early stage of development in which the child derives pleasure from his own body and its functions, and forms an idealized image of himself. This pattern of self-interest and concern may persist into adulthood. See NARCISSISTIC-PERSONALITY DISORDERS; PRIMARY N.; SECONDARY N.; DISEASE N.; BODY N.

narcissistic character a personality pattern characterized by excessive self-concern and overvaluation of the self.

narcissistic equilibrium a condition in which there is a harmonious balance between the ego and the superego.

narcissistic gain in psychoanalysis, gratification obtained solely from the functions of one's own organs without involving external objects, as in breathing, walking, and thinking.

narcissistic object choice in psychoanalysis, the investment of the libido in one's own ego, or in an individual similar to one's self.

narcissistic oral fixation a persistent tendency to seek gratification from activities involving the mouth, that is, eating, talking, smoking, biting, chewing, sucking. See ORAL EROTICISM; PRIMARY NARCISSISM.

narcissistic-personality disorder a personality disorder with the following characteristics: (a) a long-standing pattern of grandiose self-importance and exaggerated talent and achievements, (b) fantasies of unlimited sex, power, brilliance, or beauty, (c) an exhibitionistic need for attention and admiration, (d) either cool indifference or feelings of rage, humiliation, or emptiness as a response to criticism, indifference, or defeat, and (e) various interpersonal disturbances, such as feeling entitled to special favors, taking advantage of others, and inability to empathize with the feelings of others. (DSM-III)

narcissistic scar a "permanent injury to self-regard" (Freud, *Beyond the Pleasure Principle*, 1920) produced by such experiences as failure, loss of love, and physical deformity. The condition may result in a character disorder manifested by feelings of inadequacy and inferiority.

narcissistic type: See LIBIDINAL TYPES.

narcoanalysis a relatively brief form of psychoanalysis (Horsley, 1936) in which repeated injections of a narcotic drug are administered to establish rapport with the doctor, facilitate exploration and ventilation of feelings, uncover significant childhood experiences, and promote the patient's insight into unconscious forces that underlie his symptoms.

narcocatharsis a technique of narcotherapy in which the patient ventilates repressed feelings and uncovers repressed memories while under the relaxing influence of intravenous sodium Amytal or sodium pentothal.

narcohypnosis the use of narcotic drugs such as sodium Amytal and sodium pentothal as aids in the induction of hypnosis, and as a phase of hypnotherapy.

narcolepsy a disorder consisting of a sudden, irresistible urge to fall asleep. Sleep attacks are usually brief and may occur at any time or in the midst of any activity. Some cases appear to be due to organic conditions such as epidemic encephalitis or a tumor in the hypothalamus; others are apparently psychogenic, and are considered a hysterical (conversion) symptom in which loss of consciousness may be a defense against forbidden sexual or hostile impulses. The attacks often are preceded by hypnagogic illusions similar to REM-sleep dreams and brief periods of a form of paralysis in which the subject wants to move but is unable to do so. The paralysis attacks, which may last only a moment, also may occur on awakening. At other times, the patient may suddenly lose muscle tone and fall or lose his grasp, an event that usually is associated with a startle reaction or an emotional peak of anger or happiness. About ten percent of n. patients experience all of the symptoms. The sleep attacks may occur in a serious situation such as driving an automobile, and are marked by immediate entry into REM sleep without going through the usual initial stages. Some cases can be treated with drugs. Also called **paroxysmal sleep**.

narcolepsy-cataplexy syndrome a symptom pattern consisting of sudden, repeated loss of muscle tone and recurrent sleep attacks, which some investigators believe constitute a single syndrome. See CATAPLEXY; NARCOLEPSY.

narcomania a pathological desire for narcotic drugs to relieve pain or discomfort.

narcosis a state of stupor induced by narcotic drugs such as barbiturates or heroin. See STUPOR. Also see RAPTURE-OF-THE-DEEP SYNDROME; CONTINUOUS N.

narcosuggestion a technique of psychotherapy in which a narcotic drug is injected to facilitate acceptance of suggestions, such as reassurance, made by the therapist. This approach is considered strictly supportive since it does not involve uncovering the unconscious sources of the patient's problems.

narcosynthesis a treatment technique developed by R. R. Grinker and J. P. Spiegel during World War II, in which narcotic drugs (sodium Amytal, sodium pentothal) are injected to stimulate recall of repressed traumas, followed by a "synthesis" of these experiences with the patient's emotional life through discussions in the waking state.

narcotherapy psychotherapy conducted while the patient is in a stuporous or semiconscious state induced by injection of narcotic drugs such as sodium Amytal and sodium pentothal. See NARCOANALYSIS; NARCOSYNTHESIS.

narcotic a drug that produces a state of narcosis, which may be manifested as stupor or insensibility. A n. usually is a substance that is derived from opium alkaloids and has a depressant effect on the central nervous system. However, nonopiate drugs, e.g., alcohol, can also produce a narcotic effect. See N. ANALGESICS.

narcotic addiction a compulsive dependence on narcotic drugs such as barbiturates, codeine, paregoric, heroin, or morphine, with a tendency to increase the dose due to increasing tolerance. Dependence is both psychological and physiological, and withdrawal symptoms are experienced if intake is discontinued. Also called **narcotic dependence**. See OPIOID DEPENDENCE; BARBITURATE OR SIMILARLY ACTING SEDATIVE OR HYPNOTIC DEPENDENCE.

narcotic-analgesic addiction a psychological and physical dependence upon a drug such as morphine that is administered to relieve pain. A sign of n.-a.a. is the need to increase the dosage in order to obtain the same degree of relief. Withdrawal from mild n.-a.a. is marked by perspiration, watery eyes, runny nose, yawning, and sneezing. Cramps, muscle spasms, vomiting, and diarrhea occur in withdrawal from heavy n.-a.a.

narcotic analgesics substances usually but not always derived from opium alkaloids and administered to relieve pain and discomfort. Commonly used n.a. include codeine and morphine, which are opium derivatives used to relieve severe pain and to induce sleep when pain is a cause of inability to sleep; to suppress coughing; to control shock from hemorrhage; and to restrict peristalsis. Synthetic n.a. include methadone, meperidine, and phenazocine. Phenazocine has almost five times the potency of morphine, which is the standard used to measure n.a. efficacy. See OPIUM ALKALOIDS; SYNTHETIC NARCOTICS.

narcotic antagonists drugs that interfere with normal action of narcotics by competing for the same analgesic receptor sites. N.a. are produced by altering the molecular structures of morphine derivatives and are used mainly in treating the severe respiratory depression caused by narcotics. N.a. precipitate immediate severe withdrawal symptoms in narcotics addicts and are not used in the treatment of addiction. The prototype n.a. is **nalorphine**—$C_{19}H_{21}NO_3$—which was introduced in 1941. Other n.a. include **cyclazocine**—$C_{18}H_{25}NO$, **levallorphan**—$C_{19}H_{25}NO$, and **naloxone**—$C_{19}H_{21}NO_4$.

narcotic blockade the inhibition of the euphoric effects of opiates such as heroin by administration of a blocking agent, especially methadone, as maintenance treatment for drug abuse. See METHADONE.

narcotic dependence = NARCOTIC ADDICTION.

narcotic hunger a craving for narcotics, as in opioid dependence, believed to be due to a physiological and psychological need established by long-term use.

Narcotics Anonymous a mutual-support organization for present and former addicts, modeled after Alcoholics Anonymous.

narcotic stupor a state of lethargy or limited mobility and decreased responsiveness to stimulation due to the effects of narcotic drugs. N.s. usually borders on loss of consciousness and may be followed by coma.

narcotism a state of being under the influence of narcotic drugs to the extent that behavior is altered and toxic effects may occur.

narcotization the process of becoming dependent upon narcotics. N. may occur through drug abuse or through the therapeutic administration of narcotic drugs, such as morphine. Physical dependence on narcotics develops as increasingly large doses are required to produce pleasurable effects, and as interruption of regular dosage routine results in a withdrawal syndrome, marked by fever, vomiting, diarrhea, and other symptoms.

-nas-; -naso- a combining form relating to the nose (Latin *nasus*).

nasal a sound produced by letting all or most of the air pass through the nose, e.g., /ng/ in "sing," or /ôN/ in the French word *bon*; also, a letter or letters representing such a sound, e.g., *ng* in "sing," or *n* in "sink."

nasopharynx the portion of the pharynx above the level of the soft palate. An occlusion of the pharynx from the n. occurs during the normal swallowing and speaking process.

National Reference Scale: See ANCHOR TEST.

Native Americans: See BERDACHE; CASSINI LEAVES; CATNIP; CULTURE COMPLEX; DRUG CULTURE; ECHUL; HELLEBORE; INDIAN HEALTH SERVICE; KIMILUE; LAWS OF COLOR PREFERENCE; PEYOTE; POTLACH; RH BLOOD-GROUP INCOMPATIBILITY; TOLOA; WINDIGO; YOPO.

nativism the theory that mental and behavioral, as well as physical, traits are inherited. See NATURE-NURTURE CONTROVERSY.

nativistic theory: See ORIGIN-OF-LANGUAGE THEORIES.

natural aptitude: See APTITUDE.

natural childbirth a method of child delivery that generally eliminates the need for drugs and anesthetics. During the last months of pregnancy, the mother and a partner, usually the husband, learn to work as a team in training the mother to coordinate breathing efforts and relaxations between labor pains. The mother is taught to concentrate on breathing, blowing in and out to keep from pushing, and exercising the muscles needed for pushing when that stage of the process is reached during actual labor. The mother also is taught different postural positions that can be used to make the labor process more comfortable. See LAMAZE METHOD.

natural family planning controlling the number of children in a family by the use of natural birth-control techniques, such as the rhythm method, as opposed to the use of oral contraceptives, IUDs, and similar devices.

natural group a relatively stable group based on a common heritage or a deeply ingrained bond, such as a kinship group or religious cult, as contrasted with transient or loose-knit groups such as crowds or audiences.

natural homosexual period a term sometimes applied to the later latency stage when prepubertal boys seek the company of boys and men, and prepubertal girls often have crushes on each other or on teachers and counselors of the same sex.

naturalistic observation data-collection in a field setting, without laboratory controls or manipulation of variables; an observational method in which the trained observer watches and records the everyday behavior of subjects in their natural environments, e.g., an ethologist's study of the behavior of chimpanzees or an anthropologist's observation of playing children. N.o. is unselective observation under uncontrolled conditions. Also see OBSERVATIONAL METHOD.

natural monism a generalization that all sciences including psychology are ultimately reducible to physics and chemistry, and even chemistry obeys the laws of physics.

Natural Science Reading Test: See ACT ASSESS-MENT.

natural selection a theory proposed by Charles Darwin based on the fact that in nature organisms that can adapt to changing conditions are more likely to survive while individuals or species that are unable to adjust will fail to survive. The concept sometimes is known as a rule of **survival of the fittest**, because of an assumption that physically or intellectually superior individuals are most likely to survive through evolutionary processes.

nature the innate, genetically determined characteristics of an individual, particularly those making up his temperament, body type, and personality. N. is also the phenomena of the universe as a whole. See N.-NURTURE CONTROVERSY. Compare NURTURE.

nature-nurture controversy the long-standing dispute over the relative contributions of hereditary and constitutional factors (nature) and environmental factors (nurture) in the development of the individual and the etiology of abnormal behavior. Nativists emphasize (with Plato and his adherents) the role of heredity, while environmentalists emphasize (with the philosophical empiricists) sociocultural and ecological factors including family attitudes, child-rearing practices, and economic status. Also called **nature-nurture problem; nature-nurture issue**.

nausea gravidarum = MORNING SICKNESS.

Nauta stain a type of silver stain that selectively identifies axons that have been killed or are undergoing degeneration. N.s. allows an investigator to determine which nerve fibers in a histological section were nonfunctional and which target cells were innervated by the killed cells in studies of neuropathology.

nautilus eye the eye of a mollusk that is of particular value in studies of vision because it consists mainly of a spherical cavity lined with photosensitive cells responding to light that enters through a small hole at the top. The mollusk eye thus is virtually a pinhole camera made of living tissue.

nautomania a morbid fear of ships or water which not infrequently affects sailors, and is therefore also referred to as **seaman's mania**.

near-point of convergence the point nearest the eyes that an object will be perceived as a single entity, becoming double if brought closer.

nearsightedness = MYOPIA.

necessary opposition: See ENANTIODROMIA.

Necker, Louis Swiss physicist and mathematician, 1730–1804. See NECKER CUBE.

Necker cube a line drawing of a cube so that all 12 angles can be seen, as if it were transparent. It is an ambiguous figure that fluctuates when viewed from different angles. Also see RUBIN'S FIGURE.

-necr-; -necro- a combining form relating to death (**necrosis**) or dissolution (from Greek *nekros*, "dead body, corpse"). Adjective: **necrotic**.

necromania a morbid preoccupation with corpses, usually including sexual desire for the body, and a morbid interest in funerals, morgues, autopsies, and cemeteries. See NECROPHILIA; TAPHOPHILIA.

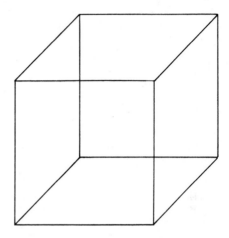

NECKER CUBE. Which face is turned toward you? Does the transparent cube shift?

necromimesis a delusion in which the patient acts as if he were dead because he believes he is.

necrophilia sexual interest in or sexual contact with dead bodies (literally, "love of corpses'). It is a perversion, or paraphilia, that appears to be confined almost completely to men, who are frequently psychotic. In some cases they may kill the victim themselves, but more frequently they remove female (or male) corpses from graves. The **necrophile** usually has no interest in normal sexual relations. See ATYPICAL PARAPHILIA; KATASEXUALITY.

necrophilic fantasies male (and, rarely, female) fantasies about viewing or having intercourse with a corpse of the opposite or the same sex as a means of achieving sexual excitement. Such fantasies are sometimes stimulated by prostitutes who satisfy necrophilic clients by simulating a lifeless appearance.

necrophobia a morbid fear of corpses; also, the fear of death. See THANATOPHOBIA.

necropsy = AUTOPSY.

necrosis; necrotic: See -NECR-.

need an internal condition of tension generated by an unsatisfied desire, urge, or wish, or an organic state of deprivation. Examples are the need for love, attention, affiliation, care, food, water, or sexual excitement. See N.-HIERARCHY THEORY; N.-PRESS THEORY; VISCEROGENIC NEEDS.

need arousal a motivational technique used primarily by propagandists, advertisers, and politicians, in which an appeal is made to the public's actual needs, such as the desire for status, health, money-saving, beauty, or security.

need-fear dilemma a conflicting set of conditions facing certain schizophrenics who need some structured control of their disorganized psyche yet have an aversion to external control or influence.

need for achievement according to McClelland, a relatively stable personality trait that is rooted in the experiences of middle childhood, and which motivates the individual to undertake tasks in which there is a reasonable probability of success and to avoid tasks that are too easy because not challenging, or too difficult because of fear of failure. Abbrev.: **n-Ach**.

need for approval a psychological need for recognition and acceptance by others, which is usually an important ingredient of self-worth. One expression of this need is the tendency to portray one's thoughts and attitudes as conforming to socially "correct" or desirable views.

need for punishment a conscious or unconscious need to be punished as a means of relieving a sense of real or fancied guilt. Some individuals feel compelled to commit crimes in which apprehension and conviction are certain. Similarly, children frequently persist in naughty behavior until they are punished, after which they appear relieved. See ACCIDENT PRONENESS.

need gratification = NEED REDUCTION.

need-hierarchy theory a theory that all human behavior is motivated by a never-ending series of needs which can be arranged in hierarchical order, starting with (a) basic physiological needs (food, water, oxygen, and the like) and progressing to (b) safety needs (protection against danger), (c) social needs (belonging, friendship, love, acceptance), (d) ego needs (self-confidence, achievement, knowledge, status, respect), and (e) self-actualization (developing one's potentialities); and beyond this range, one could place a spiritual need, (f) transcendence, the ultimate human need for higher states of consciousness beyond the quest for identity and actualization (Maslow; McGregor). Also called **hierarchy-of-needs theory**.

needle fear = BELONEPHOBIA.

need-persistent response a term used by S. Rosenzweig to characterize a reaction to frustration in which the individual focuses on the solution to a problem as contrasted with extrapunitive, ego-defensive, or other responses. See ROSENZWEIG PICTURE-FRUSTRATION STUDY.

need-press method a system of analyzing and scoring each sentence of the stories told by the subject in responding to the Thematic Apperception Test, as a means of evaluating the needs of the hero and the press of environmental factors to which he is exposed.

need-press theory H. A. Murray's explanation of behavior dynamics in terms of fundamental viscerogenic and psychogenic needs, and the stimuli and situations (presses) which are capable of arousing these preexistent needs. E.g., a piece of fruit appears desirable only when we are hungry, and the need for achievement is felt primarily when we are in a competitive situation. See MURRAY.

need reduction the reduction of a need by consummatory behavior. Also called **need gratification**.

needs assessment a term frequently applied to the identification of mental-health needs of a community, although it can also be applied to all types of needs, including the needs of an individual or group of any size. **Community n.a.** is difficult, and many methods such as household surveys and case-finding surveys of the total population fail to produce reliable results. Two other methods are more effective: canvassing the opinions of local residents and community agencies concerning community problems and the need for additional services; and airing of views on mental-health-related problems and needs in public forums. In evaluation research, n.a. means also deciding upon priorities among needs, a need being defined as a condition in which there is a discrepancy between an acceptable state of affairs and an observed state of affairs.

need tension the emotional tension associated with a need.

negation in the two-word stage of language development, the use of a negative construction to deny or contradict a statement or suggestion.

In a different sense, the term is equivalent to DENIAL. See this entry.

negation insanity: See INSANITY OF NEGATION.

negative acceleration a reduction in the rate of change or development in a given activity or function as a result of practice, e.g., a loss in learning. Compare POSITIVE ACCELERATION.

negative adaptation a gradual loss of sensitivity or weakening of response due to prolonged stimulation.

negative afterimage: See AFTERIMAGE.

negative ambition Theodore Reik's term for a type of masochistic behavior marked by avoiding competition, missing every opportunity for success, and following the line of maximum resistance.

negative attitudes in counseling, the client's feelings of rejection or disapproval of the counselor, counseling process, another person, object, or the client himself. Compare POSITIVE ATTITUDES.

negative diagnosis the identification of a disorder by excluding possible alternatives. Also called **wastebasket diagnosis**.

negative doubles: See FREGOLI'S PHENOMENON.

negative cathexis repulsion toward an object, person, or idea.

negative discriminative stimulus a stimulus that is not associated with a reinforcer and is distinct from the discriminative stimulus. If the experimental subject responds to the n.d.s. as though it were equivalent to the discriminative stimulus, reinforcement is not delivered. Abbrev.: S°; $S^\triangle$. Compare DISCRIMINATIVE STIMULUS.

negative eugenics: See EUGENICS.

negative feedback a signal from a machine or sensory receptor to reduce or arrest a function, e.g., shutting off a boiler or removing one's hand from a hot plate.

negative hallucination the failure to see a person or object while looking directly at it, as in failing to perceive a certain person in a group in response to hypnotic suggestion.

negative incentive an environmental object or condition that constitutes an aversive stimulus away from which an organism directs its behavior, e.g., extreme cold. A n.i. causes the organism to engage in avoidance behavior. Also see INCENTIVE. Compare POSITIVE INCENTIVE.

negative induction an increase in inhibition due to the effects of a preceding excitation (Pavlov).

negative Oedipus complex a reversed Oedipus complex: The son desires the father and regards the mother as rival, or the daughter is attached to the mother and regards the father as rival. Also called **inverted Oedipus complex.**

negative practice the technique in which an error is intentionally repeated for the purpose of overcoming it.

negative reinforcement a stimulus or stimulus situation that, when withdrawn or discontinued after a response, enhances the strength of that response and increases the probability of its recurrence in the same or a similar situation. E.g., the termination of shock following an animal's correct response is a n.r. Also called **negative reinforcer.** See REINFORCEMENT. Compare POSITIVE REINFORCEMENT.

negative response an abient response. See ABIENCE.

negative reward a stimulus or stimulus situation that occurs following a response or response sequence that represents a failure to perform at the expected level, e.g., a failing grade. A n.r. acts to lessen the probability that the given response will recur. It is not synonymous with negative reinforcement.

negative-state-relief model the hypothesis that helping behavior is utilized by some people in stress situations and periods of boredom and inactivity to avoid or escape negative moods.

negative suggestion a statement intended to deter or suppress a feeling, thought, or action on the part of another person.

negative tele: See TELE.

negative therapeutic reaction in psychoanalysis, an increase in neurotic behavior after a period of successful treatment. It is usually interpreted as a form of resistance due to a sense of guilt which has established a masochistic need for suffering. See SUPEREGO RESISTANCE.

negative transfer a process in which previous learning obstructs or interferes with present learning. E.g., tennis players learning racquet ball must often "unlearn" their tendency to take huge, muscular swings with the shoulder and upper arm. Compare POSITIVE TRANSFER.

negative transference in psychoanalysis, displacement to the therapist of anger or hostility experienced toward the parents or other significant individuals during childhood.

negative tropism automatic movement of an organism away from a source of stimulation.

negativism persistent resistance to the suggestions or requests of others. The reaction is considered a healthy expression of self-assertion between the ages of 18 months and four years; it is also common during adolescence. In catatonic schizophrenics, it may take the form of mutism or refusal of food or care, and is considered an expression of a need to oppose or withdraw from a threatening world; and in senile patients it is usually a regression to childish ways of expressing anger or gaining attention. Also called **command n.** See ACTIVE N.

negativistic response: See NEGATIVISM.

negotiation with God: See WIDOWHOOD CRISIS.

Nelson-Denny Reading Test: See DIAGNOSTIC EDUCATIONAL TESTS.

nemaline myopathy a congenital form of myopathy marked by the occurrence of microscopic threadlike structures throughout the fibers of the affected muscle tissue and manifested by hypotonia and generalized muscle weakness. See MYOPATHIES.

Nemiah, John Case American psychiatrist, 1918 —. See FREE-FLOATING ATTENTION.

neobehavioral viewpoint in counseling, an approach based at least in part on principles of learning. The explicit assumption is that the client's behavior is learned and that effective counseling must teach, model, or somehow impart more adaptive interpersonal patterns.

neobehaviorism a psychological approach that emphasizes the role of response and accepts molar constructs and Gestalt concepts, which some traditional behaviorists reject.

neocerebellum a dorsal portion of the cerebellum containing fibers that communicate with nuclei of the pons.

neocortex the part of the cerebral cortex that is assumed to be the most recent evolutionary stage of brain development in mammals. Also called **isocortex.**

neo-Freudian a psychoanalyst who accepts Freud's major doctrines, but with his own modifications. The term usually does not apply to Freud's contemporaries who broke away from his school in the early days, e.g., Adler. Neo-Freudians include Horney, Sullivan, and Fromm, among others. Also see CULTURALISTS.

neographism the creation of new words in writing. It is a form of neologism.

neologism a new word, such as "astronaut," coined for a purpose, or for its own sake. In psychiatry, neologisms are most often found in schizophrenia, and are generally combinations of two or more words or parts of words. Their meaning is usually highly obscure; nevertheless, they can sometimes be used as clues to the patient's inner conflicts. For an example, see CONDENSATION. Also see PORTMANTEAU N.

neologistic jargon unintelligible speech containing a mixture of inappropriate words and bizarre expressions coined by the speaker, as in the following example from Cameron, 1947: "the criminal is a birth murder because that makes him a double. . . . a birth murder is a murder that turns a cut donator extra into a double daughter-son." Also called **neologistic paraphasia**. See WORD SALAD.

neomnesis /nē·omnē′sis/ memory or recollection of the recent past.

neonatal asphyxia a condition of inadequate flow of oxygenated blood to the brain and other vital tissues because of acute blood loss or failure to breathe at the time of birth. N.a. is associated with prematurity, multiple births, prolapsed umbilical cord, maternal bleeding, maternal hypotension, or Caesarean delivery. Failure to provide immediate resuscitation can result in brain damage.

neonatal period the period from birth to approximately one month of age.

neonate the newborn infant. See NEONATAL PERIOD.

neonate differences marked differences among newborns in general personality and specific behavior such as excitability, response to noise, and vigor of cries.

neophasia a complex language system with its own vocabulary and rules of grammar invented by certain schizophrenia patients.

neophobia a morbid fear of change or of anything new, unfamiliar, or strange. Also called **kainophobia; kainotophobia**.

neoplasm literally, a new growth. The term may be applied to a benign tumor but generally is used to identify a cancerous growth, or malignant tumor. A n. usually grows rapidly by cellular proliferation but generally lacks structural organization. A **malignant n**. usually is invasive, destroying neighboring normal tissues, but like a **benign n**. it also may damage neighboring tissues by compression. Adjective: **neoplastic**.

neopsychic: See ADULT-EGO STATE.

neosleep = NREM SLEEP.

neospinothalamic pathway a component of the lemniscal system with fibers that originate in the dorsal horn, cross over to the ventrolateral tracts on the opposite sides of the spinal cord, join the medial lemniscus at the medulla and continue into the thalamus.

neostigmine bromide $C_{12}H_{19}BrN_2O_2$—a cholinergic drug used in the treatment of myasthenia gravis and glaucoma.

neostriatum a portion of the corpus striatum that evolved in the relatively recent past and includes the putamen and the caudate nucleus.

neoteny /nē·ot′ənē/ in psychology and anthropology, the process of growing young instead of growing old (Ashley Montagu, *Growing Young*, 1981); in zoology, sexual maturation in the larval state (from Greek *neos*, "new," and *teinein*, "to stretch"). Adjective: **neotenous**.

-nephr-; -nephro- a combining form relating to the kidney (Greek *nephros*).

nephrectomy the surgical procedure of removing a kidney. The excision may be made through the abdominal wall, a procedure called **abdominal n.**

or **anterior n.**, through an incision in the loin, an operation termed a **lumbar n.** or **posterior n.**, or through the side of the body, a procedure termed a **paraperitoneal n**.

nephritis: See GLOMERULONEPHRITIS; KIDNEY DISEASE; INTERSTITIAL N.

nephrogenic diabetes insipidus a form of diabetes in which the kidney is unable to produce a normal concentration of urine because the kidney tubules do not respond to the stimulus of the antidiuretic hormone. The pituitary hormone production is normal, but it does not cause the kidney to reabsorb excess water. The n.d.i. patient drinks enormous amounts of water and excretes huge volumes of dilute urine. The disorder can be critical for an infant that cannot communicate his thirst and therefore suffers water depletion leading to brain damage and mental retardation before the cause may be diagnosed.

nephron a functional unit of the kidney consisting of a renal corpuscle and the associated tubules. Each normal human kidney contains about 1,000,000 n. units, each of which filters most of the fluid and dissolved substances from the blood, then reabsorbs some of the fluid and minerals to reconstitute a purified blood while the discarded products are excreted as urine.

nephrosclerosis: See KIDNEY DISEASE.

Neri, V. Italian physician, fl. 1924. See BARRÉ-LIÉOU SYNDROME (also called **Neri-Barré syndrome**).

nerve a threadlike structure (Latin *nervus*, "sinew, cord") composed of fibers that convey electrochemical signals between organs or body areas and between the external and internal environments of the body. Kinds of n. include sensory, motor, autonomic, inhibitory, and excitatory.

nerve block the blocking of nerve impulses by drugs (e.g., anesthetics) or mechanical means.

nerve cell: See NEURON.

nerve current = NERVE IMPULSE.

nerve deafness: See SENSORINEURAL HEARING LOSS.

nerve ending any of a variety of terminals for a nerve fiber, such as annulospiral or flower-spray endings in muscle spindles, basket endings, Krause end bulbs, Meissner corpuscles, and free nerve endings.

nerve-energy doctrine = SPECIFIC-ENERGY DOCTRINE.

nerve fiber a long hairlike projection, e.g., an axon, extending from the cell body of a neuron; also, loosely, the neuron itself.

nerve impulse an electrochemical wave propagated along a neuron or chain of neurons; the means of receiving and transmitting signals in the nervous system. Also called **nerve current; nervous current; nervous impulse; neural current; neural impulse**.

nerve pathway = NEURAL PATHWAY.

nerve root the portion of a sensory or motor nerve that is connected directly to the brain or spinal cord, e.g., cranial or spinal nerves. Dorsal roots are sensory; ventral roots are motor.

nervism a Pavlovian term for the concept that all body functions are controlled by the nervous system.

nervous breakdown a lay term for mental disorder of any type, neurotic or psychotic, that has a sudden onset and produces acute distress.

nervous current = NERVE IMPULSE.

nervous energy a common term for a state of intense nervous activity or drive.

nervous exhaustion a popular term for a state of severe fatigue due to emotional strain. Also see NEURASTHENIA.

nervous habit a common term for stereotyped tension-reducing behavior, e.g., nail-biting or tics.

nervous hunger an urge to eat as a means of reducing anxiety and gratifying frustrated impulses, derived according to psychoanalysis from the oral incorporative stage of infantile development.

nervous impulse = NERVE IMPULSE.

nervousness a popular term for a state of restless tension and emotionality with a tendency to tremble and feel apprehensive.

nervous system the system of nerve tracts, cells, and receptors, which, with the endocrine organs, coordinates activities of the organism in response to signals perceived from the internal and external environments. The n.s. is sometimes considered in terms of its divisions, such as the CENTRAL N.S., PERIPHERAL N.S., or AUTONOMIC N.S. See these entries. Also see THIRD N.S.; CONCEPTUAL N.S.

nervous tissue the cell bodies and fibrous processes responsible for the various nervous-system functions. The neuroglia sometimes is included.

nervous vomiting vomiting that is functional and psychogenic, representing an expression in organ language of a desire to reject a hated idea or object. The condition occurs most commonly in young women as a physiological symbol of the idea that they "cannot stomach this situation."

nest-building a form of parental behavior observed mainly in birds and mammals. The forms of n.-b. vary widely, but generally all are associated with hormonal activity in the female, the amount of light, the temperature, and the presence of offspring. N.-b. in nonpregnant female mammals can be stimulated by introducing recently born members of the species into the lair.

net fertility the number of offspring of carriers of a specific genetic trait who reach the age category in which the trait is expressed.

network a sociometric concept employed by J. L. Moreno, who maintained that psychological networks are formed when the parts, or "social atoms," form complex chains of interrelations which shape social tradition and public opinion either spontaneously or through propaganda. The term also denotes interactions and re-lationships in a patient's environment which, according to S. H. Foulkes, play an important part in the production of psychiatric disorder. See SOCIOMETRY; N. THERAPY; SOCIAL-N. THERAPY; COMMUNICATION NETWORKS; PSYCHOLOGICAL N.

network-analysis evaluation in evaluation research, a method of studying networks of services from the vantage point of either agencies within a system or the flow of service recipients through the system. System effectiveness is defined by looking at a person's progress through the network. The proposal to apply network evaluation is significant in that it provides a conceptual framework for viewing the institution in the context of the larger system.

network biotaxis the pattern of human or animal stimulation on which the individual's fabric of interrelationships is based. Through the n.b. process, individuals influence behavior of others and are in turn influenced by the same contacts. The term applies also to the process whereby tissue cells arrange themselves in structural patterns within an organ.

network therapy a treatment approach in which an attempt is made to involve not only family members but other relatives, friends, and neighbors as sources of emotional support and possible vocational opportunity. The technique is used primarily to prevent rehospitalization of schizophrenic patients now living in the community. Also see SOCIAL-N.T.

Neumann, Isidor Edler von Heilwart /noi'män/ Austrian dermatologist, 1832–1906. See STEVENS-JOHNSON SYNDROME (also called **Neumann's aphthosis**).

-neur-; -neuro- a combining form relating to nerves or the nervous system (from Greek *neuron*, "sinew"). Adjective: **neural**.

neural arc the nerve pathway usually followed by a nerve impulse from a receptor to an effector. In the reflex arc a sensory neuron or bundle of neurons is connected directly to a motor neuron or neurons; in learned behavior the connections are more complex.

neural circuitry the pathways of nervous impulses from receptor to effector, including connector neurons.

neural conduction the passage of a nerve impulse along nerve fibers, from neuron to neuron.

neural crest a ridgelike area atop the embryonic neural plate that develops into the spinal ganglia and sympathetic nervous system.

neural current = NERVE IMPULSE.

neural excitation a state of activity or irritability, produced in a nerve fiber by stimulation.

neural fibril a component of the cytoplasm of a neuron. It is composed of ultramicroscopic filaments and tubules. Their true function has not been proved satisfactorily, and earlier theories about their role as conducting elements have not been supported by experimental evidence. Also called **neurofibril**.

neural fold the tissue layer on either side of the

embryonic neural plate that grows up and over the neural groove to enclose it.

neuralgia pain that may be recurrent, sharp, and spasmodic, occurring along a nerve or a group of nerves. The condition may be the result of injury or infection, or be due to causes that cannot be identified with any organic disorder.

neural groove a fissure in the embryonic neural plate that develops into the neural tube, whose walls evolve into the central nervous system.

neural impulse = NERVE IMPULSE.

neural induction the influence of a neuron or group of neurons on another, producing either positive or negative induction effects.

neural irritability a property of nerve tissue that makes it sensitive to stimulation and capable of responding by transmitting electrical impulses. It is dependent on polarization of ions on either side of the cell membrane.

neural parenchyma the essential functioning tissue of the nervous system as distinguished from the structural elements.

neural pathway any route followed by a nerve impulse through the nervous system. A n.p. may consist of a simple reflex arc or a complex but specific routing such as that apparently required by an impulse transmitting a specific wavelength of sound from the cochlea to the brain. Also called **nerve pathway**.

neural plate a primitive neuroectodermal region on the back surface of the embryo that develops gradually into the central nervous system. The n.p. is the first structural sign of the human nervous system and appears in the first days of embryonic life. The broad front end of the n.p. eventually becomes the brain while the rear part develops into the spinal cord. Also called **neuroplate**. Also see NEURULATION.

neural reinforcement the strengthening of a response by the simultaneous activity of a second response.

neural retina: See DETACHED RETINA.

neural reverberation: See REVERBERATORY CIRCUITS.

neural transmission the mechanism whereby a stimulus causes a release of a chemical transmitter substance or change of electrical potential, or both, that propels a nerve signal or impulse along a neural pathway.

neural tube a primitive nervous-system organ that takes shape as a longitudinal ectodermal tube in the middle of the back of a vertebrate embryo during the first days after formation of the zygote. It is formed from the neural folds which curl over and fuse. The cavity of the n.t. is retained in the ventricles of the brain and the central canal of the spinal cord when they are formed. Many of the congenital defects of the nervous system, e.g., spina bifida, originate at this stage of development. Also see NEURULATION.

neurasthenia a neurotic condition marked by fatigue, debility, insomnia, aches, and pains (from Greek *neurastheneia*, "nerve weakness"). The term originated in the 19th century with George Miller Beard, who believed these symptoms were due to exhaustion, primarily from overwork. The term is rarely used today, and the condition is now attributed primarily to emotional conflicts, tensions, frustrations, and other psychological factors. See ASTHENIC PERSONALITY; HYPOCHONDRIASIS; TRAUMATIC N.

neurasthenic helmet a type of neurasthenic headache in which the person feels as if his head was encased in a tightly fitted helmet.

neurasthenic neurosis a type of neurosis in which the patient experiences feelings of weakness, is easily fatigued, and otherwise shows signs of neurasthenia.

neuraxis the hypothetical axis formed by a line running through the spinal cord and brainstem.

neurilemma a thin membrane that covers the myelin sheath of axons. It is found mainly on white-matter fibers outside the central nervous system. The n. is composed of Schwann cells, which help in the repair or regeneration of damaged axons. Only axons surrounded by a n. appear capable of regeneration. Also called **neurolemma**.

neurilemmoma = SCHWANNOMA.

neurin the protein substance of nerve tissue; also, a term used by W. McDougall for the hypothetical energy involved in nerve excitation.

neuroanatomy the study of relationships between the various parts of the nervous system and the tissues and organs innervated by the nerve fibers.

neuroarthritism a predisposing condition that involves both nervous and rheumatoid or gouty diseases.

neuroaxonal degeneration = SEITELBERGER'S DISEASE.

neurobiotaxis the factors that influence growth of a nerve fiber toward the tissue it will innervate, an action that occurs millions of times during embryological development. The concept has been expanded to explain at least a part of the learning process as neuron-connecting points grow toward each other in response to a conditioning stimulus.

neuroblastoma a type of cancer that develops from immature nerve cells that resemble the primitive neural cells of the embryo. The n. cells are very small with very large nuclei, often arranged in sheets, clumps, or cords. About one-third of the tumors develop in the adrenal-gland region.

neurochemistry the branch of neuropharmacology and neurophysiology that deals with the roles of atoms, molecules, and ions in functions of nervous systems. Because chemical substances in a physiological system obey the same laws of nature as in other environments, activities of neurotransmitters, drugs, and other molecules in the nervous system can be explained in terms of basic chemical concepts.

neurocirculatory asthenia = DA COSTA'S SYNDROME.

neurodermatitis any form of skin inflammation that is associated with an emotional disorder. An example is urticaria (hives, or nettle rash) marked by redness and wheals on the skin that appear in periods of psychological stress in some individuals.

neuroeffector transmission the transmission of nerve impulses to the two general types of effectors, the muscles and glands. N.t. may involve stimulation through a synaptic connection or through the release of chemical transmitters, acetylcholine, epinephrine, or norepinephrine. Synaptic transmitters are found in skeletal muscles, chemical transmitters in smooth muscles.

neuroendocrinology the study of the relationship between the nervous system, especially the brain, and the endocrine system.

neuroethology a branch of psychology in which the emphasis is on the relationship between neurobiology and behavior. N. areas of research include small neural networks, visual discrimination, and the neural control of activity and motivation.

neurofibril = NEURAL FIBRIL.

neurofibrillary degeneration a pathological process of atrophy of nerve fibrils in the fifth and sixth decades of life that is associated with senile dementia and Alzheimer's disease. A secondary effect of the process, sometimes called alzheimerization of brain tissue, is reduced blood flow to the cerebrum, resulting in brain hypoxia. Abbrev.: **NFD**.

neurofibroma; neurofibromatosis: See VON RECKLINGHAUSEN'S DISEASE.

neurogenic pertaining to a condition or event that is caused or produced by a component of the nervous system.

neurogenic drive the automatic functioning of an organ or organ system because of a rhythm or pattern of discharges by nerve tissue. N.d. rhythms control automatic contractions and relaxations of heart-muscle fibers and the muscles that operate the respiratory system.

neuroglia /nyo͞orog′lē-ə/ or /nyo͞orōglī′ə/ CNS cells that serve to support other tissues. There is some inconclusive evidence that n. cells are also directly involved in nervous-system functions, based in part on recordings of electrical potentials in the cells. Also called **glia** /glē′ə/ or /glī′ə/.

neuroglial sclerosis = CHASLIN'S GLIOSIS.

neurogram an automatic or habitual response.

neurohumor a substance, such as epinephrine or serotonin, that is liberated at nerve endings to stimulate activity in a neighboring neuron, muscle cell, or gland. The specific chemical agents that transmit neural impulses across synapses and junctions at nerve endings are **neurohumoral**.

neurohypophysis the posterior pituitary gland, the portion of the hypophysis connected by the infundibulum to the hypothalamus. Hormones secreted by the n. are vasopressin, also called

the antidiuretic hormone, and oxytocin. Compare ADENOHYPOPHYSIS.

neurolemma = NEURILEMMA.

neuroleptic malignant syndrome a rare complication of therapy with phenothiazines characterized by hypertonicity, pallor, dyskinesias, hyperthermia, and pulmonary congestion, sometimes terminating in death. See PHENOTHIAZINE DEATH; AUTOPSY-NEGATIVE DEATH.

neuroleptics a group of drugs that are major tranquilizers or antipsychotic medications. They usually control psychomotor activity. N. are used mainly to treat manic states and schizophrenias. In addition to butyrophenones and phenothiazines, n. include Rauwolfia derivatives, thioxanthines, and certain opium alkaloid derivatives. See BUTYROPHENONES; PHENOTHIAZINES; RAUWOLFIA DERIVATIVES; THIOXANTHINES. Also see ANXIOLYTICS; ANTIPARKINSON DRUGS.

neuroleptic syndrome the series of effects observed in subjects who have been given neuroleptic drugs. The n.s. is characterized by reduced motor activity and emotionality, an indifference to external stimuli, and a decreased ability to perform tasks that require good motor coordination. In high-dose cases, the subject may become cataleptic.

neurological amnesia a loss or impairment of memory due to disease or injury that affects the nervous system. It includes AUDITORY AMNESIA (and WERNICKE'S APHASIA), TACTILE AMNESIA (and ASTEREOGNOSIS), VERBAL AMNESIA, and VISUAL AMNESIA. See these entries. Also see APHASIA.

neurological evaluation analysis of the data gathered by an examining physician of a patient's sensory, motor, and coordination responses. The n.e. includes speech and behavior, muscular strength, gait, deep reflexes, tests of cranial nerves, pain, temperature, discriminative senses, and sensory-organ responses.

neurological examination a systematic study of the patient's central and peripheral nervous systems covering sensory and motor functions, such as reflexes, as well as tests of his attention, levels of consciousness, memory, cognitive and related cortical functions, and observation of his behavior in general.

neurological impairment a condition marked by disruption of the nervous system or a part of the system as a result of disease, injury, or effects of a drug or other chemical. Alzheimer's form of presenile dementia, parkinsonism, and Wernicke's encephalopathy are examples of n.i.

neurology a branch of medicine that deals with the nervous system in both the normal and diseased states. The diagnosis and treatment of diseases of the nervous system is called clinical n.

neuromelanin a dark pigment similar to the pigment responsible for skin color that occurs in certain neurons of the nervous system. N. is found in cells of the locus caeruleus and the substantia nigra.

neurometrics a method of gaining quantitative data about brain functioning developed by E. Roy John and associates, involving the use of computer techniques in the analysis of EEGs and evoked potentials. Mathematical analysis of data obtained from subjects with behavioral symptoms, developmental problems, and neurologic dysfunctions yields objective, operational categories which are used in identifying different types of brain functions in individuals whose behavior manifestations are similar.

neuromuscular disease any pathologic condition that involves the nerves and muscles. Examples of a n.d. include the muscular dystrophies, myasthenia gravis, and the myopathies. A relatively common transient type of n.d. is cramps.

neuromuscular junction = MYONEURAL JUNCTION.

neuromuscular system = MOTOR SYSTEM.

neuromyelitis optica = DEVIC'S DISEASE.

neuron a nerve cell; any conducting cell of the nervous system, consisting of a cell body with nucleus and a varying number of fiber processes extending from the cell body. In addition to conductivity, a common characteristic of neurons is irritability. Also spelled **neurone**. Also see UNIPOLAR N.; BIPOLAR N.; -NEUR-.

neuronal lipidosis a disorder in which the nerve-cell cytoplasm is distended because of lipid accumulation. Variations of the condition have been observed, some with sphingolipid accumulation and some without. Most patients have ocular abnormalities and develop neurologic impairment with dementia, the age of onset varying from infancy to adulthood. Kinds of n.l. include Batten's disease, juvenile amaurotic idiocy, Kufs' disease, and Bielschowsky-Jansky disease.

neurone = NEURON.

neuroparalytic ophthalmia: See OPHTHALMIA.

neuropathic arthropathy a chronic progressive degeneration of a stress-bearing joint and a concurrent loss of sensation in the joint. More than a dozen possible causative factors have been identified, including tabes dorsalis, diabetes mellitus, syringomyelia, spina bifida with meningomyelocele, leprosy, and congenital or hereditary diseases, e.g., Riley-Day syndrome. The knee is involved most often, and the symptoms frequently are misdiagnosed as those of osteoarthritis. The joint may be swollen and deformed, and it may be filled with loose pieces of cartilage and bone chips. Although n.a. usually is painless, the patient may experience severe pain as the disease progresses. Also called **Charcot joint**.

neuropathic traits primary behavior disorders such as nail-biting, enuresis, finger-sucking, sleepwalking, nightmares, fear of darkness, and anxiety.

neuropathology the study of diseases of the nervous system. N. may include examination of the brain or other relatively large parts of the system for gross defects that may be visible to the naked eye, studies of tissue cells under a microscope, and laboratory analysis of the neurochemistry of the tissues.

neuropharmacology the scientific study of the effects of drugs on the nervous system.

neurophrenia a seldom used term for behavior disorder that can be attributed to an impairment of the central nervous system.

neurophysiology a branch of biology and medicine that is concerned with the normal and abnormal activity of nervous-system functions, including the chemical activity of individual nerve cells.

neuropil a weblike synaptic network of axon and dendrite filaments that forms the bulk of the gray matter of the central nervous system. The cell bodies of the neurons are embedded in the net of fibers.

neuroplate = NEURAL PLATE.

neuroplexus a network of nerve fibers, particularly autonomic-nervous-system fibers.

neuropsychiatry a branch of medicine that combines the studies of neurology and psychiatry, and thus deals with both organic and functional disorders involving the nervous system.

neuropsychodiagnosis the process of searching for possible organic causes for a mental disorder. N. may include careful evaluation of heredity, a review of hospital records at the time of birth for possible clues to a neonatal problem, and changes in auditory or visual abilities, altered states of consciousness, labyrinthine disorders, or lateralization deficiencies in later years.

neuropsychological assessment an evaluation of the extent of possible brain damage to a patient derived from the results of various tests of memory, coordination, and various other general and specific challenges to CNS functions.

neuropsychology a branch of medicine that combines neurology and psychology.

neuropsychosis of defense an early term applied by Freud (1894, 1896) to a group of disorders (hysteria, obsessions, phobias, hallucinatory psychosis, paranoia) that appear to have defense mechanisms (projection, conversion, displacement, etc.) and childhood sexual trauma as common denominators. The term is now obsolete.

neuropsychotropic agents any drug or other substance that produces an effect on the nervous system or a part of the system, particularly substances that affect behavior. Stimulants, depressants, and psychomimetic drugs are n.a.

neuroreceptor = RECEPTOR.

neuroscience the study of neurology and related fields, including neuroanatomy, neurophysiology, neuropharmacology, psychology, and psychiatry.

neurosis a functional mental disorder characterized by a high level of anxiety and other distressing emotional symptoms, such as morbid fears, obsessive thoughts, compulsive acts, somatic reactions, dissociative states, and depressive reactions. The symptoms do not involve gross personality disorganization, total lack of insight, or loss of contact with reality, and are generally viewed as exaggerated, unconscious methods of coping with internal conflicts and the anxiety they produce. Aso called **psychoneurosis**. In DSM-III, the term is NEUROTIC DISORDER. See this entry.

Also see ACTUAL N.; ANALYTIC N.; ANXIETY N.; CARDIAC N.; CHARACTER N.; CHRONOPHOBIA; COLLECTIVE N.; COMPENSATION N.; COMPULSIVE N.; COUNTERTRANSFERENCE N.; DEATH N.; DECOMPENSATIVE N.; DEFENSE PSYCHONEUROSIS; DESTINY N.; DYSTHYMIC DISORDER; ESOPHAGEAL N.; EXISTENTIAL VACUUM; EXPERIMENTAL N.; FAMILY N.; FATE N.; HOUSEWIFE'S SYNDROME; HYPOCHONDRIASIS; IMPULSE N.; INFINITY N.; MALIGNANT N.; MIXED N.; MONOSYMPTOMATIC N.; MOTOR N. NEURASTHENIC N.; NONCOMBAT MILITARY NEUROSES; NUCLEAR N.; OBSESSIVE-COMPULSIVE DISORDER; OCCLUSAL N.; OCCUPATIONAL N.; ORGAN N.; PAN-N.; PATHONEUROSIS; PENSION N.; PERFORMANCE N.; PERHAPS N.; PHOBIC DISORDERS; PROGREDIENT N.; PROMOTION N.; PSEUDOSCHIZOPHRENIC N.; REGRESSION N.; RETIREMENT N.; SEMISTARVATION "N."; SITUATION N.; SOCIALBREAKDOWN SYNDROME; SUCCESS N.; SUNDAY N.; SYMPTOM N.; SYMPTOM CHOICE; TRANSFERENCE N.; TRAUMATIC N.; UPROOTING N.; VAGABOND N.; VISCERAL N.; WAR N.; WERNICKE'S CRAMP.

neurosis of destiny = DESTINY NEUROSIS.

neurosyphilis: See ASYMPTOMATIC N.; PARENCHYMATOUS N.; GENERAL PARESIS; BAYLE'S DISEASE.

neurotic anxiety in psychoanalysis, anxiety that originates in unconscious conflict and is maladaptive in nature, since it has a disturbing effect on emotion and behavior and also intensifies resistance to treatment. This type of anxiety is found in the anxiety neuroses. Compare OBJECTIVE ANXIETY.

neurotic arrangement the erroneous organization by a neurotic patient of ideas and events to justify his behavior.

neurotic character: See CHARACTER NEUROSIS.

neurotic conflict in general, an intrapsychic, or internal, conflict that leads to persistent maladjustment and emotional disturbance. In Horney's approach, n.c. is a clash between neurotic needs such as an excessive need for power and independence and the need for love and dependence. See INTRAPSYCHIC CONFLICT.

neurotic defense system in Horney's approach, a pattern of "strategies" adopted to counteract "basic anxiety" arising out of disturbed relations between the child and his parents. These strategies generate insatiable neurotic needs which group themselves into three categories: moving toward people (clinging to others), moving away from people (insisting on independence and self-dependence), and moving against people (seeking power, prestige, and possessions). See NEUROTIC NEEDS.

neurotic depression; neurotic-depressive reaction: See REACTIVE DEPRESSION.

neurotic disorder as defined by DSM-III, "a mental disorder in which the predominant disturbance is a symptom or group of symptoms that is distressing to the individual and is recognized by him or her as unacceptable and alien (ego-dystonic); reality testing is grossly intact; behavior does not actively violate gross social norms (although functioning may be markedly impaired); the disturbance is relatively enduring or recurrrent without treatment and is not limited to a transitory reaction to stressors; and there is no demonstrable organic etiology or factor." See NEUROSIS; AFFECTIVE DISORDERS; ANXIETY DISORDERS; SOMATOFORM DISORDERS; DISSOCIATIVE DISORDERS; PSYCHOSEXUAL DISORDERS. (DSM-III)

neurotic fiction a term applied by Adler to a guiding fiction that is so unrealistic that its goals cannot be achieved.

neurotic guilt a feeling of guilt due to an actual, fancied, or exaggerated transgression, which creates a state of anxiety, loss of self-esteem, and internal conflict. In psychoanalysis, the conflict is between the superego and the ego, and the anxiety arises out of a conscious or unconscious fear of punishment or even annihilation. See GUILT FEELINGS.

neurotic hunger strike an Adlerian term for a fear of eating that develops in some females soon after puberty, interpreted as an attempt to retard development of a normal adult female body form and thus reject the adult female role. See ANOREXIA NERVOSA.

neurotic insanity panic a form of anxiety produced by a fear of becoming insane.

neuroticism proneness to neurosis; also, a mild condition of neurosis. N. is one of two major dimensions in Eysenck's factor theory of personality, the other being introversion-extroversion.

neurotic needs a term employed by Horney for excessive drives and demands that may arise out of the strategies we use in defending ourselves against basic anxiety and in attempts to cope with a threatening world. She enumerates ten of these n.n.: the insatiable need for affection and approval, a partner who takes over one's life, restriction of one's life, power, exploitation of others, prestige, admiration, achievement, self-sufficiency and independence, and perfection.

neurotic nucleus a personality pattern that constitutes a common denominator among neurotic individuals, according to some authorities. The n.n. consists of a high vulnerability to stress and an inability to cope with ordinary problems in effective ways. Such individuals lack ego strength, have low frustration tolerance, overreact to minor setbacks, are beset by anxiety, and overwork "favorite" defense mechanisms until they crystallize into symptoms.

neurotic paradox the tendency of the neurotic to perpetuate neurotic defenses and to resist giving them up. Presumably, this tendency constitutes a paradox because neurotic defenses prevent maximal functioning and inhibit development in one or more areas. E.g., a neurotic pattern such as an inordinate drive for sexual or business success may serve as a defense against anxiety for a time but becomes self-defeating in the end. See

NEUROSIS. Also see ANXIETY; DEFENSE MECHANISM.

neurotic personality a personality in which there is a pattern of traits and tendencies that increase susceptibility to neurosis of one type or another. The persistently tense, apprehensive, insecure individual is believed to be prone to anxiety neurosis; the overly orderly, cautious, meticulous person is more likely to develop an obsessive-compulsive disorder; a tendency toward fixed irrational fears may develop into a phobic disorder; and a susceptibility to bodily complaints may lead to a hysterical (conversion) disorder.

neurotic process the process in which an unconscious conflict comes to be expressed by neurotic symptoms and personality disturbances. In Horney's approach, the term applies to the defensive behavior and strategies employed by a neurotic individual to maintain an idealized self-image which is in conflict with the individual's real, or actual, self.

neurotic-process factor a characterological trait that is usually significant in discriminating between normal and neurotic behaviors (Cattell).

neurotic proviso = PARAPATHETIC PROVISO.

neurotic-regressive debility a personality dimension marked by such factors as rigidity, incompetence, loss of interests, and inability to mobilize habits in order to complete a task (Cattell).

neurotic resignation: See RESIGNATION.

neurotic-sleep attack a psychogenic, uncontrollable urge to sleep, usually for a few minutes or hours. The disorder is classified by some authorities as a dissociative reaction motivated by an unconscious need to escape from a distressing situation. Cases have been reported of soldiers falling asleep during a bombardment, preachers while delivering a sermon, and patients while having a tooth pulled.

neurotic sociopath a term applied by some investigators to antisocial individuals who have a high anxiety level, overdeveloped or misdirected conscience, and feelings of guilt and apprehension which they seem to ward off by engaging in outward activity that takes the form of stealing, sexual promiscuity, or other antisocial behavior. Also see PRIMARY SOCIOPATH.

neurotic solution a method of resolving a neurotic conflict by removing it from awareness.

neurotic syndromes a group of neurotic disorders comprising anxiety disorder, hysterical or conversion disorder, obsessive-compulsive disorder, dissociative disorder, depressive disorder, neurasthenic disorder, depersonalization disorder, and hypochondriacal disorder.

neurotic traits a term used in DSM-I for a group of "adjustment reactions of childhood" comprising tics, somnambulism, overactivity, stuttering, specific fears, and school phobia.

neurotic trend Horney's term for an individual's organization of tendencies toward attaining maximum security, primarily by moving toward, away from, or against people.

neurotigenesis the production or induction of a neurosis or neurotic behavior.

neurotransmitter any of several chemicals released at nerve-fiber endings to help a nerve impulse cross the synaptic gap between two neurons. Kinds of n. include acetylcholine, dopamine, and serotonin. Some investigators believe n. metabolism may be involved in the development of memory traces.

neurovegetative system the parasympathetic portion of the autonomic nervous system, which is involved in control of the body's vegetative processes.

neurulation the process of development of the primitive nervous system in the early stages of embryonic life as the neural plate forms and evolves into the neural tube which eventually becomes the spinal canal and ventricles of the brain. Also see NEURAL PLATE; NEURAL TUBE.

neutral color a color that lacks hue or saturation, e.g., a gray, white, or black.

neutral environment an environment in which the patient is subjected to no demands or rigid limits. A therapy group attempts to provide a n.e., enabling each member to modify his attitudes in his own way.

neutrality a term used by S. R. Slavson to describe the neutral role of the therapist, who remains passive and permissive and does not apply judgments of right and wrong or suggest what is proper behavior on the part of the patient.

neutralization in psychoanalysis, the utilization ("taming," "deinstinctualization") of sexual or aggressive energy in the service of the ego rather than for instinctual gratification, that is, in such functions as problem-solving, creative imagination, scientific inquiry, or decision-making. See DELIBIDINIZATION; SUBLIMATION; DEAGGRESSIVIZATION.

neutralizer a member of a therapy group who plays a role of modifying and controlling impulsive, aggressive, or destructive behaviors of other members of the group (S. R. Slavson).

neutral stimulus a stimulus that does not produce the expected response, or that does not produce the response elicited after conditioning.

Newcastle virus an acute, highly contagious disease agent of domestic fowl and other birds, causing respiratory signs and manifestations of nervous-system involvement. The agent is a paramyxovirus, and the disease is easily transmitted to humans who experience the effects as a severe conjunctivitis. It was named Newcastle for the site of its discovery in England but was later identified as the **Ranikhet disease of Asia**.

new-father blues: See MATERNITY BLUES.

newness fear = NEOPHOBIA.

nexus a connection between two variables which, if causal, makes them interdependent.

NFD = NEUROFIBRILLARY DEGENERATION.

NGU = NONGONOCOCCAL URETHRITIS.

niacin = NICOTINIC ACID.

nialamide: See MONOAMINE OXIDASE INHIBITORS.

Nicot, Jean /nikō'/ French diplomat and scholar, 1530–1600. See NICOTINE; NICOTINIC ACID; NICOTINIC-ACID DEFICIENCIES.

nicotine $C_{10}H_{14}N_2$—an alkaloid drug obtained from the tobacco plant and used for scientific purposes in physiological and pharmacologic studies. It has a stimulant effect in small doses but in large doses may function as a depressant. The effects observed in smoking tobacco are due mainly to the n. content. N. is a drug that can be used to mimic the effect of acetylcholine on ACh receptors. N. was named for the French diplomat Jean Nicot, who introduced tobacco into France in 1560. Also see TOBACCO; PSYCHOSTIMULANTS.

nicotinic acid one of the B-complex vitamins discovered in 1937 as a cure for pellagra, a vitamin-deficiency disease with neurologic complications. N.a. works with riboflavin to convert proteins and fats to glucose and oxidize glucose to release its energy. Also called **niacin; vitamin B5**.

nicotinic-acid deficiency a condition marked by weakness, lassitude, anorexia, skin disorders, and CNS symptoms, e.g., apathy, confusion, disorientation, and neuritis. Meat and milk are primary sources of nicotinic acid (niacin). Also called **pellagra**.

nictophobia = ACHLUOPHOBIA.

Nielsen, Herman Danish physician, 1882–1960. See NIELSEN'S DISEASE; BONNEVIE-ULLRICH SYNDROME; KLIPPEL-FEIL SYNDROME.

Nielsen's disease a condition named for Herman Nielsen, who first described this congenital disorder, which combines the signs and symptoms of KLIPPEL-FEIL SYNDROME and BONNEVIE-ULLRICH SYNDROME. See these entries.

Niemann, Albert /nē'män/ German surgeon, 1880–1921. See NIEMANN-PICK DISEASE; CEREBROSIDE; LIPID-METABOLISM DISORDER; SPHINGOLIPID; SPHINGOLIPIDOSES.

Niemann-Pick disease an inherited lipid-storage disorder generally marked by a deficiency of the enzyme sphingomyelinase and accumulation of phospholipids in brain tissue and visceral organs. Massive liver and spleen growths may accompany the other effects. Mental retardation, blindness, and death before adulthood are commonly associated with the disorder. Also see LIPID-METABOLISM DISORDERS.

Nietzsche, Friedrich Wilhelm /nē'chə/ German philosopher and philologist, 1844–1900. As a subtle observer of human nature, N. recognized long before Freud the extent to which sexual and unconscious factors are likely to affect even seemingly unrelated actions and our most lofty thoughts. He generally anticipated the situation of modern man. (André Gide, in 1931, went so far as to write, of N., that "nothing remains to be said and it is enough to quote him.") See EXISTENTIALISM; LISTENING WITH THE THIRD EAR; APOLLONIAN ATTITUDE; DIONYSIAN ATTITUDE; WILL TO POWER.

night blindness a visual impairment marked by

difficulty or inability to see objects in a dimly lighted environment. Also see HEMERALOPIA.

night-care program a program of psychotherapy and supportive activity such as recreational and occupational therapy provided to mental patients during the evening. The patients are in the process of recovery and in most cases live in the community and come to the hospital after working hours. Night care makes fuller and more economic use of hospital facilities and enables many patients to be released from full hospitalization sooner than usual. See NIGHT HOSPITAL.

night-eating syndrome a disorder experienced by about ten percent of obese persons, mostly women, who suffer from insomnia and eat heavily during the night. It is a form of hyperphagia precipitated by stressful circumstances and occurs every night until the stress is alleviated. See BULIMIA; HYPERPHAGIA.

night fantasy a fantasy that occurs during sleep and is not a true dream. According to Freud, a dream involves additions and alterations, whereas a n.f. is more like a daydream.

night hospital a type of partial hospitalization which originated in Montreal in 1954. Patients spend the day in the community and receive psychiatric care in the hospital at night. Also see NIGHT-CARE PROGRAM; DAY HOSPITAL.

nightmare a vivid dream depicting acutely disturbing, anxiety-provoking events. The prime motif is usually helpless terror; typically the dreamer is plunged into a threatening situation, experiences agonizing dread, makes futile attempts to escape, and awakens in a cold sweat. Some writers attribute these experiences to the emotional residue left by traumatic experiences; others, including Freud, see them as a spontaneous eruption of repressed sexual and aggressive impulses accompanied by the intense anxiety they produce. Also called **dream anxiety attacks**. See SLEEP-TERROR DISORDER.

nightmare-death syndrome = BANGUNGUT.

night phobia = ACHLUOPHOBIA.

night residue the psychic material of a previous night's dreaming that persists in the person's thoughts after he awakens. Some authors believe n.r. occurs because of a failure of repression of the dream material at the time of awakening.

nightshade poisoning the toxic effects of ingestion of the berries of the deadly nightshade plant, Atropa belladonna, a source of atropine which paralyzes the parasympathetic nervous system. The symptoms include visual hallucinations, mutism, dilated pupils, unresponsiveness, disorientation, and other effects that simulate signs of an acute schizophrenic reaction. Also see BELLADONNA ALKALOIDS; BELLADONNA DELIRIUM.

night terror = SLEEP-TERROR DISORDER.

nihilism in psychiatry, the delusion of nonexistence; the patient's fixed belief that his mind, body, or the world at large no longer exists ("I am only an empty shell," "This is a dream world," "I died twenty years ago"). Delusions of this kind occur primarily in schizophrenia, severe depression, and occasionally in general paresis, cerebral arteriosclerosis, and senile dementia. Also called **nihilistic delusion; delusion of negation**.

ninth cranial nerve = GLOSSOPHARYNGEAL NERVE.

Nirje, Bengt Swedish psychologist, fl. 1969. See NORMALIZATION PRINCIPLE.

nirvana principle in psychoanalysis, the tendency of all instincts and life processes to seek the stability and equilibrium of the inorganic state (from Sanskrit *nirvanah*, "a blowing out" [of a light], thus "extinction"). This is the goal of the death instinct, which Freud (at least late in his life) believed to be universal. Also see BUDDHISM.

Nissl, Franz German neurologist, 1860–1919. See NISSL METHODS; NISSL STAIN; TIGROID BODIES (also called **Nissl bodies; Nissl granules**).

Nissl methods techniques used to stain neurons for examination under a microscope lens. The Nissl stain contains a chemical, **toluidine blue**, which has an affinity for concentrations of RNA molecules in the membranes and inclusion bodies of nerve cells. They are used to identify the neural cell groups in brain tissue.

Nissl stain a basic dye used to stain Nissl bodies and other granulelike structures in the cytoplasm of neurons. Also called **Nissl's stain**. Also see NISSL METHODS.

nitrazepam: See BENZODIAZEPINES.

nitrogen mustard = ALKYLATING AGENT.

nitrogen narcosis: See RAPTURE-OF-THE-DEEP SYNDROME.

nitrogen poisoning the toxic effects caused by nitrogen gas bubbles that form from molecules dissolved in body tissues when a person, e.g., a deep-sea diver, moves rapidly from a region of abnormally high air pressure to one of normal, or lower, air pressure. See DECOMPRESSION SICKNESS; BENDS.

nitrous oxide: See PSYCHEDELICS.

nm: See MILLIMICRON.

NMR = NUCLEAR MAGNETIC RESONANCE.

-noci- a combining form relating to pain or injury (from Latin *nocere*, "to injure").

nociceptor a nerve receptor whose stimuli are generally painful or detrimental to the organism. Compare BENECEPTOR.

noct. an abbreviation used in prescriptions, meaning "at night" (Latin *nocte* or *noctis*).

-noct-; -nocti- a combining form relating to the night (Latin *nox*).

noctambulation = SLEEPWALKING DISORDER.

noctiphobia = ACHLUOPHOBIA.

nocturia the need to urinate during the night. The condition may simply be the result of excessive fluid intake before going to sleep. N. also can be a sign of a disease of the heart, liver, or urinary system. Renal disease in which the kidneys lose ability to concentrate urine may be a cause of n.

nocturnal emission an involuntary ejaculation

that occurs during a nocturnal dream. Studies show that nearly 80 percent of males experience a n.e. before age 21. Also about ten percent of total sexual release in a young adult male is through nocturnal emissions. Ejaculation as part of nocturnal dreams is rare among adolescent females but increases to about ten percent among mature females. A popular term for n.e. is wet dream.

nocturnal enuresis urinary incontinence at night; bedwetting during sleep. See FUNCTIONAL ENURESIS.

nocturnal hemiplegia a form of sleep paralysis in which during brief periods of falling asleep or awakening, the person is unable to move or speak but can recall the episode. The condition is due to a temporary dysfunction of the RAS and is not considered pathological. Also called **sleep paralysis**. Also see NARCOLEPSY.

nocturnal myoclonus a type of myoclonic movement of the limbs that occurs when a person is falling asleep. The involuntary spasms of muscle contractions and relaxations may happen repeatedly and can occur during sleep with sufficient activity to awaken the person. N.m. may happen occasionally to any individual and is not necessarily a sign of a nervous-system disease.

nocturnal rhythms circadian rhythms that occur during the period usually spent in sleeping. Body temperature generally declines during the rest span of a 24-hour period while sodium and calcium levels in the blood increase and the level of magnesium in the urine reaches a peak. Mitosis of epidermal cells occurs almost exclusively during the rest span. For nocturnal animals, the n.r. are generally the reverse of animals that normally sleep at night.

nodal behavior in group therapy, a period of increased activity, which may be aggressive or disorderly, followed by a relatively quiet period of antinodal behavior.

nodding spasm a disorder observed in infants and characterized by head-shaking and nystagmus, which may be continuous or intermittent, but arrhythmic and involuntary and not specifically associated with emotional disturbance.

nodes of Ranvier gaps in the myelin sheath surrounding white-matter nerve fibers. The gaps permit an ion exchange at intervals along the axon, resulting in a conductivity effect in which an impulse leaps from one node to the next, a form of nerve-impulse transmission called saltatory conduction.

noesis /nō·ē′sis/ an intellectual or cognitive process, particularly when it yields self-evident knowledge (from Greek *nous*, "mind").

Noiré, L. language theorist, 1847–89. See ORIGIN-OF-LANGUAGE THEORIES.

noise a harsh sound composed of a single frequency, as in sonic boom, or, more frequently, a nonrhythmic mixture of frequencies. Also see WHITE N.; DIFFERENTIATION THEORY.

noise abatement the application of legislation or technological skills to reduce the level of noise pollution. N.a. may require the redesign of automobile or aircraft engines, ordinances that prohibit use of airports at night, or routing of traffic patterns away from residential areas.

noise conditions in industrial psychology, the effects of different types and levels of noise on work performance, hearing, and employee comfort. In environment psychology, the term refers to the effects of traffic sounds, subway noise, jet booms, and other sources of noise pollution, on the public.

noise effects the physiological and psychological stress produced by noise, especially high levels of unpredictable noise over which the individual can exert no control. Various n.e. include diminished productivity, accuracy, and frustration tolerance, and, possibly, increased aggression.

noise fear = ACOUSTICOPHOBIA.

noise pollution: See NOISE CONDITIONS; NOISE ABATEMENT.

nomadism a pathological tendency to wander from place to place, and to repeatedly change one's residence and occupation. In milder form this tendency may be an attempt to escape from a distressing situation or from responsibility, but in extreme form it may be associated with brain damage, epilepsy, mental deficiency, or psychosis. Also see PORIOMANIA.

nomenclature a systematic classification of technical terms used in an art or science. See DSM-III; INTERNATIONAL CLASSIFICATION OF DISEASES.

nominal aphasia = AMNESTIC APHASIA.

nominalism a philosophical doctrine that only concrete particulars are real while concepts and abstractions are merely words; also, the doctrine that scientific theories are never ultimately true or false, but only more or less useful.

nominal realism a term used by Piaget for the young child's conviction that the name of an object, such as a dog, is not just a symbol but an intrinsic part of the object. This conviction is shared by many primitive peoples, and is probably the reason they believe they can either bless or curse another person by invoking his name. Also called **word realism**. Also see MAGICAL THINKING.

nominal scale a scale of measurement where data are simply classified into categories that are mutually exclusive, without indicating order, magnitude, a true zero point, etc. The data can only be enumerated, so a n.s. is the lowest form of measurement. An example would be the numbers on football jerseys. Also see ORDINAL SCALE; INTERVAL SCALE; RATIO SCALE.

nominating technique: See SOCIOMETRY.

nomological conceptual; referring, especially, to inferences about a variable. The construct validity of a test is ascertained through a n. network reflecting research and other experience with the test.

nomothetic pertaining to the formulation of general laws as the goal of scientific method, as opposed to the study of the individual case; characterizing techniques and methods used to study a single variable or norm in many subjects for the purpose of discovering general laws or principles of behavior. The **n. approach** focuses on the variation found, in many cases, on a specific trait chosen by the psychologist as an important dimension of behavior or personality that can be quantified, measured, and used for the purposes of classification and prediction. In contrast to the n. approach is the IDEOGRAPHIC APPROACH. See this entry.

nonaffective hallucination a hallucination whose content is apparently unrelated to either depression or elation.

nonaggressive socialized reaction: See CONDUCT DISORDER, SOCIALIZED, NONAGGRESSIVE.

nonaggressive societies societies whose goal is one of peaceful isolation, e.g., the Arapesh of New Guinea or the Great Whale River Eskimos. Socialization in n.s. is marked by deemphasis of achievement or power needs, disapproval of aggression, and affirmation of basic pleasures. Standards for male and female behavior are not widely divergent. The Amish, Mennonites, and Quakers represent analogous communities in technologically advanced nations.

nonaggressive undersocialized reaction: See CONDUCT DISORDER, UNDERSOCIALIZED, NONAGGRESSIVE.

nonauthoritarian rejecting-neglecting parent: See REJECTING-NEGLECTING PARENT.

noncombat military neuroses neurotic reactions arising out of the stresses of military life outside the combat situation, that is, among support troups, rear-echelon soldiers, and others who are near combat areas or waiting for combat but do not have the aggressive outlet of the soldier in battle.

noncomplementary role a role pattern that does not conform with demands and expectations of others. See ROLE. Compare COMPLEMENTARY ROLE.

non compos mentis a legal term meaning a person who is mentally defective or mentally unsound and therefore not responsible for his conduct. Compare COMPOS MENTIS.

nonconscious processes those processes that do not have the potential to reach consciousness, e.g., the buildup of cholesterol in the blood or certain autonomic functions or regulatory mechanisms. However, the eventual outcomes or consequences of n.p. may have conscious impact. N.p. must be distinguished from unconscious processes, some of which may rise to consciousness. In the past, the word **nonconscious** was used in another sense, to refer to that which is lifeless, e.g., an inanimate object.

noncontingent unrelated; describing, e.g., a control procedure in biofeedback research in which false or random feedback is given regardless of the true physiological response, so that the subject will think true biofeedback is taking place.

noncontingent reinforcement reinforcement that is not linked to or dependent on a particular response.

noncuddlers: See CUDDLING BEHAVIOR.

nondirectional test of hypothesis a statistical test that specifies only that an effect may be either greater than or less than a comparison, and therefore does not state the direction expected. A n.t.o.h. may also state that a relationship may be either positive or negative. Compare DIRECTIONAL TEST OF HYPOTHESIS.

nondirective approach an approach to counseling and psychotherapy advocated by C. Rogers, in which the patient leads the way by expressing his own feelings, defining his own problems, interpreting his own behavior, while the therapist sets up a permissive atmosphere and clarifies the patient's ideas rather than directing the process. The object of this approach is to encourage the patient to recognize his own defenses and faulty assumptions, to draw on his own reserves, and to arrive at his own solutions. Also called **nondirective counseling**.

nondirective interview: See NONDIRECTIVE APPROACH.

nondirective play therapy a form of play therapy based on the principle that even a child has the capacity to revise his own attitudes and behavior. The therapist provides a variety of play materials and either assumes a friendly, interested role without giving direct suggestions (Axline's approach) or engages the child in conversation that focuses on present feelings and present situations in his life (Allen's approach). In either case, the accepting attitude of the therapist encourages the child to try new and more appropriate ways of dealing with his problems.

nondirective teaching model a person-oriented teaching model associated with C. Rogers' approach and concerned with developing the capacity for self-instruction as well as emphasizing self-discovery, self-understanding, and the realization of innate potential.

nondirective therapy: See NONDIRECTIVE APPROACH; NONDIRECTIVE PLAY THERAPY.

nondisjunction the failure of pairs of chromosomes to separate during mitotic cell division with the result that both chromosomes move to the nucleus of one daughter cell while the other daughter cell fails to receive its normal complement.

nonexistence in the two-word stage of language development, an expression such as "gone cookie" indicating object disappearance or cessation of an activity.

nonfluency a term used to characterize motor, or expressive, aphasia involving such disturbances as DYSPROSODY, DYSARTHRIA, and AGRAMMATISM. See these entries.

nongonococcal urethritis a term applied to a group of diseases that generally are sexually transmitted and present symptoms similar to those of gonorrhea although laboratory tests usually detect another type of infectious organism, such as a strain of Chlamydia. The symptoms usually include inflammation of the urethra and sometimes a puslike discharge. Abbrev.: **NGU**. Also see NONSPECIFIC URETHRITIS.

nonjudgmental approach in psychotherapy and psychoanalysis, a neutral attitude on the part of the therapist, which encourages the patient to give free expression to his ideas and feelings, as, e.g., in free association and in the exploration of the patient's potential in nondirective therapy. Some therapists do not carry this approach to the extreme but wait for an appropriate, constructive opportunity to express their own views and interpretations.

nonlanguage test a test in which the questions or problems as well as the answers or solutions are not conveyed in words, e.g., a maze or a test that requires manipulation of objects. Also called **nonverbal test; performance test**.

nonlinear relationships two or more sets of data that cannot be described by a straight line of best fit. See CURVILINEAR REGRESSION.

nonliterate a term applied to cultures that lack a written language.

nonmarital sex = EXTRAMARITAL SEX.

nonorganic hearing loss an auditory disturbance not due to an impairment of the peripheral hearing mechanism. It is considered to be of psychogenic origin.

nonorganic speech impairment: See SPEECH IMPAIRMENT.

nonovert appeals techniques employed in consumer psychology in which the advertising message is presented by presumably ordinary people who make no deliberate attempt to persuade. N.a. may give the impression to the consumer that he is "overhearing" an independent endorsement of a product. N.a. are commonly used in "slice of life" television commercials.

nonparametric statistics statistics that do not make assumptions about parameters of the population being tested, such as normality and homogeneity of variance.

nonpathological lying: See LYING.

nonperformers those individuals in a behavior setting who have a subordinate or auxiliary role, e.g., audience members at a lecture or concert. Compare PERFORMERS.

nonperson: See PERSONALITY DETERIORATION.

non-REM sleep = NREM SLEEP.

non rep. an abbreviation used in prescriptions, meaning "do not repeat" (Latin *non repetatur*).

nonrestraint management of psychotic patients without the use of restraints such as a straitjacket.

nonreversal shift a form of discrimination learning in which the delivery of reinforcement is suddenly made contingent on another dimension of the task object. E.g., reinforcement for selecting objects according to size is shifted to reinforcement for selecting objects according to color. Also see REVERSAL SHIFT.

nonsense figure a figure that appears to have no meaning since it does not correspond to any common or familiar object and is not a recognizable geometric form such as a circle or triangle.

nonsense syllable a speech sound that is meaningless. The term was originally used by Hermann

Ebbinghaus in memory experiments. Nonsense syllables are also used in rote-learning experiments and as a mantra.

nonsense syndrome = GANSER SYNDROME.

nonspecific effects placebo factors modifying the true effects of a drug or other treatment. N.e. include, e.g., wishful thinking, the physician's enthusiasm for his treatment, and faith in science.

nonspecific urethritis an infection of the genital tract by a nonspecific disease organism. The infection may be transmitted by sexual contact and may produce symptoms resembling those of a known venereal disease, such as gonorrhea, although diagnosis often fails to identify the agent. Certain strains of mycoplasmas and Chlamydiaceae have been associated with n.u. Abbrev.: **NSU**. The term is essentially equivalent to NONGONOCOCCAL URETHRITIS. See this entry.

nonstriate visual cortex a group of neurons that surrounds the visual sensory area and appears to be involved in helping to evaluate visual sensations as they may relate to previous experiences, thereby serving the functions of identification and recognition of visual images. The n.v.c. also is associated with eye movements involved in visual impressions.

nonsyphilitic interstitial keratitis = COGAN'S SYNDROME.

nonverbal behavior actions by individuals that may communicate ideas without the use of spoken or written language. Kinds of n.b. may include eye contact, facial expression, and body angle, also sounds that are not intelligible words. N.b. may be subtle or exaggerated, depending on the interpersonal distance between the individuals and whether they are close friends or strangers. Exaggerated n.b. may be displayed by politicians, entertainers, or others who are required by occupation to appear friendly to strangers. Also called **nonverbal language; nonverbal communication**.

nonverbal intelligence an expression of intelligence that does not require language. N.i. can be measured with pictures or other performance tests. See NONLANGUAGE TEST.

nonverbal language = NONVERBAL BEHAVIOR.

nonverbal leakage: See VERBAL LEAKAGE.

nonverbal test = NONLANGUAGE TEST.

noology the science of the human mind (from Greek *nous*, "mind").

Noonan, Jacqueline Ann American cardiologist, fl. 1959, 1963. See NOONAN'S SYNDROME.

Noonan's syndrome a multiple-organ genetic disorder that involves the skin, the heart, the gonads, and the skeleton. The patients generally have short stature. Intellectual development varies, and some N.s. patients have superior intelligence, but most are mildly to moderately retarded and a few are profoundly retarded. Male patients are seldom fertile, but the opposite is true of female N.s. patients.

norepinephrine a catecholamine hormone secreted by the adrenal medulla and released by autonomic-nervous-system neurons. It is similar to epinephrine in most functions, but less potent, serving mainly to constrict blood vessels and as a nervous-system neurotransmitter. Excessive levels of n. in the brain have been associated with manic states. Also called **noradrenaline**.

norepinephrine receptors receptors in the central and sympathetic nervous systems that are sensitive to norepinephrine or substances that mimic its action. N.r. in both systems are classed in subgroups according to their sensitivities to agents that either mimic or inhibit norepinephrine activity.

norm a standard or range of values representing the typical performance of a group, or of a child of a certain age, against which comparisons can be made.

normal a value standard that represents the usual or average or near-the-central or mean for a range of values.

normal autism = AUTISTIC PHASE.

normal distribution a bell-shaped probability curve showing the expected value of sampling a random variable. It indicates the distribution of random errors of measurement. Most of the scores are grouped around the midpoint, with about 68 percent lying ± one standard deviation from the mean, about 95 percent ± two standard deviations, and more than 99 percent ± three standard deviations. Also called **Gaussian distribution; normal curve; normal probability curve**.

normality in psychiatry and psychology, a broad concept that is roughly the equivalent of mental health. Although there is no rigid yardstick for psychological normality, and the concept varies considerably from culture to culture, a few flexible criteria can be suggested: freedom from incapacitating internal conflicts; the capacity to think and act in an organized and reasonably effective manner; the ability to cope with the ordinary demands and problems of life; freedom from extreme emotional distress such as anxiety, despondency, and persistent upset; and the absence of clear-cut symptoms of mental disorder such as obsessions, phobias, confusion, and disorientation. See MENTAL HEALTH.

Normalization Principle a concept introduced in 1969 by the Swedish psychologist Bengt Nirje that mentally and physically disabled persons should not be denied social-sexual relationships merely because they are handicapped. Social-sexual relationships can include a wide range of emotional and physical contacts, from simple friendship to sexual stimulation and satisfaction.

normal-pressure hydrocephalus a syndrome involving gait apraxia, mild dementia, urinary incontinence, and enlarged ventricles with normal cerebrospinal-fluid pressure. The condition frequently benefits from shunting procedures, though complications may occur. Also see HAKIM'S DISEASE. Abbrev.: **NPH**.

normal probability curve = NORMAL DISTRIBUTION.

normative compliance the effect of perceived social influence on behavior combined with the motivation to comply with the influence. The term was introduced by A. Etzioni in 1961.

normative crisis = MATURATIONAL CRISIS.

normative-reeducative strategy in social psychology, the idea that societal change should be based on active reeducation of people within the framework of their cultural milieu. N.-r.s. holds that a program for social change based only on rational appeal is inadequate because behavioral patterns are largely determined by traditional attitudes and cultural norms. Also see EMPIRICAL-RATIONAL STRATEGY; POWER-COERCIVE STRATEGY.

normative science a science that sets norms for behavior, education, health, or other cultural or societal aspects.

normative score a person's score compared with the scores of other individuals, such as a percentile ranking in a particular group. Also see IPSATIVE SCORE.

normosplanchnic type a constitutional body type in Viola's system that corresponds roughly to Kretschmer's athletic type.

normotensive individuals persons whose blood pressure is within the normal range for their age and other factors considered. A person with abnormally low blood pressure is called hypotensive and one with abnormally high blood pressure is considered hypertensive. Also see BLOOD PRESSURE.

normotype a constitutional body type that is morphologically average, or eumorphic.

norm-referenced testing an approach to testing based on comparison of one subject's performance with others' performance on the same test. N.-r.t. differentiates among students and ranks them on the basis of their performance, e.g., a nationally standardized norm-referenced test will indicate how much better or worse than the national sample a given student performs. Compare CRITERIA-REFERENCED TESTING.

Norrie, Gordon Danish ophthalmologist, 1855–1941. See NORRIE'S DISEASE.

Norrie's disease a type of congenital blindness that is transmitted as an X-linked genetic defect affecting only males. The blindness generally is due to abnormal development of the retina before birth. Progressive loss of hearing often accompanies the blindness. About two-thirds of the patients are mentally retarded, and some experience hallucinations or other psychological difficulties.

nortriptyline; nortriptyline hydrochloride: See TRICYCLIC ANTIDEPRESSANTS.

-nos-; -noso- a combining form relating to disease (Greek *nosos*).

nosocomion a hospital or sanatorium. Also called **nosocomium**. The adjective **nosocomial** is used to refer to a hospital-induced condition unrelated to the patient's primary illness. Also see IATROGENIC ILLNESS.

nosogenesis = PATHOGENESIS.

nosological approach in psychiatry and general medicine, an approach that focuses on the naming and classifying of disorders, as well as the discovery of indicative, or pathognomonic, symptoms and their grouping into syndromes for diagnostic purposes. The n.a. contrasts with the dynamic approach which emphasizes causal factors and the inner meaning of symptoms. See KRAEPELIN.

nosology the scientific study and classification of diseases and disorders, both mental and physical. Also see PSYCHIATRIC CLASSIFICATION.

nosomania = HYPOCHONDRIASIS.

nosophobia a morbid fear of disease in general or the fear of a particular disease. Also called **pathophobia**.

nostalgia a longing to return to a place where one may be emotionally bound, e.g., home, or a native land. N. is related to a feeling of isolation in the present location. The term also is applied to a longing to return to an earlier period of life which usually is recalled as being particularly pleasant compared with the present. Also called **homesickness**.

Nothnagel, Carl Wilhelm Hermann /nōt′nägəl/ Austrian neurologist, 1841–1905. See ACROPARESTHESIA (there: **Nothnagel's acroparesthesia**).

notional word = CONTENT WORD.

not-me in H. S. Sullivan's personality theory, that part of the personified self which is based on interpersonal experiences that have evoked overwhelming anxiety, dread, and horror, and which may lead to nightmares, emotional crises, and schizophrenic reactions.

notogenesis a stage of embryonic development in which the **notocord**, or primitive backbone, and mesoderm form in the gastrula.

noumenal a term used to identify a type of intuition or knowledge derived from pure thought without regard to time or space. See NOUS.

nous the Greek word for the faculty of reason or intellect which enables human beings to perceive truth.

novelty the quality of being new and unusual. N. is one of the major determinants of attention, as in sexual attraction. The attraction to n. has been shown to begin as early as one year of age. In consumer psychology, n. is a desire for a change in the absence of dissatisfaction with the present situation. E.g., despite satisfaction with a particular product or service, studies show, 30 percent of the people occasionally switch to a different brand or company simply because they want a change. Also, 15 percent of consumers will buy a new product simply because it is new.

novelty fear = NEOPHOBIA.

NPH = NORMAL-PRESSURE HYDROCEPHALUS.

NREM sleep /en′rem/ or /non′rem/ *n*on-rapid-*e*ye-*m*ovement sleep; periods of sleep in which dreaming, as indicated by rapid eye movements

(REM), usually does not occur. During these periods, which occur most frequently in the first hours of sleep, the electroencephalogram shows only minimal activity, and there is little or no change in pulse, respiration, and blood pressure. Also called **non-REM sleep; telencephalic sleep; neosleep**. Also see DREAM STATE; DELTA-WAVE SLEEP.

NSU = NONSPECIFIC URETHRITIS.

nu /noō/ or /nyoō/ 13th letter of the Greek alphabet (N, ν).

nuclear complex a central conflict or problem that is rooted in infancy, e.g., feelings of inferiority (Adler) or an oedipal situation (Freud). N.c. is also used as an alternative term for OEDIPUS COMPLEX. See this entry.

nuclear family the core members of the family, consisting of the parents and children. See EXTENDED FAMILY.

nuclear imaging is radioisotopic encephalography, a form of imaging performed as serial exposures at one-to-two-second intervals, for the dynamic study of arterial, capillary, and venous phases. A radioactive isotope is injected into a blood vessel leading to the brain; the isotope tends to accumulate in abnormal sites, e.g., intracranial masses, which can be outlined in images produced by instruments sensitive to radiation emitted by the isotope. N.i. is said to be more specific and sensitive than the static scan. Also called **cerebral dynamic imaging**.

nuclear magnetic resonance a new imaging technique that produces pictures based on the responses of atomic nuclei in a *magnetic* field (via hydrogen-ion spin times T_1 and T_2), recreating a three-dimensional array. With n.m.r. it is unnecessary to inject anything into the body or to expose the patient to radiation, and, unlike CAT scans, this technique identifies structure as well as function. It promises to become the major diagnostic procedure of the 1990s. Abbrev.: **NMR**.

nuclear-medical technician a person who performs routine tasks in support of nuclear-medicine technologists in a hospital or similar facility. See NUCLEAR-MEDICAL TECHNOLOGIST.

nuclear-medical technologist a health professional who is responsible for the operation of brain scanners and other radioscopic equipment in a hospital or similar facility. The n.-m.t. also performs laboratory tests and analyses in connection with nuclear-medical diagnostic functions. The position usually requires a college degree in chemistry or biology plus a year of special training, but experience as a certified medical technician may be accepted in lieu of a degree.

nuclear neurosis a popular term for a pattern of complaints found among some individuals who live or work in the area of nuclear electric power plants. The behavioral effects include headaches, either anorexia or increased appetite, increased tension, distrust of authority, and worry about radiation exposure. A study by a United States Presidential Task Force following the 1979 accident at the Three Mile Island nuclear power plant (Pennsylvania) found the distress level of the general population in the vicinity of nuclear power plants nearly equal to that of patients in mental hospitals. The study also found that among some individuals the symptoms were not transient but persisted at a high level long after the triggering incident. Also called **nuclear phobia**. Also see CHINA SYNDROME SYNDROME.

nuclear problem the central conflict that is the basis of a patient's problems and the one on which therapy should be concentrated. The n.p. often is a type of maladjustment, e.g., sibling rivalry, unresolved Oedipus complex, or feelings of inadequacy.

nuclear schizophrenia = PROCESS SCHIZOPHRENIA.

nucleotides compounds consisting of a purine or pyrimidine base linked to a ribose sugar molecule and combined with phosphoric acid. Examples of n. include diphosphopyridine and triphosphopyridine.

nucleus the central portion of a tissue cell and the functional control unit of cellular activity. In most cells, the n. contains the DNA molecules and genetic templates for all anabolic and catabolic functions as well as for reproduction. The term applies also to a mass of nerve-cell bodies with the same or related functions, e.g., n. cuneatus, n. gracilis. Plural: **nuclei** /noō′klē·ī/.

nucleus cuneatus a cluster of neurons in the medulla where sensory nerves from the spinal cord terminate.

nucleus gracilis = GRACILIS NUCLEUS.

nucleus of the raphe /raf′ē/ a central complex of nuclei in the brainstem with fibers that communicate between the thalamus and the gray nuclei cells of the spinal cord. The **raphe** (a Greek word meaning "seam"), contains a high concentration of serotonin and is associated with the sleep function. Also called **central tegmental nucleus**.

nucleus pulposus a herniated intervertebral disk of the lumbar region of the spine, usually due to lifting a heavy object in a bent-forward position or to falling in this position.

nucleus ruber = RED NUCLEUS.

nucleus thoracicus = CLARKE'S COLUMN.

nuclei: See NUCLEUS.

nude-group therapy a controversial form of group psychotherapy based on the notion that psychological disclosure will be enhanced by physical disclosure. Some marathon groups have been conducted in the nude. According to I.D. Yalom (*The Theory and Practice of Group Psychotherapy*, 1975), one of the specialized techniques is to spread-eagle a member in order to achieve maximal genital disclosure.

nudism the public display of the naked human body. Various theories have been offered to explain n., including rebellion against Victorian modesty, a male's need to exhibit his masculinity as a reaction against castration anxiety, a female's need to display her body as a means of demonstrating her ability to attract men, and a "back to nature" philosophy.

null hypothesis a prediction that an experiment will find no difference between conditions or no relationship between variables. Statistical tests are then applied to the results in an attempt to disprove or reject the n.h. at a predetermined level of significance. Symbol: H_0. Also see ALTERNATIVE HYPOTHESIS.

nulliplex inheritance the inheritance of a trait determined by two recessive genes, each from one parent.

null set: See EMPTY SET.

number-completion test a test in which the subject is required to supply a missing item in a series of numbers or continue the series, e.g., 6, 9, 13, 18 . . . . (where the next answer is 24).

number factor an intelligence factor that is measured by tests of ability to handle numerical problems.

numerical ability: See PRIMARY ABILITIES.

numerology a study of the occult meaning of numbers, such as the date of one's birth or figures derived from the letters of one's name, as a means of interpreting their hypothetical influence on one's life and future. N. is sometimes considered a type of parapsychology.

nurse: See LICENSED PRACTICAL N.; NURSE'S AIDE; PSYCHIATRIC N.; PUBLIC-HEALTH N.; REGISTERED N.; REHABILITATION N.; VISITING N.

nurse's aide a person who works in a hospital or nursing home and shares the responsibility of providing personal care for patients. A n.a. usually has a minimum background education, including a high-school diploma followed by on-the-job training in a hospital or other health-care facility. Specific requirements vary with the institution employing the n.a.

nursing behavior the instinctive behavior involved in the female providing nourishment for young offspring until they are capable of obtaining their own sources of food. N.b. in mammals includes primarily the secretion of milk from the mammary glands of the mother and assisting the offspring to find the nipple so the young can suck the milk.

nursing home a long-term care facility designed to provide medical, nursing, social, psychological, recreational, and social-work support to residents afflicted with chronic illnesses or disabilities, such as rheumatic arthritis, stroke, heart disease, Parkinson's disease, atherosclerosis, Alzheimer's disease, or senile dementia.

nurturance need the need to care for, shield, defend, feed, sustain, and encourage a young child or young animal.

nurture the totality of environmental factors that influence the development and functioning of an organism throughout life. See NATURE-NURTURE CONTROVERSY. Compare NATURE.

nurturing experiences experiences that fulfill the need for nurturance, a term used by H. A. Murray to denote a fundamental need for protection, support, comfort, healing, and help.

nutmeg the seed of trees of the species Myristica acuminata and Myristica fragrans that are indigenous to the Banda Islands but are cultivated in South America, the Philippine Islands, and the West Indies. N. is the seed of a peachlike fruit and has volatile oils containing elemecin, myristicin, and other active ingredients that produce intoxicating effects that have been compared to those produced by cannabis sativa use. Also see MACE.

nutritional disorders any medical or psychological condition that results from malnutrition. Kinds of n.d. may include anorexia nervosa, obesity, pellagra, beriberi, hypervitaminosis, diabetes mellitus, or hemochromatosis.

nutritional factors nutrients required for the normal functioning of the organism, and which, if severely lacking, result in nutritional deficiency disorders. Among these requirements are a sufficient quantity of many kinds of amino acids, fatty acids, vitamins, potassium and other minerals, water, and leafy vegetables.

nux vomica the seed of a plant, Strychnos nux vomica, which grows in tropical Asia and has been used as an emetic. The name means literally a nut that causes vomiting. N.v. contains two substances, strychnine and brucine, which are CNS stimulants. N.v. also is administered in small quantities as a bitter tonic to stimulate digestion in certain cases that would not be affected by the potentially irritating effect of the drug. Also see STRYCHNINE.

NVD an abbreviation of *n*ausea, *v*omiting, and *d*iarrhea.

nyakwana = EPENA.

-nyct-; -nycto- a combining form relating to darkness or the night (Greek *nyktos*).

nyctalopia an inability to see in the dark or in a dimly lighted environment.

nyctophobia = ACHLUOPHOBIA.

nyctophonia a variation of elective mutism in which the person is able to speak at night but is mute during daylight hours.

NYD an abbreviation of *n*ot *y*et *d*iagnosed.

Nyhan, William Leo American physician, 1926—. See LESCH-NYHAN SYNDROME; AUTOAGGRESSIVE ACTIVITIES; FINGER-BITING BEHAVIOR; HYPERURICO-SURIA; HYPOXANTHINE GUANINE PHOSPHORIBOSYL TRANSFERASE; SELF-MUTILATION.

-nymph-; -nympho- a combining form relating to female sexuality (from Greek *nymphe*, "bride, maiden, nymph").

nymphomania a female disorder consisting of an excessive or insatiable desire for sexual stimulation and gratification, due to such factors as denial of homosexual tendencies, attempts to combat or disprove frigidity, a reaction to seduction in childhood, or a response to emotion-

al tension. The compulsive sex drive frequently expresses itself not only in promiscuity but in
masturbation performed several times a day.
Also called **andromania**.

nystagmus involuntary rapid movement of the
eyeballs due to a difference in orientation signals
from the semicircular canals in the left and right
inner ears. The labyrinthine disorder can be
caused by rotation of the head, damage to the
semicircular canals from injury or disease, or
electrical or thermal stimulation of the ear.
Pouring warm or cold water into the ear canal,
e.g., may upset the labyrinthine equilibrium.
The eyeball motion resulting in n. may be rota-
tory, horizontal, vertical, or a mixture. Also see
POSTROTATIONAL N.

O

oat-cell carcinoma: See CARCINOMA.

obedience a form of compliance carried out in response to direct command. Destructive o. is compliance with an authority figure, resulting in acts that are criminal, immoral, or in some way injurious to another's life. Milgram's studies were designed to measure the extent to which individuals, in an experimental setting, would obey authority if they believed they were harming another person. Based on the high level of o. found in his subjects, Milgram concluded that o. to authority is a potent determinant of behavior in American society. Also see AUTOMATIC O.; DESTRUCTIVE O.; DEFERRED O.

obesity in psychiatry, a psychogenic condition characterized by an excessive drive to eat (bulimia) and excessive weight (at least 20 percent above age and sex norms, taking individual constitution into consideration). Psychological factors frequently associated with compulsive overeating are persistent emotional tension; use of food as a substitute satisfaction in cases of sexual frustration or disappoinment; an unbearable life situation; parental overemphasis on food, or the use of food as a reward; emotional deprivation during the oral phase of psychosexual development; and a need to escape the risks and anxieties of social relationships ("Who wants a fat girl?"). See BULIMIA; HYPERPHAGIA. Also see HYPEROBESITY.

obesity treatments therapeutic efforts employed to produce substantial weight reduction, such as long-term diets, crash diets, group support, hypnotherapy, exercise programs, nutritional education, drug therapy, behavior modification of faulty eating patterns, glandular treatment where indicated, and dynamic psychotherapy focused on insight into the unconscious purposes served by excessive food intake.

object in psychoanalysis, the person, thing, or part of the body through which an instinct can achieve its aim of gratification. O. means also an aim or objective in general; anything of which the individual is aware; or a concrete entity of any kind.

object addict a description of some schizophrenia patients who cling obsessively to objects or ideas in an effort to prove they are in contact with reality.

object-assembly test a test in which the task is to reassemble an object puzzle that has been broken up or dismantled.

object attitude in structural psychology or in studies employing introspection, an attitude displayed by the type of observer who attends closely to the given object or stimulus while directing relatively less attention to the subjective processes as manifested in thoughts, feelings, and perceptions. Compare PROCESS ATTITUDE.

object blindness = VISUAL AGNOSIA.

object cathexis in psychoanalysis, the investment of psychic energy, or libido, in objects outside the self, such as a person, goal, idea, or activity. Also called **object libido**. Compare EGO CATHEXIS.

object choice in psychoanalysis, the selection of an object or person toward which psychic or libidinal energy is directed. See ANACLITIC O.C.; NARCISSISTIC O.C.

object constancy the tendency for an object to be perceived more or less unchanged despite variations in the conditions of observation.

object-finding in psychoanalysis, the process of directing the libido away from the self and toward external objects such as a friend, loved one, interest, or fetish.

objectifying attitude a tendency to react to an object, person, or event while disregarding personal feelings about it.

object-ill: See SUBJECT-ILL.

objectivation a type of defense projection in which an individual recognizes in other persons feelings or impulses that he fails to recognize in himself. O. is particularly important when it is present in a psychotherapist.

objective existing in physical reality outside the self; also, characterizing a type of observation that is free of personal bias.

objective anxiety anxiety precipitated by an external object or event, which in some instances may symbolize the original focus of anxiety, as in fear of pointed objects.

objective examination an examination in which subjective evaluation does not play a role in scoring, e.g., a multiple-choice test in which scoring standards have been formulated that allow no difference of opinion among different scorers as to the correctness of a response. In contrast, an **essay test** is a subjective examination.

objective orientation according to Piaget, moral judgment typical of children under age ten, characterized by a nearly exclusive attention to the objective, usually physical, consequences of an act, e.g., the number of cups broken rather than the child's mischievous behavior. The o.o. is a kind of literalism manifested by young children before they learn to take an individual's motives into account. Compare SUBJECTIVE ORIENTATION.

objective psychology a school of psychology that deals with observations of behavioral processes by competent persons and excludes subjective data.

objective psychotherapy a treatment procedure developed by B. Karpman primarily for use with institutionalized patients and patients with mild-to-moderate emotional disturbances. To reduce the subjectivity resulting from a personal relationship with the therapist, all therapeutic communication is carried out in writing. The patient answers written autobiographical questions, relates, and comments on dreams, and reacts to assigned readings. In return, the therapist gives interpretations and points out underlying mechanisms in written memoranda, including a "memorandum as a whole" which summarizes all the insights reached in the process.

objective reality the external world of physical objects, events, and forces that can be observed, measured, and tested. See REALITY.

objective scoring scoring a test by means of a key or formula, so that different scorers will arrive at the same score, in contrast to **subjective scoring** in which the score depends on the scorer's opinion or interpretation.

objective self-awareness a reflective state of awareness in which a person regards himself objectively, acknowledging personal limitations and the existing disparity between the "real" and "ideal" self.

objective sociogram: See SOCIOGRAM.

objective test = FORCED-RESPONSE TEST.

objective type the kind of individual who tends to view objects and events as existing in themselves rather than in relation to himself.

objectivity the tendency to base conclusions and interpretations on objective data, and to avoid judgments based on subjective factors or personal bias.

object libido = OBJECT CATHEXIS.

object loss the actual loss of a person to whom one has been deeply attached, by reason of death, illness, moving away, rejection, or other cause.
The term also refers to a threatened loss of love for one of these reasons.

object love in psychoanalysis, the investment of libidinal energy in an object or person other than the self.

object relations in psychoanalysis, relationships to persons, activities, or things that function as sources of libidinal or aggressive gratification. The gratification may occur directly or through sublimation of the psychic energy involved.

object-relations theory: See ANTILIBIDINAL EGO.

object-reversal test a learning procedure in which (a) numerous object-discrimination options may be offered, and (b), as the subject learns to make a correct choice, the problem is reversed so that the subject must learn to make a second choice, and so on until all objects can be chosen correctly.

obligations fear = PARALIPOPHOBIA.

obligatory perception the visual perception of the neonate characterized by inflexible concentration on configurations and colors of high contrast, e.g., a tendency to focus on black and white. Also see PRINCIPLE OF MAXIMUM CONTRAST; PREFERENTIAL PERCEPTION.

oblique correlated, not independent. This term is used to describe the relationship between correlated factors in a factor analysis. Also see ORTHOGONAL.

obliviscence a gradual fading of memories with the passage of time; forgetfulness.

obnubilation stupor; also, clouding of consciousness.

OBS = ORGANIC BRAIN SYNDROMES.

obscenity verbal expressions, drawings, gestures, and written material that grossly violate the norms of good taste and decency in a given society. See PORNOGRAPHY.

obscenity-purity complex a rigid set of self-imposed moral standards regarding obscene or "impure" thoughts, feelings, or actions, accompanied by a persistent dread of violating these standards. Also called **puritan complex**.

obscurantism beliefs and actions that are opposed to scientific inquiry, understanding, and the progress of knowledge; deliberate deprecation of established facts and theories, especially if these appear to contradict a given set of political, economic, social, or religious convictions; also, intentional obscurity designed to obfuscate.

observation the intentional examination of an object or process for the purpose of obtaining facts about it or reporting one's conclusions based on what was observed.

observational learning the acquisition of information or skill through watching the performance of others either directly or via films and videotapes. The term also applies to the conditioning of an animal to perform an act observed in a member of the same or a different species. An example is the o.l. by a mockingbird that results in an ability to imitate the song patterns of other kinds of birds. Also see MODELING.

observational-learning theory = SOCIAL-LEARN-ING THEORY.

observational method the scientific method in which observers are trained to watch and record animal or human behavior as precisely and completely as possible without personal bias or interpretation. Tape recorders, cameras, stopwatches, and other devices may be used to increase accuracy. Also called **observation technique**.

observation commitment in forensic psychiatry, commitment to a hospital by a court order for a limited period of observation, usually to determine fitness for trial or legal competence.

observation delusion: See DELUSION OF OBSERVATION.

observation technique = OBSERVATIONAL METHOD.

observer drift a tendency for two behavioral raters working together to begin to agree with each other in a manner that is idiosyncratic to them. O.d. results in apparent high levels of reliability but also yields data that are different from results produced by another pair of raters assigned to the same project.

observer's sociogram: See SOCIOGRAM.

obsession a thought, image, or impulse that persistently intrudes on consciousness against the individual's will. Morbid obsessions, as contrasted with benign perseverations like musical themes or meaningless phrases, have an irrational quality and may dominate consciousness and behavior to the point of interfering with work and social life. Examples are philosophical ruminations (intellectual obsessions), dread of contamination (obsessive fears), thoughts about hurting or killing others (obsessive impulses), and persistent images relating to traumatic events (obsessive fantasies). See OBSESSIVE-COMPULSIVE DISORDER.

obsessional brooding preoccupation with abstract, metaphysical questions concerning life, death, and the universe; also, a compulsion to worry about relatively trivial matters. O.b. is often interpreted as an attempt to escape from emotional problems or forbidden impulses. See INTELLECTUALIZATION; BROODING COMPULSION.

obsessional character a personality disorder characterized by such traits as excessive caution and orderliness, worry over slight errors and imperfections, and an overconscientious attitude toward the self and others. See COMPULSIVE-PERSONALITY DISORDER.

obsessionalism a term applied by H. S. Sullivan to obsessive behavior that is used as a dynamism or defense measure. See OBSESSIVE BEHAVIOR.

obsessional personality = OBSESSIVE PERSONALITY.

obsessional thoughts: See OBSESSION; OBSESSIONAL BROODING.

obsessional type: See LIBIDINAL TYPES.

obsessive attack a Rado term for the major symptoms of obsessive-compulsive psychoneurosis derived from childhood temper tantrums: spells of doubting and brooding, alternating with bouts of ritual-making and an urge to injure or kill someone. See HORRIFIC TEMPTATION.

obsessive behavior behavior characteristic of an obsessive personality or obsessive-compulsive disorder, such as persistent brooding, doubting, ruminating, worrying over trifles, cleaning up and keeping things in perfect order, or performing rituals.

obsessive-compulsive disorder an anxiety disorder in which obsessions or compulsions are a significant source of distress, and interfere with the individual's ability to function. Obsessions are persistent, recurrent ideas and impulses (e.g., thoughts of committing violence; ideas of contamination or doubt) that appear senseless or repugnant to the individual but force themselves on consciousness and cannot be ignored or suppressed. Compulsions are repetitive, stereotyped acts (e.g., hand-washing, counting, checking, touching) which must be performed in order to relieve tension even though they are recognized as excessive or senseless. Also called **obsessive-compulsive neurosis**. (DSM-III)

obsessive-compulsive personality a persistent personality pattern characterized by an extreme drive for perfection, an excessive orderliness, an inability to compromise, and an exaggerated sense of responsibility.

obsessive doubt in obsessive-compulsive disorders, a condition of obsessive brooding, doubt, and uncertainty, which may represent sexualization of thought.

obsessive fantasy a persistent image or daydream, such as a mother's recurrent mental picture of her daughter being raped.

obsessive fears persistent, irrational fears, or phobias, such as dread of contamination or fear of thinking immoral thoughts. See PHOBIA; OBSESSION.

obsessive impulse a morbid, intrusive urge to perform an inappropriate or offensive act such as shouting an obscene word or stabbing someone.

obsessive personality in DSM-I, a personality-trait disturbance characterized by excessive orderliness, perfectionism, indecisiveness, constant worry over trivia, and the imposition of rigid standards on others. Also called **obsessional personality**.

obsessive-ruminative tension state a term used by Adolf Meyer for obsessive-compulsive psychoneurosis.

obstacle sense the ability of the blind to avoid obstacles in their path.

obstinate progression movements that continue after a subject is restrained or cornered or otherwise prevented from advancing the body by leg movements. See SYNDROME OF O.P.

obstipation a form of severe constipation that usually is associated with a functional origin.

obstruction an alternative term for BLOCKING. See this entry.

obstruction box a device used in animal experiments in which the subject is required to overcome an obstacle in order to reach a reward.

E.g., in order to reach a pedal that can be pressed to deliver pleasurable brain stimulation, a rat may have to walk across an electrified grid. The o.b. helps investigators compare the values subjects place on different rewards. See OB-STRUCTION METHOD.

obstruction method a technique of determining drive dominance by pitting one drive against another, e.g., hunger versus sex. In animal experiments the subject may have to cross an electrified grid to get to the food or a mate. Also see OBSTRUCTION BOX.

obstructive = PLOSIVE.

obstructive disease any disorder that results in the obstruction of a body passageway or conduit. The term usually is applied to obstructions, e.g., enlarged prostate, tumors, or renal stones, that prevent the free flow of urine from the kidneys. A renal o.d. usually can be corrected by surgery, as an alternative to progressive degeneration leading to end-stage renal disease.

obstructive dysmenorrhea: See DYSMENORRHEA.

obtained frequency the frequency distribution observed in a set of data, and contrasted with the frequency that might be expected from various theoretical assumptions.

obtained score = RAW SCORE.

obtrusive idea an obsessive, unwanted, foreign idea that intrudes on the person's normal flow of thought.

obturation the process of closing or otherwise occluding an opening to a passageway in the body. See OBTURATOR.

obturator a prosthetic device used to close an opening in the palate. It is usually worn inside the mouth to close the opening in the hard and soft palates of cleft-palate patients, thereby improving speech production.

Occam, William of English scholastic philosopher, ca. 1280–1349. See OCCAM'S RAZOR.

Occam's razor the scientific maxim that the simplest hypothesis or explanation is always preferable. That is, given an alternative between two hypotheses, the one accompanied by the fewer assumptions should be chosen. The term is derived from the maxim of a 14th-century Franciscan monk, William of Occam. Also called **principle of economy; law of parsimony.**

occasional inversion a form of homosexual activity that may occur when the subject is deprived of the presence of persons of the opposite sex, e.g., in prison or the army. Also see SITUATIONAL HOMOSEXUALITY.

occipital lobe the part of a cerebral hemisphere that is most posterior to the rest of the cortex. The lobe is associated with the visual sense. See BRAIN.

occipitopontinus: See CORTICOPONTINE NUCLEUS.

occlusal neurosis the unconscious grinding or setting of teeth when not eating, as in nocturnal bruxism.

occlusion an obstruction or closure, as when a cerebral artery is occluded, causing a stroke; also, a phenomenon of simultaneous firing of two branches of the same neuron which may result in a total output that is less than the sum of the separate responses.

occlusive = PLOSIVE.

occult mysterious, incomprehensible, secret, especially as applied to a class of phenomena, or presumptive phenomena, that cannot be explained in either everyday or scientific terms, such as premonitory dreams, telepathic awareness, and clairvoyant communications. See EXTRASENSORY PERCEPTION; PARAPSYCHOLOGY; PSI; PSEUDOSCIENCE.

occultism the belief that natural processes can be controlled by magic or secret methods, or the attempt to control nature or people by such means.

occult myelodysplasia an abnormality in the development of the spinal cord that cannot be attributed to any particular cause, such as a genetic defect. The condition may or may not involve protrusion of nervous tissue or membranes as would occur in a case of myelomeningocele.

occupational ability the ability to perform vocational or professional tasks, generally measured by a series of occupational tests.

occupational adjustment the degree to which an individual has compatibly matched abilities, interests, and personality to job or career. The term differs from vocational adjustment in its emphasis on the interaction between an individual's personal characteristics and the objective requirements, conditions, and opportunities associated with the job. Also see VOCATIONAL ADJUSTMENT.

occupational analysis the systematic collection, processing, and interpretation of information concerning the objective work conditions found in specific occupations.

occupational cramp a psychogenic cramp, usually in the hand or arm, which prevents the individual from engaging in his occupation, such as writing, driving, sewing, playing an instrument, or shooting a gun in combat. See OCCUPATIONAL NEUROSIS.

occupational delirium = PURPOSELESS HYPERACTIVITY.

occupational drinking a pattern of consumption of above-average amounts of alcohol due in part to the nature of the imbiber's occupation, such as advertising or public relations, that requires participation in cocktail parties and similar forms of entertainment of clients or customers.

occupational family a group of jobs or vocations with similar ability requirements.

occupational hierarchy an organization of occupations in order of increasing requirements of ability or competence, and, in some cases, according to prestige.

occupational inhibition an inhibition associated with employment, which may be expressed as poor work performance or reactive symptoms of illness such as fatigue or vertigo.

occupational level an occupation or class of

occupations that requires a given degree of education or other training and competence.

occupational neurosis a neurotic reaction to one's occupation, usually in the form of extreme tension and anxiety and the development of symptoms such as cramps that make it difficult or impossible to continue the work. The symptoms are often interpreted as conversion (hysterical) reactions produced by such psychogenic factors as emotional conflict, resentment against working conditions, near accidents, or fear of failure. See OCCUPATIONAL CRAMP; SEAMSTRESS'S CRAMP; TELEGRAPHER'S CRAMP; VIOLINIST'S CRAMP; WRITER'S CRAMP; APHTHONGIA; WERNICKE'S CRAMP.

occupational norm the average or typical scores obtained from tests of abilities for a given occupational category.

occupational psychiatry = INDUSTRIAL PSYCHIATRY.

occupational rehabilitation a phase of rehabilitation in which the ability to work is restored or improved through vocational counseling and evaluation, job-finding, or work in a sheltered setting under the federal-state rehabilitation system.

occupational stability a characteristic behavior trait of an individual who rarely changes jobs.

occupational stress tension and strain experienced by workers and executives on the job, arising out of such factors as resentment against superiors, disagreeable working conditions, fatigue, occupational hazards, excessive competition, or anxiety over possible unemployment.

occupational test a test designed to measure potential ability or actual proficiency in a given occupation.

occupational therapy in psychiatry and rehabilitation, a form of supportive therapy consisting of useful tasks and activities involving skill, such as clay-modeling or gardening. Such activities help patients develop constructive interests, focus attention outside themselves, reestablish self-esteem, bring them into contact with others, and keep them from lapsing into inertia.

oceanic feeling a sense of unlimited power associated with identification with the universe as a whole. According to psychoanalytic theory, this feeling originates in the earliest period of life, before the infant is aware of the outside world or the distinction between the ego and nonego. It is accompanied by a feeling of omnipotence that is believed to arise from the infant's control over movement and the immediate satisfaction of his narcissistic needs. Oceanic feelings may be revived later in life as a schizophrenic delusion or as a religious experience. See COSMIC IDENTIFICATION; MEGALOMANIA; OMNIPOTENCE OF THOUGHT.

ochlophobia = DEMOPHOBIA.

O'Connor v. Donaldson a 1975 proceeding in which the court ruled that no nondangerous person can be custodially confined if he can survive successfully in freedom.

-ocul-; -oculo- a combining form relating to the eye (Latin *oculus*).

ocular albinism: See ALBINISM.

ocular dominance = EYE DOMINANCE.

ocular hypertelorism = MEDIUM-CLEFT-FACE SYNDROME.

ocular myopathy: MYOPATHIES.

ocular pursuit the successive fixations of an eye that is following a moving object. Also called **visual pursuit; visual tracking**.

oculoauriculovertebral dysplasia = GOLDENHAR'S SYNDROME.

oculocerebral-hypopigmentation syndrome a hereditary disorder marked by eye anomalies, absence of hair and skin pigmentation, mental retardation, and spasticity. The patients have cloudy small corneas and an apparent absence of retina and iris. The cases studied have involved children of Old Order Amish families. The syndrome is believed to be due to an autosomal-recessive trait that becomes manifested through consanguinity.

oculocerebrorenal syndrome an X-linked recessive genetic disorder affecting male children and marked by renal-tubule dysfunction, mental retardation, and a series of eye disorders including congenital glaucoma, cataracts, and distention of the eyeball because of fluid accumulation. The renal disorders include acidosis, hypophosphatemia, and excess amino acids in the urine. Neurologic deficits vary from absence-of-brain abnormalities to hydrocephalus and cerebral atrophy. Also called **o.s. of Lowe; Lowe's syndrome; Lowe's disease**.

oculogyral illusion the apparent movement of a faint light in a dark room due to rotational nystagmus produced by body movements.

oculogyric crisis a symptom of parkinsonism in which there is a prolonged fixation of the eyeballs in a single position, accompanied by tics and contraction of the cervical muscles resulting in a bizarre twisting of the neck. The patient may maintain the position for minutes to hours. The effect also is produced by certain antipsychotic drugs. Also called **oculogyric spasm**.

oculomandibulodyscephaly with hypotrichosis = HALLERMANN-STREIFF SYNDROME.

oculomotor nerve the third cranial nerve, containing both motor and sensory fibers, and innervating most of the muscles associated with movement and accommodation of the eye and constriction of the pupil (that is, all the muscles of the eye except the external rectus and superior oblique muscles). The o.n. is referred to as "cranial nerve III."

oculomotor nuclei the terminal point for most of the ascending fibers of the vestibular nerves.

O.D. an abbreviation used in prescriptions, meaning "in the right eye" (Latin *oculo dextro*).

O.D. = OVERDOSE.

odd-even reliability a method of assessing the reliability of a test by correlating scores on the odd-numbered items with scores on the even-numbered items. It is a special case of SPLIT-HALF RELIABILITY. See this entry.

oddity problem a learning task in which an animal

is required to make a choice of an object that is in some way different from other possible choices. The purpose is to test the ability of the subject to perceive relationships and differences among a number of similar objects.

-odont-; -odonto- a combining form relating to the teeth.

odontophobia a morbid fear of teeth (and perhaps of being bitten by teeth).

odor the sensory experience produced by stimulation of the olfactory nerve organ by a volatile substance. Also see SMELL; SMELL MECHANISM; OLFACTION.

odor fear = OLFACTOPHOBIA.

odorimetry the measurement of odors. Also called **olfactometry.**

odor prism a prism-shaped graphic representation of the six primary odors and their relationships: putrid, burned, spicy, resinous, ethereal, and fragrant. Also called **smell prism.**

-odyn-; -odynia a combining form relating to a specified pain (Greek *odyne*).

odynophobia = ALGOPHOBIA.

oedipal conflict = OEDIPUS COMPLEX.

oedipal phase in psychoanalysis, the phallic stage of psychosexual development, usually between ages three and seven, during which the Oedipus complex manifests itself. Also called **oedipal stage.**

oedipal situation = OEDIPUS COMPLEX.

oedipal stage = OEDIPAL PHASE.

oedipism a rarely used term for self-inflicted eye injuries. The term is derived from the mythical Oedipus, who blinded himself. Also spelled **edipism.**

Oedipus complex /ed'-/ or /ēd'-/ in psychoanalysis, the erotic feelings of the son toward the mother, accompanied by rivalry and hostility toward the father. The term is also applied to the corresponding relationship between the daughter and father, sometimes referred to as the female Oedipus complex or the Electra complex. Freud derived the name from the Greek myth in which Oedipus killed his father and married his mother. He believed the Oedipus situation is universal, dating from the phallic period of psychosexual development, between the ages of three and seven. Most anthropologists question its universality, since there are many cultures in which it does not appear. Horney claimed it was neither normal nor universal, and held that when it does occur, it is a neurotic relationship fostered by provocative behavior on the part of the parent. Freud, on the other hand, claimed that it becomes the basis for a neurosis only if it is not adequately resolved by the boy's fear of castration and gradual identification with the father. The female Oedipus complex is resolved by the threat of losing the mother's love and by finding fulfillment in the feminine role. Also called **oedipal situation; oedipal conflict.** See CASTRATION COMPLEX; ELECTRA COMPLEX; NEGATIVE O.C.; COMPLETE OEDIPUS; NUCLEAR COMPLEX.

O element = OVERLAPPING FACTOR.

oestrus = ESTRUS.

OFD I syndrome a hereditary disorder marked by cleft tongue, palate, and lip, digital anomalies, and mental retardation (*o*ral-*f*acial-*d*igital). As many as 50 percent of the cases have been found to be mentally retarded, and a few were hydrocephalic or hydranencephalic. All the patients surviving birth have been female; it is assumed the trait is lethal in male fetuses. Also called **oral-facial-digital syndrome.**

office landscaping in office design, the use of large open expanses in which work spaces are partitioned only by movable furniture, screens, plants, or accessories. Some workers find this arrangement too noisy, distracting, and lacking in privacy. Others find it helps to satisfy their need for contact and solidarity.

Ohm, Georg Simon German physicist, 1787–1854. See OHM'S LAW.

Ohm's law in audition, the principle that the ear can reduce complex tones into a series of simple sine waves.

-oid a combining form denoting resemblance.

oikiophobia = OIKOPHOBIA.

-oiko-; -oikio- a combining form relating to a house or home (Greek *oikos*).

oikofugic pertaining to an urge to travel or wander from home.

oikomania = ECOMANIA.

oikophobia a morbid fear of being in one's own house or home. Also called **oikiophobia; ecophobia.** Also see DOMATOPHOBIA.

oikotropic a tendency to be homesick when away from friends and family.

oil of wintergreen: See ASPIRIN POISONING.

oinomania an alternative term for alcoholism.

O.L. an abbreviation used in prescriptions, meaning "in the left eye" (Latin *oculo laevus*).

olfaction the sense of smell, which is activated by stimulation of receptor cells in the olfactory epithelium located in the nasal passages leading from the nostrils to the throat. See SMELL; VIBRATIONAL THEORY.

olfactometer an instrument used to regulate the amount and intensity of olfactory stimuli in threshold studies.

olfactometry = ODORIMETRY.

olfactophobia a morbid fear of odors. Also called **osphresiophobia; osmophobia.**

olfactory areas brain structures associated with the sense of smell. Experimental evidence has been compiled by excision or ablation of a number of tissues in and about the rhinencephalon with varied and often conflicting results. Only lesions of the olfactory bulb seem to produce consistently a disruption of olfactory functions.

olfactory brain: See RHINENCEPHALON.

olfactory bulb a bulblike ending on the olfactory nerve in the anterior lobe of each cerebral hemisphere.

olfactory epithelium an area of olfactory receptors or nerve endings in the lining of the nose.

olfactory eroticism pleasurable sensations, particularly of an erotic nature, associated with the sense of smell.

olfactory hallucination a false perception of odors, which are usually unpleasant or repulsive, such as poison gas or decaying flesh. It is sometimes associated with feelings of guilt, especially when accompanied by accusatory voices.

olfactory nerve the first cranial nerve; the sensory nerve of smell originating in the olfactory lobe and distributed to the nasal mucous membrane. The o.n. is referred to as "cranial nerve I."

olfactory stimulation the excitation of the spindle-shaped cells in the nasal cavity by inhalation of volatile substances called odors. There is little agreement on the precise mechanism involved.

olfactory sulcus a groove or furrow on the surface of each of the cerebral hemispheres located on the inferior side of the frontal lobes. The o.s. separates the gyrus rectus from the medial orbital gyrus.

olfactory tract a band of nerve fibers that originates in the olfactory bulb and extends backwards along the bottom side of the frontal lobe to a point called the **olfactory trigone**, at which point the tract divides into three strands leading to the medial and lateral olfactory gyri and the olfactory tubercle. Also see LATERAL O.T.

olfactory tubercle a small oval elevation near the base of the olfactory tract leading from the olfactory bulb to the brain. The o.t. occurs rarely in humans but is a common structure in animals that depend upon a sense of smell to survive. It contains auxiliary olfactory-nerve fibers and cells.

-olig-; -oligo- a combining form meaning few, scant, deficient (Greek *oligos*).

oligergasia Adolf Meyer's term for mental deficiency.

oligodactyly a congenital anomaly marked by a smaller-than-normal number of fingers or toes, as in cases of de Lange syndrome.

oligondendroglia satellite structure or support cells that are associated with neurons in the central nervous system.

oligoencephaly a form of mental deficiency associated with asymmetrical physical development and often marked by an abnormally small brain, nervous-system irregularities, and low resistance to disease.

oligohydramnios a deficiency of amniotic fluid, a condition that can result in mechanical interference with fetal movements, leading to possible congenital defects, e.g., clubfoot, torticollis, muscular dystrophy, or brain damage.

oligomenorrhea: See MENSTRUAL DISORDERS.

oligophrenia mental deficiency or mental retardation (Greek, "small mentality"). O. sometimes is used with a modifying term, as in PHENYLPYRUVIC O. See this entry.

oligospermia an abnormally low content of spermatozoa in a male semen sample. O. is one of several factors responsible for male infertility. The usually accepted minimum level of sperm needed to insure fertility is 20 million per milliliter.

olisbos = DILDO.

olivary nucleus an olive-shaped mass of gray matter in the medulla, containing nuclei of fibers that connect the cerebral cortex with other parts of the brain.

olivocochlear bundle a group of auditory-nerve fibers extending from the superior olive through the descending neural pathways to the area of the cochlear hair cells.

olivopontocerebellar atrophy a progressive hereditary neurological disease of which five types are known. Symptoms usually include varying degrees of ataxia, dysarthria, tremors, sensory loss, and in some cases retinal degeneration with progressive visual loss, facial palsy, rigidities, dementia, extrapyramidal signs, and neuronal loss throughout the cortex. In many cases onset does not occur until the second or third decade and death takes place in ten to 20 years.

-ology; -logy a combining form relating to a field of study.

ololiuqui the seed of a Latin American snake plant vine Rivea corymbosa, which contains substances chemically related to lysergic acid diethylamide (LSD), but is less potent. O. is the plant described in the 16th-century reports of the explorer Hernández as that eaten by the Aztec priests when they "wanted to commune with their gods and to receive a message from them."

olophonia defective speech due to malformed vocal organs.

Olszewski, Jerzy Polish-born Canadian neurologist, 1913–66. See STEELE-RICHARDSON-OLSZEWSKI SYNDROME.

-om-; omo- a combining form relating to the shoulder (Greek *omos*).

-oma- a combining form relating to a tumor or a swelling (from Greek suffix *-oma*, which may be derived from *onkoma*, "swelling").

ombrophobia a morbid fear of rain or a rainstorm.

ombudsman an individual appointed by an organization or legislature to hear and investigate complaints and grievances of private citizens, including patients, against government agencies, hospitals, or other facilities. The concept and term originated in Scandinavia.

omega /ōmēg'ə/ or /ōmāg'ə/ 24th letter of the Greek alphabet (Ω, ω).

omicron /om'ikron/ 15th letter of the Greek alphabet (O, o).

-omma- a combining form relating to the eye (Greek *omma*).

ommatidium a unit of a compound eye of an arthropod. The combination of the elongated **ommatidia** forms a mosaic image on the animal's retina.

ommatophobia a morbid fear of eyes.

omn. hor. an abbreviation used in prescriptions, meaning "every hour" (Latin *omni hora*).

omnibus test a test in which the items fall into several different categories; however, the items are not grouped by category but are mixed together within the test to yield a single score.

omnipotence /-nip'-/ in psychoanalysis, the infant's feeling that he is all-powerful and that all his wishes must and will be fulfilled. Later in life, patients who have lost contact with reality may experience delusions of infinite power, wealth, or potency, which some authorities interpret as a regression to infantile o. Also called **o. of the id.** See MEGALOMANIA.

omnipotence of thought the feeling that wishes can be gratified and reality changed by thought alone. Freud believed this feeling stems from infancy, when the immediate satisfaction of needs and wishes gives the child a sense of unlimited power. Later in life it may take the pathological form of grandiose ideas or magical thinking. See OCEANIC FEELING.

'omnipotent' therapist: See PRESTIGE SUGGESTION.

omn. noct. an abbreviation used in prescriptions, meaning "every night" (Latin *omni nocte*).

-omphal-; -omphalo- a combining form relating to the navel or to the umbilical cord.

omphalus = UMBILICUS.

onanism sexual withdrawal, or coitus interruptus; also, masturbation. The term is derived from the biblical passage in which "Onan went to his brother's wife" and "spilled it [his seed] on the ground" (Genesis 38:9). Also see COITUS INTERRUPTUS; MASTURBATION.

-onco- a combining form relationg to (a) a tumor, (b) volume (from Greek *onkos*, "mass").

oncology the study and treatment of benign and malignant tumors.

Oneida community: See COITUS RESERVATUS; GROUP MARRIAGE.

-oneir-; -oneira- a combining form relating to dreams (from Greek *oneiros*, "dream").

oneirism /ōnī'-/ a dreamlike state in a condition of wakefulness. Adjective: **oneiric.**

oneirodynia: See ONEIRONOSUS.

oneirogmus a nocturnal emission of semen while dreaming.

oneirology the scientific study of dreams and their interpretation. See DREAM INTERPRETATION.

oneironosus a morbid form of dreaming but distinguished from **oneirodynia,** or nightmare.

oneirophrenia a term used by Meduna and McCulloch for a psychosis resembling schizophrenia in certain symptoms, such as disturbances of emotion and associations, but distinguished from schizophrenia by a dreamlike state with clouded sensorium. See ATYPICAL PSYCHOSIS.

one-tailed probability: See ONE-TAILED TEST; TWO-TAILED TEST.

one-tailed test a statistical test of an experimental hypothesis specifying the expected direction of an effect or a relationship; half the probability of a two-tailed test. E.g., a **one-tailed probability** of .05 corresponds to a **two-tailed probability** of .10.

one-trial learning the mastery of a skill or an increment of learning on the first trial.

one-way analysis of variance a statistical test of the probability that the means of three or more samples have been drawn from the same population. With two groups, this reduces to a T TEST. See this entry.

one-way mirror a mirror or window which can be seen through only in one direction, used for the unobtrusive observation of subjects, e.g., in studying the behavior of children. Also called **one-way screen.**

oniomania an uncontrollable impulse to spend money, and to buy without regard to need or use.

on-line in computers, connected electronically and ready for, or actually, data-processing.

-onoma-; -onomato- a combining form relating to name or naming (from Greek *onoma*, "name").

onomatomania obsessive preoccupation with words or names, including persistent intrusion of certain words and sentences into one's thoughts.

onomatophobia a morbid fear of names or of hearing a particular name.

onomatopoeia /-pē'ə/ the formation of words that seem to imitate the sound of the thing or action they represent, e.g., "hiss" or "glob" (from Greek *onoma*, "name," and *poiein*, "to make"). O. may be characteristic of certain types of schizophrenia, in which case the term **onomatopoiesis** is occasionally preferred. Adjectives: **onomatopoeic** /-pē'ik/; **onomatopoetic** /-pō·et'ik/.

onomatopoeic theory: See ORIGIN-OF-LANGUAGE THEORIES.

on-the-job training vocational training provided by an employer during regular working hours for the purpose of supplying the worker with the additional knowledge or skills required for competent job performance.

on the wagon: See DELTA ALCOHOLISM.

-onto- a combining form relating to existence or being (from Greek *on, ontos*, "being, individual" or "being, existence").

ontoanalysis a form of analysis that probes the ultimate nature of being; existential analysis.

ontogenesis; ontogenetic: See ONTOGENY.

ontogenic a term used by some authorities to characterize not only the biological development of the individual but also psychological growth in terms of the stages of life and their relation to developmental processes such as learning, thinking, and expression of needs and purposes.

ontogeny /-toj'-/ the biological origin and development of the individual organism, as distinguished from phylogeny, the development of the species. Also called **ontogenesis.** Adjective: **ontogenetic.** Also see ONTOGENIC. Compare PHYLOGENY.

ontology the branch of philosophy that deals with the abstract nature of *being* as such, as distinct from material or spiritual existence, which are forms of *becoming*.

-onych-; -onycho- a combining form relating to the nails.

onychophagia; onychophagy = NAIL-BITING.

-oo- /-ō·ə-/ a combining form meaning egg, ovum (Greek *oon*).

oocyte an immature ovum in the female ovary, produced by the division of an oogonium into two daughter cells; the larger daughter cell becomes an o. and the smaller cell becomes a polar body. The first maturation division produces a primary o. and the second maturation division a secondary o. Also see POLAR BODY; PRIMARY O.; MEIOSIS.

oogenesis: See POLAR BODY.

oogonium the immature egg cell of the female before it begins dividing in the ovary into a primary oocyte and a polar body.

-oophor-; -oophoro- a combining form relating to the ovary.

oophorectomy = OVARIOTOMY.

oosperm an alternative term for the fertilized ovum.

Opalski, Adam Polish physician, 1897–1963. See WALLENBERG'S SYNDROME (there: **Opalski's syndrome**).

OPD syndrome a congenital disorder affecting males or females, believed to be X-linked and marked by short stature, mild mental retardation, bone anomalies, and a variety of other possible defects (*oto*palato*d*igital). Also called **otopalatodigital syndrome.**

open-classroom design the concept of classroom planning that provides a study environment based on results of behavioral-mapping techniques. The o.-c.d. frequently utilizes illumination by fluorescent lighting, thereby eliminating the need for traditional classroom design in which rows of desks were arranged in parallel patterns with tall windows the main source of illumination.

open-class word = CONTENT WORD.

open-cue situation a learning situation in which all the cues required to arrive at the goal are visible to the experimental subject who must comprehend the relationships that link cues to goal.

open-door hospital = open HOSPITAL.

open-door policy the policy of maintaining an open hospital or hospital unit, usually associated with the concept of a therapeutic community.

open-ended question in an examination, survey, or interview, a question that the student, subject, or respondent answers in his own words, e.g., an essay question. Compare CLOSED-ENDED QUESTION.

open fracture: See FRACTURE.

open group a counseling or therapy group that new members may join at stages during the course of therapy. Also called **continuous group.** Compare CLOSED GROUP.

open hospital a mental hospital without locked doors or physical restraints. Also called **open-door hospital.**

opening moves: See ADOLESCENT PSYCHOTHERAPY.

opening sound = PLOSIVE.

open marriage a marital arrangement, formal or common-law, in which both partners agree to accept the freedom of their spouse to have extramarital sex activity. O.m. is based on an understanding that each partner may have emotional and sexual needs that cannot be satisfied within a monogamous relationship. Success of an o.m. depends primarily upon an equal desire by both partners to maintain the arrangement.

open system a biological system in which growth can occur without conforming to laws of thermodynamics or a demonstrated constancy of energy relations.

open ward a hospital ward or unit in which the doors are not locked.

operant behavior behavior produced and maintained by its consequences, e.g., pressing a lever to obtain food; a voluntarily emitted response already within an organism's repertoire that serves to have an effect on its environment (e.g., a bird may peck the grass for food).

operant conditioning a term applied by B. F. Skinner to a process in which learning or behavioral change takes place as a result of reinforcing (rewarding) the desired behavior and withholding the reward or actively punishing undesired behavior. Examples are teaching a dog to do tricks, and rewarding behavior change in mental patients. The term is essentially equivalent to instrumental conditioning. See SHAPING; BEHAVIOR MODIFICATION.

operant learning: See OPERANT CONDITIONING.

operant level a base line of behavior as it occurs naturally prior to reinforcement, e.g., the amount of lever-pressing that occurs before an experiment begins.

operant reserve the number of responses made in an operant-conditioning program after the reinforcement has been withdrawn. It is a measure of the strength of conditioning.

operating characteristic a curve showing the probability of accepting the null hypothesis at different levels of a parameter.

operation as used by Piaget, a mental act; the derivation of logical relationships in the process of manipulating either physical objects or symbols, e.g., the manipulation of symbols to solve an equation. The process of performing operations, according to Piaget, is central in the building of intellect. See CONCRETE OPERATIONS; FORMAL OPERATIONS.

operational definition the definition of a term by referring to the operations by which it is measured, e.g., defining anxiety in terms of a test score, behavioral withdrawal, or activation of the sympathetic nervous system.

operational evaluation = PROCESS EVALUATION.

operational fatigue = COMBAT FATIGUE.

operationalism = OPERATIONISM.

operational research = OPERATIONS RESEARCH.

operationism the viewpoint that a concept's meaning and validity depends upon the procedures used to define or establish it; the viewpoint that each concept must take as its meaning a single observable and measurable operation. In concrete terms, o. might define an emotional disorder as a particular score on a diagnostic test. Also called **operationalism**.

operations research the application of scientific methods to the study of complex organizations and to the solution of complex problems involving conflicting goals, concepts, and decisions. Abbrev.: **OR**. Also called **operational research**.

operative knowledge Piaget's term for knowledge acquired in the process of performing operations. Piaget contrasts o.k. with figurative knowledge, e.g., the ability to remember facts or dates. According to Piagetians, o.k. should be more strongly emphasized in intelligence tests and schools since it is central to the development of intellect. See OPERATION. Compare FIGURATIVE KNOWLEDGE.

operators a term applied by R. Gelman to the mental processes involved in comprehending the effect of different numerical manipulations, e.g., knowing that adding an orange to a bowl of oranges changes the number while rearranging the oranges does not alter the number. Also see ESTIMATORS.

ophidiophilia an abnormal fascination with snakes (from Greek *ophis*, "snake"). Also see SNAKE SYMBOL.

ophidiophobia a morbid fear of snakes. Also called **snake phobia**. Also see SNAKE SYMBOL.

-ophthalm-; -ophthalmo- a combining form relating to the eye (Greek *ophthalmos*).

ophthalmia a severe inflammation of the eye that may affect either the conjunctiva or deeper structures. Kinds of o. include **mucous o.** or **catarrhal o.**, a form of conjunctivitis with a purulent secretion, **electric o.**, a type of irritation produced by exposure to the light of an electric welding torch, **neuroparalytic o.**, a corneal inflammation with possible ulceration associated with trigeminal-nerve lesions, and TRACHOMA. See this entry.

ophthalmia neonatorum: See SILVER NITRATE.

ophthalmic artery a branch of the internal carotid artery that arises near the point where it enters the skull. The numerous small branches of the o.a. supply blood to the various tissues of the ocular orbit, the eyeball, and the muscles of the eye, internal and external. It also supplies the eyelids and the lacrimal glands.

ophthalmoneuromyelitis = DEVIC'S DISEASE.

ophthalmoplegia: See PARINAUD'S SYNDROME; WERNICKE'S ENCEPHALOPATHY.

ophthalmoplegia externa = BALLET'S DISEASE.

ophthalmoplegic dystrophy a form of muscular dystrophy that involves the extraocular muscles controlling eye movements. The disease usually begins in adulthood and is progressive in its effects, extending to the pharyngeal muscles and other parts of the head and face. O.d. sometimes causes a drooping of the eyelids similar to the symptom observed in patients with myasthenia gravis.

ophthalmoscopy the study of the fundus of the eye

with an **ophthalmoscope**. O. may be direct, with examination of the eye at close range so as to observe an erect image, or indirect by use of a lens that produces an inverted image of the fundus. O. is also used to measure refractive errors of the eye, in which case it is termed **metric o.**

-opia; -opy a combining form relating to a defect of vision or of the eyes (from Greek *ops*, "eye").

opiates a dried and powdered opium product with addictive properties, including morphine, heroin, Dilaudid, metopon, Demerol, methadone, and codeine.

opinion a belief or attitude toward a situation, person, or activity that is not supported by verified facts and is subject to modification.

opinionaire a questionnaire that measures opinions.

opinion poll: See PUBLIC-O.P.

opioid abuse a substance-use disorder characterized by (a) pathological use, that is, intoxication throughout the day, (b) use nearly every day for at least a month, (c) episodes of overdose (impairment of respiration and consciousness), and (d) impaired functioning, as evidenced by fights, loss of friends, absence from work, loss of job, or repeated clashes with the law. (DSM-III)

opioid dependence a substance-use disorder involving either tolerance (need for an increased amount to gain the desired effect, or a decreased effect when the regular amount is taken) or a withdrawal syndrome when use is terminated or reduced. Also called **opium addiction; opium dependence**. See OPIOID WITHDRAWAL. (DSM-III)

opioid intoxication a disorder associated with recent use of natural opioids (such as heroin and morphine) or synthetics (meperidine, nonmedical methadone), and characterized by (a) pupillary changes (commonly constriction, except for dilation in cases of overdose), (b) at least one psychological sign (euphoria, dysphoria, apathy, psychomotor retardation), (c) at least one neurological sign (drowsiness, slurred speech, impaired attention or memory), and (d) disturbed behavior (impaired judgment, reduced social or occupational functioning). Serious, sometimes fatal, complications may also occur; coma, shock, or depressed or arrested respiration. (DSM-III)

opioids drugs, synthetic or natural, that produce effects similar to those of morphine and are administered primarily for the relief of pain. Although o. may affect tissues in various parts of the body, e.g., the digestive tract and respiratory system, most attention has been focused on the CNS activity, where o. interfere with the release of acetylcholine and norepinephrine of nerve fibers. See NARCOTIC ANALGESICS; OPIUM ALKALOIDS; SYNTHETIC NARCOTICS.

opioid withdrawal a pattern of symptoms produced by recent cessation or sharp reduction in opioids used for a prolonged period. The symptoms last from seven to 14 days, and include some or all of the following: tearing (lacrimation), rhinorrhea (runny nose), pupillary dilation (widened pupils), piloerection (goose flesh), sweating, diarrhea, yawning, mild hypertension, rapid heartbeat (tachycardia), fever, insomnia, and associated features such as restlessness, irritability, depression, tremor, muscle and joint pains, nausea, vomiting, and weakness. (DSM-III)

opiomania physical dependence on opium or a derivative of opium.

-opisth-; -opistho- a combining form meaning posterior or backward.

opisthotonic movements an effect observed in some cases of severe meningitis in which spasms of the back muscles cause the spinal column and limbs to arch backward. In extreme cases, the body may be raised above a level surface so that it is supported by the back of the head and the heels. Also called **tetanus posticus**.

opisthotonos a condition produced by tetanic muscle spasms, causing the spine and limbs to bend the body into a forward convex posture so that, when prone, it rests on the heels and head. Also called **tetanus dorsalis**. Also see ARC DE CERCLE; RIGIDITY.

Opitz, John Marius German-born American pediatrician, 1935—. See SMITH-LEMLI-OPITZ SYNDROME.

opium a narcotic drug produced from the resin of the unripe seed pod of the o. poppy, Papaver somniferum. O. and its derivates are eaten, smoked, injected, sniffed, and drunk. O. is the source of morphine, codeine, heroin, and other narcotic drugs. The action of o. is due mainly to its morphine content which is analgesic and euphoric and capable of producing a deep dreamless sleep from which the user can be easily aroused.

opium addiction = OPIOID DEPENDENCE.

opium alkaloids natural or semisynthetic drugs prepared from the dried juice of the oriental poppy, Papaver somniferum. The drugs are administered primarily for the relief of pain. Opium contains more than 20 alkaloids, the principal one being **morphine**—$C_{17}H_{19}NO_3$—which comprises ten percent of opium and accounts for most of the pharmacologic activity of opium. Other o.a. include **codeine**—$C_{18}H_{21}NO_3 \cdot H_2O$, **codeine phosphate**—$C_{18}H_{21}NO_3 \cdot H_3PO_4 \cdot 1/2H_2O$, heroin or DIACETYLMORPHINE (see this entry), **dihydrocodeine**—$C_{18}H_{23}NO_3$, **dihydromorphine**—$C_{17}H_{21}NO_3$, **metopon**—$C_{18}H_{21}NO_3$, **oxycodone**—$C_{18}H_{21}NO_4$, **pholcodine**—$C_{23}H_{30}N_2O_4$.

opium dependence = OPIOID DEPENDENCE.

Oppenheim, Hermann German neurologist, 1858–1919. See OPPENHEIM REFLEX; DYSTONIA MUSCULORUM DEFORMANS (also called **Oppenheim's disease**).

Oppenheim reflex extension of the great toe when the examiner strokes downward on the inside of the tibia of the lower leg. The O.r. is a diagnostic sign of pyramidal-tract disease

opponent-process theory of acquired motivation a theory which proposes that every event in life that has a strong effect has also an opposed process that fights it. In a runner's "high," pain gives way to pleasure; in the use of drugs, pleasure turns to anxiety and pain; generally, any addiction, whether to a drug or to a love object, eventually produces the opposite. The chief exponent of this theory, which contradicts the usual stimulus-response principles, is Richard Solomon.

opponents theory of color vision = HERING THEORY OF COLOR VISION.

opposites test a test in which the subject is instructed to give the opposite of the stimulus word.

oppositional disorder a persistent pattern of disobedient, negativistic, and provocative opposition to authority figures occurring between three and 18 years of age, and manifested in such behavior as temper tantrums, violation of minor rules, dawdling, argumentativeness, and stubbornness. (DSM-III)

oppositional thinking: See JANUSIAN THINKING.

-opsia; -opsy a combining form relating to a specified condition of vision (from Greek *ops*, "eye").

opsin one of the breakdown products of the exposure of rhodopsin, visual purple of the retina, to light. The other product is retinene. It is a reversible reaction in which rhodopsin reforms from retinene and opsin.

opsoclonus an ophthalmological disorder, sometimes called **dancing eyes**, marked by quick, irregular bursts of ocular movement, sometimes associated with myoclonic jerking of the limbs. The effect may be a sign of a brain tumor or damage to brain tissue caused by an infection such as encephalitis.

-opt-; -opto- a combining form relating to vision or the eyes (from Greek *optos*, "seen, visible").

Optacon a trademark for an opticon device, an electronic instrument that permits a totally blind person to visualize objects. An O. can be used by a blind person to read printed material at a rate of up to 100 words per minute, or about the same speed as the average blind individual reads words by the braille technique. The O. translates letters of the alphabet into specific vibration patterns that can be "read" tactually in a manner similar to tactual sensations produced by touching braille dots. Also see VISATONER.

optical axis a theoretical line that passes through the center of both the cornea and the lens; the center of vision.

optical defect a condition of the eye that prevents light rays from focusing properly on the retina.

optical illusion a false visual image produced by either physical or psychological factors.

optical projection the formation of a visual image by means of a slide projector or similar device; also, the localization of objects in space which correspond to the image on the retina.

optical scanner a device for the examination of small or isolated areas by means of reflected or projected light. **Optical scanning** is used in various chemical and physiological studies (e.g., the density of red blood cells in a blood sample) and in the identification of molecules of sugars or amino acids.

optic atrophy the degeneration of the optic-nerve fibers, as occurs in tabes, lead or methyl-alcohol poisoning, or multiple sclerosis.

optic atrophy-ataxia syndrome = BEHR'S SYN-DROME.

optic chiasm a flat quadrangular body in the area of the hypothalamus where tracts of optic-nerve fibers from the left and right eyes meet and separate again. Some of the fibers from each eye cross over to the cortex on the opposite side of the brain so that each hemisphere receives fibers from both the left and right eyes. Also called **chiasma** (plural: **chiasmata**). See DECUSSATION HEMIANOPIA.

optic disk an area of the retina where optic-nerve fibers gather before leaving the retina. Because the area is relatively insensitive to light, it also is known as the blind spot. See SCOTOMA.

optic-fiber regeneration a process demonstrated in lower animals, such as amphibia, whose nerve tracts grow together again after they have been cut and frayed. Functional o.-f.r. has been established in the newt even when the tract was inverted so that dorsal fibers faced ventral fibers, and vice versa. It is believed the neurons release organizer substances that help orient fibers to targets.

optic lobes a pair of elevations on the midbrain that contain visual reflex centers, that is, the upper part of the corpora quadrigemina.

optic nerve the second cranial nerve; the sensory nerve of vision originating in the occipital cortex and distributed to the receptor cells of the retina. The o.n. is referred to as "cranial nerve II."

optic neuritis a type of neuritis caused by an inflammation of the optic nerve at or near its origin in the eye. The condition may be secondary to a systemic disease (e.g., syphilis or diabetes) or carbon-monoxide poisoning. O.n. usually involves both eyes and leads to blindness.

optic radiation visual-nerve tracts that run between the lateral geniculate body and the internal capsule. Most of the fibers of the human optic tract travel this route, via the geniculate-body-internal-capsule radiation, on their way to the visual cortex in the occipital lobe. Some visual-tract fibers pass through the superior brachium and superior colliculus to the pretectal region.

optimal group size a group size that results in a comfortable level of interaction for members of a given species, that is, a group size not small enough to produce isolation but not large enough to cause a high level of undesirable interactions. Crowded conditions have been shown to yield a range of negative responses in animals.

optimal interpersonal distance the physical distance between two or more people that they judge to be comfortable while interacting. Comfortable distance varies with the type of relationship, interaction, and setting as well as with national, personality, and social-class differences.

optimal-stimulation principle = PRINCIPLE OF OPTIMAL STIMULATION.

optimism the attitude that everything happens for the best, or that wishes will ultimately be fulfilled. If these feelings are persistent in the face of adversity, they may be defenses against anxiety and disappointed expectations. See ORAL CHARACTER. Also see ORAL O.

optional stopping terminating an experiment at the whim of the experimenter, often on the basis of initial favorable results.

optogram the image of a light-reflecting object on the retina of the eye.

-or-; -oro- a combining form relating to the mouth (Latin *os, oris*). Adjective: **oral**.

OR = OPERATIONS RESEARCH.

oral administration: See ADMINISTRATION.

oral-aggressive character in psychoanalysis, a personality type resulting from sublimation of the oral-biting stage and marked by aggressiveness, envy, and exploitation. Also see ORAL CHARACTER.

oral anxiety an anxiety expressed at the oral stage of childhood by images of chewing and swallowing a loved or feared object, e.g., a parent.

oral behavior activities involving the mouth, such as thumb-sucking, smoking, eating, kissing, nail-biting, talking, and oral sex.

oral-biting period in psychoanalysis, the second phase of the oral stage of psychosexual development, from about the eighth to the 18th month, during which the child begins to feel that he is an independent person, expresses anger by biting the mother's breast or the nipple of the bottle, and derives satisfaction from chewing on anything he can put in his mouth. Also called **oral-sadistic phase**.

oral character in psychoanalysis, a pattern of personality traits derived from the oral stage of psychosexual development. If the individual has experienced sufficient sucking satisfaction and adequate attention from the mother during the oral-sucking period, he will develop an oral-receptive character marked by friendliness, optimism, generosity, and dependence on others. If he does not get enough satisfaction during the sucking and biting stage, he will develop an oral-aggressive character marked by tendencies to be hostile, critical, envious, exploitative, and overcompetitive. Also see ORAL-RECEPTIVE CHARACTER; ORAL-AGGRESSIVE CHARACTER.

oral coitus = FELLATIO.

oral-contraceptive pill a combination of synthetic estrogen and progesterone, the female sex hormones responsible for the menstrual cycle, formulated in dosages that can be taken by mouth. The synthetic hormones in the pill alter the normal menstrual activities so that ovulation and related functions are prevented. It was introduced as a contraceptive in 1960 and has been 99 percent effective in preventing pregnancies. Also called **the Pill.**

oral dependency in psychoanalysis, a tendency to be dependent on other people and to seek from them the same type of satisfaction originally experienced during the oral stage when the mother protected, nursed, and showered love and attention on the child.

oral eroticism in psychoanalysis, the pleasure derived from oral activities such as smoking, chewing, biting, talking, kissing, and oral-genital contact. Also called **oral erotism; oral gratification.** Also see ORAL-INCORPORATIVE PHASE.

oral-eroticism phase in psychoanalysis, the first phase of psychosexual development when the mouth is the principal erogenous zone and sucking is the most important source of gratification. Also called **oral-sucking period.**

oral erotism = ORAL EROTICISM.

oral-facial-digital syndrome = OFD I SYNDROME.

oral fixation in psychoanalysis, persistence of immature gratifications associated with the oral phase of psychosexual development, e.g., nail-biting, thumb-sucking, baby talk, and excessive dependence on the mother or mother surrogate.

oral-genital contact = OROGENITAL ACTIVITY.

oral gratification = ORAL EROTICISM.

oral impregnation fertilization that is rumored to occur by oral, or mouth, contact rather than genital contact. It is without scientific foundation, and circulated in many variations, but primarily as a warning that a girl can become pregnant by allowing a boy to kiss her.

oral-incorporative phase in psychoanalysis, the earliest phase of psychosexual development in which the infant unconsciously feels it is ingesting, or incorporating, the mother's being along with the milk it swallows. This phase is also believed to lay the foundation for feelings of closeness and dependence, as well as for possessiveness, greed, and voraciousness. See INCORPORATION; ORAL-EROTICISM PHASE.

oralism a method of teaching the deaf in which the primary form of communication consists of lip-reading and speaking. Also called **oral method.**

orality the oral factor in eroticism or neurosis, ranging from pleasure in biting, sucking, smoking, or oral sex to speech-making, addictions, overeating, and excessive generosity.

oral-lingual dyskinesia = BLM.

oral method = ORALISM.

oral optimism a term applied to optimism as an oral-character trait, which psychoanalysts believe stems from full oral satisfaction in infancy. This gives the child a lasting sense of self-confidence and a positive outlook on life.

oral orientation the process of interacting with the environment in terms of oral needs. E.g., an infant utilizes his mouth not only as a prime source of gratification but as a primary orientation

organ to the external world, since he learns to identify objects by placing them in his mouth.

oral-passive type: See RECEPTIVE CHARACTER.

oral personality: See ORAL CHARACTER.

oral pessimism in psychoanalysis, a pessimistic, depressive pattern believed to originate in frustration and deprivation experienced by the infant during the oral stage of psychosexual development, particularly at the hands of a cold, disinterested mother.

oral phase in psychoanalysis, the first stage of psychosexual development, occupying the first year of life, when the mouth is the principal erotic zone and gratification is achieved by sucking the nipple during the feeding process and, toward the end of the period, by biting. Also called **oral stage.** See ORAL EROTICISM; ORAL SADISM.

oral primacy the infant's first contact with the postnatal world, which is primarily with the mouth. O.p. is generally accepted as a biological fact, but the psychic significance of the oral phase depends largely on the child's experiences during this period.

oral-receptive character in psychoanalysis, a personality pattern characterized by dependence, optimism, and expectation of nourishment and care from external sources, just as the mother provided these satisfactions during the oral-sucking period. Also see ORAL CHARACTER.

oral sadism in psychoanalysis, the primitive urge to use the mouth, lips, and teeth as instruments of aggression, mastery, or sadistic sexual gratification. This impulse is believed to originate in the oral-sadistic phase of infancy.

oral-sadistic cathexis the concentration of psychic energy on oral-sadistic activities and aggressive urges, such as biting during early infancy; also, the persistence of this type of activity in adult life in the form of sexual foreplay, aggressive character traits, and neurotic symptoms.

oral-sadistic phase = ORAL-BITING PERIOD.

oral stage = ORAL PHASE.

oral-sucking period = ORAL-EROTICISM PERIOD.

oral test a type of test in which the questions are posed and answered orally.

oral triad a term applied by K. Lewin to the major desires of the infant in the early oral phase: the wish to devour, the wish to be devoured, and the wish to go to sleep.

orbital gyri a group of four gyri located about an H-shaped orbital sulcus of the frontal lobe. They are identified as **medial, anterior, lateral,** and **posterior o.g.**

orbitofrontal cortex an area of the frontal lobes that is associated with the sex drive. Lesions or ablation of the o.c. often result in hypersexuality.

-orch-; -orchido-; -orchio- a combining form relating to the testicles (from Greek *orchis*, "testis").

orchiectomy the surgical removal of one or both testes. An o. may be performed when a testis is injured or diseased, as when the male reproductive system has been invaded by cancer. O. does not necessarily eliminate coital ability but may reduce the desire for coitus. O. before puberty can affect the development of secondary male sex characteristics. Also called **orchectomy; orchidectomy**. Also see CASTRATION.

orchis = TESTIS. Also see CRYPTORCHID; MONORCHID; TRIORCHID; SYNORCHIDISM; MICROORCHIDISM.

orchitis = TESTITIS.

order effect an influence operating over time or causing a progressive change. If the order in which two experimental treatments are administered makes a difference, then this shows an o.e.

orderliness the tendency to be neat and tidy and keep everything in place. O. may express a need for security, and when extreme may be an obsessive-compulsive characteristic or a symptom of organic brain disease. Also see COMPULSIVE O.

order of magnitude an ordering of data, scores, or objects from lowest to highest so that every item but the last is followed by an item of greater value.

order of merit = MERIT RANKING.

ordinal position any place or rank as indicated by number, specifically the child's position or birth order in the family, e.g., the second child. Many relationships have been suggested between birth order and personality development. See BIRTH ORDER.

ordinal scale a scale of measurement in which the items are placed in rank order, e.g., 1, 2, 3 . . . n-2, n-1, n. This scale shows only that one item is larger than another, but not how much larger. It lacks a true zero point. Also see NOMINAL SCALE; INTERVAL SCALE; RATIO SCALE.

ordinate the vertical coordinate in a graph or data plot; the Y axis. Also see ABSCISSA.

Orestes complex in psychiatry, a son's repressed impulse to kill his mother, or the actual act of matricide. The term is derived from the myth of Orestes who killed his mother, Clytemnestra, and her lover.

orexis the affective and conative aspects of behavior, excluding its cognitive aspect (Greek, "appetite").

organ eroticism sexual arousal or sexual attachment associated with a particular organ of the body.

organic a term used in psychiatry to characterize a condition or disorder that is basically somatic or physical, as contrasted with functional or psychogenic.

organic-affective syndrome a disturbance of mood resembling a manic or depressive episode, resulting from a specific organic factor such as reserpine, methyl dopa, certain hallucinogens, viral illness, or endocrine disorder. (DSM-III)

organic amnesia a failure to register or retain experiences due to physiological changes in the nerve cells resulting from toxic conditions such as (a) lead poisoning, barbiturate poisoning, or acute alcoholic intoxication, (b) damage or destruction of nerve cells associated with head injury or brain tumors, and (c) degeneration of

brain tissue caused by cerebral arteriosclerosis or senile brain disease. Loss of memory may be fragmentary or diffuse, and recovery is usually gradual and incomplete if it occurs at all. O.a. is not recognized as a general category in DSM-III; the different organic mental disorders involving amnesia are described separately. See ALCOHOL-AMNESTIC DISORDER; MULTIINFARCT DEMENTIA; AMNESTIC SYNDROME; BARBITURATE OR SIMILARLY ACTING SEDATIVE OR HYPNOTIC AMNESTIC DISORDER; PRIMARY DEGENERATIVE DEMENTIA.

organic anxiety an anxiety linked to a painful organic disorder and attenuated in dream processes that represent efforts to cure the ailment through wish-fulfillment.

organic approach the theory that all disorders, mental and physical, have a physiological basis. In psychiatry, adherents of this view hold that all psychotic disorders, including those usually classified as functional, such as schizophrenia and manic-depressive disorder, and possibly the more severe neurotic disorders as well, result from structural brain changes or biochemical disturbances of the nervous or glandular system. The o.a. was first advocated by Hippocrates and Galen, but was not systematically developed until Wilhelm Griesinger and Emil Kraepelin launched the organic era in the latter part of the 19th century. Also called **organicism; organic viewpoint**.

organic brain syndromes acute or chronic syndromes involving impairment of brain-tissue function due to such factors as head injury, toxic conditions, encephalitis, systemic infection, brain tumor, or cerebral arteriosclerosis. The resulting symptoms include mild-to-severe impairment of memory, orientation, judgment, general intellectual functions, and emotional adjustment. In the DSM-III classification, this term refers to a pattern of organic psychological and behavior symptoms associated with transient or permanent brain dysfunction, but without reference to etiology. The category is distinguished from "organic mental disorders" (in which the etiology is known) and comprises DELIRIUM, DEMENTIA, AMNESTIC SYNDROME, ORGANIC HALLUCINOSIS, ORGANIC DELUSIONAL SYNDROME, ORGANIC-AFFECTIVE SYNDROME, ORGANIC PERSONALITY SYNDROME, INTOXICATION, WITHDRAWAL, and ATYPICAL OR MIXED O.B.S. See these entries. Abbrev.: **OBS**.

organic defect a congenital disorder that is not the result of a genetic anomaly. An o.d. that causes a mental or physical disability can result from toxemia of pregnancy, a viral infection (e.g., rubella) or a venereal disease during pregnancy, a protozoan parasite, such as toxoplasmosis during pregnancy, or dietary deficiencies or drug abuse (e.g., alcoholism) during the period of gestation.

organic-delusional syndrome a condition characterized by the occurrence of delusions, usually persecutory in nature, produced by such substances as amphetamines, cannabis (marijuana), and hallucinogens, and in some cases temporal-lobe epilepsy or cerebral lesions. The individual may appear perplexed or disheveled, and speech may be rambling, but there is no clouding of consciousness or loss of general intellectual abilities, and there are no prominent hallucinations. (DSM-III)

organic dementia an irreversible intellectual deterioration due to chronic brain disorder, as in advanced cerebral arteriosclerosis, senile brain disease, Pick's disease, and Korsakoff's syndrome.

organic disease an illness resulting from a demonstrable abnormality in the structure or biochemistry of body tissue or organs. Also called **organic disorder**. See PSYCHOGENIC DISORDERS.

organic driveness a state of hyperactivity resulting from brain damage that involves brainstem disorganization.

organic hallucinations hallucinations associated with a specific organic factor. Stimulation or irritation of a cerebral site or sensory pathway may be a factor, and precipitating causes can be an aneurysm or tumor, adverse reaction to a medication such as ephedrine or propranolol, or abuse of alcohol, cocaine, or mescaline.

organic hallucinosis a condition characterized by brief or extended hallucinations produced by hallucinogens (usually visual hallucinations), alcohol (usually auditory hallucinations), and in some cases sensory deprivation (blindness, deafness) or seizures. The syndrome does not involve clouding of consciousness, significant loss of intellectual abilities, predominant delusions, or disturbances in mood. (DSM-III)

organicism = ORGANIC APPROACH.

organicity a term used to denote organic cerebral impairment, or brain damage.

organicity assessment an evaluation of the functional effects of brain damage. Because single tests generally are inadequate, the o.a. takes into consideration a broad range of possible general and specific factors, covering deterioration of various aspects of functioning, highly specific effects, and differential damage information based on evidence of location and extent of the disorder. Also see CEREBRAL-DYSFUNCTION TESTS.

organicity tests: See CEREBRAL-DYSFUNCTION TESTS.

organic mental disorders a heterogeneous group of mental disturbances resulting from transient or permanent brain dysfunction due to specific organic factors, including alcohol, opiates, amphetamines, cocaine, toxins, infections, cardiovascular disease, trauma, neoplasm, metabolic disorders, and aging. The underlying pathology manifests itself in such organic brain syndromes as delirium, amnestic syndrome, dementia, hallucinosis, delusional syndrome, intoxication, withdrawal, affective syndrome, and organic personality. (DSM-III)

organic paralysis: See HYSTERICAL PARALYSIS.

organic personality syndrome a disorder characterized by a marked change in personality or behavior due to a specific organic factor that damages the brain, e.g., neoplasm, head trauma, vascular disease, and, less commonly, multiple sclerosis, temporal-lobe epilepsy, and Huntington's chorea. The personality change involves at least one of the following: emotional lability (temper outbursts, unprovoked crying), impulse dyscontrol (shoplifting, sexual indiscretions), marked apathy and disinterest, and suspiciousness or paranoid ideation. (DSM-III)

organic repression a form of amnesia that is retroactive and associated with a head injury. The patient may be unable to recall events prior to the injury although examiners are unable to find a personal motive for the amnesia, such as the kind of repression observed in psychogenic amnesia.

organic retardation failure of an organ or organ system to develop normally because of a genetic defect, dietary deficiency, or hormonal disorder. A failure of one or more parts of the skeletal system to grow normally could be caused by pituitary, hereditary, or dietary factors, or a combination.

organic sensations visceral sensations, which arise from deep within the body, e.g., a rumbling stomach. Also called **visceral sensations**.

organic speech impairment: See SPEECH IMPAIRMENT.

organic syndrome a pattern of symptoms that characterize a particular organic mental disorder. Typical symptoms are memory loss, impaired intellectual functions, disorientation, defective judgment, and perceptual deficit.

organic therapies somatic treatments in psychiatry, including electroconvulsive treatment, electronarcosis, electrosleep therapy, faradic shock treatment, psychopharmacology, and psychosurgery.

organic variable a process within the organism that collaborates with an immediate stimulus to produce a particular response. A headache may be an o.v. and the response may be an irritable reaction to noise in the neighborhood. Also called **O variable**.

organic viewpoint = ORGANIC APPROACH.

organ inferiority a term coined by Adler for any type of structural defect or developmental deformity, real or fancied, that produces feelings of inferiority and efforts at compensation.

organismic psychology an approach to psychology that emphasizes the total organism and rejects distinctions between mind and body. It embraces a molar, holistic approach and the interbehavior between organism and environment.

organismic variable one of the four behavioral assessment factors of the SORC system and the factor that refers to physiological and psychological influences. An example of an o.v. is the effect of alcohol or drugs of abuse. See SORC.

organization as used by Piaget, the coordinated biological activities of the organism as determined by genetic factors, interactions with the environment, and level of maturation. In human beings mental processes also become increasingly organized, developing through such stages as reflex behavior and responses to immediate stimulation, and gradually becoming self-sustaining, self-generating, and capable of reflecting the child's own thoughts.

organizational psychology: See INDUSTRIAL PSYCHOLOGY.

organized play play that is structured and supervised by a teacher, group leader, or therapist; play conducted along lines established by the leader in contrast to free play.

organ jargon an Adlerian term for symptoms used by a neurotic to express a masculine protest against feminine symptoms of weakness and expressed in terms of physical disorders, e.g., constipation.

organ language somatic expressions of emotional conflict or disturbance. E.g., difficulty in swallowing may represent an unpalatable situation; an asthmatic attack may symbolize a load on one's chest; itching may mean that something has gotten under one's skin. The term is often used interchangeably with body language. Also called **organ speech; hypochondriac language.**

organ neurosis the psychoanalytic term for a functional disorder in which a physiological change occurs, that is, for what has been called a psychosomatic or psychophysiologic disorder, a somatoform disorder, or psychological factors affecting physical condition. The term is not usually applied to conversion (hysterical) disorders but may include such conditions as migraine, peptic ulcer, hyperthyroidism, essential hypertension, bronchial asthma, and ulcerative colitis.

organ of Corti a ridge of highly specialized cells on the floor of the spiral bony cavity of the cochlea. It contains four rows of internal and external auditory-hair cells that respond to different sound frequencies and fire neural impulses which produce auditory sensations. The hair cells communicate with the vestibulocochlear, or eighth cranial, nerve. Also called **acoustic papilla; spiral organ.**

organogenesis a beginning in organic or somatic tissue. E.g., aphasia may originate in a cortical lesion in the parietal lobe. The term is also used interchangeably with SOMATOGENESIS. See this entry.

organotherapy treatment that utilizes substances normally produced by body organs, e.g., the administration of insulin in the treatment of diabetes, or the administration of hormones as replacement therapy.

organ pleasure in psychoanalysis, the pleasure and arousal associated with stimulation of the erogenous zones and organs (oral, anal, urethral, skin, muscle, breast, genital areas).

organ speech = ORGAN LANGUAGE.

organ transplants the surgical replacement of a diseased or damaged body organ or tissue by living tissue from another individual. O.t. may include blood transfusions and skin grafts as well as replacement of a cornea, kidney, heart, liver, or bone marrow tissue. The success of o.t. depends mainly on absence of immune-response rejection of the donor tissue. See EYE BANK; KIDNEY TRANSPLANT; IMMUNOSUPPRESSIVE DRUGS; TRANSPLANTATION REACTIONS.

orgasm the climax of the sex act, when the peak of pleasure is achieved by the emission of semen in the male and vaginal contractions in the female. The peak period of sexual excitement lasts less than one minute in most males and females. Besides involuntary muscle contractions, it is characterized by increased blood pressure and heart rate, and a mild clouding of consciousness. Studies show the o. potential is highest in men around the age of 18 and in women around the age of 35. Also called **climax.** Also see SEXUAL-RESPONSE CYCLE; COITUS SINE EJACULATIONE; EJACULATION; EJACULATION PHYSIOLOGY; ALIMENTARY O.; INHIBITED FEMALE O.; INHIBITED MALE O.; VAGINAL O.

orgasmic dysfunction: See INHIBITED FEMALE ORGASM; INHIBITED MALE ORGASM.

orgasmic phase: See SEXUAL-RESPONSE CYCLE.

orgasmic reconditioning a behavior-modification technique used in sex therapy, in which deviant fantasies or pictorial representations are employed to arouse the patient, who then engages in masturbation. These stimuli, however, are replaced by more conventional heterosexual representations just before orgasm, and at progressively earlier points, in order to develop normal patterns of arousal. Also called **orgasmic reorientation.**

orgastic impotence the inability of the male to achieve orgasm in spite of normal erection and ejaculation. The condition is believed to be due to anxiety, such as the unconscious fear of "letting go," or of losing an important product of the body. Also see IMPOTENCE.

orgastic potency the ability of the male or female to achieve full orgasm during the sex act. See POTENCY.

orgiastic pertaining to a situation characterized by indulgence, revelry, frenzy, and indiscriminate sexual behavior.

orgone a term coined by Wilhelm Reich for a "life energy" which he believed pervades the universe and is emitted by energy vesicles called bions, which he claimed to find in organic material. The o., he believed, was related to cosmic radiation, and he speculated that it might be responsible for the origin of life from earth and water (biogenesis), as well as the formation of hurricanes, tornadoes, and galaxies. Also see BION.

orgone accumulator a box resembling a telephone booth designed by Wilhelm Reich in which the patient sits for the purpose of capturing the vital energy Reich called orgone, and concentrating it on the sex organs as a means of restoring full orgastic potency. Also called **orgone box.**

orgone therapy the therapeutic approach of Wilhelm Reich based on the concept that the achievement of "full orgastic potency" is the key to psychological well-being. The orgasm, he believed, is the emotional-energy regulator of the body, whose purpose is to dissipate sexual tensions that would otherwise be transformed into neuroses. It derives its power from a hypothetical cosmic force termed the orgone which, he held, not only accounts for sexual capacity but for all functions of life and for the prevention of disease as well. Also called **vegetotherapy**. See CHARACTER-ANALYTIC VEGETOTHERAPY.

orgonomy the term applied by Wilhelm Reich to a new "science" based on his theory of life energy. Two aspects of this approach were the psychological or psychiatric orgone therapy (originally called character analytic vegetotherapy) and physical orgone therapy, which employed the orgone accumulator. See CHARACTER-ANALYTIC VEGETOTHERAPY.

orgy a type of social gathering marked by revelry, including unrestrained singing, dancing, drinking, and sexual indulgence. O. is also used sometimes to describe destructive activity. The word is derived from a term originally employed to identify ceremonies held by the ancient Greek and Roman populations to honor their dieties.

oriental nightmare-death syndrome = BANGUN-GUT.

orientation in psychiatry, awareness of the self and of outer reality; the ability to identify one's self and to know the time, the place, and the person one is talking to. In industrial psychology, o. is the process of introducing an applicant or employee to the job situation. In environmental psychology, the term refers to the process of adaptation to a setting, e.g., a home, neighborhood, or community: O. is established by familiarization with details of the setting so that movement and use do not depend upon the use of memory cues, such as maps. Other meanings include one's position in space; the tendency to move toward a source of stimulation; and one's general approach, ideology, or viewpoint. See ADAPTIVE BEHAVIOR. Also see DISORIENTATION; REALITY O.; RECEPTIVE O.; OBJECTIVE O.; SUBJECTIVE O.

orientation disorders confusion as to time, place, personal identity, or situation. See DISORIENTATION.

orientation illusion: See ILLUSION OF ORIENTATION.

orienting response a behavior and physiological reaction to a novel, unexpected, or threatening stimulus. Also called **general arousal**.

original response a response to a Rorschach test that occurs in no more than one percent of the records, as opposed to a popular response.

original score = RAW SCORE.

origin-of-language theories attempts to explain how human beings first developed language. Examples are the **pooh-pooh theory** (or **exclamation** or **interjectional theory**), which sees the beginnings of language in interjections that express emotions (Louis Herbert Gray, 1875–1955); the **ding-dong theory** (or **nativistic theory**), which holds that speech began with vocal expressions

that were given to the encounter of objects (Max Müller, 1823–1900); the **yo-he-ho theory**, according to which speech began as outcries under the strain of work on the environment (L. Noiré, 1847–89); the **ta-ta theory**, which sees the origin of language in combinations of gestures and tongue movements (R. Paget, 1869–1955); and the **sing-song theory**, which holds that language evolved from inarticulate chants of ritualistic nature (Otto Jespersen, 1860–1943). Among numerous other theories, most deal with human imitation of animal and other natural sounds, including the **animal-cry theory**, the **onomatopoeic theory**, the **cuckoo theory**, the **bow-wow theory**, and the **hey-nonny-nonny theory**. All these theories, however, are mainly speculative because no written records existed until about 4,000 years ago while language is probably as old as the human race.

Ferdinand de Saussure (1857–1913) demonstrated that words are very arbitrary structures; and in the 20th century, the social anthropologist Claude Lévy-Strauss emphasized that man is a structure-builder by nature and that speech is merely our most typical structure, while Noam Chomsky holds that the human brain contains something like a language-producing machine which, at least in part, operates independently of any experience.

Orne, Martin Theodore Austrian-born American research psychiatrist, 1927—. See REAL-SIMULATOR MODEL.

ornithinemia excessive ornithine in the blood possibly due to an inborn error of amino-acid metabolism, and possibly to hepatic disease. The condition sometimes occurs in siblings, who manifest mental retardation and severe speech disturbance.

ornithophobia a morbid fear of birds. Also called **bird phobia**.

orofacial dyskinesia a behavior pattern observed in aging patients who make chewing, mouthing, and tongue movements that resemble symptoms of tardive dyskinesia. The patients usually are toothless and suffer from chronic institutionalization and dementia.

orogenital activity the application of the mouth to the genitalia. The activity may be heterosexual or homosexual, as a precoital form of stimulation or as carried to orgasm. Application of the mouth to the male genitalia is called fellatio, and application of the mouth to the female genitalia is known as cunnilingus. Also called **oral-genital contact; buccal intercourse**.

oropharynx the portion of the pharynx extending from the level of the hyoid bone to the soft palate. Within this structure is the functional crossing of the alimentary and respiratory canals.

orphan virus a virus that has not been classified in one of the established categories because it lacks structural, chemical, or other identifying characteristics of other viral agents. See ECHO VIRUS.

-orth-; -ortho- a combining form meaning straight or normal (Greek *orthos*).

orthergasia an alternative term for euergasia. Adolf Meyer used both terms to denote normal psychobiological, or mental, functioning.

orthodox psychoanalysis psychoanalytic treatment that adheres without modification to Freud's basic procedures (free association, dream interpretation, analysis of resistance, and transference) as well as to his basic aim of developing insight into unconscious sources of emotional problems in order to help the patient to restructure his personality. Also see PSYCHOANALYSIS.

orthodox sleep an alternative term for NREM SLEEP. See this entry.

orthogenesis the theory that evolution has an intrinsic direction and successive generations follow the same plan irrespective of natural selection.

orthogonal at right angles to each other; independent; unrelated. In factor analysis, axes may be either oblique (correlated) or o. (uncorrelated). Also see OBLIQUE.

orthomolecular psychiatry a controversial approach to psychiatric treatment based on the theory that mental disorders are due to biochemical abnormalities that result in an increased need for specific substances. This need is determined by medical tests, and treatment consists of the administration of large doses of vitamins (**megavitamin therapy**), trace elements, or other substances.

orthonasia a term applied by K. R. Eissler to a program in which children are taught about death as a part of life, to enable them to incorporate healthy attitudes toward death in their coping repertoire. Also see DEATH NEUROSIS; ANTICIPATORY MOURNING.

orthopedic disorder any anatomical or functional abnormality of the musculoskeletal system, either congenital or acquired. Examples include torticollis, clubfoot, and scoliosis. Also see CONGENITAL ORTHOPEDIC CONDITION.

orthopnea discomfort or difficulty in breathing when the body is in any position except standing or sitting erect. O. is a common symptom of congestive-heart disease, a circulatory disorder involving the heart or lungs, or both, and marked by an inability to breathe while lying flat in bed.

orthopsychiatry an interdisciplinary approach to mental health, in which psychiatrists, psychologists, social workers, pediatricians, sociologists, nurses, and educators collaborate on the study and treatment of emotional and behavioral problems before they become severe and disabling. The approach is basically prophylactic, and the major emphasis is on child development, family life, and mental hygiene.

orthoptics an eye-exercise program designed to train patients with extraocular muscle imbalance to coordinate the vision in the left and right eyes.

orthostatic epileptoid an obsolete term referring to children who experience fainting spells and occasional convulsions after arising in the morning or maintaining a standing posture for a long period.

orthostatic hypertension: See BARBITURATE OR SIMILARLY ACTING SEDATIVE OR HYPNOTIC WITHDRAWAL.

orthotics-prosthetics the design, manufacture, and tailoring of prostheses, or orthopedic appliances for physically disabled patients. Examples may include the building of an artificial, battery-powered hand that can be controlled by voluntary nerve impulses, an electronic heart pacemaker, or a tiny metronome that can be worn as a hearing aid to help pace the speaking of a patient with a language disorder.

orthotist: See PROSTHETIST.

orthriogenesis full restoration of the ego at the moment of awakening as the cathexis, which vanished during deep sleep, has its function restored (P. Federn).

Orton, Samuel Torrey American neuropsychiatrist, 1879–1948. See STREPHOSYMBOLIA.

-osche-; -oscheo- /-os·ke(ō)-/ a combining form relating to the scrotum (Greek *oscheon*).

oscillograph an instrument that makes graphic recordings of wave forms of electrical energy produced in studies of body functions.

oscilloscope an electric device that records visually an electrical or sound wave on a fluorescent screen.

Oseretsky, N. I. Russian psychologist, fl. 1926, 1931. See BRUININKS-OSERETSKY TEST OF MOTOR PROFICIENCY; LINCOLN-OSERETSKY MOTOR DEVELOPMENT SCALE.

Osgood, Charles Egerton American psychologist, 1916—. See SEMANTIC DIFFERENTIAL.

-osis; -asis a combining form relating to (a) a diseased condition, (b) an increase, (c) a condition generally.

-osm-; -osmo- a combining form relating (a) to odor (Greek *osme*), (b) to an impulse (Greek *osmos*).

osmolarity the effect of concentrations of certain molecules on osmotic pressure. O. may be determined by such factors as the comparative sizes of molecules and their interaction with water molecules. E.g., potassium molecules are larger than sodium molecules, but sodium ions interact with water molecules which then function as molecules larger than the potassium molecules.

Osmond, Humphry British-American psychiatrist and scientific explorer, 1917—. O. is known for his studies in schizophrenia, orthomolecular psychiatry, and psychopharmacology, and his experiments with niacin and mescaline. He coined the word "psychedelic." O. developed a personality typology that consists of eight types, building on Jung's four. He has written extensively on the "dying role" and other "roles" in the human, particularly the suffering human, situation. See PSYCHEDELICS; PHANEROTHYME; MAUVE FACTOR.

osmophobia = OLFACTOPHOBIA.

osmoreceptor a receptor presumed to exist in the

brain for the purpose of measuring the concentration of various substances in the body's extracellular fluid.

osmotic pressure in physiology, the amount of pressure required to restrict the flow of water through the membrane of a cell. The pressure of water on a semipermeable membrane has a paradoxical effect in that the direction of flow is toward the side of the membrane that has the greatest concentration of dissolved substances, in order to equalize the amount of dissolved particles on both sides of the membrane.

os penis: See PENIS CAPTIVUS.

osphresiolagnia an interest in odors that is morbid or festishistic. O. is frequently associated with infantile sexuality. Some schizophrenics believe that body odors can be projected to other persons, making them ill or insane, or that they are the victims of the body odors of others. See RENIFLEUR.

osphresiophilia an abnormal attraction to odors and smells.

osphresiophobia = OLFACTOPHOBIA.

osphresis an alternative term for olfaction.

ossicles any small bones but particularly the chain of three tiny bones in the middle ear that transmit sound-wave vibrations from the tympanic membrane facing the external environment to the oval window of the inner ear, where the organ of Corti is located. The middle-ear ossicles are the MALLEUS, INCUS, and STAPES. See these entries.

-ost-; -oste-; -osteo- a combining form relating to bone (Latin *os*).

osteitis deformans a form of Paget's disease of the bone, a gradually progressive disorder marked by gross deformities of bone architecture. The bones go through phases in which original bone material is lost and new bone formed, but in bizarre patterns. See PAGET'S DISEASE.

osteitis fibrosa cystica: See BONE DISEASE.

osteoarthritis: See ARTHRITIS.

osteogenesis imperfecta a type of bone disorder marked by deformities due to the fact that the bones are fragile and plastic and fracture as a result of minor injuries. The disease may be inherited either as a dominant-autosomal trait or more rarely as a recessive-autosomal trait. Also called **Durante's disease**.

osteoma: See BONE DISEASE.

osteomalacia an adult form of rickets, or metabolic bone disease associated with vitamin-D deficiency. The disease is characterized by softening and sometimes tumors of the bones, pain, tenderness, muscular weakness, anorexia, and weight loss. Kinds of o. include **senile o.**, occurring in old age, **renal-tubular o.**, associated with a kidney disorder, and **puerperal o.**, caused by skeletal mineral depletion due to repeated pregnancies and nursing of infants.

osteomyelitis: See BONE DISEASE.

osteopetrosis: See CRANIAL ANOMALY.

osteoporosis: See CALCIUM-DEFICIENCY DISORDERS.

osteosarcoma: See SARCOMA.

osteotomy a surgical procedure that involves the cutting of a bone. The operation usually is performed to correct a deformity, e.g., knock-knee, by sawing or chiseling the affected bones to reshape them.

ostomy an artificial opening, usually between the gastrointestinal tract and the outside of the abdominal wall. The combining form is **-ostomy** or **-stomy**. See COLOSTOMY.

Ostwald, Wilhelm /ôst'vält/ German chemist and physicist, 1853–1932. See OSTWALD COLOR SYSTEM.

Ostwald color system a method of organizing chromatic and achromatic samples devised by Wilhelm Ostwald. The O.c.s. consists of 24 hues arranged around the outside of a circle with the complementary colors for each hue located along the circle's diameters. By combining adjacent colors, any color on the **Ostwald scale** can be produced.

-ot-; -oto- a combining form relating to the ear or hearing (from Greek *ous, otos,* "ear").

O.T. an abbreviation of *o*ccupational *t*herapist.

OTC drugs = OVER-THE-COUNTER DRUGS.

other-directed a term applied by D. Riesman to persons whose values, goals, and behavior stem primarily from identification with group or collective standards in contrast to individually defined standards. According to Riesman, the phenomenon of **other-directedness** is increasing in contemporary society. Also called **outer-directed**. Compare INNER-DIRECTED; TRADITION-DIRECTED.

other-directed person an individual who is readily influenced by the attitudes and opinions of other people, and who tends to be motivated by a need for approval (David Riesman). Also called **outer-directed person**.

other disorders of infancy, childhood, or adolescence (DSM-III): See REACTIVE-ATTACHMENT DISORDER OF INFANCY; SCHIZOID DISORDER OF CHILDHOOD OR ADOLESCENCE; ELECTIVE MUTISM; OPPOSITIONAL DISORDER; IDENTITY DISORDER.

other, mixed, or unspecified substance abuse or dependence a category reserved for (a) disorders involving such substances as inhaled glue and amyl nitrite not classified in the standard substance-abuse categories, (b) mixed abuse, such as amphetamines or heroin with barbiturates, and (c) abuse of an unidentified substance, also (d) a dependence on such substances as codeine or corticosteroids. The category is subtyped **other, mixed, or unspecified substance abuse** and **other specified substance dependence**. (DSM-III)

other psychosexual disorders (DSM-III): See EGO-DYSTONIC HOMOSEXUALITY; PSYCHOSEXUAL DISORDERS NOT ELSEWHERE CLASSIFIED.

others: See SIGNIFICANT O.

other specific affective disorders (DSM-III): See CYCLOTHYMIC DISORDER; DYSTHYMIC DISORDER.

other specified substance dependence: See

OTHER, MIXED, OR UNSPECIFIED SUBSTANCE ABUSE OR DEPENDENCE.

otic pertaining to the ear.

Otis, Arthur Sinton American psychologist, 1886 —. See OTIS QUICK SCORING MENTAL ABILITY TEST; OTIS SELF-ADMINISTERING TEST OF INTELLIGENCE.

Otis Quick Scoring Mental Ability Test a group intelligence test presenting verbal, spatial, and numerical items on three levels: grades 1 to 4 (Alpha test), grades 4 to 9 (Beta test), and grades 9 to 16 (Gamma test).

Otis Self-Administering Test of Intelligence a verbal intelligence test with self-contained instructions, and applicable on an individual or group basis. One form is designed for grades 4 to 9; the other, for grades 9 to 16.

otitis media an inflammation or infection of the middle ear. It is the most common cause of a conductive-hearing impairment and may originate from sinusitis, upper respiratory infections, or allergic conditions. Acute o.m. is a common occurrence in young children as a result of a viral or bacterial infection that spreads from the nasopharynx through the eustachian tube to the middle ear. It is a serious condition that can lead to brain abscess, hearing loss, vertigo, or meningitis. Also see ADHESIVE O.M.; SEROUS O.M.

otiumosis = ALYSOSIS.

otoconia = OTOLITHS.

otogenic tone a tone that arises from within the auditory mechanism rather than from an external stimulus. Also called **subjective tone**.

otohemineurasthenia a unilateral deafness for which no organic cause can be found.

otoliths tiny calcium particles in the gelatinous membrane of the acoustic macula of the inner ear. The force of gravity on the o. stimulates neighboring nerve receptors which translate the stimuli into information about the position of the animal in space, or in water. Also called **otoconia; statoconia**.

-otomy: See -TOM-.

otopalatodigital syndrome = OPD SYNDROME.

otosclerosis a formation of spongy bone that develops in the middle ear and immobilizes the stapes at the point of attachment to the oval window facing the inner ear. O. is marked by progressive deafness as the ossicles fail to transmit vibrations from the tympanic membrane to the inner ear. It is considered hereditary. Adjective: **otosclerotic**.

Ouija board /wē′jē/ a trademark for a parapsychology device consisting of a board painted with numbers and letters. A movable pointer, allegedly influenced by supernatural forces spells out messages through the hands of the person holding the pointer. The process is often seen as a form of automatic writing. (The term is a contraction of the French and German words for "yes," *oui* and *ja*.)

outcome evaluation in evaluation research, a process to decide whether the program achieved its stated goals. A randomized controlled experimental model is the ideal model generally agreed upon for evaluating the effectiveness of a program outcome. (However, in realistic evaluation situations, the degree of rigidity needed to apply these statistical methods with any confidence is rarely achieved.)

outcome research a systematic investigation of the efficacy of a single therapeutic technique, or of the comparative efficacy of different techniques, with one or more disorders.

outer boundary: See EGO BOUNDARIES.

outer-directed = OTHER-DIRECTED.

outer-directed person = OTHER-DIRECTED PERSON.

outer hair cells: See INTERNAL HAIR CELLS.

out-group persons or groups outside or excluded from membership in a specified in-group. Use of this term implies that one has or is temporarily adopting the perspective of the in-group member. Also called **they-group**. Compare IN-GROUP.

out-of-body experience in parapsychology, a dissociative experience in which the individual imagines that his soul or spirit has left his body and is acting or perceiving on its own. It is a neurologic phenomenon that may occur when death is imminent, and in some cases can be induced by the suggestion of a medium, or "sensitive,," or by the use of hallucinogens, notably phencyclidine.

out-patient an ambulatory patient whose physical or mental disorder can be treated without the need for overnight confinement in a hospital, clinic, or other facility.

out-patient services in psychiatry, services performed for ambulatory patients in hospital units, clinics, and mental-health centers. O.-p.s. include group and individual therapy, family therapy, psychological evaluation, emergency psychiatric diagnosis and treatment, home treatment, and social case work.

output the level or degree of work performance that can be completed within a given amount of time; also, a communication that conveys a signal to another person or another part of the communications system.

outreach services in psychiatry, services for the mentally ill, including aftercare for discharged mental patients living in the community, provided by a mental hospital or community mental-health center. Among the services are medication maintenance, home visits, emergency treatment, supportive psychotherapy, and social services provided by case workers and case managers.

outside density the number of persons per acre; population density within a community. Although a relationship has been found between o.d. and social pathology, the factor of inside density appears to be more significant. Compare INSIDE DENSITY.

outsider = ISOLATE.

-ov-; -ovi-; -ovo- a combining form relating to an egg, an OVUM. See this entry.

ova: See OVUM.

oval window a membrane on the surface of the

cochlea which receives sound vibrations transmitted through the middle ear. The stapes, the third bone in the chain of ossicles, is attached to the o.w. The cochlea is fluid-filled, and movements by the stapes are translated from air- to water-pressure changes by the o.w.

O variable = ORGANIC VARIABLE.

ovarian cycle the pattern of physiological functions in the ovary associated with the menstrual cycle. The major physiological change during the o.c. is the development of the egg follicle which evolves into a temporary endocrine gland, the corpus luteum, after ovulation.

ovariotomy the surgical removal of an ovary or ovarian tumor. Removal of both ovaries before or during the fertile years of a woman usually results in a sex-hormone imbalance requiring organotherapy; if the o. is performed prior to puberty, the girl is likely to develop secondary male sex characteristics. Also called **oophorectomy** /ō·ə-/.

ovary an almond-shaped female gonad, normally located on either side of the uterus, in the lower abdomen. The ovaries of the prepubertal female contain about 350,000 immature ova, of which fewer than 400 will develop into mature ova to be released at a rate of about one per month between menarche and menopause.

overachiever a person, usually a student, who achieves above his capacity as calculated by aptitude and general-intelligence tests. **Overachievement** appears to be mainly a phenomenon of the middle classes, and it has been noted far more frequently in girls than in boys. Compare UNDERACHIEVER.

overactivity excessive, restless activity especially as a defense against anxiety or as an expression of a manic state. O. is usually somewhat less extreme than hyperactivity. See FLIGHT INTO REALITY.

overage characterizing one who is beyond the average or usual age associated with a given behavior or trait. Usually, the term applies to a child or student who is chronologically older than the others in his grade. **Underage** refers to a student who is younger than his classmates.

overanxious disorder generalized and persistent anxiety or worry among children or adults, manifested in several of the following symptoms: unrealistic worry about future events; preoccupation with appropriateness of past behavior; overconcern with athletic, social, or academic competence; excessive need for reassurance about worries; somatic complaints without established physical basis; marked self-consciousness or feelings of tension. Also called **overanxious reaction**. (DSM-III)

overbreathing: See HYPERVENTILATION.

overcharged idea a conflict that continually manifests itself in a person's dreams in the form of various symbols and identifications because it is, in effect, overcharged with repressed psychic energy.

overcompensation an extreme, neurotic striving for power and self-aggrandisement motivated by an inferiority complex; overcompetitive, over-aggressive behavior in response to feelings of inadequacy. O. is a key concept of Adlerian psychology. In its original sense the term denotes a pathological need for dominance. The term is sometimes used synonomously with compensation. See INFERIORITY COMPLEX; MASCULINE PROTEST.

overcontrolled a term employed to identify a cluster of childhood behavior symptoms or behavior deficits. O. children are internalizers with feelings of shyness and being unloved, and may complain of fears and tenseness. Their symptoms are analogous to those of adults suffering from anxiety and depression.

overcrowding a higher concentration of organisms per unit of space than is customary for a given species. Experimental o. conditions significantly increase abnormal behavior and aggression in rats even when enough resources preclude the need for competition. In humans, o. is associated with stress patterns, e.g., stimulus overload. Some theorists believe that o. inevitably leads to increased aggression among humans; however, this appears to be true only in some societies. See POPULATION DENSITY. Also see INSIDE DENSITY; OVERPOPULATION.

overdetermination in psychoanalysis, the concept that several factors may collaborate to produce one symptom, dream, disorder, or aspect of behavior. Because drives and defenses operate simultaneously and derive from different layers of the personality, a dream may express more than one meaning, and a single symptom may serve more than one purpose.

overdose the administration of an excessive amount of a drug with resulting adverse effects. The precise toxic effects differ according to many factors, including the drug, the true dosage of the drug, the body weight and health of the individual, and his tolerance for the drug. Most pharmacologic agents, including caffeine, can have toxic to lethal effects if consumed in large doses. Abbrev.: **O.D.** Verb: **to O.D.** Also see HEROIN O.

overextension the tendency of very young children, as they begin to relate concepts to words, to extend a word beyond its specific meaning, e.g., to refer to all animals as "doggie." This overgeneralization is inevitable at first since a given word will enter a child's active repertoire before all the qualities to which the word refers have been learned. As these qualities are learned and the individual meanings of words become clearer, o. declines.

overgeneralization: See OVEREXTENSION.

overheating excessive ambient temperature in a behavior setting. See HEAT EFFECTS; HEAT-INDUCED ASTHENIA; HEAT EXHAUSTION; HEAT STROKE.

overinclusion failure to eliminate ineffective or inappropriate responses associated with a particular stimulus.

overinclusiveness a schizophrenic thought disturbance in which strange analogies, neologisms, obscure symbols, and irrelevant or distant associations are included in speech.

overlapping factor a common factor that influences results in at least two studies or tests. Also called **O element**.

overlapping groups in experimental psychology, groups whose distribution of scores falls to some extent within the same limits.

overlearning a type of learning that extends beyond the amount of practive actually needed for one or two repetitions. O. is often useful in rote learning tasks and skills like bicycle riding.

overload theory: See STIMULUS OVERLOAD.

overmanning a condition in which the number of persons available to perform a service or function exceeds the number required for adequate performance. Also see MAINTENANCE MINIMUM. Compare UNDERMANNING.

overmobilization an extreme activation of the psychological reserves and resources of the organism, particularly through the sympathetic nervous system, in order to meet a crisis and respond to stress. O. produces a state of tension and arousal and, if prolonged, may result in behavioral disorganization or in psychophysiologic symptoms such as ulcers and hypertension. See ADRENERGIC REACTION; GENERAL ADAPTATION SYNDROME.

overpayment payment of certain employees beyond the going rate. In industrial psychology, o. is a relatively rare form of inequity that in some cases leads to worker tension and dissatisfaction.

overpopulation a higher-than-desirable population density that may result in crowding conditions and stress. According to Konrad Lorenz, crowding inevitably leads to increased aggression and violence, and the evidence from animal behavior supports the view that crowding increases aberrant behavior and aggression. However, some human societies with very high population density have correspondingly low rates of violence and social pathology, suggesting that the negative effects of o. may have social as well as biological origins. Also see INSIDE DENSITY; POPULATION DENSITY; OVERCROWDING.

overproduction the condition in which a species reproduces too many offspring for the available food, space, and other vital resources; also, production of goods far beyond what is needed.

overproductive ideas the uncontrollable flow of ideas that is one of the primary disturbances observed in mania.

overprotection the tendency to coddle, shelter, and indulge a child to such an extent that he or she fails to become independent, cannot endure frustration or competition, and may develop a passive-dependent personality. Either parent may overprotect the child, but maternal o. is especially common.

overreaction a reaction, particularly an emotional response, that exceeds an appropriate level.

overregulation a transient error in linguistic development in which the child attempts to make language more regular than it actually is, e.g., by using "breaked" instead of "broken."

oversubmissiveness: See COMPLIANCE.

overt denoting anything that is directly observable, open to view, or publicly known.

overt behavior behavior that is explicit, or observable without instruments or expertise.

over-the-counter drugs drugs that can be purchased without a doctor's prescription, e.g., aspirin. Abbrev.: **OTC drugs**.

overt homosexuality a term applied to homosexual tendencies that are consciously recognized and expressed in sexual contact, in contrast to latent or unconscious homosexuality.

overtone a partial in a complex tone. When the frequency of an o. is an exact multiple of the fundamental tone, it is called a harmonic.

overt response any observable or external reaction, e.g., a response that can be seen or heard. The study of overt behavior is the province of behaviorists. Compare COVERT RESPONSE.

overvalued idea a false or exaggerated belief that is maintained with less rigidity or duration than a delusion, e.g., the idea that one is indispensable in an organization.

overwork fear = PONOPHOBIA.

ovulation the release of a mature ovum from its ovarian follicle. The pea-size follicle, on the surface of the ovary, ruptures when the ovum has matured, discharging the ovum into a uterine, or Fallopian, tube. Also see MITTELSCHMERZ.

ovum a single female gamete, or egg cell, that develops to maturity in the ovary. Plural: **ova**. Also see SEPARATE OVA.

own control an experimental design in which repeated measures are taken on the same group or individual. Such a design may not need an independent control group, since the subjects serve as their o.c.

oxazepam: See BENZODIAZEPINES.

oxazolidinediones a group of drugs used in the treatment of petit mal epilepsy because of their inhibiting effect on akinetic and myoclonic seizures. O. also are used to control convulsions resulting from use of convulsant drugs. Kinds of o. include **paramethadione**—$C_7H_{11}NO_3$—and **trimethadione**—$C_6H_9NO_3$.

oxycephaly = ACROCEPHALY.

oxycodone: See OPIUM ALKALOIDS.

oxygen debt an imbalance of oxygen in the body tissues that can occur when physical effort consumes oxygen in the bloodstream faster than it can be replaced by breathing. The oxygen borrowed from the bloodstream results in a "debt" that must be replaced by continued heavy breathing after the physical exertion has ended.

oxygen regulation the control of oxygen and carbon-dioxide balance in the bloodstream by chemoreceptors that measure the pH of the blood. If oxygen intake drops below a certain minimum, carbon dioxide produced by cellular metabolism increases the acidity of the blood and stimulates increased breathing to pump more oxygen into the bloodstream.

oxytocics drugs that are capable of stimulating contractions of the uterine muscles (from Greek *oxys*, "sharp, quick," and *tokos*, "childbirth"). The o. are adrenergic blocking agents and include the ergot derivatives which have been used by midwives for centuries in speeding the labor process, and as abortifacients. Also called **ecbolics**. See OXYTOCIN.

oxytocin a hormone secreted by the posterior lobe of the pituitary gland with the function of stimulating smooth muscle, particularly in the production of milk by the mammary glands and in the control of uterine contractions during labor. The uterus becomes increasingly sensitive to o. near the end of gestation. O. can be produced synthetically in a pure form that can be administered at term to help induce uterine contractions, thereby aiding in the start of labor. See OXYTOCICS.

P

P: See PRIMARY ABILITIES.

pacemakers natural or artificial devices that help establish and maintain certain biological rhythms. The term usually is applied to **cardiac p.**, which may be a natural unit, e.g., the sino-atrial node of specialized muscle fibers that sets the rhythms of heart contractions and relaxations, or an implanted electronic unit that performs the same function artificially. Other p. control uterine contractions or the rhythm of the movements of cilia. Also see THALAMIC PACEMAKER.

-pachy- a combining form meaning thick or thickening.

pachygyria a type of brain malformation in which the gyri of the cerebral cortex are abnormally thick. The condition usually is accompanied by a reduction in the fissures between the gyri. Also called **macrogyria**.

pachymeningitis an inflammation of the dura mater, or pachymeninx, the outermost layer of the three CNS protective membranes.

pachymeninx = DURA MATER.

pacification the process of soothing and quieting a restless infant by rocking, cooing, singing, patting, and using a pacifier. Infants have been found to vary widely in soothability, as well as responsiveness to different types of soothing conditions, but in most cases the activity level and heart rate decrease and respiration becomes more regular.

pacing the structuring of a learning situation or learning program so that the individual works at a comfortable rate consistent with his developmental level. P. also refers to active planning of the speed at which a sequence of behaviors or problems will be executed, e.g., planning to do ten problems per hour and allotting six minutes per problem.

Pacini, Filippo /pächē′nē/ Italian anatomist, 1812–83. See PACINIAN CORPUSCLES; ENCAPSULATED END ORGANS; SUBCUTANEOUS SENSIBILITY; VIBRATION RECEPTORS.

Pacinian corpuscles small oval bodies composed of concentric layers of connective tissue around an axon, serving as receptors for pressure sensations. Pacinian-corpuscle bodies are found in the fingers, the tendons, and abdominal membrane. A similar type of pressure receptor, called Herbst's corpuscle, is found in birds. Also called **Vater's corpuscles; corpuscula lamellosa; Pacini's corpuscles; Pacinian bodies**.

package-testing a form of product-testing in which the emphasis is on effects of the package design on consumer decisions in a test market. One p.t. study found that 30 percent of women purchasers of cosmetics changed brands when a better package for a similar product was offered and 50 percent said they would be willing to pay a higher price for the same product in a more convenient or efficient package.

packs layers of cloth, such as sheeting material, used in medical or psychiatric care of a patient when the entire body or a body area may require an application of heating or cooling effects. The p. may be hot or cold, wet or dry, depending upon the specific purpose. Also see COLD-PACK TREATMENT.

PAD: See PSEUDOCHONDROPLASTIC SPONDYLOEPIPHYSIAL DYSPLASIA.

padded cell a room in a mental hospital that is lined with mattresses or other heavy padding on the floor and walls to protect a violent or destructive patient from self-injury or from injuring others. The p.c. has been replaced in most institutions by the use of tranquilizing medications.

Paget, James English surgeon, 1814–99. See PAGET'S DISEASE; BOWING OF BONES; CALCITONIN; OSTEITIS DEFORMANS.

Paget, R. language theorist, 1869–1955. See ORIGIN-OF-LANGUAGE THEORIES.

Paget's disease a progressive disease of unknown cause occurring in middle or late life. The condition is characterized by chronic inflammation of the bones resulting in bone softening, bone thickening, and the bowing of long bones. Neurologic complications may occur due to pressure on the central nervous system or nerve roots. Also see OSTEITIS DEFORMANS.

pagophagia a craving to eat ice, believed to be related to iron-deficiency anemia, as in other forms of pica.

pain a noxious sensation due to damage to nerve tissue, stimulation of free nerve endings, or excessive stimulation such as extremely loud sounds. P. may also be a feeling of severe distress and suffering ("psychic p.") resulting from acute anxiety, loss of a loved one, or other psychological factors. Both physical p. and psychical p. are regarded as warning signals. For physical p., p. receptors occur in groups of myelinated or unmyelinated fibers distributed throughout the body, but particularly in surface tissues. P. that is experienced in surface receptors generally is perceived as sharp, sudden, and localized; receptors in internal organs send impulses that tend to be dull, longer lasting, and less localized. P. perception is partly subjective and may be experienced as distressful, agonizing, or irritating. Because of psychological factors, and previous experience and training in p. response, individual reactions vary widely. Anxiety and tension generally increase a person's sensitivity to p. Also see SUFFERING; TISSUE DAMAGE; P. MECHANISM; GATE-CONTROL THEORY OF P.; P. PATHWAYS; PLEASURE-P. PRINCIPLE; PSYCHIC P.; PSYCHOGENIC P. DISORDER; CENTRAL P.; FUNCTIONAL P.; REFERRED P.

painful intercourse discomfort that occurs during coitus and which may range from irritation if the vagina is inflamed because of a bacterial infection to severe pain by deep penetration, particularly when the uterus is retroverted. A rigid hymen, urinary tract disease, vaginal tears, loss of vaginal-lining cells during menopause, and vaginal-muscle disorders are other possible causes. Males seldom experience p.i. Also see DYSPAREUNIA.

pain mechanism a system of free nerve endings, utilizing both A and C fibers and overlapping neuron connections. Some investigators propose that prick or bright pain sensations are transmitted by A fibers and dull pain sensations by C fibers. The degree of pain also is associated with the amount of stimulation of the free nerve endings, being more intense with local tissue damage. Also see PAIN.

pain pathways the five spinal tracts that have been identified as p.p. in animal experiments. They are the medial lemniscus, the central gray matter, the reticular formation, the central tegmental fasciculus, and the spinobulbothalamic path. Some studies show that pain and temperature sensations travel in parallel paths since a lesion affecting one usually has the same effect on the other in the same body areas.

pain phobia = ALGOPHOBIA.

pain-pleasure principle = PLEASURE-PAIN PRINCIPLE.

pain sense a sensory modality, with free nerve endings on the body surface and in some internal organs, that yields a specific effect identified as pain, especially when tissue injury occurs.

pain spot any of the small areas of the skin that are especially sensitive to pain.

paired-associate learning a technique used in studying learning in which the subject learns syllables, words, or other items in pairs and is later presented with half of the pair to which he must respond with the matching half. Also called **paired-associates method**.

paired comparison a systematic procedure for comparing a set of stimuli or items for magnitude. In p.c., a pair of stimuli are compared and one is judged larger, and then the other pairs in the series are systematically compared in the same way. The method is used, e.g., in studying preference for works of art, or different personality characteristics.

palate: See CLEFT P.; CLEFT-P. SPEECH; SOFT P.

-paleo- a combining form meaning ancient or primitive (Greek *palaios*).

paleocerebellum literally, the old cerebellum, or portion of the cerebellum found in birds and lower animals for whom sensory and motor-impulse coordination is more important for survival than for some higher animals.

paleocortex the old cortex, consisting of structures on the lower surface, e.g., the limbic system, and features that represent the entire brain of lower vertebrates such as fish.

paleologic thinking prelogical thinking characterized by concrete, dreamlike thought processes found, e.g., in children. In p.t., mental activity is limited to feeling and perception and excludes logic and reasoning. Regression to this stage occurs primarily in chronic schizophrenics. See PRELOGICAL THINKING; PARALOGIA.

paleomnesis the ability to recall events from the distant past of one's life.

paleophrenia a term (meaning primitive mentality) suggested by O. Osborne as an alternative to schizophrenia to indicate a characteristic regression to a primitive type of thinking.

paleopsychology the study of those unconscious psychological processes in contemporary man that Freud and Jung believed to be inherited and to have origins in earlier stages of human and perhaps animal evolution. The term applies also to the reconstruction of the psychological reactions of prehistoric man: e.g., shackling the dead may have been due to fear that their spirits would return. See COLLECTIVE UNCONSCIOUS.

paleospinothalamic tract a group of somatosensory fibers in the ventrolateral tracts that run directly into the intralaminar nuclei of the thalamus.

paleosymbols a schizophrenic symptom in which the patient reverts to self-created idiosyncratic words or phrases, which appear to represent a return to the level of autistic expression of the young child. Remnants of common verbal symbols can frequently be detected, especially in the neologisms used by these patients.

-pali-; -palin- a combining form relating (a) to repetition, (b) to reversal of direction (from

Greek *palin*, "again, backward," and *dromos*, "course").

paligraphia the obsessive repetition of letters, words, or phrases in writing. It is the counterpart of palinphrasia.

palilalia a speech disorder in which words and phrases are needlessly repeated with increasing speed and loss of meaning. It can be frequently observed in encephalitis lethargica, Parkinson's disease, and Alzheimer's disease.

palilexia abnormal rereading of words or phrases.

palilogia an obsessive repetition of utterances or spoken phrases.

palingraphia = MIRROR WRITING.

palinlexia backward reading, e.g., "nip" for "pin," or "house my is this" for "this is my house."

palinphrasia involuntary repetition of words or phrases in speaking.

paliopsy the brief persistence of a visual image of objects no longer in the patient's visual field. P. is a diagnostic sign of a lesion in the occipital lobe.

pallesthesia sensitivity to vibration, frequently tested by placing a tuning fork in contact with a bony surface of the skin. Also called **palmesthesia; palmesthesis**.

pallidohypothalamic tract a group of nerve fibers that links the globus pallidus to the hypothalamus. It is associated with the eating behavior of animals.

pallium an obsolescent term sometimes used to identify the white-matter portion of the cerebral cortex.

palmar reflex flexion of the fingers when the palm is scratched; the grasping response of the newborn.

palm-chin reflex = PALMOMENTAL REFLEX.

palmesthesia; palmesthesis = PALLESTHESIA.

palmistry the unscientific practice of interpreting lines and other skin surface features of the palm as signs of personality traits or for predictions of the individual's future.

palmomandibular sign a reflex present in the neonate until about the tenth day of life, consisting of automatic opening of the mouth in response to pressure on the palms or forearm.

palmomental reflex a contraction of the muscles of the chin, in a twitching motion, produced by scratching the palm. The p.r. is observed in some patients with toxic brain damage but rarely occurs in normal persons. Also called **palm-chin reflex; pollicomental reflex**.

palpebral fissure the hypothetical line between the upper and lower eyelids. When the eyelids are open, the p.f. forms an elliptical space. Also called **rima palpebrarum**.

palpitation a rapid heart beat associated with an anxiety attack, excessive tension, or physical exertion.

palsy an obsolete term for paralysis. It is still used in compound expressions such as cerebral p.

-pan-; -pant-; -panto- a combining form meaning all, every, generalized.

pan-anxiety according to Hoch and Palatin, 1949, an all-pervading anxiety structure that "does not leave any life-approach of the person free of tension." It is characteristic of pseudoneurotic schizophrenia.

panarteritis a diffuse inflammation of the walls of the small and medium arteries. Arteries of the skeletal muscles, kidneys, heart, and gastrointestinal tract may be involved. The condition primarily affects men between the ages of 20 and 50, although both men and women of any age may be afflicted. The cause is unknown, but the disorder has been associated with hypertension and peripheral neuropathy.

pancreatitis an inflammation of the pancreas. Acute p. usually is marked by severe abdominal pain and caused by biliary tract disorders, e.g., gallstones, alcoholism, viral infection, such as mumps, or reaction to a drug, e.g., diuretics or azathioprine. Chronic p. is similar to the acute form in etiology and symptoms, except that alcoholism is more often the precipitating factor.

pandemic occurring universally or over a large area, as in several countries. P. is more general than EPIDEMIC. See this entry. Compare ENDEMIC.

panencephalitis a form of encephalitis that is characterized by the appearance of inclusion bodies in the nucleus or cytoplasm of the neurons of the brain. The inclusion bodies cause lesions in both gray and white matter and produce antibodies against measles virus. The evidence suggests the disease is an aftereffect of an earlier measles infection. The patients most commonly are boys, between the ages of four and 20. The onset usually is insidious, beginning with behavioral disorders and loss of interest in school work. Mental deterioration follows with myoclonus, blindness, and other neurologic disorders that may continue for months or years until death. Also called **Dawson's encephalitis; inclusion-body encephalitis**.

pangenesis a theory of heredity proposed by Charles Darwin who believed that traits were transmitted from parents by particles of each body organ or part concealed in the ovum and spermatozoon of the parents. Darwin believed all organisms were reproduced from one generation to the next by the process of p. According to the doctrine, mental traits also were inherited by p.

panglossia a type of garrulousness observed in psychotic patients, especially those in a manic state.

panic an acute reaction involving terror confusion, and irrational behavior, precipitated by a threatening situation such as an earthquake, fire, or being caught in a stalled elevator. Terror is increased by such factors as uncertainty, exhaustion, suggestion, frustration, and the hysterical behavior of other people. Also see HOMOSEXUAL P.

panic attack an episode of acute anxiety and disorganization occurring in PANIC DISORDER, MAJOR

DEPRESSION, SCHIZOPHRENIC DISORDERS, or SOMA-TIZATION DISORDER. See these entries.

panic disorder an anxiety state, or neurosis, marked by repeated panic attacks occurring unpredictably or in certain situations, such as driving a car. The attacks usually last minutes and consist of sudden, intense apprehension or terror, with such symptoms as shortness of breath (dyspnea), palpitations, chest pain, choking sensation, dizziness, sweating, trembling, feelings of unreality, or fear of dying or going crazy. Also see ANXIETY NEUROSIS; PANIC ATTACK. (DSM-III).

pan-neurosis a condition found in neurotic schizophrenia in which all types of neurotic symptoms are present at once or within a short period, including phobias, obsessions, compulsions, depression, and a wide variety of hysterical and psychophysiologic disturbances.

panophobia = PANPHOBIA.

panoramic memory the vivid recollection of long stretches of one's life during a temporal-lobe seizure or when facing possible death, as in near drowning. It is a form of HYPERMNESIA. See this entry.

panphobia a morbid fear of anything and everything. Some investigators claim this is a diffuse form of anxiety rather than a true phobic reaction. Also **panophobia; pantophobia**.

pansexualism the view that all human behavior can be explained in terms of sexuality, a theory that has been attributed to Freud. However, even though he emphasized the power of the sexual instinct, Freud also recognized nonsexual interests, self-preservative drives like hunger and thirst, the aggressive drive, and, toward the end of his life, the death instinct.

pantomime an expression of feelings and attitudes through gestures rather than words. P. is also a nonverbal therapeutic technique sometimes employed when verbal expression is blocked.

pantophobia = PANPHOBIA.

pantry-check technique an inspection of the kitchen shelves or cabinets of households to determine whether advertising-research subjects actually use the products they claim to prefer. Interviews alone often prove inadequate as evidenced by market-research control studies which show that as many as 15 percent of individuals interviewed may claim to use, prefer, or at least be acquainted with a particular product that has never been marketed or advertised. Also see RECOGNITION TECHNIQUE.

Panum, Peter Ludwig Danish physiologist, 1820–85. See PANUM PHENOMENON.

Panum phenomenon a visual illusion produced by binocular fusion of separate images presented to the left and right eyes, the fusion image appearing closer to the eyes than the stimuli.

Papanicolaou, George Greek-born American physician, 1883–1962. See PAP TEST; CERVICAL EVALUATION.

Papaver somniferum: See OPIUM; OPIUM ALKA-LOIDS.

paper-and-pencil test a test in which the problems are written, printed, or drawn and the answers are written responses.

paper chromatography: See CHROMATOGRAPHY.

Papez, James Wenceslas American anatomist, 1883–1958. See PAPEZ CIRCLE; PAPEZ'S THEORY OF EMOTIONS.

Papez circle a network of nerve centers and fibers associated with emotions. It includes the hippocampus, fornix, mammillary body, thalamus, and cingulate cortex, completing the circle through the hippocampus. See PAPEZ'S THEORY OF EMOTIONS

Papez's theory of emotions a theory that emotional experience is controlled by the Papez circle of CNS structures. The concept is a modification of CANNON'S THEORY. See this entry. Also see PAPEZ CIRCLE.

papilledema a swelling of the optic disk of the retina due to an increase in intracranial pressure. The condition may occur because the meningeal membranes of the brain are continuous with the optic-nerve sheaths, so that pressure can be transmitted to the eyeball. Also called **choked disk**.

Pappenheim, Bertha: See TALKING CURE.

Pap test a method of detecting changes in the cells of the uterine cervix that may signal the onset of cancer. The test, named for George Papanicolaou, involves the removal of a smear of loose tissue cells from the surface of the cervix and examining them under a microscope. The cells are graded from Class I, "no abnormalities," to Class V, "cancer cells observed," the intermediate grades indicating various signs of cancer potential.

-para- a combining form meaning (a) resembling, (b) beside or near, (c) abnormal or beyond.

parabiosis the temporary loss of conductivity or excitability in a nerve.

parabulia a distortion of volition, or will, in which an intended action is interrupted, or "derailed," by a "cross impulse" (Kraepelin), e.g., reaching for a cigarette, then suddenly flinging it away. The condition is an example of ambivalence, frequently found in schizophrenics.

Paracelsus, Philippus Aureolus (Theophrastus Bombastus von Hohenheim) Swiss-German physician and alchemist, 1493–1541. Though his manner was "bombastic" (our words "bombast" and "bombastic" come from his name), P. fearlessly opposed witch-hunting and held that mental illness is due to disturbing experiences and faulty development rather than demonic possession. He also introduced a pharmacological approach by using such substances as opium, mercury, iron, and sulfur in treating both mental and physical disorders, although he attributed their efficacy to magnetic forces emanating from the heavenly bodies, a theory that influenced Mesmer. See ASTROLOGY; LAUDANUM.

paracentral lobule the portion of the cerebral cortex that lies between the paracentral and marginal sulci and includes the central sulcus.

paracentral sulcus a fissure on the medial side of the cerebral hemisphere, extending upward from the cingulate sulcus between the precuneus and the paracentral lobule.

paracentral vision a form of vision that utilizes the retinal area immediately surrounding the fovea.

parachlorophenylalanine a substance that blocks the synthesis of serotonin from tryptophan. This action results in a depletion of serotonin from the brain cells and increased ergotropic activity. However, p. is not used in therapy directed toward interference with the production or release of adrenergic transmitter substances.

parachromatopsia partial color blindness. Also called **parachromopsia**.

paracusia partial deafness, especially to deeper tones. The term is also used for any abnormality of hearing other than simple deafness, e.g., impairment in determining the direction from which a sound comes.

paracyesis = ECTOPIC PREGNANCY.

paradigm a model, pattern, or diagram of the functions and interrelationships of a process. In psychological research, a p. is an experimental design or plan of the various steps of the experiment, or a model of the process or behavior under study.

paradigm clash a controversy or conflict produced when a new set of assumptions threatens to replace an established set of assumptions.

paradigm of associative inhibition = MÜLLER-SCHUMANN LAW.

paradoxical cold an effect produced in thermal-nerve endings that are sensitive to both cold and hot temperatures. The fibers have double peaks, including one for heat that is above the threshold of pain. Touching a hot object that fires a double temperature receptor can produce an illusion of cold.

paradoxical intention a method developed by V. Frankl for the treatment of phobias. The patient is instructed to magnify his fear reactions such as sweating or accelerated heart rate in an actual phobic situation. This enables the patient to achieve distance from his symptoms, especially if he is able to laugh at himself in the situation. Also see IMPLOSIVE THERAPY.

paradoxical sleep a state of sleep from which the individual cannot easily be awakened in spite of the fact that it appears to be light, according to the EEG pattern. It is observed, e.g., in cats in which EEG tracings are similar to those of wakefulness although the muscles are relaxed and it is difficult to awaken the animal. The p.s. stage lasts for about six or seven minutes in a cycle that follows an initial 25-minute period of light sleep.

paradoxical reaction a drug reaction that is contrary to the expected effect. Some patients experience excitement rather than sedation after being administered a tranquilizer, and stimulants such as amphetamines or caffeine are used to tranquilize hyperkinetic children.

paradoxical warmth a sensation of warmth produced when a cold object of approximately 30°C (86°F) stimulates a cold receptor.

paragenital pertaining to sexual intercourse in which conception is prevented.

parageusia a distorted sense of taste or a taste hallucination.

paragrammatism a form of aphasic disturbance consisting of substitutions, reversals, or omission of sounds or syllables within words, or reversals of words within sentences. Speech may be quite unintelligible if the disturbance is severe.

paragraphia a psychological distortion in written material consisting, e.g., of transposed or omitted letters and words, or insertion of incorrect and irrelevant words. The condition occurs primarily in patients with cerebral lesions, and less frequently in schizophrenia.

paragraph-meaning test a test in which the subject is asked to explain the basic point, gist, or meaning of a paragraph.

Paraguay tea an infusion made from the toasted leaves of a South American evergreen shrub, Ilex paraguayensis. The active ingredient of the leaves is caffeine, although the content usually is less than one percent. Also called **maté; yerba maté; Jesuit tea**.

parahypnosis an abnormal type of sleep that may be induced by anesthetics or hypnosis. The patient in p. may sleepwalk, be suggestible, or, when under a general anesthetic, be aware of comments made by doctors or nurses in the operating room. The overheard operating-room comments may be the cause of behavioral reactions by the patient after recovery from the surgery.

parakinesia movement executed in an awkward, clumsy, or grotesque manner. The term parakinesis is occasionally used as a synonym of p. but should properly be used only in its parapsychological sense; see PSYCHOKINESIS.

parakinesis = PSYCHOKINESIS. Also see PARAKINESIA.

paralalia any speech defect, especially the substitution of one speech sound for another; a speech disturbance in which intelligibility is affected. Examples are saying "wabbit" for rabbit, or "lello" for yellow.

paralalia literalis a difficulty in forming certain sounds correctly, usually accompanied by stammering.

paralexia a reading disorder characterized by the transposition of word order and the inclusion of further words.

paralinguistic features the formal patterns of speech that characterize the individual, including intonation and **voice quality**, e.g., "plaintive," "husky," or "falsetto." **Paralinguistics** is the study of such vocal qualifiers. P.f. are also called **paralanguage**. Also see PSYCHOLINGUISTICS.

paralipophobia a morbid fear of neglecting one's obligations. Also see HYPENGYOPHOBIA.

parallax an illusion of movement of objects in the visual field when the head is moved from side to side. Objects beyond a point of visual fixation appear to move in the same direction as the eye shift, those closer seem to move in the opposite direction.

parallel dream a Jungian term for a dream that parallels a conscious wish or attitude.

parallelism: See BODY-MIND PROBLEM.

parallel law Fechner's principle that if two stimuli of different intensities are presented to a receptor for a given time, absolute sensory intensities diminish but the difference ratio is unchanged.

parallel play the activity of at least two children who are playing next to but not with each other; autonomous play without direct interaction. P.p. is characteristic of children between 18 months and three years.

parallel processing a theory of information-processing stating that two separate sets of stimuli (information sources) can be attended to simultaneously, thus accounting for the apparent ability to carry on different cognitive functions at the same time. One information source may be processed consciously while another source is attended to subconsciously. Compare SERIAL PROCESSING.

paralog a nonsense word of two syllables.

paralogia illogical thinking and verbal expression, observed primarily in schizophrenic patients. The condition takes many forms, such as drawing false inferences, talking beside the point, or giving wrong answers to questions. Bleuler cites the example of a patient who justified his insistence that he was Switzerland by saying "Switzerland loves freedom. I love freedom. I am Switzerland." Also called **paralogical thinking; perverted thinking; perverted logic.** See GANSER SYNDROME. Also see EVASION; PALEOLOGICAL THINKING; PRELOGICAL THINKING.

paralogism an unintentional or unnoticed fallacy.

paralysis /pəral'isis/ a symptom of a wide variety of physical and psychological disorders characterized by a partial or complete loss of motor function in a body area. A common cause of physical p. is a lesion of the nervous or muscular system, due to injury, disease, or congenital factors. A nervous-system lesion may involve the central nervous system, as in a case of stroke, or the peripheral nervous system, in poliomyelitis, or damage by injury or exposure to cold. Kinds of p. include **sensory p.,** in which the sensory function is impaired although movement is not necessarily lost, **p. agitans,** a disorder that is something of a misnomer in derivation since it suggests a combination of p. and movement although the term sometimes is used interchangeably with parkinsonism, and flaccid p., a form of the disorder associated with a loss of tendon reflexes. Also see FLACCID P.

paralysis agitans: See PARKINSONISM; PARALYSIS.

paralysis of the insane: See BAYLE'S DISEASE.

paralytic dementia = GENERAL PARESIS.

parameter in psychoanalysis, a technique that de-

parts from the classical method of interpretation, such as advice, suggestion, or reassurance; in statistics, a value of a population or of a statistical universe, usually unknown, and estimated from a statistic; in mathematics, a quantity that may have various values, each fixed within the limits of a stated case or discussion; in general, a standard or determining factor; in colloquial usage, a limit.

paramethadione: See OXAZOLIDINEDIONES.

paramimia a form of apraxia in which the individual is unable to express his feelings with gestures.

paramimism a gesture or other movement that has a meaning to the patient although others may not understand its significance.

paramnesia a falsification or distortion of memory, as in the conviction that we have actually witnessed events that have only been described to us, or the illusion that we have already viewed a scene that is actually new to us. Also called **false memory.** See CONFABULATION; DÉJÀ RACONTÉ; DÉJÀ VU; JAMAIS VU; RETROSPECTIVE FALSIFICATION.

paramyotonia congenita a rare hereditary muscle disorder marked by attacks of weakness or flaccidity in the proximal muscles and myotonic cramps of the face and hands caused by exposure to cold plus lingual-muscle myotonia caused by percussion (as with a reflex hammer).

paraneoplastic limbic encephalitis a type of brain inflammation that is associated with a cancer in the viscera, such as the kidney or lungs. The inflammation occurs in the limbic cortex and is manifested by psychic disturbances, e.g., memory impairment and confusion. However, there is no evidence of cancer metastases from the viscera to the involved brain area.

paranoia insidious development of a paranoid disorder with a permanent, unalterable delusional system accompanied by preservation of clear and coherent thinking and, frequently, the belief that the patient possesses unique and superior abilities. The category includes conjugal p. and involutional paranoid state. (The literal translation of the Greek word p. is "derangement" or "madness.") See ACUTE PARANOID DISORDER; ALCOHOLIC P.; ALCOHOL-PARANOID STATE; AMOROUS P.; ATYPICAL PARANOID DISORDER; CLASSICAL P.; CONJUGAL P.; EROTIC P.; EXALTED P.; INVOLUTIONAL PARANOID STATE; LITIGIOUS P.; PROJECTIONAL P.; REFORMATORY P.; SCHIZOPHRENIC DISORDER, PARANOID TYPE; SHARED PARANOID DISORDER. (DSM-III)

paranoiac character a personality type whose primary symptom is a tendency to blame the environment for one's difficulties.

paranoia querulans = LITIGIOUS PARANOIA.

paranoia senilis a type of paranoia associated with senility and marked by delusions of being spied upon by neighbors, robbed by members of one's own family, and similar persecution fantasies.

paranoid pertaining to a mental disorder characterized by systematized or transient delusions, usually grandiose or persecutory, with few other signs of personality disorganization or deterioration. The term was first used by Karl Ludwig Kahlbaum in 1863, and paranoid disorder first became a separate clinical entity in Kraepelin's classification. It is also applied to an individual who exhibits such tendencies in lesser degree. See PARANOIA.

paranoid condition = PARANOID STATE.

paranoid disorders a group of disorders (paranoia, shared paranoid disorder, and acute paranoid disorder) essentially characterized by persistent persecutory delusions, such as being conspired against or poisoned or maligned, or delusional jealousy in which there is an unfounded conviction of unfaithfulness (conjugal paranoia). The condition lasts at least one week and is not due to a schizophrenic, affective, or organic mental disorder. See PARANOIA. (DSM-III)

paranoid erotism a form of paranoia in which the patient has delusions of a love affair that is unrequited because of circumstances or individuals that prevent the love from becoming a reality. The love object frequently is a person who is famous or powerful and the patient tries in vain to communicate with the other person by mail, telephone, or personal visits without success.

paranoid hostility anger and desire to harm others arising out of the delusion that they are persecuting or plotting against the patient.

paranoid ideation thought processes involving suspicious, persecutory, or grandiose images or ideas.

paranoid litigious state = LITIGIOUS PARANOIA.

paranoid melancholia depression accompanied by persecutory or other paranoid factors. It is a form of involutional melancholia.

paranoid-personality disorder a personality disorder characterized by (a) pervasive, unwarranted suspiciousness and mistrust (such as expectation of trickery or harm, guardedness and secretiveness, avoidance of accepting blame, overconcern with hidden motives and meanings, and pathological jealousy), (b) hypersensitivity (such as being easily slighted and quick to take offense, making mountains out of molehills, and readiness to counterattack), and (c) restricted affectivity (such as emotional coldness, no true sense of humor, or absence of soft tender feelings). (DSM-III)

paranoid psychosis a psychotic reaction pattern characterized by more or less systematized delusions without personality disorganization or deterioration. In DSM-I, p.p. is called **paranoid reaction**. See PARANOID DISORDERS; PARANOIA.

paranoid-schizoid position the hypothesis, developed by the psychoanalyst Melanie Klein, that the infant experiences birth as an attack and, by the third or fourth month, develops a fear of annihilation and persecutory anxiety. To protect himself from destruction by his death instinct, the infant (a) projects aggression onto an external object, (b) directs his own aggression against the persecutory object, and (c) introjects, or internalizes, the breast partly as a good, helpful object, and partly as a bad, hated object which is then split off and relegated to the unconscious. See BAD BREAST; GOOD BREAST. Also see DEPRESSIVE POSITION.

paranoid schizophrenia = SCHIZOPHRENIC DISORDER, PARANOID TYPE.

paranoid state a psychotic disorder characterized by transient delusions of persecution or megalomania, which are not as systematized and elaborate as in paranoia, nor as disorganized and bizarre as in paranoid schizophrenia. Also called **paranoid condition**.

paranoid trend an extreme tendency to focus anger or resentment on innocent people, and to blame them for one's problems or shortcomings even to the point of feeling persecuted.

paranormal pertaining to any phenomenon that cannot be explained by existing knowledge.

paranormal cognition = EXTRASENSORY PERCEPTION.

paranormal phenomena: See PARAPSYCHOLOGY.

paranosic gains; paranosis = PRIMARY GAINS.

para I: See PRIMIPAROUS.

parapathetic proviso an agreement or bargain a neurotic patient makes in which he justifies and accepts a neurosis as a means of preventing a personal tragedy (e.g., the death of a parent). Adler's term for p.p. is **junction**. Also called **neurotic proviso**.

parapathy a seldom used term proposed by W. Stekel to replace the term neurosis, on the ground that the latter implies a nerve disorder instead of an emotional disorder.

paraperitoneal nephrectomy: See NEPHRECTOMY.

paraphasia a speech disturbance characterized by the use of incorrect, distorted, or inappropriate words, which in some cases resemble the correct word in sound or meaning, and in other cases are completely irrelevant or absurd. E.g., a wheelchair may be called a "spinning wheel," or a hypodermic needle, a "tie pin." The disorder occurs most commonly in organic brain disorders and Pick's disease. See METONYMY; WORD APPROXIMATION; VERBAL P.; LITERAL P.; SEMANTIC P.

paraphemia a speech disorder marked by the habitual introduction of inappropriate words. The term is also used for distorted speech such as neurotic lisping.

paraphia an impaired or perverted sense of touch.

paraphilias a group of psychosexual disorders in which unusual or bizarre images or acts are necessary for sexual excitement. These disorders comprise such specific types as fetishism, transvestism, zoophilia, pedophilia, exhibitionism, voyeurism, sexual masochism, and sexual sadism. The imagery or acts may take several forms: preference for an inhuman object, such as animals or clothes of the other sex; repetitive sexual activity with humans involving real or simulated suffering or humiliation, as in whipping or bondage; or repetitive sexual activity with nonconsenting partners. Also see ATYPICAL PARAPHILIA. (DSM-III)

paraphonia an abnormal or pathologic change in voice quality.

paraphrasia = WORD SALAD.

paraphrenia an obsolete term occasionally used by Freud in place of dementia praecox and schizophrenia (1911), and later to include both schizophrenia and paranoia (1914). Kraepelin applied it to a group of paranoid states comprising **p. systematica** (roughly equivalent to paranoia), **p. confabulans** (falsification of memory involving delusions of grandeur and persecution), **p. fantastica** (auditory hallucinations and unsystematized delusions involving fantastic adventures), and **p. expansiva** (a female disorder characterized by exaltation and grandiose ideas).

paraplegia a form of paralysis that usually affects the legs and lower part of the trunk, including in some cases loss of bowel and urinary-bladder control. The condition also may be complicated by gastrointestinal and respiratory difficulties, depending upon the extent of CNS damage involved. Also see SPASTIC P.

parapraxis in psychoanalysis, behavioral errors, or "symptomatic acts," that are believed to express unconscious wishes, attitudes, or impulses, e.g., slips of the tongue or pen, forgetting significant events, mislaying objects with unpleasant associations, unintentional puns, and motivated accidents. Also called **parapraxia**. See SYMPTOMATIC ACT.

paraprofessional in psychiatry, a noncredentialed worker (that is, one not holding a postbaccalaureate professional degree) who plays a role in the improvement of mental health among clients and patients in both hospital and community settings. Three major types are (a) hospital-based workers usually from low-income backgrounds, typified by the psychiatric aide, (b) middle-class workers, typified by men or women with previous college degrees and special training in mental-health skills, and engaged in substantive therapeutic work, and (c) indigenous paraprofessionals recruited from the community, typified by men or women who do not hold college degrees and who engage in therapeutically relevant work in mental-health centers or clinics.

In general, the paraprofessions include a large number of trained and partially trained workers in psychiatry, general medicine, neurology, rehabilitation, and psychology. Among them are the homemaker-home-health aide, the teaching aide, the orientation-and-mobility instructor, the manual-arts teacher, the industrial therapist, the corrective therapist, the recreation worker, the optician, the trained volunteer worker, the respiratory-therapy assistant, the radiation-therapy assistant, the orthotist, the prosthetist, the medical or laboratory assistant, the medical-laboratory technician, the cytotechnologist, the histologic technician, the blood-bank technologist, the electroencephalograph technologist, the electrocardiograph technician, the nuclear-medical technician, the medical assistant, the dental assistant, the dental-laboratory technician, the dental hygienist, and the nurse's aide.

parapsychology the systematic study of alleged psychological phenomena that cannot be explained in terms of presently known scientific data or laws, including CLAIRVOYANCE, TELEPATHY, PRECOGNITION, PSYCHOKINESIS, POLTERGEIST, MEDIUM, DOWSING, and other "paranormal" phenomena. See these entries. Also see EXTRASENSORY PERCEPTION; ASTROLOGY; RHINE.

parareaction an abnormal or exaggerated reaction to a relatively minor incident such as tripping, which may become the basis for a delusion of persecution or a similar form of paranoia.

parasexuality any abnormal or perverted form of sexual behavior. See PARAPHILIAS.

parasitic superego in psychoanalysis, a temporary superego containing suggestions or commands that conflict with the individual's superego formed in childhood and synthesized with later influences. Control of the p.s. is exemplified by yielding to enemy propaganda or performing acts that violate one's moral code at the behest of a seductive leader. Another example of p.s. is the effect of mob-psychology influences which may be contradictory to the normal superego but which may be accepted temporarily without guilt feelings. See SUPEREGO.

parasitophobia a morbid fear of parasites; also, the illusion of having insects or other parasites in one's hair or on or under one's skin. Also see ACAROPHOBIA.

parasocial speech speech characteristic of preschool children who, in the presence of others, appear to be talking to themselves. See EGOCENTRIC SPEECH.

parasomnia disordered sleep; especially, sleep disturbances associated with brain lesions or special sleep disorders such as COMA-VIGIL and HYPERSOMNIA. See these entries.

parasuicide attempted but unsuccessful suicide, or suicidal gesture.

parasympathetic drugs = CHOLINERGIC DRUGS.

parasympathetic nervous system a division of the autonomic nervous system with preganglionic fibers that communicate with the third, seventh, ninth, and tenth cranial nerve and the first three sacral nerves. Postganglionic fibers innervate the heart, the pelvic, abdominal, and thoracic viscera, smooth muscles, and glands of the head and neck.

parasympatholytic a substance that has the effect of dilating the pupil of the eye by relaxing the ciliary muscle, e.g., atropine. Also called **mydriatic**. See MYDRIASIS.

parataxic distortion a term applied by H. S. Sullivan to distorted perceptions, judgments, and relationships resulting from earlier experiences. A prime example is misinterpretation of other people's attitudes due to feelings of unworthiness (a large "bad-me" and a small "good-me") because of parental coldness, criticism, or rejection. The distorted interpersonal relationships, such as withdrawal, serve the purpose of defense against anxiety. (The term is derived from Greek *paratassein*, "to lay side by side.") See CONSENSUAL VALIDATION; SULLIVAN.

parataxic mode a term used by H. S. Sullivan to denote the subjective, autistic interpretation and communication of experience and events characteristic of very young children who have not yet reached the stage of reasoning and logic.

parateresiomania an abnormal desire to observe, particularly sexual activities. In Freudian terms, p. is the counterpart of exhibitionism. In DSM-III, the term corresponding to p. is VOYEURISM. See this entry.

parathormone the parathyroid hormone that regulates calcium and phosphate levels in bones and extracellular fluids. A high level of p. is associated with high levels of calcium and low levels of phosphate, and vice versa. Low blood levels of blood calcium are manifested by nerve irritability, muscle twitching, and, in severe cases, convulsions. See CALCIUM REGULATION.

parathymia a distortion of mood. P. is a schizophrenic disturbance in which the patient reacts in a completely inappropriate manner, as in crying when told that he has inherited a large sum of money.

parathyroid gland a small body found, usually in pairs, in the area of the thyroid gland. It secretes a **parathyroid hormone** that controls calcium and phosphorus metabolism. See PARATHORMONE.

parathyroidism the abnormal functioning of the parathyroid glands, which secrete a hormone regulating calcium and phosphorus metabolism. Excessive activity is known as HYPERPARATHYROIDISM, and deficient activity is called HYPOPARATHYROIDISM. See these entries.

paratype the totality of environmental influences that act upon an organism to produce individual expression of a genetic trait or character.

paratypic having to do with environmental pressures and influences on the development of an organism.

paraverbal therapy a therapeutic technique developed by Evelyn P. Heimlich for children who have difficulty communicating verbally and are also beset by such disorders as hyperactivity, autism, withdrawal, or language disturbances. On the theory that these children would feel more intrigued and less threatened by a nonverbal approach, she uses the components of music such as tempo and pitch, along with mime, movement, and art in unorthodox ways to help them express themselves. The therapist participates on their level, and eventually they feel safe enough to verbalize their real feelings and participate in more conventional therapy. (*Monitor*, June 1982)

paregoric /-gôr′ik/ an opium-based medication administered for the control of severe cases of diarrhea. In addition to relieving pain and discomfort, p. reduces the peristalsis of the intestine. Besides opium, p. contains camphor, benzoic acid, glycerin, anise oil, and alcohol. P. was developed in the early 18th century, and its name was derived from the Greek word *paregorikos*, "consoling, soothing, encouraging."

parenchyma the functioning tissues of a body organ or gland, as distinguished from supporting or connecting tissues.

parenchymatous neurosyphilis a general term applied to a variety of functional effects of neurosyphilis, including paresis and tabes forms.

parental behavior in animal psychology, a three-stage process that consists of nest-building before or around the time the offspring are born, retrieving young that stray from the nest, and nursing and weaning the offspring. Avian parental behavior is similar to that of mammals except that nest-building may begin before ovulation, followed by incubation of the eggs and care of the offspring. Among humans, p.b. is less dependent on hormonal changes and more dependent on cultural factors and upbringing than among animals, but most parents want to see that the infant is well nourished, comfortable, and loved.

parental intercourse: See PRIMAL SCENE.

parental perplexity a relationship of parents to child marked by a lack of parental spontaneity, extreme indecisiveness, and an inability to sense and satisfy a child's needs. P.p. results in a child who is confused and likely to respond in a random and unpredictable manner, and may be a factor in schizophrenia.

parental rejection persistent denial of approval, affection, or care by one or both parents, sometimes concealed beneath a cover of overindulgence or overprotection. The frequent result is corrosion of self-esteem and self-confidence, a poor self-image, inability to form attachments to others, tantrums, generalized hostility, and development of psychophysical and emotional disturbances.

parent counseling professional guidance of parents on problems related to raising their children, including their roles in this process.

parent-effectiveness training client-centered discussions of principles, practices, and problems of child-rearing conducted by a psychologist, psychiatrist, or social worker on a group basis. A balance is maintained between the child's feelings and needs, and those of the parents. Abbrev.: **PET**.

parenteral drug administration any route of administration of a drug except through the digestive tract. **Parenteral** means literally not enteric, or not through the gut. P.d.a. alternatives include subcutaneous intramuscular, intravenous, vaginal, and rectal injection.

parent image a parent that exists in the mind of the individual, but not necessarily as an accurate image in general or in particulars. The term is also used for a surrogate parent.

Parents Without Partners Program: See DEATH NEUROSIS.

parergasia literally, perverted functioning. The

term was applied by Kraepelin to a schizophrenic symptom in which the patient performs an action that is not intended, as in opening his mouth when asked to close his eyes. For this meaning of p., see PARABULIA; DERAILMENT OF VOLITION.

The term was also used by Adolf Meyer to replace dementia praecox, since he believed this disorder is best described in terms of disorganized behavior and distorted thought processes.

paresis partial paralysis of the muscles. The term is also used in place of general p., in which paralysis occurs as a result of syphilitic infection of the brain. Adjective: **paretic**. See GENERAL P.; SYPHILIS.

paresthesia abnormal cutaneous, or skin, sensations, such as tingling, tickling, burning, itching, and pricking due to such factors as neurological disorder and drug side effects.

paretic: See PARESIS.

paretic curve a pattern produced in Lange's colloidal gold-reaction test when graduated amounts of cerebrospinal fluid taken from a patient with paresis are added to ten test tubes of a gold solution. About 50 percent of multiple-sclerosis cerebrospinal-fluid samples ´also show a p.c. in the test although there is no direct association between paresis and multiple sclerosis.

paretic muscles muscles that are partially but not completely paralyzed. The condition may be characterized by a weakness or loss of normal strength in an affected limb.

paretic psychosis = GENERAL PARESIS.

pargyline $C_{11}H_{13}N$—a monoamine oxidase inhibitor used in the treatment of hypertension primarily. It also may be employed as an antidepressant drug. It is believed p. causes a decline in blood pressure by enhancing the accumulation in adrenergic neurons of a substance that is a false neurotransmitter, resulting in turn in impaired adrenergic-impulse transmission.

parica = EPENA.

parietal drift = POSTURAL ARM DRIFT.

parietal lobe the portion of the cerebral cortex that occupies the upper central area of the hemispheres, between the frontal and occipital lobes but above the temporal lobes. Damage to the p.l. may cause aphasia and visual defects. P.l. functions include somatosensory activities, e.g., discrimination of size, shape, and texture of objects, as well as auditory and visual image-synthesizing. See BRAIN.

parieto-occipital sulcus a fissure that extends from a junction with the calcarine sulcus at a point posterior to the splenium, coursing upward along the medial side of the hemisphere, and forming a border between the cuneus and precuneus regions.

parietopontinus: See CORTICOPONTINE NUCLEUS.

Parinaud, Henri /pärinō'/ French ophthalmologist, 1844–1905. See PARINAUD'S SYNDROME.

Parinaud's syndrome a form of **ophthalmoplegia**, or paralysis of ocular motor nerves, in which the eyes turn upward despite efforts of the individual to control the disorder. The patient may try to break the reflex by closing the eyes and sometimes is able to force a downward gaze. The condition usually is due to a lesion at the junction of the brainstem and diencephalon and involves the posterior commissure area.

Parkinson, James English physician, 1755–1824. See PARKINSONISM; PARKINSON'S DISEASE; ANTI-PARKINSON DRUGS; AIR-POLLUTION SYNDROME; AKINESIA; AMPHETAMINE; ANTICHOLINERGICS; ANTIHISTAMINES; ANTIVIRAL DRUGS; ARTERIOSCLEROTIC DEMENTIA; BRAIN BANK; BRAIN DISORDERS; BULBOCAPNINE; CENTRAL ANTICHOLINERGIC SYNDROME; CONVENTIONAL VIRUS; CRYOGENIC METHODS; CRYOPROBE; DISEQUILIBRIUM; DOPAMINE; DOPAMINE RECEPTORS; DOPAMINERGICS; ECONOMO'S DISEASE; EXTRAPYRAMIDAL DYSKINESIA; EXTRAPYRAMIDAL SYNDROME; FACIAL EXPRESSIONS; FESTINATING GAIT; HYOSCYAMINE; LATEROPULSION; LEAD-PIPE RIGIDITY; LONG-TERM CARE FACILITIES; MARCHE À PETITS PAS; METHOCARBAMOL; MICROELECTRODE TECHNIQUE; MYDRIASIS; NEUROLOGICAL IMPAIRMENT; NURSING HOME; OCULOGYRIC CRISIS; PALILALIA; PARALYSIS; PATHOCLISIS; PHENOTHIAZINES; POSTENCEPHALITIS SYNDROME; POSTURAL HYPOTENSION; PROPULSION GAIT; PTYALISM; RETROPULSION; SINEMET.

parkinsonism any disorder that presents symptoms resembling those of Parkinson's disease. P. symptoms may occur in association with neurosyphilis, encephalitis, cerebral arteriosclerosis, or poisoning by carbon-monoxide gas or manganese products. Haloperidol, reserpine, and phenothiazines may cause drug-induced p. A term that is sometimes used synonymously with p. is **paralysis agitans**. See PARKINSON'S DISEASE. Also see PARALYSIS.

Drug-induced p. (pseudoparkinsonism) is a reversible syndrome resembling p., resulting from the dopamine-blocking action of antipsychotic drugs.

Parkinson's disease a progressive degenerative disease of the nervous system. Symptoms begin late in life with mild hand tremors and increasing rigidity, muscular weakness, and slower voluntary movements. Later symptoms include a masklike face, stooped posture, and festinating gait. P.d. is caused by damage to the extrapyramidal system of uncertain origin. Treatment usually involves surgery, drugs, and physical therapy.

parmia Cattell's term for a personality characteristic consisting of boldness, venturesomeness, and imperviousness to threats.

parole a method of maintaining supervision of a patient who has not been discharged, but who is away from the confines of a hospital, such as at a halfway house. A patient on p. may be returned to the hospital at any time without formal action by a court.

parorexia a morbid compulsion to consume unusual foods or other substances. See PICA.

parosmia any disorder of the sense of smell, either organic or psychogenic.

parosphresia a perversion or distortion of the sense of smell. Also called **parosphresis**.

parotid gland the largest of the three paired salivary glands, located below the ear under the jawbone.

paroxysm the sudden intensification or recurrence of a disorder or an emotional state; also, a spasm or seizure.

paroxysmal drinking = EPSILON ALCOHOLISM.

paroxysmal sleep = NARCOLEPSY.

parricide: See SACRIFICE.

Parry, Caleb Hillier English physician, 1755–1822. See FACIAL HEMIATROPHY (also called **Parry-Romberg syndrome**); GRAVES' DISEASE (also called **Parry's disease**).

parsimony economy or thriftiness. Scientific theories observe a principle of p. in keeping hypotheses and explanations simple. See OCCAM'S RAZOR.

-parthen-; -partheno- a combining form referring to girls or a virginal, unspoiled, or early stage or aspect (from Greek *parthenos*, "maiden, virgin").

parthenogenesis a form of sexual reproduction in which an unfertilized ovum develops into an offspring, as occurs in some lower animals, e.g., bees.

parthenophobia a morbid fear of girls or of virgins.

partial adjustments H. S. Sullivan's term for the techniques used by schizophrenic patients to reduce environmental stress during the period immediately before an acute psychotic episode, e.g., compensatory or sublimatory activities or defense reactions such as negativism and rationalization.

partial aim a pregenital form of libido satisfaction, e.g., oral eroticism.

partial correlation an estimate of a correlation between two variables with one or more additional variables held constant.

partial hospitalization in psychiatry, hospital treatment of mental patients on a part-time basis. See DAY HOSPITAL; NIGHT HOSPITAL; WEEKEND HOSPITAL.

partial insanity in forensic psychiatry, a term sometimes used to describe a borderline condition in which mental impairment is not sufficiently severe to render the individual completely irresponsible for his criminal acts. Instead, according to H. Weihofen (*Insanity as a Defense in Criminal Law*, 1933), there may be limited responsibility, with evidence that mental disorder was probably a contributing cause; or with evidence that the disorder rendered the individual incapable of deliberation, premeditation, malice, or another mental state usually requisite for first-degree offenses, and that therefore a lesser offense was committed. See M'NAGHTEN RULES. Also see LIMITED RESPONSIBILITY.

partial instinct = COMPONENT INSTINCT.

partialism a type of sexual perversion in which a person obtains sexual satisfaction from contact with a body part of the sexual partner, e.g., a leg. P. is distinguished from fetishism in which an object symbolic of the genitalia displaces the sexual partner.

partial lipodystrophy a form of fat-metabolism disorder that is usually acquired during infancy. There is a symmetric absence of adipose tissue in the face, but fat may or may not be absent from the regions above the legs. Also see TOTAL LIPODYSTROPHY.

partial reinforcement the presentation of reinforcement subsequent to some but not all occurrences of the correct response; any reinforcement schedule that is not continuous, e.g., a fixed-ratio or variable-ratio schedule. It has been experimentally demonstrated that p.r. is more effective than continuous reinforcement in maintaining responses and developing resistance to extinction. The term is used less commonly to mean the delivery of part of a reward or reinforcement, and is essentially equivalent to intermittent reinforcement.

partial sight a seriously defective visual condition, often defined as acuity of less than 20/70.

partial-thickness burns: See BURN INJURIES.

partial tone a simple component of a musical tone, e.g., a first partial or fundamental. Partial tones are responsible for the characteristic sounds of musical instruments.

participant-observation the type of observational method in which a trained observer enters the group under study as a member while avoiding a conspicuous role that would alter group processes and bias data. Cultural anthropologists become participant-observers when they enter the life of a given culture to study its structure and processes. See PARTICIPANT-OBSERVER.

participant-observer the individual who fills the role of group member while, at the same time, functioning as a scientific observer of group processes. The term was also used by H. S. Sullivan to describe a therapist who plays an active part in the therapeutic process by identifying with the patient's reactions and using his own feelings as clues to the patient's faulty patterns. See PARTICIPANT-OBSERVATION.

participation the interfacing of two or more systems that mutually influence each other. The term is also used for taking part in an activity; for the tendency of children to confuse their wishes, fantasies, or dreams with reality (Piaget); and for the primitive tendency to perceive similar things as the same.

particular complex a complex derived from a particular event in the individual's life.

part-instinct = COMPONENT INSTINCT.

part method of learning a learning technique in which the material is divided into sections, each to be mastered separately in a successive order. Compare WHOLE METHOD OF LEARNING.

partner-swapping = WIFE-SWAPPING.

part object an expression of libido in which a part of the body is the love object, e.g., the female breast.

partunate period: See BIRTH ADJUSTMENT.

-parv-; -parvi- a combining form meaning small (Latin *parvus*).

Pascal, Blaise /päskäl'/ French philosopher and mathematician, 1623–62. See EXISTENTIALISM; PRODIGY.

passion flower the flower and fruit of a climbing herb, Passiflora incarnata, that grows in the southern United States. P.f.-plant parts have been used for a variety of medicinal purposes ranging from treatment of burns and hemorrhoids to neuralgia and insomnia. **P.f. tea** has long been a folk remedy for the relief of nervous tension.

passive submissive; being acted upon rather than acting. The term was at one time used to characterize the feminine role, as in Freud's early writings.

passive-aggressive-personality disorder a personality disorder of long standing in which various means are used to resist adequate social and occupational performance, e.g., procrastination, dawdling stubbornness, intentional inefficiency, "forgetting" appointments, or misplacing important materials. These maneuvers are interpreted as passive expressions of underlying aggression. The pattern persists even where more adaptive behavior is clearly possible, and frequently interferes with job promotions, household responsibility, or academic success. (DSM-III)

passive analysis a type of psychoanalysis in which interpretations or suggestions by the analyst are minimized.

passive-avoidance learning a conditioning process in which a subject is first trained to perform an activity, then retrained to withhold that response to the same stimulus. An animal may learn to go to a particular spot to obtain food, then finds it receives an electric shock each time it goes to the food area, thereby acquiring a passive-avoidance response marked by reluctance to go to the food area.

passive castration complex: See ACTIVE CASTRATION COMPLEX.

passive-dependent personality a personality disturbance characterized by helplessness, timidity, lack of self-confidence, extreme dependence, and a tendency to express resentment and anger by making excessive demands and forcing others to take responsibility for them. This DSM-II category has been replaced in DSM-III by DEPENDENT-PERSONALITY DISORDER. See this entry.

passive immunity: See IMMUNITY.

passive introversion a type of introversion, or inward direction of the libido, that is caused by an inability to turn it outward or to restore again the libido to the object.

passive learning = INCIDENTAL LEARNING.

passive listening in counseling, attentive listening by the counselor without intruding upon or interrupting the client in any way. Also see ATTENTIVENESS.

passive mode of consciousness: See CONSCIOUS PROCESSES.

passive-receptive longing the desire to return to the infantile state where narcissistic needs are gratified without striving or reciprocation. This motive is clearly manifested in dependent individuals, masochists, and drug users.

passive recreation a form of recreational therapy in which the emphasis is on amusement or entertainment, e.g., a musical concert, as opposed to active recreation that requires physical or mental exertion.

passive therapist a nondirective therapist who plays the role of a catalyst rather than a directive guide or interpreter in group or individual psychotherapy. See NONDIRECTIVE APPROACH; CLIENT-CENTERED PSYCHOTHERAPY; ACTIVE THERAPIST.

passive transport the movement of substances across a semipermeable membrane by simple osmotic pressure, or without the assistance of enzymes or other energy systems. Compare ACTIVE TRANSPORT.

passive vocabulary the quantity of words a person can understand when he reads or hears them in context. Also called **recognition vocabulary**. Compare ACTIVE VOCABULARY.

passivism an attitude of submissiveness, especially in sexual relations. The term is often applied to unconventional sex practices, e.g., male p.

passivity a form of adaptation, or maladaptation, in which the individual adopts a pattern of submissiveness, dependence, and retreat into inaction.

pastoral counseling the application of certain psychotherapeutic principles and techniques by clergymen to parishioners who come to them with emotional difficulties. A **pastoral counselor** receives psychological training which he seeks to harmonize with his religious orientation. Usually, p.c. utilizes the techniques of supportive therapy while avoiding intensive exploration of unconscious motivation. See SUPPORTIVE PSYCHOTHERAPY.

pastoral psychiatry a branch of psychiatry that is associated with religion with the objective of offering relief from anxiety, guilt, and other emotional disorders. The term usually is extended to include the role of the clergy in providing a type of psychotherapy through marriage and family counseling.

past-pointing: See POINTING.

paternalism protective control of the behavior of individuals by an authority figure representing a political entity, business, union, or other organization.

Patau, Klaus German (?) physician, fl. 1960. See CHROMOSOME-13 TRISOMY (also called **Patau's syndrome**).

patellar reflex: See KNEE-JERK REFLEX.

paternity blues: See MATERNITY BLUES.

Paterson, Donald Gildersleeve American psychologist, 1892—. See PINTNER-PATERSON SCALE OF PERFORMANCE TESTS; MANIKIN TEST.

-path-; -patho- a combining form relating to suffering or disease (from Greek *pathos*, "suffering"). Also see -PATHY.

pathemia Cattell's term for a personality characteristic marked by emotional immaturity and inappropriately focused feelings, as opposed to realistic and objective attitudes.

pathergasia Adolf Meyer's term for psychological maladjustment due to a physical defect or malfunction.

pathetic nerve = TROCHLEAR NERVE.

pathoclisis /-klīˈsis/ sensitivity to injury or disease. The term is also used for a series of subclinical conditions, such as viral infections, arteriosclerosis, overuse of alcohol, or minor head traumas that cumulatively affect nervous-system functioning. In the opinion of some writers, p. may be responsible for Parkinsonism and senile and presenile dementias.

pathocure the displacement of a neurosis by an organic disease, a situation observed most often in moral masochists, who suffer to placate the superego. P. is the opposite of pathoneurosis.

pathogenesis the cause and course of a mental or physical disease. Also called **nosogenesis**.

pathogenic causing or leading to pathology.

pathogenic family pattern in psychiatry, family attitudes, standards, and behavior that lay the groundwork for mental disorder. Examples are parental rejection, overprotection, overindulgence, perfectionism, encouragement of sibling rivalry, marital conflict, double-bind situations, and excessively harsh, lenient, or inconsistent discipline.

pathognomonic characterizing a sign or symptom that is specifically diagnostic of a particular disease or disorder.

pathognomonic signs a constellation of symptoms that is indicative of a particular physical or mental disorder. The term is also used for Rorschach signs that point toward maladjustment.

pathognomy the recognition of feelings, emotions, and character traits, particularly when they are signs or symptoms of disease.

pathokinesis the dynamics, course, or development of an illness.

pathological drowsiness = SOMNOLENCE.

pathological fallacy a fallacy of overgeneralization in which pathological characteristics observed in abnormal individuals are attributed to the general population. E.g., many non-Freudians contend that Freud's theories are tenuous because they are based on a handful of clinical cases.

pathological gambling an impulse-control disorder consisting of a chronic, progressive failure to resist the impulse to gamble, leading to such behavior as arrest for forgery or embezzlement, defaulting on debts, borrowing from loan sharks, disruptive family life, income-tax evasion, or loss of job due to absenteeism. In spite of expressed intentions to repay debts, this rarely happens due to a persistent pattern of overspending and overconfidence in gambling as a quick solution for all financial problems. (DSM-III)

pathological grief reaction extreme or inappropriate response to bereavement, such as failure to recognize that the person has died (denial), irrational feelings of responsibility for the death, extreme guilt feelings over previous death fantasies, persistent depression and hopelessness, and excessive apathy or inertia. See GRIEF.

pathological guilt: See GUILT FEELINGS.

pathological intoxication = MANIA A POTU.

pathological lying a persistent, compulsive tendency to falsify or tell "tall tales" out of proportion to any apparent advantage that can be achieved. P.l. is found among alcoholics and victims of brain syndromes, but is most common among swindlers, impostors, con-men, and other antisocial individuals who in some cases do not seem to feel or understand the nature of a falsehood: "Perhaps such people mean for the moment to do what they promise so convincingly, but the resolution passes almost as the words are spoken" (Cleckley).

pathological mendicancy a morbid compulsion to beg regardless of whether there is a real need for financial help.

pathological sleepiness = SOMNOLENCE.

pathology the scientific study of the structural and functional changes involved in physical and mental diseases; also, a disordered condition, or disease.

pathomimicry conscious or unconscious mimicking or feigning of symptoms of disease or disorder. The simulation of disease is apparently less deliberate in CHRONIC FACTITIOUS DISORDER WITH PHYSICAL SYMPTOMS (or MUNCHAUSEN SYNDROME) than in MALINGERING. See these entries. Also called **pathomimesis**.

pathomorphism any abnormal or extreme body build.

pathoneurosis in psychoanalysis, a neurotic reaction to a physical disease and the limitations it imposes, as in denial of incapacity, or the idea that the disease was inflicted as punishment.

pathophobia = NOSOPHOBIA.

pathophysiological pattern a differential diagnostic flow chart employed to determine whether a set of signs and symptoms for a particular complaint, e.g., dizziness, headaches, or epileptic seizures, may be psychological or biochemical in origin. A p.p. may be translated into a computer program for future retrieval.

pathophysiology the study of diseases that are caused by biochemical abnormalities. Many such disorders involve sensory- or motor-nerve dysfunctions that result from chemical-messenger defects, metabolic errors, or adverse effects of drugs or environmental chemicals. Examples include excessive accumulation of magnesium or potassium in the tissues, causing heart arrhythmias and paralysis or muscle weakness.

pathopsychosis a psychotic condition that evolves

from an organic disorder, such as general paresis or brain tumor.

-pathy a combining form relating to (a) a disease, (b) therapy, that is, remedy for a disease. See -PATH-.

patient: See CLIENT.

patient-care audit evaluation and review of patient care provided by nonphysicians.

patient-centered services a term used in occupational, or industrial, psychiatry for mental-health services directly available to the workers, such as emergency psychiatric treatment, diagnosis, case-finding, and referral to clinics and social agencies. Also see ENVIRONMENT-CENTERED SERVICES.

patient government an organization of patients in a mental hospital for such purposes as making recommendations on rules and regulations, assistance with ward administration, planning social events, improving hospital décor, and orienting new patients. See THERAPEUTIC COMMUNITY.

patient obligations: See CONTRACT.

patient-oriented consultation: See PSYCHIATRIC CONSULTATION.

patients' rights: See RIGHTS OF PATIENTS; BILL OF RIGHTS.

patriarchal family a family in which the father is the final authority, decision-maker, and sole provider, while the mother plays subservient roles as full-time housewife.

patrilineal pertaining to inheritance through the male line.

patriophobia a morbid fear of inheriting something unpleasant, especially of having a hereditary disease.

pattern analysis a method of organizing items into clusters as a step in measuring a common variable such as an interest in an outdoor occupation or clerical work.

pattern discrimination the ability of humans or animals to distinguish differences in patterns such as sound frequencies and the order in which the differences occur. Examples are bird calls and other communicating sounds of various species. Also, we may respond to the visual pattern projected by a painting as opposed to responding separately to each color, texture, and shape. Also called **temporal-frequency discrimination**.

patterned interview in industrial psychology, a semistructured personnel interview predesigned to cover certain specific areas (work history, education, home situation, etc.), but at the same time to give the interviewer an opportunity to guide the dialogue into side channels and ask questions on points that need to be clarified.

patterning establishing a system or pattern of responses to stimuli, or a pattern of stimuli that will evoke a new or different set of responses. P. is used to retrain patients who have suffered a type of brain damage that disrupts normal sensory-motor activities.

patterning exercises a controversial treatment technique developed by Doman and Delacato in which mildly to severely brain-injured children are given special exercises designed to retrace the step-by-step organization of the central nervous system through the various developmental stages such as moving the arms and legs, or creeping and crawling. The object of the process is to overcome the effects of brain dysfunction by developing missing abilities that have inhibited motor, perceptual, and cognitive development.

pattern vision the ability to discriminate among shapes, sizes, and other features of objects in the environment by visual patterns. P.v. is lost following a lesion or excision of the striate cortex, as indicated by experiments with animals that bumped into objects in the environment and otherwise failed to see objects after damage to the striate cortex.

Patulin fungal toxins: See MOLDY-CORN POISONING.

Pavlov, Ivan Petrovich /päv′lôf/ Russian physiologist, 1849–1936. P. was trained in physics, chemistry, physiology, and medicine, and his major interest was in the physiology of digestion and the manner in which it is controlled by the nervous system. In the course of experiments with dogs he noted that gastric and salivary secretions occurred in connection with noise made during the preparation of food. This observation led to further experiments that yielded the concepts of unconditioned response, conditioned reflex, discrimination of stimuli, extinction of response, and production and elimination of experimental neuroses in animals. He later focused on human neuroses, developing the theory that they are due to an imbalance between the excitatory and inhibitory functions of the cortex, and advocating treatment by prolonged sleep, sedatives, and verbal and environmental therapy. Adjective: **Pavlovian** (pävlō′vē·ən/. See PAVLOVIAN CONDITIONING: ANALYZER; ASSOCIATIONISM; BEHAVIOR ANALYSIS; CONDITIONED RESPONSE; CONDITIONED STIMULUS; EXCITATORY-INHIBITORY PROCESSES; FIRST SIGNALING SYSTEM; LAMAZE METHOD; NEGATIVE INDUCTION; NERVISM; POSITIVE INDUCTION; SECOND SIGNALING SYSTEM; SIGNALING SYSTEM; TRANSCORTICAL PATHWAYS; UNCONDITIONED RESPONSE. Also see BEKHTEREV.

Pavlovian conditioning a pattern of learning discovered near the end of the 19th century by Ivan Pavlov in which a neutral, or conditioned, stimulus (CS) paired with an unconditioned stimulus (US) develops a learned, or conditioned, response (CR). In the classical conditioning experiment the ringing of a bell is the CS and food in the mouth of the dog is the US, which results in the CR, when the dog salivates. After the conditioning course is completed, ringing of the bell results in salivation by the dog in the absence of the food. Also called **classical conditioning; Type I conditioning; Type S conditioning**. See PAVLOV; CONDITIONING. Also see RESPONDENT CONDITIONING.

pavor diurnus a type of terror or fear reaction that

may occur in a small child during his afternoon nap.

pavor nocturnus = SLEEP-TERROR DISORDER.

pavor sceleris = SCELEROPHOBIA.

pay-and-don't-go a colloquial label used in transactional analysis for self-defeating patterns of behavior which, according to Eric Berne, "can be stopped just by stopping."

pay-off a colloquial label used in transactional analysis for a social "game" in which a reward of some kind is promised or bestowed, usually undeservedly.

p.c. an abbreviation used in prescriptions, meaning "after meals" (Latin *post cibum* or *post cibos*).

PCP: See PHENYLCYCLIDINE.

Pcs: See SYSTEMATIC APPROACH.

Peabody Picture Vocabulary Test a test in which sets of four pictures are presented to the subject, who selects the one that corresponds to a word uttered by the examiner. The test yields not only an estimate of the subject's vocabulary, but his grade level and IQ as well.

PeaCe Pill: See PHENCYCLIDINE.

peak clipping the elimination of a high amplitude portion of speech waves by electronic means, causing some loss of naturalness but little if any loss of intelligibility. P.c. makes it possible to reduce high-intensity noise and enable a hearing aid or public address system to utilize its power to the best advantage.

peak experiences A. Maslow's term for moments of awe or ecstasy that may at times be experienced by self-actualizers. According to Maslow, p.e. are sudden insights into life as a powerful unity transcending space, time, and the self. They may be associated with and elicited by experiences connected to mysticism, love, and the arts. See SELF-ACTUALIZATION; MASLOW'S THEORY OF HUMAN MOTIVATION.

Pearson, Karl English statistician, 1857–1936. See PRODUCT-MOMENT CORRELATION (also called **Pearson product-moment correlation; Pearson r**).

peccatophobia a morbid fear of committing a sin, usually an obsessive-compulsive symptom or associated with a paranoid delusion of sin. Also see ENOSIOPHOBIA.

pecking order a sequence or hierarchy of authority, status, and privilege which prevails in some organizations and social groups. The term originated in studies of chickens, which showed that when one of the animals aggressively pecks another, that animal pecks another in turn, and so on down the line, with each succeeding animal unable to peck the one above it.

pectus carinatum a malformation of the chest wall in which the sternum protrudes prominently like the keel of a ship, usually due to the bending inward of soft ribs. The disorder may be a symptom of rickets, the Morquio syndrome of dwarfism, or Marfan's syndrome. Also called **pigeon breast; chicken breast**.

-ped- a combining form relating (a) to children (from Greek *pais*, "child"), (b) to the feet (from Latin *pes*, "foot").

pederasty anal sexual intercourse, especially between an adult male (**pederast**) and a boy or young man (from Greek *pais*, "child, boy," and *erastes*, "lover"). Also called **pedicatio; pedication**.

pederosis an obsolete term for pedophilia.

pedestrian movement the generally regular and predictable flow of pedestrian traffic in a public area, such as a shopping mall, plaza, or street intersection. Studies show that despite an apparent random pattern of foot traffic, pedestrians usually follow the most direct route to a destination. The route may or may not conform to the pathways planned and constructed for p.m.

pediatric psychopharmacology the branch of pharmacology that is involved in the development and administration of drugs used in the treatment of psychiatric disorders of childhood. P.p. helps determine the choice of drug according to the age of the child, the diagnosis, the duration of the disorder, the severity of the illness, and the availability of the patient for behavioral and laboratory monitoring of the drug effects.

pedicatio; pedication = PEDERASTY.

pedigree method the study of family history and genealogy as a means of tracing traits that might be inherited. The method was applied with dubious results by Galton in his studies of genius and by Goddard in his studies of mental defect.

pediophobia a morbid fear of dolls.

pedolalia = BABY TALK.

pedomorphism the attribution of childish behavior characteristics to adults.

pedophilia a psychosexual disorder in which sexual acts or fantasies with prepubertal children are the persistently preferred or exclusive method of achieving sexual excitement. The children are usually at least ten years younger than the **pedophile**, or **pedophiliac**, and generally of the other sex; and the sexual activity often consists of looking and touching rather than intercourse. (DSM-III)

peduncular hallucinosis a visual hallucination associated with a lesion in the upper brainstem. The hallucination usually is recognized as such by the patient, who may see a panorama of people and events from his past life. The p.h. may be mixed with nonhallucinatory perceptions.

peeping Tom a popular term for a voyeur, derived from the name of a tailor who, according to the 11th-century legend, peeked at the virtuous Lady Godiva as she was riding naked through the streets of Coventry, for which sacrificial act her husband had promised tax relief to the people. Tom was struck by blindness for not looking discreetly away like everyone else. See VOYEURISM; TALION. Also see HYSTERICAL BLINDNESS.

peer group a group of children or adolescents with whom a young person associates; a like-aged group that influences the young person's attitudes, behavior, emotional security, and self-concept. Children begin to interact before age two, but genuine peer groups do not develop until the period of egocentrism begins to wane, usually between ages five and seven. See EGO-CENTRISM.

peer-group pressure the impact or influence of children's social groups on individual members, especially the power of the peer group to engender conformity. Studies indicate that susceptibility to p.-g.p. increases fairly steadily during grade school. Conforming behavior increases markedly at preadolescence.

peer rating the evaluation of an individual's behavior by his associates, e.g., physician peer review.

peer review professional evaluation of individual or group medical performance with the objective of maintaining or improving the quality of care and of promoting professional growth and development, as through continuing education. Also see PROFESSIONAL STANDARDS REVIEW ORGANIZATION.

PEG = PNEUMOENCEPHALOGRAM.

pegboard a performance test in which the subject inserts pegs in a series of holes as rapidly as possible. On the **Purdue p.**, one of the best known examples, manual dexterity is measured not only by inserting pegs but by adding washers and colors.

Pelizaeus-Merzbacher disease a progressive neurologic disorder marked by nystagmus, ataxia, and spasticity. Pathology shows a widespread symmetric loss of myelin. The young patient appears normal at birth, but nystagmus, tremor, and hypotonia are observed. Within four or five years, most patients have become immobile, with loss of vision, hearing, and ability to speak.

pellagra = NICOTINIC-ACID DEFICIENCY.

pellet a bit of food used in studies with rats and other experimental animals. Pellets are available in standard weights and sizes with standard contents.

pemoline a CNS stimulant.

Pende, Nicola Italian endocrinologist, 1880—. See EURYPLASTIC; HYPERGENITAL TYPE; HYPERTONIC TYPE; HYPOADRENAL CONSTITUTION; HYPOAFFECTIVE TYPE; HYPOGENITAL TYPE; REPRODUCTIVE TYPE.

pendular knee jerk an effect of the patellar knee-jerk reflex observed in patients with a lesion of the cerebellum: The leg continues to move several times after the initial reflex.

penetrance the percentage of cases in which a particular gene manifests a characteristic trait or disease in the developed organism, or phenotype.

penetration the entrance of the penis into the vagina. Legal interpretation of p. in cases of rape or illicit intercourse vary but generally regard p. to have occurred if the glans of the penis passes beyond the labia majora. Also called **immissio penis**.

penetration response a projective test response that contains a suggestion of weakness or penetrability, e.g., a "hole in the wall." Schizophrenic patients tend to include more penetration responses in testing than normal or neurotic persons.

Penfield, Wilder Graves Canadian neurosurgeon, 1891–1976. See CENTRENCEPHALIC SYSTEM; CENTRENCEPHALON; ELECTRICAL STIMULATION OF CORTEX.

-penia- a combining form relating to a deficiency.

peniaphobia a morbid fear of poverty.

penicillamine a degradation product of the antibiotic penicillin that has an ability to form chelation products by binding to toxic metals so that they can be excreted from the body. P., which is found in the urine of patients using penicillin antibiotics, is administered in the treatment of cystinuria and rheumatoid arthritis and, experimentally, in certain cases of muscular dystrophy. Also called **D-p**.

penile: See PENIS.

penile bone: See PENIS CAPTIVUS.

penilingus = FELLATIO.

penile plethysmograph: See PLETHYSMOGRAPH.

penis the male organ of coitus and urinary excretion. The p. consists of three parallel shafts of erectile tissue, the corpus spongiosum and the corpora cavernosa, bound together by skin and connective tissue. The urethra is contained in the corpus spongiosum and serves as a duct for the expulsion of semen during copulation. Adjective: **penile** /pē′nīl/. Also called **membrum virile; male member; member**. See PHALLUS; SMALL-P. COMPLEX. Also see DILDO.

penis captivus literally, captive penis, namely, held by the vaginal muscles during intercourse. While it is possible for a female to experience or deliberately produce strong vaginal muscle spasms during sexual intercourse and momentarily tighten the vagina about the male penis, true cases of p.c. are rare in the medical literature. Psychoanalysts attribute the many anecdotes involving p.c. to male castration fears and female castration impulses. P.c. may occur in cases of male animals that possess an **os penis** (a "penile bone") to help penetrate and stay long enough in the vagina.

penis envy in psychoanalysis, the desire of the female to possess a male genital organ. During the phallic stage (between three and six or seven), when the girl discovers that she lacks this organ, she feels "handicapped and ill-treated" (Freud), blames her mother for the loss, and wants to have it back. Also called **phallus envy**. See CASTRATION COMPLEX.

penis fear = PHALLOPHOBIA.

penis pride the male feeling of superiority and power associated with the possession of a phallus.

penology the scientific study of preventive treatment, punishment, and rehabilitation of criminals.

pension neurosis neurotic behavior induced by anxiety over obtaining a pension, the intense desire to obtain one, and concern over being able to obtain one, and concern over being able to live an economically secure and satisfying life during the pension years. See RETIREMENT NEUROSIS.

pentazocine: See SYNTHETIC NARCOTICS.

pentobarbital $C_{11}H_{17}N_2NaO_3$—a short-to-intermediate-acting barbiturate commonly employed as a sedative or hypnotic drug. It acts by depressing neural thresholds and reducing nervous activity. It may be used in psychotherapy to make the subject less inhibited and therefore able to express himself more effectively.

pentobarbital sodium: See BARBITURATES.

Pentothal Sodium a trademark for **thiopental sodium**—$C_{11}H_{17}N_2NaO_2S$, an intravenous anesthetic sometimes used in psychotherapy to induce a state of relaxation and suggestibility. See BARBITURATES.

pentylenetetrazol $C_6H_{10}N_4$—a powerful CNS stimulant, sometimes administered to stimulate the respiratory system. P. also may be employed in the diagnosis of hyperkinesis in children, to activate EEGs, and in the treatment of epilepsy. P. has been used as an alternative to electroshock in convulsant therapy of mental illness, particularly in cases of manic-depressive psychosis, and is used in experiments designed to test effectiveness of anticonvulsant drugs. Abbrev.: **PTZ**. Trademarks: **Metrazol; Leptazol**. See METRAZOL SHOCK TREATMENT; PSYCHOSTIMULANTS.

peonage: See INSTITUTIONAL P.

pep pills a popular name for stimulant drugs, usually containing amphetamine or caffeine as the principal ingredient, used by persons who want to stay awake under difficult conditions such as all-night highway driving. Use of p.p. has been discouraged by medical authorities because of the risk of serious accidents that may occur while using them.

pepsin: See ULCER; PEPSINOGEN.

pepsinogen a proenzyme secreted by the chief cells of the gastric glands of the stomach. P. is converted to **pepsin** (a proteolytic enzyme necessary for the catabolism of proteins) in the presence of gastric acid, also secreted by glands of the stomach.

peptic ulcer: See ULCER.

PER: See MENTAL STATUS EXAMINATION REPORT.

perceived reality a person's experience of reality; subjective experience in contrast to objective, external reality.

percentile the 100th part of a statistical distribution. One-fifth of cases fall below the 21st p.

percentile norm a norm expressed as a percentile rank rather than as a mean or average.

percentile rank a score that represents the percentage of cases that fall below the value of any given test score or result; e.g., a p.r. of 80 indicates that in 80 percent of cases tested a lower score was recorded. Also called **percentile score**.

percept the product of perception; the modification of the stimulus object as experienced by the individual. See PERCEPTION.

perceptanalysis a term used by Piotrowski for the process of inferring personality characteristics from a subject's responses to the Rorschach ink blots.

percept image a concrete image which may appear as a fantasy or memory image, and which represents a primitive level of intellectual life, commonly found in schizophrenics.

perception the awarenesss of objects, relationships, and events via the senses, including such activities as recognizing, observing, and discriminating. These activities enable us to organize and interpret the stimuli we receive into meaningful knowledge of the world.

perception deafness the inability to analyze or perceive sounds normally due to some impairment of the inner ear or auditory-nerve pathways leading to the brain. Also called **sensorineural impairment**.

perception of spatial relations an awareness of the relative position of objects in space.

perceptive referring to an individual who is sensitive and discriminating, especially in his judgment of people and works of art.

perceptive impairment and nerve loss = SENSORINEURAL HEARING LOSS.

perceptual consciousness a rarely used term of Freud's denoting the "psychic system" that receives stimuli from the external world, as distinguished from the system that records these stimuli in the form of memory traces.

perceptual constancy the ability to perceive the properties of objects such as size, shape, or color regardless of the variability of the impression these objects make on the observer. Also see CONSERVATION; SHAPE CONSTANCY; SIZE CONSTANCY; BRIGHTNESS CONSTANCY; WHITENESS CONSTANCY.

perceptual cues: See DEMAND CHARACTERISTICS.

perceptual defect = PERCEPTUAL DEFICIT.

perceptual defense the term for a form of misperception that is thought to result when anxiety-arousing stimuli are unconsciously distorted by the subject. P.d. has been the focus of studies in which taboo words are rapidly presented and misinterpreted; e.g., if the stimulus word "anal" is presented, subjects may report seeing the innocuous "canal."

perceptual deficit an impaired ability to organize and interpret sensory experience; difficulty in observing, recognizing, and understanding people, situations, words, numbers, concepts, or images. Also called **perceptual defect**.

perceptual disorders = PERCEPTUAL DISTURBANCES.

perceptual distortion an inaccurate interpretation of perceptual experience, as in the distorted images produced by dreams or hallucinogenic drugs, geometrical illusions (e.g., the Müller-Lyer illusion), visions occurring in states of sensory deprivation or dehydration, and distortions produced by expectation or suggestion.

perceptual disturbances disorders of perception, such as (a) recognizing letters but not words, (b) inability to judge size or direction, (c) confusing background with foreground, (d) inability to filter out irrelevant sounds or sights, (e) body-image distortions, and (f) difficulty with spatial relationships, e.g., perceiving the difference between a straight and a curved line. Also called **perceptual disorders**.

perceptual expansion the development of the ability to recognize, interpret, and organize intellectual, emotional, and sensory data in a meaningful way; also, the enriched understanding of one's experience that takes place in psychotherapy when defenses are relaxed.

perceptual extinction an effect of certain unilateral cortical lesions in which a stimulus, usually tactual or visual, is not detected. If a single stimulus is presented on either side of the midline, it is detected by the subject, but when two similar stimuli are presented at the same time, one on each side of the midline, the stimulus on the side contralateral to the lesion is not detected.

perceptual field the totality of the environment that a subject perceives at a given time, regardless of what actually is there, or how much it may be distorted or illusory.

perceptual filtering the process of focusing attention on a selected few of the myriad sensory stimuli that constantly bombard the body's various nerve receptors. P.f. is a necessary function for the survival of the organism which is physically incapable of responding to all of the simultaneous neural inputs.

perceptualization the process of organizing sensory inputs into a realistic and meaningful whole; also, awareness of reality as it appears to the senses rather than to the intellect, as in dreams, hallucinations, and the concrete, nonconceptual process of the schizophrenic who thinks only in terms of specific instances rather than categories.

perceptual learning training of a subject to perceive relationships between stimuli and objects in the environment. The perceptual change in the learning procedure may be associated with conditioned or instrumental responses, such as learning to discriminate among various stimuli.

perceptually handicapped a term applicable to an individual who is learning-impaired because of deficits in the perception of sensory stimuli.

perceptual maintenance in environmental design, the construction of an environment to facilitate sensory functions (e.g., seeing, hearing) and to provide an appropriate level of perceptual stimulation for the activity carried out, e.g., the lighting and soundproofing of a recording studio or the use of minimal decoration in an office in order to promote work and concentration.

perceptual masking the interference of one stimulus with another, preventing proper perception, e.g., of an object or space.

perceptual-motor disabilities combinations of handicaps that include one or more sensory and motor functions. An example would be a deaf person with cerebral palsy.

perceptual-motor learning the learning of a skill that requires both perceptual and motor responses, e.g., driving an automobile.

perceptual-motor match the ability to correlate perceptual data with a previously learned body of motor information. A child with brain damage may have to touch everything he sees because he cannot make the p.-m.m. automatically.

perceptual restructuring the process of modifying a perception to accommodate new information.

perceptual rivalry = SENSORY INATTENTION.

perceptual schema a subject's cognitive patterns that form a frame of reference for responding to environmental stimuli.

perceptual segregation the separation of one part of a perceptual field from the whole, by physical boundaries or attention-diverting methods.

perceptual set a tendency to perceive objects, people, or events according to a certain frame of reference, e.g., a prejudice.

perceptual sociogram: See SOCIOGRAM.

perceptual speed: See PRIMARY ABILITIES.

perceptual style the characteristic way an individual attends to, alters, and interprets sensory stimuli. Many authorities believe perceptual functions are distorted among schizophrenics.

perceptual synthesis the integration of experience from all the senses to establish sensory information and eliminate unessential information with respect to similarities and differences. This includes touch and perception of one's own movements.

perceptual training a method of enhancing an individual's ability to interpret perceived objects or events in concrete terms. P.t. may be employed, e.g., in accelerating the ability of a normal or retarded child to recognize letters of the alphabet by having him trace the outlines of the letters.

perceptual transformation a change in the way a problem, event, or person is perceived by the inclusion of new information or a different perspective.

percipient a person who perceives; also, in parapsychology, the alleged recipient of parapsychological messages.

perennial dream a childhood dream that recurs repeatedly during adult life.

perfectionism the compulsive tendency to demand of others or of oneself a higher level of performance than required by the situation.

perfect negative relationship; perfect positive relationship: See PRODUCT-MOMENT ORIENTATION.

performance an activity or behavior that leads to a result, e.g., a change in the environment.

performance anxiety an anxiety associated with a fear of being unable to perform a task, which often is a sexual activity, as in cases of impotence caused by a fear of failure. **Test anxiety** is another common example of p.a. Also see PERFORMANCE NEUROSIS; TESTOPHOBIA.

performance assessment an appraisal of the growth or deterioration in learning and performance through the administration of ability and achievement tests.

performance neurosis an emotional disturbance that may occur during performance of an anxiety-provoking task, usually of a severity that prevents beginning or continuing the task (e.g., taking an examination or playing before an audience). Also see PERFORMANCE ANXIETY.

performance requirements standards pertaining to the safety, structural soundness, and general operations of a building or environment.

performance test = NONLANGUAGE TEST.

performers those individuals in a behavior setting who have the central or dominant role, e.g., the musicians and conductor of an orchestra in contrast to the audience. Compare NONPERFORMERS.

perhaps neurosis a form of obsessive neurosis in which the person is preoccupied with what might have been if he had taken an alternative course of action regarding a past event.

-peri- a combining form meaning near, around, enclosing (from Greek *peri*, "around, about, beyond").

periamygdaloid cortex a part of the brain that is associated with the sense of smell. The proportion of the brain that is occupied by the p.c. varies with different animals depending upon the importance of the sense of smell in their survival. Dogs, e.g., require a larger proportion of olfactory nerve tissue than humans. Also called **pyriform cortex; pyriform lobe.**

periblepsis the wild stare of a delirious person: an expression of terror, bewilderment, and consternation.

perikaryon the portion of the neuron that includes the nucleus and cytoplasmic mass that is responsible for the growth and nourishment of the cell.

perilymph a cushion of fluid that separates the bony labyrinth and the membranous labyrinth of the inner ear.

perimacular vision a type of vision that utilizes the retinal area surrounding the macula.

perimeter the boundaries of a two-dimensional figure. In studies of an individual's visual field, e.g., a map or chart can be prepared by plotting the points of peripheral vision that can be observed when the eyes are steadily focused on the center of the chart.

perimetry the measurement of the peripheral visual field. See PERIMETER.

perinatal herpes-virus infection a complication of **herpes simplex Type 2** in which the virus in a pregnant woman may be transmitted to the fetus. The fetal infection may develop into a severe blood disorder and can also result in a fatal form of encephalitis. The complication is most likely to develop in late pregnancy. See HERPES INFECTION.

period = MENSTRUATION.

periodic drinking = EPSILON ALCOHOLISM.

Periodic Evaluation Record: See MENTAL STATUS EXAMINATION REPORT.

periodicity: See RHYTHM AND P.

periodicity theory an explanation for the ability of a person to make pitch discriminations. It maintains that the cue for pitch perception is the frequency of the impulse in the auditory system. See TELEPHONE THEORY.

periodic reinforcement: See INTERMITTENT REINFORCEMENT.

period prevalence: See PREVALENCE.

peripatologist an instructor of the blind or partially sighted who specializes in teaching the visually handicapped person to orient himself to his surroundings and to move about independently, safely, and confidently.

peripheral dysostosis with nasal hypoplasia a congenital abnormality characterized by short, wide hands and feet and a short, flat nose with nostrils bent forward. Most of the patients show some degree of mental retardation. Because of foot anomalies, they may be slow in learning to walk.

peripheralism the view of the behaviorists that emphasizes events at the periphery of an organism, such as the skeletal and laryngeal muscles, and sex organs, rather than the functions of the central nervous system. Also called **peripheralist psychology.** Compare CENTRALISM.

peripheral nervous system the portion of the nervous system that lies outside the skull and vertebral column. The p.n.s. serves the dual purpose of bringing messages from the sense organs to the central nervous system and transmitting messages from the central nervous system to the muscles and glands. Abbrev.: **PNS.** Also see SYMPATHETIC NERVOUS SYSTEM; PARASYMPATHETIC NERVOUS SYSTEM.

peripheral neuropathy a neuromuscular disorder of the extremities, usually characterized by a feeling of numbness in the hands and feet and cramplike pains in the legs. Causes may be alcohol, vitamin deficiencies, diseases such as diabetes, or toxins in the blood resulting from lead, arsenic, mercury, or other substances in the environment. The toxins can enter the nervous system through peripheral nerve endings. If p.n. is not treated at an early stage, the condition may progress to muscle atrophy and an inability to walk or maintain balance. Also see HUFFER'S NEUROPATHY.

peripheral scotoma: See SCOTOMA.

peritoneal dialysis the use of the peritoneal tissues surrounding the abdominal cavity as a membrane for dialyzing, or removing the waste products or other toxic substances from the blood when the kidneys are unable to handle that function. A dialysis fluid with a chemical content similar to that of human blood is introduced into the peritoneal cavity by catheter and allowed to remain for a specified time period, after which it is drained. The procedure removes approximately the same waste products that would be formed in urine by normally functioning kidneys, which remove waste products by a very similar type of osmosis.

peritoneal space the space between the two membranes lining the abdominal cavity. One membrane lines the inside of the body wall and the other encloses the viscera.

peritonitis an inflammation of the **peritoneum** /-nē'əm/, the protective membrane that surrounds the organs of the abdominal cavity. **Acute p.** usually results from perforation of an abdominal organ, e.g., gallbladder, appendix, or ulcerated stomach, allowing the contents to flow into the abdominal cavity. **Chronic p.**, with similar symptoms and effects, may be caused by a disease, e.g., tuberculosis, but more frequently is caused by introduction of a foreign body, such as a bullet.

Perls, Frederick (Fritz) S. German-born American psychotherapist, 1893–1970. See AWARENESS-TRAINING MODEL; CATASTROPHIC EXPECTATION; GESTALT THERAPY; HUMAN-POTENTIAL MOVEMENT; PHOBIC ATTITUDE; TOPDOG; UNDERDOG.

permanence concept recognition that objects have an independent existence, "detached from the self" (Piaget). During the first few months of life, an object out of sight is out of mind, e.g., a toy covered with a cloth ceases to exist. This idea is gradually superseded by awareness of the permanence of things, which gives rise to the concept of objective reality.

permanent planning a system of establishing a permanent home for children with their original families in order to avoid the condition in which they might be shifted continually from one foster home to another.

permeability the state of being permeable to gases, liquids, or dissolved substances that can pass through very small openings or holes. A perfect membrane has no permeability, but one with **semipermeability** may permit the passage of certain substances on a selective basis, e.g., the flow of nutrients through a cell membrane.

permissive doll play: See DOLL PLAY.

permissive environment an environment in which acting out and free expression of opinion and emotion are allowed though not necessarily approved or encouraged.

permissiveness an approach to child-rearing in which the child is given wide latitude in expressing his feelings and opinions and even in acting-out behavior. Artificial restrictions and punishment are avoided as much as possible. The laudable object is to encourage the child to assume responsibility for his own behavior; but some parents go to the extreme and refrain from giving the child the positive guidance he needs.

permissive parent according to Baumrind, a parent who disavows punitive restrictions and tries to cultivate a positive, affirmative, accepting environment in the home. A p.p. tends to make few demands and avoids exercising control while encouraging children to govern their own behavior. Rules are explained, and the children participate in decision-making. Also see AUTHORITARIAN PARENT; AUTHORITATIVE PARENT; REJECTING-NEGLECTING PARENT.

pernicious anemia: See ADDISON-BIERMER ANEMIA.

-pero- a combining form relating to a deformity or defect (from Greek *peros*, "maimed").

peroneal muscular atrophy = CHARCOT-MARIE-TOOTH DISEASE.

peroneus longus /-nē'əs/ a muscle that extends along the outside of the lower leg from a point just below the knee to a tendon that continues into the bones of the feet. The p.l. supports the arch and flexes the foot.

perplexity state a form of confusion in which the patient is bewildered and uncertain about his own thoughts. The condition is most frequently found in schizophrenia, but a similar disorder sometimes occurs in toxic, infectious, or head-injury patients.

persecution syndrome a set of symptoms associated with persons who have survived life in concentration camps or persecution in flight. The symptoms include anxiety, overreactivity, irritability, chronic depression, psychosomatic diseases, and unconscious identity with the aggressor. P.s. patients tend to marry and associate with other persons with similar life experiences. See SURVIVAL GUILT. Also see STOCKHOLM SYNDROME.

persecutory delusion = DELUSION OF PERSECUTION.

perseveration the pathological repetition of the same act, idea, word, or phrase; also, an inability to interrupt a task or shift from one task or procedure to another. Extreme p. is frequently observed in patients with brain damage or schizophrenia.

perseveration set a tendency or predisposition acquired in a previous situation which is transferred to another situation where it may facilitate or interfere with the task at hand.

perseverative error the continuing recurrence of an error, e.g., the consistent misspelling of a word.

perseverative speech a speech disorder characterized by persistent, inappropriate repetition of the same word or phrase.

persistent puberism a condition in which secondary sexual characteristics become arrested in development and the individual remains in effect pubescent for the rest of his life.

persona the mask worn by actors in Roman antiquity. Jung uses the term to refer to the "face" or "mask" one adopts in the outside world. P. pertains to conscious purposes, not to deeper layers of the personality. Jung distinguishes between **personal man**, who identifies with the p., and **individual man**, who identifies with deeper aspects of himself.

personal adjustment the adaptation by the individual to living and working conditions in his family and community, with emphasis on interfacing of the individual's personality with that of others with whom regular personal contacts are necessary.

personal attribution = DISPOSITIONAL ATTRIBUTION.

personal audit an oral or written interview or questionnaire designed to encourage the individual to assess his own personal strengths and liabilities.

personal constant = HEINIS CONSTANT.

personal construct a concept of the world from an individual's viewpoint.

personal data sheet a questionnaire designed to obtain biographical facts about the subject, including age, sex, education, occupation, interests, and health history.

personal-distance zone in social psychology, the area of physical distance adopted by persons in relationships with friends and personal acquaintances. The p.-d.z. is defined as the area from ½ to 1¼ m (1½ to 4 ft.). See PROXEMICS.

personal-document analysis examination of a subject's letters, diaries, and other personal documents as a key to his or her personality. It is a case-study technique advocated by Allport.

personal equation the difference in performance attributed to individual differences; also, historically, a difference in reaction time between two observers.

Personal Experience and Attitude Question-naire a screening test for psychopathic behavior, containing 150 items on emotional instability, sexual psychopathy, nomadism, criminalism, and other psychopathic traits.

personal-growth groups small groups that use encounter methods for self-discovery and the development of the members' potential. See EN-COUNTER GROUP; HUMAN-POTENTIAL MOVEMENT.

personal-growth laboratory a sensitivity-training institute that seeks to develop the participants' capabilities for constructive relationships, creative effort, leadership, and understanding of others through various modalities of experience and expression, such as art activities, intellectual discussions, sensory stimulation, and interactions on an emotional level.

personal-history questionnaire a guidance term for a questionnaire that records information about a pupil's special abilities, interests, extracurricular activities, family life, and any unusual medical, emotional, or other problem relating to scholastic performance or social adjustment.

personal identity =IDENTITY.

personal idiom distinguishing behavior characteristics or mannerisms of an individual.

personal image an unconscious manifestation of an individual's personal experience, as distinguished by Jung from the racial unconscious.

personalism the extent to which an individual believes that another person's actions are directed at him. P. is also the view that the individual personality should be the central subject matter of psychology.

personalistic psychology a school of psychology that originated with Edward Spranger, Wilhelm Stern, and other Europeans and was developed by Gordon W. Allport in America: The primary emphases were on the individual personality as the core of psychology (personal-

ism), the uniqueness of every human being, and the study of the individual's traits and organization of traits as the key to his personality and adjustment to the environment.

personality the configuration of characteristics and behavior that comprises an individual's unique adjustment to life, including major traits, interests, drives, values, self-concept, abilities, and emotional patterns. P. is generally viewed as a complex, dynamic integration, or totality, shaped by many forces: hereditary and constitutional tendencies, physical maturation, early training, identification with significant individuals and groups, culturally conditioned values and roles, and critical experiences and relationships.

personality assessment the evaluation of such factors as intelligence, skills, interests, aptitudes, creative abilities, attitudes, and facets of psychological development by a variety of techniques including (a) observational methods that utilize behavior sampling, interviews, and rating scales, (b) personality inventories such as the MMPI, and (c) projective techniques such as the Rorschach and Thematic Apperception tests. The uses of p.a. are manifold, e.g., in industry, research, rehabilitation, educational and vocational counseling, and clinical evaluation of children and adults.

personality cult = CULT OF PERSONALITY.

personality deterioration a progressive decline in the individual's sense of personal identity, self-worth, motivational forces, and emotional life to the point where he appears to be a "changed person" or even a "nonperson." See DETERIO-RATION.

personality development the gradual development of characteristic emotional responses or temperament, a recognizable style of life, personal roles and role behaviors, a set of values and goals, typical patterns of adjustment, characteristic interpersonal relations and sexual relationships, characteristic traits, and a relatively fixed self-image. See PERSONALITY DYNAMICS; PERSONALITY INTEGRATION; PERSONALITY STRUC-TURE; PSYCHOSEXUAL DEVELOPMENT; LIFE-STYLE.

personality disorders a group of disorders involving pervasive patterns of perceiving, relating to, and thinking about the environment and the self when these patterns interfere with long-term functioning of the individual and are not limited to isolated episodes. These disorders include PARANOID-PERSONALITY DISORDER, SCHIZOID-PERSONALITY DISORDER, SCHIZOTYPAL-PER-SONALITY DISORDER, HISTRIONIC-PERSONALITY DISORDER, NARCISSISTIC-PERSONALITY DISORDER, ANTISOCIAL-PERSONALITY DISORDER, BORDERLINE PERSONALITY DISORDER, AVOIDANT PERSONALITY DISORDER, DEPENDENT-PERSONALITY DISORDER, COMPULSIVE-PERSONALITY DISORDER, PASSIVE-AGGRESSIVE-PERSONALITY DISORDER, and ATYPI-CAL, MIXED, OR OTHER PERSONALITY DISORDER. See these entries. An individual may have more than one of these personality disorders at one time. (DSM-III)

personality dynamics the drives, emotions, and other internal forces that underlie our behavior and determine our personality and adjustment.

personality formation the organization or structure of the components of an individual's character or personality.

personality integration the unification of an individual's personality dynamics to minimize inner conflicts and achieve effective adjustment.

personality inventory a series of statements covering various characteristics and behavioral patterns to which the subject responds with "true," "false," or "?" as applied to himself or herself. The results are interpreted according to standardized norms. An example is the Minnesota Multiphasic Personality Inventory.

personality-pattern disturbance a DSM-I category comprising pervasive personality disorders that are deeply ingrained, resistant to change, and predisposed to develop into psychoses under stress. The major types include INADEQUATE PERSONALITY, SCHIZOID-PERSONALITY DISORDER, CYCLOTHYMIC DISORDER, PARANOID-PERSONALITY DISORDER, HYPOMANIC PERSONALITY, and MELANCHOLIC PERSONALITY. See these entries.

personality problem a psychological maladjustment that interferes with personal or social life but lacks the severity of a neurosis or psychosis.

personality psychology the systematic study of the human personality, including (a) its nature and definition, (b) its maturation and development, (c) the structure of the self, (d) key theories (trait theories, psychoanalytic theories, role theories, learning theories, type theories), (e) personality disorders, (f) individual differences, and (g) personality tests and measurements.

personality sphere the complete range of measurable human personality traits (Cattell). See SOURCE TRAITS; SURFACE TRAITS.

personality structure the organization of the personality in terms of its basic components and their relationship to each other. Structural theories vary widely according to their key concepts—e.g., clusters of traits (cardinal, central, secondary, as in Allport); surface and source traits (as in R. B. Cattell); the id, ego, superego (as in Freud); the individual style of life (as in Adler); the hierarchy of needs (as in Maslow); constitutional types (as in Sheldon); and the individual's inner conscious, or Eigenwelt (as in existentialism).

personality test any instrument used to help evaluate personality or measure personality traits.

personality trait a relatively stable and consistent behavior pattern which is considered to be a characteristic component of an individual's personality.

personality-trait disturbance a DSM-I category that focuses on disordered traits but with a common denominator of immaturity, emotional disequilibrium, low stress tolerance, and a tendency to revert to childish behavior when subjected to pressure. The major types include emotionally unstable personality, passive-aggressive personality, compulsive personality, hysterical personality, immature personality, and obsessive personality.

personality-trait theory: See ALLPORT'S P.-T.T.; CATTELL'S FACTORIAL THEORY OF PERSONALITY. Also see FACTOR THEORY OF PERSONALITY.

personality types a classification of human beings into specific categories determined by physique or other outstanding characteristics. Examples are Jung's division into extravert and introvert; Edward Spranger's value types (theoretical, esthetic, social, religious, active, etc.); E. Fromm's character types (exploiting, marketing, hoarding, etc.); and W. H. Sheldon's constitutional types (ectomorphic, mesomorphic, endomorphic).

personalization a term applied by D. W. Winnicott to the process of ego development based on linkage of the self with the body and its functions during infancy. See BODY-EGO CONCEPT.

personal man: See PERSONA.

personal myth distorted autobiographical memories which serve to keep threatening experiences out of consciousness, especially severe traumas that occurred in the oedipal phase (E. Kris, 1952).

personal relationship: See CONTACT BEHAVIOR.

personal-social inventory an instrument that measures various personal traits associated with emotional and social patterns and overall adjustment. The rater may be the subject in question or an outside observer, e.g., a teacher or counselor.

personal-social motive: See SOCIAL MOTIVE.

personal space the area immediately around one's body that is felt to be part of oneself or part of one's "territory." P.s. is analogous to a country's territorial waters, into which intruders may not come. See PROXEMICS.

personal-space invasion a social-psychological term for the intrusion by one person in the personal space of another. In the p.-s.i., one person inappropriately and uncomfortably crowds another and without apparent motive. See PROXEMICS.

personal unconscious Jung's term for the portion of each individual's unconscious that contains the elements of his own experience as opposed to the collective unconscious which contains the archetypes, elements universal to mankind. The p.u. consists of everything subliminal, forgotten, and repressed in an individual's life. These contents can be recalled to consciousness, and the p.u. is thus equivalent to Freud's preconscious. Compare COLLECTIVE UNCONSCIOUS.

personification the attribution of personal or human characteristics to an object or abstraction; also, Sullivan's term for the pattern of feelings and attitudes toward another person arising out of our interpersonal relations with him or her.

personified self according to H. S. Sullivan, the organization of interpersonal experiences that make up the individual's representation, or image, of himself. The p.s. is based on the acceptable and approved good-me, the unacceptable and disapproved bad-me, and the anxiety-provoking not-me. As a whole, however, the p.s. becomes a source of security and a defense against anxiety.

person in the patient a term used in relation to the psychosomatic approach to therapy, with emphasis on the role of the patient's personality, character, and emotional factors as causative agents.

personnel data information on potential employees derived from personnel tests, application forms, interviews, physical examinations, and letters of reference, to be used in matching individuals and jobs.

personnel placement the assignment of an already-employed individual to the particular job for which he or she is best qualified.

personnel psychology a branch of applied psychology that deals with testing, counseling, placement, promotion, and advising in matters relating to employment.

personnel selection the process of selecting employees according to procedures usually developed by psychologists, such as structured interviews, administration of personnel tests, assembly of biographical data, and personnel appraisal.

personnel specifications the criteria (or **predictors**) required for effective performance of a particular job, including such factors as education, training, work experience, physical characteristics, abilities, and interests. Also called **job specifications**.

personnel tests individual or group-psychological tests used in employee selection and assessment of job performance, and comprising (a) aptitude tests, which measure basic abilities and skills, (b) achievement tests, which measure job-specific abilities such as typing skill, and (c) personality and interest inventories, which are used as "predictors" of job performance.

personnel training an industrial training program designed to achieve such goals as development of knowledge and skills, orientation to the company, and modification of supervisor or employee attitudes, through such learning procedures as audiovisual aids, lectures, simulated devices, conference method, role-playing, laboratory training, case discussions, behavior-modeling, business games, and programed instruction.

personology the study of personality from the holistic point of view, on the theory that an individual's actions and reactions, thoughts and feelings, and personal and social functioning can be understood only in terms of the whole person. The term p. was applied by H. A. Murray to his theory of personality as a set of enduring tendencies that enable us to adapt to life. According to Murray, personality is also a mediator between the individual's fundamental needs

(viscerogenic and psychogenic) and the demands of the environment.

perspective the ability to view objects, events, and ideas in realistic proportions and relationships; also, the delineation of the relative position, size, and distance of objects in a plane surface as if they were three-dimensional.

persuasion therapy supportive psychotherapy in which the therapist attempts to induce the patient to modify faulty attitudes and behavior patterns by appealing to his powers of reasoning, will, and self-criticism. Adler and others (notably P.C. Dubois and Joseph Déjérine) advocated this technique as a brief alternative to reconstructive methods.

Perthes, Georg Clemens /per′təs/ German surgeon, 1869–1927. See LEGG-CALVÉ-PERTHES DISEASE.

pertussis = WHOOPING COUGH.

pervasive developmental disorders a group of disorders involving severe distortions of many psychological functions, such as language, social skills, attention, perception, reality testing, and movement. This DSM-III category consists of infantile autism, childhood-onset pervasive developmental disorder, and atypical pervasive developmental disorder. See INFANTILE AUTISM; CHILDHOOD-ONSET PERVASIVE DEVELOPMENTAL DISORDER; CHILDHOOD ONSET PERVASIVE DEVELOPMENTAL DISORDER, RESIDUAL STATE; ATYPICAL PERVASIVE DEVELOPMENTAL DISORDER. Also see DEVELOPMENTAL DISABILITY. (DSM-III)

perversion in psychiatry, a culturally unacceptable or prohibited form of behavior, particularly in the sexual sphere. The term denotes especially those practices that deviate most widely from the norm, such as sadism, masochism, necrophilia, exhibitionism, pedophilia, coprophilia, fetishism, voyeurism, and zoophilia. The preferred term in DSM-III is "paraphilia." See PARAPHILIAS. Also see POLYMORPHOUS PERVERSE; SEXUAL P.

perverted logic; perverted thinking = PARALOGIA.

pes cavus a foot with an abnormally high longitudinal arch, that is, a foot that curves upward between the heel and toes. The condition may be congenital or caused by contractures. Also called **clawfoot**. Also see HAMMER TOE.

pes equinus a foot deformity characterized by a permanent extension of the toes so that the weight of the body is carried by the ball of the foot and the heel is raised above the ground. Also called **talipes equinus; tip foot**.

pes planus = FLATFOOT.

pessimism: See ORAL P.

Pestalozzi, Johann Heinrich /pestälôt′sē/ Swiss educational reformer, 1746–1827. See CHILD PSYCHIATRY.

PET = PARENT-EFFECTIVENESS TRAINING.

PET = POSITRON-EMISSION TOMOGRAPHY.

petechial hemorrhages minute hemorrhages, often of pinpoint size, such as those occurring in

the brains of veteran prizefighters due to repeated blows to the head. See BOXER'S DEMEN-
TIA.

Peter Panism the refusal to acknowledge that one
is growing old, expressed in such ways as ignoring birthdays, dying one's hair, cosmetic
surgery, constantly proving one's prowess, and
repeatedly asserting "I'm not that old."

pethidine: See SYNTHETIC NARCOTICS.

petit mal /pətē′mäl′/ a form of epilepsy characterized by sudden, brief lapses of consciousness
during which the patient sits motionless with a
dazed, expressionless face, but does not have a
convulsion or fall (French, "small sickness").
The attacks usually develop in childhood, may
occur several times a day, and tend to subside
within a few years. The characteristic EEG
shows wave-and-spike discharges at the rate of
three per second. The symptoms may be so brief
as to be overlooked by observers or mistaken for
a few seconds of absentmindedness. Also called
p.m. epilepsy; minor epilepsy. See EPILEPSY;
GRAND MAL.

petrifaction the process of being turned into stone.
In mythology and psychoanalysis, this fantasy
may represent punishment for voyeuristic impulses or behavior.

petting behavior sexual activity of a heterosexual
nature that may lead to orgasm without intromission of the penis. P.b. is similar to foreplay
and may include stroking, kissing, and actual
placing of the genitals in apposition.

-pexy a combining form relating to a fixation.

peyote a small spineless cactus of the species
Lophophora williamsii that grows wild in Mexico. The name is derived from the Aztec word
peyotl, which describes the inside of the plant as
resembling a caterpillar's cocoon. The entire
plant is psychoactive, but only the portion above
ground is eaten, being sliced into disks called
mescal buttons. The active ingredient is the hallucinogen mescaline. P. is the only American
plant that has been used continuously in religious ceremonies from prerecorded times to the
present day; it is still incorporated into the
rituals of the Native American Church.

Pfaundler, Meinhard von /pfound′lər/ German
physician, 1872–1947. See HURLER'S SYNDROME
(also called **Pfaundler-Hurler syndrome**).

Pfeiffer, Emil /pfī′fər/ German physician, 1846–
1921. See PFEIFFER'S SYNDROME.

Pfeiffer's syndrome a familial disorder marked by
premature fusion of the cranial bones, causing a
skull deformity. The patients also have facial deformities with protruding and widely-spaced
eyes (which often show signs of strabismus),
large thumbs, and large great toes. Some but not
most of the patients observed have shown subnormal intelligence. Also called **acrocephalosyndactyly, Type VI.**

Pfropfschizophrenia /pfrôpf′-/ a form of schizophrenia superimposed, or "engrafted" (from
German *pfropfen*, "to graft"), on mental retardation, and usually involving paranoid epi-

sodes with delusions and hallucinations, which
may be followed by gradual regression to infantile, deteriorated behavior. Also widely, though
inaccurately, called **Propfschizophrenia**.

PGO spikes EEG peaks that occur during sleep
and indicate neural activity in the *p*ons, lateral
*g*eniculate, and *o*ccipital cortex. See PARADOXI-
CAL SLEEP.

PGR: See GALVANIC SKIN RESPONSE.

PGSR = PSYCHOGALVANIC SKIN-RESISTANCE AUDI-
OMETRY.

pH: See HYDROGEN-ION CONCENTRATION.

phacomatosis = PHAKOMATOSIS.

Phaedra complex incestuous love of the mother
for her son. (The term is based on the Greek
myth of Phaedra, daughter of Minos and
Pasiphaë, and wife of Theseus. When his step-
son, Hippolytus, rejected her love, she accused
him of violating her and hanged herself.) Also
see MOTHER-SON INCEST.

-phag-; -phago-; -phagia; -phagy a combining
form relating to eating (from Greek *phagein*, "to
eat").

phagomania an insatiable hunger or uncontrolled
and morbid desire to consume food.

phagophobia a morbid fear of eating. Also see
SITOPHOBIA; ANOREXIA NERVOSA.

phakomatosis a hereditary disorder characterized
by the growth of benign nodulelike tumors of
the brain, eye, and skin. Kinds of p. include
neurofibromatosis, cerebroretinal angiomatosis,
tuberous sclerosis, and encephalotrigeminal
angiomatosis. Also spelled **phacomatosis**.

phalanges /fəlan′jēz/ small bones of the fingers and
toes. Singular: **phalanx**.

phalli: See PHALLUS.

phallic character in psychoanalysis, an individual
who displays patterns of behavior arising out of
a reaction formation to castration fear. These
patterns are, typically, boastfulness, excessive
self-assurance, narcissistic vanity, and in some
cases aggressive or exhibitionistic behavior. In
women the reaction to penis envy may be in the
form of masculine behavior or antagonism
toward males. Also called **phallic-narcissistic
character**.

phallicism a reverence for the creative forces of
nature as symbolized by the phallus; phallic
worship. Also called **phallism**.

phallic love a love of the penis or the equivalent
for girls, the clitoris. P.l. may be manifested by
penile pride and interest in masturbation. The
term is also applied to love that is characteristic
of the phallic period.

phallic mother in psychoanalysis, the fantasy
among male children that the mother has a
penis. According to Freud, this belief can be so
strong that the discovery that it is false may lead
to active disgust and in some cases to future impotence, homosexuality, or misogyny.

phallic-narcissistic character = PHALLIC CHARAC-
TER.

phallic overbearance a rarely used expression signifying extreme domination by an aggressive male.

phallic phase in psychoanalysis, the stage of psychosexual development, between ages three and six or seven, when sexual feeling is first focused on the genital organs, and masturbation becomes a major source of pleasure. During this period the boy experiences sexual fantasies toward his mother and rivalry toward his father, both of which he eventually gives up due to castration fear. Similarly, the girl experiences sexual fantasies toward the father and hostility toward the mother, due to rivalry and blaming her for being deprived of the penis, but gives up these feelings when she becomes afraid of losing the love of both parents. Also called **phallic stage**. See OEDIPUS COMPLEX.

phallic pride in psychoanalysis, the sense of superiority and even omnipotence experienced by boys when they discover that they have a penis and girls do not. These feelings are believed to help master intense castration anxiety.

phallic primacy in psychoanalysis, the stage of psychosexual development which follows the pregenital period (oral and anal), and which begins in the third year, when the penis of the boy and the clitoris of the girl gradually become the central erotogenic zones.

phallic sadism aggression that is associated with the child's phallic stage of psychosexual development. The child interprets sexual intercourse as a violent, aggressive activity on the part of the male and particularly on the part of the penis.

phallic stage = PHALLIC PHASE.

phallic symbol in psychoanalysis, any object that resembles or represents the penis. Examples include not only cigars, pencils, trees, and skyscrapers, but also automobiles, airplanes, birds, snakes, and hammers. (However, even Freud is said to have said, "Sometimes a cigar is just a cigar.") See SYMBOLISM.

phallic woman a woman who is fixated at the phallic stage, and as a result consciously seeks to deny that she lacks a penis, or unconsciously wishes to castrate all men so that they will also be deprived of a penis.

phallism = PHALLICISM.

phallocentric culture a culture in which the phallus, or penis, is regarded as a sacred giver of life, source of power, or symbol of fertility. Phallic symbols have been associated with cultures throughout the world since preneolithic times, as evidenced by illustrations on cave walls. One of the Graeco-Roman gods was Priapus, a synonym for penis. Also see PRIAPISM.

phallophobia a morbid fear of the penis, especially of the erect penis.

phallus the penis or an object that resembles the form of the penis, e.g., the clitoris or the undifferentiated primordial tissue that eventually develops into either the clitoris or the penis. In psychoanalytic theory, the p. is the penis during the period of infantile sexuality. Plurals: **phalli** /fal'ī/; **phalluses**. See CLITORIS; PENIS; PRIAPISM.

phallus envy = PENIS ENVY.

phallus girl an unconscious symbolic girl with a phallus as manifested in transvestite fantasies in which the individual himself represents the girl with a penis.

phaneromania a persistent impulse to touch or stroke part of one's own body, such as the nose (which may represent the penis) or the breasts.

phanerothyme a term coined by Aldous Huxley in 1956 (from Greek *phanein*, "to reveal," and *thymos*, "mind, soul") for what was vaguely called psychotomimetic. He first used the term in a letter to his friend Humphry Osmond, who counterproposed the less unwieldy term psychedelic. See PSYCHEDELICS.

phantasm an illusion or pseudohallucination, usually of an absent person appearing in the form of a spirit or ghost, but recognized by the observer as being imaginary or illusory, as opposed to a true hallucination.

phantasmagoria the imagined process of raising or recalling the spirits of the dead.

phantasticum a term introduced in the 1920s by German toxicologist Louis Lewin to identify a category of drugs that are capable of producing hallucinatory experiences. The same drugs today are known as hallucinogens or psychedelics. Plural: **phantastica**.

phantasy = FANTASY.

phantom breast: See BREAST-PHANTOM PHENOMENON.

phantom limb the feeling, usually temporary, that an amputated limb (or other body part such as the breast or penis) is still there. The illusion is generally attributed to persistence of the intact body image, since it is not experienced by individuals born with the limb missing. The phantom is usually accompanied by paresthesias such as tingling or in some cases painful burning, itching, and twisting sensations which may be due in part to stimulation of the nerve ends and in part to psychological reactions. Also see BREAST-PHANTOM PHENOMENON; PSEUDOESTHESIA.

phantom-lover syndrome a type of delusional loving included in the category of erotomania. The patient, who is usually schizophrenic, believes an unknown, undistinguished man is in love with her.

phantom reaction: See PHANTOM LIMB; BREAST-PHANTOM PHENOMENON.

pharmacodynamic tolerance a form of drug tolerance in which the chemistry of the brain becomes adjusted to the presence of the chemical which in turn then loses its capacity for modifying brain activity. P.t. is associated with the use of all sedative-hypnotic drugs, e.g., barbiturates, and is followed by withdrawal symptoms when regular doses of the drug are interrupted.

pharmacogenetics the study of genetic factors that can influence the response of individuals to different drugs and in different dosages. The drug may be altered by the body, as occurs with half the American population in the metabolizing of the drug isoniazid because of an inherited

deficiency of an enzyme required to utilize isoniazid without adverse effects. Alteration of the
body's response to a drug occurs mainly in persons of African or Mediterranean ancestry who
lack an enzyme essential for the metabolism of
sulfa drugs, certain analgesics, and antimalaria
medications.

pharmacogenic orgasm the pleasurable sensation
obtained by some individuals in the use of drugs
of abuse. The p.o. is believed by some investigators to account for the reduced sexual and
aggressive drives that are sequelae to drug use.

pharmacokinetics the activity of pharmacological
agents within a biological system, *in vivo* or *in
vitro*, including the absorption, distribution,
metabolism, and elimination of the substance or
its metabolites.

pharmacological antagonism a form of drug
antagonism that is competitive between a receptor stimulator and a receptor blocker. P.a. may
occur, e.g., between morphine and naloxone.
The term is used to distinguish the interaction
from physiological antagonism between drugs
that have opposing actions.

pharmacomania an abnormal desire to take or
administer drugs.

pharmacophobia a morbid fear of medicine.

pharmacotherapy the treatment of a disorder by
the administration of drugs, as opposed to
surgery, psychotherapy, acupuncture, or other
methods which may include diets or faith healing. Homeopathy is a form of p. in which drugs
used are those that produce symptoms similar to
the disease; allopathy drugs produce effects
different from those caused by the disease.

pharmacothymia an obsolete term for a compelling, neurotic desire to take drugs.

pharyngeal: See GUTTURAL.

pharyngeal keratosis: See KERATOSIS.

pharynx the muscular and membranous sac between the mouth and nares (nostrils) and the
esophagus. It consists of three major sections,
the laryngopharynx, oropharynx, and nasopharynx.

phase a stage in the development of life, such as
puberty or adulthood; also, a recurrent state of
any cyclical process such as a sound wave or a p.
of the moon.

phase cue a sound localization cue in binaural
hearing. At frequencies below 800 cycles per
second, the time of arrival of sound waves
reaching the ears on opposite sides of the head is
sufficiently different to be detected.

phase difference a difference in phase sequence of
two sound waves, resulting in beats or alternating intensities.

phase sequence Hebb's term for a series of nerve-
cell assemblies linked in a functional relationship, e.g., a conscious thought process.

phase shift a type of sleep disorder caused by a disruption of the normal sleep-wake cycle, resulting in the subject being alert during a usual
sleeping period and sleepy when he should be
alert.

phasic activation attention mechanisms that are
related to the diffuse thalamic projection system
and are transitory rather than tonic or persistent
in nature.

phasic functions the transient increases of attention and arousal associated with the diffuse thalamic projection system. Longer tonic effects are
associated with the reticular activating system.

phasmophobia = DAEMONOPHOBIA.

-phemia a combining form relating to speech
(Greek *pheme*).

phenacemide: See ACETYLUREAS.

phenacetin: See ANILIDES; ASPIRIN COMBINATIONS.

phenadoxone hydrochloride: See SYNTHETIC NAR-
COTICS.

phenazocine $C_{22}H_{27}NO$—a potent analgesic which
produces the same effects as morphine, including the adverse side-effects of respiratory depression and tendency to addiction. It is more
than three times as potent as morphine and
is prescribed in a hydrobromide form—
$C_{22}H_{28}BrNO$—under the trademark of **Prinadol**. Also see SYNTHETIC NARCOTICS; NARCOTIC
ANALGESICS.

phencyclidine $C_{17}H_{25}N$—a hallucinogen of the
piperidine family chemically termed 1-1 phenyl-
cyclohexyl-piperidine HCl. Street names are,
among others, **PCP**, PeaCe Pill (hence PCP),
crystal, angel dust, rocket fuel, hog, zombie,
and superjoint. It is inhaled, injected, taken by
mouth, or most commonly sprayed over parsley,
mint leaves, or marijuana and smoked. For
effects, see P. (PCP) OR SIMILARLY ACTING ARYL-
CYCLOHEXYLAMINE ABUSE; P. (PCP) OR SIMILARLY
ACTING ARYLCYCLOHEXYLAMINE DELIRIUM; P. (PCP)
OR SIMILARLY ACTING ARYLCYCLOHEXYLAMINE IN-
TOXICATION; P. (PCP) OR SIMILARLY ACTING ARYLCY-
CLOHEXYLAMINE MIXED ORGANIC MENTAL DIS-
ORDER. Also see SERNIL; PSYCHEDELICS; PHENYL-
CYCLOHEXYL DERIVATIVES.

**phencyclidine (PCP) or similarly acting aryl-
cyclohexylamine abuse** a disorder whose distinguishing feature is pathological use of these
substances for at least one month, involving intoxication throughout the day, with episodes of
delirium or mixed organic mental disorder, and
impaired functioning, such as fights, loss of
friends or job, and repeated legal difficulties.
(DSM-III)

**phencyclidine (PCP) or similarly acting aryl-
cyclohexylamine delirium** a delirium occurring within 24 hours of use or days after overdose of these substances, and lasting up to a
week. (DSM-III)

**phencyclidine (PCP) or similarly acting aryl-
cyclohexylamine intoxication** a disorder that
develops within one hour of swallowing, or five
minutes after smoking, sniffing, or injecting
these substances. Physical symptoms include
nystagmus, increased blood pressure and heart
rate, numbness, unsteady gait, and dysarthria;
psychological symptoms include euphoria, agitation, marked anxiety, emotional lability, grandiosity, sensation of slowed time, and synesthe-

sia (such as seeing colors when hearing loud sounds). Common behavioral effects are belligerence, impulsivity, impaired judgment, and assaultiveness. Coma, convulsions, and even death may occur after a heavy dose. (DSM-III)

phencyclidine (PCP) or similarly acting aryl-cyclohexylamine mixed organic mental disorder an illness developing after recent use of these substances, in which there are features of organic brain syndromes (delusions, hallucinations, disorientation) or a progression from delirium to an organic delusional syndrome. (DSM-III)

phendimetrazine: See ADRENERGIC DRUGS.

phenelzine: See MONOAMINE OXIDASE INHIBITORS.

phengophobia a morbid fear of daylight or, generally, of any time other than night time (from Greek *phengos*, "light"). Compare FEAR OF DARKNESS.

phenmetrazine: See ADRENERGIC DRUGS.

phenobarbital: See BARBITURATES.

phenocopy imitation of a phenotype resulting from the interaction of an environmental effect and a genotype. An example is the effect of sunlight on skin or hair, resulting in variations that mimic the natural coloring or texture of other phenotypes.

phenomenal absolutism the belief that one's perceptions may be taken as objective reality. The "naive observer" equates sense perception with actual properties of a given object, expecting that independent observers will have identical perceptions.

phenomenal field = PHENOMENOLOGICAL FIELD.

phenomenalism the philosophical viewpoint that appearances, or phenomena, are the only real, accessible entities and therefore are and provide the true objects of knowledge.

phenomenal motion motion that is not real but is experienced as real; the illusion or appearance of motion as on film. See APPARENT MOVEMENT. Also see PHENOMENOLOGICAL FIELD.

phenomenal report in a nonexperimental situation, a verbal account or description of everything within one's field of awareness; in an experimental situation, a verbal account of all one's responses to a specific stimulus. See PHENOMENOLOGICAL FIELD; PHENOMENOLOGY.

phenomenal self the self as experienced by the individual at a given time. All perceptions, thoughts, ideas, images, and feelings may be said to belong to the p.s. whether or not they have direct reference to the immediate physical environment. Also see PHENOMENOLOGICAL FIELD.

phenomenistic causality a type of childish logic in which coincidences are viewed as causal relationships. E.g., the sun hides at night because it is afraid of the dark.

phenomenological analysis the method of radical empiricism in which overt behavior and immediate experience are observed and studied without concern for biographical data or reliance on a psychodynamic analysis with its assumption of unconscious mental activity.

phenomenological field one's environment as experienced by a given individual at a given time. The p.f. refers not to objective but to personal and subjective reality, including everything within one's field of awareness. Also called **phenomenal field**. Also see PHENOMENAL SELF.

phenomenology the theory that our knowledge, including psychology and psychiatry, should be based on immediate, ongoing experience, that is, on the process of attending to phenomena as they are directly presented. In other words, observation must come before analysis and interpretation: We must, e.g., attempt to get "inside the mind" of a schizophrenic patient or a person under the influence of a hallucinogenic drug in order to understand his experiences. The philosophical and psychological p. movement was initiated at the beginning of the 20th century by the German philosopher Edmund Husserl; it has greatly influenced Gestalt psychology and is the basis of modern EXISTENTIALISM. See this entry. Also see EXISTENTIAL P.

phenomenon an appearance that is associated with an implied underlying reality and is open to study.

phenomotive a term used by Wilhelm Stern for a motive that can be revealed and observed introspectively.

phenothiazine death /-*thī'*-/ sudden, unexplained autopsy-negative death occurring in patients under phenothiazine. The few cases reported appear to be associated with either cardiac arrhythmia or heat stroke. See NEUROLEPTIC MALIGNANT SYNDROME; AUTOPSY-NEGATIVE DEATH.

phenothiazines a group of neuroleptic drugs, or major tranquilizers, developed in the 1950s from a chemical originally produced as a pesticide. P. have a general inhibitory influence on catecholamine metabolism with a tranquilizing effect. P. are widely used in the treatment of manic-depressive psychoses, schizophrenias, and certain organic brain disorders, e.g., epilepsy, dementia, Huntington's chorea, and confusional states. The prototype drug of the group is CHLORPROMAZINE (see this entry), which impairs vigilance and diminishes motor activity; in large doses, it produces cataleptic effects. However, p. lack the euphoric and addicting properties of barbiturates and narcotics used previously as neuroleptic drugs. Other p. are **chlorpromazine hydrochloride**—$C_{17}H_{20}Cl_2N_2S$, **fluphenazine**—$C_{22}H_{26}F_3N_3OS$, **fluphenazine enanthate**—$C_{29}H_{38}F_3N_3O_2S$, **fluphenazine hydrochloride**—$C_{22}H_{28}Cl_2F_3N_3OS$, **thioproperazine**—$C_{22}H_{30}N_4O_2S_2$, and THIORIDAZINE (see this entry). A member of the p. that has value as an antiparkinsonism medication, **ethopropazine**—$C_{19}H_{24}N_2S$, acts as an acetylcholine antagonist. Also see ANTIMANICS.

phenotype all the manifest characteristics or attributes of an organism, especially its changing appearance, as contrasted with its underlying hereditary characteristics. See GENOTYPE.

phensuximide: See SUCCINIMIDES.

phentermine hydrochloride: See ADRENERGIC DRUGS.

phentolamine $C_{17}H_{19}N_3O$—an alpha-adrenergic blocking agent with direct action on cardiac and smooth-muscle tissues. Cardiac action is sympathomimetic in effect while gastrointestinal-tract stimulation is of a parasympathomimetic type. It is used in parenteral dosage under the trademark of **Regitine Mesylate**.

phenylalanine disorder: See PHENYLKETONURIA.

phenyl alkylamines a group of natural and synthetic drugs that can produce psychedelic effects. The original member of the group is mescaline, which was first isolated in 1896 from the peyote plant. By changing the radicals on the structural formula of mescaline, other psychedelic drugs, including some more potent than mescaline, have been produced. An example is methyl-dimethoxyamphetamine, a compound known as STP or DOM. See PSYCHEDELICS; PHENYLETHYL-AMINE DERIVATIVES.

phenylbutazone = BUTAZOLIDIN. Also see PYRAZO-LONES.

phenylcyclohexyl derivatives a category of drugs introduced around 1960 for potential use as general anesthetics but discontinued because of serious psychological disturbances affecting patients administered the p.d. The prototype drug, phencyclidine (PCP), produces sensory-deprivation effects similar to those observed in some cases of schizophrenia. Drugs of this series are considered to be psychedelics but may be employed as anesthetics and analgesics in veterinary medicine. See PHENCYCLIDINE; PSYCHEDELICS.

phenylcyclopentylglycolate: See PSYCHEDELICS.

phenylethylamine derivatives a group of drugs with psychedelic effects and a common basic structural formula. The prototype drug of the series is **mescaline**—$C_{11}H_{17}NO_3$, an alkaloid first isolated from peyote in 1896. Mescaline is one of the least potent of the psychedelic drugs, but potency is increased by adding methyl radicals to the basic molecule, thereby creating amphetaminelike variations. Other p.d. include AMPHETAMINE (see this entry) and **methyl-dimethoxyamphetamine** (**DOM**; also **STP**, for serenity, *t*ranquillity, *p*eace)—$C_{12}H_{22}NO_2$. Also called **substituted phenyl alkylamines**. Also see PHENYL ALKYLAMINES.

phenylethylhydantoin: See HYDANTOINS.

phenylisopropylamine a basic aliphatic amine molecule with adrenergic effects which vary somewhat according to the positions of different radicals on the p. structure. The prototype drug of the category is ephedrine, obtained from the ancient Chinese herb Ephedra sinica, used for the relief of symptoms of asthma and other allergic conditions.

phenylisopropylhydrazine an antihypertensive drug that also functions as a monoamine oxidase

inhibitor. P. and other hydrazine-based MAO inhibitors were among the first used for treatment of psychiatric depression. They have been replaced by other drugs that produce fewer adverse side effects such as liver disorders.

phenylketonuria an inherited metabolic disease transmitted as an autosomal-recessive trait and marked by a deficiency of an enzyme needed to utilize the amino acid phenylalanine. Untreated in early infancy by a restricted dietary intake of phenylalanine, p. leads to severe mental retardation and other nervous-system disorders. Most untreated p. patients have an IQ below 20. Abbrev.: **PKU**.

phenylpyruvic acid an intermediate product of the metabolism of phenylalanine. In patients with phenylketonuria, the phenylalanine is converted only to the p.a. stage instead of to the normal end product of tyrosine. Patients with phenylketonuria excrete p.a. in their urine.

phenylpyruvic oligophrenia a severe form of mental retardation that is associated with or due to an inborn error of metabolism of phenylalanine, as in cases of PKU. Early dietary restriction of phenylalanine may bring intelligence up to normal or near-normal. See PHENYLKETO-NURIA.

phenylthiocarbamide a compound used in human-genetics studies because it is intensely bitter to some individuals and tasteless to others. The difference is associated with an inherited trait. By determining which subjects find the substance bitter, other genetic factors can be studied in them and compared with traits in subjects who find the chemical tasteless. Abbrev.: **PTC**. Also called **phenylthiourea**.

phenyltoloxamine $C_{17}H_{21}NO$—an antihistaminic drug that is compounded with dihydrogen citrate for use as a minor tranquilizer.

phenytoin: See DILANTIN.

pheochromocytoma a small tumor that usually develops in the adrenal medulla but also may occur in tissues of the sympathetic paraganglia. Because it is composed of adrenal-tissue cells, it can secrete epinephrine and norepinephrine, producing excessive levels of the hormone, hypertension with headaches, tachycardia, visual blurring, and other symptoms. P. is believed to be an inherited disorder.

pheromone an External Chemical Messenger (ECM) released by an organism, whose odor serves to attract the other sex or to act as an alarm in case of an attack. Some investigators have hypothesized that schizophrenics are aware of and respond to odor stimuli that others ignore.

phi /fī/ 21st letter of the Greek alphabet (ϕ, $\varnothing$).

phi coefficient a measure of the degree of relationship between two continuous variables that have been dichotomized. Symbol: $\varnothing$ or $r_\varnothing = \sqrt{\chi^2/N}$.

Philadelphia chromosome disorder: See LEUKE-MIA.

-phil-; -philo- a combining form relating to love,

fondness, interest (from Greek *philos*, "loved, beloved, dear; friend"). Also see -PHILIA.

-philia in psychiatry, a combining form relating to a morbid craving or attraction.

Phillips Scale a method of analyzing the premorbid social and sexual adjustment of schizophrenia patients as part of a prediction of the chances for early recovery by the patient. The P.S. is based on questions derived by a researcher from case-history information.

philosophical psychology the study of philosophical issues related to psychology, including the body-mind problem, the nature of consciousness, the place of values in human life, the meaning of existence, and the nature and limits of scientific method. For examples, see APOLLONIAN ATTITUDE; BODY-MIND PROBLEM; BUDDHISM; CATEGORICAL IMPERATIVE; DIONYSIAN ATTITUDE; EPISTEMOPHILIA; ESSENCE; EXISTENTIALISM; HUMANISM; METAPSYCHOLOGY; MONISM; NATURE-NURTURE CONTROVERSY; NIETZSCHE; NOMINALISM; ONTOLOGY; PHENOMENALISM; PHENOMENOLOGY; POSITIVISM; PRAGMATISM; REALISM; REALITY; SENSATIONALISM; SOLIPSISM; SUICIDE; VITALISM; WELTSCHMERZ; YIN AND YANG. Also see PHILOSOPHY.

philosophy literally, love of wisdom (Greek *sophia*). Among the main meanings of p. are awareness of the principles that control and explain facts and events; the study of the basic principles of a particular field of knowledge; the practical wisdom that comes from the knowledge of general laws and principles; a system of general beliefs or views; also, composure and serenity. See PHILOSOPHICAL PSYCHOLOGY.

phimosis a condition, congenital or acquired, in which the foreskin of the penis cannot be retracted over the glans. The acquired form of p. usually is due to an infection or edema. P. may be corrected by circumcision. The condition is a frequent complication of venereal diseases.

phi phenomenon the illusion of apparent movement, seen when two lights flash on and off a fraction of a second apart, with one light seeming to jump to the position of the other light. An example is an electric advertising sign that suggests moving figures or symbols.

-phleb-; -phlebo- a combining form relating to a vein or, by way of extension, to blood.

phlebotomy = BLOOD-LETTING.

phlegmatic temperament: See HUMORAL THEORY.

phlegmatic type one of the original constitutional body types described by Galen in the second century A.D. Galen attributed the apathetic character of the p.t. to the dominance of phlegma, or mucus, over other body fluids, or humors.

phobia an excessive, unrealistic, uncontrollable fear elicited by a particular object or situation (Greek, "panic fear"). Common phobias, which Freud calls universal phobias, invoke heightened fear of phenomena arousing anxiety in most humans, e.g., snakes. Specific phobias involve those things that do not normally produce fear, e.g., cats.

This dictionary includes over 250 entries for different phobias (with another 250 cross references from alternative terms); for examples, see AICHMOPHOBIA; OPHIDIOPHOBIA; CLAUSTROPHOBIA; TRISKAIDEKAPHOBIA. Also see SIMPLE P.; PHOBIC DISORDERS; UNIVERSAL PHOBIAS.

-phobia a combining form usually relating to a morbid fear or to a fear that is out of proportion to the real danger.

phobic anxiety a term applied by Freud to a type of anxiety that stems from unconscious sources but is displaced to objects or situations (insects, telephone booths, open areas) that represent the real fear but pose little if any actual danger in themselves. P.a. was distinguished from FREE-FLOATING ANXIETY and PANIC. See these entries.

phobic attitude a term used by F. Perls to describe a behavior pattern apparently characterized by disruptions in the awareness of and attention to experience in the present, e.g., engaging in a fantasy of the future to escape a painful present reality. See GESTALT THERAPY.

phobic character a term applied by Fenichel to extremely inhibited, fearful persons. When faced with internal conflicts, these individuals resort to the defense mechanisms employed in phobic reactions, namely, projection, displacement, and avoidance.

phobic disorders a group of disorders in which the essential feature is a persistent, irrational fear and avoidance of a specific object, activity, or situation. The individual recognizes that the fear is unreasonable, but it is nevertheless so intense that it interferes with everyday functioning and is often a significant source of distress. These disorders are also called **phobic neuroses** and include, among many others, AGORAPHOBIA, SOCIAL PHOBIA, and SIMPLE PHOBIA. See these entries. Also see PHOBIA. (DSM-III)

phobic reaction a neurosis characterized by persistent irrational fears of such an intense and dominating character that they interfere with everyday life. In facing a phobic situation, such as walking through a tunnel, the individual experiences not only acute distress, but autonomic symptoms such as stomach upset, and if he continues to walk, these feelings may mount to panic proportions. While ordinary fears, such as fear of thunder, may be contracted from others, phobias arise from traumatic experiences, or symbolize unconscious conflicts and forbidden impulses. See PHOBIC DISORDERS.

phobophobia a morbid fear of fearing.

Phoenix House: See CONFRONTATIONAL METHODS.

pholcodine: See OPIUM ALKALOIDS.

phon a word element or speech sound; a unit of objective loudness or sound-level scale, based on a frequency of 1,000 cycles per second. The p. offers an arbitrary threshold or bench mark for measuring sound intensity, whereas the decibel scale has no threshold or zero but represents a ratio in loudness between two sounds of different intensities.

-phon-; -phono-; -phone; -phony a combining

form relating to voice, speech, or, generally, sound (from Greek *phone*, "sound, voice").

phonasthenia: See BREATHY VOICE.

phonation the production of voiced sounds by means of vocal-cord vibrations.

phonatory theory a fundamental concept related to voice production: The movements of the vocal cords, caused by the breath pressure, determine the intensity, the pitch, and some of the voice qualities, such as different types of hoarseness.

phoneidoscope a device that produces a visual image of sound waves by reflecting light off vibrating film.

phoneme the smallest unit of speech, distinguishing one utterance from another; e.g., /b/ and /p/ distinguish "bitch" from "pitch," and /ē/ and /i/ distinguish between "bay leaf" and "bailiff." There are about 50 phonemes in the English language. (Yet, there are over 250 English sounds. A p., strictly speaking, is not a sound, but must be "realized" through its allophones, that is, through its positional variants; e.g., the /l/ in "lamp" is different from the /l/ in "old," although the native speaker of English accepts both as "the same sound." To the native ear, only the p. has reality.) Also see GRAPHEME; MORPHEME.

phoneme-grapheme correspondence the relationship between the graphic elements of a language (such as letters and signs) and the phonological-grammatical units for which they stand (such as phonemes, syllables, and words). In most writing systems, as in English, the "fit" is far from being perfect, which is the main reason for difficulties in spelling.

phonemic disorders disturbances involving speech sounds that distinguish words from one another. E.g., in aphasic speech disorders, the patient loses those phonemes first that he has most recently acquired, which is exactly the opposite of the way phonemes are learned.

phonetic method in speech therapy, the treatment of articulation difficulties in which the therapist focuses on the specific placement and movements of the articulatory structures.

phonetics the study of speech processes, that is, the production, perception, and transcription of speech sounds, or phones, including the anatomy, neurology, and pathology of speech. See LINGUISTICS.

phonics a method of teaching reading based on the sounds of the letters in a word rather than on the word as a unit, that is, trying to match graphemes and phonemes. Also called **phonic method** or, popularly, **sounding out**. Compare SIGHT METHOD.

phonogram a graphic or symbolic representation of speech sounds or the vocal organs of speech in action.

phonology the sound system of a language (phonemes and their phonetic description); also, the history of sound changes in a language. See LINGUISTICS

phonomania the tendency to harbor or express homicidal impulses (from Greek *phonos*, "murder").

phonopathy any voice disorder.

phonophobia the fearful anticipation of failure related to singing, speaking, or acting. It is frequently noted among professional singers, speakers, and actors and reflects an emotionally-based disorder. P. is also a morbid fear of sounds, including one's own voice. Also see ACOUSTICOPHOBIA.

phonoscope any device that is used to make sound waves visible, e.g., a phoneidoscope.

phoria the turning of the eyes to view an object.

phosphene = PHOTOPSY.

phosphodiesterase an enzyme that breaks the phosphodiester bonds of molecules, including those holding nucleic-acid molecules together. The end products are subunits of the nucleic acids. P. is involved in the metabolism of cyclic AMP, which plays a role in activities of the nervous system and related hormones.

-phot-; -photo- a combining form relating to light (from Greek *phos*, "light").

photerythrosity increase in sensitivity for light near the red end of the spectrum.

photic driving the effect of certain forms of light stimuli on cortical neurons of epilepsy patients. A flickering light can trigger a seizure in epilepsy patients. Experiments indicate that controlled p.d. with flickering light can be used to study attention lapses in petit mal patients. Also see PHOTOGENIC EPILEPSY.

photic sensitivity = PHOTOSENSITIVITY.

photism a false perception or hallucination of light; also, a form of synesthesia in which light or color sensations occur through other sense modalities, e.g., perceiving a sound as a color.

photobiology the scientific study of the effects of color on the organism (color therapy, chromotherapy). Experiments have indicated, e.g., that a "bubble-gum-pink" or "passive-pink" room exerts a calming effect on manic or violent children. Different colors have also been found to affect blood pressure, pulse and respiration rates, and biological rhythms, and some physicians claim that ultraviolet light can alleviate psoriasis and prevent black-lung disease. Opinions differ as to whether the effects of color are primarily physiological or psychological.

photochemistry a branch of chemistry that deals with the relationships between chemical activity and photons or other forms of radiation.

photocoagulation the use of radiant energy, usually in the form of a laser or xenon-arc beam, to condense protein material in a tissue. P. is used in the treatment of detached retina after surgery, angioma, and degeneration of peripheral tissues.

photogenic epilepsy a form of reflex epilepsy in which seizures are precipitated by a particular kind of visual aberration, such as a flickering light. It has been found that rapid vertical movement of lines on a television screen can trigger seizures in some patients. P.e. attacks are usually, but not always, of the myoclonic type. See PHOTIC DRIVING; EPILEPSY.

photographic memory: See EIDETIC IMAGE.

photoma a visual hallucination in which sparks or light flashes are seen without external stimuli.

photomania an abnormal craving for light, particularly sunlight. The term also may be applied to the practice of sun worship.

photometrazol test a technique used in the diagnosis of hyperkinetic children, who have a lower-than-normal threshold for seizure-discharge activity. The subject is treated with the drug pentylenetetrazol, then stimulated with a stroboscopic light. The thalamic pacemaker is more easily stimulated in hyperkinetic children, and their p.t. threshold is more easily elevated with antithalamic drugs than that of normal children.

photons: See VISUAL STIMULATION.

photoperiodism the reactions of certain animals and plants to changes in the length of days or intensity of light in the environment. P. in animals accounts for seasonal migration behavior, reproductive cycles, and changes in plumage or pelage. The shedding of leaves in autumn and winter dormancy are signs of p. in plants.

photophobia an extreme and often painful sensitivity to light.

photopic luminosity the relative effectiveness of various wavelengths of light on visual acuity under light-adapted conditions.

photopic-sensitivity curve a curve plotted on a graph from data obtained as the subject adjusts the brightness of light at various wavelengths until the test light appears as bright as a standard patch of white light.

photopic vision the type of vision associated with daylight activity when the rod cells of the retina are largely ineffective because of bleaching of their rhodopsin content.

photopsin the type of opsin found in retinal cone-cell pigments.

photopsy the sensation of light flashes or sparks in the absence of actual light stimulation to the eye. It may be caused by mechanical stimulation of nerve tissue that is involved in vision. Also called **phosphene**.

photoreceptor a visual receptor; a rod or cone cell of the retina.

photosensitivity sensitivity to light, and especially to sunlight, as in cases of albinism and photogenic epilepsy; also, a common reaction to chlorpromazine and other neuroleptic drugs. The term frequently is applied to effects of sunlight on the skin and particularly to conditions of increased sensitivity, e.g., herpes simplex infection, systemic lupus erythematosus, xeroderma pigmentosum, and drugs such as thiazides, sulfonamides, and tetracyclines. P. also may represent an immune reaction in some individuals who manifest allergy symptoms after exposure to intense light. Also called **photic sensitivity**.

phototaxis a form of behavior expressed by movement toward a light source. Insects display a relationship between muscular activity and light orientation. When the left eye of a fly or bee is shaded or blinded, the legs on the side of the body with reduced vision work vigorously to keep the body turned toward the light that can be seen only with the right eye. Also see TAXES.

phototropism the automatic movement of an organism toward or away from a light source.

phrase-structure grammar the theory that structural aspects of language can best be reduced to phrase components, as meaningful units. In recall experiments, subjects made the highest number of mistakes between phrases while making fewer mistakes within phrases, indicating the tendency to remember phrases as units.

-phren-; -phreno-; -phrenia a combining form relating to the mind or the brain (from Greek *phren*, "diaphragm, heart, mind").

phrenasthenia an obsolete term for mental deficiency.

phrenic nerve a nerve that originates in the cervical plexus of the neck and sends sensory and motor branches to the heart, diaphragm, and other parts of the chest and abdomen.

phrenology a theory of personality (literally, mind science) formulated in the 18th and 19th centuries by Franz Josef Gall and Johann Kaspar Spurzheim, which claimed that traits, or faculties, such as "amativeness" and "secretiveness," can be judged by the size and location of protrusions, or "bumps," on the skull. Crude as it was, this theory had the positive effect of suggesting the idea of localization of brain functions and helped to turn the attention of physicians away from the prevailing opinion that mental illness is due to possession by the devil, and toward the view that it is due to brain disease and is treatable by medical means, a view that launched the organic era in psychiatry. Also see LOCALIZATION OF FUNCTION; PHYSIOGNOMY; CRANIOSCOPY.

phrenopraxic a term used to describe drugs that have an altering effect on the psyche, e.g., stimulants, tranquilizers, and hallucinogens.

phrenotropic pertaining to the action on the mind produced by phrenopraxic agents, e.g., the effect on neural circuits produced by psychic energizers.

phronemophobia a morbid fear of thinking or making a mental effort. Also see PSYCHOPHOBIA.

phthinoid /thin'oid/ a Kretschmer variety of the asthenic constitutional body type in which the physique is underdeveloped and usually characterized by the flat, narrow chest that is associated with the stereotype of the tuberculous patient.

phthisiomania = TUBERCULOMANIA.

phthisiophobia /thiz'-/ a morbid fear of tuberculosis. Also called **tuberculophobia**.

phyloanalysis a term used by Trigant Burrow for a means of investigating both individual and collective disorders, which, he believed, result from impaired tensional processes that affect the organism's internal balance as a whole.

phylobiology a type of behavioral science that emphasizes biological rapport with the environment as a governing, unitary force that motivates the organism.

phylogenesis; phylogenetic: See PHYLOGENY.

phylogenetic mneme the racial ancestral memory that is assumed to exist in the individual's deep unconscious. See RACIAL MEMORY.

phylogenetic principle the doctrine that ontogeny recapitulates phylogeny in human development, that is, that the individual from embryo to adult repeats the stages of organic and social evolution.

phylogeny /fīloj'-/ the origin, genealogical history, and evolutionary development of a species. P. is generally limited to biological inheritance, but has been broadened, notably by Jung, to include the development of the psyche and the storage of racial archetypes in the brain. Also called **phylogenesis**. Adjective: **phylogenetic**. See ARCHETYPE; RECAPITULATION THEORY. Compare ONTOGENY.

physiatrics = PHYSICAL THERAPY.

physiatrist a physician who specializes in PHYSICAL MEDICINE. See this entry.

physical anthropology: See ANTHROPOLOGY.

physical education in rehabilitation, the use of physical exercise to correct defects, improve the patient's physical condition, encourage socialization, and build morale.

physicalism a philosophical concept that all meaningful propositions can be stated in the language of the physical sciences and in operational definitions. See LOGICAL POSITIVISM.

physical medicine the branch of medicine that specializes in the diagnosis and treatment of disorders that cause physical disabilities, e.g., neuromotor disorders. P.m. also is involved with the rehabilitation of disabled patients through application of heat, cold, water, electricity, or mechanical devices.

physical strain: See STRESS.

physical therapy the treatment of bodily disorders by various physical or nonmedicinal means, including the use of heat, water, exercise, massage, and electric current or diathermy. P.t. is used to relieve pain and improve muscle function by the safest and most effective means. The treatment is administered by a trained **physical therapist** under the supervision of a physiatrist, a physician who specializes in physical medicine. Abbrev.: **PT**. Also called **physiatrics; physiotherapy**.

physician extender a general term for health professionals, e.g., nurse clinicians, nurse practitioners, or physician's assistants, who perform medical services under the direction or supervision of a licensed physician.

physician-originated disorder: See IATROGENESIS; IATROGENIC ILLNESS.

physiodrama: See PSYCHODRAMA FORMS.

physiogenic pertaining to a disorder that is organic in origin.

physiognomic perception a term employed by Heinz Werner (1932) to denote the child's tendency to view the world in the light of emotional and motor qualities; e.g., a diamond-shaped figure looks "cruel," or a stick may be called a "sweeping broom." The same tendency is frequently found in individuals under the influence of hallucinogenic drugs and in paranoid schizophrenics, and may also be one of the sources for abstract art.

physiognomic thinking the first stage in the process of thought development of children. It is characterized by the child's tendency to animate objects and project his ego into them ("This block is my dog"), a step called SYNCRETIC THOUGHT by Piaget. See this entry.

physiognomy the attempt to "read" personality from the facial features and expression. P. applies, e.g., to the notion that a man with a receding chin is weak, or that a woman with a high forehead is bright. The theory dates back to Aristotle and was developed into a pseudoscientific system by Johann Lavater in the 18th century and Cesare Lombroso in the 19th. Attempts are still made to judge attitudes and character from facial or other physical features, but are not considered trustworthy. Also called **physiognomics**. See SOCIAL STEREOTYPE; STIGMATA OF DEGENERACY. Also see PHRENOLOGY.

physiological age a measurement of the level of development or deterioration of an individual in terms of functional norms for various body systems.

physiological antagonism a form of drug antagonism in which two substances have opposing actions. A stimulant, e.g., caffeine, would show p.a. in combination with a barbiturate drug. See PHARMACOLOGICAL ANTAGONISM.

physiological basis of personality patterns of reaction that may have a biochemical or genetic basis. A pattern may be associated, e.g., with amounts of endocrine secretions, or it may be genetic, as in examples of the familial incidence of schizophrenia or certain inborn errors of metabolism.

physiological dependence a state of tissue tolerance to a substance of abuse usually marked by a gradual need to increase the dosage in order to achieve the same effect and by withdrawal symptoms following sudden interruption of the usual level of intake of the substance. P.d. also is characterized in some instances by a craving that leads to crime or other socially unacceptable behavior in order to satisfy the craving for the substance. P.d. usually is associated with drugs that have a depressant effect, e.g., alcohol, barbiturates, and opium-based narcotics. P.d. is a term recommended by the World Health Organization as a less ambiguous substitute for the word ADDICTION. See this entry.

physiological feedback a form of conditioning in which the response of an organ or organ system of the body influences the nervous system. In animal experiments, the subject may be trained to respond to a stimulus while the involved body area is paralyzed. Through p.f. the conditioned response is developed and can be demonstrated after normal neuromuscular activity is restored. Also called **internal feedback**.

physiological limit a theoretical limit beyond which continued practice would produce no gains.

physiological maintenance the design and construction of an environment so that it proves safe and comfortable with respect to such variables as safety hazards, ventilation, temperature, and noise level.

physiological memory a memory for somatic experiences outside conscious awareness, e.g., the memory of a conditioned-automatic-system response; also, storage of memory traces by means of RNA.

physiological motive a motive based on a bodily need, e.g., sex, thirst, or a circadian rhythm.

physiological needs the lowest level of A. Maslow's hierarchy of needs, comprising food, water, air, sleep, and other survival needs. See NEED-HIERARCHY THEORY. Also see PRIMARY NEEDS.

physiological paradigm the concept that mental disorders are caused by abnormalities of brain anatomy and physiology. The p.p. includes the viewpoint that mental disorders can be treated with drugs, surgery, or other techniques ordinarily used to correct bodily malfunctioning.

physiological psychology a branch of psychology that deals with the physical and chemical factors involved in the processes of behavior.

physiological response specificity the principle that an individual who responds physiologically to a stimulus in one system will respond in the same system to other stimuli. Thus, some individuals tend to respond to many different stimuli with heart-rate increases, others with breathing changes, others with sweaty palms, etc. This principle was proposed by Lacey.

physiological self-regulation the ability of a subject to learn to control his internal organs and vital functions such as blood pressure, dilation of the arteries of the brain, and brain-wave activity through the use of biofeedback or operant reinforcement.

physiological zero the temperature at which an object in contact with the skin feels neither warm nor cold, a reading of about 32°C (90°F) for the hands and feet.

physiology the science of the chemical and physical activities of the cells and organs of plants and animals, as opposed to static anatomical or structural factors.

physiopathology the study of disorders of physiology, both functional and organic, including their causes and how they may affect the total personality and the various activities of the individual.

physiotherapy = PHYSICAL THERAPY.

physique type the basic physical structure, build, and body type of an individual, particularly as related to his CONSTITUTIONAL TYPE. See this entry.

-physo- a combining form relating to gas or air.

physostigmine an alkaloid derived from the dried seed of an African vine and used as a cholinergic agent that prevents the natural destruction of acetylcholine. As a medication, p. is employed as a topical miotic that causes the pupils to contract. Under the name **eserine** it is also employed as a cholinesterase inhibitor to antagonize the CNS toxic effects of tricyclic antidepressant medications.

pi /pī/ 16th letter of the Greek alphabet (π, π).

Piaget, Jean /zhäN pē·äzhe'/ Swiss psychologist, 1896–1980. P. devoted his long intellectual life primarily to the study of cognitive development, showing how the child gradually abandons animistic explanations; acquires such concepts as cause and effect, space and time, and number; and gradually learns to apply them in thinking logically, using imagination, and forming hypotheses. Adjective: **Piagetian** /pē·äzhā'tē·ən/.

See ADAPTATION MECHANISM; ANIMISTIC THINKING; AUTONOMOUS STAGE; CATEGORICAL THOUGHT; CIRCULAR REACTION; CLASS INCLUSION; CODIFICATION-OF-RULES STAGE; COGNITIVE DEVELOPMENT; COGNITIVE PSYCHOLOGY; COGNITIVIST; CONCRETE OPERATIONAL STAGE; CONCRETE OPERATIONS; CONSERVATION; CONSTRUCTIONISM; COORDINATION OF SECONDARY SCHEMES; DECENTER; DECENTRATION; DEVELOPMENTAL TEACHING MODEL; DISCOVERY METHOD; DISEQUILIBRIUM; DISTRIBUTIVE JUSTICE; EGOCENTRIC; EGOCENTRIC SPEECH; EQUILIBRIUM; EXPIATORY PUNISHMENT; FIGURATIVE KNOWLEDGE; FORMAL OPERATIONS; FUNCTIONAL INVARIANTS; HETERONOMOUS STAGE; HETERONOMY; HYPOTHETICO-DEDUCTIVE REASONING;

IMMANENT JUSTICE; INDISSOCIATION; INTENTIONAL BEHAVIOR; INTERNALIZED SPEECH; INTERIORIZED IMITATION; LOGO; MAKE-BELIEVE; MORAL INDEPENDENCE; MORALITY OF CONSTRAINT; MORALITY OF COOPERATION; MORAL JUDGMENT; MORAL REALISM; MORAL RELATIVISM; NAIVE REALISM; NOMINAL REALISM; OBJECTIVE ORIENTATION; OPERATION; OPERATIVE KNOWLEDGE; ORGANIZATION; PARTICIPATION; PERMANENCE CONCEPT; PRECAUSAL THINKING; PREOPERATIONAL STAGE; PRIMARY CIRCULAR REACTION; RECIPROCAL PUNISHMENT; REPRESENTATIONAL SKILLS; REPRESENTATIONAL STAGE; REVERSIBILITY; RULES OF THE GAME; SCHEMA; SCHEMES; SECONDARY CIRCULAR REACTION; SENSORIMOTOR INTELLIGENCE; SENSORIMOTOR STAGE; SYNCRETIC THOUGHT; SYNCRETISM; TERTIARY CIRCULAR REACTION; TOPOLOGY; VERBAL PROPOSITION.

pia mater a delicate membrane that covers the surface of the brain and spinal cord and the innermost layer of the meninges. The cranial portion of the p.m. is richly supplied with blood vessels and follows the contours of the cortex, extending into the fissures and sulci. The spinal p.m. is thicker and firmer, and consists of two separate layers. At the bottom of the spinal cord, the p.m. fuses with the dura mater and periosteum to form a ligament.

piano theory = PLACE THEORY.

p.i. basis: See COUPON-RETURN TECHNIQUE.

piblokto a culture-specific syndrome believed to be a hysterical state of dissociation that has been observed among Eskimos, particularly female Eskimos (first reported by Admiral Peary). The patient screams, tears off her clothing, and runs about naked in the subzero ice and snow emitting the sounds of wild animals or birds. The attacks ends in less than two hours; the patient collapses into unconsciousness, and has amnesia for the event. Friends and relatives of the patient avoid offering assistance during an attack because of superstition associated with p., which many Eskimos believe to be caused by supernatural factors. The true cause of the disorder is believed to be long-standing repressions and frustrations due to the fact that women are considered the property of men, who can buy, sell, and exchange them at will. Also called **piloktoq**.

pica a rare eating disorder found primarily in young children and pregnant women, and marked by a persistent craving for unnatural, nonnutritive substances, such as plaster, paint, hair, starch, or dirt. Also see DYSGEUSIA. (DSM-III)

Pick, Arnold Prague psychiatrist, 1851–1924. See PICK'S DISEASE; NIEMANN-PICK DISEASE; AGRAMMATISM; ALEXIA; AUTOMATISM; BRAIN ATROPHY; BRAIN DISEASES; CEREBROSIDE; DEMENTIA; ECHOLALIA; HALLUCINATION; HYPOKINESIS; LIPID-METABOLISM DISORDER; ORGANIC DEMENTIA; PARAPHASIA; SENIUM PRAECOX; SPHINGOLIPID; SPHINGOLIPIDOSES.

Pick's disease a rare degenerative disease of the brain occurring between the ages of 45 and 50 among more women than men. The higher associative areas of the cortex atrophy, and the disorder is therefore progressive, involving increasing difficulty in thinking, concentrating, dealing with new situations and abstractions, followed by bewilderment, rambling talk, inability to read, write, or speak, paralysis, incontinence, and debility. Death usually occurs four to six years after onset. See the DSM-III category PRIMARY DEGENERATIVE DEMENTIA.

Pickwickian syndrome a syndrome characterized by grotesque obesity associated with hypersomnolence, cyanosis, congestive heart failure, muscle twitching, and general debility. These symptoms are usually believed to result from respiratory disability induced by extreme obesity. (The term is derived from the "fat boy" in Dickens' *Pickwick Papers*, 1836–37.)

picrotoxin a CNS stimulant derived from the berries of an East Indian shrub, Anamirta cocculus. P. originally was used as a fish poison but acquired neuropharmacologic value in the 1930s when it was introduced as therapy for barbiturate poisoning. It is believed to act by blocking presynaptic inhibition. P. is toxic to normal persons but can be tolerated in large doses by individuals in a coma.

pictorial imagery: See IMAGERY.

picture-anomalies test a nonverbal test of social intelligence that depends upon the ability of a patient to detect absurdities in cartoon pictures. The test also aids in the diagnosis of right temporal-lobe lesions, since patients with such disorders are likely to find the absurd figures logical and logical items ridiculous.

picture-arrangement test a subtest of the Wechsler intelligence scales, in which the subject is required to arrange in proper order a series of sketches that tell a brief story.

picture-completion test a test consisting of simple line drawings of familiar objects with significant features missing. The task is to recognize and specify the missing parts. Also see INCOMPLETE-PICTURES TEST.

picture-frustration study: See ROSENZWEIG P.-F.S.

picture-interpretation test a test in which the subject must interpret a pictorial situation.

picture world test a children's projective test in which the subject composes a story about realistic scenes, adding objects or figures as he or she wishes. The child is instructed to picture either a world that actually exists or one that he would like to exist.

Piderit, Th. German anatomist and psychologist, fl. 1859–1915. See PIDERIT DRAWINGS.

Piderit drawings a large series of simplified drawings of the human face showing a wide assortment of emotional expressions. The drawings are cut into interchangeable pieces that can be rearranged in various alternative composite illustrations to show the variety of possible facial expressions, and the influence of one part of the face on the overall expression.

Pierre Robin's syndrome a congenital disorder with anomalies that include micrognathia, cleft palate, and glossoptosis. Serious eye disorders occur in most patients, with a small receding chin, and a tongue that falls backward into the pharynx, interfering with breathing and feeding. Various studies have found an incidence of mental retardation ranging from five to 50 percent.

Pigem's question a question designed to elicit projective responses by a patient undergoing a mental-status examination. The question usually is a variation of "What would you like most to change in your life?"

pigeon breast = PECTUS CARINATUM.

pigmentary retinal lipoid neuronal heredodegeneration a juvenile form of amaurotic familial idiocy that is not limited in incidence to members of an ethnic group but may affect any child between the ages of five and ten. A common symptom is a "salt-and-pepper" type of retinal pigmentation.

pil. an abbreviation used in prescriptions, meaning "pill" (Latin *pilula*; plural: *pilulae*).

-pil-; -pilo- a combining form relating to hair.

Pill = ORAL-CONTRACEPTIVE PILL.

pilocarpine an alkaloid derived from several tropical American plants but mainly from Pilocarpus jaborandi. P. is a powerful parasympathomimetic agent, affecting postganglionic cholinergic receptors. P. also stimulates secretion of epinephrine from the adrenal medulla and aids in the transmission of impulses across autonomic-ganglia synapses.

piloerection goose flesh, or goose pimples, or goose skin; a temporary roughness of the skin because of cold, fear, or sexual or other excitation.

pilot study a preliminary research project designed to evaluate and correct procedures in preparation for a subsequent research project. Pilot studies are designed to reveal information about the viability and potential outcomes of a proposed experiment or series of studies.

-pimel-; -pimelo- a combining form relating to fat.

piminodine: See SYNTHETIC NARCOTICS.

pineal body a small, cone-shaped structure in the epithalamus, between the superior colliculi. The anterior portion of the p.b. in certain animals, e.g., lampreys, lizards, and tadpoles, contains photosensitive neurons and is regarded as a possible third eye, the **pineal eye**. Also called **epiphysis; epiphysis cerebri.** See PINEAL GLAND.

pineal gland a small gland attached by a stalk to the posterior wall of the third ventricle of the cortex. In amphibians and reptiles, the gland appears to function as a part of the visual system. In mammals, the gland is believed to function as a source of melatonin, a substance that inhibits estrus and ovarian growth. In view of its central location, Descartes believed it was the "seat of the rational soul" and the connection between mind and body. The term is essentially synonymous with PINEAL BODY. See this entry.

Pinel, Philippe /pēnel'/ French physician, 1745–1826. P., the most revolutionary psychiatrist of the 18th century, served as head physician of the Bicêtre Hospital, and later of the Salpêtrière Hospital in Paris. Shocked by the prevailing public belief that the mentally ill are "wild beasts" possessed by the devil, and even more by the practice of keeping them in chains and confined to dungeons, he declared that "the mentally deranged, far from being guilty people deserving of punishment, are sick people whose miserable state deserves all the consideration that is due to suffering humanity." Defying both the public and the government, he not only had their chains removed, but compiled case histories, and gradually replaced such inhuman methods as blood-letting, purging, and beatings with "moral treatment" consisting of talks between physician and patient, kindliness and empathy, and occupational therapy. See PINEL'S SYSTEM; PINEL-HASLAM SYNDROME; MORAL TREATMENT; IDIOTISM; SALPÊTRIÈRE. Also see ESQUIROL.

Pinel-Haslam syndrome a form of schizophrenia first described by Pinel and characterized by diminished expression of feelings, difficulty in forming abstractions, dissociation of mood and content of thinking, and inattention and withdrawal.

Pinel's system a classification of mental disorders

and symptoms outlined by Pinel in the 18th century. The four major categories were melancholias, manias with delirium, manias without delirium, and dementia or mental deterioration.

pink disease = ACRODYNIA.

pink puffer the common name for a type of chronic-bronchitis patient, characterized by a pink complexion or skin color and a respiration pattern of scanty coughing and breathlessness. The p.p. may also have several distinctive physical features, including a barrel-chested rib cage, slim body build, and abdominal, chest, and neck muscles that reflect the constant effort required to maintain breathing. Also called **Type A; Type PP.** Also see BLUE BLOATER.

pink spot a common name for a reaction that occurs when a chemical, **3,4-dimethoxyphenethylamine (DMPEA)**, is treated with reagents, yielding a pink color. Because the chemical has been found in the urine of schizophrenic patients, it has been proposed that the p.s. test might be a diagnostic clue for schizophrenia.

pinna the part of the ear that projects beyond the head (Latin, "wing").

pinocytosis a metabolic transport mechanism within the central nervous system. Fluids are trapped by the folds of cellular membranes and absorbed, moving through the cytoplasm in vacuoles.

Pintner, Rudolf English-born American psychologist, 1884–1942. See PINTNER-PATERSON SCALE OF PERFORMANCE TESTS; MANIKIN TEST.

Pintner-Paterson Scale of Performance Tests a series of 15 performance tests for subjects ranging in most instances from four to 15 years. It is particularly applicable to individuals who do not speak English or who have hearing and speech defects. The Pintner-Paterson scale, as an early intelligence test, was developed in 1917.

Piotrowski, Zygmunt American psychiatrist, fl. 1937. See PERCEPTANALYSIS.

Piper, Hans Edmund /pē'pər/ German physiologist, 1877–1915. See PIPER'S LAW.

piperidinediones hypnotic drugs that act on subcortical centers for use as a daytime sedative for anxiety-tension-state patients and for the induction of sleep in cases of simple insomnia. P. resemble short-acting barbiturates in structure and function; however, they produce greater cardiac compression, and less respiratory depression. The prototype of the p. is **glutethimide** (trademark: **Doriden**)—$C_{13}H_{15}NO_2$. Other p. include **methyprylon**—$C_{10}H_{17}NO_2$—and THALIDOMIDE (see this entry). While thalidomide has been withdrawn from use because of its known teratogenic effects, glutethimide and methyprylon are believed to be free of teratogenic activity because they are metabolized in a different manner.

piperidyl derivatives antidepressant drugs that have psychedelic effects because of a potent central anticholinergic action. The benzilic acid forms of p.d. produce increased heart rate and blood pressure, distortions of space and time, ataxia, confusion, and delirium.

Piper's law the principle that for a uniformly stimulated retinal area, the threshold for luminance is inversely proportional to the square root of the area stimulated.

pipradrol: See ANALEPTICS.

Piptadenia peregrina a South American legume that is roasted, powdered, and snuffed. The snuff, variously identified as yopo and niopo, reportedly enables the user to suppress hunger and thirst for long periods. The effects of the agents, which include dimethyltryptamine, have been compared to those produced by the use of fly agaric. The plant species sometimes is identified as a member of the Anadenanthera genus.

piriform area = PYRIFORM AREA.

pitch the sound quality of highness or lowness, which is mainly dependent upon the frequency of vibrations stated in cycles per second, that is, the number of times a wave of air alternates between positive and negative pressure in a single second. P. may also depend to some extent on loudness, or intensity.

pitch discrimination the ability to detect changes in sound frequencies. In humans, because of the design of the cochlea, higher frequencies can be analyzed with less difficulty than lower frequencies.

pithiatism a term coined by Babinski for removal of hysterical symptoms by persuasion (from Greek *pithanotes*, "persuasiveness"), on the theory that these symptoms are produced by suggestion and can therefore be eliminated by suggestion.

Pitres, A. French neurologist, fl. 1895. See PITRES' RULE.

Pitres' rule a generalization that when a multilingual person recovers from aphasia caused by a stroke or cerebral injury, he recovers his language ability in an order that usually begins with the language in which he was most fluent or familiar at the onset of aphasia. Other previously learned languages are reestablished in a slower and often less complete manner.

pituitarism a disorder of pituitary-gland functioning. Overactivity is identified as either p. or hyperpituitarism, and deficient activity as hypopituitarism.

pituitary cachexia = HYPOPHYSEAL CACHEXIA.

pituitary gland /pityoo′iterē/ a pea-sized gland at the base of the brain, connected by a stalk to the hypothalamus. The p.g. is divided into an anterior and a posterior lobe. The anterior lobe, the adenohypophysis, produces seven hormones, six of which control other endocrine glands. They are the thyroid-stimulating, follicle-stimulating, melanocyte-stimulating, adrenocorticotrophic, growth, luteinizing, and luteotrophic hormones. The posterior lobe, the neurohypophysis, secretes two hormones, vasopressin and oxytocin. The pituitary's role of releasing hormones that stimulate the production of other hormones has resulted in its identification as the "master gland

of the endocrine system." Also called **hypophysis** /-pof′-/; **hypophysis cerebri**.

Pituitrin a trademark for a substance extracted from the posterior lobe of the pituitary gland and composed of a mixture of two hormones, vasopressin and oxytocin. It functions as a vasoconstrictor and in controlling water balance. P. is produced from the pituitary glands of cattle.

pituri a shrub of the species Duboisia hopwoodii or Duboisia myoporoides that grows in Australia and is the source of a psychotropic herb used by members of aboriginal tribes. The p. leaves are roasted, moistened, then rolled into a quid to be chewed. The primary active ingredient of p. is scopolamine, which may have stimulating and hallucinogenic effects. Since the introduction of tobacco into their lives, the tribesmen have learned to smoke p. as well as chew it.

pity a feeling of sorrow and compassion for persons in distress, especially those who are weak or defective. According to some investigators, a persistent tendency to pity others may arise from masochistic identification with their suffering, or may be a reflection of the pitier's own need to be loved and assisted.

PK = PSYCHOKINESIS.

PKU = PHENYLKETONURIA.

placebo an inert substance, such as a bread or sugar pill, which superficially resembles an active drug but is administered either as a control in testing new drugs or as a psychotherapeutic agent, as in relieving pain or inducing sleep by suggestion (Latin, "I shall please"). Also called **dummy**. See P. EFFECT.

placebo effect a clinically significant response to a therapeutically inert substance or nonspecific treatment. Appearance of a p.e. suggests the absence of an organic basis for the symptoms. It also must be assumed that remission of symptoms does not occur at the same time, as could occur in conditions such as rheumatoid arthritis marked by symptoms that may peak and wane regardless of therapy. See PLACEBO.

placebo reactor a person who tends to react to a placebo as if the inert substance actually had a pharmacologic effect. Various studies indicate that p.r. individuals are suggestible, or chronic liars, or possess other traits that account for their responses. However, a p.r. generally does not react to all placebos.

place fear = TOPOPHOBIA.

place learning E. C. Tolman's term for learning of locations or physical positions of goals, e.g., where food can be found. Also see RESPONSE LEARNING.

placement the assignment of a student to the appropriate class or section, or the assignment of an individual to a job. In high school and college, p. often refers to the process of assisting students to choose a suitable curriculum on the basis of demonstrated ability or achievement. For referral of the disabled or handicapped, see P. COUNSELING.

placement counseling in rehabilitation, a vocational-placement service that provides advice to disabled persons about job opportunities for which they may be qualified. P.c. may in some agencies include coaching or training of disabled persons for job interviews, procedures for filling out applications properly, and other details that may be psychological obstacles for disabled job hunters. P.c. with the nondisabled is similar.

placement test a test used by educational institutions to place students in classes appropriate to their abilities, achievements, and interests.

placenta the organ formed in the lining of the uterus by the union of the uterine membranes with the membranes of the fetus. The p. provides osmotic transmission of food products and respiratory gases between the blood of the fetus and that of the mother, as well as elimination of fetal waste products into the mother's bloodstream.

placental hormones hormones produced by the placenta after the zygote becomes implanted in the uterine wall of a mammalian female. The hormones are gonadotrophins similar to those secreted by the anterior pituitary.

placental immunity a function of the placenta that protects the fetus from many but not all types of infectious agents. The spirochete of syphilis and the smallpox virus cross the placenta barrier, as examples of exceptions. The mother's own antibodies, meanwhile, also can cross the placenta to confer temporary immunity against certain common infections for the first few months following birth.

placental infection an involvement of the placenta in a contagious disease complication. Viruses or other pathogenic microorganisms can invade the placental tissues to cause placentitis or septicemia, resulting in fetal damage or death. High fever or toxic effects of the infection also can trigger premature uterine contractility and spontaneous abortion.

placenta praevia a placenta that develops in the lower part of the uterus so that it blocks the birth canal, as opposed to a normal position higher on the uterine wall. A p.p. can be life-threatening to both mother and fetus because pressure on the cervical walls can cause the placental tissues to tear with hemorrhaging. The condition may require correction by Caesarean section. Also spelled **placenta previa**.

placentitis: See PLACENTAL INFECTION.

place theory an explanation for pitch perception, proposed by Helmholtz, based on the assumption that the place of stimulation on the basilar membrane determines the sound frequency perceived by a subject, since this membrane was believed to consist of a series of resonating fibers, each tuned to a different frequency. Also called **p.t. of hearing; piano theory; harp theory**. Also SEE TELEPHONE THEORY; HEARING THEORIES.

placing a reflex movement in which a baby lifts his foot onto a surface during the first three months of life.

placing reaction a postural reaction of an animal

held so that its feet hang free. It will attempt to place the feet on any solid surface it can see. P.r. is one of several possible limb adjustments directed toward firm support of the body.

planchette an automatic-writing device consisting of a small tripod, one of whose legs rests on a writing surface. The subject's hand, hidden behind a screen, rests lightly on the p., which records the involuntary movements.

planophrasia an obsolete term for a flight of ideas as manifested in cases of manic-depressive psychoses.

plaque a small patch or area on the surface of a body tissue that is abnormal and usually differentiated in appearance from the surrounding normal tissue. Kinds of p. include **atherosclerotic p.**, consisting of lipid deposits on the lining of arterial walls, **dental p.**, caused by bacterial activity on the surface of a tooth, and **demyelination p.**, which develops on the protective nerve sheaths of multiple-sclerosis patients.

-plasia a combining form relating to formation or development.

-plasm-; -plasmo- a combining form relating to blood plasma.

plastic-arts therapy the use of plastic media such as clay, finger paint, play dough, and papier mâché in play therapy and rehabilitation. These materials are believed to have multiple values, such as stimulating fantasy, giving vent to hostile impulses, expressing the urge to smear and mess, improving manual coordination, and increasing self-esteem by producing objects admired by others.

plasticity flexibility and adaptability, as opposed to rigidity; also, the modifiability of the nervous system which makes it possible to learn and register new experiences. See RIGIDITY. Also see FUNCTIONAL P.

plastic surgery a branch of surgery that specializes in the removal, transfer, and repair of damaged or diseased tissue so that a body area can be restored in a normal or near-normal form. P.s. is commonly employed in reconstruction of the female breast, facial features such as the nose or a harelip, and genital features, e.g., vaginalplasty or reconstruction of a penis following amputation of the original organ. P.s. was practiced by ancient Hindus and Egyptians. P.s. has been recognized as a medical specialty in the United States since 1939.

plastic tonus a type of plasticity observed in catatonic patients who do not move a limb from a position set by an observer.

plateau a period in learning when the learning curve flattens because the rate of increase has stopped temporarily, often because of fatigue, boredom, loss of motivation, or a change in the level of skill required.

Plateau, Joseph Antoine Ferdinand /plätō'/ Belgian physicist, 1801–83. See TALBOT-PLATEAU LAW.

plateau phase: See SEXUAL-RESPONSE CYCLE.

plateau speech a type of speech observed in

patients with certain CNS disorders such as epilepsy or multiple sclerosis and characterized by a monotonal quality. The effect results from a loss of normal pitch characteristics of vowel sounds.

Plato Greek philosopher, 428 (or 427)–348 (or 347) B.C. Though primarily a social philosopher, P. contributed to the history of psychology by founding the Academy, the first center for the study of physical and human sciences, and by developing concepts that anticipated later developments. Among these were the doctrine of formal discipline, the introspective method (the process of "reminiscence"), faculty psychology (the division of the soul into three parts: reason, spirit, and appetite), the importance of abstract concepts in scientific method, the efficacy of tests in selecting candidates for education, and his view that the goal of society is to enable all citizens (not slaves) to fulfill their needs and realize themselves. See PLATONIC LOVE; PLATONIZATION; DIALECTICAL METHOD; HUMOR; NATURE-NURTURE CONTROVERSY. Also see ARISTOTLE.

Platonic love a type of love in which there is no overt sexual behavior or desire.

platonization the maintenance of a nonerotic relationship between two persons of opposite sex, or the converting of erotic affect into contemplation of the ideal—or other nonerotic activities—as a defense mechanism.

-platy- a combining form meaning broad, flat.

platycephaly a head whose crown is abnormally flat.

platykurtic a distribution of scores flatter than a normal distribution, that is, having more scores at the extremes and fewer in the center than in a normal distribution. Also see MESOKURTIC; LEPTOKURTIC.

play activities that are freely sought and pursued for the sake of individual or group enjoyment. Studies indicate that the urge to play is as natural as the urge to eat or sleep, and is an indispensable instrumentality for growth, contributing immeasurably to practically every phase of development, physical, mental, social, and recreational. It is also a prime means of exploring the self and the world, as well as a means of maintaining mental health and achieving a balanced life. Some theorists have gone so far as to define civilized man as *homo ludens*, "the human being that plays." Also called **ludic activity**.

play acting dramatic play in which children, teenagers, or adults (including group-therapy patients) take different roles, and in the process test out relationships, rehearse different ways of dealing with situations, identify with important figures, realize their wishes in imagination, and play out feelings of anger, jealousy, or fear within the safe realm of make-believe.

players: See GAME THEORY.

play-group psychotherapy a therapeutic technique on the preschool level introduced by S. R. Slavson in 1943. Materials of many kinds (clay, toys, blocks, figurines) are used to stimulate the expression of conflicts and fantasies, and to give the therapist an opportunity to ask questions and help the children in a group understand their feelings, behavior, and relationships. Also see GROUP PSYCHOTHERAPY.

playing dead: See DEATH-FEIGNING.

play therapy the use of play activities and materials (clay, water, blocks, dolls, puppets, role-taking, drawing, finger paint) in child psychotherapy and mental hygiene. Play techniques are based on the theory that such activities mirror the child's emotional life and fantasies, enable him to "play out" his feelings and problems, and to test out new approaches and relationships in action rather than words. This form of therapy is usually nondirective and nonpsychoanalytic, but may be conducted on a more directive or on a more analytic level. It is occasionally termed **ludotherapy**. Also see DIRECTIVE-P.T.

pleasure ego a term used by Freud in 1911 in distinguishing between two ego processes: a p.e., which acts on behalf of unconscious mental processes, and a **reality ego**, which utilizes consciousness, reality-testing, judgment, and activity to "strive for what is useful and guard itself against damage." The distinction later crystalized into the structural distinction between the id, ego, and superego.

pleasure fear = HEDONOPHOBIA.

pleasure-pain principle in psychoanalysis, the view that human beings are governed by the two-pronged desire for instinctual gratification (pleasure) and for the discharge of tension that builds up as pain or "unpleasure" when gratification is lacking. Also called **pain-pleasure principle**.

pleasure principle in psychoanalysis the psychic force that motivates us to seek immediate gratification of our instinctual, or libidinal, impulses, such as sex, hunger, thirst, and elimination. Freud said that when these needs or drives are unsatisfied, we are in a state of tension, and when they are fulfilled, the reduction in tension evokes the experience of pleasure. The p.p. dominates the early life of the child but is gradually "tamed" and modified by the REALITY PRINCIPLE. See this entry.

-pleg-; -plegy; -plegia a combining form relating to paralysis (from Greek *plege*, "stroke, blow").

-pleio; -pleo- a combining form meaning multiple, excessive, or greedy.

pleniloquence a compulsion to talk incessantly.

pleonasm a form of redundancy in which an excess of words is used to express an idea.

pleonexia an abnormal greediness or desire for the acquisition of objects. The term also is used to describe a symptom of air hunger or abnormal intake of oxygen.

plethysmograph a device for measuring and recording volume or volume changes in organs or body tissues, such as the blood supply flowing through an organ. Examples include **penile p.**, which records change in the size of the penis and thus measures blood flow and erection, and **vaginal p.**, which records the amount of blood in the walls of the vagina and thus measures arousal.

-pleur-; -pleuro a combining form relating to (a) the **pleura** (the covering of the lungs and of the inside of the chest wall), (b) the inside of the body. Adjective: **pleural**.

plexiform molecular layer of Cajal: See CELLULAR LAYERS OF CORTEX.

plexus a network of nerves or blood vessels; also, in general, an intricately interwoven combination of elements.

plosive a speech sound made by building pressure in the air tract and suddenly releasing it. A p. may be voiced, e.g., /b/, /d/, /g/, or voiceless, e.g., /p/, /t/, /k/. Also called **explosive; opening sound; obstructive; occlusive; stop**. Also see LABIAL; ALVEOLAR.

plumbism an alternative term for lead poisoning (from Latin *plumbum*, "lead").

Plummer, Henry Stanley American surgeon, 1874–1936. See THYROTOXICOSIS (there: **Plummer's disease**).

pluralism in psychiatry, the concept that behavior is causally related to a multiplicity of interrelated conditions rather than a single dominant factor. In Freud, e.g., these conditions may reflect both conscious and unconscious forces, and both current and past conflicts and experiences. In Adolf Meyer, they reflect interdependent relationships between biological, social, and psychological forces.

plural marriage: See GROUP MARRIAGE.

plutomania an inordinate striving for money and possessions.

PMS an abbreviation of *prem*enstrual *s*yndrome or *prem*enstrual-*s*tress syndrome. See PREMENSTRUAL TENSION; PREMENSTRUAL DISORDER.

-pnea; -pneo- /-nē·ə-; -nē·ō-/ a combining form relating to breathing (from Greek *pnoia*, "breath").

-pneum-; -pneumo- /-nyo͞om-/ a combining form relating to air or gas, or to the lungs (from Greek *pneumon*, "lung").

pneumococcal meningitis an inflammation of the meninges of the brain and spinal cord due to an infection by the pneumococcus bacterium commonly associated with bacterial pneumonia. It is the third most common form of bacterial meningitis and usually begins with respiratory distress or sore throat, followed by fever, headache, stiff neck, and vomiting. P.m. generally responds to antibiotic therapy.

pneumoencephalogram a radiographic picture of the normally fluid-filled spaces of the brain enhanced by withdrawing small amounts of cerebrospinal fluid from the lumbar area of the spinal cord and injecting a gas into the spaces. The gas may be ordinary air or oxygen or an inert gas such as helium. Abbrev.: **PEG**. For use of **pneumoencephalography** as a diagnostic technique, see AIR ENCEPHALOGRAPHY.

pneumogastric nerve = VAGUS NERVE.

pneumograph a record of examination of the lungs, either by electric monitoring of the rate and extent of respiratory movements or by producing an X-ray photograph of the lungs after they have been injected with a gas to help improve the visual contrast between tissue areas.

pneumonia an inflammation of the lungs. P. may be caused by a viral, bacterial, or fungal infection, inhalation of a toxic gas, inhalation of droplets of an oily or fatty substance, blood stagnation from lying in the same position for a long period, an infarction following embolism in a pulmonary artery, or a severe blow to the chest.

pneumophonia a voice disorder characterized by excessive breathiness.

pneumotaxic center a mechanism in the central nervous system that controls breathing. Also called **autonomous respiratory center**.

pneumothorax the presence of air or gas in the pleural cavity that separates the membrane layers between the inside of the chest wall and the organs of the chest. P. may be produced therapeutically to introduce an inert gas to collapse a diseased lung, accidentally through a wound that punctures the chest wall to admit air, or as a complication of a disease, e.g., emphysema or a lung abscess.

pnigerophobia /nījērō-/ a morbid fear of smothering.

pnigophobia /nigō-/ a morbid fear of choking or suffocating. Also called **anginophobia**. Also see SUFFOCATION FEAR.

PNS = PERIPHERAL NERVOUS SYSTEM.

Poggendorf, Johann Christian /pôg'-/ German physicist and chemist, 1796–1877. See POGGENDORF ILLUSION.

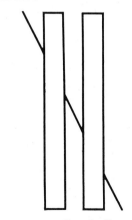

POGGENDORF ILLUSION. Does the diagonal line look straight?

Poggendorf illusion a visual illusion in which a straight diagonal line looks jagged when it appears to pass behind parallel lines or figures.

poiesis in psychiatry, the creation of a word or phrase, particularly a type of neologism constructed by schizophrenics to express their wishes and assure themselves that these wishes have been fulfilled (from Greek *poiein*, "to make").

-poiesis a combining form relating to production or formation.

poikilotherms animals, e.g., reptiles, whose body temperature varies with the temperature of their environment (from Greek *poikilos*, "varied," and *therme*, "heat"). Also called **cold-blooded animals**. Adjective: **poikilothermic**. Compare HOMOIOTHERMS.

poinephobia a morbid fear of punishment.

point biserial correlation a measure of the degree of relationship between two variables, with one variable a true dichotomy (e.g., male versus female), and the other a continuous variable (e.g., anxiety level). Also see BISERIAL CORRELATION.

point estimate a single numerical value used to estimate a parameter, without allowing for the band of uncertainty around the number. Also see INTERVAL ESTIMATE.

point fear = AICHMOPHOBIA.

point-for-point correspondence a relationship in which for every point in one variable there is a corresponding point in a second variable.

pointing a test for vestibular function in which the patient, first with the eyes open and again with the eyes closed, touches his extended index finger to the closely held index fingers of the examiner as they stand facing each other. Knowing the location of the examiner's fingers, the subject should be able to touch them with his eyes closed. Failure is called **past-p.**

pointing the bone: See VOODOO DEATH.

point-localization test a somatosensory test in which a skin area, usually on the hand, is touched twice with an intervening period of one second. The subject is required to determine whether the points touched were in the same place.

point mutation mutation of a single gene.

point of regard a visual fixation point on a line of sight that terminates on the retinal fovea.

point of subjective equality the value of a comparison stimulus that, for a given observer, is equally likely to be judged as higher or lower than a standard stimulus. Abbrev.: **PSE.**

point prevalence: See PREVALENCE.

point scale a test in which each item has a point value and the score is rated in total points earned.

Poisson, Siméon-Denis /pô·äsôN'/ French mathematician, 1781–1840. See POISSON DISTRIBUTION.

Poisson distribution a theoretical statistical distribution that shows the probability of occurrence of rare events that are randomly distributed in time or space. It is useful for quality control, for estimating numbers of infrequent accidents, and for similar purposes.

polar body a small, incomplete ovum that is produced during the process of **oogenesis**, or egg formation, in the human ovary. Normally, as the oocyte is being formed during the meiosis stage

of gamete-cell division, the division occurs unequally. One small cell, the p.b., is pinched off and allowed to degenerate, while the larger cell proceeds to yield the oocyte, or regular ovum. The p.b. contains the haploid set of 23 chromosomes.

polar continuum a series whose end points are completely opposite, as with ascendance-submission.

polarities in psychoanalysis, the opposing forces that govern all mental life: (a) subject (ego) and object (the external world), (b) pleasure and unpleasure, or pain, (c) active and passive. In neuroses, the balance between some or all of these antitheses is disturbed, and one of the major aims of psychoanalysis is to restore this balance.

polarization a principle in which a difference in electrical potential develops between two surfaces or two sides of one surface because of chemical activity. P. occurs normally in electric batteries and also in neurons which maintain an equilibrium of a positive charge on one side of the cell membrane and a negative charge on the other. P. also denotes a condition in which light waves travel in parallel paths along one plane.

-poli-; -polio- a combining form relating to the gray matter of the nervous system.

policy analysis in evaluation research, a collection of techniques of synthesizing information (a) to specify alternative policy and program choices in cost-benefit terms, (b) to assess organizational goals in terms of inputs and outcome performance, and (c) to provide additional information as a guide for future decisions concerning research activities.

polio = POLIOMYELITIS.

polioencephalitis an inflammation of the brain, due to an infectious disease, involving primarily the gray matter. One form of p. is marked by changes in the motor centers of the medulla oblongata. Symptoms include paralysis of the lips, tongue, and throat muscles.

poliomyelitis an acute contagious viral disease of the central nervous system, resulting in destruction of nerve cells associated with control of the muscles. The paralysis can affect the muscles controlled by autonomic nerves as well as skeletal muscles so that breathing, swallowing, or similar functions are disrupted. More specifically, there are three types of paralytic p.: **spinal p.** (weakness of trunk, neck, extremities, and possibly chest muscles), **bulbar p.** (impairment of facial movements, phonation, swallowing, respiration, circulation), and **bulbospinal p.** (diffuse involvement including loss of respiratory independence). Abbrev.: **polio.** Also called **infantile paralysis.**

political genetics the incorporation of genetic principles and practices into politics and government policy.

political psychiatry the application of psychiatric principles and knowledge to the formation of public policy, especially as it relates to mental-health services, treatment of the mentally ill, questions of medical ethics, prosecution and rehabilitation of criminals, and attempts at thought or behavior control. See PSYCHOPOLITICS.

poll: See PUBLIC-OPINION P.

pollicomental reflex = PALMOMENTAL REFLEX.

Pollyanna mechanism an attitude that all is well and life is good despite the reality that it is not (from the fatuous heroine of Eleanor H. Porter's novel *Pollyanna*, 1913).

poltergeist /pōlt'ərgīst/ an alleged paranormal phenomenon (from German *Poltergeist*, "noisy ghost") consisting of an unseen person who is believed to occupy a "haunted house," disturbing the peace with such pranks as slamming doors, rapping on walls, upsetting furniture, and breaking crockery. Investigations indicate that these events often are reported in homes where there is a preadolescent child.

-poly- a combining form meaning many, multiple, excessive, generalized.

polyamino acid = POLYPEPTIDE.

polyandry marriage of a woman to more than one husband at the same time, which is an accepted custom in certain cultures.

Polycrates complex in psychoanalysis, an unconscious feeling of guilt, anxiety, and need for punishment occasionally observed among patients who have enjoyed great success. The concept is based on a story related by Herodotus: The tyrant Polycrates believed that his successful exploits aroused the envy of the gods and to appease them threw his signet ring into the sea; but he realized he was doomed when the ring was found in the belly of a fish served to him the next day. Also called **polycratism**. Also see SUCCESS NEUROSIS.

polycyesis a multiple pregnancy (from Greek *poly*, "many," and *kyesis*, "pregnancy").

polycystic kidney disease a kidney disorder marked by the formation of numerous cysts in the kidney tissues, enlarging the size of the organs while compressing the functioning units until the patient dies of uremia. P.k.d. occurs in an infantile and adult form; both are hereditary, but the genetic patterns are different. The adult form is slowly progressive and may not begin until middle age; it is associated with hypertension and brain hemorrhage. See INFANTILE POLYCYSTIC DISEASE.

polycystic renal disorder: See INFANTILE POLYCYSTIC DISEASE.

polycythemia a blood disease marked by an excess of red cells in the blood. The excessive red cells, which may be twice the normal concentration, thicken the blood so that it cannot circulate freely. The p. patient may feel fatigued, be forgetful and unable to concentrate, and suffer from dizzy spells and headaches. Thrombosis and hemorrhage are complications. The symptoms usually begin after middle age, and men are affected more often than women.

polydactylism the possession of supernumerary digits on the hands or feet. Also called **polydactyly; polydactylia**.

polydipsia excessive, pathological thirst. See PSYCHOGENIC P.

polydrug abuse: See POLYDRUG ADDICTION.

polydrug addiction the physical or psychological dependence on more than one type of drug of abuse. A user may, e.g., self-administer a sedative and also a stimulant such as cocaine or amphetamines. Other combinations may include opiated hashish, alcohol and marijuana, or alcohol and methaqualone. P.a. may develop from therapeutic administration of more than one drug. See POLYPHARMACY.

polydystrophic oligophrenia = SANFILIPPO'S SYNDROME.

polyestrous: See ESTRUS.

polygamy marriage to more than one spouse at the same time, which is an accepted custom in certain cultures.

polygenic traits traits that are determined by numerous sets of genes rather than only one, e.g., normal intelligence. The majority of human traits are polygenic.

polyglot amnesia the tendency to forget one's current language and speak a language spoken at a much earlier period, after a severely traumatic experience of an organic or functional nature.

polygyny /-lij'-/ marriage of a man to more than one wife at the same time, which is an accepted custom in certain cultures.

polyglot neophasia a variation of neologism in which a patient, usually in a manic or paranoiac state, creates one or more languages which may be structured with their own vocabulary, grammar, and syntax.

polyglot reaction recovery from aphasia in which a multilingual person first uses a language other than his mother tongue, as opposed to the usual reaction in which recovery of the mother tongue comes first.

polygraph: See KEELER P.; LIE DETECTOR.

polyideic somnambulism: See MONOIDEIC SOMNAMBULISM.

polylogia = LOGORRHEA.

polymatric having many mothers. The term pertains to a family or household in which the child-rearing responsibilities are shared by two or more persons. Compare MONOMATRIC.

polymorphic fusiform layer: See CELLULAR LAYERS OF CORTEX.

polymorphous perverse a psychoanalytic term referring to being capable of responding to many kinds of sexual excitation, such as touching, smelling, sucking, viewing, masturbating, exhibiting, rocking, defecating, urinating, hurting, and being hurt. According to Freud, this capacity stems from early infancy, is expressed in some degree in normal sexual activity, and takes pathological form in practices that are often characterized as perversions. See FOREPLAY; PARAPHILIAS.

polymyositis: See MYOSITIS.

polyneuritis an inflammation of several nerves at the same time, usually involving peripheral nerves as a result of infection or poisoning. Symptoms include intense pain, muscle atrophy, and paralysis. Also see ACUTE P.

polyopia formation of more than one image on a retina due to a refractive error of the eye, or, in some cases, hysterical disorder.

polyorchid a male have one or more supernumerary testes.

polyp any mass of tissue that extends outward from the normal surface of a tissue and is visible without the aid of a microscope. A p. usually appears as a mound or as a round object at the end of a slender stalk. It may be a tissue malformation or a tumor. The presence of numerous polyps in an organ, especially the intestinal tract, is a pathological condition termed **polyposis**.

polypeptide a series of two or more amino acids linked by peptide bonds. A p. usually is identified by the number of amino acids in the chain, as dipeptide, tripeptide, tetrapeptide. The synthesis of polypeptides that become neural tissues is controlled by hereditary messages in DNA molecules. Also called **polyamino acid**.

polyphagia = BULIMIA.

polypharmacy the simultaneous use of a variety of drugs of the same or different kinds in the treatment of psychiatric patients. The need for p. may arise in special cases as when an epilepsy patient is admitted to an institution for the treatment of schizophrenia. P. also may be practiced as a matter of controlling adverse side effects of primary drugs.

polyphasic activity: See TYPE A BEHAVIOR.

polyphasic sleep rhythm a sleep pattern in which sleep occurs throughout a 24-hour period in relatively short naps. A human infant may begin life with a p.s.r. that consists of a half-dozen sleep periods. The rhythm becomes monophasic, with one long daily sleep period, about the time the child is ready for school. Also see SLEEP-WAKE CYCLE. Compare MONOPHASIC SLEEP RHYTHM.

polyphobia a morbid fear of many things.

polyphrasia = LOGORRHEA.

polypnea an abnormal increase in the rate and depth of breathing, which may be deep, labored, and rapid. Also called **hyperpnea**.

polyposis: See POLYP.

polysensory units neurons that normally respond to more than one type of stimulus. E.g., cutaneous sensory units that produce prick-pain impulses also produce sensations of itching.

polysomnography a recording of various physiological processes—such as eye movements, brain waves, heart rate, or penile tumescence—throughout the night, for the diagnosis of sleep-related disorders.

polysurgical addiction a compulsive drive to undergo one surgical procedure after another even when organic pathology cannot be found. The condition may be a manifestation of chronic factitious disorder with physical symptoms, hypochondriasis, or somatization disorder.

polysynaptic arc = MULTISYNAPTIC ARC.

polytoxicomanics individuals with an abnormal desire to consume various toxic substances, including narcotics or other drugs of abuse.

polyvitamin therapy the administration of a combination of vitamins, usually of the B complex, in large doses. P.t. is commonly used in the treatment of alcoholism. The vitamin-B deficiency associated with chronic alcoholism contributes to a form of cardiomyopathy called beriberi heart disease and to CNS symptoms, e.g., Korsakoff's psychosis.

Pompadour fantasy /pôNpädo͞or'/ a variation of the hetaeral fantasy in which the woman fantasizes that she is the mistress of a king or emperor. The term is derived from the name of Madame Jeanne Antoinette Pompadour (1721–64), a mistress of King Louis XV of France.

Pompe, J. C. Dutch physician, fl. 1932. See POMPE'S DISEASE; TARUI'S DISEASE.

Pompe's disease an autosomal-recessive disorder marked by deposits of glycogen in the heart and other muscle tissues. Nervous-system effects include loss of motor skills acquired during early infancy, absence of tendon reflexes, facial palsy, and mild mental retardation. Enlarged heart and muscular hypotonia are among the symptoms that begin in the first few months of life, and death usually occurs within a year. P.d. is due to a carbohydrate-enzyme deficiency. Also called **glycogenosis Type II**.

POMR: See PROBLEM-ORIENTED RECORD.

ponophobia a morbid fear of being overworked. Also called **work phobia**.

pons a part (Latin, "bridge") of the central nervous system between the midbrain and the medulla oblongata, appearing as a swelling on the ventral surface of the brainstem. It consists of bundles of transverse and ascending and descending nerve fibers and nuclei, including facial-nerve nuclei. As the name implies, it serves primarily as a bridge, or transmission structure, between different areas of the nervous system. It also works with the cerebellum in controlling equilibrium and with the cerebral cortex in smoothing and coordinating voluntary movements. Adjective: **pontine**.

pontine hemorrhage: See INTRACRANIAL HEMORRHAGE.

pontine sleep: See DREAM STATE.

pontocerebellar-angle syndrome a condition of persistent tinnitus, progressive deafness, and vertigo caused by acoustic neuromas. Cerebellar involvement results in ataxia with staggering, while the pontine effect is one of contralateral hemiplegia and hemianesthesia. If the facial nerve is involved, there is facial anesthesia and loss of corneal reflex on the same side of the body as the neuromas.

pooh-pooh theory: See ORIGIN-OF-LANGUAGE THEORIES.

pooling the combining of data, scores, or test results and treating them as a single variable.

popular response a term used in scoring Rorschach tests for responses that are given most frequently by normal subjects, as opposed to original or unique responses that occur rarely.

population the total number of individuals, humans or other organisms, in a given geographical area. In statistics, p. is a universe with certain unknown characteristics; a p. is sampled statistically for the purpose of describing its parameters. Also see SAMPLE.

population density the number of individuals per acre or other measure. In many countries, high p.d. is significantly related to various forms of social pathology; this is not true in all countries, e.g., Japan. See OVERCROWDING; OVERPOPULATION; POPULATION RESEARCH.

population research studies of population-related issues and problems. E.g., reports published in the 1970s showed that (a) 70 percent of an estimated 500 million women at risk of having an unwanted pregnancy did not use any contraceptive method, (b) only half of the 150 million who used contraceptive methods relied on the most effective techniques (the Pill, an IUD, sterilization, abortion), (c) in 1971 there were an estimated 55 million induced abortions worldwide, four for every ten live births, and (d) 46 percent of unmarried women had intercourse by age 19, and at that age the general level of knowledge about the period of greatest likelihood of conception during the menstrual cycle was found to be low. See FAMILY PLANNING; POPULATION DENSITY.

population standard deviation: See STANDARD DEVIATION.

POR = PROBLEM-ORIENTED RECORD.

porencephaly: See CEREBRAL DYSPLASIA.

poriomania an irresistible, apparently aimless impulse to run away or wander off, either consciously or in a state of amnesia during which an irresponsible act or a crime may be committed. The condition occurs in epileptic and senile patients. Also called **poriomanic fugue**. Also see FUGUE; NOMADISM.

pornographomania a morbid impulse to write obscene letters.

pornography writings or illustrations that are likely to cause sexual arousal in some individuals; the creation or the study of such works. Legal interpretations vary. (The term is derived from the Greek, meaning "description of prostitutes.") Also called **psychological aphrodisiacs**. Also see EROTICA.

pornolagnia an attraction to prostitutes as sexual objects.

porphyria a metabolic disorder involving excessive or abnormal **porphyrins** (breakdown products of hemoglobin) in the urine. The acute intermittent type is characterized by abdominal pain, nausea, weakness or paralysis of the extremities, and psychiatric symptoms such as irritability, depression, agitation, and delirium.

porphyropsin a visual pigment that is similar to rhodopsin except that its vitamin-A component has a different carbon-ring bonding. The vitamin-A molecule in p. sometimes is identified as A_2, while that in rhodopsin is identified as A_1.

porropsia a visual disorder in which objects appear to be more distant than they actually are, though their size is unchanged.

portal-systemic encephalopathy a type of metabolic encephalopathy marked by disorders of consciousness, tremors with increased muscle tone, hyperventilation with alkalosis, and psychiatric disturbances. It is associated with liver disease and an accumulation of ammonia products in the blood and other tissues.

Porter, Eleanor Hodgman American novelist, 1868–1920. See POLLYANNA MECHANISM.

Porter, Thomas Cunningham English scientist, fl. 1892, 1899. See PORTER'S LAW.

Porter's law the principle that the critical flicker frequency increases with the logarithm of the brightness of the stimulus independent of the stimulus wavelength. Also called **Ferry-Porter law**.

Porteus, Stanley David Australian-born psychologist in Hawaii, 1883—. See PORTEUS MAZE.

Porteus maze one of the original paper-and-pencil intelligence tests designed to assess ability to plan ahead and apply reasoning to the solution of a problem. In its various forms, a P.m. consists of a complex set of straight pathways that turn abruptly at right angles and run into numerous blind alleys. Only one pathway leads directly through the maze.

portmanteau neologism an artificial word formed by condensing several other words, e.g., "stagflation," from "*stag*nation" and "in*flation*." See NEOLOGISM.

port-wine stain a symptom of the Sturge-Weber syndrome consisting of a diffuse discoloration of the face, ranging from pink to bluish-red. See STURGE-WEBER SYNDROME.

position the location in space of an object in relation to a reference point or other objects; also, the social standing or rank of a person in a social group, or one's stand on an issue.

Position Analysis Questionnaire: See JOB-COMPONENT METHOD.

positive acceleration an improvement in the rate of change or development in a given activity or function as a result of practice, e.g., a gain in learning. Compare NEGATIVE ACCELERATION.

positive afterimage: See AFTERIMAGE.

positive attitudes in counseling, the client's feelings of acceptance and approval of the counselor, counseling process, another person, object, or the client himself. Compare NEGATIVE ATTITUDES.

positive cathexis the investment of positive emotions such as love or approval in an object, idea, or activity.

positive conditioned reflex a phase of a differential-conditioning system in which a subject is trained to respond in different ways to two different stimuli. E.g., an animal may be conditioned to lift a leg on one cue, a positive conditioned stimulus, and fail to lift the leg on a second, a negative conditioned stimulus. See INHIBITORY REFLEX.

positive eugenics: See EUGENICS.

positive feedback a signal from a machine that its speed or output should be increased, or from a receptor that a reaction or activity should be enhanced. As another example, p.f. in the form of applause usually has a stimulating effect on a speaker.

positive incentive an environmental object or condition that constitutes a goal toward which an organism directs its behavior, e.g., food or warmth. A p.i. results in approaching behavior. Also see INCENTIVE. Compare NEGATIVE INCENTIVE.

positive induction a Pavlovian term for increased neural activity in a stimulated area due to preceding inhibition in neighboring areas.

positive motivations: See RESPONSE-HOLD MECHANISM.

positive regard according to C. Rogers, a parent's warm, caring, accepting feelings for a child. P.r. is considered necessary for the child to develop a consistent sense of self-worth. Rogers also uses the term to refer to the counselor's feelings for the client as a separate individual whom he cares for and values. Also see CONDITIONAL P.R.; UNCONDITIONAL P.R.

positive reinforcement a stimulus or stimulus situation that, presented after a response, enhances the strength of that response and increases the probability that the response will appear again, given the same or a similar stimulus situation, e.g., the presentation of food to a hungry chimpanzee following a correct response. Also called **positive reinforcer; reward**. See REINFORCEMENT. Compare NEGATIVE REINFORCEMENT.

positive retroaction = RETROACTIVE FACILITATION.

positive spike pattern an EEG pattern observed in examination of epilepsy patients, marked by spikes that occur at frequencies of 14 to 16 per second. The p.s.p. may be associated with behavioral changes that may range from hostility and rage to complaints of aches and pains which might appear to be psychosomatic in nature except for verification by EEG analysis.

positive tele: See TELE.

positive transfer the improvement or enhancement of present learning by previous learning. E.g., learning to type on a manual machine facilitates learning on an electric machine. Compare NEGATIVE TRANSFER.

positive transference in psychoanalysis, displacement to the therapist of attachment, love, idealization, or other positive emotions originally experienced toward the parents or other significant individuals.

positive tropism automatic orientation of an organism toward a source of stimulation e.g.,

the attraction of a moth to the flame or a plant to the sun.

positivism a philosophical viewpoint that knowledge is limited to observed facts and what can be deduced from those facts; the approach that underlies empiricism and behaviorism and rejects metaphysical speculation.

positron-emission tomography a new technique to evaluate cerebral metabolism using radioactive trace elements such as 2-deoxyglucose and CAT. Abbrev.: **PET**.

possession in the two-word stage of language development, an expression of ownership, as in "Mommy dress."

Also see DEMONIC P.

postambivalent phase the culminating stage of psychosexual development, when genital primacy is reached and genuine love is possible. Such love is, potentially at least, unmixed with hateful or destructive feelings, as in prior stages in which the process of achieving satisfaction destroys the object, e.g., in swallowing and biting. The p.p. requires the ability to achieve full satisfaction through genital orgasm. It is the ultimate stage of object love. Also called **real love; postambivalent stage**.

postcentral area a sensory area of the parietal lobe with fibers involved in touch and taste sensations.

postconcussion syndrome personality changes observed in a small number of posttraumatic cases. The less severe reactions are characterized by anxiety plus headache, oversensitivity to stimuli, vertigo, insomnia, inability to concentrate, sudden emotional changes, reduced tolerance for alcohol, and "head consciousness." For the more severe reactions to head injury, see POSTTRAUMATIC PERSONALITY DISORDER.

postconventional level Kohlberg's third and highest level of moral reasoning characterized by commitment to valid moral principles sustained independently of any identification with family, group, or country. The earlier stage (stage 5) reflects legalistic, utilitarian concerns with individual rights in relation to the needs of society. The later stage (stage 6) is concerned with the application of self-determined, rational principles that have universal validity. For the first two levels, see PRECONVENTIONAL LEVEL; CONVENTIONAL LEVEL.

postconventional stage of moral development the stage at which moral values are no longer determined by tradition or social groups but are defined in terms of their application to situations as well as the individual's conscience and ethical principles.

postdental an alternative term for ALVEOLAR. See this entry.

postdisaster adaptation the range of responses following the crisis phase of a disaster. In addition to the constructive responses involved in rebuilding and reconstruction, long-term psychological consequences may ensue or preexisting disorders may be aggravated. Common psychological problems associated with disasters include grief, anxiety, and psychosomatic complaints. Also see DISASTER SYNDROME; PREDISASTER ADAPTATION.

postemotive schizophrenia a type of schizophrenia in which symptoms are triggered by an emotional crisis. The patient in such cases usually is predisposed to the disorder because of an existing condition, such as schizoidism. The emotional crisis may be one that threatens his sex life, self-preservation, or a similar basic psychological aspect of his life.

postemployment services in vocational rehabilitation, follow-up services provided by agency personnel to help a recently employed disabled person adjust to the new job situation.

postencephalitic amnesia a form of severe memory disorder that occurs in some patients who have recovered from an attack of viral encephalitis. The symptoms include a gross defect of recent memory, partial retrograde amnesia, and difficulty in following ongoing events. However, the brain infection causes no other significant intellectual deficits in patients experiencing the memory disorder.

postencephalitis syndrome a pathological condition that occurs following or as a result of encephalitis. An example is a type of parkinsonism that developed in patients who recovered from an epidemic of Economo's disease, or encephalitis lethargica, from 1919 to 1926. The onset of symptoms in some cases was not observed until ten years after the encephalitis attack.

postepileptic twilight state a twilight state that follows an epileptic attack. It may last for a variable period of time during which the patient may perform activities which he is unable to recall later. See TWILIGHT STATE.

posterior cerebral artery a branch of the basilar artery that begins near the oculomotor nerve and sends out branches that supply blood to the third ventricle area, including the thalamus and choroid plexus, the posterior surface of the occipital lobe, and the lingual, fusiform, and inferior temporal gyri.

posterior commissure a large bundle of nerve fibers that crosses from one side of the cerebrum to the other, composed mainly of myelinated tracts connecting oculomotor and related cells of the midbrain.

posterior communicating artery an artery that runs backward from the internal carotid artery and merges with the posterior cerebral branch of the basilar artery. Branches of the p.c.a. supply the genu and parts of the internal capsule, the third ventricle, and the thalamus.

posterior diencephalon an area of the forebrain that contains the thalamus and epithalamus along with the pineal body. Lesions in the p.d. of laboratory animals result in changes in sleep patterns.

posterior forceps a forceps-shaped band of fibers of the corpus callosum near the part of the brain marked by a cleft between the left and right occipital lobes. Also called **forceps major**.

posterior fossa: See FOSSA.

posterior nephrectomy: See NEPHRECTOMY.

posterior nucleus a subcortical station in the thalamus for nerve fibers of the visual system. Lesions in this area affect brightness discrimination and, to a lesser extent, form discrimination, thereby disrupting conditioning that depends upon visual cues.

posterior orbital gyrus: See ORBITAL GYRI.

posterior parietal area a region of the cerebral cortex along the postcentral sulcus containing neural tracts associated with tactile and kinesthetic functions.

posterior parietal lobe an area of the cerebral cortex generally posterior to the postcentral sulcus. The p.p.l. contains the angular and supramarginal gyri. P.p.l. lesions in some animals result in impairment of weight-discrimination ability.

posterior rhizotomy: See RHIZOTOMY.

posterior subarachnoidean space = CISTERNA MAGNA.

posterior thalamus the portion of the thalamus in the area of the epithalamus and pineal body and the site of the posterior nuclei, which are associated with auditory and vestibular functions.

posterolateral sclerosis a subacute degeneration of the spinal cord associated with a nutritional deficiency of the intrinsic factor, a cofactor of vitamin B_{12}. The disorder is marked by demyelination of the posterolateral columns of the spinal cord and of the peripheral nerves, with loss of sensations of touch, pain, position, and vibration. Treatment includes administration of vitamin B_{12}.

postexperimental inquiry a control procedure for demand characteristics, in which the subject is asked about the responses he gave in an experiment.

postfigurative culture a term used by M. Mead for a society or culture in which children learn chiefly from their parents, grandparents, and other adults. Also see CONFIGURATIVE CULTURE. Compare PREFIGURATIVE CULTURE.

postganglionic autonomic neurons nerve cells of the autonomic system that innervate certain target organs such as the kidneys, ovaries, and salivary glands. Compare PREGANGLIONIC AUTONOMIC NEURONS.

posthypnotic amnesia the subject's incapacity to remember what transpired during the hypnotic trance. Typically, the subject is instructed to forget the hypnotic experience until receiving a prearranged cue from the hypnotist; at that point, memory of the experience returns.

posthypnotic suggestion a suggestion made to a hypnotized subject and carried out upon awakening from the hypnotic trance. Usually, the p.s. is acted upon in response to a prearranged cue, and the subject does not know why he is performing the act.

postictal /pōstik'təl/ after a stroke, such as an acute epileptic seizure.

postictal depression a state of depression that follows a seizure, as in cases of epilepsy attacks. The p.d. phase of an epileptic attack appears as a distinctive phase of the seizure pattern on EEG records.

post-mortem examination = AUTOPSY.

postnatal sensorineural lesions an impairment of the inner ear, or auditory-nerve pathways, acquired sometime during life. This results in loss of hearing. It may be due to such agents as injury, drug toxicity, viral infections, diseases such as mumps, measles, or scarlet fever, and simply old age.

postoedipal /-ed'-/ or /-ēd'-/ referring to the period following the resolution of the Oedipus complex, approximately between ages six and 12. It is a rarely used term, suggested by L. E. Peller, to replace latency, which he believed to imply falsely that sexual interest is completely latent. See LATENCY.

postoperative disorders neurotic or psychotic reactions following surgery. Neurotic reactions include anxiety; occasionally, hysterical symptoms; and in some cases (as in removal of cataracts) panic. Children who have not been properly prepared for an operation may become phobic, negativistic, and extremely dependent. Psychotic reactions include disorientation, hallucinations, delusions, and acute manic, depressive, or schizophrenic episodes in predisposed patients.

postpartal eclamptic symptoms: See ECLAMPTIC SYMPTOMS.

postpartal period the period of time following childbirth during which the mother's reproductive system gradually returns to its prepregnancy state.

postpartum blues = MATERNITY BLUES.

postpartum emotional disturbances transient emotional disorders following childbirth, including depression ("maternity blues"), indifference or hostility toward the child or father, feelings of anxiety and apprehensiveness, and disturbed sleep patterns. For more extreme reactions, see POSTPARTUM PSYCHOSIS; PUERPERAL DISORDERS. Also see MATERNITY BLUES.

postpartum psychosis a psychotic episode associated with childbirth, usually schizophrenic but sometimes depressive in nature. The disorder is believed to be a reaction to the physiological and psychological stresses of the puerperium, but the condition may be caused or aggravated by such factors as preexisting personality defects and maladjustments, marital instability, inability to assume responsibility, lack of desire for the baby on the part of the wife or husband, and financial burdens. Because p.p. occurs in the month after delivery, it has been suggested that endocrinological phenomena may be among the causative factors. Also called **puerperal psychosis**.

postreconstructive surgery surgery performed on an arm, leg, or other body part subsequent to the original reconstructive procedure. Such surgery is often required to achieve optimum functioning, and may involve the transfer of muscle or tendon fibers between body areas, or redirecting nerve fibers.

postremity principle a generalization that the most recent response learned by an organism is the one most likely to be made when the situation is repeated (from Latin *post rem*, "after the thing").

postrotational nystagmus the nystagmus that occurs when rapid rotation of the body ceases.

postschizophrenic depression a period of depression that may follow an acute schizophrenic episode. P.d. is viewed by some authors as a routine event in recovery from schizophrenic decompensation, as a mood disturbance that existed previously and was masked by the schizophrenic episode, or as a side effect to drug treatment for schizophrenia.

postsynaptic potential the electric potential at a dendrite or other surface of a neighboring neuron after an impulse has crossed a synapse from a communicating axon. A p.p. may have either an excitatory or inhibitory effect. Abbrev.: **PSP**.

posttetanic potentiation a condition in which an overabundance of transmitter substance accumulates at the synaptic knobs of a spinal motor network following a period of rapid firing of impulses through the synapses. The p.p. may continue for about 60 seconds after the build-up of transmitter substance. Abbrev.: **PTP**.

posttraumatic amnesia a period of amnesia following a blow to the head or an acute psychological trauma. The traumatic event may be forgotten (retrograde amnesia), or events following the trauma may be forgotten (anterograde amnesia).

posttraumatic communicating hydrocephalus a form of hydrocephalus involving the frontal lobes after a head injury. There may or may not be a lesion, and diagnosis usually is based on a CAT or radioisotope scan or pneumoencephalography. The disorder occurs most commonly in older individuals and is characterized by dementia, an abnormal gait, and incontinence.

posttraumatic constitution a number of syndromes that are varied in character, often involving both neurotic and psychotic manifestations. One of the more common types, **Friedmann's complex**, is believed to be due to cerebral vasomotor disturbance resulting in headache, irritability, fatigability, and insomnia.

posttraumatic disorders emotional or other disturbances whose symptoms appear after a patient has endured a traumatic experience. Examples include symptoms of amnesia, personality disorders, epileptic attacks, headaches, and gastrointestinal effects such as constipation.

posttraumatic epilepsy epileptic seizures precipitated by a blow to the head severe enough to cause brain damage. The seizures may occur soon after the injury, or in some cases months or years later.

posttraumatic headache a headache following a severe trauma, often accompanied by vivid, terrifying nightmares and startle reactions that symbolize the threat to survival experienced during the event.

posttraumatic neurosis: See POSTTRAUMATIC STRESS DISORDER; TRAUMATIC NEUROSIS.

posttraumatic personality disorder a personality disorder occasionally observed after a severe head injury. Some patients become indifferent and withdrawn, but they are more likely to be irritable, impulsive, petulant, extremely selfish, and irresponsible. Older patients and those suffering from frontal-lobe damage may show impaired memory with confabulation. Also see POSTCONCUSSION SYNDROME.

posttraumatic-stress disorder an anxiety disorder produced by an uncommon, extremely stressful event (assault, rape, military combat, flood, earthquake, death camp, torture, car accident, head trauma), and characterized by (a) reexperiencing the trauma in painful recollections or recurrent dreams or nightmares, (b) diminished responsiveness (emotional anesthesia or numbing), with disinterest in significant activities and with feelings of detachment and estrangement from others, and (c) such symptoms as exaggerated startle response, disturbed sleep, difficulty in concentrating or remembering, guilt about surviving when others did not, and avoidance of activities that call the traumatic event to mind. Subtypes are **acute p.s.d.** and **chronic or delayed p.s.d.** (DSM-III)

posttraumatic syndrome a term sometimes applied to a reaction pattern that may develop days or weeks after a catastrophe. The major features are mild-to-acute anxiety attacks, recurrent nightmares, irritability, and persistent tension with tremors, restlessness, and insomnia.

postural alignment a phase of orthopedic rehabilitation in which emphasis is given to symmetrical alignment of muscles, bones, and joints so that physical stresses of sitting or standing will not result in pain, discomfort, or added wear and tear during the lifetime of the patient.

postural arm drift a test result that suggests certain types of brain damage: The patient is required to hold the arms outstretched and in a static position, with the eyes closed; if the arms drift from the original position, it may be an indication of a parietal lesion. The drift, if it occurs, is usually toward the midline. Also called **parietal drift**.

postural control a landmark in development when, at about three weeks of age, the infant lying on his stomach is first able to lift his head and raise his chin. Within a few weeks, further steps in p.c. are achieved, such as holding the head erect, turning it, and sitting with and then without support. These abilities expand the child's psychological field immeasurably.

postural hypotension an abnormal drop in blood pressure that may occur when an erect posture is assumed. P.h. involves a complex rerouting of blood flow through arteries and veins but is basically the result of a sudden pull of gravity on blood to lower body areas with a resultant impaired blood flow to the brain, producing a brief dizziness or even loss of consciousness. P.h. can be caused by a number of psychoactive drugs as well as diseases such as diabetes mellitus, amyloidosis, and Parkinson's disease.

postural reflex any of a variety of tonic reactions or complex limb movements needed to support the body, shift weight, grasp objects, or maintain balance.

postural set a positioning of the body with increased muscle tonus in readiness for a response, e.g., when a batter is getting set for the next pitch.

posture the position or bearing of the body. Kinds of p. may include erect p., recumbent p., prone p., or supine p. Like gesture and facial expression, p. can be expressive of underlying attitudes toward the self or external world. E.g., a rigid p. is frequently observed in obsessive compulsives, and a bent, in-drawn p. in schizoids.

posturing maintaining a bizarre body position or attitude for an extended period of time. It is commonly observed in catatonia.

postventral nucleus one of the relay nuclei in the thalamus for fibers from sensory receptors in the skin and muscles.

pot a street name for marijuana.

potamophobia a morbid fear of rivers.

potassium cyanate KCNO—a white soluble solid produced commercially by the reaction of lead monoxide and potassium cyanide. Lead metal also is produced by the reaction. P.c. is a basic form of the family of cyanates, and is a component of certain garden chemicals. A toxic effect of exposure to p.c. is falling blood pressure resulting in a reduced flow of blood to brain tissues and cerebral ischemia. P.c. also is associated with the destruction of red blood cells, an effect that may in turn result in a form of cerebral anoxia similar to that produced by carbon monoxide.

potassium deprivation the lack of potassium in the diet, a situation that can disrupt sodium metabolism, causing muscular weakness, respiratory paralysis, and damage to the heart and kidneys. It is postulated that in rats p.d. may cause a sodium hunger which may in turn be manifested as a potassium preference when it again becomes available in food or beverage. It also is assumed that because of similarities in the taste of potassium and sodium salts, the animal may use them interchangeably.

potassium nitrate KNO_3—a chemical compound sometimes administered as a diuretic or as an agent to induce sweating. At one time, p.n. was combined with jimson-weed leaves in the treatment of asthma. P.n. is one of the oldest known pharmacological substances and was included in prescriptions recorded on a Sumerian tablet of 2100 B.C. Also called **saltpeter**.

potassium permanganate $KMnO_4$—a strong oxidizing chemical sometimes used as an antiseptic and deodorant in the treatment of certain pus-forming ulcers and tumors. P.p. also is used as a gastric lavage in cases of poisoning by substances such as aconite, morphine, picrotoxin, and strychnine.

potency the ability of the male to perform sexual intercourse, maintaining an erection and achieving ejaculation. Also called **potentia coeundi** /kō·ā·ōōn'dē/. Compare IMPOTENCE.

potential an electrochemical charge that builds up between the inner and outer sides of a neural membrane. Generally, there is an excess of negative charge inside and an excess of positive charge on the outside when the inner and outer ions are in equilibrium. The p. difference has been measured as a range of 50 to 100 millivolts. For kinds of p., see RESTING P.; SPIKE P.; GRADED POTENTIALS; POSTSYNAPTIC P.

potential-stress score: See LIFE-CHANGE UNITS.

potlatch /pot'lach/ a ceremony among Native Americans of the Northwest (especially the Kwakiutl nation) which consists in establishing prestige by giving away or destroying one's possessions, usually with the goal of outdoing a visitor in being able to make such sacrifices.

Pott, Percival English surgeon, 1713–88. See ANKYLOSING SPONDYLITIS (there: **Pott's disease**).

Pötzl, Otto /pœts'əl/ Austrian psychiatrist, 1877—. See PÖTZL PHENOMENON; PÖTZL'S SYNDROME.

Pötzl phenomenon the appearance in dreams of parts of a tachistoscopically viewed picture not reported at the time of the experiment.

Pötzl's syndrome a form of pure alexia associated with visual-field defects and disturbances of the color sense. The syndrome is believed to be due to a lesion in the medullary layer of the lingual gyrus of the dominant hemisphere, with damage to the corpus callosum.

poverty fear = PENIAPHOBIA.

poverty of content of speech speech that is adequate in quantity but too vague, repetitious and lacking in content to be qualitatively adequate. It is frequently observed in schizophrenic patients.

poverty of ideas a thought disturbance found in schizophrenic, senile, and severely depressed patients who are limited to repeating a few simple or meaningless phrases over and over. The term is sometimes used interchangeably with intellectual impoverishment. Also see LACONIC SPEECH.

poverty of speech = LACONIC SPEECH.

power-coercive strategy in social psychology, a strategy based on the uses of economic, social, and political power to effect societal change, usually through nonviolent measures, e.g., organized boycotts, strikes, sit-ins, demonstrations, registration drives, and lobbying. Also see EMPIRICAL-RATIONAL STRATEGY; NORMATIVE-REEDUCATIVE STRATEGY.

power complex a term used by Jung to denote "all those ideas and strivings whose tendency it is to range the ego above other influences . . . quite irrespective of whether they have their source in men and objective conditions, or spring from one's own subjective impulses, feelings, and thoughts."

power factor a general intellectual factor that energizes other mental functions and determines the general efficiency of the brain.

power figure an individual who represents power or authority.

power of a test the ability of a statistical test to detect effects of a given size.

power test a type of test intended to calculate the subject's level of mastery of a particular topic under conditions of little or no time pressure. The test is designed so that items are progressively more difficult. Compare SPEED TEST.

practice curve a graphic representation of progress in learning with trials plotted on the horizontal axis and successes or errors on the vertical axis.

practice effect in learning, any change or improvement that results from practice or repetition of task items. The p.e. is a potentially invalidating factor in certain tests if some subjects receive coaching. However, the p.e. is more pronounced in specific areas such as vocabulary; and through systematic control measures it can be minimized.

practice limit in any learning situation, the point at which continued practice yields no more results; the optimal level that can be achieved by practice on a given task by a given subject at a given time.

practice material in experiments or tests, the introductory items or examples that illustrate test procedure and acquaint the subject with the nature of the problems. P.m. is not scored.

practice period in experiments or tests, the introductory period in which the subject is provided with practice material and allowed time to acquaint himself with the nature of the problems. The term is also used to mean a **learning session**.

practice theory of play a generalization that children's play prepares them for adult roles.

Prader, Andrea /prä'dər/ Swiss pediatrician, 1919—. See PRADER-LABHART-WILLI SYNDROME.

Prader-Labhart-Willi syndrome a congenital disorder marked by mental retardation, short stature, muscular hypotonia, hypogonadism, obesity, and short hands and feet. It is believed to be transmitted as an autosomal-dominant trait and is observed most frequently in males, perhaps because the gonadal abnormality is more easily detected in males. When diabetes mellitus is associated with the condition, it is called **Royer's syndrome**. From the initials of the words *h*ypomentia, *h*ypotonia, *h*ypogonadism, and *o*besity, this syndrome is also called **HHHO** /tripəlāchō'/.

praeputism = PREPUTIUM.

pragmatism William James' philosophical theory that the truth of an idea depends upon its practical consequences, and the main purpose of thinking is to achieve a better adjustment to the environment.

Prägnanz: See PRINCIPLE OF P.

prandial drinking the ingesting of water or other fluids with meals.

praxernia a personality quality marked by practical, conforming behavior (Cattell).

praxiology Dunlap's term for a science of psychology that deals mainly with actions and overt behavior, to the exclusion of consciousness and metaphysical concepts.

praxis motor activity; performance of an action.

preadolescence /prē·ad-/ the developmental period preceding puberty, comprising approximately the two years between the ages of ten and 12 in girls and 11 and 13 in boys. Also called **prepuberty; prepubescence; prepubertal stage**.

preanimistic: See PRIMITIVE.

precausal thinking a term applied by Piaget to the tendency of the young child (below age eight) to perceive natural events such as rain, wind, and clouds in terms of intentions and willful acts, that is, in anthropomorphic rather than mechanical terms.

precentral area = MOTOR AREA.

precipice fear = CREMNOPHOBIA.

precipitating cause the particular factor, usually a traumatic or stressful experience, that is the immediate cause of a mental disorder. The onset of a behavioral disturbance is usually associated with more than one stressor that predisposes the patient to a mental disorder, but one precipitating event turns a latent condition into the manifest form of the disorder.

precision law: See LAW OF PRECISION.

preclinical psychopharmacology the area of psychopharmacology that precedes the actual clinical application of a new drug on an individual patient or patient population. P.p. usually includes laboratory studies of the pharmacological mechanisms of the drug, extrapolation of research data into human-use terms, and evaluation of possible interactions with drugs in use or with patient idiosyncrasies.

precocious puberty abnormally early development of sexual maturity, usually before the age of eight in a female and ten in a male. True p.p. is marked by mature gonads capable of ovulation or spermatogenesis, adult levels of female or male sex hormones, and secondary sex characteristics. Also called **pubertas praecox. Pseudoprecocious puberty** is a condition usually caused by an endocrine-gland tumor that results only in premature development of secondary sex characteristics.

precocity a very early, often premature, development in a child of physical or mental functions and characteristics.

precognition the purported foreknowledge of an occurrence or experience, supposedly through nonrational channels. See PARAPSYCHOLOGY; EXTRASENSORY PERCEPTION.

preconception a conclusion that is reached before the facts are known and evaluated.

preconditioning the presentation of two stimuli consecutively without reinforcement to determine if the subject will respond to both stimuli when conditioned to respond only to the first.

preconscious in psychoanalysis, the division of the personality that contains thoughts, feelings, and impulses not presently in awareness, but which can be more or less readily called into consciousness. Examples are the face of a friend, a verbal cliché, and the memory of a recent event. The term is sometimes used as an adjective characterizing the mental contents themselves. Also called **foreconscious**.

preconscious thinking a term introduced by Fenichel to identify the pictorial, magical, fantasy thinking of children that precedes the development of logical thinking. Later, types of p.t. can be found in the daydreaming of hysterics, the concepts of compulsive-neurotics, and the thinking processes of schizophrenics.

preconventional level Kohlberg's first level of moral reasoning characteristic of children and marked by obedience, unquestioning acceptance of parents' moral definitions, and evaluation of an act's material consequences only. The earlier stage (stage 1) reflects concern with punishment and reward. In the later stage (stage 2), an act is appraised for its potential for self-gratification although awareness of others' needs does exist. For the later two levels, see CONVENTIONAL LEVEL; POSTCONVENTIONAL LEVEL.

precuneus an area of the parietal lobe that is located between the parieto-occipital fissure and the cingulate sulcus. Immediately behind the p. is the wedge-shaped cuneus lobule of the occipital lobe. Also called **quadrate lobule**.

predation a form of behavior characterized by the stalking, capturing, and killing of other animals for food. The behavior is exhibited by animals that are **predatory**, or **predacious**. See PREDATORY BEHAVIOR.

predatory aggression: See ANIMAL AGGRESSION.

predatory behavior behavior in which one animal preys on another. P.b. has been described in terms of food deprivation and eating, but some animals will hunt and kill another of the same or a different species but avoid eating the prey. A hungry cat, e.g., may leave a meal to hunt and kill a mouse without then eating the mouse.

predelay reinforcement a delayed-response test in which an animal is rewarded at a certain place, but prevented for a time from returning to the place, to determine whether it will return to the place after the delay.

predementia praecox an early stage of schizophrenia when the patient becomes preoccupied with fantasies and daydreams and loses his capacity for coping with difficulties. The overt symptoms of schizophrenia may appear when the p.p. patient encounters a stress that a normal person would be able to handle without great difficulty.

predicate thinking a thought process in which objects are considered identical only because they bear some resemblance to each other.

prediction the foretelling of future events. In psychiatry it may be possible to predict the general behavior or prognosis of patients whose personality pattern is known, but not their specific behavior, since so many factors are involved. In parapsychology, the term is essentially equivalent to PRECOGNITION. See this entry.

predictive efficiency the number or proportion of correct predictions that a test can make.

predictive validity = CRITERION VALIDITY.

predictive value the validity of a test as a predictor of accurate information.

predictor-cell assemblies a theoretical model of motoneurons in a network that allows for evaluation of inputs so that an appropriate response is predictable. The mechanism resembles an electronic computer flow chart.

predictors: See PERSONNEL SPECIFICATIONS; PERSONNEL TESTS; FRAMINGHAM STUDY.

predisaster adaptation the range of responses to disaster warnings. Most people appear to be passive when confronted with warnings of disaster, e.g., earthquake warnings. On the whole, there are few adaptive responses. A few individuals may stock up on food; others engage in alarmist activities, e.g., buying expensive insurance policies. Also see CRISIS EFFECT; LEVEE EFFECT; POSTDISASTER ADAPTATION.

predisposing cause a factor that increases the probability that a mental disorder or hereditary characteristic will develop.

predisposition in genetics, any hereditary factor that, given the necessary conditions, will lead to the development of a certain trait, characteristic, or disease.

preeclampsia: See TOXEMIA OF PREGNANCY; ECLAMPTIC SYMPTOMS.

preestablished harmony Leibniz' doctrine that psychological and physiological processes follow parallel harmonious paths without interaction.

preference behavior a type of behavior marked by a preference or an aversion for an object when the choice has been induced by conditioning. The subject may have been conditioned with or without rewards for making the "correct" decision.

preference method a research technique in which a subject chooses one of several possible stimuli, e.g., a food choice by animals, or various preferences by human subjects such as paintings, activities, or vocations.

preferential perception in infants, the visual perception characterized by a certain flexibility as the child no longer appears fixated on high contrast areas but begins to focus on, differentiate, and favor certain colors and configurations. Obligatory perception precedes p.p. See OBLIGATORY PERCEPTION.

prefigurative culture a society or culture in which adults learn from children. Because of the extremely rapid rate of social change and the resulting isolation of many adults, M. Mead has proposed that contemporary society may be moving toward a p.c. in which children will possess a keener intuition of the present and thus will have to "navigate the future." Also see CONFIGURATIVE CULTURE. Compare POSTFIGURATIVE CULTURE.

preformism the doctrine that development consists of the emerging into adult form of the traits and capacities that exist in prototypical form in the germ cell. An early example of p. is the 16th- and 17th-century notion of the homunculus, a minute but completely formed human body in the spermatozoon. P. contrasts with the epigenetic principle of successive differentiation in complex and cumulative stages of development. Also see HOMUNCULUS. Compare EPIGENESIS.

prefrontal areas the parts of the cerebral cortex that are anterior to the frontal lobes. The p.a. contain association areas involved in integrating problem-solving and related activities.

prefrontal lobotomy = LEUCOTOMY.

preganglionic autonomic neurons neurons of the autonomic nervous system that are located in the central nervous system and innervate internal organs such as the bladder and heart. Their impulses are relayed through ganglia to POSTGANGLIONIC AUTONOMIC NEURONS. See this entry.

pregenital love in psychoanalysis, the phase before dominance of the genital zone, when the libido is directed toward anal, urethral, and oral satisfactions.

pregenital organization a Freudian term for libido functions in the developmental phase preceding genital primacy.

pregenital phase in psychoanalysis, the stages of psychosexual development that precede the stages of phallic primacy, when the penis and clitoris become central erogenous zones, and genital primacy, when the sex organs begin to exert a dominant influence. The p.p. comprises the first stages of sexuality, when the libido is concentrated on the mouth, anus, and urethra rather than the genital organs.

pregnancy the period of embryonic and fetal development in the female between conception and the birth or abortion of the offspring. A p. normally involves a developing offspring within the uterus, but the p. may be extrauterine, or ectopic, occurring in the Fallopian tube, the abdominal cavity, or the cervical canal. If the p. involves twin offspring, it may be called bigeminal. The term false p. is usually applied to a condition due to psychogenic factors, but signs of p. may also be due to a tumor, or a hormonal disorder. Also called **cyesis** /sī·ē′sis/ (Greek *kyesis*); **cyophoria** /sī·ō-/; **fetation; gravidity**. See ADOLESCENT P.; ECTOPIC P.; FALLOPIAN-TUBE P.; FALSE P.; GESTATION; P. FANTASY; TOXEMIA OF P.

pregnancy fantasy fantasies about pregnancy, which take many forms, e.g., that the baby will be a gift from the father, or that it will be born through the anus, mouth, or umbilicus. Underlying them all, according to psychoanalysis, is the identification of the baby with the breast, the feces, or the penis, all of which are highly desired objects that have been viewed as part of the self, but painfully taken away. Neurotic symptoms, such as fear of mutilation, vomiting, or fear of being devoured by the fetus, may develop during pregnancy due to revival of pregenital fantasies. See FALSE PREGNANCY.

prehension the act of grasping, clasping, or seizing, usually with an appendage adapted for that purpose. The hands of humans and primates and the tails and toes of certain species of monkeys are **prehensile**, or adapted for prehension.

prejudice in social psychology, a persistently held attitude toward a certain group or individual, more often negative than positive, formed in advance of sufficient evidence (literally, prejudgment). Krech and colleagues, 1962, have described such attitudes as "highly stereotyped, emotionally charged, and not easily changed by contrary information." Typically, prejudicial attitudes are acquired from parents, friends, and social groups, and are frequently perpetuated for psychological reasons, such as deriving a sense of power from lording it over others, or using minority groups as scapegoats. Also see STEREOTYPE; RACISM.

prelinguistic period the stage preceding the development of actual speech, roughly the first year of life. The p.p. comprises the earliest infant vocalizations as well as the babbling stage characteristic of the second half of the first year. Holophrases (single-word expressions) usually emerge near the beginning of the second year.

preliterate referring to a culture or population group that has not yet acquired a written language.

prelogical thinking in psychoanalysis, primitive or primary thinking that is characteristic of early childhood, when thought is under the control of the pleasure principle rather than the reality principle. Examples are daydreaming, in which wish fulfillment is dominant, and the concrete thinking of schizophrenics. For a case cited by Bleuler, see PARALOGIA. Also see PALEOLOGIC THINKING; PRIMARY PROCESS.

premarital counseling educational and supportive guidance provided to individuals planning marriage. The p.c. may be offered by a clergyman, sex-education specialist, or therapist, who are prepared to provide advice and answers to questions covering a wide range of matters, such as rights and responsibilities of husband and wife in marriage, birth-control methods, and sexual compatibility.

premarital sex sexual relations before marriage. See FORNICATION.

premature ejaculation a psychosexual disorder in which ejaculation occurs before the individual wishes it, due to recurrent and persistent absence of reasonable voluntary control, taking into account such factors as age, novelty of the sexual partner, and the frequency and duration of intercourse. The term only applies if the disturbance is not due to another mental disorder.

Also called **ejaculatio praecox**. Also see SQUEEZE TECHNIQUE. (DSM-III)

prematurity a state of underdevelopment, as in the birth of an offspring before it has completed the normal fetal processes of development.

premeditation a legal term applied to crimes, particularly violent crimes, that are planned rather than spontaneous acts.

premenstrual disorders transient emotional disturbances associated with glandular imbalance preceding menstrual flow, especially tension, irritability, anxiety, and general upset. More severe disturbances, such as depression, disgust, guilt feelings, self-depreciation, and migraine may be experienced if the mother has denigrated the feminine role or has characterized sexual activity as repugnant and menstruation as an illness or "curse." Also see PREMENSTRUAL TENSION.

premenstrual-stress syndrome: See PREMENSTRUAL DISORDERS; PREMENSTRUAL TENSION.

premenstrual tension a syndrome of irritability, headache, bloating, and abdominal discomfort that develops in many menstruating women about a week before the menstrual period. P.t. is associated with effects of progesterone secretion and fluid retention. The symptoms diminish with the onset of the menstrual period. Also see PREMENSTRUAL DISORDER.

premise a statement from which a conclusion is drawn or which contributes in part to a conclusion.

premoral stage stage 0 of L. Kohlberg's stages of moral reasoning. This stage corresponds to infancy (birth to roughly 18 months) and is followed by stage 1 of Kohlberg's PRECONVENTIONAL LEVEL. See this entry. Also see CONVENTIONAL LEVEL; POSTCONVENTIONAL LEVEL.

premorbid characterizing the patient's condition before the onset of disease or disorder.

premorbid adjustment a measure of the ability of a schizophrenia patient to make adequate social and sexual adjustments before the onset of symptoms of the disorder. The p.a., as used in the Phillips Scale, has been found to be valuable in predicting the rate of recovery from schizophrenia.

premorbid personality previously existing personality defects that predispose the individual to one or another mental disorder, determining, e.g., that he or she will become depressive rather than schizophrenic.

premotor area = INTERMEDIATE PRECENTRAL AREA.

premotor cortex an area of the frontal lobes that contains cells concerned with the organization of motor impulses. The p.c. cells contribute to coordinated movements of body parts. After suffering a lesion in the p.c., a patient may have difficulty in manipulating the fingers, as in fastening buttons on clothes, or playing a musical instrument.

premsia Cattell's term for a personality characteristic consisting of emotional sensitivity, absence of aggressiveness, and dependence.

prenatal developmental anomaly a congenital abnormality that originates in the course of prenatal development. Examples are cleft palate, hydrocephalus, phocomelia, osteogenesis imperfecta, hypertelorism, and arthrogryposis.

prenatal influences any influence on the developing organism between conception and birth. Early theories cited such "old wives' tales" as the notion that strawberry-colored birthmarks may be acquired by the child if the mother watches a fire. Today the emphasis is on radiation effects, maternal diseases such as rubella, fetal alcohol syndrome, blindness due to gonorrhea, barbiturate poisoning, drug abuse, lead poisoning, blood incompatibility, nutritional deficiency, and prematurity associated with excessive smoking or maternal vitamin deficiency, as well as the effects of maternal emotional stress.

prenatal period the developmental period between conception and birth, commonly and roughly divided into the germinal period (approximately the first two weeks), the embryonic period (the first two months), and the fetal period (from two months to birth). Also see GESTATION PERIOD.

prenatal sensorineural lesions a congenital abnormality of the inner ear, or of the auditory nerve, resulting in loss of hearing associated with damage to the embryo *in utero*, or maternal illness during the first three months of pregnancy, e.g., rubella.

preoccupation a state of being self-absorbed and "lost in thought," ranging from transient absent-mindedness to a symptom of autistic schizophrenia in which the patient withdraws from external reality and turns inward upon the self. Also called **p. with thought**.

preoedipal /prē·ed′-/ or /prē·ed′-/ in psychoanalysis, referring to the first stages of psychosexual development when the mother is the exclusive love object of both sexes and the father is not yet considered either a rival or a love object.

preoperational stage a Piagetian term for the period of cognitive development between ages two and seven when the ability to record experience symbolically emerges along with the ability to represent an object, event, or feeling in speech, movement, drawing, and the like. During the later two years of the p.s., egocentrism diminishes noticeably with the emerging ability to adopt the point of view of others. Also called **symbolic stage**. For Piaget's other stages of cognitive development, see CONCRETE OPERATIONAL STAGE; FORMAL OPERATIONS; SENSORIMOTOR STAGE. Also see REPRESENTATIONAL STAGE.

preorgasmic characterizing the state before orgasm, which usually extends over a period of 30 seconds to three minutes following foreplay. It is characterized by increased breathing, heart rate, blood pressure, semispastic muscle contractions, and maximum increase in the size of the glans penis, testes, and upper vaginal walls.

preparation the state or process of increasing readiness for an activity, e.g., compiling data needed to solve a problem.

preparatory interval the time period between a warning signal and actual stimulus presentation.

preparatory set a special alertness or preparedness to respond in a particular manner to an expected stimulus, action, or event. A p.s. may be manifested physically and experienced mentally; e.g., a tennis player set to receive a serve graphically demonstrates a p.s., while a chess player anticipating an opponent's next move experiences a p.s. mentally. Postural set and motor set are narrower terms, referring mainly to physiological responses. Also see MENTAL SET; POSTURAL SET; MOTOR SET.

preparedness a conditioning predisposition in which the individual has a biological sensitivity to certain stimuli which are associated in turn with an unconditioned stimulus.

prepartal eclamptic symptoms: See ECLAMPTIC SYMPTOMS.

preperception a readiness state before a stimulus is received, possibly including imagery, e.g., anticipating what it will be like to make a deep-sea dive.

prephallic a stage of psychosexual development preceding the phallic stage. The p. stage includes the oral and anal phases of development.

prephallic masturbation equivalents in psychoanalysis, autoerotic activities occurring before sexuality is centered in the genital organs; autoerotic pleasure derived from the mouth, anus, urethra, skin, musculature, or from motor activity, sensation, and perception.

prepotent response a response that has higher priority than other responses, e.g., a pain response.

prepsychotic panic a stage in the development of schizophrenia in which the patient's self-image is disordered and he feels guilty, unlovable, humiliated, or otherwise different, but has not yet acquired symptoms of delusions and hallucinations.

prepsychotic personality a marginally adjusted individual who displays characteristics and behavior that may later develop into psychosis, e.g., eccentricities, withdrawal, litigiousness, apathy, hypersensitivity, or grimacing.

prepsychotic psychosis = LATENT PSYCHOSIS.

prepubertal stage; prepuberty; prepubescence = PREADOLESCENCE.

prepuce = PREPUTIUM.

prepuce of clitoris = PREPUTIUM CLITORIDIS.

prepuce of penis = PREPUTIUM PENIS.

preputial glands = TYSON'S GLANDS.

preputium a covering fold of skin, e.g., the preputium clitoridis. Also called **prepuce; praeputium**. See P. PENIS; P. CLITORIDIS; FORESKIN. Also see REDUNDANT PREPUCE.

preputium clitoridis a fold of skin formed by the union of the labia minora anterior and the clitoris. Also called **prepuce of clitoris**.

preputium penis the fold of skin covering the glans penis. P.p., also called **prepuce of penis**, is essentially synonymous with FORESKIN. See this entry.

prepyriform area the olfactory projection area at the base of the brain.

prerecognition hypothesis a theory that an unverbalized expectation of an event comes as the result of previous experiences in similar situations.

prerelease anxiety state a type of anxiety experienced by prison inmates who fear being released and having to compete in the real world again. Also see FURLOUGH PSYCHOSIS.

-presby-; -presbyo- a combining form relating to old age (from Greek *presbys*, "old, venerable").

presbycusis the gradual diminution of hearing acuity associated with aging.

presbyophrenia a senile psychosis characterized by confusion, disorientation, defective memory, confabulation, misidentification, agitation, poverty of ideas, and puerile but generally amiable behavior. Also called **Wernicke's dementia; Kahlbaum-Wernicke syndrome**.

presbyopia a visual impairment of aging due to decreased lens elasticity and accommodation that causes the near point of distinct vision to become farther removed from the eye. P. is usually correctible with bifocal lenses.

preschizophrenic ego a condition of impaired ego synthesis that is observed in the prepsychotic personality of the schizophrenic patient, who lacks the normal characteristic of an integrated person. Typical symptoms are withdrawal into fantasies, dreams of his own death, aimless overaggressiveness, and bizarre somatic sensations.

preschool programs educational curriculums for children who are below the required minimum age for participation in regular classroom work. P.p. for mentally retarded or disturbed children are designed to help develop social skills and provide stimulation at levels appropriate for the individual children.

presenile degeneration = SENIUM PRAECOX.

presenile dementia: See PRIMARY DEGENERATIVE DEMENTIA.

presenile gangrene = BUERGER'S DISEASE.

presentation the act of exposing a subject to stimuli or learning materials during an experiment; also, in psychoanalysis, the means or vehicle through which an instinctual drive is expressed.

Present State Examination a structured interview comprising about 400 items, including a wide range of symptoms likely to be manifested during an acute episode of one of the functional neuroses or psychoses. The **PSE**, as it is usually called, was developed for the WHO-supported **International Pilot Study of Schizophrenia (IPSS)**.

prespeech development the earliest forms of perceptual experience, learning, and communication that precede actual speech and are requisite for its development, e.g., an infant's attention to sound, perceptual discriminations, and limitation and production of sounds. Babies attend to sound at birth and can differentiate the human voice from other sounds within the first month. Cross-cultural studies reveal that mothers routinely use techniques that help their infants acquire language; e.g., they shorten their expressions, stress important words, simplify syntax, and speak louder and with exaggerated distinctness. For prespeech sounds, see BABBLING; BABY TALK; INFANTILE SPEECH.

press a term applied by H. A. Murray to an environmental stimulus, person, or situation that arouses a psychogenic or viscerogenic need. Examples are the birth of a sibling, parental discord, feelings of social inferiority, or the sight of food when we are hungry.

Pressey, Sidney L. American psychologist, 1888—. See X-O TEST.

press-need pattern the relationship between needs, or motives, and presses, or environmental situation, e.g., the activities performed in winning a wife or husband (H. A. Murray).

pressor effect the effect of constricting blood vessels, mainly arterioles, leading from the arteries so that blood pressure is raised. The p.e. generally is controlled by the vasopressin hormone, which is secreted by the posterior pituitary.

pressure in abnormal psychology, excessive or stressful demands made on an individual. P. may vary with different persons depending upon their own educational, occupational, family, and other demands, e.g., parental p. for achievement.

pressured speech = PRESSURE OF SPEECH.

pressure gradient a gradual reduction in pressure extending in all directions when a stimulus is applied to the skin.

pressure of activity compulsive hyperactivity characteristic of the manic phase of bipolar disorder. The patient talks "a mile a minute," moves restlessly about, pours forth an endless flow of unrealistic ideas, and, in cases of hypermania, may also decorate himself with badges, break up furniture, and make indiscriminate sexual advances.

pressure of ideas = THOUGHT PRESSURE.

pressure of speech accelerated, uncontrollable talking which includes, in some cases, ordering other people about or declaiming in theatrical tones. It is a symptom of hypomania, acute mania, and some cases of schizophrenia and organic brain syndrome. Also called **pressured speech**. See LOGORRHEA. Also see HAPLOLOGY.

pressure sense the sensation of stress or strain, compression, expansion, pull, or shear, usually caused by a force in the external environment. Receptors for the p.s. may interlock or overlap with the pain receptors so that one sensation is accompanied by the other.

pressure sores: See DECUBITI.

pressure spot any of the points on the body surface that are particularly sensitive to pressure stimuli.

pressure testicular atrophy: See TESTICULAR ATROPHY.

pressure-threshold test a sensory test in which pressure sensitivity is measured with a series of hairs of graded stiffness.

prestige the state of being held in high esteem by one's peers or the whole community, particularly when others are influenced by one's position.

prestige motive the drive to acquire prestige.

prestige suggestion supportive, symptomatic psychotherapy that depends upon the prestige of the therapist in the eyes of the patient. The "omnipotent" therapist may abolish the symptoms, at least temporarily, by suggestion.

prestriate area a visual-association center in the occipital portion of the cerebral cortex. Also called **Brodmann's areas 18 and 19; prestriate cortex**.

presuperego phase the early stage of life before the superego is formed. The p.p. includes the oral, anal, and phallic stages of approximately the first five years of life, at which time the superego replaces the Oedipus complex, according to psychoanalysts.

presynaptic inhibition a mechanism whereby an impulse is blocked at a synapse by reduced release of a transmitter substance associated with a partial depolarization. The effect is most likely to occur at an axo-axonal synapse. See HYPERPOLARIZATION.

pretend situations: See DIRECTIVE-PLAY THERAPY.

pretest: See BEFORE-AFTER DESIGN.

pretraumatic personality the personality traits of a person before an injury that may have resulted in a psychiatric disorder. The p.p. is important for the proper diagnosis and prognosis of a posttraumatic personality disorder and for administration of the appropriate therapy.

prevalence in epidemiology, the total number of cases of a disease existing in a given population at a given point in time (**point p.**) or during a specified time (**period p.**). Also see INCIDENCE.

prevention efforts to control the occurrence or reduce the severity of undesirable phenomena such as mental disorder, birth defects, delinquency and crime, environmental disasters, drug addiction, accidents, and physical disease. Also see PRIMARY P.; SECONDARY P.; TERTIARY P.

preventive intervention active, immediate efforts undertaken by a psychiatrist, clinical psychologist, or other professionally trained individual to deal with emergencies such as suicidal threats or attempts, psychotic breaks, cyclothymic crises, or dyscontrol episodes. See EMERGENCY PSYCHOTHERAPY.

preventive psychiatry a branch of preventive medicine concerned with measures (a) to forestall mental disorders (primary prevention), (b) to limit the severity of illness through early case-finding and treatment (secondary prevention), and (c) to reduce disability resulting from disorder (tertiary prevention). P.p. overlaps with the fields of community psychiatry, industrial or occupational psychiatry, and social psychiatry.

preverbal construct a concept that may have developed during the prespeaking stage and which is still maintained, but without a verbal symbol.

prevocational training rehabilitation programs that emphasize basic work skills. P.t. usually is offered disabled adolescents and adults who have not had actual work experience in a competitive job market. It usually takes place in sheltered workshops.

priapism /prī′ə-/ persistent penile erection that occurs independently of sexual arousal. The condition is associated with leukemia and sickle-cell anemia and is usually painful. Immediate causes may be thrombosis, cancer, hemorrhage, inflammation, or lesions involving nerve tracts between the brain and the urethra. (P. is named for Priapus the Greco-Roman god of procreation and of the generative force in nature. He was the son of Dionysus and Aphrodite and the basis of a cult that worshiped the phallus.) The term p. may also be used as a synonym for SATYRIASIS. See this entry. Also see PHALLOCENTRIC CULTURE.

Pribram, Karl Harry Austrian-born American physician and medical researcher, 1919—. See EXTRINSIC CORTEX; INTRINSIC CORTEX.

Prichard, James Cowles English ethnologist and physician, 1786–1848. See MORAL INSANITY.

prick experience the sensation produced when a pin, needle, or small electrical stimulus is applied to a receptor area of the skin. A p.e. may appear as a variation of other somatic sensations, such as itch, tickle, pain, or pressure, depending upon how the stimulus is applied.

pride a feeling of self-esteem which may be exaggerated or unfounded (conceit, false p.) or a reflection of admirable self-assurance and determination (as in setting high standards and doing one's best). The psychoanalyst Rado applied the term **domesticated p.** (also known as **moral p.**) to overvaluation of the self in obsessive patients, which he interpreted as a reaction to guilt, fear, and repressed feelings of humiliation. This type of p. has been distinguished from **real p.** or **brute p.** based on self-assertive rage. Also see PENIS P.

primacy effect the tendency for facts, impressions, or items that are presented first in formal learning situations to be better learned or remembered than others. The p.e. appears to have special bearing on information of high interest and familiarity. Also called **law of primacy; principle of primacy**. Compare RECENCY EFFECT.

primacy zone the erotogenic area that dominates others in the libido organization. According to Freud, one p.z. succeeds another in the order of oral, anal, phallic, and, finally, genital.

primal anxiety in psychoanalysis, the most basic form of anxiety, first experienced when the infant is separated from the mother at birth and suddenly has to cope with the flood of new stimuli.

primal depression depression experienced in early childhood, due primarily to disappointment stemming from lack of "emotional supplies" of security and love which the child needs in order to maintain his self-esteem. Fenichel, among others, traced cases of adult depression to this type of childhood experience.

primal fantasies in psychoanalysis, fantasies often employed by children to fill gaps in their knowledge of sexual experience, especially fantasies about conception, birth, parental intercourse, and castration. Such fantasies are most clearly revealed in dreams and daydreams, and are also called **unconscious fantasies**.

primal father the hypothetical head of a primitive tribe whom Freud pictured as slain and devoured by his sons, and later revered as a god. The crime has a tragic effect on the son who killed him, and becomes enshrined in the culture of the tribe (*Totem and Taboo*, 1913). See PRIMAL-HORDE THEORY.

primal-horde theory Freud's speculative reconstruction of the original human family comprised of a dominant male holding sway over a subordinate group of females and probably younger men. Freud used the theory to account for the origin of exogamy, the incest taboo, guilt, and totemism.

primal ictal automatism a form of psychomotor epilepsy in which semipurposeful activities are automatically performed without preceding aura and followed by amnesia.

primal pain: See PRIMAL THERAPY.

primal repression = PRIMARY REPRESSION.

primal sadism a Freudian term for a part of the death instinct that is identical with masochism and remains within the person, partly as a component of the libido and partly with the self as an object.

primal scene in psychoanalysis, the child's first observation—in reality or fantasy—of parental intercourse or seduction. The fragmentary or illusory recollection of this event may play a part in neuroses.

primal therapy a technique developed by A. Janov, which seeks to treat neurosis by encouraging the patient to relive basic, or "primal," traumatic events and discharge painful emotions associated with them. The events frequently involve feelings of abandonment or rejection experienced in infancy or early childhood, and during the enactment the patient may sob, cry, scream, or writhe in agony. Afterwards he experiences a sense of release and rebirth and, freed from "primal pain," is believed to be better able to divest himself of the defenses with which he has been seeking to escape or anesthetize the pain. Also called **primal-scream therapy**.

primal trauma an original painful situation to which an individual was subjected in early life and which is presumed to be the basis of a neurosis in later life.

primary abilities according to L. L. Thurstone, the unitary factors revealed by factor analysis to be essential components of intelligence. There are seven p.a.: verbal meaning (V), word fluency (WF), numerical ability (N), spatial relations (S), memory (M), perceptual speed (P), and reasoning (R). These factors are measured by the **Primary Mental Abilities Test**. Also called **primary mental abilities**.

primary aging: See SECONDARY AGING.

primary amenorrhea: See AMENORRHEA.

primary amyloidosis: See AMYLOIDOSIS.

primary area: See METASTASIS.

primary attention attention that does not require conscious effort, e.g., attention to an intense, powerful, or arresting stimulus. Compare SECONDARY ATTENTION.

primary behavior disorders a general term applied to psychiatric disorders in children and adolescents, including habit disturbances (nail-biting, temper tantrums, enuresis), conduct disorders (vandalism, fire-setting, alcohol or drug use, sex offenses, stealing, glue-sniffing), certain neurotic symptoms (tics, somnambulism, stuttering, overactivity), and school-centered difficulties (truancy, school phobia, disruptive behavior).

primary cause a term used to identify a condition or event that predisposes a disorder which probably would not have occurred in the absence of the p.c. Sexual contact, e.g., is a common p.c. of a venereal disease.

primary circular reaction the type of repetitive action that, according to Piaget, represents the earliest nonreflexive infantile behavior; e.g., in the first months of life, a hungry baby may repeatedly attempt to put his hand in his mouth. A p.c.r. does not result in effective goal-oriented behavior, but it indicates a primitive link between goal (easing hunger) and action (attempting to suck on hand). This is sensorimotor substage 2, the first substage consisting of the activation of reflexes like sucking, swallowing, crying and moving the arms and legs. Also see SECONDARY CIRCULAR REACTION; TERTIARY CIRCULAR REACTION.

primary cognition the manner of perceiving the world in infancy when there are no ways of distinguishing between the self and the nonself. Some authors believe schizophrenia represents a regression to a state of p.c.

primary colors the basic colors from which all the various hues can be produced by mixing in different combinations. Some investigators believe human color perception involves combinations of three p.c., blue, green, and red; others contend that yellow and/or violet should be included because of findings of visual color sensitivity peaks at those wavelengths.

primary cortex a region of the cortex that is located about midway through the cytoarchitectual layers and containing cells that are highly specific in projection functions associated with sensations from particular receptors. The p.c. cells, e.g., are organized so that specific cells receive only certain tones from auditory sources or certain parts of the visual field from visual receptors.

primary cortical zone: See CORTICAL ZONES.

primary data the original experimental or observational data prior to statistical treatment and analysis.

primary degenerative dementia a syndrome of insidious onset and no specific cause, usually starting after age 65. Its principal features are a gradual, progressive loss of intellectual ability, including memory, judgment, and abstract thought, together with changes in personality and behavior, such as apathy, withdrawal, and irritability. Subtypes are **p.d.d., senile onset**, and **p.d.d., presenile onset**, each (a) **with delirium**, (b) **with delusions**, (c) **with depression**, or (d) **uncomplicated**. P.d.d. is also called **senile dementia**. See DEMENTIA. Also see ALZHEIMER'S DISEASE; PICK'S DISEASE. (DSM-III)

primary drive a species-specific drive that is unlearned, universal, and has an organic basis. Compare SECONDARY DRIVE.

primary dysmenorrhea: See DYSMENORRHEA.

primary empathy an approach in the C. Rogers system of client-centered therapy in which the therapist tries to restate to clients their thoughts, feelings, and experiences from the client's point of view.

primary environment an environment that is central in a person's life and in which personal or family interactions can be sustained, e.g., a work place or apartment. The term is similar to primary territory. Also see SECONDARY ENVIRONMENT.

primary erectile dysfunction a form of male sexual impotence characterized by a condition in which the man has never been able to achieve penile erection sufficient for heterosexual or homosexual intercourse. Also called **primary impotence**. Also see IMPOTENCE.

primary familial xanthomatosis = WOLMAN'S DISEASE.

primary gains the basic psychological benefits derived from neurotic symptoms: relief from anxiety generated by conflicting impulses or threatening experiences. Also called **paranosis; paranosic gains**. See SECONDARY GAINS. Also see TERTIARY GAINS.

primary groups face-to-face groups characterized by relatively strong, enduring, intimate, and complex relationships, e.g., a family, partnership, or long-term therapy group. P.g. are associated with mutual cooperation, problem-solving, protection, and companionship. In contrast to secondary groups, they tend to be smaller, more cohesive, and more meaningful to the individual.

primary hue an alternative term for primary color.

primary identification the first form of identification, which occurs in the oral stage of development when the infant takes the mother's breast into his mouth and regards it as part of himself. After weaning he begins to differentiate between the self and external reality. Also called **primary narcissistic identification**.

primary impotence = PRIMARY ERECTILE DYSFUNCTION.

primary integration the realization by a child that his own body is separate from the environment.

primary masochism in psychoanalysis, the first, covert, expression of the death wish, or destructive impulse, which is presumed to occur in the early narcissistic stage before the libido is directed to objects of the external world. Later it becomes a "lust of pain" as a condition for sexual gratification. Also called **erotogenic masochism**.

primary memory image = EIDETIC IMAGE.

primary mental abilities; Primary Mental Abilities Test: See PRIMARY ABILITIES.

primary mental deficiency subnormal intelligence due to genetic factors.

primary microcephaly a congenital disorder in which microcephaly is the primary, and usually the only, evidence of an anomaly of fetal development. The most common characteristic is a normal-size face combined with a small cranium. The forehead is low and narrow but recedes sharply. The back of the head is flat, and the vertex often is pointed. Mental retardation and spasticity of limbs are neurologic deficits.

primary motivation the drives related to unlearned body needs, e.g., hunger, thirst, or sex.

primary narcissism in psychoanalysis, the earliest type of self-love, in which the young child's libido is directed toward his own body and its satisfaction rather than toward the environment, or "object relations." At this stage the child forms a narcissistic ego ideal stemming from his own perfection and omnipotence arising partially out of the fact that his slightest gesture leads to satisfaction of his need for food, partially out of increasing abilities, and partially as a reaction formation to feelings of helplessness and anxiety. Compare SECONDARY NARCISSISM.

primary narcissistic identification = PRIMARY IDENTIFICATION.

primary need an unlearned need that arises out of biological processes and leads to physical satisfaction: the need for air, water, food, rest, sleep, urination, defecation, and sex. The expression primary needs is essentially equivalent to H. A. Murray's term VISCEROGENIC NEEDS. See this entry. Also see PHYSIOLOGICAL NEEDS.

primary oocyte the first stage in the development of an ovum from a cell of germinal epithelium in the ovary. The process is similar to that of the development of spermatozoa from a primordial germ cell in the male, except that instead of dividing equally, the female germ cell divides into one large primary oocyte and one small polar body. In the next stage, the step is repeated to produce a secondary oocyte and secondary polar body.

primary orgasmic dysfunction a form of female sexual insufficiency in which the woman is unable to achieve a normal sexual orgasm under any known condition of stimulation.

primary personality the original personality, as opposed to a secondary personality or secondary personalities, of a multiple-personality case.

primary physician generally, a family physician or general practitioner to whom the patient first comes for help, whatever the nature of the illness or disorder.

primary prevention in psychiatry, efforts directed to laying a firm foundation for mental health so that mental disorder will not develop. In general, three types of preventive measures are used: (a) **biological measures**, such as eugenic measures to prevent birth defects, prenatal care of the mother, obstetrical techniques designed to prevent birth injury, and health, safety, and nutritional measures during childhood, (b) **psychological measures**, including adequate mothering, approval, and encouragement, firm but kind discipline, freedom to explore, experiment, and express feelings, emotional support during periods of stress, and promotion of constructive interpersonal relations, (c) **sociological measures**, reduction of social stresses that lead to personality distortion, creation of a healthy social environment, and development of community resources that help to maintain mental health. Also see PREVENTIVE PSYCHIATRY.

primary process in psychoanalysis, unconscious mental activity in which there is free, uninhibited discharge of the instinctual, or id, impulses without regard to reality or logic. Examples are the dreams, fantasies, and magical thinking of young children, and the distorted logic, neologisms, and bizarre gestures of regressed schizophrenics. Also see PRELOGICAL THINKING.

primary-process thinking thought processes dominated by the mechanisms of the primary process, or "first phase of repression," that screens out unconscious material, such as infantile or "primordial" wishes and impulses that the schizophrenic.

primary quality a fundamental and indispensable property of an object, e.g., spatiality.

primary-reaction tendencies the characteristic ways in which individuals react to stress. The p.-r.t. appear to be constitutional since they can be observed in babies, as in cases of infants that may react to a routine change by developing a fever, experiencing sleep disturbances, or showing signs of digestive distress.

primary reinforcement in operant conditioning, a stimulus that increases the probability of a response without a need to value the value of the reinforcer; a stimulus that possesses inherent, or rewarding, characteristics, such as food. Also called **primary reinforcer**. See REINFORCEMENT; SECONDARY REINFORCEMENT.

primary repression in psychoanalysis, the mental process, or "first phase of repression," that screens out unconscious material, such as infantile or "primordial" wishes and impulses that have never become conscious, as contrasted with "repression proper" or "afterexpulsion," in which the repressed material has already been in the realm of consciousness. Also called **primal repression**. See REPRESSION.

primary sex characteristics: See SEX CHARACTERISTICS.

primary signaling system; primary signal system = FIRST SIGNALING SYSTEM.

primary social unit: See SOCIUS.

primary sociopath a term applied by some investigators to antisocial individuals who exhibit a low anxiety level and an undeveloped conscience, and who engage in criminal activities as a way of life or as a form of rebellious, egocentric behavior. Also see NEUROTIC SOCIOPATH.

primary stuttering the neuromuscular spasms and dysfluencies in the speech of young children without accompanying irrelevant movements of the face or body, and with absence of awareness or anxiety related to speaking. Also see SECONDARY STUTTERING.

primary symptoms: See FUNDAMENTAL SYMPTOMS.

primary territory in social psychology, a space controlled by and identified with a person or group who uses it exclusively and to whom it is essential, e.g., an apartment or house. The term is similar to primary environment. Also see SECONDARY TERRITORY; PROXEMICS.

primary thinking: See PRELOGICAL THINKING.

primary thought disorder a disorder primarily observed in schizophrenia, characterized by incoherent and irrelevant intellectual functions and peculiar language patterns that include bizarre syntax, neologisms, and word salad.

primary tumor a tumor located at its point of origin. The tumor may be caused by any of a number of factors, e.g., a chemical carcinogen in the environment, a carcinogenic food substance, a viral infection, exposure to sunlight, or exposure to radioactivity. Cells with a high rate of proliferation, such as those in the liver and intestinal tract, are common p.t. sites.

primidone $C_{12}H_{14}N_2O_2$—a barbituratelike drug administered in the treatment of certain convulsive disorders. It functions in a manner similar to that of phenobarbital in controlling epileptic seizures although it has only about one-tenth the potency of the barbiturate antiepileptic and often is administered as an adjunct to one of the hydantoins. P. has a formula with a barbituratelike structure; however, it is technically a pyrimidine molecule. Also see BARBITURATES.

primiparous /-mip′-/ bearing or having borne only once. The term is derived from the Latin words *prima*, "first," and *parere*, "to produce." Thus, a woman who has had only one pregnancy resulting in a child, regardless of whether it was a single or multiple birth, is identified as a **primipara** /-mip′-/, or **para I**. A woman who is pregnant for the first time is designated as a **primigravida** /-grav′-/, or **gravida I**. P. is also called **uniparous** /-nip′-/.

primitivation = PRIMITIVIZATION.

primitive in anthropology, pertaining to the earliest stage of human development, before the advent of social organization, as we know it, and usually characterized—from the Western perspective—as savage or uncivilized. In psychoanalysis, the term was used by Freud to characterize the two earliest stages in the development of the psyche: the preanimistic, in which human life is more or less directly at tne mercy of the external world, and the animistic, in which the world is populated by demons and souls which have power over external events and human life. He interpreted the latter forces as projections of man's narcissistic belief in the power of his own thought. See ANIMISM.

primitive superego according to some psychoanalysts, such as Bychowski, the primary image of the self, which at an early age instilled narcissism and grandiosity in the ego and thus compensates for the infant's feelings of weakness and passivity. According to others, such as Laforgue, the term also applies to a superego that antedates parental influences and is responsible for organizing and differentiating the cells of the fetus in accordance with hereditary factors.

primitive thinking: See PRELOGICAL THINKING.

primitivization a loss of all higher ego functions such as objective thinking, reality testing, and purposeful behavior, together with regression to the primitive stage of development characterized by magical thinking, helplessness, and emotional dependence. P. occurs primarily in traumatic neuroses in which higher functions are blocked by the overwhelming task of meeting the emergency; and in advanced schizophrenia, in which the ego breaks down and psychic energy is withdrawn from external reality and concentrated on a narcissistic fantasy life. Also called **primitivation**.

primordial /prīmôrd′ē·əl/ earliest formed, primitive, existing from the beginning, original.

primordial image as used by Jung, an archetypal idea, such as the original, unconscious mother image in the mind of the child, which Jung believed to be ultimately derived from the racial, or collective, unconscious. See ARCHETYPE.

primordial image of hero birth a concept of Jung that the unconscious contains a pregnancy dream in which the hero to be born represents and molds the individuality, or soul, of the dreamer.

primordial impulse in psychoanalysis, the first instincts, or drives, manifested in life, such as sucking and biting.

primordial nanosomia a type of dwarfism characterized by normal mental development, normal reproductive ability, and a well-proportioned dwarf body. The condition is hereditary.

primordial panic a reaction observed in some schizophrenic children who express fright and anger with disorganized motor responses similar to the startle responses of infants. Also called **elementary anxiety**.

Prinadol: See PHENAZOCINE.

Prince, Morton American psychologist, 1854–1929. P., a significant contributor to the dynamic approach, obtained his medical degree at Harvard Medical School, studied with Charcot and Janet in Paris, and returned to teach and establish a psychological clinic at Harvard University. As a result of his studies abroad, he developed a lasting interest in dissociation, which he believed was due to unconscious conflicts that split the personality apart. This in turn led to the theory that a fragmented personality could be integrated through analysis, interpretation, and hypnosis. He believed this process could best be illustrated in the treatment of multiple personality, as vividly described in his celebrated work *The Dissociation of a Personality*, 1906. See CO-CONSCIOUS PERSONALITY; DEPERSONALIZATION.

principal factors a widely-used form of factor analysis in which each factor extracts a maximum amount of variance.

principled level the level of moral reasoning in which the individual adopts principles and values that appear to have universal validity and application.

principled stage stage 6 of L. Kohlberg's seven stages of moral development. The p.s. represents the concern with individual principles, conscience, and consistent, universal, ethical standards. See POST-CONVENTIONAL LEVEL. For the seventh stage, see GURU STAGE.

principle-learning learning of the nature of the relationships that bind concepts, facts, and principles together; learning of the meaningful links or associations between facts within a larger conceptual framework.

principle of anticipatory maturation a generalization that nearly all functions of organisms can be evoked experimentally at some time prior to the normal appearance of the function, since the structures develop before they are actually needed for interaction with the environment.

principle of belongingness Thorndike's principle of learning which states that connections between items are more readily formed if the items are closely related in some way, so that one may elicit the other, e.g., "Coney" and "Island."

principle of constancy = LAW OF CONSTANCY.

principle of economy = OCCAM'S RAZOR.

principle of equipotentiality = LAW OF EQUIPOTENTIALITY.

principle of independent assortment; principle of independent segregation: See MENDELIAN MODES OF INHERITANCE.

principle of inertia a form of repetition-compulsion but with a greater emphasis on automatic action (Franz Alexander).

principle of mass action = LAW OF MASS ACTION.

principle of maximum contrast the tendency of the infant and very young child to gravitate to perceptual opposites and striking contrasts rather than subtle contrasts. Also see OBLIGATORY PERCEPTION.

principle of optimal stimulation a theory that organisms tend to learn those responses that lead to optimal stimulation or excitation. Also called **optimal-stimulation principle**.

principle of Prägnanz /preg·nänts'/ a Gestalt concept that perceptions tend to assume forms that are meaningful, stable, and complete when evaluated in the mind from sensory inputs (German *Prägnanz*, "terseness"). The principle applies not only to grouping letters into words, but grouping separate notes into melodies, and rounding out a story by supplying missing details. Also called **law of Prägnanz**. Also see CLOSURE; GOODNESS OF CONFIGURATION.

principle of primacy = PRIMACY EFFECT.

principle of recency = RECENCY EFFECT.

principle of the irresistible impulse: See IRRESISTIBLE IMPULSE.

principles transfer: See TRANSFER BY GENERALIZATION.

prior-entry law: See LAW OF PRIOR ENTRY.

prism a triangular lens with the property of bending light waves passing through it so that they are broken down into their component wave lengths in spectral order.

prisoner-of-war reactions situational personality disturbances occurring in individuals subjected to the physical and psychological strains of P.O.W. experience. The reactions vary greatly from individual to individual, but include depression due to loss of freedom and identity; personality changes such as sullen withdrawal and suspiciousness; inertia and loss of interest due to confinement and debilitating conditions; loss of ego strength; and, occasionally, death. The disturbance has been compared to the anaclitic depression observed in hospitalized and deprived children. Also called **prisoner-of-war syndrome**.

prisoner's dilemma a game situation used in social-psychological studies in which subjects must choose between competition and cooperation. It derives from a standard detective ploy (used when incriminating evidence is lacking) in which two suspects are first separated and then told that the one who confesses will go free or receive a light sentence. The prisoner may choose silence, hoping that his partner does the same (a cooperative motive) or he may confess, hoping to improve his own situation (a competitive motive). The game is used in studies investigating the motives associated with competition and cooperation.

prison neurosis: See CHRONOPHOBIA.

prison psychologist: See CORRECTIONAL PSYCHOLOGY.

prison psychosis a severe emotional disturbance precipitated by actual or anticipated incarceration. The types of disturbance vary, and in many cases are due to long-standing tendencies toward schizophrenia or paranoid reactions released by the stress of imprisonment. Symptoms include delusions of innocence, pardon, ill treatment, or persecution; periods of excitement; or rage and destructiveness. See GANSER SYNDROME.

privacy as used in psychology, "selective control of access to the self and one's group" (J. Altman, 1975) by regulation of input from others through use of barriers (doors, curtains, "Keep out" signs), and regulation of our own output in the form of communication with others. As used in psychiatry, the term refers to the right of the patient to control the amount and disposition of the information he divulges about himself.

private mental hospital a hospital for patients with mental disorders, organized and run by a group of psychiatrists and other administrators. Private mental hospitals are considerably smaller than most public mental institutions, usually have a far higher doctor-patient ratio, and generally offer specialized, intensive treatment rather than chronic care.

privates = GENITALS.

privation a lack of the necessities of life; absence of the means required to satisfy needs. In psychoanalysis, p. is the philosophy or rule which prescribes sexual abstinence on the theory that the energy of the dammed-up libido would be used to release early emotional experiences and thereby contribute to the therapeutic process. See RULE OF ABSTINENCE.

privilege in forensic psychiatry, the legal right of a patient to prevent his physician from testifying about information obtained in the course of treatment, as recognized in most states. See PRIVILEGED COMMUNICATION.

privileged communication confidential information, that is, professional information regarding a patient, which is obtained by a clinical psychologist, psychiatrist, or other physician, and cannot be divulged without the patient's consent. Also see PRIVILEGE.

p.r.n. an abbreviation used in prescriptions, meaning "as occasion arises," "as needed" (Latin *pro re nata*).

proactive inhibition interference of prior learning with subsequent learning, e.g., the study of French may in many cases interfere with learning Spanish. A similar effect, termed **proactive interference**, occurs in tests involving two or more types of stimuli, such as color discrimination and nonsense figures. During new trials the subject tends to confuse the new stimuli with those in previous trials. Compare RETROACTIVE INHIBITION.

probabilism the concept that events or sequences of events can be predicted with a high, though not perfect, degree of probability and validity on the basis of rational and empirical data. Also see STOCHASTIC.

probabilistic functionalism the view that behavior is best understood in terms of its probable success in attaining goals.

probability the degree to which an event is likely to occur as compared with alternatives. Also see TRANSITIONAL P.

probability curve a graphic representation of the expected frequency of occurrence of a variable.

probability learning a principle of choice behavior in which the probability of a response tends to approach the probability of the reinforcement.

probability table a chart or table showing the relative frequency of an occurrence under specified conditions.

probable error of the mean a statistic showing the range within which 50 percent of sample means will fall. This statistic has now been supplanted by the standard error.

proband the individual with an apparent inherited disorder who forms the baseline for the construction of a pedigree. By tracing the same or similar traits in other members of the family, the inheritance factor may be determined. Also called **index case**.

probe in psychology, a follow-up question in an interview or survey; also, as a verb, to investigate or explore in depth.

probenecid: See BENEMID.

probing in counseling, the counselor's use of direct questions intended to stimulate additional discussion with the hope of uncovering relevant information or helping the client come to a particular realization.

probing technique a short-term-memory test in which a subject is asked to recall one of a series of items.

problematic characterizing a situation or problem in which the outcome is uncertain.

problem behavior behavior that is maladjustive, destructive, or antisocial; also, behavior that is perplexing to the individual or others.

problem box a problem-solving test consisting of a box with latches, strings, or other fastenings that the subject must learn to manipulate in such a way as to get in or, in some cases, get out.

problem check list a type of self-inventory listing various personal, social, educational, or vocational problems. The individual indicates the items that apply to his or her situation.

problem child a general term for any child whose behavior either brings him into an unusual degree of conflict with others or in some way deviates from the norm. The term is nonspecific as to causes; it merely indicates a child whose difficulties are great enough to call for some form of professional evaluation and treatment.

problem drinking: See ALPHA ALCOHOLISM.

problem-oriented record a method devised by L. L. Weed for organizing a medical chart into (a) data base (standardized information on history, physical examination, mental status, etc.), (b) problem list, based on the data base, (c) treatment plan for each problem, (d) progress notes as related to the problems, and (e) discharge summary recording the patient's response to each treatment. Abbrev.: **POR**. Also called **problem-oriented medical record (POMR)**.

problem-solving behavior the step-by-step process through which we attempt to overcome difficulties and to reach a conclusion through the use of higher mental functions such as reasoning and creative thinking. John Dewey's four-stage outline (*How We Think*, 1910) in terms of motivation (or challenge), delimitation (or defining the problem), hypotheses (or tentative solutions), and testing (or verification) still holds today. It even seems to apply, though in simpler form, to animal behavior that involves the use of mazes, delayed-response techniques, or problem boxes that require pressing a lever or performing a similar act in order to receive a reward.

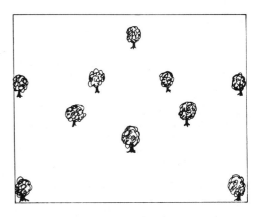

PROBLEM-SOLVING BEHAVIOR. Solution to the task of planting ten trees in five rows of four trees each. (The first step was to give up the common idea of making the five rows parallel.)

problem-solving interview in industrial psychology, a technique used on both the employee and supervisory level, in which an interview is focused on specific issues, usually of a human-relations nature, with the aim of encouraging the worker to become more sensitive to the needs and aims of fellow workers.

procaine a local anesthetic applied in solution for infiltration, nerve block, or as a spinal anesthetic. It may be used in studies of neural activity to suppress electrical excitability of an axon without affecting depolarizing processes. P. was introduced in 1905 as the first synthetic substitute for cocaine.

process analysis in evaluation research, an analytic procedure that focuses on the internal elements of an evaluation program; a qualitative approach in evaluation with emphasis on identifying ways of improving program operations and designs.

process attitude in structural psychology or in studies employing introspection, an attitude displayed by the type of observer who attends closely to subjective experience as manifested in perceptions, feelings, and thoughts while directing relatively less attention to a specific object or stimulus. Compare OBJECT ATTITUDE.

process evaluation in evaluation research, an in-house function in which the evaluator quickly moves into the situation to be evaluated, conducts the evaluation, feeds back findings to the program administrator for immediate program modification (if necessary), then repeats the process. Also called **operational evaluation**.

processing error an error that takes place during the measuring, recording, computation, or interpretation of data.

process observer in groups, the member whose role is to observe and later report on the group's functioning, e.g., an organization's secretary. A p.o. usually concentrates on goal-oriented behavior, e.g., decision-making, debate, and voting.

processomania a term introduced by Bianchi to describe a mania for litigation.

processor in information theory, any device or system that can perform specific operations on data that have been presented to it in proper quantified format.

process psychosis a chronic progressive form of schizophrenia that tends to terminate in permanent dementia. Many specialists believe there is a constitutional predisposition in these cases.

process-reactive referring to the distinction between gradual and acute onset of schizophrenia symptoms. Process schizophrenia is marked by a long-term gradual deterioration before the disease is manifest whereas reactive schizophrenia is associated with a rapid onset of symptoms after a relatively normal premorbid period.

process research the study of various psychological mechanisms or processes of psychotherapy that produce a positive prognosis.

process schizophrenia a term applied by some specialists to schizophrenic cases that begin early in life, develop gradually, and are believed to be due to endogenous factors, possibly of a constitutional nature. These patients are withdrawn (into an "inner world"), socially inadequate, and indulge in excessive fantasies, even though they have never been subjected to any special situations of stress. (The term was used prominently by some psychiatric consultants in the 1982 trial of John W. Hinckley, Jr.) Also called **nuclear schizophrenia**. Compare REACTIVE SCHIZOPHRENIA.

prochlorperazine = CARPHENAZINE.

procreational behavior any behavior pattern that is normally associated with sexual reproduction.

procreation fantasy an imagined participation in sexual reproduction. The condition is observed occasionally in women who experience a false pregnancy. A male p.f. may manifest itself as playing the role of a father who begets a famous offspring.

-proct-; -procto- a combining form relating to the anus or the rectum (from Greek *proktos*, "anus").

proctophobia a morbid fear of anything having to do with the rectum.

procursive epilepsy = DROMOLEPSY.

procyclidine: See ANTICHOLINERGICS.

prodigy the rare person who shows an extraordinary talent in one or more areas, usually at a very early age, and quite often in mathematics

or music, e.g., Pascal and Mozart. If superior endowment is the cause of their exceptional abilities, prodigies still require the opportunities to train and develop their gifts.

prodromal: See PRODROME.

prodromal myopia: See MYOPIA.

prodrome an early symptom of a mental or physical disorder that frequently serves as a warning or premonitory sign which may, in some cases, lead to preventive measures (from Greek *prodromos*, "running before"). Examples are the aura that often occurs before epileptic seizures, or the headache, fatigue, dizziness, and insidious impairment of ability that precede cerebral arteriosclerosis. Also called **prodromic phase**. Adjectives: **prodromic; prodromal**.

prodromic dream a dream that contains a warning of impending disorder. In the fourth century, Hippocrates suggested that the symptoms of illness may appear in dream symbolism long before they manifest themselves in waking life. In this century, Jung revived this concept and cited dreams he believed to be prodromic. Also see PROPHETIC DREAMS.

prodromic phase: See PRODROME.

product appeals advertising appeals directed toward a specific type of consumer personality. E.g., for a conservative family car p.a. would be directed toward married businessmen with young children, while p.a. for a foreign sports car might be directed toward younger or older men with fewer family responsibilities and a possibly suppressed desire to appear sexually attractive to women.

product image the unique identity of a product, or special brand of product, established usually by careful psychologic studies to create a receptive feeling for the product in the mind of the consumer. Coffees often are given the image of being mountain-grown in Latin America, hand-picked by experts with Hispanic names, and carefully roasted to yield a rich, warm, dark beverage, although the brand may actually contain coffees from Africa or Indonesia.

productive love according to E. Fromm, a feature of healthy individuals who are able to establish close, interdependent relationships without abridging their individuality. Respect, care, responsibility, and knowledge of the other are essential components. According to Fromm, p.l. is accomplished through active effort and is an aspect of the PRODUCTIVE ORIENTATION. See this entry.

productive memory the theory that most remembering involves reconstruction, in contrast to the idea that memory is chiefly a function of retrieval. In the process of reconstruction, it is assumed that alterations of memory occur that reflect the individual's personal and cultural background. Also see RECONSTRUCTION.

productive orientation a term applied by E. Fromm to a personality pattern in which the individual is able to develop and apply his potentialities without being unduly dependent on outside control. Such an individual is highly active in feeling, thinking, and relating to others, and at the same time retains the separateness and integrity of his own self.

productive thinking according to E. Fromm, the form or style of thinking in which a given question or issue is considered with objectivity as well as respect and concern for the problem as a whole. P.t. is a feature of the PRODUCTIVE ORIENTATION. See this entry.

productivity the capacity to produce goods and services having exchange value. Vocational rehabilitation programs use the p. of disabled patients as a major measure of the effectiveness of the programs. P. is also, according to Roger Brown, one of the three formal properties of language, consisting of the ability to combine individual words to produce an unlimited number of sentences. See SEMANTICITY.

product-moment correlation a measure of the degree of relationship between two variables, ranging from −1.00 (perfect negative relationship) through .00 (no relationship) to 1.00 (perfect positive relationship). Also called **Pearson r; Pearson p.-m.c.** Symbol: $r_{xy} = \dfrac{\Sigma_{(xy)}}{N\sigma_x\sigma_y}$.

product scale a scale of products or performance samples assigned numbered merit values, against which a product or performance can be judged.

product-testing the testing of consumer response to a new product before or after it has been offered for sale. P.-t. usually is conducted on a limited scale in certain test markets, such as Omaha, Nebraska, or Rochester, New York, which have been studied intensively as populations with known consumer characteristics. Large-scale advertising campaigns are based on results of the localized p.-t., which also may influence changes in product or package design.

proestrogenic: See PROGESTOGENS.

proestrous /prō·es′-/ the period immediately preceding estrus, a phase of cyclic sexual behavior in nonprimate female mammals.

professional-aptitude tests tests designed for use in selecting candidates for professional training by measuring the mental capacities, types of information, skill, and approaches needed for higher education and for effectiveness in such areas as medicine, law, nursing, engineering, dentistry, accounting, theology, and teaching.

professionalization the process in which professional guidelines and rules of conduct are established and enforced in a given occupation. Specific concerns focus on criteria for professional training, minimal qualifications for entrance into practice, and guidelines for fees, general business practices, and ethical relations between professional members, colleagues, and clients or patients.

professional neurasthenia a form of occupational neurosis in which the patient feels so debilitated that he cannot use the organ or organs normally required for performing his work.

Professional Standards Review Organization an organization of physicians authorized by federal law in a given region as a means of reviewing the quality of health-care services, and determining whether the in-patient services rendered are medically necessary. Abbrev.: **PSRO.** Also see PEER REVIEW.

profile a graphic representation of scores or other data by means of curves or histograms.

profile analysis a method of evaluating a person in terms of his traits judged against a set of norms or standards.

profile chart a curve uniting points that represent an individual's scores on various tests.

profoundly retarded: See IDIOCY; IDIOT; PROFOUND MENTAL RETARDATION.

profound mental retardation a diagnostic category applying to persons with IQs below 20, comprising about one percent of the retarded population. Due to sensorimotor abnormalities as well as intellectual deficit, they do not achieve more than rudimentary speech and limited self-care, and require a highly structured environment with constant aid and supervision all through life. (DSM-III)

progeria a rare familial disorder marked by premature aging, dwarfism, loss of subcutaneous fat, and birdlike features. Mental retardation is not a part of the syndrome. Many of the patients die by the age of ten to 15 of coronary-artery disease. Also called **Hutchinson-Gilford syndrome.** Also see WERNER'S DISEASE.

progeria adultorum = WERNER'S DISEASE.

progerism a premature state of resignation to old age. E.g., "a man in his fifties, who has lost all hope of attaining financial success, wards off feelings of depression or anxiety by accepting the role of the useless old man (although still in good health)" (Eidelberg, *Encyclopedia of Psychoanalysis*, 1968).

Progestasert a trademark for a medicated intrauterine device that releases small amounts of the hormone progesterone onto the endometrial lining of the uterus, thereby preventing implantation of a fertilized ovum.

progesterone the hormone of pregnancy, secreted by the corpus luteum of the ovary and carried to the uterus where it stimulates tissue changes needed for implantation of the embryo after fertilization of the ovum. It protects the embryo and enhances development of the placenta. P. also aids in the function of prolactin in preparing the mammary glands for the role of nursing the offspring.

progestin any of a group of natural or synthetic progestational agents. The term originally was used to identify a hormone produced by the corpus luteum, now called progesterone.

progestogens substances that produce physiological effects similar to those of the corpus luteum hormone progesterone. Most p. are synthetic steroids and may be derived from progesterone or testosterone. While the natural progesterone hormone has an antiestrogenic action, synthetic

p. may have different effects such as proestrogenic activity. They are used in oral contraceptives and medications for menstrual disorders.

prognosis in psychiatry and general medicine, prediction of the future course, duration, severity, and outcome of a disease or mental disorder.

prognostic test a test that forecasts the results of education or training for a specific skill.

programed instruction a learning technique used in academic, industrial, and government settings, in which the material is presented in a series of sequential, graduated steps, or **frames**. The learner is required to make a response at each step; if it is correct, it leads to the next step, and if it is incorrect, it leads to further review. Also called **programed learning**.

program evaluation in evaluation research, a process whose purpose it is (a) to contribute to decisions on installing programs; continuing, expanding, or certifying programs; and modifying programs; (b) to obtain evidence to rally support for a program or opposition to a program; and (c) to contribute to basic knowledge.

program impact in evaluation research, the effects of a program designed to produce some type of good or service, measured in terms of success or failure in achieving the goals or objectives established before the program was implemented.

program-impact evaluation in evaluation research, an assessment of the overall effectiveness of a national program in meeting its objectives, or an assessment of the relative effectiveness of two or more programs in meeting common objectives.

programing the process of feeding coded instructions into a computer which will direct it to perform a specific set of operations in language that it can read and understand. Once the computer is programed, it can repeat the same operations indefinitely. The term is also used for preparation of a sequential operation in such areas as social organization or experimental research.

progredient neurosis a form of neurosis in which the patient is unable to adopt adequate defenses or discharge his impulses, which accumulate to cause progressively severe symptoms. The patient may become increasingly withdrawn and phobic so that, e.g., a fear of travel gradually evolves into a fear of leaving the house and eventually into a fear of getting out of bed. Some cases of p.n. may stabilize for a period, then become progredient again.

progression law: See LAW OF PROGRESSION.

progressive bulbar palsy a variation of amyotrophic lateral sclerosis in which chewing, swallowing, and talking are difficult because of involvement of muscles innervated by cranial nerves and corticobulbar tracts. The nerve tracts undergo progressive degeneration, also causing inappropriate emotional responses.

progressive degenerative subcortical encephalopathy any of a group of progressive diseases of demyelination of the cerebral cortex that begin in childhood, e.g., Balo's disease, Krabbe's disease.

progressive diaphyseal dysplasia = ENGELMANN'S DISEASE.

progressive education a broad educational approach associated with John Dewey's philosophy. It includes an emphasis on experimentalism as opposed to dogmatism in teaching, "learning by doing," recognition of individual differences in the rate of learning, latitude in choosing areas of study according to interest, and a closer relationship between academic learning and experience in the world outside the classroom.

progressive infantile cerebral poliodystrophy = ALPER'S DISEASE.

progressive lipodystrophy: See LIPODYSTROPHY.

Progressive Matrices a nonverbal test of mental ability consisting of abstract designs, each of which is missing one part. The subject chooses the missing component from several alternatives in order to complete the design. Scales of different levels of difficulty are available (for children, average adults, and superior adults), but all require some degree of logic and analytic ability.

progressive-multifocal leukoencephalopathy a degenerative disease of the central nervous system marked by destruction of the white matter of the brain. Demyelination is followed by degeneration of the axon cylinders and may be extended to the cerebellum and basal ganglia. Because of its multifocal nature, p.-m.l. is characterized by a variety of ambiguous symptoms, including loss of vision and hearing, ataxia, convulsions, or laughing attacks.

progressive muscular atrophy = AMYOTROPHIC LATERAL SCLEROSIS.

progressive myopia: See MYOPIA.

progressive relaxation a technique developed by E. Jacobson in which the patient is trained to relax his entire body by becoming aware of tensions in various muscle groups, and then relaxing one muscle group at a time.

progressive spinal-muscular atrophy any of a group of related disorders that may begin in childhood or as late as the fifth decade and be characterized by skeletal-muscle atrophy associated with degeneration of nerve cells in the anterior horn of the spinal cord. The group includes **infantile p.s.-m.a.**, also known as Werdnig-Hoffmann disease, **juvenile p.s.-m.a.**, also called Wohlfart-Kugelberg-Welander disease, and **adult spinal-muscular atrophy**, or Aran-Duchenne disease. The p.s.-m.a. disorders also are related to peroneal muscular atrophy, or Charcot-Marie-Tooth disease, and amyotrophic lateral sclerosis, or Lou Gehrig's disease, which also involve muscle weakness and wasting due to denervation of the anterior horn cells. Rehabilitation efforts yield limited results in all these diseases.

progressive subcortical encephalopathy = BINSWANGER'S DISEASE.

progressive teleologic regression a term coined

by S. Arieti for the schizophrenic's purposive return to the primary-process level, in an attempt to cope with the world and a self-image that are bizarre, threatening, and frightening. The regression, however, is progressive, since it fails to accomplish its purpose and becomes more extreme and may lead to total dilapidation.

progressive total a cumulative or running total; the sum of all scores or values that have been gathered or computed up to a particular point.

prohibited behavior a behavior that usually is prohibited in any of a wide range of cultures. Examples of p.b. include incest, murder, treason, stealing, harming food, laziness, inviting bad luck, deceiving others, adultery, and assuming the prerogatives of another person. Compare COMPELLED BEHAVIOR.

projected jealousy a type of behavior in which a male or female sex partner who is unfaithful, or who represses impulses to be unfaithful, accuses the partner of being unfaithful, thereby projecting his or her own impulses.

Project Head Start = HEAD START PROJECT.

projection a defense mechanism in which unacceptable impulses are attributed to others or personal failures are blamed on others. These patterns are often used to justify prejudice or evade responsibility, and in some cases may develop into paranoid delusions in which, e.g., an individual who blames others for his problems may come to believe that they are plotting against him.

projectional paranoia the classical form of paranoia in which unacceptable feelings and impulses are projected onto others, e.g., attributing to others one's own hostility or tendency to cheat.

projection areas areas of the cerebral cortex that are associated with a particular sense organ. Each sense has two or more cortical areas where its inputs are projected. Each projection area is identified with a Roman numeral, such as Visual I, Visual II. Also see LOCALIZATION OF FUNCTION.

projection fibers nerve fibers that carry impulses between the cerebral cortex and the deeper brain structures, such as the thalamus, hypothalamus, brainstem, cerebellum, and spinal cord. The fibers are myelinated axons of neurons.

projection therapy a term sometimes applied to a form of psychotherapy in which the child plays out his problems, anxieties, and fantasies with toys of his own choosing. Some therapists participate and make interpretations, others remain on the sidelines as observers. See PLAY THERAPY.

projective device in consumer psychology, a word-association technique employed in motivation research. Key words are mixed with neutral background words and subjects are asked to make associations without being aware of which terms are the key words. Such projective devices enable advertisers to learn which words are likely to be most attractive to consumers when used in advertising copy.

projective doll play: See DOLL PLAY.

projective method = PROJECTIVE TEST.

projective play a variation of play therapy in which dolls and other toys are used by children to express their unconscious feelings, which can be helpful in diagnosing their mental disturbances.

projective psychotherapy a treatment procedure developed by M. Harrower, in which selected responses on various projective tests are "fed back" to the patient, who associates with them in much the same way that analytic patients make free associations to dreams.

projective test a personality test in which the subject reveals his characteristic traits, feelings, attitudes, and behavior patterns through responses to relatively unstructured stimuli such as ambiguous pictures, ink blots, or play materials. The method is based on the unconscious tendency of the subject to attribute his own thoughts and feelings to others, and to impose his own interpretations on what he sees. Also called **projective method; projective technique**.

projectivity a personality trait marked by the disavowal of unacceptable and feared impulses that are projected onto other persons and groups, especially weaker minority groups outside the conventional social milieu. P. was identified by Adorno and Frenkel-Brunswik as one of the traits associated with the authoritarian personality. See PROJECTION. Also see AUTHORITARIANISM.

project method a teaching method in which students work alone or together to initiate, develop, and carry through a project with a minimal amount of direct guidance from the teacher.

prolactin a hormone secreted by the anterior pituitary gland to stimulate the development and production of milk by the mammary glands. Also called **lactogenic hormone; luteotrophic hormone; mammotrophic hormone**.

prolapse the herniation or protrusion of an organ through surrounding tissues, usually because of a failure of structural tissues supporting the herniated organ. E.g., a colostomy may p. through the stoma in the abdominal wall or a uterus may p. into the vagina. Also see PTOSIS.

proliferative phase the portion of the menstrual cycle when the endometrium thickens and becomes enriched with a blood supply in anticipation of the arrival of a fertilized ovum to be implanted in the tissue. If the next ovum is not fertilized, the enriched endometrial layer is shed, resulting in the process of menstruation.

prolonged-sleep treatment: See CONTINUOUS-SLEEP THERAPY; SLEEP TREATMENT.

promazine: See ALIPHATIC PHENOTHIAZINES.

Promethean will a factor trait expressed as irreverence, aggressiveness, determination, resourcefulness, and egotism (Cattell).

promiscuity transient, casual sexual relations with a variety of partners. Behavior of this kind may be traced to such factors as a disorganized family life, parental rejection or neglect, rigid or loose parental morality, the impact of a delinquent subculture, lack of impulse control, fear of becoming involved, or psychosexual disorders such as frigidity, impotence, nymphomania, or satyriasis. Adjective: **promiscuous**.

promotion neurosis a condition occasionally associated with obsessional neurosis: The patient is unable to function when given added responsibilty or authority.

prompting method; prompts: See ANTICIPATION METHOD.

prone: See POSTURE.

pronoun reversal a speech phenomenon observed in cases of infantile autism in which a child refers to himself in the second or third person while identifying others by first person pronouns. Thus, the child may refer to himself as "you" and another person as "me."

proofreader's illusion a visual misperception in which a misspelling, omission, extra letter, transposition, or faulty syntax is overlooked, probably due to the fact that the transformation of the stimulus word into mental image relies on context and other subtle cues that may outweigh the impact of the word or phrase as literally spelled or mispelled. In other words, it is easy to miss minor errors embedded in a familiar context and to read for meaning, not words, seeing, e.g., a manuscript as it should be rather than as it actually is. For this reason a writer is said to be his own worst proofreader.

propaedeutic task a task that is used as a teaching aid, particularly in teaching the mentally retarded. A p.t. usually is a simpler form of another task, such as sorting.

propaganda an intentional effort to influence the beliefs and actions of others; deliberate persuasion primarily, though not entirely, through an appeal to emotion that is designed to win support for an idea or course of action or to belittle or disparage the ideas or programs of others. P. may be overt or covert, that is, its aim may be openly expressed or it may be hidden, especially behind a façade of "rational" argument. To **propagandize** means to engage in the various techniques of p. Also see BANDWAGON EFFECT; BRAINWASHING; CARD-STACKING; FEAR APPEAL; FLOGGING THE DEAD HORSE; GLITTERING GENERALITIES; SUGGESTION.

propaganda analysis a study of the techniques, appeals, content, and effectiveness of propaganda.

propagandize: See PROPAGANDA.

propanediols a group of anxiolytics derived from propyl alcohol with pharmacologic actions that include skeletal muscle relaxation, CNS depression, and a calming effect through interference with autonomic reactions. In addition to their use as minor tranquilizers, p. are administered for control of tremors and spasticity and in the treatment of alcoholism. The prototype p. is **meprobamate** (trademark: **Miltown**)—$C_9H_{18}N_2O_4$—which can block neuronal circuits with minimal loss of alertness. Wakefulness is maintained by sensory-feedback impulses.

Other p. include **mephenesin**—$C_{10}H_{14}O_3$—and **carisoprodol**—$C_{12}H_{24}N_2O_4$.

propanolol = PROPRANOLOL.

propensity a strong tendency or inclination toward a certain action or type of behavior, arising out of habit or hereditary predisposition.

Propfschizophrenia = PFROPFSCHIZOPHRENIA.

prophetic dreams dreams alleged to predict future events, as in warning of a natural catastrophe or invasion by an enemy. P.d. are found in the religious writings of the Egyptians, Assyrians, Hebrews, Muslims, and Greeks. Jung felt that "dreams can be anticipations, irrational experiences, even telepathic visions" which throw light on the influence of the collective unconscious on the future behavior of the individual; and W. Stekel used symbolic-dream material in forecasting the wishes of the dreamer. Also see PRODROMIC DREAM.

prophylactic = CONDOM.

prophylactic maintenance the administration of drugs that tend to prevent or reduce the risk of recurrence of symptoms of a disorder. Methysergide is used in p.m. of migraine headaches; lithium may be administered as part of the p.m. regimen for manic-depressive disorders.

prophylaxis the use of systematic preventive methods in avoiding disease or disorder, either mental or physical.

propinquity the nearness of two or more people to each other. In environmental psychology, p. is associated with group territorial behavior. E.g., the closest social contacts identified by persons interviewed usually are people who live in the same neighborhood, or even in the same apartment building. Also see PROXEMICS.

proposita: See PROPOSITUS.

proposition a statement put forward for acceptance or rejection; a proposal or scheme to be acted upon. In grammar, a p. is a sentence or part of a sentence that contains an assertion or declaration about the subject, that is, one subject plus one predicate. Also see VERBAL P.

propulsion gait a type of gait observed in parkinsonism patients, marked by short, shuffling steps that begin slowly but increase in rapidity while the body leans forward to maintain balance.

propositus a male proband or index case. The female counterpart is called a **proposita**.

propoxyphene: See SYNTHETIC NARCOTICS.

propranolol $C_{16}H_{21}NO_2$—a beta-adrenergic blocking drug derived as a substituted propylamine rather than as an ethylamine product like other beta-adrenergic blockers. P. is more potent than the ethylamine derivatives and has virtually no beta-stimulant activity of its own. P. is used primarily in the control of heart arrythmias and some forms of aortic stenosis. P. is unique in its ability to alter the electrical activity of cardiac cell membranes, which appears to account for the antiarrhythmic effect. Also called **propanolol**.

propriate striving G. W. Allport's final stage in the development of the proprium, or self, emerging in adolescence with the search for identity. P.s. includes the experimentation common to adolescents before making long-range commitments. Because Allport believed in the independence of adult motivation, in contrast to childhood motivation, adolescence is considered especially significant as the time when conscious intentions and future-oriented planning begin to motivate the personality. See FUNCTIONAL AUTONOMY; PROPRIUM.

proprietary drug any chemical used for medicinal purposes that is formulated or manufactured under a name that is protected from competition by trademark, also through patent or secret process. The ingredients, however, may be components of generic drugs that have the same or similar effects. See TRADEMARK.

proprioception the sense of body movement and position; the reception of stimuli from nerve endings or organs located in the muscles, tendons, and joints and the labyrinth of the ear. The sensations are mediated by the fifth cranial nerve and enable the body without visual clues to determine its spatial orientation through effects of changes in muscle tension or muscle stretching as body positions change, coupled with the labyrinthine stimuli which react to gravitational changes. Also called **proprioceptive sensation**.

proprioceptor a receptor sensitive to body and position movement including motion of the limbs. See PROPRIOCEPTION.

proprium G. W. Allport's term for the self; that which is consistent, unique, and central in the individual. The p. incorporates body sense, self-identity, self-esteem, self-extension, rational thinking, self-image, propriate striving, and knowing. It develops from infancy through adolescence and seven cumulative stages. Development at each stage rests on the achievements of earlier stages. However, the mature p. is far more than an echo of the past; it is an integrated biosocial entity with its own aims and motives.

proptriptyline hydrochloride: See TRICYCLIC ANTIDEPRESSANTS.

prosencephalon = FOREBRAIN.

prosocial aggression any act of aggression that has socially constructive and desirable consequences, as in intervening to prevent a holdup or rape, or demonstrating against nuclear weapons. See AGGRESSION. Compare ANTISOCIAL AGGRESSION.

prosocial behavior any act, deed, or behavioral pattern that is socially constructive or in some way beneficial to another person or group. The term applies to a broad range of behavior including simple everyday acts, e.g., providing assistance to an elderly person crossing the street. Compare ANTISOCIAL BEHAVIOR.

prosopagnosia an inability to recognize faces. In some cases it is a congenital condition, in others a result of brain injury or disease. See AGNOSIA.

prospective research research that is planned well in advance, often making use of controls and other features of good experimental design. Also see RETROSPECTIVE RESEARCH; EX POST FACTO RESEARCH.

prostaglandins a group of chemically related substances that occur naturally in the tissue cells of humans and other organisms. P. occur in four basic types, designated by the letters A, B, E, and F, with subscripts $_1$, $_2$, and $_3$, to indicate the degree of saturation of fatty-acid side chains. Through stimulation, vasodepression, and other functions, P. affect mainly smooth-muscle tissues of reproductive organs and other body systems such as the gastrointestinal, cardiovascular, nervous, and respiratory systems.

prostatectomy the surgical removal of a part or all of the prostate gland. P. may be performed through an abdominal or perineal incision, or by transurethral resection in which prostate tissue is removed via the urethra. P. usually is performed because of cancer or prostatic hypertrophy that results in blockage of normal urinary flow.

prostate gland a walnut-size male reproductive organ that surrounds the urethra immediately beneath the urinary bladder. The p.g. secretes a thin alkaline fluid that increases in volume during sexual stimulation and becomes a part of semen during ejaculation. In the absence of sexual activity, excess p.g. fluid is excreted in the urine.

prosthetist a health professional who makes and fits artificial limbs for amputees, as distinguished from an **orthotist**, who makes and fits braces for orthopedic patients.

prostitution a sex service that is based on the payment of money or exchange of other property or valuables. P. applies to heterosexual or homosexual services, performed by male or female prostitutes, professional or nonprofessional prostitutes. The sex service may be simple coitus or performance of acts leading to gratification of paraphilias. Also see MALE HOMOSEXUAL P.

protanomaly a kind of red-color blindness in which the red-sensitive retinal receptor does not function normally although there is evidence that some red sensitivity is present.

protanopia a type of color-blindness in which the loss of color perception is in the red area of the spectrum. The cause of the visual malfunction may be a deficiency of red receptors in the retina or the absence of a receptor process required for normal perception of red. The term may be used to distinguish a complete lack of red-color vision from a deficient red-color vision, or protanomaly.

protein deficiency lack of a normal quantity of proteins, particularly complete proteins, in the diet or body tissues. Complete proteins contain the essential amino acids, which must be acquired from the external environment in meals since they cannot be synthesized by the body's own chemistry. In addition to the need for certain amino acids for basic structural and functional processes, several amino acids are required for learning and other mental activities. These include glutamic acid, lysine, and cystine. P.d. also may occur as a result of a lack of carbohydrates or fats in the diet, a condition that causes the body to consume its own proteins as a source of energy. If the self-digestion process of protein-burning is not controlled, irreversible damage to vital organs results. Also see KWASHIORKOR.

protein hunger a preference for protein or other amino-acid sources exhibited in experimental animals on various deficiency diets. E.g., when an amino-acid solution in a rat diet is diluted, the animal increases its intake of the diluted protein source until the deficiency has been compensated. Even when the amino acids are made less palatable by the addition of quinine, the animal consumes the needed amount.

protein synthesis the production of a protein molecule by combining certain amino acids in a particular sequence. Information for p.s. is contained in genetic material in an individual's DNA. The p.s. process is performed in specialized tissue cells, such as cells of the liver.

protein-synthesis inhibitors substances that interfere with the normal production of proteins and thus presumably retard learning ability if long-term memory involves storage of learning experiences in protein molecules. P.-s.i. may include sedative-hypnotic and tranquilizing drugs, which seem to cause learning deficits.

protension Cattell's term for a personality trait consisting of jealousy, suspicion, and rigidity in defense.

protest psychosis a brief reactive psychosis observed among black persons charged with aggressive crimes. Onset is abrupt and the symptoms resemble those of some forms of schizophrenia: mutism, bizarre speech and mannerisms, incoherence, auditory or visual hallucinations. The term p.p. is used because the manifestations often include ideology of Muslim or African origin and hostility to whites.

-proto- a combining form meaning first, early, primitive, preceding.

protocol the original notes of a case, study, or experiment recorded during or immediately after a particular session or trial. In psychiatry, p. may refer to a case history and workup. The term may also refer to any account or transcript of a subject's thoughts, feelings, or ideas as verbally reported.

proton-beam radiography a device or process of producing a radiogram, or photographic image, by directing a beam of protons, the positively charged elementary particles of atoms, through an organ or area of tissue to be studied or examined. Also called **heavy-particle radiography**.

proton irradiation the use of radioactive particles that consist of the nuclear fragments of disintegrating atoms and are capable of penetrating living tissue to produce therapeutic or other changes. P.i. may be produced by the decay of uranium atoms, which release two protons and two neutrons per atom.

protopathic system a subsystem of the somatosensory system. The p.s. carries fibers from receptors for cold, warmth, pain, and crude applications of touch. (The term protopathic denotes primary sensitivity.) Also see EPICRITIC SYSTEM; EPICRITIC SENSATION.

protophallic phase a term applied by Ernest Jones to a presumptive first phallic stage in which the child assumes that "the rest of the world is built like itself and has a satisfactory [sex] organ— penis or clitoris—as the case may be." The term is rarely used today. See DEUTEROPHALLIC PHASE.

protoplasm a complex semifluid substance which is the living matter of all plant and animal cells and tissues. Also see CYTOPLASM.

protopsyche a term applied by Ferenczi to a primitive stage of development to which the psyche regresses when it makes the "puzzling leap" from the mental to the somatic that occurs when conversion symptoms develop.

prototaxic mode a term applied by H. S. Sullivan to chaotic, undifferentiated, fleeting, and uncommunicable mental states that occur in the infantile period when self-awareness and concepts of time and space are lacking.

prototheory an incomplete, untested theory or initial working hypothesis. The term is sometimes used to characterize an explanation offered as a justification of a clinical strategy.

proverb test a verbal test in which the subject attempts to explain the meaning of proverbs.

provisional try the trial-and-error behavior of an animal engaged in a problem situation such as a maze in which alternate pathways are tried out in the process of finding the correct course. Humans often engage in similar behavior when faced with problems.

proxemics in social psychology, the study of interpersonal spatial behavior. P. is concerned with territoriality, interpersonal distance, spatial arrangements, crowding, and other aspects of physical environment that affect behavior, such as an inquiry as to whether areas with high population density have a greater incidence of mental illness than other areas. See BODY BUFFER ZONE; BUBBLE CONCEPT OF PERSONAL SPACE; CIGARETTE-SMOKE POLLUTION; CROWDING; DISTANCE ZONES; ETHOLOGICAL MODELS OF PERSONAL SPACE; GROUP SPACE; INSIDE DENSITY; INTERACTION TERRITORY; INTERPERSONAL DISTANCE; INTIMATE ZONE; OPTIMAL INTERPERSONAL DISTANCE; OUTSIDE DENSITY; PERSONAL-DISTANCE ZONE; PERSONAL SPACE; PERSONAL-SPACE INVASION; PRIMARY TERRITORY; PROPINQUITY; PUBLIC-DISTANCE ZONE; PUBLIC TERRITORY; SECONDARY TERRITORY; SOCIAL DISTANCE; SOCIAL ZONE; SOCIOFUGAL SPACE; SOCIOMETRIC DISTANCE; SOCIOPETAL SPACE; TERRITORIALITY.

proximal nearer, or closer. E.g., one part of an organ or organism is p. (closer) to the center than other parts. Compare DISTAL.

proximal receptors sense-organ receptors that detect stimuli that are in direct or near-direct contact with the body, e.g., taste and touch.

proximal response a response that occurs in or on the boundary of an organism, specifically, a glandular reaction or muscular activity. See DISTAL RESPONSE.

proximal stimulus the changes in or the activity of a sense organ in contrast to the distal stimulus, the object or energy that causes this activity to take place. In reading, e.g., p.s. refers to the chemical changes occurring in the retina whereas the distal stimulus is the light energy reflected by the print.

proximity principle the Gestalt principle which states that objects or stimuli that are close together will be perceived as a unity. E.g., a series of notes become a melody, and a series of unconnected lines in a neon sign become a word or sentence. Also called **law of proximity**.

proximodistal development the progression of physical and motor development from the center of the organism toward the periphery. E.g., the child learns to control shoulder movements before he controls arm and finger movements.

prudery the quality of being excessively modest or priggish, particularly in sexual matters.

pruritus /prŏŏrī′təs/ an itching dermatitis due to sensory-nerve irritation and resulting from organic or functioning conditions. Also see PSYCHOGENIC P.

PSE = PRESENT STATE EXAMINATION.

psellism /sel′-/ a term for stammering, stuttering, or other speech defects, e.g., indistinct or faulty pronunciation (from Greek *psellisma*, "stammer").

-pseud-; -pseudo- /-sŏŏd-/ a combining form meaning false, spurious, falsely imitating.

pseudesthesia = PSEUDOESTHESIA.

pseudoachondroplastic spondyloepiphysial dysplasia a type of dwarfism characterized by a normal shape and size of the head, a relatively normal trunk, and abnormally short arms and legs. Abbrev.: **PAD**. See BONE DISEASE; DWARFISM.

pseudoaffective behavior a response to a stimulus in which the reaction is influenced or controlled by experimental lesions of the cortex, and therefore may not represent a true, natural reaction. Also see SHAM RAGE.

pseudoaggression a neurotic reaction in which masochistic tendencies are denied by transforming them into aggression toward others. Also see REVERSAL.

pseudoamok syndrome a syndrome, probably hysterical in nature, in which all the symptoms observed in amok are simulated—withdrawal, brooding, sudden emotional outburst—except that the patients do not hurt anyone, and meekly give themselves up when cornered. See AMOK.

pseudoanhedonia a common psychiatric reaction among the aged, especially those suffering from chronic brain syndrome. These patients act as if "Nothing matters; just leave me alone," whereas they are actually acting out of a variety of motives such as resistance to pressure, punishment of others for their own deficiencies, self-punishment, and a bid for sympathy.

pseudochondroplasia: See BONE DISEASE.

pseudochromesthesia a color sensation that is experienced when hearing a tone.

pseudocollusion as defined by Freedman, Kaplan, and Sadock, a "sense of closeness, relationship or cooperation that is not real but is based on transference" (*Comprehensive Textbook of Psychiatry*, 1980). See TRANSFERENCE.

pseudocommunication distorted attempts at communication, or vestiges of communication in the form of fragments of words, apparently meaningless sounds, and unfathomable gestures. The condition is characteristic of hebephrenic (disorganized) schizophrenia.

pseudocommunity a term applied by N. Cameron to a paranoid delusion in which a group of real or imagined persons are believed to be organized for the purpose of conspiring against the patient.

pseudoconditioning elicitation of a response to a previously neutral stimulus when it is presented following a series of conditioned stimuli; e.g., if the fire siren sounds three times in one day, the first two sounds may not produce a reaction, but the third is almost certain to have an effect. The response is probably a form of sensitization and not conditioning, because there is no pairing of a new stimulus with an old stimulus. Also called **false conditioning**.

pseudoconversation a form of egocentric, unsocialized speech (sometimes called a "collective monologue") in which two- or three-year-old children talk without endeavoring to communicate with others or to share or exchange ideas with them.

pseudoconvulsion a type of seizure associated with hysteria in which the subject may collapse and experience muscular contractions, although other signs, such as pupillary signs, loss of consciousness, and amnesia are not observed. A p. may be a conscious or unconscious act intended to gain sympathy.

pseudocopulation bodily contact between a male and female with liberation of gametes but without actual sexual union.

pseudocyesis = FALSE PREGNANCY.

pseudodebility = PSEUDOIMBECILITY.

pseudodementia a condition in which the patient has developed his capacities to a normal degree but suddenly appears to deteriorate, without physical impairment, and acts as if he were retarded. He is usually unable to answer the simplest questions or give a coherent account of himself. The condition may occur, reversibly, in depression, or manifest itself in hysterical form.

See HYSTERICAL P.; HYSTERICAL PUERILISM; GANSER SYNDROME.

pseudoepilepsy = PSEUDOSEIZURE.

pseudoesthesia an illusionary sensation, e.g., a feeling of irritation in a limb that has been amputated. Also called **pseudesthesia**. See PHANTOM LIMB.

pseudofamily a foster family or other substitute for a biological family, which tends to the needs of an infant or child.

pseudofeeblemindedness = PSEUDORETARDATION.

pseudogeusia a taste sensation that is not appropriate to the stimulus or a taste sensation that occurs without a stimulus, that is, a false perception of taste.

pseudogiftedness an apparent talent in a child that develops not from any inborn ability or motivation but rather from an ability to imitate others.

pseudohallucination a vivid hallucination, usually visual, which the individual recognizes as hallucinatory and pathological. P. is observed primarily in schizophrenia and organic psychosis, and is considered a step toward a true hallucination.

pseudohermaphroditism a form of hermaphroditism caused by a hormonal disturbance, e.g., adrenal virilism in females resulting in a large hooded clitoris, fusion of the labia, and changes in the voice and hair distribution. The same hormonal abnormality in males results in precocious puberty. Another form of p. may occur in animals after injecting pregnant females with male hormones in an effort to produce female offspring with male characteristics.

pseudohomosexuality aspects of homosexual behavior that are not specifically sex-oriented. P. factors can include feelings of isolation, loneliness, insecurity, and not being fully accepted by society. Also see SITUATIONAL HOMOSEXUALITY.

pseudohydrocephalus: See SILVER-RUSSELL SYNDROME.

pseudohydrophobia: See CYNOPHOBIA.

pseudohypertrophic muscular dystrophy: See DUCHENNE'S P.M.D.

pseudohypoparathyroidism a condition resembling hypoparathyroidism, but failing to respond to parathyroid hormone treatment. Patients have a round face and thick-set figure, and seem to have impaired senses of smell and taste. In most cases they are mildly to moderately retarded. The disease is believed to be due to a genetic defect that blocks normal response to parathyroid hormone by receptor tissues. Also called **Albright's hereditary osteodystrophy**.

pseudoidentification a defense mechanism in which the individual adopts the opinions of others in order to protect himself against attack or criticism. If challenged, he maintains that he knows his own mind but only pretends to agree with other people; therefore the identification is termed pseudo, or false.

pseudoimbecility consciously or unconsciously simulated mental defect, as opposed to actual mental retardation; a neurotic pattern in which a child or infantile adult uses the appearance of stupidity as a defense against anxiety, as an escape from retaliation for aggression (a stupid person is not punished), or in some cases as a means of satisfying sexual curiosity (being allowed to watch parental intercourse, since he or she would not understand what is going on). Also called **pseudodebility**. See PSEUDORETARDATION.

pseudoindependent personality an individual who presents a façade of extreme independence, self-reliance, and aggressive self-assertion, but who harbors, and denies, strong underlying dependent needs such as the need to be cared for and supported by others.

pseudoinsomnia a complaint of insomnia by a patient who actually sleeps an adequate number of hours. The reason for the complaint is often obscure, and may involve a subtle misperception of sleep or the use of the complaint as a symptom when the patient is anxious or depressed.

pseudoisochromatic charts a set of color plates used for testing color vision.

pseudolalia the production of meaningless speech sounds.

pseudologia fantastica a clinical syndrome characterized by elaborate fabrications which are usually concocted to impress others, get out of a tight situation, or give the individual an ego lift. Unlike confabulations, these fantasies are believed only momentarily and are dropped as soon as they are contradicted by evidence. Typical examples are the "tall tales" told by sociopaths, though the symptom is also found in neuroses and psychoses.

pseudomania a mental state in which the person exhibits a shame psychosis by accusing himself of committing crimes of which he actually is innocent.

pseudomature syndrome a pattern occasionally found in children around ten years of age who behave in a semimature manner by taking over some of the responsibilities of the home. This occurs most clearly in children of alcoholic or psychotic parents, and in children with a disabled brother or sister.

pseudomemory a false memory, such as a spurious recollection of events that never took place. At one time p. was called **pseudomnesia**. See PARAMNESIA.

pseudomental deficiency = PSEUDORETARDATION.

pseudomnesia = PSEUDOMEMORY.

pseudomotivations a term introduced by Bleuler for the reasons some patients create after the fact to justify earlier behavior. The patient, usually a schizophrenic, may or may not be aware of the inconsistencies in the excuse, or may be indifferent to them.

pseudomutuality a family relationship that has a superficial appearance of mutuality, openness, and understanding although in fact the relationship is rigid and depersonalizing. Investigators have found that schizophrenic relationships often exhibit p.

pseudoneurotic schizophrenia a type of schizophrenia characterized by all-pervasive anxiety (pan-anxiety) and a wide variety of neurotic symptoms (pan-neurosis), but with underlying psychotic tendencies (autistic withdrawal, inappropriate emotional responses, anhedonia, subtle thought disturbances) which at times develop into brief psychotic episodes termed **micropsychoses**.

pseudonomania an abnormal urge to lie or falsify information.

pseudoparkinsonism: See PARKINSONISM.

pseudopersonality a fictitious characterization contrived by a subject in an effort to conceal facts about the true self from other persons. E.g., a prostitute may contrive a p. for business reasons and to maintain a certain amount of anonymity. The p. usually evolves into a character defense and is treated as such by the therapist.

pseudophone an instrument used in studying the localization of sound. The p. diverts to the left ear those sounds that would normally enter the right ear, and vice versa.

pseudoprecocious puberty: See PRECOCIOUS PUBERTY.

pseudoprodigy an individual who develops an exceptionally high degree of skill or knowledge usually at an early age, primarily as a result of overtraining by overzealous parents or teachers.

pseudopsychology an approach to psychology that utilizes unscientific or fraudulent methods, e.g., palmistry, phrenology, physiognomy, or biorhythm. Also see PSEUDOSCIENCE.

pseudopsychopathic schizophrenia a type of schizophrenia in which psychotic tendencies are masked or overlaid by antisocial tendencies such as pathological lying, sexual deviations, and violent or other uninhibited behavior.

pseudoreminiscence: See CONFABULATION.

pseudoretardation retarded intellectual development due to adverse cultural or psychological conditions rather than congenital mental deficiency. Among these conditions are maternal deprivation, intellectual impoverishment, severe emotional disturbance, and perceptual deficits. Also called **pseudomental deficiency; pseudofeeblemindedness**. Also see PSEUDODEMENTIA; SIX-HOUR RETARDED CHILD.

pseudoschizophrenias: See ACUTE DELUSIONAL PSYCHOSIS.

pseudoschizophrenic neurosis a term introduced by M. Roth for a phobic anxiety-depersonalization neurosis, a form of mixed neurosis, which some consider an endogenous depression and others a temporal-lobe or limbic-system disorder.

pseudoscience a system of theories and methods that claims falsely to be scientific or that is falsely regarded as scientific. For examples and related entries, see ASTROLOGY; BIORHYTHMS; CHARACTEROLOGY; CLAIRVOYANCE; DIANETICS; DOWSING; EXORCISM; EXTRASENSORY PERCEPTION; MEDIUM; NUMEROLOGY; OBSCURANTISM; OCCULT; ORGONOMY; OUIJA BOARD; OUT-OF-BODY EXPERIENCE; PALMISTRY; PARAPSYCHOLOGY; PHRENOLOGY; PHYSIOGNOMY; POLTERGEIST; PRECOGNITION; PSEUDOPSYCHOLOGY; PSI; PSYCHOKINESIS; SEANCE; SUPERSTITION; TELEPATHY.

pseudoscope an optical instrument designed to create visual illusions by transposing images between the left and right eyes and inverting distance relations so that solid objects appear hollow and hollow objects solid.

pseudoseizure a seizure that has the outward appearance of an epileptic attack but lacks the clinical characteristics of a true epileptic seizure, such as EEG dysrhythmia. Moreover, the patient can suddenly end the seizure on command or when it is ignored by observers. Also called **pseudoepilepsy**.

pseudosenility an acute, reversible confusional state or depression in the elderly resulting from such factors as drug effects, malnutrition, diminished cardiac output, fever, alcoholism, intracranial tumor, an unreported fall, or a metabolic disturbance.

pseudotrisomy 18 a congenital disorder, believed to be due to an autosomal-recessive trait, marked by the same general anomalies found in chromosome-18-trisomy patients. However, chromosome studies of the patients have failed to show signs of chromosome-18 trisomy, translocation, or other abnormalities. All of the patients observed have been mentally retarded. See CHROMOSOME-18 TRISOMY.

psi /sī/ 23rd letter of the Greek alphabet (ψ, ψ).

psi /sī/ denoting unspecified mental functions believed to be involved in telepathy and other parapsychological processes which at this time defy scientific explanation. The term is usually explained as an abbreviation of psychic.

psilocin; psilocybin: See PSYCHEDELICS; TRYPTAMINE DERIVATIVES.

psittacism /sit'-/ a form of neologism that is completely lacking in content.

psopholalia /sof-/ infantile babbling; incomprehensible speech.

psoriatic arthritis: See ARTHRITIS.

PSP = POSTSYNAPTIC POTENTIAL.

PSRO = PROFESSIONAL STANDARDS REVIEW ORGANIZATION.

psychagogy a method of reeducational psychotherapy that emphasizes the relationship of the patient to the environment, particularly the social environment.

psychalgalia; psychalgia = PSYCHIC PAIN.

psychasthenia literally, weakness of the mind; a term applied by Janet to a type of neurosis characterized by anxiety states, phobias, obsessions, and compulsions, all of which he attributed to lack of conscious control which he believed occurs when our "psychic tension" or energy is diminished by constitutional deficiency, fatigue, stress, or internal conflict. The term is obsolete.

psychataxia a form of mental confusion in which the patient is unable to make a sustained mental effort or maintain attention.

psyche /sīk′ē/ in psychology and psychiatry, the mind in its totality, as distinguished from the physical organism; also, the self, or soul. The term is Greek, meaning breath and, by way of extension, life, spirit, human soul, mind (also see -PSYCHRO-).

psychedelic experience reactions to hallucinogenic or other mind-altering drugs, including bizarre images, distorted perceptions, visual hallucinations, terrifying visions, time expansion or contraction, synesthesias, alternating with periods of kaleidoscopic colors, feelings of oneness with the universe, and transcendental ecstasy. Similar experiences have been known to occur without the use of drugs.

psychedelics drugs that are capable of producing altered states of awareness, which may be marked by an unstable flow of ideation and affect, distorted perception, hallucinations, or symptoms that mimic signs of mental disturbances observed in psychotic patients. The term psychedelic (from Greek *psyche* and *delos*, "visible, manifest") was coined by Humphry Osmond in 1956 in a letter to his friend Aldous Huxley ("To fall in Hell or soar angelic, you'll need a pinch of psychedelic," in response to Huxley's proposed coinage "phanerothyme"). Some investigators disagree on the scope of drugs that warrant classification as p., suggesting, e.g., that **tetrahydrocannabinols** (marijuana, hashish)—$C_{21}H_{30}O_2$—are actually sedatives while amphetamine-derived substances, e.g., **methyldimethoxyamphetamine (DOM, STP)**—$C_{12}H_{22}NO_2$—should be identified as stimulants, despite their mind-altering effects. Among the designated categories of "true" p. are the substituted indole alkylamines, which include **lysergic acid diethylamide (LSD)**—$C_{20}H_{25}N_3O$, **lysergic acid amide** (from morning-glory seeds)—$C_{16}H_{17}N_3O$, BUFOTENINE (see this entry), **psilocin**—$C_{12}H_{16}N_2O$, **psilocybin**—$C_{12}H_{17}N_2O_4P$, and **diethyltryptamine**—$C_{14}H_{19}N_2$, some of which may also be classified as indole derivatives or **tryptamines**, according to chemical or pharmacologic designations. Substituted phenyl alkylamines include **mescaline**—$C_{11}H_{17}NO_3$, methyldimethoxyamphetamine (see above), and **methylenedioxy-5-methoxyphenylisopropylamine**—$C_{10}H_{16}NO_3$, which is ten times as potent as mescaline. The phenylcyclohexyl-derivatives category has on important psychedelic member, PHENCYCLIDINE (see this entry). Miscellaneous p. include AMYL NITRITE, BENACTYZINE (see these entries), **benzene**—C_6H_6, **carbon tetrachloride**—CCl_4, **phenylcyclopentylglycolate** (trademark: **Ditran**)—$C_{20}H_{29}NO_3$, **muscarine**—$C_9H_{20}NO_2$, **myristic acid**—$C_{14}H_{28}O_2$, **naphtha**—$C_{10}H_8$, **nitrous oxide**—N_2O, and **toluol**—C_7H_8. Also see HASHISH; CARBON-TETRACHLORIDE POISONING; PHENYLETHYLAMINE DERIVATIVES; PHENYLCYCLOHEXYL DERIVATIVES; TRYPTAMINE DERIVATIVES; PSYCHOTOMIMETICS; LSD PSYCHOTHERAPY; PSY-

CHOTOGENS; PHENYL ALKYLAMINES; ERGOT ALKALOIDS.

psychedelic therapy the use of psychedelic drugs in the treatment of some types of mental or physical illness. P.t. has been used in Europe in the treatment of alcoholism and autism, and to ease the suffering of terminally ill patients.

psychelytic a term that means literally mind releasing or mind-loosening and is used to identify certain substances, such as psychedelic drugs, that have an effect on mental and emotional processes.

psychergograph an apparatus that presents a stimulus for discrimination as soon as the subject makes a correct response to the preceding stimulus. Also called **serial discriminator**.

psycherhexic a term sometimes used to describe drugs that are psychotropic or psychedelic.

psychiatric aide a trained individual who tends to the personal needs of psychiatric patients, providing physical care (dressing, bathing, feeding) when they require it, and psychological care when they need companionship, understanding, and encouragement, as well as a calming influence if they become overwrought. Since psychiatric aides are in more direct and continuous contact with the patients than any other member of the psychiatric team, the aides of today play a crucial part in the "therapeutic community" of the hospital, and can often contribute information and insight of great value to the psychiatrist and other staff members. Their role is therefore more professional than that of the old-time attendant.

psychiatric anaphylaxis: See ANAPHYLAXIS.

psychiatric classification the grouping of mental disorders into diagnostic categories, as in DSM-I, DSM-II, and DSM-III. Also called **psychiatric nosology**. See DSM-III.

psychiatric consultation a process in which the psychiatrist functions as a specialist, giving advice, information, or guidance to the attending physician (**patient-oriented consultation**), to one or more colleagues (**colleague-centered consultation**), to an entire agency or organization (**agency-centered consultation**), or to the non-psychiatric units of a general hospital (liaison psychiatry). All these functions fall within consultation psychiatry. Also see CONSULTATION-LIAISON PSYCHIATRY.

psychiatric diagnosis: See CLINICAL DIAGNOSIS.

psychiatric disability chronic loss or impairment of function due to a mental disorder, resulting in a severe handicap in meeting the demands of life.

psychiatric disorder = MENTAL DISORDER.

psychiatric emergency a situation in which immediate psychiatric care is required, as in a suicidal attempt, an acute psychotic break, a panic attack, a state of furor, an amnesic episode, a natural or man-made disaster, or a sudden loss of control (explosive disorder).

psychiatric epidemic a term sometimes applied to instances of mass hysteria, such as dancing mania and biting mania, which sweep through an entire population. See MASS HYSTERIA.

psychiatric epidemiology the study of the incidence, distribution, and techniques for controlling mental disorders in a given population. See EPIDEMIOLOGY.

psychiatric examination a comprehensive evaluation, or diagnostic formulation, of an individual from a psychiatric point of view, for such purposes as clarification of the symptom picture, at least a tentative understanding of the development and dynamics of the individual's disorder, classification for treatment purposes, formulation of a tentative treatment plan, and prognosis. The examination includes a clinical interview, history-taking, medical examination, and administration of psychological tests as needed.

psychiatric history information gathered by a psychiatric social worker, psychiatrist, or psychologist from members of the patient's family or from the patient himself, including such data as age, sex, marital status; an account of the general nature and development of the disorder; the patient's conception of his illness, the family history in terms of hereditary conditions, child-rearing methods, sibling relationships, parental relationships, and environmental factors; the developmental history of the patient; and a description of his personality tendencies, attitudes, interests, and interpersonal relationships. Also see ANAMNESIS.

psychiatric hospital = MENTAL HOSPITAL.

psychiatric illness = MENTAL DISORDER.

psychiatric interview a general term for any one-to-one session with a psychiatrist for diagnostic or therapeutic purposes. H. S. Sullivan applied the term to a four-stage therapeutic interview consisting of (a) formal inception, in which the therapist quietly observes the patient as he explains why he is seeking help, (b) reconnaissance, in which the therapist questions the patient about himself and his family, (c) detailed inquiry, in which periods of acute anxiety in the patient's life are closely examined in order to reveal characteristic "security operations," and to formulate and test hypotheses regarding his problems, and (d) termination, in which the whole process is summarized in terms of the patient's past and future interpersonal relationships.

psychiatric nosology = PSYCHIATRIC CLASSIFICATION.

psychiatric nurse a registered nurse, usually with a master's degree, who has received special training in psychiatry, and generally works in a hospital setting supervising the administration of medication, giving supportive and sometimes group therapy, participating in staff conferences, discharging administrative responsibilities, and assisting the psychiatrist in applying electroshock and other treatments.

psychiatric rehabilitation the process of restoring mental patients to full, active participation in the community. In a hospital organized as a thera-

peutic community, this process starts before they are fully recovered, and consists of activity programs, patient government, and discussion groups aimed at preparing them for a constructive, independent life. After discharge from residential treatment, transitional facilities provide aftercare programs, the Federal-State rehabilitation system comes into play, and readjustment to the community is achieved with the aid of vocational counselors, employment specialists, and social workers.

psychiatric screening: See SCREENING.

psychiatric services diagnostic, therapeutic, and prophylactic services offered in a variety of settings, including general hospitals, colleges, adult homes, health-related facilities (HRFs), skilled-nursing facilities (SNFs), intermediate-care facilities, halfway houses, residential facilities, and community-health centers.

psychiatric social treatment therapy directed to the adjustment of a patient to social life in his community. The treatment may require increased insight, emotional retraining, and modification of the environment so that the patient can adapt more easily to it.

psychiatric social work a field of specialized social work concerned primarily with psychiatric patients and their families. Psychiatric case work is performed in mental hospitals and clinics, general hospitals, courts, health departments, and rehabilitation centers, and consists primarily of evaluation of (a) family, environmental, and social factors in the patient's illness, (b) collaboration on intake, orientation, and development of a treatment plan, (c) conducting group and family counseling, (d) planning for discharge and follow-up care, and (e) maintaining relationships with community agencies.

psychiatric team a multidisciplinary group of professionals and paraprofessionals who work together under the leadership of a psychiatrist in a mental hospital, psychiatric unit, mental-health center, or clinic. The team usually consists of psychiatrists, clinical psychologists, psychiatric social workers, psychiatric nurses, and adjunctive therapists such as dance, music, art, and recreation specialists.

psychiatric unit a unit of a general hospital organized for treatment of acutely disturbed psychiatric patients on an in-patient basis. Such units usually include provision for emergency coverage and admission; treatment with psychotropic drugs or ECT; group therapy; psychological examinations where indicated; and use of adjunctive modalities such as social-work services, occupational therapy, art therapy, movement therapy, and music therapy, as well as discussion groups. Many authorities regard the general hospital as the logical gate for patients entering the mental-health delivery system.

psychiatrist a physician who specializes in the diagnosis, treatment, prevention, and study of mental and emotional disorders. In the United

States, education for this profession consists of premedical training in a four-year college, a four-year course in medical school, a one-year hospital internship, a three-year residency in an American Medical Association approved hospital or agency, and at least two additional years of experience followed by an examination for certification by the American Board of Psychiatry and Neurology.

psychiatry the medical specialty concerned with the study, diagnosis, treatment, and prevention of mental and emotional disorders. Training for psychiatry includes the study of psychopathology, biochemistry, psychopharmacology, neurology, neuropathology, psychology, psychoanalysis, genetics, social science, and community mental health, as well as the many theories and approaches advanced in the field itself. (This Dictionary lists 42 headwords ending in "psychiatry.")

psychic a general term for all phenomena associated with the mind; also, as a noun, a medium.

psychic apparatus a term applied by Freud to mental structures and mechanisms, which he first (1900) divided into unconscious, preconscious, and conscious areas or "systems," and later (1923) into the id, ego, and superego, in which the id is described as unconscious, and the ego and superego as partly conscious, partly preconscious, and partly unconscious. Also called **mental apparatus**. See STRUCTURAL MODEL; SYSTEMATIC APPROACH.

psychic determinism the doctrine that all mental, or psychic, events obey the law of cause and effect and are not subject to free will or pure chance. See DETERMINISM; DYNAMIC APPROACH.

psychic driving the continuous replaying of psychodynamically significant material. The recorded material contains the patient's own verbal cues that help penetrate his or her defenses and bring deeply repressed material to the surface.

psychic energizer a drug that has an antidepressant effect. The term was introduced in the late 1950s by N. S. Kline to identify monoamine oxidase inhibitors derived from iproniazid, which had been developed for control of tuberculosis. The iproniazid drug was discontinued as a tuberculosis drug because of its powerful effects on the central nervous system.

psychic energy in psychoanalysis, the dynamic force behind all mental processes. According to Freud, the basic source of this energy is the id, or instinctual needs of the individual, which seek immediate gratification: "These instincts fill it [the id] with energy, but it has no organization and no unified will, only an impulsion to obtain satisfaction for the instinctual needs, in accordance with the pleasure principle" (*New Introductory Lectures on Psychoanalysis*, 1933). Jung also believed there is a reservoir of p.e., termed libido, but objected to Freud's "endless repetition of instinctual themes," and placed primary emphasis on channeling this energy into the de-

velopment of the personality and the expression of cultural and spiritual values rather than pleasurable gratification of biological instincts. Also called **mental energy**. See ID; LIBIDO.

psychic equivalent an alternative term for psychomotor epilepsy.

psychic helplessness a state of helpless anxiety which Freud believed to be first experienced during the birth process due to respiratory and other physiological changes occurring at that time. He believed the p.h. state to be the prototype of all later anxiety states.

psychic impotence a functional inability of the male to perform normal sexual intercourse despite intact genitalia and sexual desire. P.i. may be manifested in many forms including premature ejaculation, inability to achieve erection, or the need for certain conditions in order to perform coitus.

psychic inertia in psychoanalysis, fixation at an infantile stage, which acts as a form of resistance and impedes therapeutic progress. Freud and Jung both recognized that inertia is a basic characteristic of neurosis.

psychic isolation a term introduced by Jung to identify withdrawal from social contacts in order to prevent unconscious material from being revealed; also, a feeling of estrangement when material from the collective unconscious erupts into consciousness.

psychic masochism = IDEAL MASOCHISM.

psychic masturbation the achievement of orgasm through sexual fantasies without physical manipulation of the genitals or other erogenous zones.

psychic mobility the movement of a population from previously established social norms, concepts, or attitudes toward new ones. P.m. is an expression of the freedom of humans to manifest desires that may have been previously dormant in new or novel ways, e.g., in clothing styles, designs of homes and home furnishings, or popular music. P.m. is more active in periods of affluence when the people have greater discretionary income.

psychic norm a standard for mental health—an individual who may be described as in harmony with himself and the environment, in conformance with cultural mores, and suffers no impairment of reasoning, judgment, or intellectual abilities.

psychic pain psychological, or emotional, pain associated especially with feelings of acute anxiety and in some cases with hallucinations, obsessions, or depressive thoughts. P.p. is usually localized in the head. Also called **psychalgia; psychalgalia**. Also see ALGOPSYCHALIA.

psychic paralysis of visual fixation = BALINT'S SYNDROME.

psychic reality in psychoanalysis, the inner, or internal, reality of fantasies, wishes, fears, dreams, memories, and anticipations, as distinguished from the external reality of actual events and experiences.

psychic reflex arc the term assigned by Ferenczi to the Freudian autoplastic stage of development when adaptation is achieved by simple motor discharge, e.g., the whimpering of an infant, which modifies himself rather than the environment.

psychic research an alternative term for parapsychology.

psychic scar the residual symptoms of a mental disorder that may remain after completion of appropriate therapy; e.g., a delusion may remain after delirium.

psychic seizure a seizure occurring in psychomotor epilepsy, during which the patient experiences psychological disturbances such as vivid panoramic memories or a "twilight state" during which he is disoriented and utters unintelligible sounds or performs automatic activities. See PSYCHOMOTOR EPILEPSY.

psychic suicide a form of self-destruction in which the individual decides to die and actually does so without resorting to a physical agency. Also see VOODOO DEATH.

psychic tension a sense of emotional strain experienced in emergency situations or situations that generate inner conflict or anxiety. See STRESS; TENSION.

psychic tone: See ATONIA.

psychic trauma an experience that inflicts damage to the personality, often of a lasting nature. Examples are sexual assault, discovery of adoption under adverse circumstances, child abuse, and abandonment by a parent.

psychic vaginismus a painful vaginal spasm that represents repugnance to the sexual act and prevents sexual intercourse. For the corresponding DSM-III term, see FUNCTIONAL VAGINISMUS.

psychoacoustics an interdisciplinary study of sound and hearing with contributions from physics, psychology, and physiology.

psychoactive drug any chemical compound that affects the normal mental functioning of an individual, altering either the mood or thought processes, or both. A p.d. may be a tranquilizer as well as a psychedelic drug, a stimulant, or a sedative.

psychoanaleptica: See PSYCHOLEPTICA.

psychoanalysis the theory of dynamic psychology developed by Sigmund Freud, and the therapeutic technique based upon that theory. P. focuses primarily on the influence of unconscious forces such as repressed impulses, internal conflicts, and childhood traumas on the mental life and adjustment of the individual. The foundations on which it rests are the concept of infantile sexuality; the Oedipus complex; the theory of instincts; the pleasure and reality principles; the three-fold division of the psyche into id, ego, and superego; and the central importance of anxiety and defenses against anxiety in neurotic reactions. P. as a form of therapy is directed primarily to psychoneuroses, which it seeks to eliminate by bringing about basic modifications in the personality. This is done by establishing a constructive therapeutic relationship, or transference, with the analyst, which will enable him to elicit and interpret the unconscious experiences and impulses that have produced the neurosis. The specific methods used to achieve this goal are free association, dream interpretation, analysis of resistances and defenses, and working through the feelings and experiences revealed in the transference process. (This Dictionary lists 47 headwords ending in "psychoanalysis" or related "analysis.")

psychoanalyst a psychiatrist or clinical psychologist who has undergone special training in psychoanalytic theory and practice, and who applies the techniques developed by Freud to the treatment of mental disorders. The American Psychoanalytic Association requires graduation from a medical school and three years of psychiatric training at an approved hospital, but these requirements are not universally followed. All recognized training centers, however, require a thorough study of the works of Freud and others in the field, supervised clinical training, and a personal psychoanalysis.

psychoanalytic anthropology the application of principles and insights gained from the treatment of neurotic individuals to the understanding of unconscious factors responsible for behavior in primitive societies. Among the subjects dealt with are the psychic function of taboos, the handling of aggression, the importance of the leader, the study of myths and rituals, and the interpretation of customs and mores found in different cultures. This general approach was introduced by Freud in *Totem and Taboo* (1913), and further elaborated in *The Future of an Illusion* (1927), *Civilization and Its Discontents* (1930), and *Moses and Monotheism* (1939).

psychoanalytic development psychology a description of the internalization of interpersonal relations in psychoanalytic terms; also, the effect of human object relationships on the organization and structure of the psyche.

psychoanalytic group psychotherapy group therapy in which basic psychoanalytic concepts and methods, such as free association, analysis of resistances and defenses, and dream interpretation, are utilized in modified form. One example is A. Wolf's approach in which the group members act as cotherapists and free-associate with each other. A second example is W. R. Bion's approach in which the focus is on the emotional states of the group in relation to a central problem. A third is H. Thalen's approach in which the emphasis is on the emotional and cognitive relations between the individual and the group culture.

psychoanalytic psychiatry the branch of psychiatry that applies psychoanalytic techniques to the diagnosis, treatment, and prevention of mental problems, as contrasted with psychoanalysis as a theory of the structure and dynamics of the mind.

psychoanalytic setting a setting designed to encourage the psychoanalytic patient to attend to the inward world of feeling, fantasy, and early experience, and to say whatever comes to mind. The session is therefore held in a private study free from distracting influences; the patient reclines on a couch, and the therapist sits out of sight where he can unobtrusively take notes, observe significant gestures, facial expressions, and postural changes; but above all the analyst serves as a shadowy figure to whom the patient may direct, or "transfer," intense feelings originally directed to significant individuals in his life.

psychobioanalysis an alternative term for BIO-ANALYSIS. See this entry.

psychobiogram a type of personality profile developed by Kretschmer that includes data concerning the patient's heredity and history, plus information about intelligence, temperament, and attitudes, combined with somatotype evaluation.

psychobiological factors the multiple determinants of personality and behavior—biological, psychological, and sociological—which Adolf Meyer cited in his holistic, multidisciplinary approach. See PSYCHOBIOLOGY.

psychobiology the holistic approach developed by Adolf Meyer, in which the individual is viewed as an integrated unit, and both normal and abnormal behavior are explained in terms of biological, sociological, and psychological determinants. Symptoms are seen as real but distorted attempts at adjustment which can be understood by observing the patient in concrete, everyday activity and by compiling a biographical report, or anamnesis, based on all phases of his or her history, physical and mental, conscious and unconscious. Meyer believed that this study, which he termed distributive analysis and synthesis, would reveal assets out of which a more effective personality could be developed. The term may be used interchangeably with ERGASIOLOGY. See this entry.

psychochemistry a field of chemistry that is concerned with the relationships between chemicals and behavior, including genetic or metabolic aspects of behavior. As an example, different individuals may react in different ways to the same stimulant, because of inherited traits that affect metabolism of the drug.

psychochemistry intelligence the effects of biochemical factors such as drugs, hormones, and nutritional factors on intelligence, learning, or performance. Examples include caffeine, which may improve mental performance temporarily, while a dietary deficiency of niacin can result in lowered performance of mental tasks.

psychocultural stress cultural factors that generate significant psychological tension or anxiety, and, in many cases, mental illness. E. D. Wittkower and R. Prince (in *American Handbook of Psychiatry*, 1974) classify these factors under (a) cultural content, including frustrating rules and taboos, values such as vain pursuit of success and racial discrimination, (b) social organization, including anomie and rigidity that demands adherence to prescribed social norms, and (c) sociocultural change, as in rapid technological development or migration from a rural to an urban area.

psychodance: See PSYCHODRAMA FORMS.

psychodiagnostics the study of an individual's personality through observation of his behavior and mannerisms as well as test results.

psychodietetics application of nutritional principles and nutritional supplements in the treatment of mental and neurologic disorders, e.g., pellagra, beriberi, PKU.

psychodometer an instrument that uses a tuning fork in the measurement of response time.

psychodrama a technique of psychotherapy developed by J. L. Moreno, in which patients achieve new insight and alter faulty patterns of behavior through spontaneous enactment of life situations. The process involves (a) a protagonist, or patient, who presents and acts out his or her emotional problems and interpersonal relationships, (b) trained "auxiliary egos" who play supportive roles representing significant individuals in the dramatized situations, and (c) a director or therapist, who guides this process and leads an interpretive session when it is completed. Various special techniques are used to advance the therapy, among them exchanging roles, soliloquy, enactment of dreams, and hypnotic dramatizations. See HYPNODRAMA.

psychodrama forms the various types of psychodrama developed by J. L. Moreno to explore the private worlds of patients and provide them with therapeutic experiences, including (a) sociodrama, which deals with the active structuring of social worlds and collective ideologies, (b) **physiodrama**, which blends physical conditioning with psychodrama, (c) **axiodrama**, which deals with ethics and the eternal verities such as truth, justice, and beauty, (d) hypnodrama, which combines psychodrama with hypnosis, (e) **psychomusic**, in which spontaneous music is a part of psychodrama, and (f) **psychodance**, which utilizes spontaneous dance in psychodrama. See PSYCHODRAMA. Also see SOCIODRAMA; HYPNODRAMA.

psychodramatic shock a form of psychotherapy in which a patient is encouraged to relive a psychotic attack in order to achieve a cathartic effect. E.g., the patient may be asked to revive a hallucinatory experience by acting it out, using members of the staff to recreate the situation as a psychodrama.

psychodynamics the pattern of motivational forces, conscious or unconscious, that gives rise to a particular psychological event or state, such as an attitude, action, symptom, or mental disorder. These forces include drives, wishes, emotions, and defense mechanisms, as well as biological needs such as hunger and sex. Also called **dynamics**. See DYNAMIC APPROACH.

psychodynamic theory: See DYNAMIC APPROACH; PSYCHODYNAMICS.

psychodysleptica: See PSYCHOLEPTICA.

psychoeducational diagnostician a specialist trained in the diagnosis and remediation of children with learning disabilities.

psychoeducational problems: See SCHOOL PSYCHOLOGY.

psychoendocrinology the study of the hormonal system in order to discover sites for the manifestation of biochemical abnormalities that play a significant role in the production of mental disorders.

psychoexploration any of a group of psychotherapeutic techniques that include catharsis, hypnosis, abreaction, narcoanalysis, and narcosynthesis.

psychogalvanic reflex = GALVANIC SKIN RESPONSE.

psychogalvanic skin-resistance audiometry a procedure adapted for audiology by Bordley and Hardy (1949) for testing the auditory acuity of young children and suspected malingerers. The dermal-sweating responses to controlled test tones are graphically recorded. Abbrev.: **PGSR**. See KEELER POLYGRAPH; LIE DETECTOR; GALVANIC SKIN RESPONSE.

psychogalvanometer an ultrasensitive galvanometer used in measuring electrical changes in the skin surface. See PSYCHOGALVANIC SKIN-RESISTANCE AUDIOMETRY.

psychogender a term used in the treatment of intersexed patients to distinguish between psychological sex identification and biological sex.

psychogenesis the origin and development of mental or psychic processes. See PSYCHOGENIC.

psychogenic resulting from psychological, mental, or emotional factors, as contrasted with organic or somatic factors. Also called **functional**.

psychogenic amnesia a dissociative disorder marked by a sudden inability to recall important personal information that is too extensive to be explained by ordinary forgetfulness. The amnesia is not due to an organic brain disorder, such as alcohol intoxication, and is most commonly localized or circumscribed, as in failure to recall the first few hours after a profoundly disturbing event. Other forms of amnesia, also due to stress, are the **selective** type (a failure to recall some but not all of the event), the **generalized** type, in which there is a failure to recall one's entire life, and the **continuous** type, in which events are not recalled after a specific time up to and including the present. (DSM-III)

psychogenic aspermia a form of psychogenic impotence in which emission of semen does not occur.

psychogenic constipation: See CONSTIPATION.

psychogenic disorders functional disorders; disorders that do not have an organic basis and are believed to be due to psychological factors such as emotional conflicts or stress. The term applies to all types of psychoneuroses, psychophysiologic and somatoform disorders, personality disorders, and functional psychoses. There is disagreement about schizophrenic and manic-depressive disorders, since some investigators claim to have found evidence of hereditary factors, constitutional predisposition, or physiological factors, at least as contributory causes. Also called **functional disorders**.

psychogenic fugue a dissociative disorder characterized by (a) sudden, unexpected travel away from home or work with inability to recall one's past identity, (b) partial or complete assumption of a new identity that usually contrasts with the former personality. Also see FUGUE. (DSM-III)

psychogenic hallucination a hallucination arising from psychological factors such as a need to enhance self-esteem, or relief from a sense of guilt, as opposed to hallucinations produced primarily by physiological conditions such as intoxication.

psychogenic hypersomnia sleep attacks or sleep of excessive duration, precipitated by psychological factors such as a wish to escape from a threatening or other anxiety-provoking situation. See NARCOLEPSY.

psychogenic mutism: see MUTISM.

psychogenic needs: See NEED-PRESS THEORY.

psychogenic pain disorder a somatoform disorder characterized by severe, prolonged pain (e.g., chest pain or sciatica) for which there is evidence of psychological involvement but no evidence of an adequate physical basis. Though involuntary, the pain may serve such psychological ends as avoidance of distasteful activity or gaining extra attention or support from others. (DSM-III)

psychogenic polydipsia excessive fluid ingestion for no observable physiological reason. It has been suggested that the behavior is related to food displacement as it develops in experimental animals required to wait for food after pressing a lever. However, p.p. behavior also occurs in humans with immediate access to food.

psychogenic pruritus one of a group of psychosomatic dermatological disorders, characterized by a functional itching that resists treatment. P.p. occurs in obsessive-compulsive individuals who are rigid, defensive, and not easily suggestible.

psychogenic-purpura-and-painful-bruising syndrome = GARDNER-DIAMOND SYNDROME.

psychogenic stupor a state of extreme unresponsiveness without loss of consciousness, associated with functional rather than organic syndromes, as in catatonic and depressive states, combat exhaustion, and extreme panic. See BENIGN STUPOR; MALIGNANT STUPOR; STUPOR.

psychogeriatrics: See GEROPSYCHIATRY.

psychograph = TRAIT PROFILE.

psychographics a branch of psychology that deals with the study of life-styles of a population on a quantitative basis. The term was introduced by E. Demby in the 1970s to describe an extended form of demographics that surveys activities, interests, and opinions of the population, in addition to such factors as income, education, and place of residence. Also called **AIO (Activity, Interest, Opinion)**. Also see ETHICAL HIGHBROW.

psychography the natural history and description of mental phenomena, as in psychoanalysis and psychobiology.

psychohistory the interpretation of historical events, trends, and personalities in psychological or psychoanalytic terms. Also see APPLIED PSYCHOANALYSIS.

psychoinfantilism the appearance in an adult of psychic qualities normally associated with a child. P. is not regarded as a disease state but a reaction to a severe crisis or a difficult decision characterized by uncertainty, mental weakness, dependence on stronger persons, and inability to cope on one's own.

psychokinesis in parapsychology, the alleged ability to control external events and move or change the shape of objects through the power of thought, e.g., to influence the roll of dice or bend a piece of metal by exerting "mind over matter." Abbrev.: **PK**. Also called **telekinesis; parakinesis**.

psycholepsy a sudden depressive state, marked by a dramatic decline in the level of mental tension, and generally associated with individuals who lack emotional stability. The abrupt psycholeptic crisis usually follows an experience of ecstasy or triumph during which psychic tension is at a peak.

psycholeptica the kinds of psychotropic drugs that have their primary effect on the psyche rather than the psychomotor areas of the nervous system. P. drugs include the minor tranquilizers. **Psychoanaleptica** include the antidepressant drugs and **psychodysleptica** the hallucinogens that cause a disintegration of psychic functions.

psycholinguistics the study of the psychological functions of language and of the effects of language on individual and group relationships. Its primary functions are to promote communication, to enable us to use concepts as tools of thought, to study language as a medium for the expression of feelings and emotions, and to enable us to build a body of literature that enriches human life. See LINGUISTICS; PSYCHOLOGICAL LINGUISTICS; PHONOLOGY; SIGN LANGUAGE; DEVELOPMENTAL P.; ILLINOIS TEST OF PSYCHOLINGUISTIC ABILITIES.

psychological aphrodisiacs = PORNOGRAPHY.

psychological autopsy the study of possible reasons for an individual's suicide by processes such as examination of his letters and interviewing his friends and relatives.

psychological counseling: See COUNSELING PSYCHOLOGIST.

psychological deficit the performance of any significant psychological process at a level that is below that of a normal person.

psychological dependence a state of dependence upon a psychoactive substance for the sense of well-being provided by use of the substance. The dependence generally lacks the factors of increasing tissue tolerance and withdrawal symptoms observed in cases of physiological, or physical, dependence. P.d. is associated with marijuana, nicotine, amphetamines, and caffeine. Tolerance is likely to occur but not in significant degree, and withdrawal symptoms are mild compared with those associated with alcohol and narcotic drugs.

psychological esthetics a branch of psychology that deals with the psychological effects of different art forms, patterns, colors, composition, and other aspects of visual stimuli contained in paintings, sculpture, photographs, architecture, natural landscapes, and the like. Certain colors or patterns, e.g., may excite viewers while others may have a calming effect. P.e. also may be applied to the study of political, social, economic, or other influences on the work of artists.

psychological examination examination of a patient by means of interviews, observations of behavior, and administration of psychological tests, with the purpose of evaluating his personality adjustment, abilities, interests, and functioning in important phases of life. The purpose of the p.e. may be to determine his needs, identify his difficulties and problems, and contribute to the diagnosis of mental disorder and determination of the type of treatment required.

psychological factors functional factors—as opposed to organic (constitutional, hereditary) factors—that contribute to the development of personality and the etiology of mental disorder. P.f. include, among others, childhood experiences, faulty role models, rejection or overprotection, and traumatic experiences.

psychological factors affecting physical condition a clinical category comprising psychological conditions and stimuli that contribute to the initiation or aggravation of physical conditions or single symptoms. Examples of the psychological stimuli are serious arguments and the death of a loved one; examples of the physical conditions and symptoms are tension headaches, obesity, angina pectoris, asthma, rheumatoid arthritis, gastric ulcer, ulcerative colitis, nausea, vomiting, and sacroiliac pain. Conversion disorders and somatoform disorders are not included in this category, which replaces psychosomatic and psychophysiologic disorders in previous classifications. (DSM-III)

psychological field the individual's life space or environment as he perceives it at any given moment (K. Lewin).

psychological geography the pattern of an entire community showing the location and interrelations of groups within it, with emphasis on the "psychological currents" flowing between them (J. L. Moreno).

psychological invalidism the attitude of a patient who refuses to accept the fact that he has been cured of a physical disorder and insists on continuing to live as a sick person with all the restrictions as well as all the benefits (attention, concern, care) that accompany invalidism.

psychological linguistics a general term for different approaches to language from the point of view of psychology. By observation and experiment, p.l. explores how we acquire language, how we behave in producing and perceiving speech, how we use language to learn other skills, how the use of language is related to memory, and how language interrelates with thinking. Also see PSYCHOLINGUISTICS; LINGUISTICS; ORIGIN-OF-LANGUAGE THEORIES.

psychological measures: See PRIMARY PREVENTION.

psychological motive any motive that is not believed to arise from purely physiological need, that is, a learned motive or a motive that has a mental, emotional, or cultural origin; also, a motive, such as competition, that arises from our interactions with others. A p.m. may be universal, culture-specific, or individual.

psychological need a need that is fostered by environmental interactions with the individual. An example is social-approval need.

psychological network the loose but cohesive interrelationship of individuals, families, and social groups that helps form social traditions and emotional support for the participants.

psychological rapport Jung's term for transference, which he describes as "the intensified tie to the physician which is a compensation symptom for the defective relationship to present reality," and "inevitable in every fundamental analysis."

psychological rehabilitation the development or restoration of an effective identity in the disabled client through psychological approaches such as counseling, individual or group therapy, ability assessment, and medications. The object is to help the client improve his or her self-image, cope with emotional problems, and become a more competent, autonomous person.

psychological scale a measuring device for a psychological function, e.g., intelligence and attitudes.

psychological statistics mathematical methods that describe, summarize, or lead to inferences about data dealing with the behavior or cognition of individuals or groups. These methods include measures of central tendency, variability, correlation, significance, probability, and the like. Also see STATISTICAL PSYCHOLOGY.

psychological stress: See STRESS.

psychological test a standardized instrument (test, inventory, scale) used in measuring intelligence, specific mental abilities (reasoning, comprehension, abstract thinking, etc.), specific aptitudes (mechanical aptitude, manual coordination, dexterity, etc.), achievement (reading, spelling, arithmetic, etc.), attitudes, values, interests, personality, and personality disorders. Also see the Appendix for TESTS.

psychological testing the use of objective or projective tests to assess behavior, attitudes, motives, or traits, for purposes such as psychodiagnosis, research, or personnel and educational assessment. P.t. makes use of questionnaires, in-

terpretation of ambiguous stimuli, ratings of self and others, intellectual problems, and the like. P.t. also comprises the development and construction of tests, and their validity, reliability, and standardization.

psychological time subjective estimation of time based on such factors as the ocurrence and nature of events, experience with the time taken by regularly-occurring events, and physiological rhythms. Also see TIME SENSE.

psychological tremor: See TREMOR.

psychological type a category of individuals classified according to certain characteristics, e.g., intuitive type.

psychological warfare a type of warfare in which propaganda and other techniques are used to lower the morale of the enemy and to heighten the support of the war effort by one's own population.

psychological zero the level at which a sensation (temperature, pressure, sound) is not experienced. The p.z. for the temperature of the skin is about 90°F (32°C) for most of the body, but 82°F for the ear and 98°F for the armpit.

psychologist a professionally trained individual who devotes himself or herself to research, teaching, writing, or practice in one or more branches of behavioral science. Training includes a wide variety of courses leading to at least an M.A. degree, but preferably a Ph.D. obtained at a university or school of professional psychology. In most states of the United States certification or licensing is required for participation in the profession. The psychologist's activities are carried out in a variety of settings: schools, colleges, social agencies, hospitals, clinics, the military, industry and business, prisons, or the government.

psychologist's fallacy the projection by a psychologist of what he believes to be appropriate thoughts or behavior into the mind of the client.

psychology the science of human and animal behavior as part of the total life process, including the bodily systems associated with behavior, sensory and motor functions, social interactions, the sequence of development, hereditary and environmental forces, conscious and unconscious mental processes, mental health and disorder, the dynamics of behavior, the observation, testing, and experimental study of behavior, and the application of psychological knowledge to such fields as employment, education, psychotherapy, and consumer behavior. (This Dictionary lists 82 headwords ending in "psychology.")

psycholytic therapy a technique of LSD therapy developed by H. Leuner, but almost completely discarded today because of difficulty in controlling the drug reactions. Out-patients were given small doses of the drug in groups or individually, and psychological material elicited under its influence was analytically interpreted. Also see LSD PSYCHOTHERAPY.

psychometric examination a series of psychological tests administered to determine intelligence, manual skills, personality characteristics, interests, or other mental factors.

psychometric function = PSYCHOPHYSICAL FUNCTION.

psychometrician a specialist in the administration of mental tests and in the evaluation of results, also in the development and use of statistical and mathematical procedures. Also called **psychometrist**.

psychometry the science or the process of measuring abilities and personality through psychological tests and statistics. The term is also used in the field of parapsychology for the reputed ability of some persons to hold an object in their hands and become aware of facts about its history or about people who have been associated with it. In its first sense, p. is also called **psychometrics**.

psychomimetics: See PSYCHOTOMIMETICS.

psychomimic syndrome a condition in which a patient develops symptoms of an illness actually suffered by another person, who may have died of the disorder. The patient lacks any organic evidence of the illness, and the person who experienced the actual disease was ambivalently related to the patient. The symptoms usually occur around the anniversary of the death of the other person.

psychomotility a motor action or habit that is influenced or controlled by a mental process, e.g., tics, handwriting, gait, stammering, or dysarthria, which may be signs of psychomotor disturbance.

psychomotor action an action or reaction that is the result of an idea or perception.

psychomotor agitation a state of tense, restless physical and mental overactivity, as in agitated depression, during which the patient wrings his hands and paces the floor while bemoaning his fate.

psychomotor attack a brief temporal-lobe seizure involving extreme, sometimes violent, activity, for which there is complete amnesia.

psychomotor disorder a disturbance in the psychological control of movement; a motor disorder precipitated by psychological factors. Examples are epileptic seizures brought on by stress, temporal-lobe seizures (psychomotor epilepsy), psychomotor retardation associated with depression, and hyperactivity exhibited during a manic episode.

psychomotor epilepsy a type of epilepsy characterized by a brief, trancelike, "dreamy" state accompanied by paramnesias (déjà vu, jamais vu), ill-defined hallucinations, chewing and swallowing movements, repetitive automatic activities, and in some cases feelings of rage or terror which may lead to violent behavior. The EEG reveals characteristic spike discharges in the temporal lobe, hence the condition is also called **temporal-lobe epilepsy**. See FUROR.

psychomotor excitement a state of physical and mental overactivity characterized by extreme restlessness, flight of ideas, and pressure of speech. The condition is most frequently found in the manic phase of bipolar disorder.

psychomotor hallucination the sensation that parts of the body are moving or being moved to different areas of the body.

psychomotor retardation a general slowing down (motor inhibition) of mental and physical activity most frequently observed in major depressions and catatonic schizophrenia. The patient sits for hours with folded hands, speaks haltingly if at all, finds it hard to concentrate and think, and feels that an enormous burden is holding him back.

psychomotor stimulants agents that stimulate the motor neurons of the cerebrum to produce increased psychomotor activity. Examples of p.s. include amphetamine, caffeine, and methylphenidate.

psychomotor tests skill tests requiring a coordination of sensory processes with motor activities as in the Crawford Small Parts Dexterity Test, and the Minnesota Rate of Manipulation Test.

psychomusic: See PSYCHODRAMA FORMS.

psychoneural parallelism = PSYCHOPHYSICAL PARALLELISM.

psychoneurosis = NEUROSIS.

psychonomic denoting an approach to psychology that emphasizes quantitative measurement, experimental control, and operational definitions.

psychonomics the science of the laws governing the mind, also of the environmental factors that influence development.

psychonosology the systematic classification of mental disorders.

psychopathia sexualis a term used by Richard von Krafft-Ebing for psychosexual perversions and as the title of his classic work on the subject.

psychopathic personality: See ANTISOCIAL REACTION.

psychopathologist a medical or psychological professional person who studies the causes of mental disorders. **Psychopathology** is a broad field of study and may involve biochemistry, pharmacology, psychiatry, neurology, cytology, experimental psychology, and other related subjects.

psychopathy /-kop'-/ a broad term for any psychological disorder or mental disease, usually of an unspecified nature. Also see CONSTITUTIONAL PSYCHOPATH; AUTISTIC P.

psychopedics a branch of psychology that specializes in the psychological treatment and guidance of children.

psychopenetration test a test of emotional flexibility or rigidity of a patient based on reactions to five questions during carbon-dioxide-inhalation therapy. The questions are designed to elicit evidence of the degree of unconscious resistance to the concepts of sex, killing, attention, deceiving, and showing all feeling; and the reactions are used as a guide to therapeutic procedures.

psychopharmacological drugs any medications used in the treatment of mental disorders.

psychopharmacology the study of pharmacology as it relates to psychology. P. is concerned primarily with the mode of action of various substances that affect different areas of the brain and nervous system, including drugs of abuse. P. research may explore the reasons why an animal may turn left in a maze after receiving one type of drug but turn right in the same maze after being administered another drug.

psychopharmacotherapy the use of pharmacologic agents in the treatment of mental disorders. As an example, p. for acute or chronic cases of schizophrenia might include antipsychotic drugs and major tranquilizers, which will not cure the disorder but will provide significant relief from symptoms so that social rehabilitation and psychotherapeutic techniques may be employed with greater effectiveness.

psychophobia a morbid fear of the mind, of thinking about the mind, or simply of thinking. Also see PHRONEMOPHOBIA.

psychophysical dualism the doctrine that mental processes have both an organic and psychic aspect but that there is no interaction or causal relation between them. Also see PSYCHOPHYSICAL PARALLELISM.

psychophysical function a psychometric relationship between a stimulus and judgments about the stimulus, as expressed in a mathematical formula. Also called **psychometric function**.

psychophysical law a mathematical relationship between a sensation and the intensity of the stimulus. The relationship shows that a neural receptor generates an impulse frequency that is proportional to the logarithm of the stimulus. The data, when plotted, should follow a straight line curve. Also called **psychophysical relationship**.

psychophysical methods the standard techniques used in investigating psychophysical problems, e.g., the method of average error, the method of equal-appearing intervals, and the method of limits.

psychophysical parallelism the doctrine that for every mental event there is a corresponding event in the nervous system. It is a variation of psychophysical dualism. Also called **psychoneural parallelism**.

psychophysical relationship = PSYCHOPHYSICAL LAW.

psychophysics a branch of psychology that deals with relationships between stimulus magnitudes, stimulus differences, and corresponding sensory processes. See WEBER, ERNST HEINRICH.

psychophysiologic cardiovascular reaction a DSM-I term for psychophysiologic disorders involving the cardiovascular system, including hypertension, Raynaud's disease, migraine, tachycardia, vascular spasm, coronary disease, and general anginal syndrome.

psychophysiologic endocrine reaction a DSM-I term for psychophysiologic disorders involving the endocrine system, including diabetic reactions, obesity, and hyperthyroidism.

psychophysiologic gastrointestinal reaction a DSM-I term for psychophysiologic disorders involving the gastrointestinal system, including anorexia nervosa, colitis, peptic ulcer, bulimia, constipation, gastritis, hyperacidity, and "heartburn."

psychophysiologic genitourinary reaction a DSM-I term for psychophysiologic disorders involving the genitourinary system, including frigidity, impotence, menstrual disorders, menopause, false pregnancy, infertility, painful urination, vaginismus, urethritis.

psychophysiologic hemic and lymphatic reaction a DSM-I term for psychophysiologic disorders involving the blood and lymph systems, such as anemia.

psychophysiologic musculoskeletal reaction a DSM-I term for psychophysiologic disorders involving the musculoskeletal system, including arthritis, tension headache, backache, muscle cramps, and psychogenic rheumatism.

psychophysiologic nervous-system reaction a DSM-I term for psychophysiologic disorders involving the nervous system, including asthenic reaction (neurasthenia), phantom reaction, anxiety reaction, certain convulsive disorders, and body-image disturbance.

psychophysiologic respiratory reaction a DSM-I term for psychophysiologic disorders involving the respiratory system, including asthma, breath-holding, common cold, hyperventilation syndrome, tuberculosis, hayfever, sinusitis, and recurring bronchitis.

psychophysiologic skin reaction a DSM-I term for psychophysiologic disorders involving the cutaneous system, including neurodermatitis, hives, acne, allergic eczema.

psychophysiologic special-sense reaction a DSM-I term for psychophysiologic disorders involving organs of the special senses including conjunctivitis, glaucoma, photophobia, and disorders of taste, hearing, and smell.

psychophysiology the study of physiological relationships in normal and abnormal behavior. Also see PSYCHOSOMATIC MEDICINE; PHYSIOLOGICAL PSYCHOLOGY.

psychopolitics research and action on the psychological aspects of political behavior, such as the effects on society of different types of leadership (democratic, fascist, socialist); also, the use of psychological tactics or strategies by politicians. Also see POLITICAL PSYCHIATRY.

psychorrhea a symptom of hebephrenic (disorganized) schizophrenia consisting of a stream of vague, bizarre, and usually incoherent theories of philosophy.

psychorrhexis a war-time variation of anxiety neurosis in which the patient expresses anguish and perplexity rather than fear or excitement. Symptoms include a rapid pulse and slow breathing rate, fever, jaundice, restlessness, facial spasms, and automatic movements. The condition tends to affect persons with a previous labile sympathetic system who experience severe mental trauma while physically exhausted. Death may occur within a few days in some cases.

psychosciences sciences that deal with the mind and mental behavior, with mental diseases and disorders, and with their treatment and cure—in particular, psychology, psychiatry, and psychoanalysis.

psychose passionnelle = CLÉRAMBAULT'S SYNDROME.

psychosexual development in psychoanalysis, the step-by-step growth of sexual life as it affects personality development. The impetus for p.d. stems from a single energy source, the libido. According to Freud, the human being is sexually "polymorphous," since sexuality takes many forms and goes through many stages—oral, anal, phallic, latency, and genital. Each stage gives rise to its own characteristic erotic activities, e.g., sucking and biting in the oral stage, and the early expressions may lead to "perverse" activities later in life, such as sadism, masochism, voyeurism, and exhibitionism. Moreover, the different stages leave their mark on the individual's character and personality, especially if sexual development is arrested, or "fixated," at one particular stage. Also called **libidinal development**.

psychosexual disorders a group of disorders of sexual functioning stemming from psychological rather than organic factors, and comprising gender-identity disorders (discomfort with one's own anatomic sex, or behavior associated with the opposite sex), paraphilias (arousal by unusual sexual objects or situations), psychosexual dysfunctions (disturbances in sexual desire or response), and other p.d. (ego-dystonic homosexuality; psychosexual disorders not elsewhere classified). See GENDER-IDENTITY DISORDERS; PARAPHILIAS; PSYCHOSEXUAL DYSFUNCTIONS; EGO-DYSTONIC HOMOSEXUALITY; PSYCHOSEXUAL DISORDERS NOT ELSEWHERE CLASSIFIED. (DSM-III)

psychosexual disorders not elsewhere classified a residual DSM-III category comprising psychological sexual disturbances not covered by the specific categories, including, e.g., marked feelings of inadequacy associated with the size and shape of the sex organs or with sexual performance, confusion about preferred sexual orientation, or distress over repeated sexual conquests, as in Don Juanism and nymphomania. See DON JUAN; NYMPHOMANIA.

psychosexual dysfunctions a group of sexual disorders characterized by inhibition in one or more phases of the complete sexual response cycle, which comprises the appetitive phase (sexual fantasies and desire), excitement (sexual pleasure accompanying such physiological changes as tumescence and vaginal lubrication), orgasm (the peaking of sexual pleasure, with release of sexual tension), and resolution (a sense of general relaxation and well-being). P.d. include INHIBITED SEXUAL DESIRE, INHIBITED SEXUAL EXCITEMENT, INHIBITED FEMALE ORGASM, INHIBITED MALE ORGASM, PREMATURE EJACULATION, FUNCTIONAL DYSPAREUNIA, FUNCTIONAL VAGINISMUS, and ATYPICAL PSYCHOSEXUAL DYSFUNCTION. See these entries. (DSM-III)

psychosexual stages: See PSYCHOSEXUAL DEVELOPMENT.

psychosexual trauma a frightening, degrading, or otherwise traumatic sexual experience in earlier life that is related to a current psychosexual dysfunction. Examples include incest or other forms of child abuse.

psychosis a severe mental disorder of organic or functional origin characterized by gross impairment in reality testing. That is, "the individual incorrectly evaluates the accuracy of his or her perceptions and thoughts and makes incorrect inferences about external reality, even in the face of contrary evidence" (DSM-III). Specific symptoms indicative of psychosis are delusions, hallucinations, markedly incoherent speech, disorientation, and confusion. Psychotic individuals have little or no insight into their symptoms, and are so impaired that they cannot meet the usual demands of life.

See ACUTE DELUSIONAL P.; ACUTE PSYCHOTIC BREAK; ACUTE SHOCK P.; AFFECTIVE P.; AKINETIC P.; ALCOHOLIC PARANOIA; ALCOHOLIC PSYCHOSES; ALLOPSYCHOSIS; ALTERNATING P.; ANTIPSYCHOTICS; ATYPICAL P.; AUTISTIC P.; AUTOPSYCHOSIS; BARBED-WIRE P.; BIOGENIC P.; BORDERLINE P.; BRIEF REACTIVE P.; BROMIDE INTOXICATION; BUFFOONERY P.; CANNABIS P.; CARDIAC P.; CIRCULAR P.; CIRCULATORY P.; COLLECTIVE P.; DEGENERATIVE PSYCHOSES; DEPRESSIVE P.; DETERIORATIVE P.; DRUG-INDUCED P.; EXOTIC P.; FAMILIAL P.; FOLIE A DEUX; FUNCTIONAL P.; FURLOUGH P.; GENERAL PARESIS; GERIOPSYCHOSIS; GOVERNESS P.; HYPOPSYCHOSIS; HYSTERICAL P.;

IATROGENIC P.; INDUCED P.; INFECTIVE-EXHAUSTIVE P.; INTERMITTENT P.; INVOCATIONAL P.; INVOLUTIONAL PSYCHOTIC REACTION; LATENT P.; MALIGNANT P.; MANIC-DEPRESSIVE ILLNESS; MODEL P.; MONOSYMPTOMATIC P.; MOOD-CONGRUENT PSYCHOTIC FEATURES; MOOD-INCONGRUENT PSYCHOTIC FEATURES; NEUROPSYCHOSIS OF DEFENSE; PARANOID P.; PATHOPSYCHOSIS; POSTPARTUM P.; PRISON P.; PROTEST P.; PSEUDONEUROTIC SCHIZOPHRENIA; SCHIZOAFFECTIVE P.; SEMANTIC P.; SENILE PSYCHOSES; SEPTICEMIA P.; SHOCK P.; SITUATIONAL P.; SOMATOPSYCHOSIS; SYMBIOTIC P.; SYMPTOMATIC P.; TABETIC P.; TOXIC-INFECTIOUS P.; TOXIC P.; UNIPOLAR MANIC-DEPRESSIVE P.; UNIPOLAR P.

psychosis with cardiorenal disease an organic brain syndrome associated with heart disease. Psychotic symptoms include delirium, confusion, hallucinations, attention deficits, and memory impairment.

psychosis with cerebral arteriosclerosis: See MULTIINFARCT DEMENTIA.

psychosis with mental retardation the episodes

of excitement, depression, hallucinations, or paranoia that occur occasionally in mentally retarded persons but are usually temporary.

psychosocial deprivation lack of adequate opportunity for social and intellectual stimulation. It may be a significant factor in emotional disturbance and retarded mental development in children. See PSEUDORETARDATION.

psychosocial dwarfism reversible retardation of growth associated with behavioral symptoms that are also reversible upon change from an adverse living situation to a benign, salutary environment.

psychosocial factors social situations, relationships, and pressures that have psychological effects, e.g., business competition, rapid technological change, work deadlines, and changes in the roles and status of women.

psychosocial stressor a life situation that creates such severe stress that it may contribute to the development or aggravation of a psychiatric disorder, e.g., divorce, death of a child, prolonged illness, change of residence, a natural catastrophe, or a highly competitive work situation.

psychosocial system a term introduced by Masters and Johnson to describe the various social, psychological, and cultural attitudes toward sexual responses.

psychosocial therapy psychological treatment techniques designed to help the individual with emotional or behavioral disturbances to adjust to situations that require social interfacing with other members of the community. P.t. generally is more important in city settings where the individual encounters large numbers of persons with different backgrounds and personalities than in a rural or village setting.

psychosomatic characterizing an approach or type of disorder that involves both the mind (psyche) and the body (soma), especially illnesses that are primarily physical with at least a partly emotional etiology.

psychosomatic disorder a disorder characterized by physical symptoms resulting from psychological factors, usually involving one system of the body, such as the gastrointestinal, respiratory, or genitourinary. It is termed "psychophysiologic disorder" in DSM-I and "psychological factors affecting physical condition" in DSM-III. Also called **psychosomatic illness**.

psychosomatic medicine a branch of medicine that evaluates an illness in terms of its organic and psychological components. As most illnesses incorporate both organic and psychological factors, each case must be considered on the basis of the specific nature and relative importance of these factors.

psychosomatic suicide a self-destructive impulse occasionally observed in patients with ulcerative colitis and bronchial asthma, and believed to be caused by intense frustration. Repression of this impulse may lead to a fulminant attack which resists medical treatment.

psychostimulants stimulant drugs that affect primarily the central nervous system. P. include drugs that may or may not be a member of a specific group of stimulants, e.g., PENTYLENE-TETRAZOL (see this entry), a laboratory tool that can produce convulsions that mimic a petit mal seizure. **Doxapram**—$C_{24}H_{30}N_2O_2$—acts on the medulla to increase the rate of breathing. NICOTINE (see this entry), is a ganglionic stimulating drug which in large doses produces effects of p. whereas in small doses the effects involve mainly the peripheral nerves. **Ephedrine** —$C_{10}H_{15}NO$, an ancient Oriental alkaloid, also produces effects on the autonomic nervous system as well as the central nervous system in a manner that mimics the action of epinephrine. Both ephedrine and COCAINE (see this entry) have relationships to the amphetamines, ephedrine has a structural formula similar to amphetamine, and cocaine produces mood effects that are almost identical to those of the amphetamines.

psychosurgery the treatment of a mental or CNS disorder by surgical techniques that require invasion of the brain tissues. Examples include prefrontal lobotomy and the use of supercold temperature to freeze certain brain tissues.

psychosynthesis an attempt to unify and harmonize various components of the unconscious, such as dreams, fantasies, and instinctual strivings with the rest of the personality. This principle was advocated by Jung and termed **constructive approach**, in contrast to Freud's **reductive approach**.

psychotechnics the application of psychological principles to alter or control behavior; also, the practical application of psychological principles in economics, sociology, and business.

psychotechnology the body of psychological facts and principles involved in the practical applications of psychology.

psychotherapist an individual professionally trained to treat mental, emotional, and behavioral disorders.

psychotherapy the treatment of personality problems, maladjustments, and mental disorders by psychological means. Wolberg (*The Technique of Psychotherapy*, 1954) defines p. as "a form of treatment for problems of an emotional nature in which a trained person deliberately establishes a professional relationship with a patient with the object of removing, modifying or retarding existing symptoms, of mediating disturbed patterns of behavior, and of promoting positive personality growth and development." For examples of *traditional psychotherapies*, see PSYCHOANALYSIS; ANALYTIC PSYCHOLOGY; ADLER. For examples of *human-potential therapies*, see CLIENT-CENTERED PSYCHOTHERAPY; GESTALT THERAPY; BIOENERGETICS; HUMAN-POTENTIAL MOVEMENT; THIRD-FORCE THERAPY. For examples of *group therapies*, see PSYCHODRAMA; FAMILY THERAPY; TRANSACTIONAL ANALYSIS; GROUP PSYCHOTHERAPY. For examples of *cognitive-behavioral therapies*, see COGNITIVE THERAPY; BE-

HAVIOR THERAPY; BIOFEEDBACK TRAINING. Also, more than 200 cross references are listed in the Appendix on THERAPIES.

psychotherapy by reciprocal inhibitions a type of behavior therapy in which emphasis is placed on weakening of the bond between anxiety responses and anxiety-provoking stimuli by conditioning the anxiety-provoking response to an incompatible response such as muscle relaxation. See RECIPROCAL INHIBITION; SYSTEMATIC DESENSITIZATION.

psychotic pertaining to a psychosis or psychoses; also, an individual afflicted with a psychosis.

psychotic character a borderline psychotic disorder in which the pathological individual is able to maintain a relationship with others who remain unaware of his disorder due to the fact that he gratifies their repressed wishes. E.g., a group may elevate a megalomanic individual to a position of leadership because of their need for hero worship. The term is seldom used.

psychotic-depressive reaction a psychosis involving a depressed mood, generally precipitated by situational factors in an individual who does not have a history of recurrent depression. See MAJOR DEPRESSION.

psychotic disorder an alternative term for psychosis.

psychotic disorders not elsewhere classified (DSM-III): See SCHIZOPHRENIFORM DISORDER; BRIEF REACTIVE PSYCHOSIS; SCHIZOAFFECTIVE DISORDER; ATYPICAL PSYCHOSIS.

psychoticism a factor developed by Eysenck for distinguishing the three groups of normal, schizophrenic, and manic-depressive individuals from each other. The system uses tests of judgment of spatial distance, reading speed, level of proficiency in mirror drawing, and adding rows of numbers.

psychotogenic an agent that induces psychosis or signs and symptoms that resemble manifestations of psychoses. Hallucinogenic drugs may be capable of producing a p. state marked by sensory illusions, distortions, and hallucinations, accompanied by a loss of control, paranoid delusions, intense depression, or an overwhelming flood of anxiety. See PSYCHEDELICS.

psychotogens psychotomimetic drugs such as LSD that were used experimentally at one time in an effort to induce signs or symptoms of psychoses. The term is essentially equivalent to PSYCHEDELICS. See this entry.

psychotomimetics drugs now classed as psychedelics but originally used in laboratory experiments to determine if they could induce psychoses, or states mimicking psychoses, on the basis of their psychogenic effects. The group includes LSD. P. also may include amphetamine drugs which in cases of chronic abuse can lead to compulsive behavior patterns, violence, paranoia, and other psychotic symptoms. A term that is often used interchangeably with p. is **psychomimetics**. See PSYCHEDELICS; PHANEROTHYME.

psychotropic drug any drug that has a primary effect on behavior, experience, or other psychological functions. Kinds of p.d. include sedatives, hypnotics, stimulants, narcotics, antidepressants, psychedelics, and major and minor tranquilizers. Generally excluded are substances that may have mind-altering effects although that is not their primary function.

-psychro- a combining form meaning cold (from Greek *psychein*, "to breathe, blow, make cold," hence also *psyche*, "breath, mind").

psychrophobia a morbid fear of the cold or a cold object. Also called **cryophobia; cheimaphobia**.

PT = PHYSICAL THERAPY.

PTC = PHENYLTHIOCARBAMIDE.

P technique a type of factor analysis for data varying over time. See also Q METHODOLOGY; R METHODOLOGY.

pteronophobia a morbid fear of feathers.

ptosis /tō′sis/ the sinking or dropping of an organ or part of the body. The term is usually applied to a drooping eyelid associated with paralysis of the third cranial nerve and a diagnostic sign of myasthenia gravis (the condition may also occur in anemic or neurotic persons on awakening). Also see PROLAPSE.

PTP = POSTTETANIC POTENTIATION.

-ptyal-; -ptyalo- /-tī·əl-/ a combining form relating to saliva.

ptyalism the excessive production of saliva. Normal daily production of the parotid, submaxillary, and sublingual glands is between 1,000 and 1,500 milliliters per day for an adult human. P. may be associated with epilepsy, encephalitis, certain medications, high blood pressure, deep emotion, or high anxiety. The term also is applied to cases in which saliva production is normal but the patient is unable to swallow the saliva as fast as it is secreted, as in cases of parkinsonism, bulbar or pseudobulbar paralysis, or bilateral facial-nerve palsy. Certain drugs, such as pilocarpine, can be a cause of p. Also see SALIVARY GLANDS.

PTZ = PENTYLENETETRAZOL.

puberism = PUBERTY.

pubertal sexual recapitulation a generalization that the beginning of adult sexuality development at puberty involves a recapitulation of the stages of infantile sexuality. The concept assumes that sexuality at puberty first must regress toward the infantile state in order to recapitulate.

pubertas praecox = PRECOCIOUS PUBERTY.

puberty the stage of development when the genital organs reach maturity and secondary sex characteristics begin to appear. The period extends from about 11 to 13 in females and 12 to 14 in males, and is marked by ejaculation of sperm in the male, onset of menstruation and development of breasts in the female, and growth of pubic hair and increasing interest in the opposite sex in both. Also called **puberism**. Also see PRECOCIOUS P.; PERSISTENT PUBERISM.

puberty rites the initiation into adult life of a pubescent member of a community through ceremonies, cultural-lore indoctrination, and similar customs. Also see PUBIC RITE.

pubescence the period or process of reaching puberty. Adjective: **pubescent**.

pubic rite a type of puberty rite in which a part of the ceremony may involve mutilation or scarification of the genitalia. Also see PUBERTY RITES.

public-criticism fear = HOMILOPHOBIA.

public-distance zone in social psychology, the area of physical distance between persons in formal, official, or ceremonial interactions. The p.-d.z. is defined as the area from 3½ to 7½ m (11½ to 24½ ft.). Also see PROXEMICS.

public-health approach an approach to mental and physical health revolving around three prime concepts: (a) the host, or vulnerable individual (in terms of general health, past history, genetic makeup, etc.), (b) the relevant environment (including its stressful aspects, both physical and psychological), and (c) the agent (the specific modality or sequence of environmental events that results in an identifiable disease or disorder, e.g., mosquitoes causing malaria, or a syphilitic infection producing general paresis). The approach also focuses on various levels of prevention (primary, secondary, tertiary), prevalence of different diseases, and identification of high-risk groups.

public-health nurse a graduate of a professional nursing school who has received additional special training in public-health services—in a government or community agency, or as undergraduate- or graduate-college field experience. A p.-h.n. is concerned with the health of individuals or populations in their own environment, such as home, work, or school. A p.-h.n. often has a graduate degree in public-health science.

public mental hospital a hospital for patients with mental disorders organized and run by the state, the county, or the Veterans Administration. Public mental hospitals are considerably larger than most private mental hospitals, usually have a lower doctor-patient ratio, and, though focusing increasingly on intensive treatment and rehabilitation, have a considerably higher percentage of chronic patients. See DEINSTITUTIONAL-IZATION.

public opinion the general attitude of a population toward a specific issue or group of issues.

public-opinion poll an attitude test or survey administered to a representative sample of a given population to discover the distribution of beliefs or opinions on a particular social or political issue. The validity of polls is affected by such factors as sampling techniques, wording of questions, interviewer effects, and respondents' needs for social desirability. Also called **public-opinion survey**.

public-service psychology an area of psychology that focuses on problems encountered by psychologists employed full-time in federal, state, and local government agencies.

public territory in social psychology, a public space temporarily used by a person or group, e.g., a park bench or bus seat. Also see PROXEMICS.

pubococcygeus a muscle of the pelvic area that draws the anus toward the pubic area when it contracts. The muscle is employed when a person wants to interrupt the flow of urine after it has started. P. muscle contractions are a part of the KEGEL EXERCISES. See this entry.

pudendal nerve a combined sensory and motor nerve that carries fibers to the muscles and skin of the perineal region from branches of the second, third, and fourth sacral nerves. The p.n. usually is involved in painful disorders of the penis, scrotum, and testes.

pudendum = VULVA.

puella publica /poo-el′ä/ a seldom used term for prostitute (Latin, "public girl").

puer aeternus /poo′ər īter′noos/ a Jungian term for the archetype of eternal youth (Latin, "eternal boy").

puerilism immature, childish behavior characteristic of the stage between the infantile and puberty (puberism) phases of development; a behavior pattern frequently observed in immature personalities. Also see HYSTERICAL P.; IMMATURE PERSONALITY.

puerperal disorders disorders occurring during the puerperium, which extends from the termination of labor to the return of the uterus to its normal condition. P.d. include schizophrenic and depressive reactions and, occasionally, manic episodes or delirious states precipitated by infection, hemorrhage, exhaustion, or toxemia. See POSTPARTUM PSYCHOSIS; POSTPARTUM EMOTIONAL DISTURBANCES.

puerperal osteomalacia: See OSTEOMALACIA.

puerperal psychosis = POSTPARTUM PSYCHOSIS.

puerperal sepsis: See SEPSIS.

puerperium the period of time immediately following childbirth. For most women, the p. lasts about six weeks. During the p., the female reproductive system gradually returns to its normal prepregnancy condition and usually is followed by the return of menstruation.

Puerto Rican syndrome a culture-specific syndrome occurring in Puerto Rico under the name of **mal de pelea** (Spanish, "fighting sickness"). As in amok, the individual goes off by himself and broods, then suddenly and apparently without provocation becomes violent and strikes out at anyone near him. But unlike amok, the attack usually subsides before anyone is killed.

-pulmo-; -pulmono- a combining form relating to the lungs.

pulmonary disorders diseases or injuries that involve the lungs. Kinds of p.d. may include tuberculosis, pneumonia, emphysema, chronic bronchitis, and lung cancer.

pulmonic stenosis a constriction of the pulmonary

artery that restricts the flow of blood from the right ventricle of the heart, thereby diminishing the amount of blood that can receive fresh oxygen in the alveoli of the lungs.

pulse reactor a person whose reaction to a stressful situation is manifested by changes in the circulatory system, as indicated by altered pulse strength and rate. Some pulse reactions are a normal fight-or-flight type of autonomic response.

pulv. an abbreviation used in prescriptions, meaning "powder," "powders," or "powdered" (Latin *pulvis, pulveres,* or *pulveratus*).

pulvinar a structural feature of the thalamus, appearing as a rounded, cushionlike prominence on the posterior of the diencephalon unit. The pineal gland is situated between the pulvinar surfaces of the thalami.

pun a play on words based on a double meaning (double entendre). Puns range from the lowest form of humor ("Upun my word") to an incisive and creative form of wit, as in Benjamin Franklin's statement "We must all hang together, or assuredly we shall all hang separately." From a pathological point of view, puns are a common product of the flight of ideas that occurs in manic episodes. Like other forms of humor, puns frequently "let the cat out of the bag," releasing latent hostilities or sexual impulses. See HUMOR; JOKE.

punch-drunk: See BOXER'S DEMENTIA.

punctate pertaining to a part of the skin that contains points that are sensitive to a tactile stimulus.

punctate sensitivity the variable distribution of sense receptors in the skin with the result that some points are more sensitive to certain types of stimuli than others. On most parts of the skin, pain spots are more thickly distributed than touch, cold, and warmth spots in that order.

pundning compulsive, stereotyped, purposeless searching and grooming behavior of individuals who use amphetamines.

punishment in operant conditioning, a stimulus that inflicts pain or discomfort for failure to make the proper response, resulting in a decreased probability that the improper response will recur. See BEHAVIOR MODIFICATION; REINFORCEMENT. Also see NEED FOR P.; SELF-P.

punishment fear = POINEPHOBIA.

pupillary reflex the automatic change in size of the pupil in response to light changes or a change of fixation point. Also called **light reflex**.

pupil of eye the aperture, or opening, through which light passes on entering the eye. It is located immediately in front of the lens but at the back of the anterior chamber containing aqueous humor. The size of the opening is controlled by a circle of muscle innervated by fibers of the autonomic nervous system.

puppetry therapy the use of puppets as a projective form of play therapy.

puppy love a common term for a highly romantic type of love that flourishes during adolescence but is unstable and transient. P.l. is regarded as a manifestation of emotional maturation. Also called **calf love**.

Purdue Pegboard: See PEGBOARD.

pure line a genetic line of organisms descended from a common ancestor through self-fertilization, which continue to breed true regardless of environmental differences.

pure meaning L. Vigotsky's term for the final union of language and thought in adult reasoning. According to Vigotsky, language and thought begin as independent processes but coalesce around age two, leading to the development of egocentric speech, inner speech, verbal thought, concept development, and eventually p.m. (Gardner, *Developmental Psychology,* 1978).

pure microcephaly a condition marked by an abnormally small cranium in the absence of other congenital anomalies. Pure-microcephalic individuals usually have a face of normal size and are mentally retarded. They may be smaller than average in height and in many cases are affected by spasticity of the limbs. Also called **true microcephaly; microcephalia vera**.

pure research research designed to answer a theoretical or academic question, or to develop a theory. Compare APPLIED RESEARCH.

pure-stimulus act an act that does not move an organism toward its goal although it does activate proprioceptive stimuli that initiate the appropriate operant response (Hull).

pure tone a tone produced by a simple vibration, e.g., a tuning-fork tone.

pure-tone audiometry a technique of measuring hearing loss using an instrument with electronically generated tones whose intensity is controlled by an attenuator. Hearing loss is expressed as the number of decibels in excess of the lowest intensity at which the normal ear can detect the tone. The tones are presented to each ear via head phones, at controlled frequencies.

purified delta-9-tetrahydrocannabinol: See CANNABIS ORGANIC MENTAL DISORDERS.

puritan complex = OBSCENITY-PURITY COMPLEX.

puritanical attitude inflexible adherence to a rigid moral code, including the tendency to hold others to perfectionistic standards. A p.a. is characteristic of individuals with compulsive personalities. See OBSCENITY-PURITY COMPLEX.

Purkinje, Jan Evangelista Czech physiologist, 1787–1869. See PURKINJE CELL; PURKINJE FIGURES; PURKINJE SHIFT; PURKINJE-SANSON IMAGES; BIDWELL'S GHOST (also called **Purkinje afterimage**); BIEMOND'S ATAXIA; CORPUSCLE; GABA.

Purkinje cell a heavily branched cell in the cerebellum that receives incoming signals about the position of the body and transmits signals to spinal nerves for coordinated muscle actions. P.c. degeneration is associated with tremors, shuffling gait, and other neuromuscular disorders.

Purkinje figures the shadowy images on the retina created by its blood-vessel network.

Purkinje-Sanson images three reflected images of a fixated object produced by the surface of the cornea and the front and back of the lens.

Purkinje shift a visual phenomenon in which colors appear to change with the level of illumination. A rose, e.g., may appear a bright red and its leaves a bright green at the beginning of twilights, then gradually change to a black flower with light gray leaves as the level of daylight declines, affecting the brilliance of the red end of the spectrum before the blue end.

puromycin an antibiotic used primarily as an anticancer medication and as a drug effective against some trypanosomes. Because it is a protein-synthesis inhibitor, p. has been used in some learning experiments to determine a possible molecular basis for memory.

purposeless hyperactivity a symptom of certain forms of organic brain disease characterized by exaggerated emotional responses or prolonged periods of excessive activity that has no purpose. Also called **occupational delirium**.

purposive accident an accident believed to be motivated by unconscious factors such as unacknowledged wishes or needs. Among these are the urge to express resentment, punish oneself, and seek sympathy. Also called **intentional accident**. See PARAPRAXIS.

purposive psychology = HORMIC PSYCHOLOGY.

pursuitmeter an instrument that measures the ability of a subject to follow a moving target by manipulating a pointer.

putamen a part of the lenticular nucleus that is lateral to the globus pallidus, associated with the corpus striatum, which supports the basal ganglia.

puzzle box an experimental box in which an animal subject must manipulate some type of device to get a reward. It was originally used by Thorndike in studying animal learning and intelligence.

puzzling leap: PROTOPSYCHE.

-py-; -pyo- a combining form relating to pus.

-pycn-; -pycno-: See -PYKN-.

pycnodysostosis an autosomal-recessive syndrome characterized by dense but defective bones, open skull sutures, and short stature. The patients rarely reach an adult height of five feet, and about 20 percent are likely to be mentally retarded. Also spelled **pyknodysostosis**.

pyelitis: See KIDNEY DISEASE.

pyelonephritis an inflammation of the pelvic area of the kidney, where the ureter receives the urine secreted by the nephrons. P. is usually due to a bacterial infection, which may begin in the bladder and spread upward through the ureter to the kidney or may develop as a complication of an obstruction in the ureter that diminishes the flow of urine from the renal pelvis. Also see KIDNEY DISEASE.

-pyg-; -pygo- a combining form relating to the buttocks (Greek *pyge*).

Pygmalion effect = ROSENTHAL EFFECT.

pygmalionism the act of falling in love with one's own creation (from Pygmalion in Greek mythology who fell in love with his own statue of Aphrodite). Also see ROSENTHAL EFFECT.

pygmyism a constitutional anomaly consisting of a dwarfed but well-proportioned body, roughly equivalent to the primordial **nanosomia body type** that is hereditary. It is a typical body build for certain groups of people, particularly in central Africa. Communities of similar small people have been described in myths and ancient literatures of Europe.

-pykn-; -pykno-; -pycn-; -pycno- a combining form relating to thickness or density.

pyknic type the short, thickset, stocky type of individual who, according to E. Kretschmer, tends to be jovial, extraversive, and subject to mood swings (cyclothymic temperament). See CONSTITUTIONAL TYPE.

pyknodysostosis = PYCNODYSOSTOSIS.

pyknolepsy a form of petit mal epilepsy, or a condition related to it, in which children below the age of seven experience frequent, brief clouding or interruption of consciousness, with the eyes turning upwards and the arms and trunk suddenly stiffening. The condition usually clears up spontaneously.

pyloric stenosis: See STENOSIS.

-pyr-; -pyro-; -pyret-; -pyrex- a combining form relating to fire, burning, or fever (from Greek *pyr*, "fire").

pyramidal system a network of motor-nerve tracts that originate in the cerebral-cortex-motor areas and extend to the brainstem and spinal cord uninterrupted by synapses. The tracts communicate with fibers extending to the peripheral muscles. The system is called pyramidal because the fibers form a pyramid in the medulla as they cross from the left hemisphere toward the right side of the body, and vice versa. Also see EXTRAPYRAMIDAL MOTOR SYSTEM.

pyramidal tract descending motor neurons that originate in the motor area of the cortex, the premotor area, somatosensory area, and the frontal and parietal lobes. The p.t. fibers communicate with fibers that innervate the peripheral muscles. Because of the contralateral relationship between left and right hemispheres and motor activity on the opposite sides of the body, p.t. fibers cross in the pyramidal system of the medulla.

pyrazolones a group of nonnarcotic analgesics with antipyretic effects that result from action on the thermoregulatory center of the brain. The prototype drug, **antipyrine**—$C_{11}H_{12}N_2O$—was introduced in 1884 for the treatment of malaria. Other p. include **aminopyrine**—$C_{13}H_{17}N_3O$—and **phenylbutazone**—$C_{19}H_{20}N_2O_2$. Also called **pyrazolines**. See ANTIPYRETICS. Also see BUTAZOLIDIN.

-pyret-; -pyrex-: See -PYR-.

pyrexeophobia; pyrexiophobia = FEBRIPHOBIA.

pyridostigmine $C_9H_{13}BrN_2O_2$—a cholinesterase

inhibitor used in the treatment of myasthenia gravis. P. frequently is an alternative drug to neostigmine for patients who experience side effects from that medication. Also called **p. bromide**. Trademark: **Mestinon**.

pyridoxine: See GLUTAMIC ACID; GLYCINE.

pyriform area a pear-shaped region of the rhinencephalon containing clumps of stellate and pyramidal cells. It receives olfactory tracts of the second order and relays impulses to the hippocampal formation. Also spelled **piriform area**.

pyriform cortex; pyriform lobe = PERIAMYGDA- LOID CORTEX.

pyrogen any agent that causes an increase in body temperature. Injections of serotonin into the third ventricle of cats increases their body temperature by stimulating the anterior hypothalamus. Injections of fever-producing bacteria are used as pyrogens for treating certain human diseases in which it is necessary to elevate the body temperature.

pyrolagnia the arousal of sexual excitement by large fires or conflagrations. Also called **erotic pyromania**.

pyromania a disorder of impulse control characterized by (a) a repeated failure to resist impulses to set fires and watch them burn, without monetary, social, political, or other motivations, and (b) a sense of increased tension before starting the fire, and intense pleasure, gratification, or release while committing the act. An older term is **incendiarism**. Also see PYROLAGNIA. (DSM-III)

pyrophobia a morbid fear of fire. Also called **fire phobia**.

pyrosis a burning sensation in the esophagus and stomach, sometimes identified as heartburn.

pyruvic acid a waste substance formed in body tissues during the metabolism of carbohydrates. The body's chemistry can rebuild the molecule into glycogen, or body starch, or metabolize it further into carbon dioxide to be excreted through the lungs.

Q

Q an abbreviation of *q*uantitative test. See ACE TEST.

Q data data gleaned from responses to *q*uestionnaires.

q.h. an abbreviation used in prescriptions, meaning "every hour" (Latin *quaque hora*).

q.i.d. an abbreviation used in prescriptions, meaning "four times daily" (Latin *quater in die* /dē′ā/).

Q method the use of *q*uestionnaires to obtain information.

Q methodology factor analysis across individuals rather than across tests. Q m. will show how individuals cluster together in their ratings or responses, but it does not show how traits, abilities, or other test patterns cluster together. Compare R METHODOLOGY.

qq. hor. an abbreviation used in prescriptions, meaning "every hour" (Latin *quaque hora*).

qq. 2 hor. an abbreviation used in prescriptions, meaning "every two hours" (Latin *quaque secunda hora*).

q.s. an abbreviation used in prescriptions, meaning "a sufficient quantity" (Latin *quantum sufficiat*).

Q-sort a technique used in personality evaluation in which the subject or a rater observing the subject sorts cards which stand for personal traits into piles ranging from "most characteristic" to "least characteristic." The traits can then be assigned numerical values and compared. Ordinarily, the responses are sorted along a normal distribution. Also see SELF-IDEAL Q-S.

Q technique = INVERTED FACTOR ANALYSIS.

q. 2h an abbreviation used in prescriptions, meaning "every two hours" (Latin *quaque secunda hora*).

Quaalude: See METHAQUALONE.

quadrangular therapy marital therapy involving the married couple and each spouse's individual therapist, usually conducted on a group basis.

quadrantanopsia a type of visual-field defect in which one-fourth, or one quadrant, of the normal field is lost because of a lesion involving half the optic radiation fibers. The lost quadrant is related to the area of the lesion; e.g., a lesion in the lower fibers of the right hemisphere will produce a loss of visual field in the upper left quadrant. Also called **quadrantic hemianopsia**.

quadrate lobule = PRECUNEUS.

quadriparesis a form of weakness or partial paralysis due to loss of motor-nerve functions in all four limbs. Q. occurs in certain cases of cerebral palsy. Also called **tetraparesis**. Also see QUADRIPLEGIA.

quadriplegia paralysis of all four limbs, a condition that usually is associated with severe cerebral palsy or a spinal injury that results in paralysis from the neck down. Also called **tetraplegia**. Also see QUADRIPARESIS; PARAPLEGIA.

quale /kwä′lə/ a sense datum or item of experience (Latin, "what kind") that is observed without reference to its context or significance. Q. is an aspect of structural psychology that is rejected by Gestalt principles.

qualitative approach = SYSTEMATIC APPROACH.

qualitative judgment: See VALUE JUDGMENT.

quality the character or characteristics of a sensation or other entity that makes it unique; a difference in kind rather than quantity, as between various sounds of the same note played on different instruments.

quality assurance in psychiatry, evaluation of the quality of services in terms of effectiveness, appropriateness, acceptability, efficacy, adequacy of diagnostic evaluation, length of stay, and measures of outcome. Also called **quality assessment**.

'quality of life' on the job: See JOB ENRICHMENT.

quantal hypothesis = QUANTUM THEORY.

quantitative approach the doctrine, advanced by Freud, that mental processes such as tensions, obsessions, pleasure, and unpleasure, differ in quantity as well as quality. Even though the amounts cannot be measured as exactly as in the physical sciences, they nevertheless exist. E.g., the amount of tension existing in the psyche at one time can be compared with the amount at another time.

quantitative electrophysiological battery a term used in neurometrics for a computer analysis of evoked brain potentials recorded as the subject is confronted with a series of changes in his environment, called challenges. See NEUROMETRICS.

quantitative judgment: See VALUE JUDGMENT.

quantitative score: See ACE TEST.

quantitative semantics: See CONTENT ANALYSIS.

quantum theory in psychology, the concept that changes in sensation occur in discrete steps and not along a continuum, based upon the all-or-none law of neural activity. Also called **quantal hypothesis**.

quartile one-fourth of a distribution of scores. E.g., the first q. of a distribution would be the lowest 25 percent of scores, the second q. would range from 26 percent to 50 percent, and so on.

quasi-experimental design experimentation in which full control of standard procedures is not possible, e.g., in which assignment to groups cannot be made at random.

quasi-experimental research research in which the investigator cannot control or manipulate the independent variable but can determine how the dependent variable is measured. Examples of q.-e.r. are studies that deal with the responses of large populations to such variables as natural disasters or sweeping social-policy changes that directly affect many lives.

Quasimodo complex a personality disorder arising out of the subject's concern about a defect in his physical appearance. (The term is derived from the name of the deformed bellringer in Victor Hugo's novel *The Hunchback of Notre Dame*, 1831).

quasi need K. Lewin's term for a tension state that initiates goal-directed activity with an origin in intent or purpose rather than a biological deficit.

quat = KHAT.

quaternity a unit of four components, a term sometimes applied to Jung's four-fold concept of personality: feeling, thinking, intuiting, and sensing. For Jung the q. is an archetype exemplified in myriad ways, such as the four points of the compass, four-dimensional thinking, and the four points of the cross.

querulent a quarrelsome, complaining, irritable, suspicious individual. Also see LITIGIOUS PARANOIA.

questionnaires lists of questions asked subjects in order to obtain information that may reveal lifestyles, attitudes, and other patterns of data important in psychological research. Most q. are carefully designed to avoid responses that may be biased in favor of the study objective and thus use an indirect approach of VISUALIZATION, a PROJECTIVE DEVICE, or a DEPTH INTERVIEW. See these entries.

question stage in the two-word stage of language development, the transformation of all types of sentences into questions through rising intonation on question words, as in "when go?" Generally, the q.s. is the so-called "questioning age," in which an often overwhelming number of questions are asked by the child, beginning at about three years of age and reaching a peak at around six. What and who questions usually precede questions about why and how, but in any case there are likely to be multiple motives, especially a desire to maintain social contact, to gain attention, to practice language, and to satisfy curiosity.

Quick Test a brief intelligence test (Ammons and Ammons) used for screening purposes and for the severely disabled, since the subject may respond by pointing or nodding without using words.

Quincke, Georg /kwing′kə/ German physicist, 1834–1924. See QUINCKE TUBES.

Quincke, Heinrich Irenaeus /kwing′kə/ German physician, 1842–1922. See ANGIONEUROTIC EDEMA (also called **Quincke's disease**).

Quincke tubes a set of glass tubes that produce very high-pitched sounds when air is blown across the open ends. Q.t. are used in the study of hearing thresholds.

quota control a survey-sample technique in which the quota of certain elements is proportional to the distribution in the general population. See QUOTA SAMPLING.

quota sampling a method of selecting respondents for interview in public-opinion research, in which an interviewer selects individuals with specific background characteristics, such as a particular age, race, sex, or education.

R

R: See PRIMARY ABILITIES. Also see MULTIPLE COR-RELATION.

rabies one of the infectious viral diseases that can be transmitted from animals to humans. R. usually is communicated through a bite of an infected animal although the virus may enter through any break in the skin. The r. virus travels along nerve fibers until it reaches the brain. It causes pain, fever, mental derangement, and paralysis of muscles, particularly those of the respiratory tract, and suppresses urinary function. Antirabies-vaccine treatment must be started before the virus reaches the brain. Otherwise, the infection may cause death within two to five days. The term is essentially equivalent to HYDROPHOBIA. See this entry.

rabies encephalitis a virus inflammation of the central nervous system transmitted by the bite of a rabid animal, and characterized by fever, chills, nausea, vomiting, headache, vertigo, hydrophobia, and, in most cases, death.

rabies fear = HYDROPHOBOPHOBIA. Also see CYNOPHOBIA.

race an unscientific term sometimes used to designate a portion of the human population with common ancestry and physical characteristics, and also loosely applied to cultural, religious, or other groups.

race differences differences between racial groups with regard to such factors as intelligence, temperament, and sensory acuity. As cited by Klineberg (1935), studies indicate that any differences in IQ between blacks and whites tend to decrease in size when both groups have approximately the same socioeconomic status and educational opportunities. Similarly, Japanese and Chinese children educated in the United States make the same average scores as native-born Americans. Klineberg also found (1957) that "the correlations between traits of intelligence or temperament...and anatomical characteristics...have almost invariably yielded results of no predictive value." There is also no truth to the idea of inborn differences or even group differences in sensory acuity, as proved by Woodworth's extensive studies. Probably the most insistent, and controversial, advocate of the view that blacks as a whole are in-herently inferior to whites in intelligence is Arthur R. Jensen.

-rachi-; -rachio- a combining form relating to the spine.

rachischisis /rakis′kəsis/ a congenital fissure of the spinal column. An example of r. is SPINA BIFIDA. See this entry.

racial memory thought patterns, feelings, and traces of experiences believed to be transmitted from generation to generation, and to have a basic influence on our minds and behavior. Jung and Freud both embraced the concept of a phylogenetic heritage, but focused on different examples. Freud cited the primal-horde theory, religious rituals designed to relieve feelings of anxiety and guilt, and fantasies connected with parental coitus and castration fear. Jung cited the archetypes of the collective unconscious, and images, symbols, and personifications which spontaneously appear in different cultures. Also see RACIAL UNCONSCIOUS.

racial unconscious the division of the unconscious that, according to Jung, comprises "contents that do not originate in personal acquisitions but in the inherited possibility of psychic functions in general, namely, in the inherited brain-structure. These are the mythological associations—those motives and images that can spring anew in every age and clime, without historical tradition or migration" (*Contributions to Analytical Psychology*, 1928). Though he did not develop the concept as far as Jung, Freud recognized "psychical processes that continued from one generation to another" (*Totem and Taboo*, 1913), and in *Moses and Monotheism*, 1939, he stated that children respond instinctively "in a manner that is only explicable as phylogenetic acquisition." See COLLECTIVE UNCONSCIOUS; RACIAL MEMORY.

racism the fixed attitude that one "race" is superior to all others by nature, accompanied by prejudicial attitudes and discriminatory behavior toward members of "races" labeled inferior. Also see AVERSIVE R.; STEREOTYPE; PREJUDICE; RACE DIFFERENCES.

-rad- a combining form relating (a) to a root (Latin *radix*), forming the adjective **radical,** (b) to a rod or a ray (Latin *radius*), forming the adjective **radial.**

radial reflex a deep extension reflex in which the forearm flexes when the lower end of the radius is tapped. If the fingers also flex, it is a sign of hyperflexia.

radiant energy energy that generally radiates outward from a source, e.g., electromagnetic light waves from a lamp.

radiation in medicine, the transmission of light, electromagnetics waves (e.g., short radio waves), or nuclear particles for diagnostic, therapeutic, or experimental purposes. R. may include X-rays, ultraviolet light, or beta rays of radioactive chemicals. The term r. applies also to the spreading of excitation to adjacent neurons. Also see COBALT TREATMENT; RADIO-THERAPY.

radiation sickness a condition that results from overexposure to sources of radioactivity, which may be therapeutic doses. Onset of symptoms may be marked by headache and general malaise, nausea, vomiting, and anorexia. The severity of r.s. depends upon the physical condition of the subject, the intensity and duration of the exposure, the body area affected, and the type of radiation.

radiation-therapy technologist a type of health professional concerned with several subspecialties associated with the use of radiologic and nuclear technologies in diagnostic and therapeutic procedures. The category includes diagnostic X-ray technologist, nuclear-medical technologist, radiation-therapy technologist, and nuclear-medical technician. A r.-t.t. is also called a **radiologic technologist**.

radical: See -RAD-.

radical characterizing behavior that is associated with motivation directed toward sudden, extreme, and fundamental changes.

radical behaviorism the theory of conditioning developed by B. F. Skinner. Also see DESCRIPTIVE BEHAVIORISM. See BEHAVIOR ANALYSIS.

radical hysterectomy: See HYSTERECTOMY.

radical mastectomy: See MASTECTOMY.

radical therapy a therapeutic approach focused on changes in the social structure as a whole, as contrasted with the standard individual, group, family, and community approaches. R.t. is based on the idea that individual pathology often reflects social pathology, and that the major factors that produce psychological problems are not internal conflicts but social conflicts, as well as social roles and environmental conditions that hamper individual expression and personal growth. It is therefore the structure more than the person that needs changing. If, e.g., the rate of schizophrenia is to be reduced, we must eliminate poverty and deprivation, since the incidence of schizophrenia is highest in poor communities. And if the "housewife syndrome" is to be avoided, society must find ways to enable women to achieve a greater sense of fulfillment in the outside world.

radiculitis an inflammation of a spinal-nerve root, particularly the portion between the spinal cord and the intervertebral canal.

radiculopathies disorders of the spinal-nerve roots. R. include various myopathies produced by vertebrae compressing the nerve roots, such as the condition commonly known as slipped disk.

radioactive-iodine therapy the use of radioisotopes of iodine in the treatment of thyroid-gland disease. The isotopes, radioiodine ^{125}I or ^{131}I, are injected into the bloodstream and taken up by cells of the thyroid gland which requires iodine for the synthesis of thyroxine. The radiation damages or destroys thyroid tissue, thereby reducing the excess production of thyroid hormone.

radioactive isotopes variations of chemical elements that have the same number of nuclear protons but different numbers of neutrons, and which also emit radiation in the form of alpha particles or beta or gamma rays. The radiation is produced as the isotopes decay into simpler atoms and lose energy while gaining stability. Because r.i. affect photographic film, produce an electric charge in the surrounding air and fluorescence with certain other substances, and have the ability to destroy or alter cells or microorganisms, they are used widely in diagnostic and therapeutic techniques.

radioactive tracers chemical compounds that are prepared with a radioactive isotope, such as calcium (^{45}Ca) or carbon (^{14}C), so that their metabolic pathways can be traced through body tissues. R.t. may be used for diagnostic, therapeutic, or research purposes. For tobacco research, nicotine molecules can be tagged with r.t. and the path of the alkaloid traced through the lungs and bloodstream of cigarette smokers.

radioautography = AUTORADIOGRAPHY.

radiograph an apparatus for making a **radiogram**, or photographic image produced by X-rays or radioactive isotopes. Also see PROTON-BEAM RADIOGRAPHY.

radioimmunoassay /-as'ā/ an immune-system study procedure in which an antigen, which may be a hormone or other substance, is tagged with a radioactive isotope and allowed to react with a specific antibody. It is applied in determining abnormal hormone levels, allergies and infections, and drug overdoses.

radioisotope an isotope of an atom that is radioactive. A r. may be used in diagnosis, therapy, or research because of its radioactive properties, e.g., in encephalography (**radioisotopic encephalography**).

radiologic technologist = RADIATION-THERAPY TECHNOLOGIST.

radiomimetic drugs substances that produce effects similar to those of radioactive materials. Examples include the alkylating agents such as nitrogen mustards, cyclophosphamide, and chlorambucil, used in the treatment of lymphomas and leukemias.

radiotherapy the use of radiant energy, e.g., X-rays and radioactive isotopes, in the treatment of diseases. R. is employed mainly in the destruction of cancer cells by implanting radioactive isotopes or directing beams of radiant energy so that a known dose of radiation can be delivered to a specific tissue area. Localizing the effect is important since the radiation can damage or destroy surrounding tissue as well as the cancer cells.

radix in physiology, a bundle of nerve fibers at the point of entry or departure from the central nervous system (Latin, "root").

Rado, Sandor Hungarian-born American psychoanalyst, 1890–1972. See ADAPTATIONAL APPROACH; ALIMENTARY ORGASM; EMERGENCY DYSCONTROL; HORRIFIC TEMPTATION; MOOD-CYCLIC DISORDERS; OBSESSIVE ATTACK; PRIDE; RETROFLEXION; RIDDANCE PHENOMENON; RITUAL-MAKING; UNEMOTIONAL THOUGHT.

rage an intense, violent anger during which the body mobilizes itself for attack, which may or may not be carried out. R. is a primitive response to frustration resembling the overwhelming temper reactions of young children. The pattern may vary with different species, but generally includes rapid respiration, thrusting and jerking of limbs, and clawing, biting, and snarling. Also see SHAM R.

railroad fear = SIDERODROMOPHOBIA.

railway spine = ERICHSEN'S DISEASE.

rain phobia = OMBROPHOBIA.

Raman, Sir Chandra-Sekhara Venkata Indian physicist, 1888–1970. See RAMAN SHIFT; INFRARED-THEORY OF SMELL; VIBRATION THEORY.

Raman shift a shift in the frequency of light caused by the interaction of a photon and the energy-level changes of an atom or molecule exposed to the photon. The R.s. is the basis for one of several theories used to explain the olfactory phenomenon. Also called **Raman effect**.

Ramón y Cajal, Santiago Spanish histologist, 1852–1934. See CELLULAR LAYERS OF CORTEX (there: **plexiform layer of Cajal**).

Ramsay Hunt's syndrome = HUNT'S SYNDROME.

ramus a branch of a nerve or vein, or a neural tract linking the sympathetic ganglia to the spinal cord and visceral or peripheral organs (Latin, "branch, bough").

random activity behavior that has no apparent goal or purpose or specific stimulus, e.g., infant's movements.

random assignment: See RANDOMIZED-GROUP DESIGN.

random error an error due to chance alone, and randomly distributed around a true score. R.e. may be contrasted to constant error or systematic bias. Also called **chance error; variable error**.

randomized clinical trial an experimental design in which a group of patients is randomly divided into a group that will receive an experimental treatment and a second group that will receive a comparison treatment or placebo.

randomized-group design an experimental design in which subjects are assigned at random to experimental or control groups without matching on a background variable. Compare MATCHED-GROUP DESIGN.

random model an experimental paradigm used in the analysis of variance, in which the experimenter randomly samples the independent variables. Also called **components-of-variance model**. Also see FIXED MODEL; MIXED MODEL.

random numbers a set of numbers generated by chance alone, without a predictable pattern. In order to avoid biased assignment to experimental conditions, a table of r.n. is often used.

random observation any observation that occurs spontaneously or by chance, is uncontrolled, and is not part of a schedule of organized observation.

random sample a sample drawn from a population in such a way as to insure that every unit in the population has an equal chance of being selected, and that only chance dictates which unit is selected. A r.s. may be contrasted with a casual or haphazard sample in which no systematic means is used to insure that only chance governs selection. Compare SELECTED GROUP. Also see HAPHAZARD SAMPLING.

random variable a variable whose value depends upon chance.

range in statistics, a measure of dispersion, obtained by subtracting the lowest score from the highest score in a distribution. Also see MEASURE OF VARIATION.

range effect in pursuit or tracking, a tendency to make movements too large when the target motion is small and too small when the target motion is large.

range of audibility the span of sound frequencies an individual can hear, a range that for a young adult covers frequencies from 20 to 20,000 cycles per second.

range-of-motion exercises exercises that test and train the ability of the patient to move a joint through a hypothetical path that can be measured in degrees of a circle. R.-o.-m.e. for the cervical spine involve rotating the head as far to the left and right as possible without moving the trunk, leaning the head as far backward and forward as possible, and moving the head alternately toward the left and right shoulders.

range restriction selection of a limited portion of a sample, e.g., studying subjects with IQs between 90 and 100 and neglecting more extreme cases. In practice, this often leads to lower correlations with other measures.

Ranikhet disease of Asia = NEWCASTLE VIRUS.

Rank, Otto /rängk/ Austrian psychoanalyst, 1884–1939. R. began his professional career as a member of Freud's coterie, but broke away because of his emphasis on short-term therapy and on the birth trauma, which he believed to be at the root of neuroses. His therapy was aimed at eliminating the effects of the trauma, especially anxiety and dependence, and helping the patient to achieve constructive independence and trusting relationships. See BIRTH EXPERIENCE; BIRTH FEAR; BIRTH TRAUMA; TRUE SYMBOLISM; WILL THERAPY.

rank-difference correlation: See RANK-ORDER CORRELATION.

ranked distribution a method of distributing scores or values in an order from highest to lowest or lowest to highest.

Rankian therapy = WILL THERAPY.

rank order the arrangement of a series of items, e.g., scores or individuals, in an order of magnitude or merit.

rank-order correlation a measure of the degree of relationship between two variables that have each been placed in ranks. Also called **rank-difference correlation; Spearman's rho; Spearman r.-o.c.** Symbol: $\text{rho} = \dfrac{6\Sigma D^2}{N(N^2-1)}$

rank-order method a technique of arranging a series of items (scores, individual cases) according to an order of merit.

Ranvier, Louis Antoine /räNvē·ā'/ French pathologist, 1835–1922. See NODES OF RANVIER; SALTATORY CONDUCTION.

rape forced sexual intercourse, usually by a man with a woman, but also with a man or boy (homosexual rape), mainly in prisons. The act is interpreted, especially by psychoanalysts, as a means of gratifying both libidinal (sexual) and aggressive impulses. The need to humiliate the victim may also be involved. Local laws define specific variations, such as the absence or presence of genital penetration, the married or unmarried status of the parties, or the interpretation of the term "valid consent." Also see STATUTORY R.

rape counseling provision of guidance and support for victims of rape. **Rape crisis centers** are located in many communities to offer expert counseling in the psychiatric emergency that usually follows a sexual attack accompanied by violence and humiliation.

rape-trauma syndrome a symptom complex consisting of confusion, fear, guilt, humiliation, rage, and shame experienced by a rape victim. The symptoms, which may include fear of being alone, phobic attitudes toward sex, vaginismus, male impotence, or repeated washing of the body, may persist for a year or more after the rape. The r.-t.s. may be aggravated by an attitude of others that the victim "invited" rape by her dress or other behavior (or by his behavior).

rap group a form of group interaction in which the members engage in an informal dialogue about their current problems with or without a professional leader. E.g., a group of women may meet periodically to discuss their own roles, the status of women in Western society, and various ways they can achieve a greater sense of fulfillment. Also called **rap session.** The purpose of such groups is often described as CONSCIOUSNESS-RAISING. See this entry.

raphe: See NUCLEUS OF THE R.

rapid-change theory a theory concerning the position of the aged in society, which states that their status tends to be high in static societies and to decline in proportion to rapid social change.

rapid eye movement: See REM SLEEP.

rapid-smoking treatment a behavior-modification treatment for cigarette-smokers in which the patient is instructed to puff rapidly and smoke the cigarettes faster than usual to intensify the aversive effect.

rapport /rəpôr'/ a warm, relaxed relationship that promotes mutual acceptance, e.g., between therapist and patient, or between teacher and student. R. implies that the confidence inspired by the former produces trust and willing cooperation in the latter.

rapprochement a state of cordial relations between individuals or groups. In M. S. Mahler's theory of separation-individuation, r. is a phase of the process in which the child, after about 18 months of age, makes active approaches to the mother, as contrasted with the preceding stage in which the child was relatively oblivious of her.

rap session = RAP GROUP.

rapture a state of extreme joy or pleasure, often identified with mystical or spiritual ecstasy.

rapture-of-the-deep syndrome an acute, transient psychosis experienced by scuba and deep-sea divers, believed to be precipitated by an excessively high blood-nitrogen level (**nitrogen narcosis**), in combination with sensory deprivation.

raptus action a reaction to extreme, unbearable tension, in which the individual is suddenly seized (Latin *raptus*, "seized") by a destructive, or self-destructive, impulse to commit suicide, castrate himself, set a fire, or commit a violent crime. Other examples are the sudden disorganized movements and periods of cataleptic rigidity observed in catatonic schizophrenics, both of which appear to be attempts to relieve tension.

RAS = RETICULAR ACTIVATING SYSTEM.

ratee the individual who is rated.

rate of first admissions the ratio of the number of first admissions to a hospital for treatment of a mental disease during a year to the population of the area, such as a city, county, or state. The figure may be expressed as the number per 100,000 population or a percentage, or both.

rate of occurrence: See INCIDENCE; PREVALENCE.

rate score the number of tasks finished in a defined period of time.

rating a rank or score assigned to an item, e.g., an individual, test result, or mechanical device; also, the process of assigning ranks or scores.

rating scale an instrument used by teachers, counselors, and interviewers to assess selected characteristics of a given individual. Usually, a r.s. consists of short phrases describing the variables to be evaluated; e.g., graduate-school applicants are rated by former professors on dimensions reflecting intellectual and social development.

ratio any relationship between two quantities expressed as a quotient or the product of a mathematical division, e.g., the IQ is the r. of the mental age divided by the chronological age.

rational-emotive therapy = RATIONAL PSYCHO-THERAPY.

rationalization the defense mechanism in which questionable reasons are given to justify unacceptable behavior or personal shortcomings. Examples are: "Doesn't *everybody* cheat?"; "An expensive car saves money in the end"; "You have to beat children to toughen them up." Excuses of this kind are used to ward off feelings of guilt, maintain self-respect, and protect ourselves from criticism.

rational learning meaningful learning, involving a clear understanding of the learned material and the relationship among its components.

rational psychotherapy a cognitive-behavioral approach developed by Albert Ellis, based on the view that emotional problems and disorders stem from faulty, distorted attitudes and self-defeating beliefs. These ideas are repeatedly expressed in the form of "internalized sentences" such as "It is better to avoid than to face difficulties." In the process of therapy, the irrational attitudes are unmasked by direct confrontation, and altered by first showing how they produce the patient's problems and then indicating how they can be changed through behavior-therapy techniques. Also called **rational-emotive therapy (RET)**. Also see COGNITIVE BEHAVIOR MODIFICATION.

rational type one of Jung's major categories of psychological types. It is composed of the thinking and feeling functional types, as distinguished from the irrational functional types of intuitive and sensational.

ratio reinforcement reinforcement that is made contingent on the subject's behavior. In operant conditioning, r.r. is presented after the subject has made the prearranged number of correct responses, in contrast to reinforcement delivered on the basis of a time schedule only. Also see FIXED-R.R. SCHEDULE; VARIABLE-R.R. SCHEDULE; INTERVAL REINFORCEMENT.

ratio scale in statistics, a scale of measurement that has a true zero point and which allows operations of multiplication and division, as well as addition and subtraction. Also see INTERVAL SCALE; NOMINAL SCALE; ORDINAL SCALE.

Rat Man a landmark case of Freud's (1907), in which a 30-year-old lawyer's obsessional fear of rats was traced to repressed death wishes toward his father generated by oedipal conflicts. One example of his obsession was his belief that a rat that appeared to come out of his father's grave had eaten the corpse; another was a fantasy that a rat had been placed in his father's anus and had eaten through his intestines. Analysis of these reactions laid the groundwork for the

psychoanalytic interpretation of obsessional neurosis.

Rauwolf, Leonhard /rou'vŏlf/ German botanist, died 1596. See RAUWOLFIA DERIVATIVES; NEUROLEPTICS; RESCINNAMINE.

Rauwolfia derivatives alkaloid substances obtained from a plant of the genus Rauwolfia, primarily R. serpentina, the ancient Hindu snakeroot. R.d. have sedative, antihypertensive, and pulse-depressant actions and are used as neuroleptics. Rauwolfia had been used as a tranquilizer since about 1000 B.C. by Hindu doctors and was given its botanical name in honor of the German botanist Leonhard Rauwolf who discovered its use for Europe in 1575 while traveling in India. The prototype drug of the group is **reserpine**—$C_{33}H_{40}N_2O_9$—which acts by depleting central- and peripheral-nervous-system stores of amines. R.d. are used mainly in treatment of certain severely disturbed psychotic patients and in Huntington's chorea. Also see DESERPIDINE.

raving madness a term used in the Middle Ages for a mental illness, or insanity, that was believed to threaten the security of other citizens. The raving individuals were divided into two classes: criminals, who violated legal conventions and were subject to incarceration or other forms of punishment, and the possessed, who violated social conventions and were sent on pilgrimages to seek cures at holy places.

raw score the original test score before it is converted to other units or another form. Also called **crude score; obtained score; original score**.

Ray, Isaac American physician, 1807–81. One of the most influential psychiatrists of his time, R. helped to create the Association of Medical Superintendents of American Institutions for the Insane, the forerunner of the American Psychiatric Association. He also contributed to the development of forensic psychiatry, and collaborated with Thomas Kirkbride in developing policies and plans for well-built and well-managed mental hospitals, in which patients would have "abundant means for occupation and amusement," though he also insisted on advocating physical restraint. See MORAL TREATMENT.

Rayleigh equation a statement of the proportion of red and green stimuli needed for a normal human eye to perceive yellow. Persons who are red-weak or green-weak require different proportions.

Raynaud, Maurice /rānō'/ French physician, 1834–81. See RAYNAUD'S DISEASE; PSYCHOPHYSIOLOGIC CARDIOVASCULAR REACTION.

Raynaud's disease spasms of the arteries or arterioles, particularly in peripheral areas such as fingers or toes, with pallor or cyanosis of the associated skin surfaces. The phenomenon may be spontaneous or secondary to a disease (e.g., myxedema) or drug intoxication, e.g., ergot.

Spontaneous attacks of R.d. are often precipitated by exposure to cold or by an emotional disturbance, and occur most frequently in young women. The condition may be aggravated by use of nicotine, which constricts peripheral circulation. Chronic R.d. may be marked by smooth, shiny skin on the digits, with loss of subcutaneous tissue. Also called **Raynaud's phenomenon**.

reactance the theory that restrictions on any type of object or behavior add to its desirability.

reaction a response to a stimulus; or a response pattern such as a psychiatric disorder or personality type; also, a negative attitude to a person, or to a party on the political scene.

reactional biography in industrial psychology, an applicant' account of himself in terms of the way he reacts to the events of his life. A skillful interviewer attempts to elicit these reactions in addition to the usual factual data.

reaction formation a defense mechanism in which unacceptable or threatening impulses are denied by going to the opposite extreme. To conceal prejudice, we may preach tolerance; to deny feelings of rejection, a mother may be overindulgent toward her child; and, as pointed out by R. M. Goldenson, *The Encyclopedia of Human Behavior* (1970), "the outward behavior may, at least in some cases, provide a disguise or unconscious outlet for the tendencies it seems to oppose. The professional defender of public morals may get a good deal of satisfaction from reading the literature or seeing the shows he so roundly condemns."

reaction products: See SUBSTRATE.

reaction range the potential or limits of an individual's reactions as determined by genetic factors. Genetic conditions define the mental and physical boundaries of an individual; environment and experience determine whether those boundaries can be reached.

reaction time = RESPONSE TIME.

reaction-time test any test designed to measure the interval between the application of a stimulus and the start of the subject's response.

reaction type a syndrome classified in terms of predominating symptoms, as in Adolf Meyer's affective, delirious, deteriorated, disguised-conflict, organic, and paranoid reaction types. In reaction-time experiments, the term applies to a particular type of set or readiness: motor, sensory, or mixed.

reactivation process: See MIRROR TRANSFERENCE.

reactive characterizing an episode, such as depressive or schizophrenic, that is secondary to a traumatic event in the life of the patient. A r. episode generally has a more favorable prognosis than a similar episode that is endogenous in origin and unrelated to a specific happening.

reactive alcoholism = ALPHA ALCOHOLISM.

reactive-attachment disorder of infancy a disorder characterized by lack of responsiveness associated with absence of affectional care, as in gross emotional neglect or social isolation in an institution. Common signs are absence of visual tracking, of smiling, of visual or vocal reciprocity, of turning toward a caretaker's voice, of reaching for the mother, or of participation in playful games, as well as a weak cry, excessive sleep, disinterest in the environment, hypomotility, poor muscle tone, weak rooting and grasping in feeding attempts, or weight loss or failure to gain when not due to physical disorder. (DSM-III)

reactive confusion a term used in the ICD-8 (eighth edition of the International Classification of Diseases) for a state of bewilderment and disorientation occurring as a reaction to a stressful event such as removal of an elderly person to a nursing home. R.c. is an acute psychotic episode which may or may not mark the onset of a chronic illness. The term **reactive excitation** is also used in a similar sense.

reactive depression a transient, nonrecurrent depression precipitated by an intensely distressing event such as loss of a loved one, loss of a job, or a financial setback. R.d. is usually treated with antidepressant drugs, and in some cases with electroshock as an emergency measure. Also called **exogenous depression; neurotic-depressive reaction; depressive reaction**. Compare ENDOGENOUS DEPRESSION.

reactive disorder a mental disorder which is apparently precipitated by severe environmental pressure or a traumatic event. Examples are reactive depression and reactive schizophrenia.

reactive ego alteration the expenditure of energy in repressing libidinal or aggressive impulses in which the ego is altered by a reaction-formation against the impulses. An example is that of a hysterical woman who treats with excessive tenderness children she actually hates.

reactive excitation: See REACTIVE CONFUSION.

reactive inhibition a tendency for response magnitude to decrease with increasing practice or fatigue (Hull).

reactive mania a form of hypomania that represents a reaction to an external event.

reactive measures measurements that alter the variable under investigation. E.g., if a subject is conscious of being observed, his reactions may be influenced more by the observer and the fact that he is being observed than by the stimulus object or situation to which he is ostensibly responding. Compare UNOBTRUSIVE MEASURES.

reactive psychosis = SITUATIONAL PSYCHOSIS.

reactive schizophrenia an acute form of schizophrenia which develops in response to predisposing or precipitating environmental factors such as extreme stress. The patient has a history of better adjustment in childhood, and has usually shown an interest in the opposite sex during adolescence. The prognosis is generally more favorable than for schizophrenia that originates endogenously. Compare PROCESS SCHIZOPHRENIA.

reactivity the condition in which an object being observed is changed by the fact that it is the object of observation. See REACTIVE MEASURES.

readability level the level at which a child is able to read successfully. It is a relative measure of skills in terms of grade level. The degree of readability is measured in terms of such factors as legibility of the printed page, vocabulary, sentence length and structure, human interest, and general intelligibility.

readership-survey technique an advertising-research method of determining how thoroughly a consumer may have read the copy in a print-media advertisement. The subject is shown a list of products, brand names, or company names. If the subject claims to have seen an ad for any of them in a particular magazine or newspaper, he is asked to recall information about the content of the advertising copy.

readiness the state of preparedness to respond to a stimulus; in learning, the degree of preparation necessary for a specific task or subject to represent meaningful learning. R. embraces all aspects of development, e.g., physical, intellectual, and social.

readiness law: See LAW OF READINESS.

readiness test a test designed to predict how well an individual is prepared to profit from instruction in a particular field, especially reading, mathematics (arithmetic, algebra, geometry), and foreign languages.

reading disability deficiency in reading skill associated with such conditions as perceptual deficit, faulty habit patterns (mouthing words, backtracking), poor comprehension, inadequate word analysis, deficient vocabulary, defective auditory perception, directional confusion, minimal brain dysfunction, emotional problems, or environmental deprivation. Corrective or remedial programs are usually recommended. Also see DYSLEXIA; PARALEXIA.

reading disorder: See DEVELOPMENTAL R.D.; DYSLEXIA.

reading epilepsy a type of reflex epilepsy in which reading precipitates myoclonic jaw movements. If reading continues after the initial symptom, a general convulsion may occur.

reading-fear = BIBLIOPHOBIA.

reading quotient a child's reading ability as determined by dividing his reading-age test score by his chronological age.

reading readiness the development of early language skills, auditory and visual discrimination, cognitive abilities, and fine motor coordination which are the prerequisites of reading.

reading retardation a term applied to a category of individuals whose reading-achievement level is two or more years below their mental age.

reading span = RECOGNITION SPAN.

readmission the admission to a mental hospital or other institution of a patient who had been admitted previously. The rate of readmissions has tended to increase in recent years, a factor attributed to policies of early discharge of first admissions, resulting in a pattern sometimes called a revolving-door phenomenon.

Realangst: See REAL ANXIETY.

real anxiety the *Realangst* /rä·äl'ängst/ of Freud, who used the term to identify anxiety caused by a true danger posed by the external world of reality. Also called **reality anxiety.** The term is essentially equivalent to OBJECTIVE ANXIETY. See this entry.

realism the philosophical doctrine that objects have an existence independent of the observer (in contrast to idealism). The term applies also to the older philosophical doctrine that abstract concepts have a greater genuine reality than the physical objects to which they refer (in contrast to nominalism).

realism factor in psychological esthetics, the effect of independent and objective influences on art judgments, in contrast to judgments dominated by subjective or idealistic factors.

realistic stage: See CRYSTALLIZATION.

realistic thinking thinking that is based or focused on the objective qualities and requirements that pertain in different situations. R.t. permits adjustment of thoughts and behavior to the demands of a situation; it is predicated on the ability to interpret external situations in a fairly consistent, accurate manner. This, in turn, is based on the capacity to distinguish fantasy and subjective experience from external reality. Also see REALITY TESTING.

reality the universe as a whole; or the actual as opposed to the illusory. In psychoanalysis, r. is the environment, or external world, as contrasted to the internal world of thoughts, feelings, and fantasies. "To a large degree reality is whatever the people who are around at the time agree to" (Milton H. Miller, *Psychiatry: A Personal View*, 1982). Also see PSYCHIC R.; RELATIVITY OF R.; SOCIAL R.; OBJECTIVE R.

reality anxiety = REAL ANXIETY.

reality assumptions the assumptions about how things really are and what kind of persons we are that are fundamental to the functioning of the self-structure.

reality denial: See DENIAL.

reality ego: See PLEASURE EGO.

reality life of ego in psychoanalysis, the practical everyday life of the patient and its reality problems, which the therapist may help to improve indirectly in carrying out his main task of treating the patient's conflicts by analyzing his impulses and resistances.

reality orientation in psychiatry, a form of re-motivation that aims to reduce the confusion of a patient who lacks full orientation to time, place, or person. The technique consists of continual reminders to the patient of who he is, what day it is, where he is, and what is happening or is about to take place. In attribution theory, r.o. consists of trying to comprehend the relationships that link environmental events and interactions between persons so that one may predict outcomes and successfully mold one's own behavior to the existing conditions.

reality principle in psychoanalysis, the regulatory mechanism that represents the demands of the external world and requires us to forego or modify gratification or postpone it to a more appropriate time. In contrast to the pleasure principle, which governs the life of the infant and child, and represents the id or instinctual impulses, the r.p., represents the ego, which controls our impulses and enables us to deal rationally and effectively with the situations of life.

reality testing in psychoanalysis, the objective evaluation of sense impressions, which enables us to distinguish between the internal and external world, and between fantasy and reality. Defective r.t. is the major criterion of psychosis.

reality therapy a treatment technique developed by William Glasser, which focuses on present behavior and the development of the patient's ability to cope with the stresses of reality and take greater responsibility for the fulfillment of his needs. To achieve these purposes, the therapist plays an active role in "examining the patient's daily activities and suggesting better ways for him to behave."

real love = POSTAMBIVALENT PHASE.

real pride: See PRIDE.

real self a term applied by Horney to the individual's potential for further growth and development.

real-simulator model an experimental design in which some subjects are instructed to simulate hypnosis, or some other psychological state, while other subjects are genuinely experiencing it. The experimenter is usually unaware of whether he is dealing with a real case or a simulator. This model was originated by Orne.

real time a term referring to a calculation or simulation taking place while an outside event is occurring. If statistics are calculated on physiological responses as they take place, they are performed in r.t.

real-world setting: See FIELD EXPERIMENT; MUNDANE REALISM; STRESS TEST.

reasoning a type of thinking that depends upon logical processes of an inductive or deductive character.

reassociation a process of renewing or reviewing a forgotten or repressed traumatic event in hypnoanalysis, so that the experience will be integrated with the person's normal personality and consciousness.

reassurance in psychotherapy, a supportive approach that encourages the patient to believe in himself and the possibilities of improvement. It is used frequently in supportive therapy and occasionally in reconstructive therapy to encourage a patient as he explores new relationships and feelings. R. is also used to diminish anxiety, e.g., by explaining to a patient that a period of heightened depression or tension is temporary and not unexpected.

rebelliousness resistance to authority, especially parental authority or its equivalent; in adolescence, an expression of the need for independence. If persistent and indiscriminate, r. may be a sign of immaturity or neurotic aggressiveness.

rebirth fantasy in psychoanalysis, the fantasy of being born again, usually expressed in dreams involving emergence from water. R.f. is variously interpreted as a desire to return to the tranquillity of the womb; an unconscious incestuous wish for the mother; an attempt to deny death; and an expression of the religious belief in resurrection.

rebound eating an effect of stimulating the ventromedial hypothalamus, which contains neurons that have been associated with glucose utilization: The stimulus is believed to override a mechanism that inhibits the urge to eat.

rebound phenomenon a test for ataxia which shows that the patient has lost the ability of the cerebellum to control coordinated movement: If he attempts to extend his forearm against resistance and then suddenly lets go, the hand or fist will snap back against the mouth or shoulder. Also called **r.p. of Gordon Holmes; Holmes' phenomenon; Gordon Holmes r.p.**

recall the process of bringing learned material or past experiences into consciousness. Also see FREE R.

recall method a technique of evaluating memory in terms of the percentage of learned material that can be correctly reproduced after an interval. Also called **recall test.**

recapitulation theory the theory that the growing organism passes through all the stages of evolutionary development characteristic of the species, that is, ontogeny repeats phylogeny. Also called **biogenetic law.** Also see FORMAL PARALLELISM.

recathexis in psychoanalysis, an attempt by the schizophrenic to restore, or "reconstitute" the lost object world (that is, regain contact with reality) through delusions and hallucinations.

receiver in communication theory, a device or process that translates a signal into a message, e.g., the sensory apparatus of vision or hearing, or a radio r.

receiving hospital a health facility that is specially equipped and staffed to handle new patients requiring diagnosis and preliminary treatment, e.g., cases of suspected mental disorder.

recency effect the tendency for the most recently presented facts, impressions, or items in formal-learning situations to be learned or remembered best. The r.e. appears to have special relevance to information of low interest and familiarity. Also called **law of recency; principle of recency.** Compare PRIMACY EFFECT.

receptive amimia: See AMIMIA.

receptive aphasia a communication disorder, usually due to brain damage, in which the subject can hear words but does not understand them or can see words but is unable to read. Such patients once were identified as word-deaf or word-blind. The condition, however, concerns all forms of language, not just words. Also called **receptive dysphasia; sensory aphasia; impressive aphasia; logagnosia; logamnesia**. Also see EXPRESSIVE APHASIA.

receptive character Fromm's term for a passive, dependent, and compliant personality type, roughly equivalent to the oral-passive or passive-dependent types described by others. Also see RECEPTIVE ORIENTATION.

receptive dysphasia = RECEPTIVE APHASIA.

receptive field the area of the surface of a sensory organ that is served by a single nerve fiber. A r.f. can be very small or as large as several square inches, depending upon the distribution of dendritic branches. Also called **receptor field**.

receptive language language that is received and understood through gestures or spoken or written symbols. A disturbance in the central nervous system may disrupt the normal r.l. process.

receptive orientation a term employed by E. Fromm for a personality pattern characterized by dependence on others, inability to make decisions or take responsibility, the search for a "magic helper," and a need to conform. Also see RECEPTIVE CHARACTER; ORAL CHARACTER.

receptor any of several different types of nerve cells that are specialized to receive appropriate stimuli. Kinds of r. include chemical, light, mechanical, and thermal. A r. type may be specialized further, such as mechanical receptors that are sensitive to sound, touch, or balance. Also called **neuroreceptor**.

receptor field = RECEPTIVE FIELD.

receptor potential the electrical potential across the membrane of a receptor cell of a sense organ. The potential may vary with the intensity of a stimulus. Potentials in the retina, e.g., change with the light falling upon the eye.

recess a rest or recreation interval between trials, practice sessions, or work periods.

recessive gene a gene or hereditary trait that will be transmitted to an offspring only if it is present on two homologous chromosomes or on a hemizygous chromosome. See DOMINANT GENE; GENE.

recessive inheritance transmission of a genetic trait that is recessive. A r.i. is expressed as a physical trait only when it is contributed at conception by gametes of both parents.

recessive trait a genetic trait that will not be expressed in an offspring in the presence of a dominant trait for the same characteristic. If both parents have the r.t., it will appear in the offspring.

recidives in schizophrenia a form of schizophrenia in which there are intermittent, recurring, acute episodes after a long period of remission. The attacks usually duplicate past episodes, but with new features.

recidivism /-sid'-/ repetition of delinquent or criminal behavior, especially as applied to habitual criminals, or "repeaters," who have been convicted several times. The term is also occasionally applied to mental patients who have had many relapses.

reciprocal determinism a concept that opposes the radical or exclusive emphasis on environmental determination of responses and asserts that a reciprocal relation exists between environment, behavior, and the individual. That is, instead of conceptualizing the environment as a one-way determinant of behavior, r.d. maintains that the environment influences behavior, behavior influences the environment, and both influence the individual who also influences them. This concept is associated with social learning theory.

reciprocal inhibition the inhibition of one spinal reflex when another is elicited (C. S. Sherrington); or a mechanism that prevents opposing muscles from contracting at the same time. R.i. is also the inability to recall two associated ideas because of their interference with each other. In behavior therapy, r.i. is the technique in which the strength of response to an anxiety-provoking stimulus can be weakened or suppressed if a response antagonistic to the anxiety occurs while the stimulus is being presented; e.g., the patient is taught to relax while facing a situation that has habitually elicited fear. See SYSTEMATIC DESENSITIZATION; PSYCHOTHERAPY BY R.I.

reciprocal innervation the principle of motoneuron activity which states that when one set of muscles receives a signal for a reflex action, the antagonistic set of muscles receives a simultaneous signal that inhibits reaction. See RECIPROCAL INHIBITION.

reciprocal overlap a mechanism whereby afferent nerve fibers branch at every synapse level and communicate with several neighboring higher-order cells.

reciprocal punishment Piaget's term for the type of punishment advocated by children age eight and older in which the punishment is made to fit the crime. E.g., a child who consistently neglects to feed his pet would himself go without a meal. In this way, the culprit gains insight into the consequences of his act. Compare EXPIATORY PUNISHMENT.

reciprocity norm the social standard that persons should assist and not harm those who assist them.

recitation method a memorizing technique in which the subject devotes a portion of the learning time to the oral or silent repetition of the material.

Recklinghausen: See VON R.

recognition a sense of awareness and familiarity experienced when we encounter people, events, or objects we have encountered before, or when we come upon material we have learned in the past. Also, r. is acknowledgment of an achievement by bestowing awards or words of praise. Also see VISUAL PERCEPTION.

recognition method a technique of measuring the amount of material learned in a session by testing the subject's recognition of the content, usually by presenting new items along with those presented in the session. Also called **recognition test**.

recognition span the number of words a subject can grasp in reading during a single fixation, that is, in the interval in which the eyeball does not move. Also called **reading span**.

recognition technique a type of readership-survey technique employed in consumer-psychology research. The subject is asked to recall information about a product he claims to recognize from previous exposure to its advertisements. The subject also may be asked questions about ads that have never appeared to determine his suggestibility, or false recognition level. Also see PANTRY-CHECK TECHNIQUE.

recognition test = RECOGNITION METHOD.

recognition vocabulary = PASSIVE VOCABULARY.

recollection the act of recalling past events and experiences, a process that occurs spontaneously in ordinary life and during free association, but which can also be stimulated by hypnotic suggestion, pictures, or visits.

recombinant DNA a term applied to the process of creating artificial genetic material by removing pieces of genes from one species and implanting them in the chromosomes of another species. The process was developed initially to develop strains of bacteria that could produce natural substances of therapeutic value. See DNA; GENE SPLICING.

recombination a natural occurrence in genetic reproduction in which material contained in homologous chromosomes is exchanged during the first meiotic division, resulting in new gene combinations. The exchange of genetic material is called a **crossover**.

recommencement mania: See MANIA OF RECOM-MENCEMENT.

recompensation an increase in the ability of an individual to adapt to the environment and alleviate stressor situations. It is the opposite of decompensation.

reconditioning the process of strengthening or reestablishing a conditioned response that has weakened or been extinguished. R. may be brought about by additional reinforcement or by additional presentation of the unconditioned stimulus.

reconditioning therapy a form of behavior therapy in which the patient is conditioned to replace undesirable responses with desirable responses; e.g., male transvestites are sometimes treated by giving them a nauseating drug and then showing them photographs of themselves wearing feminine clothing. See AVERSIVE THERAPY.

reconstitution reconstruction; revision of one's attitudes or goals; also, the final stage of the grieving process experienced by patients with catastrophic illnesses resulting in disability. After going through the stages of denial, ventilation, and defensiveness, the patient may (or may not) be able to cope with his handicap by helping others with a similar condition or by achieving some degree of rehabilitation in a sheltered workshop.

reconstruction in psychoanalysis, the revival and interpretation of past experiences that have been instrumental in producing present emotional disturbance. More generally, r. is the form of recollection marked by the imaginative or logical recreation of an experience or event that has been only partially stored in memory.

reconstruction method a memory-study technique in which a subject tries to restore disarranged items to the order in which they were originally presented.

reconstructive psychotherapy psychotherapy directed toward basic and extensive modification in the patient's character structure, through enhancing insight into his or her personality development, unconscious conflicts, and adaptive responses. Examples are Freudian psychoanalysis, Adlerian individual psychology, Jungian analytic psychology, and the approaches of Horney and H. S. Sullivan.

reconstructive surgery: See PLASTIC SURGERY.

Recovery, Inc.: See SELF-HELP GROUPS; DIDACTIC GROUP THERAPY.

recovery of function the renewed ability of motor function following a lesion of the pyramidal tract, which is enhanced by fibers from extrapyramidal neurons. R.o.f. often is accompanied by abnormal muscle tonus and sensitivity to reflex stimuli, manifested by spasticity.

recovery ratio the ratio of the number of patients discharged during the year, or another period, to the total number in the original group.

recovery stage: See DISASTER SYNDROME.

recovery time the time required for a neural unit to recover from a response before it is capable of responding to a stimulus again; the time required for a physiological process to return to a normal state after it has been altered by the response to a stimulus. An example of the latter is the refractory interval required after a male orgasm before the reproductive organism can respond again to sexual stimulation.

recovery wish in psychoanalysis and other forms of psychotherapy, the wish, and will, to get well, which varies from patient to patient, and is an important element in determining the prognosis. Many factors tend to perpetuate neurotic illness and nullify the r.w.: an unconscious need for punishment (moral masochism); an unstable ego and superego; secondary gains derived from the disorder; lack of self-esteem; and narcissistic gratification derived from talking about one's problems.

recreational therapy the use of recreational activities (clubs, bowling, excursions, athletics, hobbies) as an integral part of the rehabilitation or therapeutic process. The purpose is to increase enjoyment of life, stimulate activity and self-expression, enhance socialization, and counterbalance self-concern. See ARTS AND CRAFTS; ART THERAPY; DANCE THERAPY; MUSIC THERAPY.

recreation specialist an individual who has obtained a college degree in recreational therapy and is prepared to plan and direct a program of activities for patients in mental hospitals, health agencies, nursing homes, or facilities for the retarded. In addition to in-service training, the recreation aide usually needs an associate degree; a recreation leader, a B.A. from an accredited college; and a recreation director, an M.A.

recruiting system = INTRALAMINAR SYSTEM.

recruitment a rapid increase in the sensation of loudness once the threshold of hearing has been reached. It is characteristic of sensorineural impairment due to inner-ear problems.

rectal administration: See ADMINISTRATION.

rectangular axes: See ORTHOGONAL.

rectangular distribution a statistical distribution in which each score occurs with the same frequency, so that its plot consists of a flat horizontal line.

rectum fear = PROCTOPHOBIA.

recumbent: See POSTURE.

recurrence in the two-word stage of language development, an expression indicating presence, absence, and repetition, as in "cookie again."

recurrent circuits a network of neurons and synapses which make it possible for a nerve impulse to make a complete circular path back to its starting point. Neural networks in the third nucleus of the midbrain make such reverberatory nerve circuits possible in theory and help explain certain types of spontaneous activity, such as repeating a poem.

recurrent collateral inhibition a negative-feedback system in the motoneuron system that prevents rapid repeated firing of the same neuron. The mechanism depends upon one branch of a motoneuron axon that loops back toward the cell body and communicates with an inhibitory Renshaw cell. The Renshaw cell in turn communicates with the motoneurons, including the cell with the feedback loop.

recurrent depression: See MAJOR DEPRESSION.

recurrent dreams repeated dreams, which Freud described as punishment rather than wish-fulfillment dreams, arising from a masochistic need for self-criticism for fantasies of excessive ambition. Jung regarded r.d. as more revealing than single dreams, and found that in a dream series the later dreams often throw light on the earlier ones. R.d. may also be an attempt to come to terms with disturbing experiences.

recurring-figures test a test of memory in which the subject is shown a series of cards featuring generally nonsensical figures or geometric forms. Some figures appear on more than one card, and the subject must try to recall whether a figure has appeared on a previous card.

red-color fear = ERYTHROPHOBIA.

Red Dye No. 3 one of several synthetic food colorings associated with hyperactivity because of their effects on brain-cell structure and function. R.D. No. 3 has been shown experimentally to cause oxidative reactions in brain-cell membranes and to affect dopamine transport. Other food dyes, **Yellow Dye No. 5** and **6** and **Red Dye No. 40**, have been shown to interact with cell-membrane lipids.

red-green blindness a form of color blindness in which certain shades of red and green are confused.

red-green responses a concept of color vision in which responses of certain retinal receptors are excitatory while others are inhibitory to the same wavelength. Since red and green are at opposite ends of the spectrum, it is assumed that a red excitatory response is accompanied by a green inhibitory response, each representing a different receptor process.

redintegration the process of organizing mental processes after they have been disorganized by a psychotic disorder; also, the process of recovering or recollecting memories from partial cues, or reminders, as in recalling an entire song when a few notes are played. R. is also the classical conditioning process in which a sensory stimulus associated with a second stimulus becomes capable of arousing the same response that the second stimulus arouses. Also called **reintegration**.

Redlich, Emil Austrian neurologist, 1866–1930. See ECONOMO'S DISEASE (also called **Redlich's encephalitis**).

red nucleus a structure of the extrapyramidal system that receives fibers from the cerebellum. It is located in the anterior part of the tegmentum and extends into the hypothalamus. Although it consists of gray matter, the nucleus is reddish in fresh specimens, hence its name. Also called **nucleus ruber**.

reduced cue a learning principle that after repeated S-R trials, a response can be elicited by only a portion of the original stimulus. Also see MINIMAL CUE; CUE REDUCTION.

reductionism the theory that all phenomena can be best understood by analyzing them into their simplest components. In psychology, r. is an attempt to discover irreducible mental contents, and behaviorism tends to explain complex activities in terms of responses to stimuli. Also see ATOMISM; STRUCTURALISM.

reduction division the process of gamete production, or meiosis, in which a cell containing the full complement of chromosomes divides into two cells each of which has half of the normal number.

reductive approach: See PSYCHOSYNTHESIS.

reductive interpretation a Jungian concept that behavior can be interpreted as a sign or symptom of an unconscious process affecting the psyche.

redundancy the condition of a message or category of information containing needlessly repeated data that can be deleted without loss of meaningful content; the duplication, recurrence, or repetition of elements within a communication. R. is built into grammatical rules and syntactic conventions, constituting roughly 50 percent of most spoken and written language. Duplication reinforces the intended meaning of a communication by enhancing the probability of correct interpretation. Also called **T function**. Also see DISTRIBUTIONAL R.

redundant prepuce an excessive growth of prepuce, or foreskin. The condition may be pathologic if the excess foreskin prevents the prepuce from being drawn back over the glans as may be necessary to prevent inflammation from trapped smegma or urine.

reduplicative memory deception a false memory observed in patients with organic brain disease who insist they already have experienced an event, such as a medical examination, when in fact the situation has not occurred before.

reeducation a form of psychological treatment in which the patient learns more effective ways of dealing with problems and relationships through one or another form of nonreconstructive therapy, such as relationship therapy, behavior therapy, hypnotic suggestion, counseling, persuasion therapy, nonanalytic group therapy, and reality therapy. Also called **reeducative therapy**.

reenactment the process of reliving traumatic events, repressed experiences, and past relationships while reviving the original emotions associated with them. This technique is used in psychodrama, primal therapy, and an early form of psychoanalysis. See ABREACTION.

reentry the return of a patient to the real world after experiencing the relatively open and honest environment of an encounter group.

reevaluation counseling a therapeutic approach developed by Harvey Jackins in which mutual "cocounseling" by ordinary people is practiced, that is, each individual is counselor for one hour and client for one hour. The two sit holding hands and maintain eye contact, and the process starts with the counselor asking a provocative question such as "Whom do I remind you of?" (which usually carries the client back to childhood experiences), and continues with other steps such as asking the client to cite two or three minor upsets that recently occurred. The client is encouraged to react emotionally in his responses, to work through his emotions, and then to reverse roles and act as the counselor for the other person.

reference: See DELUSION OF R.

referenced cognitive test a test of cognitive function or dysfunction that has been standardized so that results can be compared objectively.

reference groups formal or informal groups of people who influence the attitudes, behaviors, and self-conceptions of other persons. R.g. may include a family, a group of classmates, religious organizations, professional associations, trade unions, and political clubs which serve as a point of reference for life-styles and behaviors.

reference-group theory the concept that our attitudes, including our prejudices, are largely determined by the normative, or reference, group from which we derive our social and interpersonal standards. See REFERENCE GROUPS.

referential attitude an expectancy attitude observed in certain schizophrenia patients who believe they are targets of hostility and are seeking justification for their belief.

referral the act of directing a patient to a therapist, agency, or institution for evaluation, consultation, or treatment. The term is also applied to the individual who is referred.

referred pain pain that is felt in a part of the body other than the site of the pain stimulus.

referred sensation a sensation that is localized at a point different from the area stimulated.

refined mode a statistical term for an estimate of the mode of the universe from which a sample was taken.

reflection = MEDITATION.

reflection of feeling a counselor's statement that is intended to highlight the affective content of a client's communication, that is, the feelings or attitudes implicitly expressed. According to C. Rogers, r.o.f. consists of understanding and communicating the essence of the client's experience from the client's point of view so that hidden or obscured feelings can be brought to light for clarification.

reflex any of a number of automatic, unlearned, relatively fixed responses to stimuli which do not require conscious effort to complete. R. actions often involve a faster response to a stimulus than might be possible if a conscious evaluation of the input was required. A common example is that of the series of self-preservation acts required instantly when a hand is placed on a hot stove. Serious injury could occur in the time needed to make a conscious response. (This Dictionary lists about 80 entries whose headwords include the terms "reflex" or "reflexes.")

reflex act a term used by Freud in pointing out that all psychic activities follow the same general pattern as neurological reflexes. Like the reflex arc, they begin with stimulation from an external or internal source, proceed to a central regulatory system (the mind or psyche), and discharge through efferent channels. He termed this process r.a. as opposed to reflex arc.

reflex arc a neurological unit which, in its simplest form, consists of an afferent, or sensory, neuron that conducts an impulse from a receptor to the spinal cord, where it connects directly or via an interneuron to an efferent, or motor, neuron that carries the impulse to an effector, that is, a muscle or gland. Also see PSYCHIC R.A.

reflex circle a tendency for muscle contractions to activate proprioceptive reflex loops, thereby strengthening the muscle contraction.

reflex epilepsy a type of epilepsy marked by convulsions that are triggered by sensory input, such as sound, touch, or light. The attack often is controlled by reflexive inhibition in the form of another strong stimulus. Photogenic epilepsy is an example of a r.e.

reflex excitability a term referring to the gradations of reflex thresholds during periods of sleep versus wakefulness. Tendon reflexes, such as the knee jerk, have an increased threshold during sleep while cutaneous stimuli such as touching the skin produce a normal reaction of brushing away the stimulus or perhaps scratching the area if the stimulus causes an itching or tickling sensation.

reflex figure a pattern of reflexes involved in a complex action such as walking or running. Some four-legged animals extend the right forelimb while the right hindlimb undergoes a flexion reflex and the left hindlimb undergoes a crossed extension reaction, the pattern alternating with each step of the r.f.

reflex latency the amount of time that elapses between application of the stimulus and the start of the reflex response. Also called **central reflex time**.

reflexology the study of involuntary automatic responses to stimuli, particularly as they affect the behavior of humans and other animals. See BEKHTEREV.

reflex-sensitization principle the principle that after a response has been repeatedly elicited by a stimulus, it can be elicited by a neutral stimulus.

reformatory paranoia a type of megalomania expressed as a personality trait in persons who concoct plans to reform the world and try to convince others to follow their ideas.

refraction index: See INDEX OF REFRACTION.

refractory mental illness: See TOPECTOMY.

refractory period a rest period after a nerve or muscle cell has undergone excitation. As the cell is being repolarized, it will not respond to any stimulus during the early part of the r.p., called the absolute r.p. As it phases into a relative r.p., it may respond only to a strong stimulus. Also called **refractory phase**.

refrigerator parents Kanner's term for parents of autistic children whom he believed (usually mistakenly) to be cold, intellectual, and relatively uninterested in stimulating their children.

Refsum, Sigvald Bernhard Norwegian physician, 1907—. See REFSUM'S SYNDROME.

Refsum's syndrome a disorder believed to be an inherited defect of lipid metabolism, causing pigmentary retinitis, deafness, chronic polyneuritis, ataxia, and other cerebellar disturbances. The syndrome may also be marked by cardiovascular, skin, and skeletal abnormalities.

The onset of symptoms usually is between childhood and early adulthood. Also called **heredopathia atactica polyneuritiformis**.

regeneration of nerves the ability of certain nerve cells to repair themselves after their death or injury. Nerves of the central nervous system of amphibia are able to perform this function, but warm-blooded animals do not have the ability. Some myelinated nerves, those beyond the central nervous system, are able to perform a self-repair function, however.

regimen a detailed treatment program, including a schedule, for regulation of diet, exercise, rest, medication, and other therapeutic measures.

regional anesthetics: See ANESTHETICS.

registered nurse a professional nurse who has completed an accredited educational program and has successfully passed a required state-supervised licensing examination. Education programs are hospital-based or university-or college-based with practical experience in affiliated hospitals. Hospital-based programs were established in the United States in 1873, and the University of Minnesota introduced academic-based training of nurses in 1910. Abbrev.: **RN**.

registration the first step in learning and memory, in which stimuli make an impression or record on the central nervous system. One of the major symptoms of Korsakoff's patients is inability to integrate new material into their memory, leaving a gap that is frequently filled with fabrications, or confabulations.

Regitine Mesylate = PHENTOLAMINE.

regnancy H. A. Murray's term for the briefest unit of experience, often used in the plural form because of the difficulty of recording a single r. or **regnant process**, since it integrates many physiological and psychological activities.

regression a defense mechanism consisting of reversion to immature behavior when the individual is threatened with overwhelming external problems or internal conflicts. The revival of earlier reactions such as weeping, pouting, thumb-sucking, or temper tantrums is usually an unconscious attempt to gain special attention and sympathy, or force others to solve one's problems. In psychoanalysis, the emphasis is on a return to one of the earlier stages in psychosexual development. In chronic schizophrenia, patients sometimes regress to a completely infantile level where they have to be washed, dressed, and fed, and in some cases assume a fetal position. Also see HYPNOTIC R.

regression analysis a statistical technique for predicting one score from another score; e.g., a regression equation $(Y = a + bX)$ might be used to predict a student's college grades from his high-school grades. Also see MULTIPLE REGRESSION.

regression line a straight or curved line fitting a set of points.

regression neurosis a neurosis characterized by behavior appropriate for an earlier stage of life when responsibilities could be avoided and wishes could be easily fulfilled.

regression time the amount of time expended by a reader in returning to preceding words and re-reading them.

regression toward the mean a statistical effect in which scores that were extreme on an initial measurement become less extreme on a subsequent measurement, that is, they move closer to or revert to the mean. This can be due to the action of random errors. Also called **statistical regression**.

regressive alcoholism = GAMMA ALCOHOLISM.

regressive electroshock therapy electroconvulsive therapy administered several times a day to schizophrenic patients when other treatment methods have failed and the prognosis is poor. The patients regress to a point where they are incontinent, out of contact, and have to be spoon-fed. It takes a week to a month for them to recover from this state.

regressive-reconstructive approach a psychotherapeutic technique in which the patient is encouraged to regress to an earlier stage of life and to revive and reproduce a traumatic situation that occurred at that time, as a means of bringing about personality change and achieving greater emotional maturity.

regressive schizophrenia a form of schizophrenia in which the symptoms represent a regression, primitivization, or loss of mental processes acquired through mental development. The symptoms may include depersonalization, archaic speech and thought, delusions, and certain symptoms of both hebephrenia and catatonia.

regularity: See CONSTIPATION.

regulatory behavior behavior that helps keep an organism in balance by fulfilling primary needs.

regulatory system any system that helps maintain homeostasis, or balance, in an organ or organism.

regurgitation: See VOMITING.

rehabilitation the restoration of an individual with a physical or mental disability to his or her fullest possible functioning in all aspects of life. R. is often described as the fourth phase of medical practice, the others being prevention, diagnosis, and treatment. In psychiatry, it is recognized that residuals of mental disorder may remain after treatment, and the r. process is designed to keep them from interfering with social and occupational activities. R. consists of such measures as vocational counseling and retraining, social and recreational activities, ex-mental-patient clubs, and living in a halfway house or other group residence during the readjustment period. Also see HABILITATION; PSYCHIATRIC R.; PSYCHOLOGICAL R.; SEXUAL R.; SOCIAL R.

rehabilitation center an organization devoted to the restoration of individuals with mental or physical disorders and disabilities, including the multihandicapped, to an adequate level of functioning. Rehabilitation centers use such techniques as vocational training, work in a shel-tered situation, occupational therapy, physical therapy, educational therapy, social therapy, recreational therapy, and psychological counseling.

rehabilitation counselor a professional worker who is trained and equipped to evaluate and guide physically, mentally, and emotionally handicapped individuals in all major phases of the rehabilitation process: vocational, educational, personal, psychological, social, recreational. The r.c. helps to coordinate the various services offered by the rehabilitation team, and focus them on individual needs. Preparation for the field is essentially on a graduate level leading to the M.A. degree.

rehabilitation medicine the branch of medicine that specializes in the restoration of a mentally or physically disabled person to an active, independent life in the community. If the goal cannot be realized, r.m. tries to enable the individual to make the best possible use of his residual capacities.

rehabilitation nurse a nurse who specializes in the restoration of mentally or physically disabled patients to social, vocational, and economic usefulness to the community. The r.n. provides personalized care in cooperation with other members of the rehabilitation team.

rehabilitation program the overall system of rehabilitation services provided in support of medical-surgical therapy for physically disabled persons and psychiatric therapy for the mentally disabled. The total r.p. includes subdivisions of physical, recreational, and occupational-therapy, psychological, social-service, educational, and vocational programs, as well as appropriate special areas such as speech and hearing or mobility training for the blind.

rehabilitation psychologist a psychologist who devotes much or all of his professional time to the emotional and behavioral therapy needs of patients, regardless of the cause of their disability. The responsibility also requires evaluating the patients' capacities through appropriate tests, and encouraging them to cope realistically and constructively with the limitations, frustrations, and uncertainties associated with their impairment.

rehabilitation team the group of various health-professional specialists who coordinate their efforts in the rehabilitation of patients on an individual basis. A r.t. may include plastic surgeons, orthopedic surgeons, neurologists, psychiatrists, physical therapists, occupational therapists, and psychologists, among others, depending upon the needs of the patient.

rehearsal an aid for storing a complex piece of information in one's long-term memory. By repeated recall, the memory trace is strengthened.

rehospitalization in psychiatry, the return of the patient to a mental hospital due to relapse. Studies conducted by the Massachussetts Mental Health Center have shown that even though total time spent in the hospital during a five-year follow-up period was shorter in 1967 than in 1947, more patients in the 1967 group tended to relapse and be rehospitalized. One explanation is that the 1967 patients had become dependent on psychotropic drugs which retarded their social recovery.

Reich, Wilhelm /rīsh/ Austrian-American psychoanalyst, 1897–1957. R. was a member of the psychoanalytic movement who broke with Freud by refusing to accept the death instinct and by developing his own theory that the achievement of "full orgastic potency" is the single measure of psychological well-being. See BIOENERGETICS; BION; CHARACTER ANALYSIS; CHARACTER-ANALYTIC VEGOTHERAPY; CHARACTER ARMOR; LIFE ENERGY; ORGONE; ORGONE ACCUMULATOR; ORGONE THERAPY; ORGONOMY.

Reid, Thomas Scottish philosopher, 1710–96. See FACULTY PSYCHOLOGY.

reification the treating of an abstraction, concept, formulation, etc., as though it were a real object or static structure rather than a symbol which stands for a dynamic process. In psychiatry, r. is a type of thinking frequently observed in schizophrenics in which they confuse the abstract with the real.

Reik, Theodor /rīk/ Austrian-born American psychoanalyst, 1888–1970. See LISTENING WITH THE THIRD EAR; MASS MASOCHISM; NEGATIVE AMBITION; SOCIAL MASOCHISM; VERBAL MASOCHISM.

Reil, Johann Christian /rīl/ German physician, 1759–1813. See ISLAND OF REIL.

reindoctrination: See DEPROGRAMING.

reinforce to enhance or increase a response or to increase the probability of a response. See REINFORCEMENT.

reinforcement a procedure that changes the frequency or probability of a response; a procedure or incentive that increases the strength of a conditioning or other learning process. The term refers also to the use of devices such as reward or punishment in learning situations to produce contiguous firing of cognitive and motivational cell complexes; it is believed by some investigators that r. can affect the rate at which neural connections develop. In classical conditioning, r. is the repeated association of the conditioned stimulus (e.g., bell) with the unconditioned stimulus (e.g., food); in operant conditioning, the term denotes the reward given after a correct response, or the punishment that follows an incorrect response. Also, r. refers to knowledge of results or recognition of the correctness of the response, as in programed learning. Also called **reinforcer**. See INTERMITTENT R.; PARTIAL R.; PRIMARY R.; SECONDARY R.; SCHEDULE OF R.; POSITIVE R ; NEGATIVE R.; MIXED R.; SERIAL R.

reinforcement analysis the system of evaluating negative versus positive reinforcement factors. In environmental psychology, positive reinforcement leads to rewards, e.g., development of community land for recreational purposes, good schools, and consumer markets; whereas negative reinforcement factors have negative effects,

such as deterioration of areas into ghettos or slums. As used in environmental psychology, r.a. is also called **functional analysis of environments**.

reinforcement counseling a behavioral approach to counseling based on the idea that behavior is learned and can be predictably modified by various reinforcement techniques that strengthen or weaken specific types of behavior through schedules of positive or negative reinforcement.

reinforcement gradient: See GRADIENT OF REINFORCEMENT.

reinforcer = REINFORCEMENT.

reinforcing cause a condition that tends to maintain maladaptive behavior in a patient. An example is the special attention given a person who is ill, which can in fact contribute to a delayed recovery.

reinforcing stimulus a stimulus that acts to maintain a response or to enhance its strength. In classical conditioning, the r.s. is the unconditioned stimulus; in operant conditioning, it is the reward stimulus presented after the correct response. Also see NEGATIVE REINFORCEMENT; POSITIVE REINFORCEMENT.

reintegration = REDINTEGRATION.

Reissner, Ernst /rīs'nər/ German anatomist, 1824–78. See REISSNER'S MEMBRANE; SCALA VESTIBULI.

Reissner's membrane a cochlear membrane that separates the scala vestibuli and the scala media. Also called **vestibular membrane**. See BASILAR MEMBRANE.

Reiter, Hans Conrad Julius /rī'tər/ German physician, 1881—. See REITER'S SYNDROME.

Reiter's syndrome a symptom complex grouped by some authorities with Behcet's syndrome, and possibly caused by a virus or an allergy. The major symptoms are arthritis, conjunctivitis, and nonspecific urethritis.

rejecting-neglecting parent a parent who generally discourages emotional dependency and fails to enrich the child's environment. Baumrind distinguishes between the **nonauthoritarian r.-n.p.** who may minimally encourage independence, and the **authoritarian r.-n.p.** who exercises control and demands obedience. Also see AUTHORITARIAN PARENT; AUTHORITATIVE PARENT; PERMISSIVE PARENT.

rejection denial of love, attention, interest, or approval; also, an antagonistic or discriminatory attitude toward a minority group. In psychoanalysis, the term is applied to deliberate denial of gratification of an instinct or impulse.

rejection fear = FEAR OF REJECTION.

rejuvenants substances that are claimed to have the effect of restoring strength, vigor, or youthful qualities to a cell, tissue, or organism.

relapse the recurrence of symptoms of a disease after a period of improvement or apparent cure.

relapse rate the incidence of patients who have recovered or improved that later suffer a recurrence of their disorder.

related model = SEGREGATED MODEL.

relatedness a reciprocal relationship of empathy, trust, and oneness between two or more persons.

relatedness needs: See EXISTENCE, RELATEDNESS, AND GROWTH THEORY.

relational word = FUNCTION WORD.

relationship therapy any form of psychotherapy, from direct guidance to psychoanalysis, in which the relationship between patient and therapist is a key factor, serving such purposes as providing emotional support, creating an accepting atmosphere that fosters personality growth, or eliciting past attitudes and experiences to be studied during the sessions. In a more specialized sense, the term was applied by F. H. Allen and J. Taft to the use of warm, friendly contact with troubled children as a means of accelerating their capacity to change.

relative pitch the pitch of a tone that is higher or lower than a given standard.

relative position = INTERPOSITION.

relative refractory period: See REFRACTORY PERIOD.

relative risk in epidemiology the ratio of the frequency of a certain disorder in groups exposed and groups not exposed to a specific environmental or hereditary factor.

relativism a generalization that concepts, such as mental disorder, right, and good have no absolute definition, but depend for their meaning on the individual's perspective, or on circumstances such as time, place, or the cultural environment.

relativity of reality variations in the concept of the external world. Many psychoanalysts have maintained that normal individuals frequently distort reality through wishful thinking and various defense maneuvers. Neurotics and psychotics, however, tend to distort reality even more, due to their pathological defenses against internal conflicts and repressed impulses. Also see REALITY.

relaxation a tension-free state in which internal conflicts and disturbing feelings of anxiety, anger, and fear are eased and a state of tranquility prevails. R. is also the return of a muscle to its normal state after a period of contraction.

relaxation principle a modification of the psychoanalytic technique, developed by Ferenczi, who found that a loving, tender, permissive approach to his patients was more effective in releasing their repressed impulses and making them accessible to analysis than a strict application of Freud's privation philosophy, which he found to arouse hostility and other forms of resistance. See PRIVATION.

relaxation therapy the use of muscle-relaxation techniques as an aid in the treatment of emotional tension, especially when the tension is associated with such conditions as peptic ulcer, asthma, spastic colitis, and tachycardia. For details, see DIFFERENTIAL RELAXATION; MUSCLE RELAXANTS.

relaxation training: See AUTOGENIC TRAINING; PROGRESSIVE RELAXATION.

relaxed flatfoot: See FLATFOOT.

relay nuclei neural cells in the thalamus that relay impulses from one tract to another. The lateroventral nuclei receive fibers from the cerebellum and send fibers to the frontal lobe.

relearning method a technique measuring retention by learning again material previously learned but forgotten. Savings in time or trials over the original learning indicate the amount of retention. Also called **savings method**.

release inhibitors substances that prevent or interfere with the release of hormones or other agents from glands or tissue cells that normally release a physiologically active chemical. Somatostatin is a r.i. that prevents the normal rate of release of the somatotrophin growth hormone.

release phenomenon unrestricted activity of a lower brain center when a higher center with inhibitory control is damaged or excised.

releaser a key stimulus or environmental cue that routinely evokes a specific response or pattern of responses specific to a particular species; e.g., the sight or presence of a mother hen elicits a following-reaction in chicks. Also called **releasing stimulus; sign stimulus**. Also see INNATE RELEASING MECHANISM; IMPRINTING.

release therapy a form of therapy developed by D. M. Levy in which young children "play out" anxieties, frightening experiences, and traumatic events with such materials as figurines, toy animals, and water guns.

releasing stimulus = RELEASER.

reliability index: See INDEX OF RELIABILITY.

reliability sampling a statistical measure or assessment of the extent of correspondence or agreement between at least two samples drawn from the same population.

reliable stable or consistent. A test is r. if it gives the same result on a second measurement, or if different parts of the test measure the same thing. Also see SPLIT-HALF RELIABILITY; ODD-EVEN RELIABILITY.

relief-discomfort quotient; relief-distress quotient: See DISTRESS-RELIEF QUOTIENT.

religious delusions delusions associated with religious beliefs, such as delusions of sin and damnation, and grandiose ideas in which the patient pictures himself as the Messiah who can cure all illness and save all humankind or (as in Krafft-Ebing's cases) rape "Marys" to beget Jesus.

religious faith the belief in a Supreme Being or other spiritual force that sets standards of conduct, responds to prayer, and often assures the ultimate triumph of good over evil. It is usually but not always accompanied by a system of ceremonials and doctrines and an institution organized to put them in practice. Freud regarded religion as a collective neurosis, which mankind would eventually outgrow. See FAITH HEALING; RELIGIOUS THERAPY; MAGICAL THINKING.

religious healers: See FAITH HEALING.

religious mania a state of acute hyperactivity, agitation, and restlessness accompanied by hallucinations of a religious nature. Also see STIGMATA.

religious-objects fear = HIEROPHOBIA.

religious therapy supportive psychotherapy provided by pastoral counseling, Bible classes, church-sponsored community activities, and the confessional.

remake memory = LONG-TERM MEMORY.

remedial reading specialized instruction for individuals whose reading quotient is significantly subnormal, or who have developed faulty reading patterns.

remedial therapy treatment of learning disorders such as reading disability through audiovisual devices, programed learning, study in a resource room, tutoring, or the use of the reading laboratory.

remembering the process of consciously reviving or bringing to awareness previous events, experiences, or information. R. is also the process of retaining such material, which is essential to learning, since without it we would not profit from training, practice, or past experience. For different forms of remembering, see RECALL; RECOGNITION; RECOLLECTION; RELEARNING METHOD.

reminiscence the recollection of previous experiences, especially those of a pleasant nature; dwelling on the past. R. is also a temporary, and not fully explained, rise in the retention curve after an interval.

remission a significant abatement of symptoms, or an improvement, in a mental or physical disorder. R. may be temporary or permanent, partial or complete. Also see SPONTANEOUS R.

remorse anguish caused by a sense of guilt, which may have a real or fancied basis. Various methods are used to relieve, or "undo," feelings of guilt, ranging from bestowing gifts to doing penance. For examples, see UNDOING.

remote association in verbal learning, an association between one item in a list or series with another item that does not adjoin it on the list.

remote-association test a creativity test in which the subject is asked to suggest a fourth word that links three apparently unrelated words, such as rat-blue-cottage.

remote memory recall or recognition of experiences or information dating from the distant past. It is characteristic of many elderly individuals. See LONG-TERM MEMORY.

remotivation efforts directed toward stimulating chronic, withdrawn persons in mental hospitals, e.g., by involving them in poetry-reading groups or conversation groups in which a "bridge to reality" is established by discussing current topics such as space flight.

REM sleep /rem/ *r*apid-*e*ye-*m*ovement sleep, accounting for one-quarter to one-fifth of total sleep time; the stage in which dreaming occurs

and the electroencephalogram shows activity characteristic of wakefulness except for inhibition of motor expression other than conjugate (that is, coordinated) movements of the eyes. See DREAM STATE.

-ren-; -reni-; -reno- a combining form relating to the kidney. Adjective: **renal**.

renal cortex: See CORTEX.

renal disorder = KIDNEY DISEASE.

renal threshold: See THRESHOLD.

renal-tubular osteomalacia: See OSTEOMALACIA.

Rendu, Henri Jules Louis Marie /räNdē′/ French physician, 1844–1902. See STEVENS-JOHNSON SYNDROME (also called **Fiessinger-Rendu syndrome**).

renifleur /reniflœr′/ a person with a morbid interest in body odors, especially as a means of sexual excitement. See OSPHRESIOLAGNIA.

Renpenning's syndrome a condition involving mental retardation that is inherited as X-linked recessive and lacking any associated physical abnormality.

Renshaw cells inhibitory cells that communicate with motoneuron axons near the spinal cord. R.c. are a part of the negative-feedback system that prevents rapid repeated firing of motoneurons.

renunciation in psychoanalysis, a refusal of the ego to follow impulses of the id; also, in religion, the surrender of one's own will to a deity.

Renwick, T. K. English physician, fl. 1956. See FISCH-RENWICK SYNDROME.

reorganization principle a Gestalt theory that new learning or perception disrupts old cognitive structures, requiring a reorganized structure.

repeaters: See RECIDIVISM.

repetition-compulsion a term used by Freud to describe the unconscious need to reenact early traumas in the attempt to overcome or master them. In r.-c. the early painful experience is repeated in a new situation symbolic of the repressed prototype. R.-c. acts as an unconscious resistance to therapeutic change since the goal of therapy is not to repeat but to remember the trauma and to see its relation to present behavior. Also see ACTING OUT.

repetition law: See LAW OF FREQUENCY.

repetitive pattern a persistent attitude or form of behavior that becomes a typical part of the individual's personality, and is repeatedly expressed automatically and unconsciously, e.g., thriftiness, deliberateness, or use of a particular gesture. See MANNERISM.

replacement memory the substitution of one memory for another, as in a screen or cover memory.

replacement therapy in psychiatry, the process of replacing abnormal thoughts or behavior with healthy reactions through the use of occupational therapy that focuses on constructive activities and interests. The term applies also to a treatment technique in which a natural or synthetic substance is substituted for one that is deficient in the body of the patient; e.g., a cystic-fibrosis patient can obtain some relief from symptoms of the disease by replacement of pancreatic enzymes that are lacking in the digestive system.

replication the repetition of an original experiment or a trial in an experiment to gain information about its internal validity or application in other settings. In **exact r.**, procedures are identical to the original experiment. In **modified r.**, alternate procedures and additional conditions may be incorporated. In **conceptual r.**, different techniques and manipulations are introduced to gain theoretical information.

replication therapy a behavior-therapy technique in which the therapist evokes and reinforces behavior patterns resembling those in the patient's environment.

representation in psychoanalysis, the process of using a symbol or image to stand for an object, act, or unconscious impulse; in psychology, an idea or concept ("democracy," "horse") that takes the place of external reality.

representational skills as used by Piaget, cognitive skills involved in understanding the world of people, objects, and events, including the ability to use images, words, and at least rudimentary concepts and elementary logic.

representational stage according to Piaget, the period of cognitive development that begins with the PREOPERATIONAL STAGE and ends with the CONCRETE-OPERATIONAL STAGE. See these entries.

representative design an experimental design in which a stratified or representative sample of subjects is included.

representative factors the activities that are assumed to permit an organism to continue or renew a response when the original stimulus is discontinued; also, the verbal symbols and imagery that serve as mediators of ideation.

representativeness the close correspondence between a sample and the population from which it is drawn so that the sample accurately symbolizes its population. A representative sample reproduces the essential characteristics and constitution of a population in correct number and proportions. R. is the foundation of scientific sampling.

representative sampling the selection of a survey sample that will insure a valid representation of the total population. See REPRESENTATIVENESS.

repressed ancestors: See FAMILIAL UNCONSCIOUS; FATE ANALYSIS.

repressed complex a group of emotional factors or ideas that have been repressed, thereby becoming the source of abnormal behavior.

repression in psychoanalysis, the basic defense mechanism, which consists of excluding painful experiences and unacceptable impulses from consciousness. R. operates on an unconscious level as a protection against anxiety produced by objectionable sexual wishes, feelings of hostility, and ego-threatening experiences of all kinds. It

also comes into play in most of our other defenses, e.g., when we fail to perceive unpleasant realities (denial) or conceal shameful impulses by going to the opposite extreme (reaction formation). Also see PRIMARY R.; AFTEREXPULSION; STRANGULATED AFFECT.

repression proper = AFTEREXPULSION.

repression-resistance the resistance displayed by the ego in order to maintain the repression of unacceptable impulses. R.-r. may manifest itself by forgetting events, by an impeded flow of free associations, or by applying the analyst's interpretation to others but not to the patient himself. Also called **ego resistance**.

repressive approach an attempt to eliminate symptoms by command, persuasion, or suggestion, without exploring their unconscious sources or attempting to bring about basic personality change.

repressive-inspirational group psychotherapy an approach which is repressive in the sense of strengthening the individual's defenses instead of breaking through them to elicit unconscious material, and inspirational in the sense of using various measures to encourage the members, such as testimonials, socializing, sharing of experiences, reassurance, and esprit de corps. For an example, see ALCOHOLICS ANONYMOUS.

reproduction in learning, the repetition of a task in the manner in which it was learned originally; in biology, the process by which organic life is transmitted as a means of preserving the species.

reproductive behavior activity that leads to propagation of the species. The mechanism varies somewhat with the type of organism, ranging from simple cell division in a unicellular organism to a merger of chromosomes contributed by the male and female parents and supervision of the offspring until they are able to survive in the external environment.

reproductive facilitation an improvement in reproducing a formerly learned response or behavioral sequence. The enhancement may be due to one of several factors, e.g., the chance to rest between the time of original learning and the reproduction.

reproductive function the total process of creating a new organism, or a specific act of the process, such as sexual intercourse.

reproductive instincts behavioral drives or impulses as expressed in courtship, nest-building, and parental activities.

reproductive strength in learning, the totality of factors that increase the probability that a specific response will occur.

reproductive type a constitutional type in the Rostan system, characterized by a dominance of the reproductive system over other body systems. It is roughly comparable to Pende's hypergenital type.

REP Test = ROLE CONSTRUCT REPERTORY TEST.

repulsion in genetics, a process whereby genes of different parents show an aversion to entering the same gametes, resulting in an excess of parental gene combinations and a deficiency of new combinations as might be expected according to the Mendelian principle of independent assortment.

required behavior behavior that is strongly reinforced either by law or social convention; predictable, expected behavior, as in matters of speech, dress, manners, and the various amenities appropriate to personal, social, and business relationships.

rescinnamine a Rauwolfia alkaloid that is similar to but less potent than reserpine. Effects include sedation and a mild decrease in blood pressure. Serotonin and other amines are released from brain cells and dopamine is depleted, thereby interfering with the synthesis of norepinephrine and epinephrine neurotransmitters, which helps account for the sedative activity of r.

res cogitans: See CARTESIAN DUALISM; CONARIUM.

rescue fantasy in psychoanalysis, the fantasy of saving the life of a parent or another important person who represents the parent. This fantasy is believed to be based on a desire to overcome infantile helplessness and display almost magical power. It is often one of the elements in the FAMILY ROMANCE. See this entry.

research the systematic effort to discover or confirm facts by scientific methods of observation and experiment, usually including investigation of previous reports and studies in libraries or computerized sources.

reserpine: See RAUWOLFIA DERIVATIVES.

res extensa: See CARTESIAN DUALISM; CONARIUM.

residence rate the ratio of the number of patients residing in institutions of a given type on a given date to the total population of the city, county, state, or another area.

residential care care that is provided physically or mentally disabled persons, including mentally retarded patients, in a foster home or group home, as opposed to a large institution. Treatment-oriented r.c. provides staffing and supervision by specialized health professionals in a homelike atmosphere.

residential schools special educational facilities for retarded children that are a part of a residential facility.

residential treatment facilities small institutions in which disturbed children, adolescents, and in some cases adults reside and participate in a total program which usually includes group therapy or counseling, social and recreational activities, and work experiences.

residual a condition in which acute symptoms have subsided, but chronic or less severe symptoms remain. Also, r. means either a remaining ability, as in r. hearing, or a remaining disability, as in r. loss of vision after a trauma or surgery. In statistics, the term denotes the difference between an observed and a computed value; also, the variance left over after the variance of all factors has been extracted.

residual schizophrenia = SCHIZOPHRENIC DISORDER, RESIDUAL TYPE.

resignation in general, an attitude of apathetic surrender to one's situation or symptoms, frequently occurring in institutionalized patients. To Horney, neurotic r. is extreme withdrawal and avoidance of situations and activities that might produce anxiety or bring an internal conflict into awareness. The withdrawal may take the form of total inactivity, or overactivity in other areas.

resistance in psychiatry and psychoanalysis, "everything in the words or actions of the [patient] that obstructs his gaining access to his unconscious" (LaPlanche and Pontalis, *The Language of Psychoanalysis*, 1973). Conscious r. is the withholding of information due to embarrassment or fear; unconscious r. arises in the ego's struggle to maintain repression of the anxiety-evoking unconscious material as it gradually rises to consciousness in the course of treatment. Also see ANALYSIS OF THE R.; ANALYTICAL INSIGHT; CONSCIOUS R.; ID R.; REPRESSION R.

resistance stage = STAGE OF RESISTANCE.

resistance to extinction the endurance or persistence of a conditioned response during extinction trials; or, the number of trials required to bring about extinction. R.t.e. provides a standard for judging the strength of conditioning.

resistance to stress the second stage of H. Selye's general adaptation syndrome. It follows the alarm reaction which is marked by psychosomatic or physiological changes related to emotional stress. In r.t.s. the organism attempts to adjust to the stressful situation in order to endure and survive.

resocialization the process of restoring social relationships and skills that will enable the hospitalized mental patient to participate in community life.

resolution phase: See SEXUAL-RESPONSE CYCLE.

resolving power the ability of the eye to perceive two distinct objects when both are viewed simultaneously or when two images are in close proximity on the retina.

resource person an individual with either professional training or special skills, talent, or knowledge who acts as adviser or consultant to a group.

resource teacher a specialist who works with learning-disabled children from a centralized resource room within the school, and acts as a consultant to other teachers.

respirator a mechanical device that assists a patient in breathing by providing an appropriate inhalation pressure or specified respiratory gases, e.g., an adjustable mixture of oxygen and nitrogen or other gases. A r. also may be a resuscitator or artificial respiration machine.

respiratory depression a reduced rate of oxygen intake produced by narcotic drugs such as morphine. Narcotics raise the threshold level of the respiratory center that normally would react to increased carbon dioxide in the tissues by increasing the rate and depth of breathing. R.d. is a primary hazard of morphine use, including therapeutic administration in hospitals.

respiratory disorders any disease, injury, or congenital defect that interferes with the normal exchange of oxygen and carbon dioxide between the body tissues and the environmental atmosphere. R.d. can involve any part of the respiratory system, from the nasopharynx to the body cells, which have an internal respiration function. In addition to pulmonary disorders, r.d. may include disorders of the abdominal, intracostal, and diaphragm muscles, and CNS-breathing factors. Also see RESPIRATORY FAILURE.

respiratory-distress syndrome: See HYALINE-MEMBRANE DISEASE.

respiratory eroticism in psychoanalysis, the gratification of libidinal drives through use of the respiratory apparatus, as in smoking.

respiratory failure any condition in which the respiratory function is inadequate to maintain the body-tissue cells' requirements for a continuing supply of fresh oxygen and removal of carbon dioxide. R.f. can result from a number of respiratory disorders and is marked by difficult breathing, wheezing, apprehension, mental confusion, drowsiness, and, in extreme cases, loss of consciousness. See RESPIRATORY DISORDERS.

respiratory therapy the treatment of cardiopulmonary disorders by administration of oxygen and therapeutic gases or mists that relieve breathing difficulties, as in emphysema, tuberculosis, asthma, and cardiac conditions. An inhalation therapist handles oxygen masks, respirators, positive-pressure breathing machines, and various gases and mists used in r.t. Also called **inhalation therapy**.

respirograph a graphic representation of an individual's respiratory cycle.

respondent the organism that responds to a stimulus. The term is also applied to a person who is interviewed or who replies to a survey or questionnaire.

respondent behavior behavior that is evoked by a specific stimulus and will consistently and predictably occur if the stimulus is presented. Also called **elicited behavior**. Also see OPERANT BEHAVIOR; EMITTED BEHAVIOR.

respondent conditioning a term introduced by B. F. Skinner to identify classical conditioning as contrasted with operant conditioning or instrumental learning, which requires no specifiable conditioned stimulus.

response any glandular, muscular, neural, or other reaction to a stimulus; a unit of behavior defined either by its result (such as pressing a lever) or by its topography (e.g., raising an arm).

response acquiescence the tendency of a subject to agree with a question regardless of its content.

response amplitude the measure in a given dimension of the magnitude of a response, e.g.. the increase in blood pressure measured in millimeters of mercury.

response-by-analogy principle the generalization that a subject in an unfamiliar situation will react in a manner similar to the way he would in a similar and familiar situation.

response circuit the neural pathway or loop from a receptor to an effector.

response cost a procedure in operant conditioning in which a subject who misbehaves is punished by a loss of previously earned reinforcers.

response-cost contingencies an operant-conditioning technique in which stimuli from the subject's environment are removed to weaken preceding responses.

response deviation the tendency of a subject to answer items on a questionnaire in an unconventional way, regardless of their content.

response dispersion a succession of responses displayed by an organism when its progress toward a goal is obstructed. The responses appear random, irregular, aimless, and haphazard.

response equivalence the similarity between two or more responses that are elicited by the same or similar stimuli. The term is related to response generalization, the chief difference being that generalization refers to quite similar or nearly identical responses made to very similar stimuli whereas equivalence usually refers to responses that are less similar but still closely allied.

response-executing function: See DUAL-AROUSAL MODEL.

response-generalization principle the principle that when a conditioned stimulus regularly elicits a specific response, that stimulus will also evoke different, related responses. E.g., if a rat is conditioned to press a bar at the sound of a buzzer, the buzzer will be able to evoke similar responses in associated situations such as pressing a trap door to obtain reinforcement. Also see STIMULUS GENERALIZATION.

response hierarchy the ranking of a group of responses or response sequences in the order in which they are likely to be evoked by a specific stimulus or stimulus situation; an ordering of responses from the most likely to occur to the least likely to occur.

response-hold mechanism a drive-gate filter system that restricts the flow of stimuli to those compatible with a certain response pattern, such as those for positive motivations. A r.-h.m. works in a reciprocal relationship with a response-switch mechanism so that only one controls the subject's behavior at any moment. Positive motivations are those considered necessary for survival of the individual and the species.

response intensity: See RESPONSE RATE.

response latency = LATENCY OF RESPONSE.

response learning learning to perform specific movements or responses. R.l. is contrasted, in E. C. Tolman's writings, to place learning (finding locations) and to learning that involves the following of given principles. Also called **movement learning**.

response magnitude the response strength as measured in terms of amplitude, duration, frequency, or intensity. Also called **response strength**.

response-oriented theories or systems the systems of psychology that emphasize responses as primary-study data, e.g., operant conditioning, stimulus-response psychology, functionalism, and act psychology.

response prevention = DELAY THERAPY.

response rate the number of responses that occur within a specified time interval. R.r., response intensity, and response time may be used as criteria in calculating the strength of learning or conditioning.

response set a tendency to respond in a particular style regardless of the question; a readiness to respond or a state of concentration as one prepares to react to a stimulus. In social psychology, as an example, a r.s. is a tendency to respond to questionnaire items in a way that is influenced more by the social implications of one's answers than by the question content, e.g., the tendency to give answers that do not reflect true attitudes but seem socially acceptable. Also, some individuals show r.s. by tending, e.g., to answer "Yes" to the items on any questionnaire.

response strength = RESPONSE MAGNITUDE.

response system any body system associated with motor-nerve terminals, e.g., the muscles and glands; also, the totality of processes, physiological and psychological, involved in a response.

response threshold the minimal value of all internal and external determinants that will elicit a particular response.

response time the elapsed time between the onset of a stimulus (e.g., red light) and the beginning of the subject's response (e.g., depressing a brake). R.t. measures the speed of response, which differs in different sense modalities, and is affected by such factors as intensity of stimulus, motivation, drugs (alcohol, caffeine, etc.), gravitational forces, age, sex, and set. R.t. can be measured with inputs from potentials in the cortex and in the muscles. Motor-cortex activity may be detected several seconds before muscle contractions begin. The motor-cortex potential can be observed until the response occurs or the subject abandons the intention to respond, in which case the potential fades away. Also called **reaction time**.

response-switch mechanism a variation of the response-hold mechanism that operates with noxious or damaging stimuli and may be dominant in the absence of positive stimuli. Noxious or damaging stimuli might include drug abuse, which could eventually become accepted as positive in helping the organism survive in a stressful environment.

response variable the changes in reaction of the subject to an experimental stimulus, or stimulus variable.

responsibility fear = HYPENGYOPHOBIA.

restatement in counseling, a statement by the counselor that repeats or rephrases a client's statement in identical or similar terms. The purpose is not only to confirm that the client's remarks have been understood, but to provide a mirror in which the client can see his feelings and ideas more clearly. Also see CLARIFICATION; INTERPRETATION.

rest-cure technique a treatment approach developed by Silas Weir Mitchell for victims of nervous disorders he attributed to the hectic pace of life in the "railroad age." His regimen consisted not only of extended rest, but also physical therapy, massage, environmental change, mild exercise, and a nutritious diet.

rest home a facility for convalescent care, or for the elderly who do not need continuous medical or nursing care. It is sometimes called **adult home**.

resting potential the potential difference in electrical charge across the membrane of a neuron before it is irritated, or stimulated to release the charge. The r.p. usually is about 50 to 100 negative millivolts, representing in that amount an excess of negatively charged ions on the inside of the membrane. The charge outside a neural membrane normally is positive.

restitution in psychoanalysis, a defense in which an individual makes amends not merely for actual damage done but for thoughts or behavior fraught with a deep sense of guilt. The wrongdoing is usually greatly exaggerated (or completely imaginary), and the acts of restitution are equally exaggerated, e.g., a compulsive drive to "do for others," or a persistent pattern of martyrdom.

restitutional schizophrenia a condition observed in schizophrenic patients who are regaining reality and mental processes lost by regression. The symptoms may include delusions or hallucinations, social and speech characteristics typical of schizophrenia, and some symptoms of catatonic behavior. Also see SCHIZOPHRENIC SURRENDER.

restitutive therapies short-term therapies based on the induction of altered states of consciousness (ASC). Pharmacologic agents are used in most of these therapies, either to enable the patient to achieve a peak or transcendental experience, which is believed to have a salutary effect in itself; or to render the patient more amenable to other techniques and modalities such as narcoanalysis and narcosynthesis, in which greater integration of the personality is achieved through ventilation, abreaction, and release of inhibitions and conflicts. Among the agents used are mescaline, psilocybin, marijuana, carbon dioxide, trichloroethylene, nitrous oxide, Methedrine, sodium Amytal, and, in the recent past, LSD.

restless-legs syndrome = EKBOM'S SYNDROME.

restlessness a form of bodily activity that may appear purposeless and limited in time or intensity. A human being may constantly move, become distractible, or pace the floor. An animal may move about its cage, change positions, or look around, but without walking any significant distance or exercising, e.g., in a running wheel. Also see LOCOMOTOR ACTIVITY.

restoration therapy treatment that is directed toward the establishment of normal or near-normal structure and function in a body part or system that has suffered a damaging loss or deficiency because of disease or injury. R.t. may be employed in restoring the structure of the voice box and the function of speech after a throat-cancer operation, or the use of the affected leg for walking after a paralyzing stroke.

Restorff: See VON R.

rest periods brief pauses in work activity taken on a regularly scheduled or discretionary basis for purposes of rest, refreshment, and avoidance of overfatigue or boredom.

restraint the use of control measures, e.g., straitjacket, or camisole, to protect a violent patient from injuring himself or others.

restricted affect emotional expression that is reduced in range and intensity. It is common in depression, inhibited personalities, and schizophrenia. See FLAT AFFECT.

resymbolization the redefining by a recovered patient of all of his conceptions, especially those related to his conflicts.

-ret- a combining form relating to a net or netlike formation (from Latin rete, "net").

RET: See RATIONAL PSYCHOTHERAPY.

retained-members method a retention-measuring technique in which a subject tries to remember as many items of a series as possible.

retaliation: See TALION.

retardation slowing down of any mental or physical activity, as in psychomotor r. occurring in depression; or slow intellectual development, as in mental retardation. Also, r. applies to a delay in the appearance of a conditioned response due to presentation of the unconditioned stimulus several minutes after the start of the conditioned stimulus.

retardation psychopathology learning difficulties, slow development, and other disorders that may accompany intellectual impairment. The emotional manifestations often include nonpsychotic autism, repetitiousness, impaired differentiation of ego function, immaturity, inflexibility, and passivity.

retarded depression a type of depression in which the patient wears a despondent look, sits with bowed head, speaks slowly in a toneless voice, moves as if he were carrying a heavy burden, loses his appetite, has a coated tongue and foul breath, and may sink into a state of stupor.

retarded schizophrenia a schizophrenic state in which the patient speaks, moves, and responds slowly and with great difficulty, if at all. See PSYCHOMOTOR RETARDATION.

rete mirabile /ret'ə mērä'bilə/ a network of blood vessels that is derived from a nearby artery or vein. The term sometimes is applied to the web of small arterial vessels in the kidney or the rete (Latin, "net") of small veins in the liver. A cranial r.m. is found in the brains of certain domestic animals but is seen as a congenital lesion in humans.

retention persistence of learned behavior or experience during a period when it is not being performed or practiced, as indicated by the ability to recall, recognize, reproduce, or relearn it. R. means also the inability or refusal to defecate or urinate.

retention curve a graphic representation of the subject's retention of material over a period of time. Also called **memory curve**.

retention hysteria a term used by Freud early in his career (1895), but later discarded. It denoted a type of hysteria in which a traumatic experience is suppressed, or "retained," resulting in conversion of the emotion associated with it into somatic symptoms. He therefore attempted to cure this condition by getting the patient to "abreact," or relive, the experience.

retention of affect: See STRANGULATED AFFECT.

reticular activating system a network of cell bodies and fibers extending from the hindbrain to the midbrain and hypothalamus. It serves as an indirect route for sensory impulses being transmitted to the cerebral cortex. Functions of the r.a.s. involve arousal, attention, and sleep. Abbrev.: **RAS**. Also called **reticular formation**.

Rétif de la Bretonne, Nicolas Edmé French educator and novelist, 1734–1806. See RETIFISM.

retifism a form of fetishism in which sexual excitement is achieved through contact or masturbation with a shoe or foot, particularly the shoe since it represents the female genitals. The term is derived from the name of an 18th-century French educator, Rétif de la Bretonne.

retina /ret'-/ a complex network of light-sensitive nerve receptors and other neurons organized in several microscopic layers in a lining that covers about two-thirds of the inner surface of the eyeball. The layers contain rod and cone cells, bipolar cells, and ganglia whose fibers extend to a collecting point at the back of the eyeball where they form the optic nerve. Also see DETACHED R.; DIABETIC RETINOPATHY.

retinal bipolar cells neurons in the second layer of the retina that collect inputs from rod and cone cells near the surface and relay the impulses to the ganglion cells in the third layer of the retina. R.b.c. have multiple dendrites that may communicate with several different rod or cone cells.

retinal cones receptors in the first layer of the retinal neurons containing photo-sensitive chemicals that react to certain colors. R.c. are concentrated near the center of the retina and are involved in space perception and visual acuity, in addition to color perception. Although originally named for their shape, cone cells now are identified by function since some cone cells resemble rod cells, and vice versa.

retinal detachment: See DETACHED RETINA.

retinal disparity the slight difference between the right and left retinal images. When both eyes focus on an object, the different position of the eyes produces a disparity of visual angle, and a slightly different image is received by each retina. The two images are automatically compared and fused; this unconscious comparison yields an important cue to depth perception. Also called **binocular disparity**. Also see DEPTH PERCEPTION.

retinal fields the distribution of retinal receptors (rods and cones) that fire under various conditions of illumination and color stimuli. The r.f. generally increase in the peripheral areas as illumination diminishes and decrease as illumination increases. R.f. also demonstrate a reciprocal effect in that peripheral receptors usually fire in the opposite way from those near the center.

retinal ganglion cells cells in the third, or inner, neuron layer of the retina that collect inputs from bipolar cells and transmit them along fibers that form the optic nerve. R.g.c. may communicate with more than one bipolar cell so that they may collect inputs from a number of different rod or cone cells.

retinal hemorrhage bleeding from ruptured aneurysms of the retinal capillaries. The condition is a common cause of detached retinas and the loss of vision in diabetes mellitus. R.h. also is a cause of a form of glaucoma.

retinal horizontal cells association cells in the retina that collect inputs from some receptor cells and feed impulses back to others.

retinal image the image formed on the retina of an eye focused on an external object. The resolution of the image varies with the diameter of the pupil, the focus becoming sharper as illumination of the object increases and the aperture of the pupil decreases. Also called **retinal picture**.

retinal light a sensation of light in the absence of any type of stimulation, apparently due to intrinsic activity within the visual system.

retinal macula a yellowish depressed area on the retina at a point lateral to and below the optic disk. At its center is the fovea centralis, the area of maximum visual acuity containing only cones. Also called **macula lutea**.

retinal mixture: See COLOR MIXTURE.

retinal oscillations the excitation effect of a brief visual stimulus experienced in persistent aftersensations or alternating dark and light bands.

retinal picture = RETINAL IMAGE.

retinal rivalry an effect of alternating visual images in the left and right eyes when each is focused on a different field and the images cannot be fused to produce a single interpretation. Also called **binocular rivalry**.

retinal rods light-sensitive receptors in the first neuron level of the retinal layers. R.r. are not color-sensitive but transform gray values of images into impulses according to the light inten-sity. R.r. are more sensitive than cones to variations in light levels and for peripheral vision.

retinal size the dimensions of the retinal image. R.s. diminishes in proportion to a reflected object's distance from the eye. Size perception is a compromise between r.s. and an object's actual size.

retinene /ret′inēn/ a form of vitamin A that is a component of the visual pigment rhodopsin. When rhodopsin is exposed to light, it breaks down into opsin and r.

retinitis an inflammation of the retina.

retinoblastoma a type of eye tumor that develops from cells of the retina. R. is a rare disorder that apparently is hereditary and unusual in that it generally occurs in persons of above-average intelligence, as opposed to the frequent association of below-normal intelligence with many other inherited neurological disorders.

retinodiencephalic degeneration = LAURENCE-MOON-BIEDL SYNDROME.

retinoscope a mirrored device with a small aperture that permits a study of the interior of the eye when light is projected into it from the mirror.

retirement counseling individual or group counseling of employees for the purpose of helping them to prepare for retirement. Discussions usually include such topics as mental and physical health, recreational activities, part-time or consultant work, finances, insurance, government programs, and problems related to residence.

retirement neurosis a persistent state of maladjustment among retirees, characterized primarily by feelings of emptiness, uselessness, and meaninglessness, as well as general apathy and loss of initiative. Individuals most susceptible to r.n. have depended solely upon work as their major source of satisfaction and self-esteem, and have not developed absorbing interests or productive activities to pursue during the later years of life. See ROLE DEPRIVATION; DISENGAGEMENT THEORY; PENSION NEUROSIS.

retrieval the process involved in recovering or locating information stored in memory or in a computer or other storage device.

retrieving behavior a pattern of animal activity related to parental behavior and characterized by picking up and carrying to the nest, or lair, young offspring that may have wandered away or, in some cases, may have been born outside the nest.

retroactive pertaining to an action or experience that modifies or alters something that occurred in the past, as in retroactive inhibition (the negative influence new learning may have on prior learning).

retroactive association a learned association between one item on a list and a preceding item.

retroactive facilitation the strengthening of a learned association by a previously learned association. Also called **positive retroaction**.

retroactive inhibition the removal from the memory of recently learned material by the introduction of new stimuli. R.i. occurs when new learning partially or extensively interferes with the ability to remember material or carry out activities previously learned, especially if the two sets of material are similar, as in studying French and Latin in quick succession. R.i. is one of the processes that account for forgetting. Also called **retroactive interference**. Compare **proactive inhibition.**

retroactive therapy a form of therapy or rehabilitation undertaken to relieve a condition after it becomes evident, with particular reference to a condition that is experimentally induced. E.g., in studies of learned helplessness, r.t. was employed to reverse the effects of aversive conditioning.

retroflexion a psychoanalytic term used by S. Rado to characterize rage turned back on the self (literally, turning backward).

retrogasserian rhizotomy: See RHIZOTOMY.

retrograde amnesia loss of memory for events and experiences that occurred before the situation that precipitated the amnesia. E.g., a soldier may forget events preceding the bursting of a shell that threw him to the ground. Also see AMNESIA. Compare ANTEROGRADE AMNESIA.

retrograde ejaculation the ejaculation of semen in a reverse direction. The effect is a possible result of surgery of the prostate gland. The semen is ejaculated into the urinary bladder, from which it is excreted later. R.e. also happens when the penis is squeezed just before ejaculation—a misguided attempt at preventing impregnation.

retrogression the return to behavior appropriate to an earlier stage of maturation when more-adult techniques fail to solve a conflict. (The term is used in lieu of regression, a word that is closely identified with psychoanalysis.)

retrogressive formation = BACK-FORMATION.

retrolental fibroplasia a disorder of the tissues behind the lens of the eye, marked by the presence of an opaque substance that causes detachment of the retina and blindness. R.f. occurs mainly in premature infants and is associated with excessive administration of oxygen that leads to exudation of blood and serum through the walls of retinal blood vessels.

retropulsion running backward with short steps, observed in some parkinsonism patients. Also see RETROPULSIVE EPILEPSY.

retropulsive epilepsy epilepsy in which a major symptom is a sudden impulsive running backward.

retrospection an observation or review of an experience from the recent past, as opposed to a report on a current experience, which is termed introspection.

retrospective falsification an unconscious distortion of memory to conform to wishes and expectations; also, the addition of false details about past experiences to support a delusional system in paranoid schizophrenia. Also see PARAMNESIA.

retrospective medical audit: See MEDICAL AUDIT.

retrospective report a report of a past event that is based on the memory of the event by an individual.

retrospective research research that starts with the present and tries to explain it in terms of past events. R.r. cannot usually manipulate variables or make use of a true experimental design. Also see EX POST FACTO RESEARCH; PROSPECTIVE RESEARCH.

return of the repressed the return to the conscious level of ideas or impulses that had been repressed into the unconscious level.

return sweep in reading, the shift of the eyes back from the end of one line to the beginning of the next line.

re-uptake the return of a transmitter substance to the neuron that released it. R. is controlled by a pumping action of the presynaptic neuron utilizing a driving force powered by cellular energy. See ACTIVE TRANSPORT.

revealed-differences technique a method of studying the behavior of members of a family in a laboratory setting by posing a question and observing how the members reach agreement on an answer.

revenge in psychoanalysis, a retaliation for real or fancied wrongs, which may in turn lead to a neurotic fear of retaliation from the target of aggression.

reverberatory circuits neural circuits that recycle information inputs more or less continuously so that retrieval on demand is possible. A theory of r.c. has been proposed to explain learning and memory processes. Although r.c. have been demonstrated only in the autonomic system, they are also believed to exist in the central nervous system. Also called **reverberating circuits**.

reverie daydreaming or musing; ideation carried out on a fantasy level.

reversal in psychoanalysis, the change in the aim of an instinct into its opposite, as in transforming a masochistic impulse to hurt the self into a sadistic impulse to hurt others, or vice versa. Also called **r. of affect; inversion of affect**. Also see PSEUDOAGGRESSION.

reversal design = CROSSOVER DESIGN.

reversal learning a conditioning technique in which an animal must adapt to making correct selections that previously were the wrong choices. That is, the subject is trained to respond in exactly the opposite way to a learning stimulus. E.g., an animal that has been trained to run a maze in a particular manner must learn to run a pattern that is the reverse of the original. A similar technique is used to test the mental flexibility of children.

reversal of affect = INVERSION OF AFFECT.

reversal shift a form of discrimination learning in

which the delivery of reinforcement is suddenly made contingent on responses to the opposite pole of a given dimension. E.g., reinforcement for selecting white objects is changed to reinforcement for selecting black objects. Also see NONREVERSAL SHIFT.

reverse tolerance an effect of certain drugs, particularly psychoactive substances, in which repeated use alters the body's sensitivity so that a smaller dose will produce the same effects previous caused by a large dose.

reversibility a term applied by Piaget to the ability to think of a transformation that would reverse the sequence of events or restore the original condition. E.g., the child realizes that a glass of milk poured into a bottle will remain the same in amount when poured back into the glass. Also see CONSERVATION.

reversible figure an ambiguous figure in which the perspective is easily reversed. For examples, see NECKER CUBE; RUBIN'S FIGURE.

reversible perspective: See AMBIGUOUS FIGURE; REVERSIBLE FIGURE; NECKER CUBE; RUBIN'S FIGURE.

reversion in genetics, the expression of a hereditary trait that was not manifested in a parent. The offspring may resemble a remote ancestor more closely than a member of the immediate family. R. is also used as an alternative term for REGRESSION. See this entry.

review assessment of medical care and services, including (a) peer review, the professional evaluation of individual and group performance, with application of screening criteria for measuring quality of care, (b) emphasis on continuing education as a means of improving methods of practice and quality of care as well as profession growth and development, (c) claims review, focused on cost containment and medical necessity, and (d) utilization review, in which admissions are analyzed to determine medical necessity for the level of the particular services provided and for the duration of stay in the institution. Also see ADMISSION CERTIFICATION; CONTINUED-STAY REVIEW.

revival an obsolete term for recall.

revivification a hypnotic technique in which suggestion is used to induce the subject to revive and relive forgotten or repressed memories.

revolving-door phenomenon a term used to describe the repeated readmission of patients to hospitals or other institutions because they are apparently discharged before they have adequately recovered.

reward = POSITIVE REINFORCEMENT.

reward by the superego in psychoanalysis, a feeling of satisfaction for attitudes or behavior which unconsciously elicit the approval of the superego, e.g., for renouncing guilty sexual or aggressive impulses. The inner reward is based on the satisfaction experienced by the individual when, as a child, his parents approved his actions.

reward conditioning: See OPERANT CONDITIONING.

reward delay: See DELAY-OF-REWARD GRADIENT; DELAYED REWARD.

reward expectancy Tolman's term for a response-readiness set that develops when a subject expects to be rewarded as he has been in a similar situation in the recent past.

reward system a set of interrelated factors that link a particular stimulus with some form of tangible or intangible satisfaction. In animal self-stimulation experiments, a r.s. may consist of the animal pressing a lever that allows an electric current to flow to electrodes implanted in cells of its thalamus or limbic system, apparently giving the animal a pleasurable sensation. See SELF-STIMULATION MECHANISM.

rhabdomancy /rab'-/ the practice of divination by rod or wand, as in dowsing (from Greek *rhabdos*, "rod," and *manteia*, "divination"). See DOWSING.

rhabdophobia a morbid fear of being punished with a rod, or of a rod in general.

rhathymia a term applied to a carefree, happy-go-lucky attitude, a characteristic revealed by factor analysis.

Rh blood-group incompatibility an immune-reaction disorder that may be caused by any of eight different genetically determined antigens on the surface of red blood cells. The antigens, called Rh factors (for *rhesus* monkeys used in early studies), produce an antigen-antibody reaction similar to those of ABO blood-group conflicts when mixed during transfusion or pregnancy with red blood cells tagged with antibodies to reject the Rh antigens. An individual with Rh blood factors is labeled Rh-positive while one whose blood does not carry one of the antigens is classed as Rh-negative. Blacks, Native Americans, and Orientals are about 99 percent Rh-positive, as are 85 percent of Caucasians. The Rh b.-g.i. conflict in pregnancy arises when an Rh-negative mother bears a child that has inherited Rh-positive blood and the Rh antigens pass through the placental membrane and her antibodies react through the placenta to destroy the red blood cells of her own child. The damaged blood cells yield bilirubin which the fetus cannot detoxify and kernicterus may result. Also called **Rhesus incompatibility**. Also see RH REACTION.

rheobase the least amount of current that will produce contraction of a muscle, or excitation of a nerve.

rheotropism the orientation of an organism in the direction of flow of a stream of water. Also called **rheotaxis**.

Rhesus incompatibility = RH BLOOD-GROUP INCOMPATIBILITY.

rheumatism an indefinite term generally used by laymen to describe a variety of painful, motion-limiting disorders of the musculoskeletal system. The same conditions may be diagnosed as rheumatoid arthritis, osteoarthritis, bursitis, sciatica, myalgia, myositis, or fibrositis.

rheumatoid arthritis: See ARTHRITIS.

Rh factor any of at least eight different kinds of antigens, each determined genetically, that may be attached to the surface of an individual's red blood cells. A person whose blood cells carry an Rh f. is said to be Rh-positive. One whose blood cells lack an Rh f. is Rh-negative. See RH BLOOD-GROUP INCOMPATIBILITY.

-rhin-; -rhino- a combining form relating to the nose or the sense of smell (from Greek *rhinos*, "nose").

Rhine, Joseph Banks American parapsychologist, 1895–1980. A leader in parapsychology research, R. began by investigating the possibility of life after death, and continued with studies of CLAIRVOYANCE, PRECOGNITION, PSYCHOKINESIS, and TELEPATHY. See these entries. Also see PSI; PARAPSYCHOLOGY; MCDOUGALL.

rhinencephalon a portion of the brain that includes the olfactory nerves, bulbs, tracts, and related structures and the limbic system. The name, r., literally translates as "smell brain" because early anatomists assumed it was an olfactory organ itself.

rhinolalia the speech quality characterized by abnormal nasal resonance due to obstruction in the posterior part of the nasal passages, or inadequate velopharyngeal closure.

rhinorrhea a persistent running of watery mucus from the nose; a runny nose.

rhizomelic a disorder involving the hip or shoulder joint, an abnormality that is associated with certain congenital defects that are observed in mentally retarded patients. A patient may, e.g., have one leg shorter than the other or contractures of the hip and shoulder joints.

rhizotomy a surgical procedure in which a spinal-nerve root is severed within the spinal canal. R. may be performed for the relief of pain or other discomfort or to control a disorder such as hypertension. **Anterior r.** is a term applied to cutting of an anterior spinal nerve and **posterior r.** to the procedure involving a posterior spinal nerve. Transection of the sensory root fibers of the trigeminal nerve is called **retrogasserian r.**

rho /rō/ 17th letter of the Greek alphabet (P, ρ).

rhodopsin /-dop'-/ a visual pigment associated mainly with functions of the retinal rod cells. When activated by photons, r. breaks down into retinene and opsin and loses its own purple pigmentation. Usually, retinene and opsin rejoin almost immediately as new molecules of r.

rhombencephalic sleep the second phase of sleep (the first is telencephalic sleep, or neosleep) during which dreaming occurs as the subjective concomitant of a distinctive physiologic state termed the D-state, during which rapid eye movements occur (REM sleep). R.s. depends physiologically on the inhibitory action of the caudal pontine nucleus on the pontobulbar reticular system and on the limbic system.

rhombencephalon = HINDBRAIN.

rhonchus a coarse rattling in the throat or bronchial tubes caused by an obstruction, such as mucus. The term also is applied at times to a wheezing sound in the respiratory tract.

Rh reaction an adverse effect that can occur in blood transfusions and pregnancies when an Rh-negative person's blood is mixed with Rh-positive blood from another individual. The Rh r. is similar to an immune reaction to an invasion of the body tissues by a foreign agent. In pregnancy, an Rh-negative mother may carry an Rh-positive fetus, her body forming anti-Rh antibodies that destroy the red blood cells of the fetus. Also see RH BLOOD-GROUP INCOMPATIBILITY.

rhyming delirium an occasional symptom of the manic phase of manic-depressive reactions, consisting of speaking or declaiming in rhymes.

rhypophobia = DIRT PHOBIA.

rhythm and periodicity the regular repetition that characterizes not only biological processes such as pulse, respiration, hunger, menstruation, urination, and metabolic changes, but behavioral phenomena as well, such as thumb-sucking, nursing, masturbation, mood changes, and rhythmic games, dances and songs. Many pathological manifestations are also rhythmic or periodic: the manic-depressive cycle, the tendency to repeat traumatic experiences in recurrent dreams, and the repetitive activities of obsessive-compulsives, all of which Freud sought to explain by the single principle of the REPETITION-COMPULSION. See this entry.

rhythm disorders: See TIME AND R.D.

rhythmic sensory-bombardment therapy a form of sensory-overloading treatment in which certain types of psychotic and psychoneurotic patients are bombarded with sonic, photic, or tactile stimulation applied intermittently and rhythmically for one hour.

rhythmic stimulation an automatic effect of a flickering light characterized by synchronization of the EEG pattern to the frequency of the flicker. The effect of light flicker on brain waves may vary with different species of animals. Flickering lights may precipitate seizures in predisposed individuals.

rhythm method a technique of contraception in which the female abstains from coitus during the days of the month in which she is most likely to become pregnant, usually just before and after ovulation. The r.m. is only about 80 percent effective because of the difficulty in making advance predictions of the precise time of ovulation. The predictions are made by daily charting of rectal or vaginal temperature changes, or by testing changes in the sugar content of the cervical mucus.

riboflavin $C_{17}H_{20}N_4O_6$—a vitamin in the B-complex group, functioning as a coenzyme of protein metabolism. A deficiency of r. is marked by skin eruptions, slow healing of wounds, cracks around the corners of the mouth and nose, and extra blood vessels in the corneas. R. was named for its ribose sugar component and yellow pigment, for which the Latin word is *flavus*.

ribonuclease an enzyme that breaks down ribonucleic-acid molecules into smaller units.

ribonucleic acid = RNA.

ribosomal RNA a form of RNA found in intracellular nucleoprotein particles, or ribosomes, where it plays a role in linking amino acids into protein molecules.

ribosome structures that occur in the cytoplasm of living cells where they function as protein factories. They may be found singly or in clusters, bound to a cell membrane or floating freely in the cytoplasm.

Richardson, John Clifford Canadian neurologist, 1909—. See STEELE-RICHARDSON-OLSZEWSKI SYNDROME.

Richardson, Marion Webster American psychologist, 1891—. See KUDER-RICHARDSON FORMULAS.

rickets a calcium-deficiency disease occurring in infants and young children, characterized by softening of the bones and skeletal deformities such as bowed legs. Also see OSTEOMALACIA.

riddance phenomenon a term used by S. Rado for various reflexes that help to eliminate annoying or painful agents from the body, including scratching, spitting, vomiting, sneezing, and shedding tears.

Ridgway, Robert American ornithologist, 1850–1929. See RIDGWAY COLOR SYSTEM.

Ridgway color system a method of organizing more than 1,100 hues based on the natural colors of bird feathers.

ridicule fear = CATAGELOPHOBIA.

Rieger, Herwigh /rē′gər/ German ophthalmologist, 1898—. See RIEGER'S SYNDROME.

Rieger's syndrome an autosomal-dominant disorder marked by dental and eye abnormalities. The dental anomalies may include missing teeth and enamel hypoplasia. Visual disorders usually involve anomalies of the iris and cornea. Mental retardation is sometimes present. Also called **hypodontia; iris dysgenesis**.

Riesman, David American social scientist, 1909—. See INNER-DIRECTED; OTHER-DIRECTED; OTHER-DIRECTED PERSON; TRADITION-DIRECTED.

rifampin $C_{43}H_{58}N_4O_{12}$—a semisynthetic antibiotic used mainly in the treatment of tuberculosis but also employed occasionally in cases of acute bacterial meningitis and leprosy. Also called **rifampicin**.

right-and-wrong-cases method an alternative term for the METHOD OF CONSTANT STIMULI. See this entry.

right-and-wrong test a test of criminal responsibility derived from the M'NAGHTEN RULES. See this entry.

right angles: See ORTHOGONAL.

right-handedness preferential use of the right hand for major activities, such as eating, writing, and throwing. It is a component of dextrality, and applies to about 90 percent of the population. See DEXTRALITY; LATERALITY; DEXTRALITY-SINISTRALITY; CEREBRAL DOMINANCE; HANDEDNESS.

righting reflex an automatic tendency of an organism to return to an upright position when it has been thrown off balance or placed on its back. The reflexes involved are optic, vestibular, and kinesthetic, but different sensory stimuli and subcortical structures may become recruited into the reflex action. Also called **righting reaction**. Also see VISUAL-RIGHTING REFLEXES.

right-left disorientation a disorder characterized by general difficulty in distinguishing between the right and left sides. The r.-l.d. condition has been linked to aphasia and other disorders of comprehension despite evidence that it also occurs in the absence of such disorders. R.-l.d. also occurs to a mild degree in presumably normal adults.

right of the first night = JUS PRIMAE NOCTIS.

right-or-wrong test: See RIGHT-AND-WRONG TEST.

right-side fear = DEXTROPHOBIA.

rights of disabled the basic constitutional rights guaranteed all individuals in the United States and reinforced by special legislation and court rulings to protect patients in mental institutions. E.g., retarded children are protected against corporal punishment and inadequate medical care, mental patients are allowed to refuse treatment administered primarily for the benefit of the hospital staff, and confidentiality of psychiatric records is assured. Also see INSTITUTIONAL PEONAGE; BILL OF RIGHTS.

rights of patients the doctrine that a patient who is involuntarily hospitalized (that is, legally committed) has the right to communicate with persons outside the facility, to keep clothing and personal effects, to vote, to follow his religion, to be employed if possible, to execute wills or other legal instruments, to enter into contractual relationships, to make purchases, to be educated, to marry, to retain licenses and permits, to sue or be sued, and not to be subjected to unnecessary restraint.

rights of the mentally retarded mentally retarded persons' rights as stated by the United Nations Declaration on the Rights of Mentally Retarded Persons (1971): The mentally retarded have the same rights to the maximum degree of feasibility as other human beings including the right to receive proper medical care, physical therapy, education, training, rehabilitation, and guidance; the right to economic security; the right to work; the right to live with one's own family or foster parents or, if this is not feasible, to live in an institution under circumstances as close as possible to family life; and protection from abuse and exploitation.

right temporal lobectomy: See TEMPORAL LOBECTOMY.

right to refuse treatment the view that mental patients have a r.t.r.t. that may be potentially hazardous or intrusive, including electroshock therapy and psychotropic drugs, particularly when such treatments appear to be administered for the convenience of the hospital staff rather than for the benefit of the patient. Various state laws and court rulings support the rights of patients to receive or reject certain treatments, but there is a lack of uniformity in such regulations. Also see FORCED TREATMENT.

right to treatment in forensic psychiatry, the principle that a facility that has assumed the responsibility to provide treatment for a patient is legally obligated to provide adequate treatment.

rigid control the use of inner restraints, such as inhibitions, repression, suppression, and reaction formation in coping with environmental stressors.

rigid flatfoot: See FLATFOOT.

rigidity in psychiatry, a personality trait characterized by inability or strong resistance to changing one's behavior, or to altering one's opinions and attitudes. In physiology, r. is a condition of extreme and persistent muscular contraction, as in certain neuromuscular disorders such as cerebral palsy. See AFFECTIVE R.; OPISTHOTONOS; INTELLECTUAL R. Also see DECEREBRATION.

Riley, Conrad Milton American pediatrician, 1913—. See FAMILIAL DYSAUTONOMIA (also called **Riley-Day syndrome**); NEUROPATHIC ARTHROPATHY.

rima palpebrarum = PALPEBRAL FISSURE.

Rimbaud, Arthur /reNbō'/ French symbolist poet, 1854–91. See VERBOCHROMIA.

ring chromosome a defective chromosome that results from breakage in both arms of a chromatid which then fuses at the ends to form a circle. Ring chromosome abnormalities tend to involve one of the X chromosomes.

ring chromosome 18 a congenital disorder characterized by microcephaly, ear and eye abnormalities, and severe mental retardation. Cause of the condition is not hereditary but due to breakage of arms of chromosome 18 which fuse to form one or more rings of varying sizes. The less severely retarded children may qualify for special education classes.

ring D syndrome: See CHROMOSOME 13, DELETION OF LONG ARM.

ring-finger dermatitis a form of cutaneous disease involving an area of a finger where a ring usually is worn. The condition may be marked by itching, redness, eruption of small blisters, or similar effects. In the absence of evidence that the skin eruption is caused by chemical irritation of substances in the ring or soap or detergents trapped beneath the ring, r.-f.d. may be a cutaneous reaction to an emotional problem.

Rinné test a tuning-fork test used to aid in differentiating between a conductive and sensorineural hearing loss.

risk: See AT R.; HIGH-R. STUDIES; MORBIDITY R.

risk hypothesis: See ETHICAL-R.H.

risk-rescue rating a formula, devised by A. Weisman and J. W. Worden (1972), for assessing the lethality of suicide attempts: $(A \times 100)/(A + B)$, where A is the risk score (the agent used, impairment of consciousness, toxicity, lesions, reversibility treatment required) and B is the rescue score (site of attempt, person initiating rescue, probability of discovery by rescuer, accessibility to rescue, delay until discovery).

risk-taking a pattern of taking unnecessary risks, which may be motivated, usually unconsciously, by masochistic needs; bravado and the desire to prove oneself or tempt fate. R.-t. may involve superstitious attitudes, as with the gambler who risks his entire fortune on a hunch. See PATHOLOGICAL GAMBLING.

Ritalin a trademark for a form of methylphenidate hydrochloride used to treat hyperactivity in children. The drug is a mild CNS stimulant that is more effective than caffeine but less effective than amphetamine in increasing mental and motor performance.

ritualistic behavior: See RITUALS.

ritual-making Rado's term for obsessive attacks in which the patient goes through repetitive sequences of a daily-life routine, e.g., bathing or dressing, in a stereotyped ceremonial manner. The routine may be continued until the patient is exhausted.

rituals a series of acts repeatedly and compulsively carried out as a defense against anxiety, or for release of tension. Among children and obsessive-compulsive adults, these "ceremonials" are usually interpreted as a kind of magic unconsciously adopted to ward off feelings of guilt generated by forbidden wishes and impulses. Freud cites the example of an 11-year-old boy who could not go to sleep until he had recited all the events of the day to his mother, pushed his bed to the wall with three chairs beside it, and kicked a certain number of times (*The Neuro-Psychoses of Defense*, 1894).

river fear = POTAMOPHOBIA.

R methodology factor analysis across tests rather than across individuals. R m. shows how traits, abilities, etc., fall into patterns called factors, but it does not show how individuals cluster together. Compare Q METHODOLOGY.

RN = REGISTERED NURSE.

RNA *ribo*nucleic *a*cid, a nucleic acid that controls the synthesis of protein molecules in living cells, and in some cases may have other special functions. Kinds of RNA include messenger RNA, which carries the genetic code from the cell nucleus to the cytoplasm; ribosomal RNA, which is found in ribosomes where it forms proteins from amino acids; and transfer RNA, which carries a specific amino acid for protein synthesis. Each of 20 amino acids has a corresponding RNA to place the amino acid in the proper sequence in protein building. RNA is similar to DNA in structure except for differences in a sugar unit and one base unit. Also see MESSENGER RNA; TRANSFER RNA; RIBOSOMAL RNA.

robber fear = HARPAXOPHOBIA.

Robertson: See ARGYLL-R.

Robert's syndrome an autosomal-recessive disorder in which the child is born with abnormally short arms and legs as well as a cleft lip and palate. Microcephaly and genital hypertrophy accompany the other anomalies. Few of the patients survive early infancy, and those that do are likely to be severely mentally retarded. Also see TETRAPHOCOMELIA.

Robin, Pierre /rōbeN'/ French physician, 1867–1950. See PIERRE ROBIN'S SYNDROME.

Robinson, Edward Stevens American psychologist, fl. 1919, 1937. See KJERSTED-ROBINSON LAW; SKAGGS-ROBINSON HYPOTHESIS; FATIGUE STUDIES.

Robinson Crusoe age = INDUSTRY VERSUS INFERIORITY.

robot a machine that performs functions similar to those of a human (e.g., a spot-welding r.); also, a human whose rigid behavior resembles that of a machine. (The term is derived from the Czech word *robotnik*, "slave," and became known from the title of a play by Karel Capek, 1920.)

rocket fuel: See PHENCYCLIDINE.

rocking a form of stereotyped motor behavior observed primarily in some severely or profoundly retarded children, in children with infantile autism, and also among chimpanzees reared in isolation. In some instances, r. may be a form of masturbation.

Rocky Mountain spotted fever an acute rickettsial infection, marked by a sudden fever reaching 104°F (40°C) and remaining high for more than two weeks in many cases. A major target of the infection is the central nervous system. Neurologic symptoms include headache, insomnia, delirium, and coma. The disease is commonly transmitted by the wood tick, Dermacentor andersoni, which also is a disease vector for tularemia and Q fever.

rodding operation a surgical procedure performed in the treatment of osteogenesis imperfecta in which steel rods are inserted in the long bones. The hollow central portion of the bones is cut into segments and the rods are inserted so that space is left between segments for new bone tissue to form. The limb is then placed in a cast while the segments grow together. For a small child the r.o. must be repeated at intervals of about three years. Also called SHISH-KEBAB OPERATION.

rod fear = RHABDOPHOBIA.

rods of Corti the pillarlike structures that form an arch in the organ of Corti.

rod vision vision that depends solely upon the rod cells of the retina, as in twilight (scotoscopic) vision.

Roentgen, Wilhelm /rent'gən/ German physicist, 1845–1923. R. won the first Nobel Prize in physics (1901), for his discovery of Roentgen rays, or X-rays. Also spelled **Röntgen**. See ROENTGENOGRAM; X-RAY (also called **Roentgen ray**).

roentgenogram a photographic record produced by X-ray exposure. A r. may be identified specifically with a particular perspective or technique; e.g., a **Towne projection r.** shows a midfacial view of the skull bones, a **Waters view r.** produces a shadow picture of the maxillary sinuses of both sides for comparison. R. is named for the German physicist Wilhelm Roentgen who developed the technique. Also see X-RAY.

Rogerian therapy: See CLIENT-CENTERED PSYCHOTHERAPY; ROGERS.

Rogers, Carl American psychologist, 1902—. R. originated client-centered psychotherapy and the nondirective approach, which he conceived as providing the patient with a warm, accepting climate that would foster personality growth and the realization of inner potentialities. Adjective: **Rogerian** /rōjer'-/. See CLIENT-CENTERED PSYCHOTHERAPY; CONDITIONAL POSITIVE REGARD; CONDITIONS OF WORTH; CONGRUENCE; EXISTENTIAL LIVING; FULLY FUNCTIONING PERSON; GROWTH PRINCIPLE; HELPING RELATIONSHIP; HUMANISTIC PERSPECTIVE; NONDIRECTIVE APPROACH; NONDIRECTIVE TEACHING MODEL; POSITIVE REGARD; PRIMARY EMPATHY; REFLECTION OF FEELING; SENSITIVITY TRAINING; THERAPEUTIC ATMOSPHERE; UNCONDITIONAL POSITIVE REGARD; UNCRITICALNESS.

Rolandic fissure = FISSURE OF ROLANDO.

Rolando, Luigi Italian anatomist, 1773–1831. See FISSURE OF ROLANDO; SPINAL-TRIGEMINAL NUCLEUS.

role the functions adopted by an individual, or assigned to him, in a social structure; or the characteristic attitudes and patterns of behavior that determine the part he plays in specific situations or life in general. Examples are the role of teacher, foreman, or peacemaker, or the masculine role in a particular culture. See SOCIAL R.

role behaviors; role categories: See SOCIAL ROLE.

role conflict a state of tension or conflict that arises when an individual fills two or more functions that clash or compete. **Intrarole conflict** means that the source of tension can be located within one role, e.g., the parental role when two children have incompatible needs. **Interrole conflict** arises in the clash between two different roles, e.g., that of parent and that of employee.

role confusion masculine behavior in a female or feminine behavior in a male. R.c. may result from mistaken assignment of sex roles in infants with ambiguous genitalia, cross dressing during early childhood, separation from the mother or father during infancy, or other environmental influences. Sex-role identity usually is established by the age of three years. Feminine behavior in boys after that age generally is more difficult to correct than tomboyishness in girls. Also called **identity confusion; identity diffusion**. Also see GENDER IDENTITY; GENDER-IDENTITY DISORDER OF CHILDHOOD; TRANSGENDERISM; IDENTITY VERSUS R.C.

Role Construct Repertory Test a technique devised by G. A. Kelly for use in clinical practice based on the idea that the concepts of constructs used by an individual to perceive objects or events influence his or her behavior. The test is designed to help the clinician identify the client's important constructs, such as the roles other people play in his or her life. Abbrev.: **REP Test**.

role-construct theory a cognitive theory of human behavior stating that people attempt to select constructs or concepts that can make their environments understandable and predictable while providing clues to behavior. According to r.-c.t., an individual seeks to sustain and substantiate a construct system once it has been developed.

role deprivation denial of culturally and psychologically significant statuses and roles to certain individuals or groups, usually producing some degree of psychopathology. Examples are mandatory, indiscriminate retirement, discrimination against minority groups, and exiling individuals who criticize the prevailing political system.

role diffusion a term used by Erikson to denote an adolescent's inability to define his identity. See ROLE CONFUSION.

role distortion a change in role behavior from what is expected to an undesirable form.

role-divided therapy = MULTIPLE THERAPY.

role-enactment theory a theory of hypnosis stating that the subject under hypnosis unconsciously assumes or takes on whatever role the hypnotist assigns, and behaves in accordance with this role while in the hypnotic trance.

role expectations: See SOCIAL ROLE.

role model a person or group serving as a pattern for the goals, attitudes, or behavior of an individual. The individual identifies with the r.m. and seeks to imitate him or her.

role obsolescence a condition in which the social role of an individual or type of individual has diminished importance within the group or population.

role-playing a technique of human-relations training and psychotherapy in which the individual acts out social roles of other people, or tries out new roles for himself. Originally developed as a psychodrama procedure, r.-p. is now widely used in industrial, educational, and clinical settings for such purposes as training employees to handle sales problems, testing out different attitudes and relationships in group and family psychotherapy, and rehearsing different ways of coping with stresses and conflicts. Special techniques are often used, such as exchanging roles with another person, or acting out one's last marital quarrel. R.-p. is also an alternative term for visualization in motivation research. See VISUALIZATION.

role reversal a technique of psychodrama in which the protagonist exchanges roles with an auxiliary in acting out a significant interpersonal situation. R.r. is also used in management development programs, in which, e.g., the supervisor and the employee exchange roles.

role shift in any two-person relationship, the adop-

tion by each partner of the characteristic behavior of the other. E.g., an ordinarily dominant partner may consciously or unconsciously exchange roles with the usually submissive partner. Also see ROLE REVERSAL.

role specialization in consumer psychology, the relative decision-making influences of husband and wife. The role structures fall into four categories: husband dominant; wife dominant; autonomous, in which decisions are made independently by either spouse; and syncratic, in which decisions are made jointly. Autonomous decisions might involve use of alcoholic beverages in the home. Syncratic decisions involve, e.g., choice of housing or vacation plans.

role-taking the ability to take the role or viewpoint of another person. It is an essential process in cognitive and social development.

role theory of personality a theory that describes personality development in terms of (a) gradual acquisition of roles (boy, girl, gang member, "brain"), (b) the individual's role models, (c) the role behavior prescribed by the particular culture, and (d) the individual's ability to select his own roles and develop them in his own way.

Rolf, Ida American physical therapist, 1896–1979. See ROLFING.

rolfing a deep-massage technique developed by the biochemist Ida Rolf at the Esalen Institute in California. The technique is based on a theory that muscle massage will relieve both physical and psychic pain.

romance: See FAMILY R.

romanticism factor: See CLASSICISM FACTOR.

Romberg, Moritz Heinrich von German neurologist, 1795–1873. See ROMBERG'S DISEASE; ROMBERG'S SIGN; FACIAL HEMIATROPHY (also called **Parry-Romberg syndrome**); DISFIGUREMENT.

Romberg's disease a form of facial hemiatrophy or disfigurement marked by atrophy of the tissues of one side of the face. Also called **facial trophoneurosis**. Also see FACIAL HEMIATROPHY.

Romberg's sign a diagnostic symptom of locomotor ataxia consisting of a swaying motion when the patient stands with his eyes closed and feet together.

Röntgen: See ROENTGEN.

rooming-in a practice in some hospitals whereby the mother and her newborn child share the same room so that the mother can feed, care for, and establish a close relationship with the baby as soon after birth as is feasible.

root conflict a nuclear problem with roots in infancy that affects later personality development.

rootedness need according to Fromm, the human need to establish bonds or ties with others that provide emotional security and serve to reduce the isolation and insignificance Fromm believed to lie at the heart of human existence. The r.n. is manifested positively in BROTHERLINESS, negatively in INCESTUOUS TIES. See these entries.

rooting reflex a reflex in which the healthy newborn infant turns his head toward a gentle stimulus applied to the corner of his mouth or cheek, e.g., a finger or nipple.

Rorschach, Hermann /rôr′shäkh/ Swiss psychiatrist, 1884–1922. R. was the originator of the widely-used projective test of personality that bears his name, which arose out of experiments on hallucinations in which ink blots were utilized. See RORSCHACH TEST; BEHN-RORSCHACH TEST; ACHROMATIC RESPONSE; AFFECTIVE RATIO; BODY BOUNDARIES; CHROMATIC RESPONSE; FACTOR-LOADING; INQUIRY; ORIGINAL RESPONSE; PATHOGNOMONIC SIGNS; PERCEPTANALYSIS; PERSONALITY ASSESSMENT; POPULAR RESPONSE.

Rorschach test a projective technique developed by Hermann Rorschach in which the subject is presented with ten unstructured ink blots (in mostly black and gray, but sometimes in color) and is asked "What might this be?" or "What do you see in this?" The examiner classifies the responses according to such factors as color (C), movement (M), detail (D), whole (W), popular or common (P), animal (A), form (F), and human (H). Various scoring systems, either qualitative or quantitative, are used. The object is to interpret the subject's personality structure in terms of such factors as emotionality, cognitive style, creativity, bizarreness, and various defensive patterns.

Rosanoff, Aaron Joshua American psychologist, 1878–1943. See KENT-ROSANOFF TEST; WORD-ASSOCIATION TEST.

Roscoe, Henry Enfield English chemist, 1833–1915. See BUNSEN-ROSCOE LAW.

Rosenbach, Ottomar /rō′zənbäkh/ German physician, 1851–1907. See ROSENBACH'S SIGN; GMELIN TEST (also called **Rosenbach-Gmelin test**).

Rosenbach's sign the inability of a patient to close his eyes immediately and completely on command, a diagnostic sign of neurasthenia.

Rosenberg Draw-a-Person Technique a projective test in which the subject draws a human figure and is asked what the person is like, after which he is required to redraw the figure; and if there are any changes, the examiner asks questions designed to reveal the psychodynamics behind the changes.

Rosenman, Ray H. American physician, 1920—. See TYPE A PERSONALITY; TYPE B PERSONALITY.

Rosenthal, Curt /rō′zəntäl/ German psychiatrist, fl. 1927. See ROSENTHAL EFFECT; MELKERSSON-ROSENTHAL SYNDROME; PYGMALIONISM; SELF-FULFILLING PROPHECY.

Rosenthal effect a form of self-fulfilling prophecy or expectancy effect, in which, e.g., the expectation that a student will succeed or fail leads to that result, or in which an experimenter unconsciously biases his data. Also called **Pygmalion effect**. See SELF-FULFILLING PROPHECY; PYGMALIONISM.

Rosenzweig, Saul American psychologist, 1907—. See ROSENZWEIG PICTURE-FRUSTRATION STUDY; IMPUNITIVE RESPONSE; INTROPUNITIVE RESPONSE; NEED-PERSISTENT RESPONSE; STRUCTURED STIMULUS.

Rosenzweig Picture-Frustration Study a projective test in which the subject reveals patterns of responses to 24 frustrating situations depicted in line drawings. E.g., a driver who splashes a pedestrian apologizes, and the subject is asked to indicate what the pedestrian would reply. The responses are interpreted in terms of three types of aggression: extrapunitive (directed outward: "I am going to sue you"), intropunitive (directed inward: "I should have noticed the puddle"), and impunitive (making light of the problem: "It was an accident").

Ross, Sir George William Canadian physician, 1841–1931. See ROSS-JONES TEST.

Ross-Jones test a test for the amount of globulin in a patient's cerebrospinal fluid. Also called **ammonium-sulfate test**.

Rössle, Robert /res′lə/ German pathologist, 1876–1956. See URBACH-WIETHE DISEASE (also called **Rössle-Urbach-Wiethe lipoproteinosis**).

rostral indicating the front or anterior portion of an organ or organism.

rostrum a beak-shaped structure, such as the r. of the corpus callosum in the area where it curves backward under the frontal lobe.

rotary-pursuit test a reaction test that requires a subject to follow an irregularly moving target with a pointer or other indicator.

rotation perception sensitivity to motion produced by rotation of the body, due to fluid in the semicircular canals, followed by the sensation of rotating in the opposite direction when the actual rotation is stopped.

rotation system a technique of group psychotherapy in which the therapist works with each individual patient in sequence in the presence of other group members.

rotation treatment: See GYRATOR TREATMENT.

rote learning the type of learning in which acquisition occurs in the absence of comprehension. The student can answer correctly but does not understand the reasoning behind or the logical implications of his response.

rote recall precise recollection of information that has been stored in its entirety, e.g., an address, chemical formula, color pattern, or piece of music. Also called **verbatim recall**.

Rothmund, August von, Jr. /rōt′mo͞ont/ German physician, 1830–1906. See ROTHMUND-THOMSON SYNDROME.

Rothmund-Thomson syndrome an autosomal-recessive disorder characterized by skin lesions that form a marbelized pattern. Many of the patients also have cataracts, and some are mentally retarded.

roughness discrimination a test of somesthetic sensitivity in which a subject is expected to determine by touch which of a choice of surfaces has a greater roughness. The surfaces may be grades of sandpaper. The ability is sometimes lost following a lesion in a brain area related to the sense of touch.

round window a membrane-covered opening in

the cochlea which helps relieve the fluid pressure in the inner ear. When the stapes bone of the middle ear vibrates the oval window in transmitting sound impulses, the displaced cochlear fluid might damage delicate inner-ear structures if they are not protected by the flexible surface of the r.w.

Rouse v. Cameron: See LEAST-RESTRICTIVE ALTERNATIVE.

Roussy, Gustave /roosē'/ French pathologist, 1874–1948. See ROUSSY-LÉVY SYNDROME.

Roussy-Lévy syndrome a form of Friedreich's ataxia involving peroneal atrophy, or wasting of the lower calf or thigh.

routes of administration: See ADMINISTRATION.

Royer, Pierre /rô·äyä'/ French pediatrician, 1917– . See PRADER-LABHART-WILLI SYNDROME (there: **Royer's syndrome**).

R-R conditioning a type of conditioning in which one *re*sponse is a prerequisite for a second *re*sponse.

-rrhagia; -rrhage a combining form relating to excessive flow or discharge (from Greek *-rrhagia*, "a bursting forth").

-rrhea /-rē'ə/ a combining form relating to flow or discharge (from Greek *rhoia*, "flow, flux").

rubber = CONDOM. Also see FROTTAGE.

rubella = GERMAN MEASLES. Also see CONGENITAL R.-SYNDROME.

rubeola: See EXANTHEMATA.

rubidium a silvery metal (symbol: Rb) of the alkali group which some specialists claim to have an antidepressant effect. During the 1880s, r. was used in the treatment of epilepsy and syphilis.

Rubin, Edgar J. Danish phenomenologist, 1886–1951. See RUBIN'S FIGURE.

Rubin's figure an ambiguous figure that may be perceived either as one goblet or as two facing profiles. Also called **goblet figure**. Also see NECKER CUBE.

Rubinstein, Jack Herbert American child psychiatrist, 1925– . See RUBINSTEIN-TAYBI SYNDROME.

Rubinstein-Taybi syndrome a familial disorder marked by facial abnormalities, including microcephaly and hypertelorism, broad thumbs and toes, and mental retardation. Hypotonia and a stiff gait are common. One study of intelligence of the patients found more than 80 percent had IQs of less than 50. Also called **broad-thumb-hallux syndrome**.

rubospinal tract: See CORTICOSPINAL TRACT.

Ruffini, Angelo /roofē'nē/ Italian anatomist, 1864–1929. See RUFFINI PAPILLARY ENDINGS; RUFFINI'S CORPUSCLES.

Ruffini papillary endings nerve endings in the papillary layer of the skin that are associated with pressure sensations.

Ruffini's corpuscles sensory nerve endings in the subcutaneous tissues of human fingers, believed to mediate warmth sensations.

rule of abstinence in psychoanalysis, the rule that the patient should abstain from all gratifications which might distract from the analytic process or drain off instinctual energy, anxiety, and frustration that could be used as a driving force in the therapeutic process. Examples of such gratifications are smoking, engaging in idle conversation, or acting out during the sessions, and unlimited sexual activity, absorbing interests, and other pleasures pursued outside the sessions. Also called **abstinence rule**.

rules of the game a term that refers to children's changing attitudes toward rules. According to Piaget, when children first learn the meaning of rules, they view them as utterly binding. Even then they break rules, they tend not to challenge their validity. However, as they approach adolescence (beginning around age ten), children tend to shift their attitude and view rules as social conventions or laws that can be questioned and modified under conditions of mutual consent. According to Piaget, this shift is a sign of the child's growing maturity because it represents a more realistic cognitive assessment of the social nature of rules while encompassing an emotional attitude of cooperation.

rum fits generalized grand mal seizures that occur in some cases of alcohol-withdrawal syndrome. The patient may experience one or two r.f. during withdrawal, but not all patients suffer the symptom. Also called **alcoholic epilepsy**.

rumination the act of persistently pondering or meditating about a problem, and in some cases an insoluble metaphysical question, for an excessive period of time. It is a common symptom of obsessive-compulsive disorder. R. is also used as a briefer term for R. DISORDER OF INFANCY. See this entry.

rumination disorder of infancy a rare disorder in which infants between three and 12 months of age repeatedly regurgitate all food, with ejection or reswallowing but without nausea. These infants may develop potentially fatal weight loss and malnutrition. (DSM-III)

Rumpf, Theodor /roompf/ German physician, 1851–1923. See RUMPF'S SIGN.

Rumpf's sign a reaction in cases of neurasthenia in which pressure over a point of pain increases the pulse rate by as much as 20 beats per minute.

run amok: See AMOK.

runs test a test for the deviation from randomness of a series with only two possibilities, such as aaabbaaaaaab.

runway the pathway that leads from a starting box to a goal box or to the main part of a maze.

rupophobia = DIRT PHOBIA.

rural environment an environment characterized by open land and a relatively sparse population that depends full- or part-time on agricultural activities as a means of livelihood. In environmental psychology, the r.e. often is used as a basis for comparison of physical and social conditions that produce stressors, e.g., air-pollution levels, crowding, and crime of urban environments.

rush an effect experienced by a person who receives an intravenous injection of amphetamine.

The sensation sometimes is described as a sudden awakening or alertness accompanied by a degree of euphoria or pleasure. Also called **flash**.

Rush, Benjamin American physician, 1745–1813. A man of varied interests and accomplishments, R. spent the first 20 years of his professional life as professor of chemistry, member of the Continental Congress (he was a signer of the Declaration of Independence), and Physician General in the Revolutionary War. He then turned his attention to psychiatry, establishing a separate wing of the Pennsylvania Hospital for the active treatment and intensive study of mental patients, on the theory that insanity is a disease and essentially treatable. His treatment methods, however, included not only calming patients through kindness, but bloodletting, purging, keeping them awake and on foot for 24 hours, intimidation, and, if all else failed, whirling them in a "gyrator" or strapping them into a "tranquilizing chair." See AMENOMANIA; ANOMIA; GYRATOR TREATMENT; MORAL TREATMENT; TRANQUILIZER CHAIR.

Russell, Alexander English pediatrician, fl. 1935, 1964. See SILVER-RUSSELL SYNDROME (also called **Russell's dwarf**).

Russian fly = SPANISH FLY.

rut = ESTROUS BEHAVIOR.

S

s. an abbreviation used in prescriptions, meaning "write on label" (Latin *signa*).

S = SPATIAL RELATIONS; SPATIAL RELATIONSHIPS. Also see PRIMARY ABILITIES.

S^D = DISCRIMINATIVE STIMULUS.

S°; S$^\triangle$: See NEGATIVE DISCRIMINATIVE STIMULUS.

saccadic movement the movement of the eye from one fixation point (target) to another. Also called **saccadics.**

-sacchar-; -saccharo- a combining form relating to sugar.

saccule a part of the vestibular mechanism of the inner ear which along with the utricle and the three semicircular canals maintains the mechanism of balance. It contains sensory hair cells embedded in a gelatinous substance that also contains crystals of calcium carbonate. When the head is moved from any normal position, the movement exerts a momentum pressure on the hair cells, which then fire impulses indicating a change in body position in space.

Sacher-Masoch, Leopold von /zäkh′ər mäz′ôkh/ Austrian lawyer and writer, 1836–95. The term masochism /mas′əkizəm/ is derived from the kind of eroticism that is typical in his later novels. See MASOCHISM; FEMININE MASOCHISM; IDEAL MASOCHISM; MASOCHISTIC CHARACTER; MASOCHISTIC FANTASIES; MASOCHISTIC SABOTAGE; MASOCHISTIC WISH-DREAM; MASS MASOCHISM; MORAL MASOCHISM; PRIMARY MASOCHISM; SADOMASOCHISTIC RELATIONSHIP; SEXUAL MASOCHISM; SOCIAL MASOCHISM; VERBAL MASOCHISM; ABASEMENT; ALGOLAGNIA; ALGOPHILY; ASCETICISM; BONDAGE AND DISCIPLINE; COUNTERTRANSFERENCE NEUROSIS; DEMONIC CHARACTER; HUMILIATION; ILLNESS AS SELF-PUNISHMENT; NEGATIVE AMBITION; NEGATIVE THERAPEUTIC REACTION; PATHOCURE; PERVERSION; PITY; PRIMAL SADISM; PSEUDOAGGRESSION; PSYCHOSEXUAL DEVELOPMENT; RECOVERY WISH; RECURRENT DREAMS; REVERSAL; RISK-TAKING; SELF-INJURIOUS BEHAVIOR; SELF-PUNISHMENT; SKIN-EROTICISM; STIGMATA; SUCCESS NEUROSIS; SUFFERING; SUPEREGO RESISTANCE; SWINGING; SYMBIOTIC RELATEDNESS; WHIPPING.

Sachs, Bernard Parney American neurologist, 1858–1944. See TAY-SACHS DISEASE; AMAUROTIC IDIOCY; AUTOSOMAL ABERRATIONS; BATTEN'S DISEASE; BIRTH DEFECT; CEREBROMACULAR DEGENERATION; CNS ABNORMALITY; DOLLINGER-BIELSCHOWSKY SYNDROME; GANGLIOSIDOSIS; HEXOSAMINIDASE A; INBORN ERROR OF METABOLISM; SPHINGOLIPID; SPHINGOLIPIDOSES.

sacral division the parasympathetic portion of the autonomic nervous system located in the sacral area of the spine.

sacral nerves: See SPINAL NERVES.

sacred disease an early term for epilepsy used by the Greeks, based on the belief that seizures were evidence of divine visitation. Hippocrates, however, rejected this view, saying "Surely it, too, has its nature and causes whence it originates, just like other diseases, and is curable by means comparable to their cure."

sacrifice in psychoanalysis, the tendency of the patient to deprive himself of things he really needs, as an unconscious attempt to bribe the superego or to make restitution for guilty thoughts or actions. Freud interpreted s. of human beings in primitive societies in oedipal terms, claiming that it was a form of symbolic parricide. See UNDOING.

saddle-back: See LORDOSIS.

Sade, Donatien Alphonse François, Comte de /säd/ French soldier, writer, and libertine, 1740–1814. The term sadism /sad′izəm, säd′izəm/ is derived from the name, writings, and personal practices of the "Marquis de Sade." See SADISM; ANAL SADISM; ANAL-SADISTIC STAGE; ID SADISM; INFANTILE SADISM; LARVAL SADISM; ORAL SADISM; ORAL-SADISTIC CATHEXIS; PHALLIC SADISM; PRIMAL SADISM; SADOMASOCHISTIC RELATIONSHIP; SEXUAL SADISM; SUPEREGO SADISM; ALGOLAGNIA; BITING ATTACK; BONDAGE AND DISCIPLINE; BRAID-CUTTING; COMPONENT INSTINCT; DEATH INSTINCT; HUMILIATION; LUST MURDER; MASOCHISTIC CHARACTER; ORAL-BITING PERIOD; PERVERSION; PSYCHOSEXUAL DEVELOPMENT; REVERSAL; SUFFERING; SWINGING; SYMBIOTIC RELATEDNESS; SZONDI TEST; VAMPIRISM; WHIPPING; ZOOSADISM.

sadism a sexual deviation in which gratification is obtained by inflicting pain or humiliation on a sexual partner. The term also is used to denote cruelty in general. The practice may be extended beyond the sexual partner to include animals.

Although technically a deviation, s. is an accepted part of foreplay in many cultures. See SADE.

sadomasochistic relationship a complementary interaction, usually sexual in nature, based on the enjoyment of suffering by one individual and the enjoyment of inflicting pain by the other. A common abbreviation for **sadomasochism** is **S-M.**

safety and health education the instruction of pupils in health-related matters, including the causes and prevention of malnutrition, alcoholism, drug addiction, and venereal disease, as well as safety on the roads, in shopwork, at home, and on the playing field. Also see ACCIDENT PREVENTION.

safety device a Horney term for any means used in protecting oneself from threats, particularly the hostile elements of the environment.

safety motive a Horney term for indirect neurotic behavior in which an individual tries to protect himself from threats in the external world, as in protecting himself from failure by avoiding competition.

safety needs the second level in A. Maslow's hierarchy of needs (after physiological needs) consisting of needs for freedom from illness or danger and the need for a secure, familiar, predictable environment. See NEED-HIERARCHY THEORY.

safety psychology the study of the human and environmental factors involved in accidents and accident prevention. Environmental measures include such factors as safe highway construction, safe working conditions, reduction of overcrowding, redesign of signs, noise abatement, use of seat belts, and improved design of kitchens and bathrooms. The human approach includes an investigation of safe and unsafe attitudes, stress conditions, safety habits, relevant personality and physiological factors, parental guidance, and the techniques of safety education. See ACCIDENT PREVENTION; ACCIDENT PRONENESS; ACCIDENT REDUCTION.

sagittal a plane or theoretical slice of a body that would divide the left and right sides from top to bottom. The term may be modified by a directional adjective, as in **medial s.,** for a vertical slice at the center of the organ or organism.

saggital axis in vision, a straight line extending from the center of the retina through the center of the lens and pupil to the center of the object viewed.

sagittal fissure the longitudinal fissure that divides the cerebrum into left and right hemispheres.

SAI the *social-a*dequacy *i*ndex representing the degree of handicap related to hearing and understanding of speech based upon the results of speech audiometry and articulation tests.

Saint Anthony's dance: See CHOREA.

Saint Anthony's fire a name given in the Middle Ages to the symptoms of ergot poisoning which causes agonizing burning sensations of the limbs as they become blackened with gangrene. Other effects include headaches, vertigo, convulsions, hallucinations, and in some cases suicidal acts. Relief reportedly was obtained by a trip to the shrine of Saint Anthony (founded by the Congregation of the Antonines in 1095) because the monks fed victims meals that were free of grain contaminated by ergot fungus, the cause of ERGOTISM. See this entry.

Saint Dymphna's disease an early term for mental disease based on the name of the patron saint of the insane, a medieval Irish princess who, according to legend, fled to Belgium to escape the incestuous advances of her mad father, who later put her to death near a shrine at Gheel. See GHEEL COLONY.

Saint John's dance: See CHOREA.

Saint Mathurin's disease a term sometimes used to identify epileptic psychosis and also severe mental retardation. The term is derived from the name of Saint Mathurin, the patron saint of idiots and fools.

Saint Vitus' dance; Saint With's dance: See CHOREA.

Sakel, Manfred Polish-born Austrian-American psychiatrist, 1900–57. See INSULIN-COMA THERAPY.

salaam convulsions = WEST'S SYNDROME.

sales-aptitude tests tests developed as an aid in sales-personnel selection, by measuring understanding of sales principles or by appraising interests and drives related to salesmanship.

sales-survey technique a method of testing the effectiveness of advertising appeals by analyzing sales of a product after it has been advertised in one or several communities and comparing the results with sales of the same product in areas where it was not advertised. The method requires consideration of various extraneous factors, such as weather conditions, that may have affected shopper behavior during the period studied.

salicylates /-lis'-/ a group of chemical compounds that includes salicylic acid, its sodium salt, and other derivatives produced by molecular manipulation. S. have been used since ancient times as a nonnarcotic analgesic and antipyretic. They apparently act on the central nervous system at the thalamic level but also mimic in some respects the adrenal hormones, particularly when used in the treatment of rheumatic fever. S. have been used primarily in aspirin compounds, combined with a form of acetic acid, since the drug was introduced in 1899 to replace a sodium-salicylate medication. S. originally were obtained from the bark of the willow tree, Salix alba, which gave its name to the drug. Because of a belief in the **Doctrine of Signatures,** which claimed that a cure for a disease could be found with its cause, the willow tree (which grows in moist places) seemed to the ancients to be a logical source for a cure for fevers and rheumatism, disorders thought to be caused by dampness. Kinds of s. include **acetylsalicylic acid (aspirin)**—$C_9H_8O_4$, **salicylamide**—$C_7H_7NO_2$, and **salicylic acid**—$C_7H_6O_3$. Also see ASPIRIN EFFECTS; ASPIRIN POISONING.

salicylism = ASPIRIN POISONING.

salivary glands glands located throughout the mouth that secrete a fluid containing a digestive enzyme, ptyalin. The major s.g. are the parotid, submaxillary, and sublingual glands. Smaller s.g. are scattered over the cheeks and tongue. The s.g. are controlled by the nervous system, responding by reflex action to stimuli associated with food.

salivary-gland virus one of several cytomegaloviruses associated with cytomegalic-inclusion disease, a major cause of birth defects of the central nervous system. Malformed infants often exhibit signs of the viral inclusions. Mental retardation, deafness, blindness, and hydrocephaly are among the effects of the infection acquired from the mother, who may be asymptomatic. Also see CYTOMEGALIC DISEASE.

salivation the secretion of saliva by the salivary glands. The salivary glands of a human produce about three pints of saliva daily. See SALIVARY GLANDS.

Salpêtrière an institution for women founded in Paris in 1656, and transformed by Philippe Pinel from an asylum for the infirm, aged, and insane into a hospital when he was appointed director in 1795. At one time it contained nearly 10,000 people, and treatment was proverbially brutal. In the 1860s, the hospital became the center for Charcot's school of psychopathology based on the use of hypnosis.

-salping-; -salpingo- a combining form relating to (a) the Fallopian tube, (b) the auditory tube (meatus).

salpingectomy the surgical removal of a Fallopian tube. The excision may be performed as a sterilization measure or because of an infection or malignant growth in the female reproductive tract. Psychosexual conflicts often are associated with the procedure.

salpingitis the inflammation of a tubular structure of the body, e.g., the Fallopian tube or Eustachian tube.

-salt- a combining form referring to jumping or a leap (from Latin *saltare*, "to dance, jump"). Adjective: **saltatory**.

saltatory conduction a type of nerve-impulse transmission that occurs in myelinated fibers. A s.c. theory contends that impulses along a myelinated fiber get a boost at the nodes of Ranvier along the fiber after losing momentum between the nodes.

saltatory spasm a type of muscle spasm of the lower extremities, manifested by jumping or skipping movements. The condition is usually of hysterical origin.

salt balance the system in which the body's homeostatic mechanisms maintain a favorable relationship between the amounts of fluid and sodium ions in the body tissues. Sodium is an essential mineral, but excess amounts normally are excreted through the kidneys as an alterna-

tive to accumulating water in the tissues in order to hold the excess salt, or sodium, in solution.

saltpeter = POTASSIUM NITRATE.

salt taste a gustatory sensation stimulated in the taste buds at the edge of the tongue by ions of certain chemical compounds. Although the sensation is associated subjectively with table salt, or sodium chloride, the same or similar sensations can be produced by a number of other chemical salts including nitrates and sulfates as well as chlorides, iodides, and bromides.

sample in statistics, a portion of a population of elements or subjects. A s. is drawn in order to generalize about or to describe the population as a whole. See also POPULATION; RANDOM S.

sample bias any factor or method of sampling that makes the sample nonrepresentative and is therefore likely to distort results.

sample standard deviation: See STANDARD DEVIATION.

sampling in surveys and experimental studies, the process of selecting a limited number of respondents or subjects who are presumed to be representative of the population as a whole.

sampling distribution a set of estimates of a parameter, obtained by repeatedly taking samples from a population.

sampling error an error in the selection process that renders a sample nonrepresentative; or the error in an interpretation based on a nonrepresentative sample. The term is also used to mean the predictable margin of error that occurs in studies of sampling populations.

sampling population in experimental studies or surveys, the population from which a sample is selected. The sample consists only of those cases actually studied whereas the population is the entire group of cases within a specified area from which the sample is taken. If the sample is truly representative, the experimental findings should apply to the population as a whole.

sampling stability a state in which repeated samplings from the same population yield consistent results and are therefore reliable.

sampling theory the principles of drawing survey samples that accurately represent the population.

sanatorium an institution for the treatment and convalescence of individuals with chronic diseases such as rheumatism, tuberculosis, neurological disorders, or mental disorders. Also called **sanitarium**.

sand fear = AMATHOPHOBIA.

sane society: See FROMM.

Sanfilippo, Sylvester I. American pediatrician, fl. 1963. See SANFILIPPO'S SYNDROME; MUCOPOLYSACCHARIDOSES.

Sanfilippo's syndrome a form of severe mental retardation associated with bone and joint defects and a tendency toward dwarfism. The patient also may show signs of corneal opacities. The disease is transmitted as an autosomal-recessive trait that causes a systemic form of mucopolysaccharidosis. After normal early mental development, the child shows mental regression. The ability to speak deteriorates and eventually is lost. Motor control also degenerates until the patient reaches his teens as a demented bedridden individual. Also called **MPS III; polydystrophic oligophrenia; heparitinuria**.

-sangui-; -sanguino- a combining form relating to blood (Latin *sanguis*).

sanguine type one of the four constitutional and temperamental types established by Galen, who believed that the humor and enthusiasm displayed by such individuals was due to the predominance of the blood over other body fluids.

sanitarium = SANATORIUM.

Sanson, Louis Joseph /säNsôN'/ French surgeon, 1790–1841. See PURKINJE-SANSON IMAGES.

Sapir-Whorf hypothesis = WHORF'S HYPOTHESIS.

Sapphism = LESBIANISM.

-sapr-; -sapro- a combining form relating to decay, putrefaction.

Sarason, Seymour Bernard American psychologist, 1919—. See ANXIETY SCALES (there: **Sarason Test Anxiety Scale**).

-sarc-; -sarco- a combining form relating to flesh or muscle tissue (from Greek *sarkos*, "flesh").

sarcasm a caustic, derisive remark. S. is a form of verbal aggression.

sarcoma a tumor that develops from cells that are derived from the mesodermal layer of early embryonic tissue, e.g., bones, muscles, blood, cardiovascular and lymphatic tissues, connective tissue, and parts of the urogenital system. A s. usually is highly malignant. The term often is combined with the name of the tissue involved, such as lymphosarcoma, osteosarcoma, or leukocytic s. See CANCER.

Sartre, Jean-Paul /särt'(r)/ French philosopher and writer, 1905–80. See EXISTENTIALISM.

SAT = SCHOLASTIC APTITUDE TEST.

satanophobia a morbid fear of the devil. Also see DAEMONOPHOBIA.

satellite clinic a psychiatric facility operated on an outreach basis by a psychiatric or general hospital. Satellite clinics are located in the inner city, in suburbs, and in rural areas, and usually provide crisis services, out-patient treatment, precare, and aftercare.

satellite housing apartments or single-family homes where patients can live without direct supervisory care but with access to emergency treatment.

satellitosis an accumulation of neuroglia cells that forms around a damaged neuron.

satiation a condition of being satisfied or gratified regarding a need for food, fluid, sexual stimulation, or a psychic goal such as disposable income.

satiety center = VENTROMEDIAL NUCLEUS.

satisfaction of instincts in psychoanalysis, the gratification of basic needs (hunger, thirst, sex, aggression), which discharges tension, eliminates unpleasure, and restores the organism to a balanced state. Satisfaction may occur on a conscious, preconscious, or unconscious level. Also called **gratification of instincts**.

satisfier Thorndike's term for a reward or circumstance that leads to satisfaction.

satori: See ZEN BUDDHISM.

saturated test in factor analysis, a test that is shown to have a high degree of correlation with a given factor.

saturation in color theory, the degree of color purity; hue intensity; the degree to which a hue is weakened by gray. Highly saturated colors have little if any gray and appear to be pure hue, but colors of low saturation are more akin to gray; e.g., a highly saturated blue is vividly blue while a low saturated blue will have much gray. The term may also be used to denote the extent to which a test is correlated with a factor.

saturnine pseudogeneral paralysis a form of chronic encephalopathy caused by lead poisoning. Also called **saturnism**.

satyriasis /-rī'ə-/ a male psychosexual disorder consisting of an excessive or insatiable desire for sexual gratification. This gratification is usually incomplete, and the obsessional drive is therefore believed to mask impotence. S. is not due to being "oversexed" in the physiological sense but arises from unconscious emotional needs, such as (a) the need for reassurance of potency, (b) a compensation for failures, frustrations, or a poor self-image, (c) a means of warding off anxiety stemming from emotional conflicts, or (d) an attempt to deny homosexual tendencies. Also called **Don Juan syndrome**. See DON JUAN; EROTOMANIA.

sauce Béarnaise effect /bernäz'/ a popular term for a type of learning response that is an exception to the usual laws of conditioning. It is characterized by an association to a highly specific stimulus, with learning after a single trial, and a delayed negative reinforcement. The s.B.e. represents an analogy to becoming ill some hours after a meal that included sauce Béarnaise. Regardless of the cause of the illness, the sauce will be identified with it.

Saussure, Ferdinand de /sôsēr'/ Swiss linguist, 1857–1913. S. was perhaps the most influential pioneer in modern linguistics. See ORIGIN-OF-LANGUAGE THEORIES.

savage: See PRIMITIVE.

savings method = RELEARNING METHOD.

saw-tooth waves bursts of sharp EEG waves occurring during REM sleep.

S-B = STANFORD-BINET INTELLIGENCE SCALE.

scabiophobia a morbid fear of scabies.

scalability the characteristic of an item that allows it to fit into a progression.

scala media one of the three **scalae**, or canals, in the bony cavity of the cochlea, or inner ear. It is the middle scala, or canal, located between the scala vestibuli and the scala tympani. The s.m. contains the organ of Corti, regarded as the true organ of hearing.

scalar analysis the process of determining where an item fits or is located on a scale, e.g., to determine the strength of a motive.

scala tympani one of the three **scalae**, or canals, in the cochlea, or inner ear. It is located immediately below the scala media and contains a fluid, perilymph. The s.t. also contains the round window of the cochlea, which relieves fluid pressure on cochlear structures resulting from vibrations by the middle-ear bones on the oval window of the cochlea.

scala vestibuli one of the three **scalae**, or canals, in the cochlea, or inner ear. It is separated from the scala media by Reissner's membrane. The s.v. opens at the basal end of the cochlea into the vestibule of the labyrinth, where the oval window receives sound vibrations transmitted by the stapes, one of the middle-ear bones. The air vibrations are converted here to fluid vibrations.

scale a system of arranging items in a progressive series according to their magnitude or value (from Latin *scala*, "ladder, staircase").

scaled test a test in which the items are arranged in order of increasing difficulty; also, a test in which the items are assigned a value, or score, according to a principle.

scale value the number that indicates or represents the value of a reference point on a scale.

scaling the process of designing or constructing a scale to show the distribution of scores or other items, e.g., psychological test results.

scalloping a response pattern characteristically associated with fixed-interval reinforcement schedules in which appropriate or meaningful responses diminish sharply or stop altogether after reinforcement but dramatically increase directly before the next reinforcement is scheduled to occur. S. gets its name from the wavy, "scalloped" appearance of the fixed-interval curve. Also called **scallop pattern**.

scalogram = CUMULATIVE SCALE.

scanning rapidly examining a situation, such as a football configuration, before making a response; also, skimming written material to identify the main ideas or to search for specific information. In medicine, the term refers, e.g., to a brain-scan or CAT-scan procedure in diagnosing a patient.

scanning speech drawling, slurred, monotonous or singsong speech, such as occurs in some cases of multiple sclerosis.

scapegoating the process whereby anger and aggression are displaced onto other, usually less powerful, groups or persons not responsible for the aggressor's frustration. The true source of frustration lies in someone or some entity that cannot be directly confronted, or in the psychological deficiencies of the attacker. In the latter case, the defense mechanism of projection is at work. Also called **scapegoat mechanism**. See DISPLACEMENT; PROJECTION.

scarlet fever an acute contagious disease caused by a strain of streptococcus bacteria and affecting mainly children. S.f. usually follows a strepto-coccal infection of the skin or nasopharynx area, and may be transmitted by direct or indirect contact with an infected person, e.g., by handling contaminated toys, clothing, or dishes. Complications may include otitis media and mastoiditis.

Scarpa, Antonio Italian anatomist and ophthalmologist, 1747–1832. See SCARPA'S GANGLION.

Scarpa's ganglion the vestibular ganglion which is the source of the fibers of the vestibular nerve that supplies the utricle, the saccule, and the ampullae of the semicircular ducts. The axons of S.g. form a part of the eighth cranial nerve.

SCAT = SCHOOL AND COLLEGE ABILITY TEST.

-scat-; -scato- a combining form relating to feces or filth (from Greek *scatos*, "dung, feces").

scatologia preoccupation with obscenities, lewdness, and filth, mainly of an excremental nature. The term, derived from the Greek word for dung, is usually associated with anal eroticism. Also called **scatology**. Adjective: **scatological**. Also see TELEPHONE S.; COPROPHEMIA.

scatophagy /-tof'-/ the eating of excrement.

scatophobia = COPROPHOBIA.

scatter the tendency for an individual's test profile to show a pattern of high and low points rather than a single overall level. Compare ELEVATION.

scatter analysis the study and evaluation of the relationships among subtest scores.

scatter child a popular term for MINIMAL BRAIN DAMAGE. See this entry.

scatter diagram: See SCATTERPLOT.

scattering a type of thinking observed in schizophrenic patients who make tangential or irrelevant associations that may be expressed in speech that is incomprehensible.

scatterplot a chart tallying the relationship between two variables, with both variables determining the placement of each tally mark. Also called **scatter diagram**.

scavenging behavior in animal psychology, feeding on dead organic matter, such as carrion or scraps left by other animals. It is a type of behavior found in many species such as vultures, hyenas, jackals, and chimpanzees.

Schaeffer, Max German neurologist, 1852–1923. See SCHAEFFER REFLEX.

Schaeffer reflex the dorsal flexion of the great toe induced by pinching the Achilles tendon. The effect is observed in cases of pyramidal tract lesions when the lower motor centers are released from normal inhibition controls.

schedule an operational plan for a series of tests, experiments, or other activities, usually designed to include a time frame for various stages; also, a questionnaire.

schedule of reinforcement in operant conditioning, a program of periodic reinforcement in which a response is rewarded or punished according to a schedule based either on the number of responses or the passage of a certain amount of time. See CONTINUOUS REINFORCEMENT; FIXED-RATIO REINFORCEMENT SCHEDULE;

FIXED-INTERVAL REINFORCEMENT SCHEDULE; INTERMITTENT REINFORCEMENT; REINFORCEMENT; VARIABLE-INTERVAL REINFORCEMENT SCHEDULE; VARIABLE-RATIO REINFORCEMENT SCHEDULE.

Scheerer, Martin German-born American psychologist, 1900–61. See GOLDSTEIN-SCHEERER TESTS; WEIGL-GOLDSTEIN-SCHEERER TEST; CONCEPT-FORMATION TESTS.

Scheffé, Henry American mathematician, 1907—. See SCHEFFÉ TEST.

Scheffé test a statistical test comparing the differences between means in the analysis of variance; an after-F test. This test is more appropriate for post-mortem comparisons of means in the analysis of variance than a number of t tests. Also called **test for contrasts**.

Scheie, Harold Glendon American ophthalmologist, 1909—. See SCHEIE'S SYNDROME; MUCOPOLYSACCHARIDOSES.

Scheie's syndrome a form of mucopolysaccharidosis inherited as an autosomal-recessive disorder and characterized by cloudy corneas, skeletal abnormalities, and excessive chondroitin sulfate in the urine. Mental retardation is not a significant factor in this syndrome. Also called **MPS V**.

schema according to Piaget, a forerunner and "functional equivalent" of a concept in the first phase of intellectual development, which occurs before age two. The early schemas are sensorimotor in nature (seeing, handling, sucking, etc.), and the child fits more and more new things into them through the processes of assimilation and accommodation. Plurals: **schemas; schemata**.

schematic image a mental picture or representation of a given object composed of that object's most conspicuous features. Once formed, the s.i. is the model against which similar perceptual configurations are judged. According to J. Kagan, the ability to construct schematic images is fundamental once the infant is able to perceive complete forms.

schemes Piaget's term for the cognitive structures that develop as infants and young children learn to adapt their behavior to environmental conditions. S. are "specific ways of knowing the world" that generalize to other situations and link means to ends. ". . . the scheme is not bound up in any specific motor action. Rather, it is . . . that set of features which holds constant across different instances of a specific physical action." (H. Gardner, *Developmental Psychology*, 1978)

Schilder, Paul /shil′dər/ Austrian-born American psychiatrist, 1886–1940. A man of wide-ranging professional interests, S. made significant contributions to neurology and psychiatry in Vienna, including a classic description of encephalitis periaxialis diffusa, and studies of the dynamics of schizophrenia. Later, at Bellevue Hospital in New York, he focused his efforts on the concept of body image, the dreams of epileptics, the psychology of mania, applications of psycho-

analytic concepts to organic psychoses, and the development of group therapy. See ADRENO-LEUKODYSTROPHY (also called **Schilder's disease**); BALO'S DISEASE; BODY-IMAGE DISTURBANCE; SIGN SYSTEM.

Schiotz, Hjalmar /shē′ets/ Norwegian physician, 1850–1927. See TONOMETRY (there: **Schiotz indentation tonometer**).

-schisis; -schisto-; -schiz-; -schizo- a combining form relating to a split or fissure (from Greek *schizein*, "to split").

schistosomiasis an infectious disease caused by parasitic flatworms, or flukes, that live in the blood vessels of humans and other animals. The fluke usually enters the body through the digestive tract in the form of ova and travels through the veins to the liver. A complication is **hepatic encephalopathy**, which may produce symptoms ranging from disturbances of consciousness and psychiatric changes to deep coma or tremors. Also called **bilharziasis**.

-schiz-; -schizo-: See -SCHISIS.

schizencephalic pertaining to structural abnormalities of the brain that are manifested as divisions or clefts in the brain tissues. The structural deformities may appear as cavities that result from maldevelopment during fetal life or early infancy or from destructive lesions of the brain area.

schizoaffective disorder a controversial category sometimes used when a differential diagnosis between AFFECTIVE DISORDERS and either SCHIZOPHRENIFORM DISORDER or SCHIZOPHRENIC DISORDERS cannot be made. See these entries. (DSM-III)

schizoaffective psychosis a form of schizophrenia in which the initial symptoms are those of mania or depression, sometimes leading to a misdiagnosis of the true nature of the disorder. As the disease progresses, the schizophrenic factors become dominant. See SCHIZOAFFECTIVE DISORDER.

schizocaria an obsolete term for an acute, malignant form of schizophrenia in which the patient's personality rapidly deteriorates. Also called **catastrophic schizophrenia**.

schizoid character: See SCHIZOID-PERSONALITY DISORDER.

schizoid disorder of childhood or adolescence a disorder where major criteria are absence of close friends other than relatives or isolated children, no apparent interest in making friends, no pleasure from peer interactions, general avoidance of social contacts, lack of interest in team sports and other activities that involve other children, and a duration of at least three months. (DSM-III)

schizoidism a complex of behavioral factors that includes seclusiveness, quietness, and other introversion traits indicating a separation by the person from his surroundings, the confining of psychic interests to himself, and in many cases a tendency toward schizophrenia. Also called **schizoidia**.

schizoid-manic state a psychotic state cited by

Adolf Meyer, A. A. Brill, and Bleuler, combining features of both manic and schizophrenic excitement. Also called **schizomania**.

schizoid-personality disorder a personality disorder characterized by long-term emotional coldness, absence of tender feelings for others, indifference to praise or criticism and to the feelings of others, close friendships with no more than one or two persons, and absence of eccentricities of speech, behavior, or thought such as are characteristic of schizotypal disorder. (DSM-III)

schizokinesis a drug effect involving dissociation of visceral and motor functions.

schizomania = SCHIZOID-MANIC STATE.

schizophasia jumbled speech, observed in advanced schizophrenia. See WORD SALAD.

schizophrenia: See SCHIZOPHRENIC DISORDERS. Also see ACUTE SCHIZOPHRENIC EPISODE; AMBULATORY S.; BORDERLINE S.; BURNED-OUT; CHILDHOOD S.; CHRONIC S.; CHRONIC UNDIFFERENTIATED S.; HEBEPHRENIA; LARVAL S.; MIXED S.; PARANOID-SCHIZOID POSITION; PFROPFSCHIZOPHRENIA; POST-EMOTIVE S.; PROCESS S.; PSEUDONEUROTIC S.; PSEUDOPSYCHOPATHIC S.; REACTIVE S.; RECIDIVES IN S.; REGRESSIVE S.; RESTITUTIONAL S.; RETARDED S.; SCHIZOCARIA; SIMPLE S.; SYMPTOMATIC S.; THREE-DAY S.; UNDIFFERENTIATED S.

schizophrenic disorder, catatonic type a type of schizophrenia characterized by a marked psychomotor disturbance consisting of (a) catatonic stupor (the patient does not react or move spontaneously, and may be mute), (b) catatonic negativism (resists instructions or attempts to be moved), (c) catatonic rigidity (has rigid posture in spite of attempts to be moved), (d) catatonic excitement (is excited, shows apparently purposeless motor activity), or (e) catatonic posturing (assumes inappropriate or bizarre postures, often with waxy flexibility). Also called **catatonic schizophrenia**. (DSM-III)

schizophrenic disorder, disorganized type a type of schizophrenia characterized by (a) frequent, marked incoherence, (b) absence of systematized delusions, though fragmentary delusions and hallucinations may be present, and (c) blunted, inappropriate or silly affect frequently associated with grimaces, mannerisms, and extreme social withdrawal. Also called **disorganized schizophrenia**. Also see HEBEPHRENIA. (DSM-III)

schizophrenic disorder, paranoid type a type of schizophrenia usually with onset later in life than other types, with one or more of the following manifestations: delusions of persecution or grandeur, delusional jealousy, and persecutory or grandiose hallucinations, but without gross disorganization of behavior. Also called **paranoid schizophrenia**. (DSM-III)

schizophrenic disorder, residual type a disorder in which the individual has experienced at least one episode of schizophrenia with prominent psychotic symptoms (especially delusions and hallucinations) which are no longer present,

although signs of illness persist in the form of blunted or inappropriate affect, social withdrawal, eccentric behavior, illogical thinking, or loose associations. Also called **residual schizophrenia**. (DSM-III)

schizophrenic disorder, undifferentiated type a disorder that does not meet the criteria for other types of schizophrenia, or meets the criteria for more than one type. There are, however, prominent psychotic features, such as delusions, hallucinations, incoherence, or grossly disorganized behavior. See UNDIFFERENTIATED SCHIZOPHRENIA. (DSM-III)

schizophrenic disorders a group of mental disturbances essentially characterized by (a) one or more psychotic features during the active phase, including bizarre or absurd delusions (such as being controlled or thought-broadcasting), (b) somatic, grandiose, religious, or nihilistic delusions, (c) delusions of persecution or jealousy with hallucinations, (d) incoherence with marked loosening of associations, illogical thought, or poverty of speech together with either blunted, flat, or inappropriate affect, (f) delusions or hallucinations, or (g) grossly disorganized behavior, such as catatonia. Other common characteristics are deterioration from a previous level of job, social, or self-care functioning, and onset before age 45, with a duration of at least six months. A common term for schizophrenic disorder is **schizophrenia**. See SCHIZOPHRENIC DISORDER, CATATONIC TYPE; SCHIZOPHRENIC DISORDER, DISORGANIZED TYPE; SCHIZOPHRENIC DISORDER, PARANOID TYPE; SCHIZOPHRENIC DISORDER, RESIDUAL TYPE; SCHIZOPHRENIC DISORDER, UNDIFFERENTIATED TYPE. Also see BLEULER. (DSM-III)

schizophrenic excitement a state of acute hyperactivity, impulsivity, and in some cases elation, occurring most frequently in the catatonic form of schizophrenia. See SCHIZOPHRENIC DISORDER, CATATONIC TYPE.

schizophrenic personality: See SCHIZOID-PERSONALITY DISORDER; SCHIZOTYPAL-PERSONALITY DISORDER.

schizophrenic spectrum a term applied by S. S. Kety and associates to a hypothetical range of schizophrenic states that appear to have a genetic etiology that is similar to classic schizophrenia. There are wide differences in intensity in these states, due, it is believed, to environmental or genetic modification of the common genetic diathesis.

schizophrenic states: See ACUTE DELUSIONAL PSYCHOSIS.

schizophrenic surrender a term first applied by C. M. Campbell (1941) to regressive symptoms characteristic of the breakdown of the ego in schizophrenic patients who are no longer able to make efforts at restoration or "restitution." These patients withdraw further and further from reality and may experience feelings of depersonalization, fantasies of world destruction, and delusions of grandeur. The regressive pattern reaches its most extreme form in hebephrenia. Also see RESTITUTIONAL SCHIZOPHRENIA; SCHIZOPHRENIC DISORDER, DISORGANIZED TYPE.

schizophreniform disorder a disorder that meets all the criteria for schizophrenia except for shorter duration (two weeks to six months), and a greater likelihood for emotional turmoil, acute onset and resolution, and recovery to a preillness level of functioning. See SCHIZOPHRENIC DISORDERS. (DSM-III)

schizophrenogenic denoting a factor or influence that is the cause of or contributes to the onset of schizophrenia. The term sometimes is applied to a family member, particularly the mother, whose attitude toward the patient is believed to have been a causative factor. See S. MOTHER.

schizophrenogenic mother a term applied to a mother who is believed to contribute to the development of schizophrenia, particularly in one or more male children. Studies indicate that she herself is emotionally disturbed and tends to be cold, rejecting, dominating, perfectionistic, and insensitive. At the same time, however, she is overprotective, fosters dependence, and is both seductive and rigidly moralistic. As a result, her male children tend to be immature, helpless, anxious, and sexually conflicted.

schizotaxia a genetic predisposition to schizophrenia which may become overt if environmental stresses are severe.

schizothymia: See SCHIZOTHYMIC PERSONALITY.

schizothymic personality a personality pattern characterized by schizoid behavior such as introversion and seclusiveness, but within the limits of normality.

schizotypal-personality disorder a personality disorder characterized by various oddities of thought, perception, speech, and behavior that are not severe enough to warrant a diagnosis of schizophrenia. The symptom picture comprises at least four of the following: magical thinking; ideas of reference; social isolation; recurrent illusions (e.g., feeling that a dead relative is present) or depersonalization (things are not real); vague or metaphorical speech without incoherence; inadequate rapport with others due to aloofness or lack of feeling; suspicious or paranoid thoughts; and undue sensitivity to real or imagined criticism. (DSM-III)

Schnauzkrampf /shnouts'krämpf/ a term introduced by Kahlbaum to describe the snoutlike protrusion of lips observed in some catatonic patients (German, "snout cramp").

Schneider, Kurt /shnī'dər/ German psychiatrist, 1887–1967. See FIRST-RANK SYMPTOMS.

scholastic acceleration = EDUCATIONAL ACCELERATION.

scholastic achievement test any test that measures the subject's knowledge and ability in a specific area of academic study, such as chemistry, history, mathematics, Spanish, or literature.

Scholastic Aptitude Test a set of verbal and mathematical questions with heavy emphasis on abstract intelligence, used in selecting candidates for college admission. Abbrev.: **SAT**.

School and College Ability Test an academic aptitude test extending, in three levels, from the end of grade 3 through grade 12. All levels yield a verbal score based on a verbal analogies test; a quantitative score based on comparison involving fundamental number operations; and a total score. Abbrev.: **SCAT**.

school phobia a neurotic reaction in primary-school children characterized by persistent resistance to attending school, accompanied by acute anxiety that may reach panic proportions. The disorder is considered a form of separation anxiety, which is usually caused or aggravated by the mother's overprotectiveness and fear of "losing her baby." See SEPARATION-ANXIETY DISORDER.

school psychology a field of psychology concerned with psychoeducational problems arising in primary and secondary schools. Among the responsibilities of the school psychologist are pupil-behavior problems, involvement in curriculum-planning, administration of psychological tests, interviews with parents concerning their child's progress and problems, counseling of teachers and students, and in some cases research on educational questions and issues.

Schreber case a landmark case of Freud's based on his analysis of *Memoirs of a Neurotic* by Daniel Paul Schreber, 1903. His notes on this case, published in 1911, contained an interpretation of paranoid processes and ideas and their relation to repressed homosexuality, at least in the male.

Schüller, Artur /shil'ər/ Austrian neurologist, 1874—. See HAND-CHRISTIAN-SCHÜLLER SYNDROME; XANTHOMATOSIS.

Schultz, J. H. German neurologist, fl. 1970. See AUTOGENIC TRAINING.

Schumann, Friedrich German psychologist, fl. 1887, 1932. See MÜLLER-SCHUMANN LAW.

Schwann, Theodor /shvän/ German anatomist, 1810–82. See SCHWANN CELLS; SCHWANNOMA; METACHROMATIC LEUKODYSTROPHY; NEURILEMMA.

Schwann cells neurilemma, or satellite cells, which form a sheath over most of the length of an axon of a peripheral nerve. The S.c. are named for the German 19th-century anatomist Theodor Schwann, who also was founder of the cell theory of animal structure.

schwannoma a tumor that develops from the Schwann cells that form a sheath over the axons of peripheral nerves. Also called **neurilemmoma**.

scelerophobia a morbid fear of bad people such as thiefs, swindlers, or kidnapers. Also called **pavor sceleris**.

sciascope = SKIASCOPE.

scieropia a visual anomaly in which objects appear to be in a shadow. The visual defect may be due to an emotional or psychological disorder, in which case the condition is identified as **scierneuropsia**.

scientific attitude an attitude characterized by an objective and impartial approach and the use of empirical methods in the search for knowledge.

scientific illiteracy: See COMPUTER ILLITERACY.

scientific management an application of scientific methods to achieve improved worker efficiency and work conditions.

scientific method the use of carefully planned naturalistic observation and experimentation in obtaining and verifying data and in discovering laws and principles that govern phenomena.

SCII = STRONG-CAMPBELL INTEREST INVENTORY.

scintillating scotoma: See SCOTOMA.

scintillator: See COMPUTERIZED AXIAL TOMOGRAPHY.

sciosophy /sī·os′-/ any system of thought that is not supported by scientific methods, e.g., astrology or theology (from Greek *skia*, "shade, shadow").

scissors gait a type of gait observed in some cerebral-palsy patients who must cross their legs in scissors fashion in taking steps.

-scler-; -sclero- a combining form meaning hard, hardening, thickening.

sclera the tough, white outer coat of the eyeball which is continuous with the cornea at the front and the optic-nerve sheath at the back of the eyeball. Also called **sclerotic coat.**

sclerosing encephalitis = SUBACUTE SCLEROSING PANENCEPHALITIS.

sclerosis: See DIFFUSE S.

sclerotic coat = SCLERA.

scoliosis an abnormal curvature of the spinal column. A simple lateral deviation form of s. usually is postural and can be corrected by extreme spinal flexion. An S-shaped or other more complex curve is a sign of **compensatory s.,** which may be due to torticollis, a shortened leg, or a hip disorder. **Structural s.** is associated with congenital defects or paralysis of muscles of the trunk of the body. S. sometimes is complicated by kyphosis.

-scop-; -scopo-; -scopy a combining form relating to observation, watching, or inspection (from Greek *skopein*, "to look at").

-scope a combining form relating to an instrument for observing.

scopic method a technique of measuring scores or data by direct observation rather than by graphic representation in which instruments are used.

scopolamine $C_{17}H_{21}NO_4$—an anticholinergic drug derived as an alkaloid from various plants. It can produce EEG synchronization and apparently can inhibit the stimulatory effect of acetylcholine. Small doses can have a sedative effect, but large doses may cause restlessness and agitation. S. is sometimes employed in labor to produce twilight sleep and amnesia for the event. Also called **hyoscine.** Also see ANTIHISTAMINES; ANTICHOLINERGICS.

scopophilia sexual pleasure derived from watching others in a state of nudity, disrobing, or engaging in sexual activity. If s. is persistent, the term is essentially equivalent to VOYEURISM. See this entry. S. is also called **scoptophilia** or **scotophilia.**

scopophobia a morbid fear of being looked at. It is usually a sign of extreme shyness.

scoptophilia = SCOPOPHILIA.

score a quantitative value assigned to test results, or other measurable responses or judgments.

-scot-; -scoto- a combining form relating to darkness and, by way of extension, to blindness (from Greek *skotos*, "darkness").

scoterythrous vision a type of color blindness in which reds appear darkened because of a deficiency in perceiving the red end of the spectrum.

scotoma an area of depressed vision within the visual field. An **absolute s.** is an area in which perception of light is lost completely. Other kinds of s. include **color s., peripheral s.,** and **scintillating s.** The alternative term "blind spot" is mainly used in psychiatry and psychoanalysis. Also see OPTIC DISK.

scotomization the tendency to ignore or be blind to impulses or memories that would threaten the individual's ego. S. is a defense mechanism and may also be a form of resistance. Also called **scotomatization.** Also see BLIND SPOT.

scotophilia = SCOPOPHILIA.

scotophobia = ACHLUOPHOBIA.

scotopic pertaining to dark adaptation or the ability of the eye to adjust to darkness.

scotopic vision a form of visual perception in dim light that utilizes rod-cell function. Also called **twilight vision.**

scotopsin a protein substance in the rod cells of the retina that combines with retinene to form rhodopsin, the light-sensitive visual pigment.

scratch fear = AMYCHOPHOBIA.

scratch reflex a stimulus response that requires an intersegmental arc of neural conduction. E.g., stimulating the skin of a dog at its shoulder sends an impulse to the spinal cord where an interneuron connection must be made with a motor nerve of another spinal segment so a hindleg muscle group will get the message to scratch the shoulder.

screen defense in psychoanalysis, a defensive device in which a memory, fantasy, or dream image is unconsciously employed to conceal the real but disturbing object of one's feelings.

screening in psychiatry, the initial patient evaluation based on a medical and psychiatric history, mental-status examination, and diagnostic formulation, to determine the patient's suitability for the facility and for a particular type of treatment. Also, the term refers to the process of selecting items for a psychological test; and to the process of determining, through a preliminary test, whether or not an individual requires a more thorough evaluation.

screening audiometry a technique of rapidly sweeping across low and high frequencies at a controlled, fixed volume, usually 20 to 25 decibels, to determine if the subject is responding at each frequency for each ear being tested.

screening programs organized efforts to identify individuals with certain disorders such as hypertension or genetic diseases through the use of tests and other diagnostic and evaluative procedures.

screen memory the memory of an unacceptable experience, often of a trivial or harmless nature, which unconsciously serves the purpose of concealing or screening out an associated experience of a more significant nature. S.m. is a form of resistance frequently encountered in psychoanalysis. Also called **cover memory**.

script analysis in transactional psychotherapy, the analysis of the patient's unconscious life plan, or script, in its totality. The **script** is, in Eric Berne's opinion, always based on fantasies, attitudes, and "games" or ploys derived from the individual's early experiences. Also see LIFE SCRIPT; SEXUAL SCRIPT.

scrotum the pouch of skin that contains the testes and parts of the spermatic cords. A ridge on the surface is continuous with the skin on the undersurface of the penis.

scrupulosity overconcern with questions of right and wrong and meticulous attention to detail. S. is a common characteristic of the obsessive-compulsive personality.

scrying = CRYSTAL GAZING.

sculpting a group-therapy technique in which, e.g., a family group and a therapist first discuss the functioning position of each member, then create a "living sculpture" in which the members assume the position decided upon, such as submissive, bossy, clinging, or detached. The object is to help them become more aware of themselves and their relationship to each other.

SDAT an abbreviation of *s*enile *d*ementia of the *A*lzheimer *t*ype, an alternative term for ALZHEIMER'S DISEASE. See this entry.

seaman's mania = NAUTOMANIA.

seamstress' cramp a neurotic symptom consisting of an inability to perform such manual operations as threading a needle and using scissors in cutting cloth. See OCCUPATIONAL NEUROSIS.

seance /sā′äns/ a parapsychology practice in which individuals sit in a darkened room trying or believing to observe psychic phenomena such as communications from deceased persons (from French *séance*, "session").

sea phobia = THALASSOPHOBIA.

Seashore, Carl Emil American psychologist, 1866–1949. See SEASHORE MEASURES OF MUSICAL TALENT.

Seashore Measures of Musical Talent a series of recorded tests of the components of musical aptitude, including tonal memory, time sense, rhythm sense, pitch discrimination, timbre sense, and loudness discrimination.

seasonal cycle: See GONADAL CYCLE.

sebaceous glands /sibāsh′əs/ glands in the skin that secrete oily matter, mainly to lubricate the skin and hair (from Latin *sebum*, "tallow").

-sec-; -sect- a combining form relating to a cut or cutting (from Latin *secare*, "to cut").

Seckel, Helmut Paul Georg German physician, 1900—. See SECKEL'S BIRD-HEADED DWARFISM.

Seckel's bird-headed dwarfism a familial disorder, possibly due to gene mutations, marked by microcephaly, a beaklike nose, prominent eyes, narrow face, and short stature. Abilities of patients studied have ranged from inability to care for themselves to IQ's in the 70s. Also called **nanocephalic dwarfism**.

seclusion need H. A. Murray's term for the need for privacy, the need to be alone.

seclusiveness the tendency to isolate oneself from social contacts or human relationships.

secobarbital sodium: See BARBITURATES.

secondary aging aging processes accelerated by disabilities resulting from disease, as distinguished from **primary** or **biological aging** that is governed apparently by inborn and time-related processes but also influenced by stress, trauma, and environment.

secondary amenorrhea: See AMENORRHEA.

secondary amyloidosis: See AMYLOIDOSIS.

secondary area: See METASTASIS.

secondary attention active attention that requires conscious effort, e.g., the attention needed to analyze a painting or sculpture. Compare PRIMARY ATTENTION.

secondary autoerotism a type of erotic pleasure produced by indirect association with the erogenous zones, e.g., sexual arousal from contact with urine.

secondary cause a contributing factor to the onset of mental-disorder symptoms although the factor in itself would not be sufficient to cause the disorder.

secondary circular reaction according to Piaget, a repetitive action, usually emerging around the age of four to five months, that signifies the infant's aim of making things happen. The infant repeats actions such as rattling the crib that have yielded results in the past but is not able to coordinate them so as to meet the requirements of a new situation. This forward step occurs during the sensorimotor period. Also see PRIMARY CIRCULAR REACTION; COORDINATION OF SECONDARY SCHEMES; TERTIARY CIRCULAR REACTION.

secondary cortical zone: See CORTICAL ZONES.

secondary defense symptoms a set of defensive measures employed by an obsessional neurosis patient when his primary defenses against repressed memories no longer offer protection. The secondary defenses usually include obsessional thinking, folie du doute, and speculations, which may be expressed as phobias, ceremonials, superstitions, or pedantry.

secondary deviance the term used in connection with the idea that maladjustment or emotional disturbance experienced by those whom society labels "deviant" may stem more from social oppression than from deep-seated emotional conflict arising from a given condition. An example is the idea that emotional difficulties experienced by some homosexuals arise from the experience of discrimination and social rejection.

secondary drive a learned drive such as the desire for a particular kind of food or drink. See ACQUIRED DRIVE. Compare PRIMARY DRIVE.

secondary elaboration in psychoanalysis, the process of altering the memory and description of a dream to make it more coherent and less fragmentary or distorted. Also called **s.e. of dreams**.

secondary environment an environment that is incidental or marginally important in a person's life and in which interactions with others are comparatively brief and impersonal, e.g., a bank or shop. Also see PRIMARY ENVIRONMENT.

secondary erectile dysfunction a condition in which a man is no longer capable of producing or maintaining a penile erection as needed for successful heterosexual or homosexual intercourse although he was previously capable of performing intercourse successfully. Also called **secondary impotence**. Also see IMPOTENCE.

secondary evaluation in evaluation research, a process that occurs "when the data and/or the reports of an evaluation are studied and reported upon by another evaluator. S.e. is sometimes referred to as metaevaluation because it is a process that occurs 'above and beyond' the primary evaluation." S.e. may simply be a critical review of the primary evaluation. (S. Anderson, S. Ball, and T. Murphy, *Encyclopedia of Educational Evaluation*, 1975) Also see METAEVALUATION.

secondary extinction the extinction or weakening in rate or intensity of a conditioned response as a result of its association with another response that has been or is in the process of being extinguished.

secondary gains in psychoanalysis, advantages derived from a neurosis, other than the primary gain of relieving anxiety or internal conflict. Examples are extra attention, sympathy, avoidance of work, personal service, and domination of others. All these gains are reactions to the illness instead of causal factors, and are therefore called secondary. They often prolong the neurosis and create resistance to therapy. The term is essentially equivalent to epinosic gains. See PRIMARY GAINS. Also see TERTIARY GAINS.

secondary groups social groups characterized by relatively weak, superficial interpersonal relationships, e.g., large lecture classes. Compare PRIMARY GROUPS.

secondary identification in psychoanalysis, a pathological form of identification occurring after the stage of primary identification. It consists of incorporating the traits of another person into the self for defensive purposes, e.g., unconsciously attempting to restore a deceased loved one to life by adopting his or her characteristics. The term is also applied to identification with admired figures other than the parents. See PRIMARY IDENTIFICATION.

secondary impotence = SECONDARY ERECTILE DYSFUNCTION.

secondary integration in psychoanalysis, the normal evolution of pregenital psychic components into an integrated psychosexual unit on an adult, genital level.

secondary mental deficiency a type of subnormal intelligence due to disease or brain injury rather than congenital factors.

secondary motivation acquired or learned drives that lack a bodily basis, e.g., an urge to learn classical music or to become a movie star.

secondary narcissism self-love that develops later in life, after the original infantile primary narcissism. An example is narcissism in the form of a delusion of grandeur, which frequently occurs in schizophrenia when the libido is withdrawn from the external world and centered on the self. Compare PRIMARY NARCISSISM.

secondary oocyte: See OOCYTE; PRIMARY OOCYTE.

secondary personality a second self that has its own behavior patterns, attitudes, name, and way of speaking and dressing, all of which are usually in sharp contrast to the original, or primary, personality. See MULTIPLE PERSONALITY.

secondary prevention in psychiatry, early case-finding, prompt care and treatment, with the aim of arresting mental disorders in their incipient stages. Also see PREVENTIVE PSYCHIATRY.

secondary process in psychoanalysis, conscious mental activities under control of the ego and the reality principle. These thought processes, which include problem-solving, judgment, and systematic thinking, enable us to meet the external demands of the environment, and the internal demands of our instincts, in rational, effective ways. Also called **s.p. thinking**.

secondary quality a property of an item that is not necessary for its existence, e.g., the color of a toy.

secondary reinforcement a process of conditioning by the use of a learned reinforcer, e.g., teaching a subject the value of a token needed to obtain a reward. Also called **secondary reinforcer**. See REINFORCEMENT; PRIMARY REINFORCEMENT.

secondary repression = AFTEREXPULSION.

secondary reward a reward with a learned value that is needed to retrieve, in turn, the primary reward. A s.r. could be a map showing the location of buried treasure, the primary reward.

secondary sensation = SYNESTHESIA.

secondary sex characteristics: See SEX CHARACTERISTICS.

secondary signaling system; secondary signal system = SECOND SIGNALING SYSTEM.

secondary stuttering the neuromuscular spasms and speech dysfluencies accompanied by anxiety and habitual movements to conceal or alter speech blockages. Also see PRIMARY STUTTERING.

secondary symptoms a term applied by Bleuler to

symptoms, such as apathy and loss of initiative, that stem from the hospital environment rather than from the disease itself. He also contrasted secondary, or accessory, symptoms of schizophrenia with fundamental or pathognomonic symptoms. For details, see ACCESSORY SYMPTOMS; SOCIAL-BREAKDOWN SYNDROME. Compare FUNDAMENTAL SYMPTOMS.

secondary territory in social psychology, a space routinely used by a person or group who do not control or use it exclusively, e.g., the local tennis court. Habitués may harbor feelings of possession but they will acknowledge others' claims. Also see PRIMARY TERRITORY; PROXEMICS.

secondary tumor a tumor that develops by metastasis from cells of a primary tumor in another part of the body. Secondary tumors often follow patterns of migration and in many instances provide the first diagnostic clue as to the presence of a primary tumor which may develop silently. A lung cancer may not be detected until it produces a s.t. at a site that causes more painful symptoms.

second childhood a lay term for the hypothetical tendency of the aged to regress to a childish state of mind. The term is sometimes used as a synonym for senility.

second cranial nerve = OPTIC NERVE.

second-degree burns: See BURN INJURIES.

second-messenger hormonal accessories: See CYCLIC NUCLEOTIDES.

second negative phase the resurgence of resistant or negative behavior in adolescence, usually associated with the adolescent's efforts to achieve autonomy. The term **first negative phase** refers to the no-saying so prevalent during the child's second and third years, a period associated with the toddler's struggle for independence.

second-order language = METALANGUAGE.

second signaling system a term used by Pavlov to refer to the system of human language and symbolic knowledge that is based, according to Pavlov, on the first signaling system. The s.s.s. derives from individual experience within a culture. It depends on language, abstraction, generalization, analysis, and synthesis. Also called **secondary signaling system; secondary signal system.** See SIGNALING SYSTEM; FIRST SIGNALING SYSTEM.

secret control: See DELUSION OF INFLUENCE.

sect a group whose members actively follow a doctrinal leader or adhere to a set of doctrines, beliefs, and rituals. Often the term is used to describe a dissenting faction that breaks away from a larger religious, political, or other social organization. Adjective: **sectarian.**

sector therapy a therapeutic procedure developed by Felix Deutsch, in which chains of association that have produced emotional problems are broken up and replaced by more realistic and constructive patterns. Unlike psychoanalysis, this process, which Deutsch describes as **goal-limited adjustment therapy**, is focused on specific "sectors" revealed by the patient's own autobiographical account, or anamnesis. The procedure enables the patient to understand his faulty associations and gradually establish new ones with the aid of the therapist. See ASSOCIATIONISM.

secular pertaining to that which is not religious in nature. E.g., in secular society, many religions may exist, but they exist independently of the laws and governing institutions over which they ostensibly exert no influence.

secular trend the main trend or direction of a time series, as distinguished from temporary or seasonal variations.

security a sense of safety, confidence, and freedom from apprehension, which is believed to be engendered by such factors as warm, accepting parents and friends, development of age-appropriate skills and abilities, and experiences that build ego strength.

security blanket: See TRANSITIONAL OBJECT.

security operations a term applied by H. S. Sullivan to a variety of defensive measures, such as arrogance, boredom, or anger, which are used as a protection against anxiety or loss of self-esteem, usually at the expense of harmonious interpersonal relationships.

sedative any substance that relieves excitement or irritability by depressing the central nervous system. The degree of **sedation** depends upon the agent, the size of the dose, the method of administration, and the condition of the patient. A s. that sedates in small doses may be a hypnotic in larger doses and may be used as such to induce sleep. Barbiturates are commonly used as sedative-hypnotic drugs.

sedative-hypnotics drugs that can be utilized both as sedatives and hypnotics. Generally, a small dose is administered for a sedative effect and a large dose to produce sleep. An example is phenobarbital, one of the barbiturates, which often is administered in a 30-milligram dose as a sedative but in a 100-milligram dose as a hypnotic. In addition to the BARBITURATES, s.-h. include certain ANTICHOLINERGICS and ANTIHISTAMINES, ALCOHOL DERIVATIVES, BENZODIAZEPINES, CHLORAL DERIVATIVES, METHAQUALONE, and PIPERIDINEDIONES. See these entries.

sedative occupation an activity that has a soothing or sedating effect because of its monotonous repetition, e.g., certain occupational-therapy tasks such as weaving.

seduction the inducement of a person to participate in sexual intercourse, without the use of force. Local laws vary in interpretation of the term, and common law does not recognize s. as a crime. However, some laws regard s. as a crime if it involves a promise by a man to marry a woman in the near future if she will submit to intercourse now. Also see CASANOVA.

seed psychosurgery = STEREOTACTIC TRACTOTOMY.

Seeing Eye dog = GUIDE DOG.

SEG = SONOENCEPHALOGRAM.

segmental insufficiency a defect or inferiority of a

segment of the body as manifested by a tumor or other disorder of the skin of that segment. S.i. is a term introduced by Adler, who also termed such skin disorders as **external stigmata**.

segmental reactions: See SUPRASEGMENTAL REFLEXES; SPINAL REFLEXES.

segregated model in evaluation research, one possible administrative relationship used in formative evaluation between the program director, the production unit, and the evaluation unit, as three distinct units, in which the production unit and the evaluation unit share equal importance and improved access to the program director. Also called **related model**. See INTEGRATED MODEL.

segregation the isolation of items with a minimum of interfacing between them. The items may be mental processes, ethnic groups, or a pair of gametes. Some segregated entities, such as genes, can give rise to new combinations.

Seguin, Edouard French-American physician, 1812–80. S. acquired an interest in the mentally retarded from Jean Itard, who had attempted to teach the "wild boy of Aveyron." Noting that the boy was able to master a few social habits, he concluded that mentally defective children could be trained, and proceeded to devise a wide variety of materials and methods designed to develop their motor and sensory capacities, including climbing ladders, walking a straight line, and exposure to varied colors, sounds, and shapes. The principal effect of these efforts was to encourage institutions to adopt an educational instead of an exclusively custodial approach. See WILD BOY OF AVEYRON.

Seitelberger, Franz /zī′təlbergər/ Austrian neuropathologist, 1916—. See SEITELBERGER'S DISEASE.

Seitelberger's disease a condition of spastic paraplegia, impaired sense of equilibrium, ocular tremor, and mental retardation. It is caused by demyelination of the pyramidal tracts, development of rounded masses in the gray matter, and other neurologic defects. Also called **neuroaxonal degeneration**.

seizure a sudden onset of symptoms of a disease condition, including convulsions, palpitations, dizziness, or other disagreeable sensations. The term also is applied to a specific pattern of signs or symptoms of an epileptic disorder, e.g., grand mal epilepsy, in which the s. is interpreted in terms of neural discharges within a certain area of brain tissues. Also see CONVULSION; EPILEPSY.

seizure disorders = CONVULSIVE DISORDERS.

seizure dyscontrol an extreme form of dyscontrol occasionally occurring immediately after a grand mal seizure, and characterized by indiscriminate acts of aggression such as assaulting the nearest person or terrorizing other patients.

selaphobia a morbid fear of a flash.

selected group an experimental group selected with respect to specified criteria related to the purpose of the experiment, e.g., a sample of citizens age 65 and over for a study of attitudinal patterns in the elderly. Also called **selected sample**. Compare RANDOM SAMPLE.

selection the process of choosing an item, e.g., an individual or object, for a purpose, such as study, testing, classifying, or working (employee s.).

selection bias bias in selecting subjects for experimentation, as in selecting specially motivated subjects, or in differential assignment to groups.

selection index a mathematical formula used to determine the discriminatory power of a test or test item.

selective amnesia: See PSYCHOGENIC AMNESIA.

selective analysis a pseudopsychoanalytic approach in which aspects chosen for interpretation reflect the therapist's own interests and problems rather than the patient's needs and conflicts.

selective-answer test a type of test in which two or more alternative answers accompany question items and the subject is directed to choose the best answer, e.g., multiple-choice or **true-false tests**. Also see MULTIPLE-CHOICE TEST.

selective attention = CONTROLLED ATTENTION.

selective inattention a term coined by H. S. Sullivan for a perceptual defense in which anxiety-provoking or threatening experiences are ignored or forgotten.

selective migration a doubtful term used in reference to possible reasons for the superior scores of Asian-American children on intelligence tests. S.m. is the white, racist speculation that Oriental emigrants to the United States may have been a superior group, that is, a nonrepresentative sample of their native populations. See RACE DIFFERENCES.

selective response a response that has been differentiated from a group of possible alternative responses.

selective retention a general term referring to the fact that the capacity to remember varies greatly from person to person with respect to the vividness, accuracy, quantity, and specific contents of memory. The selectivity, however, is usually determined by such factors as interest, experience, motivation, and emotional factors more than by basic capacity. Also see REPRESSION.

self in psychoanalysis, the total concept of the individual, consisting of all characteristic attributes, conscious and unconscious, mental and physical. Jung maintained that the self gradually develops by a process of individuation which is not complete until late maturity is reached. Adler identified the self with the individual's life-style, the manner in which he seeks fulfillment. James believed we have not one but many selves, since we are called upon to adapt to many different situations. Horney held that our real self, as opposed to our idealized self-image, consists of our unique capacities for growth and development. G. W. Allport substituted the word proprium for self, and conceived it as the essence of the individual, consisting of a gradually developing body sense, identity, self-estimate, and set of personal values, attitudes, and intentions. Also see BAD S.; CREATIVE S.; DEFORMATION OF THE S.; DESUBJECTIVIZATION OF THE S.; DISORDERS OF THE S.; LOOKING-GLASS S.; PERSONIFIED S.; PHENOMENAL S.; REAL S.; SENSE OF S.; SENSORY S.-STIMULATION; SOCIAL S.; TRUE S.

self-abasement = SELF-DEBASEMENT.

self-absorption: See GENERATIVITY VERSUS S.-A.

self-abuse a euphemism sometimes used for masturbation. The term is without scientific foundation and apparently evolved from an 18th-century attempt by certain religious and medical writers to identify masturbation as "the sin of Onan" and to substantiate unscientific claims that a number of diseases were produced by masturbation, including blindness and mental retardation.

self-acceptance recognition of our abilities and achievements, together with acknowledgment and acceptance of our limitations. S.-a. essentially means that we recognize our real qualities and are at peace with them. Lack of genuine s.-a. is one of the major characteristics of emotional disturbance.

self-accusation the process or habit of blaming oneself, usually unjustifiably and out of a false sense of guilt. It is often a factor in depression. Also called **intropunitiveness**. See INTROPUNITIVE RESPONSE; ANGER-IN.

self-actualization according to A. Maslow, the "full use and exploitation of talent, capacities, potentialities" such that the individual develops to maximum self-realization, ideally integrating physical, social, intellectual, and emotional needs. The process of striving toward full potential is fundamental according to Maslow; however, s.-a. can only be fully realized if the basic needs of survival, safety, love, belongingness, and esteem are fulfilled. See NEED-HIERARCHY THEORY. Also see HUMANISTIC PERSPECTIVE.

self-administered test a type of test in which the instructions are sufficiently self-evident to preclude further clarification by the tester. Also called **self-administering test**.

self-alienation a state in which the individual feels he is a stranger to himself and is unaware of his own intrapsychic processes.

self-analysis an attempt to apply the principles of psychoanalysis to a study of one's own drives, feelings, and behavior. It was proposed by Freud early in his career as part of the preparation of an analyst but later dropped in favor of a training analysis. See DIDACTIC ANALYSIS.

self-appraisal; self-assessment = SELF-CONCEPT.

self-awareness = SELF-UNDERSTANDING.

self-blaming depression a depression in which the individual derogates himself and accuses himself of faults or misdeeds, usually to an unwarranted degree.

self-care the activities of daily life, e.g., eating, dressing, grooming, or the handling of objects, that can ordinarily be managed by the individual without the assistance of others.

self-censure an individual's conscious self-blame, condemnation, or guilt in judging his own behavior to be inconsistent with personal standards of moral conduct.

self-concept the individual's conception and evaluation of himself, including his values, abilities, goals, and personal worth. Also called **self-appraisal; self-assessment; self-evaluation; self-rating**. See SELF-IMAGE; SELF-PERCEPTION.

self-concept tests personality tests designed to determine how the individual views his own attitudes, values, goals, body concept, personal worth, and abilities. Three types of techniques are most frequently used: checking of adjectives that apply to oneself; interpretation of personality inventory responses on the MMPI or other tests; and the Q-sort technique. See ADJECTIVE CHECK LIST; MINNESOTA MULTIPHASIC PERSONALITY INVENTORY; Q-SORT.

self-confidence self-assurance; trust in one's own abilities, capacities, and judgment.

self-consciousness an extreme sensitivity about one's own behavior, appearance, or other attributes; overconcern about the impression one makes on others.

self-consistency a term applied to behavior or personality that has a high degree of internal harmony and stability; also, the compatibility of all aspects of a theory or system.

self-control the ability to be in command of one's behavior, and to restrain or inhibit one's impulses.

self-control techniques a behavior-therapy approach in which clients are trained to evaluate their own behavior, and reinforce desired behavior with appropriate material or social rewards.

self-correlation the correlation of any test or measuring instrument with aspects of itself. The correlation may be between separate administrations of the test, between different sections of the test, or between the entire test and an equivalent instrument.

self-criticism the ability to scrutinize and evaluate one's behavior, and to recognize one's weaknesses, errors, and shortcomings.

self-debasement the act of degrading or demeaning one's self; also, extreme submission to the will of another person. Also called **self-abasement**.

self-deception a failure to recognize one's own limitations; the development of a false or unrealistic self-concept.

self-defeating behavior behavior that blocks the individual's own goals and wishes. Examples are the tendency to compete so aggressively that we cannot hold a job; or the tendency of an antisocial individual to take such great risks that he is almost bound to get caught.

self-demand schedule a feeding schedule regulated by the infant's needs, in contrast to a fixed or rigid schedule. Feedings are in response to the baby's hunger cry or other demonstration of hunger. Most mothers and infants on the s.-

d.s. eventually develop regular patterns of feeding. Also called **demand feeding**.

self-denial the act of suppressing desires and foregoing satisfactions. It is often a form of self-punishment for real or fancied guilt.

self-derogation a tendency to disparage oneself, often as a result of false expectations or aspirations, or an exaggerated sense of self-blame. S.-d. is frequently found in depression. See SELF-HATE.

self-desensitization a behavior-therapy procedure in which the individual, when confronted with fear-eliciting objects or situations, engages in coping strategies designed to reduce anxiety, e.g., coping self-statements, rehearsal strategies, and muscle relaxation.

self-destructiveness: See DESTRUCTIVE BEHAVIOR; DEATH INSTINCT.

self-determination the control of one's behavior by internal convictions and decisions rather than external demands. Also called **self-direction**.

self-development the growth or improvement of one's own qualities and abilities.

self-differentiation a measure of the uniqueness of an individual with respect to other members of his group.

self-direction = SELF-DETERMINATION.

self-discipline the control of one's own impulses and desires; foregoing immediate satisfaction in favor of long-term goals.

self-disclosure the ability to reveal and express one's personal, innermost feelings, fantasies, experiences, and aspirations. S.-d. is believed by many to be a requisite for therapeutic change and personal growth in group psychotherapy.

self-discovery in existentialism, the process of finding one's unique self; the "quest for identity"; in psychoanalysis, the freeing of one's repressed ego, including one's aims and goals, from limitations imposed by submission to others.

self-dynamism according to H. S. Sullivan, the pattern of motivations or drives that comprise our self-system, including especially our pursuit of biological satisfaction and our pursuit of security and freedom from anxiety.

self-effacement a Horney term for a neurotic idealization of compliancy, dependency, and selfless love as a reaction to identification with the hated self.

self-efficacy a comprehensive sense of one's own capability, effectiveness, strength, or power to attain desired results.

self-employment the conducting and earning of income directly from one's own business or profession, as opposed to working for specified wages or salary paid by a corporation, government agency, or other employer.

self-esteem an attitude of self-acceptance, self-approval, and self-respect. A feeling of self-worth is an important ingredient of mental health; a loss of self-esteem and feelings of worthlessness are common depressive symptoms. In psychoanalysis, having s.-e. means being on good terms with one's superego.

self-evaluation = SELF-CONCEPT.

self-examination: See BREAST S.-A.

self-expression free expression of one's feelings, thoughts, talents, attitudes, or impulses through such means as verbal communication, poetry, arts and crafts, dancing, and dramatic activities.

self-extension a term applied by G. W. Allport to an early stage in the development of the proprium or self, beginning roughly at age four and marked by the child's emerging ability to incorporate people, objects, and abstractions into the self-concept. As used by Allport, s.-e. is the investment of ego in those objects outside the self with which the individual feels affinity or identification. See PROPRIUM.

self-extinction a Horney term for a form of neurotic behavior in which the patient lacks experience of himself as an entity and identifies vicariously with the experiences and lives of others.

self-feeding being able to feed oneself without direct assistance of others. A severely retarded person may not be capable of feeding himself whereas a quadriplegic patient may be able to perform the task of s.-f. with the help of certain DAILY-LIVING AIDS. See this entry.

self-fulfilling prophecy a belief or expectation that helps to bring about its own fulfillment, e.g., Rosenthal's findings that teachers' preconceptions about their students' abilities can influence the children's achievement for better or worse. S.-f. p. is essentially equivalent to ROSENTHAL EFFECT. See this entry.

self-fulfillment the process of developing and expressing one's basic capacities and aspirations. Also see SELF-ACTUALIZATION; SELF-REALIZATION.

self-gratification the satisfaction of one's own needs, particularly needs associated with our appetites and our drive for self-enhancement through prestige, boasting, and display.

self-handicapping strategy a psychological ploy by means of which a person lessens his chances of performing well at a task in which he is ego-involved and at which he expects to possibly fail or do poorly, e.g., neglecting to rehearse before an audition. The purpose is to create an acceptable excuse for an anticipated poor showing so that shortcomings can be attributed to circumstance and not to lack of ability.

self-hate an extreme loss of self-esteem in which the patient despises and derogates himself, as in a self-blaming depression.

self-help groups groups or programs in which victims of disorders, and in some cases members of their families, band together for purposes of emotional support, morale-boosting, and practical assistance. Examples are Alcoholics Anonymous, Narcotics Anonymous, Gamblers Anonymous, Weight Watchers, and Recovery, Inc. (for ex-mental patients). A growing number of self-help groups are developing among the physically disabled, many of which are coordinated by the American Coalition of Citizens with Disabilities (ACCD).

self-hypnorelaxation a form of self-hypnosis in which the patient is trained to respond to his own relaxation suggestions.

self-hypnosis the process of putting oneself in a trance or trancelike state through autosuggestion. See AUTOHYPNOSIS; AUTOSUGGESTION.

self ideal = EGO IDEAL.

self-ideal Q-sort a personality test designed to measure the discrepancy between an individual's self-concept and his or her self-ideal. See Q-SORT TECHNIQUE.

self-image an individual's picture or concept of himself, including a self-evaluation of his abilities, personal worth, goals, and potential. Whether the self-image is idealized or realistic, it is bound to be a basic component of the personality.

self-injurious behavior actions that inflict damage upon one's own body, such as head-banging, face-slapping, lip-biting, or tripping and falling "accidentally on purpose". S.-i.b. frequently occurs in mentally retarded children, schizophrenics, drug abusers, alcoholics, compulsive gamblers, and masochistic adolescents and adults.

self-instructional training a form of cognitive behavior modification (Meichenbaum, 1977) in which the therapist identifies maladaptive thoughts, or "self-statements," such as "Everybody hates me," and models appropriate behavior while verbalizing constructive **self-instructions**. The client then engages in the behavior while repeating these instructions aloud.

self-inventory a questionnaire or series of statements on which the subject checks characteristics or traits that apply to himself or herself.

self-love excessive self-regard; a narcissistic attitude toward one's own body, abilities, or personality. See NARCISSISM; EGOTISM.

self-managed reinforcement self-regulation of one's own reinforcement. S.-m.r. essentially means that the individual determines the relationships between his or her behavior and the time and amount of reinforcement. E.g., "How much or how long must I work before I can rest (and how long can I rest before I go back to work)?"

self-management a behavior-therapy program in which the patient is trained to apply techniques that will help him modify his own behavior, such as smoking, excessive eating, or aggressive outbursts. The individual learns to pinpoint the problem, set realistic goals, use various contingencies to establish and maintain the desired behavior, and monitor his own progress.

self-marking test a type of test that automatically scores a subject's responses as correct or incorrect.

self-maximation the drive to maintain feelings of personal adequacy through competitive situations, such as competition for status at home, at school, or at work.

self-mutilation a destructive act in which the individual disfigures himself or herself. It has been observed in some neurological disorders, such as the Lesch-Nyhan syndrome, and among schizophrenics in a state of catatonic excitement. In some cases the individual appears to be inflicting self-punishment in order to relieve intense and (usually exaggerated) feelings of guilt. Also see CUTTING.

self-objectification as used by G. W. Allport, objective knowledge about the self; self-understanding.

self-observation self-scrutiny, either of the body and its functioning or of the psyche and its functioning. In psychoanalysis, the examination of one's own feelings, impulses, motives, and behavior is regarded as one of the prime functions of the ego. See INTROSPECTION.

self-perception awareness of the various components that constitute the self, that is, one's unique feelings, impulses, aspirations, and personality characteristics. The term is often used interchangeably with **self-percept** and SELF-CONCEPT. See this entry.

self-preservation instinct a general term for the basic impulse to insure the continuation of the individual as a living organism.

self psychology a system of psychology that is focused upon the self, that is, the interpretation of all behavior in reference to the self.

self-punishment inflicting harm on oneself for real or fancied misdeeds, usually to relieve a sense of guilt. S.-p. is particularly common in depression and takes many forms, such as verbal castigation of oneself, extreme self-denial, martyrdom, masochistic infliction of pain, and, in extreme cases, self-mutilation and suicide. See EGO SUFFERING; EXPIATION. Also see ILLNESS AS S.-P.

self-rating = SELF-CONCEPT.

self-rating scale any questionnaire, inventory, or other instrument used by a subject to rate or assess his own characteristics, attitudes, interests, or performance.

self-realization the process or goal of fulfilling one's full potentialities, including aptitudes, goals, and capacities. S.-r. is a major objective in many therapeutic approaches, such as psychodrama, client-centered counseling, K. Goldstein's organismic theory, and A. Maslow's humanistic psychology. Also see SELF-ACTUALIZATION.

self-recitation a learning technique in which study time is at least partially spent in reciting or recalling learned material.

self-reference a persistent tendency to direct a discussion or the attention of others back to one's self.

self-regulation the control of one's own behavior through a process of (a) self-monitoring of the conditions that evoke desired and undesired behavior, (b) structuring of the personal environment to facilitate desired behavior and circumvent situations that tend to elicit undesired behavior, and (c) self-evaluation and self-reinforcement, including self-administration of punishments and rewards. Self-regulatory processes are stressed in behavior therapy.

self-reinforcement the rewarding of oneself for appropriate behavior, a part of cognitive-behavioral therapy. S.-r. has a record of more consistent effects over a wide range of population and behaviors than self-monitoring.

self-report inventory a questionnaire on which the subject indicates personality characteristics and behavior that apply or do not apply to him. See WOODWORTH-MATTHEWS PERSONAL DATA SHEET; GUILFORD-ZIMMERMAN TEMPERAMENT SURVEY; ALLPORT A-S REACTION STUDY; MOONEY PROBLEM CHECK LIST; BELL ADJUSTMENT INVENTORY; MINNESOTA MULTIPHASIC PERSONALITY INVENTORY.

self-respect a feeling of self-worth and self-esteem especially a proper regard for one's own values, character, and dignity. The term is essentially equivalent to SELF-ESTEEM. See this entry.

self-schema a cognitive framework comprising organized information about the self in a specific realm of experience; a component of identity that is organized and well-defined, e.g., a clear conception of oneself as parent or worker.

self-selection of diet the concept that animals, including humans, will tend to select foods that maintain them in good health when they are offered food in cafeteria style. The theory is supported by experiments with human infants and also with animals offered essential nutrients in unfamiliar forms. Also see SPECIFIC HUNGER; SUGAR SELF-SELECTION; APPETITE CONTROL; CAFETERIA FEEDING; FOOD PREFERENCES.

self-statements: See SELF-INSTRUCTIONAL TRAINING.

self-stimulation mechanism a system of electrodes inserted in certain brain areas so that the subject can stimulate neurons that are associated with pleasurable sensations. Rats with electrodes implanted in the septal area have pressed a bar as many as 5,000 times an hour to administer a shock to this "pleasure center." See LIMBIC SYSTEM; REWARD SYSTEM. Also see SENSORY SELF-STIMULATION.

self-synchrony: See SYNCHRONY.

self-system a term used by H. S. Sullivan for the relatively fixed personality of the individual resulting from relationships with the parents and other significant adults, in which approved attitudes and behavior patterns tend to be retained, and disapproved actions and attitudes tend to be blocked out.

self-talk a term used by Albert Ellis for an internal dialogue in which we repeatedly utter "internalized sentences" to ourselves. The sentences often confirm and reinforce faulty beliefs and attitudes, such as fears and false aspirations, which have a disturbing effect on our feelings and reactions. One of the tasks of the therapist is to encourage the patient to replace self-defeating s.-t. with more constructive s.-t. See RATIONAL PSYCHOTHERAPY. Also see INTERNALIZED SPEECH.

self-theory a viewpoint that the individual's own sense of his identity, worth, and capabilities is the key factor in personality organization and function.

self-transcendence the term used by V. Frankl to refer to the state in which an individual transcends preoccupation with self and is able to devote himself or herself fully to another person, work, or cause or other activity. In common with other humanistic psychologists, Frankl maintains that deep commitment or absorption in something beyond the self is a central feature of the healthy individual.

self-understanding the attainment of insight into one's attitudes, motives, reactions, defenses, strengths, and weaknesses. The achievement of s.-u. is one of the major goals of psychotherapy. Also called **self-awareness**.

self-worth an individual's evaluation of himself as a worthwhile human being. If he has positive feelings of s.-w., he tends to have a high degree of self-acceptance and self-esteem.

Selye, Hans /sel'yə/ Austrian-born Canadian endocrinologist and psychologist, 1907–82. S. founded the International Institute of Stress, having introduced the concept of stress to psychology around 1940. See EXHAUSTION STAGE; EUSTRESS; GENERAL ADAPTATION SYNDROME; RESISTANCE TO STRESS; STAGE OF RESISTANCE; STRESS; STRESS THEORY.

sem. an abbreviation used in prescriptions, meaning "half" (Latin *semi* or *semis*).

-sem- a combining form relating to signs or meaning (from Greek *sema*, "sign").

semanteme = CONTENT WORD.

semantic aphasia a form of aphasia in which the patient is unable to comprehend the meaning of words even though he may be able to utter them. Also see LOGICOGRAMMATICAL DISORDERS.

semantic code the encoding of an object, idea, or impression in terms of its conceptual or abstract components. E.g., if the item "typewriter" is remembered in terms of its functional meaning or properties, a s.c. is said to be employed. In contrast, an imagery code would encode "typewriter" in memory as a mental picture. See IMAGERY CODE.

semantic conditioning a variety of classical conditioning in which a concept in the form of a word, phrase, or sentence functions as a conditioned stimulus, as a result of pairing with an unconditioned stimulus or as a result of generalization. E.g., the word delicious, when paired with actual food, will eventually elicit the response of salivation. After "delicious" is establishd as a conditioned stimulus, related words or phrases may elicit the same or similar responses through generalization.

semantic counseling a type of counseling in which emphasis is placed on interpretations of meanings, particularly those related to adjustment and maladjustment.

semantic dementia an inability to feel or appreciate the full meaning of emotional concepts such as love, grief, and shame. According to Cleck-

CURIOSITY

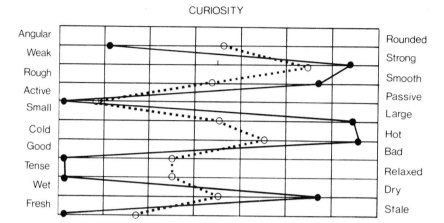

SEMANTIC DIFFERENTIAL. Two profiles of the concept "curiosity." (Note that the two responses—the solid and the broken lines—differ more in degree than in kind.)

ley, this is a major feature of the psychopathic personality.

semantic differential a technique developed by Osgood and his associates for measuring the connotation for the individual of any given concept by rating it on a seven-point scale with reference to pairs of opposites such as strong-weak, cruel-kind, or good-bad. The concepts, or opposites, are chosen to fit the problem being investigated, which may be to rate oneself, family members, friends, employers, public figures, recreational activities, abstract ideas such as democracy or peace, product names, or television programs.

semantic dissociation a distortion between symbol and meaning. S.d. includes **semantic dissolution**, marked by a complete loss of meaning and communication; **semantic dispersion**, in which meaning and syntax are lost or reduced; **semantic distortion**, in which meaning may be transferred to neologisms; or enlarged **semantic halo**, marked by coherent but vague and ambiguous language. All these distortions can be found in schizophrenics.

semanticity the learning of meanings of words and the process of communicating meaning through language. According to Roger Brown, s. is one of the three formal properties of language. See DISPLACEMENT; PRODUCTIVITY.

semantic jargon a form of Wernicke's (receptive, or sensory) aphasia associated with a lesion of the posterior-middle and superior-temporal gyrus, either bilateral or unilateral. The patient utters actual words and sentences, but with defective meaning; e.g., one patient said "My wires don't hire right," when asked about his poor vision.

semantic paraphasia a semantic disorder in which conversational speech is fairly fluent but objects are misnamed, though some association connection may exist. E.g., a pipe may be called a

"smoker," and glasses a "telescope." The condition occurs in cases of diffuse disease, confusion, drowsiness, and Korsakoff's syndrome. Also see PARAPHASIA.

semantic psychosis a term applied by H. Cleckley to the tendency of the antisocial individual to distort the meaning of words: he might say "I shouldn't have done that" when he merely means "I'll say that because that's what he wants to hear, and then he'll let me go."

semantics the study of the meanings of words and their historical development. (The term was coined by Michel Bréal in 1897—French *sémantique*—from Greek *semantikos*, "significant.") Also see SEMASIOLOGY; GENERAL S.

semantic therapy a form of psychotherapy in which the patient is trained to rectify faulty word habits and distorted ideas so that he can think more clearly and critically about his aims, values, and relationships. This approach is based on an active search for the meaning of the key words the patient uses, and on practice in the formation of clear abstractions, as well as on uncovering of hidden assumptions and increased awareness of the emotional tone behind the words he has been using. Chief exponents of this approach are Alfred Korzybski and Wendell Johnson. Also see GENERAL SEMANTICS.

semantogenic disorder a mental disorder originating in a misinterpretation of the meanings of emotion-colored words.

semasiology the study of development and changes in the meanings of words. Also called **historical semantics**. Also see SEMANTICS.

semeiology /semē·ol′-/ the art of using and interpreting signs or sign language. In medicine, s. means symptomatology, that is, the combined symptoms of a disease and their study. Also spelled **semiology**.

Semelaigne, Georges /semelen′yə/ French pediatrician, fl. 1934. See DEBRÉ-SEMELAIGNE SYN-DROME; KOCHER-DEBRÉ-SEMELAIGNE SYNDROME.

semen a fluid discharged through the penis during ejaculation, containing spermatozoa and secretions needed to sustain the viability of the spermatozoa within the female reproductive tract. The secretions originate in the prostate gland, the seminal vesicles, and other glands of the male reproductive system. Adjective: **seminal**.

semen fear = SPERMATOPHOBIA.

semenuria = SPERMATURIA.

semicircular canals a set of three structures in the vestibular system that monitor the position in space of the head, and indirectly the rest of the body. One of the three s.c. is approximately horizontal when the head is held in a normal position. The others are vertical but at right angles to each other. The s.c. also are positioned at about a 45-degree angle to the principal axes of the head so that nearly any possible change in the position of the head will alter the orientation of one or more of the s.c. Each canal is filled with fluid which shifts with the pull of gravity as the head is moved, thereby stimulating sensory-nerve fibers in a gelatinous crysta at the end of each canal. See CRYSTA; CUPULA.

seminal: See SEMEN.

seminal discharge the discharge of semen or seminal fluid. S.d. normally occurs during coital ejaculation, nocturnal emission, or masturbation.

seminal duct = DUCTUS DEFERENS.

seminal vesicles two membranous pouches, approximately three inches long, located between the bladder and the rectum. The s.v. secrete a fluid that enters the ejaculatory duct at the base of the prostate gland. The fluid mixes with secretions of the prostate gland to form the bulk of the content of semen.

semination = INSEMINATION.

seminiferous tubules /-nif'-/ minute convoluted tubules in the lobules of the testis. The s.t. contain layers of cells in which spermatozoa evolve and mature from primordial male gametes. Each lobule of a testis may contain from one to several s.t., and a single testis may contain as many as 400 lobules.

semiology = SEMEIOLOGY.

semiotic movement a trend toward formalization of systems of visual communication by the use of signs or symbols that are not a part of the standard alphabet. The s.m., which has been particularly popular in the United States, promotes the acceptance of "rules of grammar" for symbolic logic, mathematical formulas, or other symbolic systems that may be analogous to language. In a more general sense, the s.m., or **semiotics**, is the study and application of codes through which people communicate.

semipermeability: See PERMEABILITY.

semiplosive = AFFRICATE.

semistarvation 'neurosis' a descriptive term applied to reactions experienced by experimental subjects who volunteered to live for six months on a diet typical of the famine areas during World War II. The symptom pattern consisted primarily of apathy, dejection, withdrawal, irritation, and preoccupation with the subject of food.

semivowel: See SONANT.

-sen-; -senil- a combining form meaning old or aging (from Latin *senex*, "old, aged," *senescere*, "to grow old").

senescence the process of growing old; also, the period during which this process occurs. Also see SENILITY.

senile brain disease a DSM-I category replaced in DSM-III by PRIMARY DEGENERATIVE DEMENTIA. See this entry. Also see SENILE PSYCHOSES.

senile chorea severe, progressive dyskinesia in the elderly, involving stereotyped or disorganized movements of an involuntary nature.

senile delirium a type of senile psychosis in which the patient experiences clouding of consciousness, hallucinations, insomnia, restlessness, and wandering. The symptoms often follow a head injury, infection, or exposure to surgical anesthesia.

senile dementia = PRIMARY DEGENERATIVE DEMENTIA.

senile dementia of the Alzheimer type: See SDAT.

senile deterioration a syndrome associated with the effects of aging on the brain, e.g., demyelination and cerebral atherosclerosis, and characterized by such symptoms as memory gaps and confabulation, apathy, irritability, suspiciousness, hoarding, disorientation, attention deficits, and a tendency to wander from home.

senile keratosis: See KERATOSIS.

senile osteomalacia: See OSTEOMALACIA.

senile plaques areas of brain-tissue degeneration found in older persons. The plaques are composed of granular material and filaments that can be identified pathologically with a silver stain. S.p. are associated with symptoms of Alzheimer's disease.

senile psychoses a group of psychoses resulting primarily from degeneration of the brain in old age (senile dementia, or senile brain disease). Various clinical types are cited in DSM-I, but overlap considerably. They comprise, in order of prevalence, the simple-deterioration, paranoid, depressed and agitated, delirious and confused, and presbyophrenic types.

senilism the appearance of symptoms of senility in old age or before.

senility advanced age involving moderate-to-severe loss of physical strength and decline in mental functions such as memory, alertness, and flexible thought processes. For extremes, see PRIMARY DEGENERATIVE DEMENTIA. Also see PSEUDO-SENILITY.

senior citizen a popular term used to identify a person who has reached the age of retirement, which is usually 65, whether or not one is employed.

senium the period of old age.

senium praecox premature senility (usually before age 55), associated primarily with the two major forms of presenile dementia, PICK'S DISEASE and ALZHEIMER'S DISEASE. See these entries. S.p. is also called **presenile degeneration**.

sensa: See SENSE DATUM.

sensate-focus-oriented therapy the Masters and Johnson approach to sexual-incapacity problems, in which the individual is trained to focus attention on his or her own natural, biological sensual cues, and gradually achieves the freedom to enjoy sensory stimuli. Therapy is conducted by coequal male-female cotherapy teams in joint interviews with the partners. Steps in the process include a detailed history of the patients' attitudes and patterns; a contract specifying appointments, homework, etc.; reassurance and support; improvement in communication between partners; and prescribed body-massage exercises designed to give and receive pleasure, first from noneroticized areas of the body, then from eroticized areas.

sensation an irreducible unit of experience produced by stimulation of a receptor, or sense organ, and the resultant activation of a specific brain center; basic awareness of a sound, odor, color, shape, taste, temperature, pressure, pain, muscular tension, position of the body, or changes in the internal organs associated with such processes as hunger, thirst, bladder and bowel distention, stomach distress, nausea, and sexual excitement. Experimental evidence indicates that in the absence of a completed neural conduction from a sensory area to the cortex, as may result from a nerve injury, no s. is experienced. Also, direct stimulation of certain brain cells by electrodes produces s. effects without stimulation of a sensory organ.

sensationalism the theory that all knowledge originates in sensations, that even reflective ideas and intuitions can be traced back to elementary sense impressions.

sensation increment a psychophysical term for an increase in the intensity of a sensory experience.

sensation level the intensity level of a particular stimulus or sensation, e.g., the intensity of electric shock as measured in volts, or the intensity of auditory stimuli, in which case s.l. is measured in number of decibels.

sensation threshold: See ABSOLUTE THRESHOLD.

sensation type a Jungian personality category characterized by behavior that is dominated by sense perception, as contrasted with thinking, feeling, and intuition. This type of individual lives a life of sense experience and enjoyment.

sensation unit a discriminable sensory experience; also, the just-noticeable difference, or j.n.d.

sense a general term with many possible meanings, including (a) a neural organ or system, (b) a perception based on a s.-organ function, (c) a special kind of awareness, (d) a personality trait, (e) **good s.**, meaning good judgment or intelli-

gence, and (f) a consensus ("the s. of the meeting").

sense datum a sensation or unit of information conveyed by a receptor organ. Also called **sense impression; sensum** (plural: **sensa**).

sensed difference a clearly perceived difference between two stimuli that are introduced simultaneously or consecutively.

sense distance the interval between two distinct sensations along a given dimension, e.g., the distance between C and G on the musical scale.

sense experience awareness produced by stimulation of a sense receptor.

sense feeling a pleasant or unpleasant affect associated with a sense experience.

sense impression = SENSE DATUM.

sense modality a category of sensation: vision, hearing, taste, pressure, pain, smell, temperature, kinesthesis, vestibular. Each s.m. has its own receptors, responds to characteristic stimuli, and has its own pathways to a special part of the brain.

sense of equilibrium the ability of the person to maintain balance while sitting, standing, walking, or otherwise maneuvering the body. The s.o.e. is controlled by cells in the semicircular canals of the inner ear where the fluid endolymph detects motions of the head because of the effect of gravity on the fluid. Also called **labyrinthine sense; vestibular sense; static sense**.

sense of guilt painful feelings of culpability associated with a violation of the individual's moral, social, or religious code. Such feelings may exist on a conscious or unconscious level, and in some cases may have an imaginary basis. In psychoanalysis, feelings of guilt are indicative of a conflict between the ego and the superego and, if they are repressed, or stem from unconscious sources, usually give rise to neurotic anxiety and depression. The term is essentially equivalent to GUILT FEELINGS. See this entry.

sense of identity awareness of being a separate and distinct person. The first signs of a sense of identity are believed to appear when the infant experiences separation from the mother and begins to be aware of his ability to move and perceive the environment. As he grows and matures, he gradually perceives himself as a unique person with his own feelings, impulses, aims, and personality characteristics. The term is essentially equivalent to IDENTITY. See this entry. Also see SELF; SEPARATION-INDIVIDUATION.

sense of self an individual's feeling of identity, uniqueness, and self-direction. See SELF-IMAGE; SENSE OF IDENTITY.

sense organ a sensory receptor and the specialized cells and associated structures that support its functions.

sense perception the process of assimilating inputs from sense organs and interpreting the information as knowledge about objects or events.

sense-ratios method a system of scaling sensory

magnitudes by selecting stimuli that form equal intervals along the scale.

sensibility the capacity to be stimulated by sensory inputs; also, a capacity for intense feeling.

sensitive in parapsychology, a person who allegedly is capable of receiving supernormal messages or knowledge. As an adjective, the term means easily affected or hurt.

sensitive period a stage in development when an organism can most advantageously form specific attachments or acquire necessary skills. E.g., in humans, the first year of life is considered sensitive or critical for the development of a secure attachment bond or basic trust. A stage may be considered a s.p. or a critical period depending on the writer's point of view. The essential difference is the implication that the consequences for the organism may not be irreversible if the s.p. passes and the given acquisition has not fully occurred. For an example of s.p., see IMPRINTING. Also see CRITICAL PERIOD.

sensitive zone any point on the body that is highly responsive to a particular type of stimulus, such as touch or pain.

sensitivity the capacity to be receptive to stimuli; also, emotional and esthetic awareness; and responsiveness to the feelings of others.

sensitivity training a group process, originated by Kurt Lewin and Carl Rogers, focused on the development of self-awareness, productive interpersonal relations, and sensitivity to the feelings, attitudes, and needs of others. The primary method used in s.t. is free, unstructured discussion with a leader functioning as an observer and facilitator, though other techniques such as roleplaying may be used. S.t. is employed in human-relations training in industry and general life, with various types of groups (workers, executives, married couples) meeting once a week or over a weekend. See ACTION RESEARCH; HUMAN-RELATIONS TRAINING; LABORATORY TRAINING; PERSONAL-GROWTH LABORATORY; T-GROUP.

sensitization the process of becoming sensitive, or susceptible, to a given stimulus; also, the theory that a synaptic knob that has been fired repeatedly eventually becomes sensitized so that it can fire without other synaptic knobs on the same cell also firing. Also see NEUROBIOTAXIS; COVERT S.

sensor a sense organ, or a sensitive device that responds to energy changes.

sensorimotor pertaining to a function that involves sensory (afferent) and motor (efferent) nerve routes; as a noun, the integration of sensation and output of motor activity. The human being obtains data about the world around him through six intake channels: sight, sound, touch, muscle feeling, smell, and taste.

sensorimotor aphasia a combination of sensory, or receptive, and motor, or expressive aphasia, in which there is impairment or loss of ability to perceive and understand as well as to use language. Also called **global aphasia; total aphasia.**

sensorimotor intelligence according to Piaget, knowledge that is obtained from sensory perception and motor actions involving objects in the environment.

sensorimotor stage the first major stage of cognitive development, extending, according to Piaget, from birth through the first two years of life. The s.s. is characterized by the development of sensory and motor processes, and by the infant's first knowledge of the world acquired by interacting with the environment. Some rudimentary awareness of the reality of time, space, and cause and effect is present. For Piaget's other stages of cognitive development, see CONCRETE OPERATIONAL STAGE; PREOPERATIONAL STAGE; FORMAL OPERATIONS.

sensorineural hearing loss the loss or absence of hearing function due to pathology in the inner ear, or along the nerve pathway from the inner ear to the brainstem. Also called **perceptive impairment and nerve loss; sensorineural deafness; nerve deafness.**

sensorineural impairment: See PERCEPTION DEAFNESS.

sensorium the sensory and perceptual mechanism as a whole. The state of the s. is tested during the psychiatric examination to see if it is clear or cloudy, by asking such questions as "Where are we now?", "What are you doing here?", "Who am I?" The term is sometimes used interchangeably with consciousness. Also see CLEAR S.; CLOUDED S.

sensory pertaining to a part or all of the neural apparatus, including supporting structures, involved in the experience of sensation.

sensory acuity the ability to react to stimuli of minimal intensity or duration, and to discriminate minimal differences among stimuli.

sensory adaptation any alteration in a receptor due to increased, decreased, or prolonged stimulation.

sensory amimia: See AMIMIA.

sensory amusia an impairment or loss of the ability to perceive and comprehend musical tones and sequences. See AMUSIA.

sensory aphasia = RECEPTIVE APHASIA.

sensory apraxia = IDEATIONAL APRAXIA.

sensory area an area of the cortex that receives inputs from sensory nerves. Kinds of sensory areas include auditory, somatic, olfactory, and visual.

sensory awareness the ability to perceive sense data, or stimuli, received through the sense organs, such as sights, sounds, and cutaneous sensations.

sensory-awareness groups human-potential groups primarily concerned with increasing the members' awareness of their own feelings and the feelings of others through such means as embracing, learning to "listen with the third ear," free expression of emotion (including punching a pillow or shouting epithets), reenactment of traumatic or peak experiences, and reporting their feelings and bodily sensations at a given moment. See ENCOUNTER GROUP; GESTALT THERAPY.

sensory-awareness procedures the methods used in sensate-focus and similar therapies to help a patient become more acutely aware of his own feelings and sensations and to accept new ways of experiencing feelings and sensations.

sensory capacity the ability of a subject to receive and evaluate inputs from a sense organ. Discriminative learning usually depends upon freedom from any impairments along the sensory pathways, such as the visual sensory system.

sensory conditioning a method of developing stimuli that can be substituted for each other by repeating them as paired stimuli until either will elicit the same response.

sensory-conditioning system = FIRST SIGNALING SYSTEM.

sensory conformance: See CONFORMANCE.

sensory conversion symptoms: See CONVERSION SYMPTOMS.

sensory cortex the parts of the cerebrum that are terminal areas for sensory neurons.

sensory cues stimuli that evoke a response or a behavior pattern. Stimuli that would normally evoke sexual behavior might include visual, tactual, olfactory, or auditory cues. In some instances, only one of the s.c. may be needed as a stimulus.

sensory deficit the loss, absence, or marked impairment of a normal sensory function, such as vision, hearing, or the sense of taste, touch, or smell. The term may also refer to a drive, behavior pattern, or response that seems to result from the lack or absence of stimuli. An example is the nest-building behavior of a bird that appears to be stimulated by nothing more than the lack of a nest. If a nest is removed, it builds another. But it will not build a nest as long as one already exists for it.

sensory deprivation the reduction of sensory stimulation to a minimum; the absence of normal contact with the environment. S.d. may be an experimental procedure to test reactions of subjects in underwater chambers or lightproof and soundproof cubicles; or a real-life situation such as occurs in solitary confinement, deep-sea diving, or loss of eyesight. In any case, such reactions as hallucinations, delusions, panic, hypersuggestibility, and incoherent fantasies may occur. The effects of s.d. vary with the species or organism. A frog may suffer a loss of normal sexual function after visual sensory deprivation, but a human usually would retain the sexual function after loss of vision. Previous learning also can be a factor in effects of s.d.

sensory discrimination the ability to differentiate stimuli; particularly, the degree to which one can distinguish closely related sensory stimuli, e.g., the differentiation among very similar shades of green.

sensory disorders anatomical or physiological abnormalities that interfere with optimum transmission of information from a sense organ to its appropriate reception point in the brain or spinal cord. An auditory sensory disorder, e.g., may be due to an accumulation of ear wax, an infection that involves the middle-ear ossicles, or damage from injury or disease to the cochlear structures. The term refers also to organic or psychogenic disorders of sensory functions, such as anesthesias, paresthesias, or blindness. Also called **sensory disturbances**.

sensory epilepsy a type of petit mal epilepsy usually caused by a temporal-lobe lesion and manifested by paresthesias of all or a part of the opposite side of the body. The seizure may occur without loss of consciousness.

sensory-evoked potentials electrical potentials that can be detected in the cortex when a sensory organ of an anesthetized animal is stimulated. The mapping of s.-e.p. in the cortex helps locate sensory-projection areas for the various sense organs.

sensory exploration: See CURIOSITY.

sensory extinction in neurology, failure to report one of two simultaneously presented sensory stimuli, usually visual or tactile, even though either stimulus presented alone is correctly reported. It is a defect that is likely to occur in occipital-parietal brain lesions. Also see SENSORY INATTENTION.

sensory feedback = BIOFEEDBACK.

sensory field the totality of the stimuli that impinge on a receptor or subject at a given time.

sensory gating = GATING.

sensory habit a learned behavior in which the subject must differentiate between stimuli rather than respond to any of them.

sensory homunculus an imaginary organism that is drawn to the proportional scale of its sensory areas. An animal with a huge olfactory sensory area, e.g., would be shown with a huge nose.

sensory inattention an inability to perceive a stimulus when an identical or similar stimulus is applied to a corresponding part of the body but on the opposite side. The patient may be able to identify a tactual or visual stimulus on either side when only one stimulus is presented. The recognition failure is for the stimulus on the side of the body opposite a brain lesion. The phenomenon of s.i. is utilized in neurological tests. Also called **perceptual rivalry**. Also see SENSORY EXTINCTION.

sensory-information store the memory "storehouse" that processes sensory stimuli utilized in perception. It is believed that most sensory inputs are preserved in storage for only a second or two at the most; e.g., visual inputs are probably stored for less than a second.

sensory input the stimulation of a sensory organ, causing an impulse to travel to its appropriate destination in the brain or spinal cord.

sensory-integrative functioning the normal neural processes involved in perceiving and evaluating sensory inputs from the environment before responsive impulses are transmitted through the motor nerves. Most bodily activities require a combination of motor and s.-i.f.

sensory interaction the integration of sensory processes in performing a task, as in listening to a lecture while looking at the blackboard.

sensory isolation a situation in which sensory stimulation is reduced to such an extent that interpersonal communication is curtailed or absent. See SOCIAL-ISOLATION SYNDROME.

sensory nerve a nerve or bundle of neurons that carry impulses from a receptor to the central nervous system.

sensory organization the process of organizing nerve impulses from receptors into a meaningful perception.

sensory paralysis: See PARALYSIS.

sensory pathways the routes followed by nerve impulses traveling from sense-organ receptors to sensory areas of the brain or other points in the body. Some s.p. can be traced in a living animal by placing electrodes in nerve structures between a sense organ and the brain, then stimulating the receptor while observing potential changes from the electrodes.

sensory polyneuropathy a form of nervous-system disorder that occurs almost exclusively in cases of bronchogenic cancer. It begins as symptoms of peripheral pains and paresthesias and advances progressively toward the central body areas. Eventually, the patient loses all sensation.

sensory-projection area a region of the cerebral cortex where afferent fibers from sense organs terminate.

sensory roots the areas of the spinal cord where sensory-nerve fibers enter the cord. The s.r. are located on either side of the vertebral column, between the vertebrae. As the fibers approach the cord, they come together as a single nerve representing all the sensory receptors for one dermatome or body segment.

sensory self-stimulation the act of stimulating sensory areas of the cortex by control of a device such as a lever that completes an electrical circuit with electrodes implanted in the brain. Also see SELF-STIMULATION MECHANISM.

sensory spots skin spots or locations of high sensitivity to tactile, thermal, or pain stimuli.

sensory stimulation arousal of a sense organ by physical energy, such as light waves which stimulate the retina, sound waves which stimulate the cochlear membrane, or odors which stimulate the olfactory membrane.

sensory system the total structure involved in sensation, including the sense organs, afferent nerves, and sensory areas in the cerebral cortex in which these tracts terminate. These networks may range from rather simple reflex arcs of somatic senses to very complex mechanisms of color vision.

sensory tests tests designed to measure various sensory abilities, such as visual acuity, depth perception, color discrimination, and auditory acuity.

sensual referring to satisfaction obtained from indulging or overindulging in activities that involve the appropriate senses, e.g., sex or food.

sensuous referring to the sensory aspect of an experience or something that is capable of arousing the senses.

sensum = SENSE DATUM.

sensus communis literally, common sense (Latin); according to Aristotle, that which integrates the various sense modalities and enables us to perceive such qualities as unity, motion, rest, time, and shape. He believed the integrating organ was the heart.

sentence-completion test a test in which the subject must complete an unfinished sentence by filling in the missing word or phrase. A specific word or phrase is required if the test is used as an ability test. However, the term also refers to a type of projective test in which the subject is presented with an introductory phrase to which he may respond in any way. As a projective technique, the s.-c.t. is an extension of the word-association test in that responses are free and believed to contain psychologically meaningful material. Also called **incomplete-sentence test**.

sentence-repetition test a test in which the subject must repeat sentences of increasing difficulty and complexity directly after the examiner reads them.

sentience the simplest or most primitive form of cognition, or barely sensing without associating or perceiving.

sentience need H. A. Murray's term for a need to enjoy sights, sounds, and other sensuous experiences.

sentiment an attitude or expression of soft, gentle, subdued emotions.

separate ova a term applying to the release of two or more female gametes from the ovary, or ovaries, at the same time. Simultaneous fertilization of the s.o. usually results in the birth of dizygotic twins.

separation anxiety the normal alarm or fear in a young child separated or facing the prospect of separation from his mother or surrogate mother. S.a. is usually first noted at six months and is most active between six and ten months. Separation from loved ones in later years may elicit similar anxiety, but if excessive fear exists, neurotic attachment is indicated.

separation-anxiety disorder a disorder characterized by excessive anxiety lasting at least two weeks during which separation from attachment figures occurs or is anticipated. The disorder involves such reactions as worry about possible harm to these figures; fear of being lost or kidnaped; reluctance or refusal to go to school, sleep alone, or stay alone; repeated nightmares involving separation; physical complaints on school days; temper tantrums, crying, or pleading; and social withdrawal, sadness, apathy, or difficulty in concentrating. (DSM-III)

separation distress discomfort and anxiety felt by an infant when it loses contact with its attachment figure, usually the mother or mother surrogate. See SEPARATION ANXIETY.

separation-individuation a term used by the psychoanalyst M. S. Mahler for the process in which the infant gradually differentiates himself from the mother and attains the relatively autonomous status of a toddler.

-seps-: See -SEPT-.

sepsis a condition of blood or other tissues contaminated by the presence of pus-forming and other types of pathogenic organisms or the toxic substances produced by such microorganisms. Kinds of s. include **puerperal s.,** in which the source of infection is matter absorbed from the birth canal during childbirth, **intestinal s.,** associated with intestinal sources of toxins, and septicemia, marked by proliferation of bacteria in the blood. See BLOOD-POISONING

sept a subdivision of a clan or a segment of a larger family unit (probably derived from *sect*). A Celtic clan may be composed of several septs which may be affiliated through a common interest rather than a common ancestor. See CLAN.

-sept-; -septi-; -seps- a combining form relating to (a) a partition, (b) putrefactive destruction (sepsis). Adjective: **septic**.

septal area an area of the brain where a triangular double membrane (the septum pellucidum) separates the anterior horns or the lateral ventricles. It contains several nuclear groups and nerve fibers that run to the hypothalamus. Lesions in the s.a. result in a temporary display of very aggressive behavior.

septic: See -SEPT-.

septicemia = BLOOD-POISONING.

septicemia psychosis a form of toxic psychosis associated with a severe infection and characterized primarily by delirium. S.p. technically is an organic brain syndrome with psychotic symptoms secondary to a systemic infection.

septum pellucidum a two-layer membrane separating the two lateral ventricles. It communicates with the corpus callosum and the body of the fornix. See SEPTAL AREA.

Sequard: See BROWN-S.

sequela the residual effects of an illness or injury, particularly effects in the form of persistent or permanent impairment. An example is paralysis that may be the s. of an attack of poliomyelitis. Plural: **sequelae**.

sequence the temporal order in which a series of events occurs. Also see DEVELOPMENTAL SEQUENCE.

sequence preference the tendency of a subject to respond in a particular direction or distinctive manner, e.g., the tendency of an experimental animal to make right turns first and then to alternate left and right turns.

sequential analysis an analysis that is carried out in sequences, usually at each step of a procedure, to determine the acceptability of the data.

sequential design a research design in which subjects of different but overlapping ages are observed and tested for a number of years. By studying several individuals of overlapping ages, the s.d. reduces the amount of time required by a longitudinal study while improving generalizability. In addition, the design is intended to provide greater depth than a cross-section approach.

sequential memory the memory of the proper order of things or concepts. Also called **serial memory**.

sequestration the process of separating the unacceptable or pathological aspects of one's personality from the normal part. E.g., a patient who cannot control his impulses and desires may isolate them from the rest of his self and become totally unaware of them.

-ser-; -sero- a combining form relating to (a) serum, (b) a serous membrane.

serendipity the faculty for making fortunate discoveries by accident; the knack of finding something valuable while looking for something else. S. is often considered a characteristic of a creative scientist. The word was coined by Horace Walpole in 1754, from the title of his earlier story "The Three Princes of Serendip." (Serendip was an old Arabic name for Ceylon—now Sri Lanka—whose princes were said to have had this amiable inclination.)

serenity, tranquillity, peace: See PHENYLETHYLAMINE DERIVATIVES.

serial-anticipation method an alternative term for ANTICIPATION METHOD. See this entry.

serial association a learning technique in which verbal items are learned in a specific order.

serial behavior an integrated sequence of responses that elicit each other in fixed order, e.g., playing music. The individual responses that comprise the sequence are referred to as **serial responses**, that is, responses that occupy specific positions within the behavioral sequence.

serial discriminator = PSYCHERGOGRAPH.

serial-exploration method a method of determining the smallest difference that can be perceived. For details, see JUST-NOTICEABLE-DIFFERENCES METHOD.

serial interpretation a psychoanalytic technique in which the analyst studies a series of consecutive dreams which, when taken as a group, provide clues that would be overlooked in interpretation of a single, isolated dream.

serialization the process of organizing objects along a quantified dimension, e.g., by weight, size, or volume.

serial learning the learning of a sequence of responses in the precise order of their presentation. Each response elicits (becomes a stimulus for) the next response in the series; e.g., actors employ s.l. as they learn their parts. **Serial memorization** refers to memorizing a sequence of responses in precise order. Also called **serial-order learning**.

serial memory = SEQUENTIAL MEMORY.

serial-memory search a retrieval process in which

each item in short-term memory is examined in the order in which it was encoded.

serial-order learning = SERIAL LEARNING.

serial-position effect in serial learning tasks, the effect of an item's position on how well or how fast it is learned. Items near the beginning of a list are usually remembered most effectively while items in the middle are usually learned least well.

serial processing a theory of information processing stating that very rapid shifting between different information sources accounts for the apparent ability to carry on separate cognitive functions simultaneously. According to this view, two sets of stimuli cannot be processed simultaneously. Also called **intermittent processing**. Compare PARALLEL PROCESSING.

serial reinforcement a serial-learning technique in which each correct response increases the probability of the correct response occurring again.

serial responses: See SERIAL BEHAVIOR.

seriation the process of arranging data into an ordered series for analysis and interpretation.

sermon fear = HOMILOPHOBIA.

Sernyl a trademark for a brand of phencyclidine hydrochloride, an anesthetic with hallucinogenic properties sometimes taken as a drug of abuse. See PHENCYCLIDINE.

serotonergic neurons neurons that contain serotonin or are activated by the substance.

serotonin a neurotransmitter substance derived from the essential amino acid tryptophan and found in the blood, nerve cells, and other tissues. S. also functions as a smooth-muscle stimulator and a constrictor of blood vessels. Brain levels of s. have been associated with mental disorders such as schizophrenia. Also called **hydroxytryptamine; 5-hydroxytryptamine**.

serotonin inhibitors adrenergic blocking agents that are useful in the control of migraine symptoms because they exert an antiserotonin action. Like the ergot derivatives, the s.i. administered for migraine analgesia are related chemically to lysergic acid. The group includes **methyergol carbamide maleate**—$C_{24}H_{30}N_4O_5$—and METHYSERGIDE. See this entry.

serotonin receptors receptors found in the brain and in peripheral areas, with sensitivities that vary according to blocker susceptibility. Some brain s.r. are, e.g., blocked by lysergic acid diethylamide and some are not. One type of brain s.r. also mediates postsynaptic potentials while the other kind does not. Different types of s.r. also are found in the smooth muscles of the intestine.

serous otitis media the result of an inflammatory process whereby fluid, or serum, collects in the middle ear due to a lack of normal pressure in the middle ear which forces serum to exude from the mucous membrane. It produces a conductive-hearing impairment; and it may involve as the main symptom a blocked Eustachian tube.

Sertoli, Enrico Italian histologist, 1842–1910. See SERTOLI CELLS; SUSTENACULAR CELLS.

Sertoli cells elongated supporting cells of the lining of the seminiferous tubules. As the spermatozoa approach maturity, they become oriented in the seminiferous tubules so that they are partly imbedded in the S.c.

serum glutamic oxalacetic transaminase: See GLUTAMIC OXALACETIC TRANSAMINASE.

servomechanism a mechanism in which control is effected by a device or devices that automatically change or correct, or help to change or correct, the performance of certain functions according to a predetermined setting or manipulation. E.g., a torpedo keeps itself on beam by utilizing stimuli, or input, coming from the target as well as information from its own output.

set a fixed pattern of behavior or responses, such as a predictable sequence of motor-neuron activity; also, a temporary readiness to respond in a certain way to a specific situation or stimulus. A motorist gets set to move ahead when the light changes (motor set); a sleeping mother is set to awaken when her baby cries (perceptual set); a bridge player is set to obey the rules of the game—a mental set. See MOTOR SET; PERCEPTUAL SET; MENTAL SET.

seventh cranial nerve = FACIAL NERVE.

severe mental retardation a diagnostic category applying to persons with IQs of 20 to 30, comprising about seven percent of the retarded population. These individuals cannot acquire any academic skills and frequently have sensory and motor defects. However, they are able to talk, and can be taught to dress and feed and take of themselves, and can be trained to perform simple work under close supervision. (DSM-III)

sex the physical and mental traits that distinguish between males and females; also, the physiological and psychological processes related to procreation and erotic pleasure. (The term is derived from the Latin word *sexus*, with the original meaning of "division, *section*," and related to *secare*, "to cut.")

sex-appropriate behavior: See SEX-TYPING.

sex change the alteration of a patient's sex characteristics in order to make them resemble as closely as possible the physical traits of the opposite sex. S.c. is accomplished with surgery and hormone treatments. The changes are limited to external appearances and do not affect the patient's inherent reproductive role or genotype, which were determined before birth. Also see METAMORPHOSIS SEXUALIS PARANOICA.

sex characteristics the traits associated with gender identity. **Primary s.c.** include traits directly involved in reproduction of the species, e.g., gonads. **Secondary s.c.** are features not directly concerned with reproduction, such as the presence or absence of facial hair, voice quality, and breasts.

sex chromatin a chromatin mass that is observed in the nucleus of tissue cells of females during interphase. The substance represents X-chromosome material that is not involved in tissue-cell metabolism. The presence of sex chromatin in tissue cells is generally regarded as proof of the sexual identity of females. Also called **Barr body**.

sex-chromosomal aberrations structural or functional disorders, or both, that are associated with the complete or partial absence of a sex chromosome or with extra sex chromosomes. Examples include hermaphrodites with XX and XY mosaicism, Klinefelter's syndrome, and males with XYY sex-chromosome combinations rather than a normal XY complement.

sex chromosomes the chromosomes that carry the traits identifying males and females. An individual usually is considered to be a female if the body cells contain the XX combination of chromosomes, and male if the cells contain the XY combination, regardless of physical traits or signs of hermaphroditism.

sex counseling = SEXUAL COUNSELING.

sex determination the genetic mechanism that determines the sex of the offspring. E.g., in humans a fertilized egg with two XX chromosomes becomes a female, and an egg with one X and one Y becomes a male.

sex differentiation the process of acquiring distinctive sexual features during the course of development. Human s.d. is determined genetically at the time of fertilization although the anatomical differences do not begin to appear until the seventh week of development. Because bisexual behavior is common among animals regardless of levels of male or female sex hormones, it is assumed that nervous structures for both sexes are present in all members of a species.

sex discrimination as usually interpreted, discrimination against women in hiring practices, work roles, and wage levels, and acceptance of mothers in the work force. Many aspects of this situation are being reevaluated and are changing under the impact of such factors as the women's liberation movement, postponement of marriage, availability of day-care facilities, increased educational opportunities, role changes in the home, and manpower shortages in certain industries.

sex distribution = SEX RATIO.

sex drive = SEXUAL DRIVE.

sex education a formal course of instruction in reproductive processes presented in a classroom setting. S.e. ideally supplements information about sexual functions as explained by parents and peers and is handled in a frank, open communication manner that permits young adolescents to obtain authoritative and objective information about both the psychological and physical aspects of sex.

sex fear = GENOPHOBIA.

sex feeling the pleasurable feeling associated with coitus or other sexual contact.

sex hormones the hormones that stimulate various reproductive functions. Primary sources of the s.h. are the pituitary gland and the male and female gonads. Kinds of s.h. include androsterone, testosterone, estrone, estriol, estradiol, progesterone, and prolactin.

sex hygiene the health-maintenance procedures, including disease prevention, related to sexual activity, e.g., venereal-disease control.

sex identification the gradual adoption of the attitudes and behavior patterns associated with one or the other sex. A clear concept of sexual identity gradually develops out of a perception of physical sex differences, starting during the first three or four years of life, and, somewhat later, awareness of psychological differences determined by the particular culture and particular family. Confusion about sexual identity may give rise to serious psychological problems. See SEX ROLES.

sex identity = SEXUAL IDENTITY.

sex-influenced character an inherited trait that is dominant in one sex but recessive in the other, e.g., male balding patterns.

sex instincts = SEXUAL INSTINCTS.

sex interest a readiness to engage or participate in discussions, viewing, or other activities related to or leading to sexual contact.

sexism discriminatory and prejudicial beliefs and practices directed against one of the two sexes, usually against women. A **sexist** culture assigns predetermined economic, social, familial, and emotional roles to men and women not on the basis of individual skills but rather on the basis of sexual stereotypes that are inculcated by sex-role socialization, reinforced by economic and social organization, and justified by reference to women's reproductive role as child-bearer.

sex-limited characteristic of a trait or anomaly that affects only one sex.

sex object = SEXUAL OBJECT.

sex offenders persons who have been apprehended and convicted of committing a sex act that is prohibited by local laws. S.o. are not necessarily sexual deviates or psychologically disturbed individuals since the local law may ban fornication, obscenity, or discussing the "facts of life" with children, which in a different culture or community would be considered as normal activities, as opposed to more serious SEX OFFENSES. See this entry.

sex offenses sex acts that are prohibited by laws in most countries of the western world. Examples of s.o. include forcible and statutory rape, incest, adultery, prostitution and pimping, bestiality, sodomy, sex murder, and forcible sexual assault without coitus. Also called **sexual offenses**. Also see MOLESTATION.

sexological examination the study of an individual's sexual behavior in terms of physiological, psychological, sociological, and specific genetic and environmental influences.

sexology the study of sexual relations, particularly among humans, including the anatomy, physiology, and psychology of sexual activity and reproduction. Also see SIECUS.

sex perversion = SEXUAL PERVERSION.

sex preselection predetermination of the sex of offspring through sex-control technology.

sex ratio the proportion of male and female infants born in a given population. The average s.r. is about 106 boys per 100 girls at birth; because of the higher mortality ratio of males, the proportion becomes reversed in later life. Also called **sex distribution**.

sex rehabilitation = SEXUAL REHABILITATION.

sex reversal a procedure in which the physical features of one sex are established in an adult hermaphrodite, usually by surgery supported by hormones and other techniques. See SEX CHANGE.

sex rivalry any behavior that tends to favor one sex as superior to the other; also, the competition between a parent and child of the same sex for the affections of the other parent.

sex-role inversion an abnormal behavior pattern marked by female-to-male or male-to-female transfer of gender roles. Severe gender-identity problems generally result from the psychological absence of the mother during early development of a girl or psychological absence of a role-model father during early development of a boy. A parent may be physically present but fail to provide the role-model guidance of a "father image" or "mother image."

sex roles the behavior and attitudinal patterns characteristically associated with masculinity and femininity as defined in a given society. S.r. reflect the interaction between biological heritage and the pressures of socialization. Usually, the term refers to overt behavior and must be distinguished from gender or psychosexual identity, although the two usually match. The extent to which an individual manifests typical sex-role behavior varies greatly according to familial and cultural influences. See GENDER IDENTITY.

sex-role stereotypes fixed, simplified concepts of the traits and behavior patterns believed to be typical of each sex.

sex selection = SEXUAL SELECTION.

sex sensations the effects of tactile stimulation of the genitalia and other erogenous zones.

sex service: See PROSTITUTION.

sex therapy the treatment of psychosexual disorders with techniques that vary with the problem and its severity. S.t. generally requires psychological or psychiatric treatment, often including behavior-therapy methods, as well as correction of misinformation and teaching the patient the basic facts about sex anatomy, physiology, and techniques.

sex trauma = SEXUAL TRAUMA.

sex-typed denoting the labeling process whereby certain characteristics or responses are categorized as masculine or feminine in accordance with prevailing sex-role stereotypes. See SEX-TYPING.

sex-typing any form of behavior or any attitude that results from social programing regarding appropriate male and female behavior. S.-t. studies reveal that young children of both sexes favor masculine games and toys, but girls increasingly direct their interests to feminine activities as they grow older. Boys consistently show greater concern for **sex-appropriate behavior**, presumably due to stronger cultural prohibitions against behavior that appears to undermine or contradict cultural definitions of masculinity.

sexual adjustment the process of establishing a satisfactory relationship with one or more sexual partners. S.a. may depend upon varied psychological as well as physical factors, e.g., female characteristics in the voice of a virile male could affect his s.a.

sexual aggression: See ANIMAL AGGRESSION.

sexual anesthesia an absence of normal sensation associated with coitus. S.a. usually is psychogenic and associated with unpleasant heterosexual intercourse experiences. Evidence of the functional nature of s.a. is observed in the fact that most patients report they obtain sexual pleasure in masturbation. Also see FRIGIDITY.

sexual anomaly a congenital or developmental abnormality of the reproductive system, e.g., the presence of both male and female gonads in an infant.

sexual arousal stimulation of the reproductive organs by mental influences such as sexual dreams or fantasies, by erotic odors, or by sexual contact resulting in CNS impulses transmitted to the sacral region of the spinal cord. The impulses also trigger the release of sex hormones, dilation of the arteries supplying the genital areas, and inhibition of vasoconstrictor centers of the lumbar nerves. The s.a. effects are mediated through the hypothalamus, which can be stimulated in monkeys to produce sexual behavior including penile erection in males. Lesions in the anterior hypothalamus usually eliminate sexual interest. See SEXUAL-RESPONSE CYCLE.

sexual assault the forced participation of an unwilling party in sexual activity by the use of physical violence or direct or implied threats. S.a. may involve actual physical contact such as rape or acts of exhibitionism or indecent exposure between adults and children.

sexual attitudes a conscious or unconscious predisposition or readiness to act or react in specific ways toward sex, usually manifested in a person's individual sexual behavior which in turn has evolved from his or her sex education, both formal and informal, and from prior sexual experience.

sexual behavior a pattern of activity related to reproduction of the species or to stimulation of the sex organs for pleasurable satisfaction without the objective of reproduction. S.b. may include orientation of the partners in some form of courtship, postural accommodations for intercourse, and genital reflexes. In some species, s.b. may occur only at certain seasons or at specific stages of estrus cycles. The onset of s.b. in humans usually occurs during puberty.

sexual change = SEX CHANGE.

sexual characteristics = SEX CHARACTERISTICS.

sexual contact any person-to-person contact that involves touching or connection of genital or erogenous skin or membrane surfaces, as in kissing, biting, coitus, or fondling.

sexual counseling guidance provided by therapists to sex partners in such matters as impotence, frigidity, birth control, infertility, and general feelings of inadequate sexual performance.

sexual curiosity a form of curiosity that comprises an integral part of the forepleasure phase of the sexual act, though in the neurotic it may be sufficient to produce sexual gratification, or end-pleasure, by itself. Some psychoanalysts claim that s.c. can be sublimated into a drive to acquire knowledge, and that if it is repressed it might inhibit intellectual curiosity.

sexual delusion a false belief maintained despite evidence to the contrary regarding one's sexual identity, appearance, practices, or attitudes.

sexual development the progressive steps toward sexual maturity, including attitudes and behavior as well as physical characteristics, from infancy through puberty. Also see PSYCHOSEXUAL DEVELOPMENT.

sexual deviancy any sexual behavior that is regarded as significantly different from the standards established by a local culture or subculture. Deviant forms of sexual behavior may include homosexuali.y, voyeurism, fetishism, bestiality, necrophilia, transvestitism, sadism, and exhibitionism. In the Shaker subculture, all sexual activity was considered deviant. The corresponding term in DSM-III is "psychosexual disorders.' Also called **sexual deviation**. See PARAPHILIAS; PERVERSION; PSYCHOSEXUAL DISORDERS.

sexual differentiation = SEX DIFFERENTIATION.

sexual discrimination = SEX DISCRIMINATION.

sexual disorders any physical or psychological impairment of the ability to perform coitus or produce offspring. The term usually is applied to functional disorders, such as impotence or frigidity, but not to psychosexual behaviors such as rape, incest, sadism, or sodomy.

sexual drive a primary drive, or impulse, directed to sexual gratification and, ultimately, to reproduction. Unlike other drives described as primary, such as hunger and thirst, the individual's survival does not depend on it, though survival of the species does; also, s.d. is more dependent on experience, learning, and external stimulation. In higher species, such as man, this drive is less seasonal, less dependent on the estrous cycle, more varied in expression, more subject to cortical control, and aroused by a wider variety of stimuli than in the lower species. Also called **sex drive**. See SEXUAL INSTINCTS.

sexual dysfunction a lack or loss of ability to participate in normal sexual activity, such as coitus. Causes of s.d. may be psychological or physiological, or both.

sexual education = SEX EDUCATION.

sexual expectations: See SEXUAL SCRIPT.

sexual feeling = SEX FEELING.

sexual functioning the performance of sexual intercourse; or the capability of performing sexual intercourse.

sexual history the collection of information relating to a patient's sexual behavior as a part of developing a case history. Because many cases of mental disorder involve a disturbed sexual relationship, the s.h. often leads to an understanding of the patient's conflicts.

sexual hygiene = SEX HYGIENE.

sexual identification = SEX IDENTIFICATION.

sexual identity the individual's biologically determined sexual state; the internal sense of maleness or femaleness. Also see GENDER IDENTITY.

sexual infantilism the tendency of a mature person to engage in sexual behavior characteristic of a small child. S.i. may be manifested in certain forms of psychosexual disorders such as voyeurism, fetishism, or lovemaking that is limited to foreplay acts of kissing, biting, or stroking the skin.

sexual inhibition an unconscious suppression of the sexual impulse; especially the inability to feel sexual desire, to perform sexually, or to experience sexual gratification, due to such factors as fear of inadequacy or feelings of guilt implanted by parents. See INHIBITED SEXUAL DESIRE; INHIBITED SEXUAL EXCITEMENT; INHIBITED FEMALE ORGASM; INHIBITED MALE ORGASM.

sexual instincts in psychoanalysis, a term applied to all erotic drives and sublimations of these drives, including not only genital sex, but anal and oral manifestations, the self-preservative impulses of hunger, thirst, and elimination, and the channeling of erotic, or libidinal, energy into artistic and scientific pursuits.

sexual intercourse = COITUS.

sexual interest = SEX INTEREST.

sexual inversion = INVERSION.

sexuality the capacity to derive pleasure from sexual stimulation, and particularly from sexual intercourse. In psychoanalysis, the term is broadly applied to "organ pleasure" derived from all erogenous zones and processes of the body, including the mouth, anus, urethra, breasts, skin, muscles, and genital organs, as well as such functions as sucking, biting, eating, defecating, urinating, masturbation, and intercourse. In addition, s. includes all types of behavior into which sexual energy is sublimated, as in creative art and scientific investigation.

sexualization in psychoanalysis, the process of investing sexual energy in an organ or function. In the course of development, different parts of the body (mouth, nipples, hands, ears) and different activities (dancing, joking, clay-modeling) may become sexualized. The process may also occur on a completely indirect and unconscious level: Some psychoanalysts interpret in sexual terms the satisfaction we experience from obsessional thinking, exhibitionistic public speeches, and masochistic atonement for our errors.

sexual life-style the individual pattern of sexual behavior that evolves from early childhood observations and experiences with male and female contacts, modified by additional observations and experiences acquired through adolescence and early maturity.

sexually transmissible disease = VENEREAL DISEASE.

sexual masochism a psychosexual disorder in which sexual excitement is repeatedly or exclusively achieved through being humiliated, bound, beaten, or otherwise made to suffer, or through intentional participation in an activity that involves being subjected to physical harm or threat to life. (DSM-III)

sexual maturation the stage of development of the reproductive system at which coitus and reproduction can be achieved.

sexual negativism a term introduced by Magnus Hirschfeld to identify a lack of interest in sex that could be attributed to a deficit of sexual hormones.

sexual object a person, animal, or inanimate object toward which the sexual energy of an individual is directed. The s.o. is an object that is external to the individual's own body or psyche. Also called **sex object**.

sexual offenders = SEX OFFENDERS.

sexual offenses = SEX OFFENSES.

sexual orgasm: See ORGASM.

sexual orientation the dominant sexual behavior pattern of an individual, specifically, a preference for sexual activities with persons of the same or opposite sex, or both.

sexual-orientation disturbance an obsolete diagnostic category replaced in DSM-III by EGO-DYSTONIC HOMOSEXUALITY. See this entry.

sexual perversion any sexual practice that is regarded by the community or subculture as an abnormal means of achieving orgasm or sexual arousal. In some cultures, s.p. is applied to any practice other than penile-vaginal intercourse between an adult female and her husband. See PARAPHILIAS.

sexual reflex penile erection produced by stimulation of the male genitalia; clitoral and secretion response produced by stimulation of the female genitalia; also, reflex activity involved in orgasm. Also see SEXUAL REFLEXES.

sexual reflexes components of sexual behavior, such as the cremasteric reflex, that are not under direct control of the higher brain levels and may be stimulated through spinal or bulbar neural connections. Also see SEXUAL REFLEX.

sexual rehabilitation restoration of an individual's ability to enjoy normal sexual activity following

correction of a dysfunction, such as impotence or rape-trauma syndrome.

sexual response reaction to sexual stimulation. Initial s.r. in a female is marked by erection of the nipples. In the male, the most noticeable s.r. is erection of the penis.

sexual-response cycle both men and women exhibit a four-stage s.-r.c., differing mainly in manifestations characteristic of the sex. The stages include **excitement phase**, lasting several minutes to hours, **plateau phase**, 30 seconds to three minutes, **orgasmic phase**, 15 seconds, and **resolution phase**, lasting from 15 minutes to one day, the shorter period being associated with absence of an orgasm. Also see SEXUAL AROUSAL; ORGASM.

sexual rivalry = SEX RIVALRY.

sexual roles = SEX ROLES.

sexual sadism a psychosexual disorder in which sexual excitement is achieved by intentional infliction of physical or psychological suffering on another person. The harm may be inflicted on a nonconsenting partner or, in the case of a consenting partner, may take the form of either simulated or mildly injurious bodily suffering combined with humiliation; or it may involve extensive, permanent, or possibly fatal bodily injury when practiced with nonconsenting partners. The latter activity is likely to be repeated until the individual is apprehended; and in the most severe cases the individual may rape, torture, or kill the victim. (DSM-III)

sexual script the expectations an individual has about sexual feelings, roles, behavior, and relationships; the associated attitudes that define one's general orientation to sexuality. Sexual expectations are learned or acquired in the process of socialization and thus reflect the influences of culture, family, and individual experience.

sexual selection the selection of individuals of the opposite sex for the purpose of producing offspring who will continue the survival of the species. Among animals and many humans, the process tends to favor the reproduction of individuals with traits that are most likely to prove attractive to members of the opposite sex.

sexual sensations = SEX SENSATIONS.

sexual stimulation = GENITAL STIMULATION.

sexual synergism the sexual arousal that results from a combination of stimuli experienced at the same time. The term may be applied to situations in which the stimuli might appear to be somewhat contradictory, such as love and hate, fear, pain, or fright.

sexual tension a condition of anxiety and restlessness associated with the sex drive and a normal desire for release of sexual energy. S.t. may be complicated by fear of inadequate performance, fear of an unwanted pregnancy, fear of discovery, or other concerns.

sexual trauma any disturbing experience associated with sexual activity. Rape, incest, and other sexual offenses may be a cause of s.t. in older children and adults. Freud associated childhood s.t. with psychoneurosis in later life.

sexual-value system the system of sexual stimulation and response that an individual feels is necessary for a satisfactory sexual relationship.

sexual vandalism a morbid impulse to destroy the erogenous zones of figures portrayed in illustrations and statues.

s factor a designated *specific* or *special* factor found in factor analysis of ability tests. The s f. for a particular test represents the specific ability required to do well in that area.

SGOT: See GLUTAMIC OXALACETIC TRANSAMINASE.

shadow according to Jung, an archetype that represents instincts inherited from lower organisms, mainly sexual and aggressive instincts, which tend to be unacceptable to the conscious ego and are therefore repressed into the personal unconscious where they may form complexes.

Shaker subculture: See SEXUAL DEVIANCY.

shaking palsy an obsolescent term for paralysis agitans, or PARKINSONISM. See this entry.

shallowness of affect impaired ability to react emotionally; extreme apathy and indifference even in situations that usually arouse intense feeling. It is a common symptom of schizophrenia.

shallow side: See VISUAL CLIFF.

shaman /shä′mən/ a "medicine man" or priest, mainly of one of the religions of northern Asia, who uses allegedly supernatural or magical powers to cure mental or physical illness. Also called **witch doctor**.

sham disorders: See FACTITIOUS DISORDERS.

shame a painful feeling of humiliation associated with guilt, immodesty, dishonorable behavior, or not living up to one's own expectations. Psychoanalysts believe s. frequently stems from an unconscious fear of sexual exposure or is a defense against exhibitionistic tendencies which conflict with the superego or might bring scorn or ridicule from society.

shame-aversion therapy a type of behavior therapy in which the behavior, usually a sexual deviation, is demonstrated before a neutral audience with the assumption that the patient will feel shame.

shamelessness a character trait that is interpreted by Fenichel and others as a reaction formation to unconscious feelings of shame, that is, going to the opposite extreme in order to deny shame. Extreme s. and immodesty are frequently observed in mania and general paresis, disorders in which normal cortical control is suspended.

sham operation in animal research, a control surgical procedure similar to the experimental operation, but leaving intact a structure removed by the experimental operation. This procedure controls for the stress of the experimental operation.

sham rage manifestations of rage such as growling, spitting, scratching, or biting that are elicited from an animal without emotional inputs. The behavior can be demonstrated in animals that have undergone surgical interruption of neural control above the middle brain. It is assumed that higher CNS influence is required for true rage. Also see PSEUDOAFFECTIVE BEHAVIOR.

shape the spatial form of an object as it stands out from its background.

shape constancy the type of perceptual or object constancy in which an object is perceived as having the same shape when viewed at different angles, e.g., the common observation that a plate viewed at an angle still appears circular, not elliptical. Also see PERCEPTUAL CONSTANCY.

shaping an operant-conditioning procedure in which behavior is modified by the step-by-step reinforcement of closer and closer approximations to the desired response. It is a behavior therapy technique devised by B. F. Skinner. Also called **approximation conditioning; behavior-shaping**. See BEHAVIOR THERAPY. Also see METHOD OF SUCCESSIVE APPROXIMATIONS.

shared paranoid disorder a disorder characterized by a persecutory delusional system that develops as a result of a close relationship with another person or persons who have this disorder. The delusional beliefs usually diminish or disappear if the relationship is terminated. Although more than two persons may be involved, s.p.d. is often called FOLIE À DEUX. See this entry. (DSM-III)

sharpening a phenomenon in which some details of a memory are omitted while others are more sharply defined and accentuated than in the original experience.

Sheehan, Harold Leeming English pathologist, fl. 1937, 1964. See HYPOPHYSEAL CACHEXIA (there: **Sheehan's syndrome**).

Sheldon, Joseph Harold English pediatrician, fl. 1920, 1964. See FREEMAN-SHELDON SYNDROME.

Sheldon, William H. American psychologist, 1898–1970. S. developed a constitutional typology in which individuals are rated according to three dimensions of physique (endomorphic, mesomorphic, ectomorphic) and three dimensions of temperament (viscerotonic, somatotonic, cerebrotonic), which he then related to psychiatric categories and delinquency. See SHELDON'S CONSTITUTIONAL THEORY OF PERSONALITY; APOPLECTIC TYPE; CEREBROTONIA; CONSTITUTIONAL TYPE; ECTOMORPH; ENDOMORPH; MESOMORPH; PERSONALITY STRUCTURE; PERSONALITY TYPES.

Sheldon's constitutional theory of personality a concept by W. H. Sheldon that every person possesses some degree of three primary temperamental components that relate to three basic body builds, or somatotypes, measured along a seven-point scale. The three body types, ectomorphy, endomorphy, and mesomorphy, are correlated with the three components of temperament, termed cerebrotonia, viscerotonia, and somatotonia. Constitution provides a substructure, but nutrition and early experiences also influence the physique and temperament, respectively.

shell shock an obsolete World War I term for an acute mental disorder resulting from combat experience, and characterized by such symptoms as tremors, paralysis, and confusion. The disorder was attributed solely to minor brain hemorrhages or brain concussion due to exploding shells and bombs, without involving psychological factors. For later terms, see COMBAT FATIGUE; WAR NEUROSIS.

shelter care provision of a placement unit for the custody, care, and management of children considered unmanageable in the community, and involved in court and child-welfare services. Such facilities are usually operated by private organizations under contract with a government agency, but are often inadequately staffed and pay little attention to emotional problems. Other shelter services are provided by sheltered workshops, halfway houses, and ex-patient clubs such as Alcoholics Anonymous.

sheltered workshop a work-oriented rehabilitation facility with a controlled working environment and individual vocational goals, which utilizes work experience and related services for assisting the handicapped person to progress toward normal living and a productive vocational status.

Sherrington, Charles Scott English physiologist, 1861–1952. Sherrington's research, carried out at Cambridge, is responsible for most of our basic knowledge of nerve activity, including the many types of reflexes, the functions of the synapse, the summation of stimuli, and the effects of drugs and fatigue on nerve impulses. See RECIPROCAL INHIBITION.

shift work work scheduled during the swing shift (usually 4 P.M. to 12 A.M.) or night shift 12 to 8 A.M.). Studies show wide variations in the attitudes of employees and their ability to adjust their circadian rhythms and adapt to changes in sleep, meals, digestion, and social patterns during these work shifts. See CIRCADIAN RHYTHMS.

shinecock: See CATNIP.

shish-kebab operation = RODDING OPERATION.

Shneidman, Edwin S. American thanatologist and suicidologist, 1918—. See MAKE A PICTURE STORY.

shock fear = HORMEPHOBIA.

shock psychosis a war-time reaction of combat soldiers who are overcome by shock or fright and experience delusions in which everything and everybody in the environment is regarded as hostile. Wild motor activity, mutism, sleep disturbances, depression, and immobility were among the effects observed after hospitalization. Rehabilitation included relearning sphincter control and ability to speak and feed themselves.

shock reaction an acute emotional disturbance occurring immediately after a traumatic event, such as a car accident or natural catastrophe. During this so-called "shock stage" (Raker, 1956), the victim is usually so dazed and stunned that he is unaware of the extent of his injuries, and in extreme cases may become stuporous, disorganized, and amnesic for the precipitating event. Also see DISASTER SYNDROME.

shock stage: See SHOCK REACTION; DISASTER SYNDROME.

shock treatment in psychiatry, treatment of severe mental disorders by administering a drug such as insulin or an electric current to the brain to induce loss of consciousness or convulsions. Also called **shock therapy.** See ELECTROCONVULSIVE TREATMENT; INSULIN-COMA THERAPY.

shoe anesthesia: See GLOVE ANESTHESIA.

shoe fetishism: See RETIFISM.

shook yong = KORO.

short-acting barbiturates: See SHORT-TO-INTERMEDIATE-ACTING BARBITURATES.

short-answer test an objective test utilizing such techniques as multiple choice, fill-in, true-false, and matching alternatives instead of requiring lengthy or complex answers.

short-circuit appeal the use of emotional rather than intellectual appeals to arouse an audience.

short-circuiting the development of a shorter neural pathway as a result of practice which lowers its excitability threshold.

short-stare epilepsy one of three subdivisions of petit mal epilepsy, the others being myoclonic and akinetic epilepsy. The patient stops and stares uncomprehendingly for a moment or two.

short-term memory the reproduction, recognition, or recall of a limited amount of material after a period of about ten seconds. It is frequently tested in intelligence or organicity evaluations. Abbrev.: **STM.** See IMMEDIATE MEMORY; LONG-TERM MEMORY.

short-term therapy brief psychotherapy aimed at assistance with emotional problems and maladjustments during a period of weeks rather than months. Short-term approaches may be applied on a deeper level, as in hypnoanalysis and narcosynthesis; on a level of emotional reeducation; or on a more symptomatic level, as in reconditioning and other forms of behavior therapy. Also called **brief psychotherapy.** See BEHAVIOR THERAPY; DIRECTIVE COUNSELING; GOAL-LIMITED THERAPY; HYPNOTHERAPY; NARCOTHERAPY; REALITY THERAPY; SECTOR THERAPY.

short-to-intermediate-acting barbiturates a category of barbiturates based on rates of action, including onset of effect, absorption, and excretion. A short-acting barbiturate may produce effects in as little as one or two minutes whereas an intermediate-acting barbiturate may require five to ten minutes to achieve the same effect, and long-acting barbiturates may take more than 20 minutes. Thiopental sodium and pentobarbital are ultrashort-acting and short-acting, aprobarbital and vinbarbital are intermediate-acting barbiturates. Classifications of the barbiturates as to rate of action are based on animal experiments and radioactive-tracer studies and may not be fully applicable to clinical use with individual patients.

shrink: See HEAD-SHRINKING.

shunting the diversion of blood or cerebrospinal fluid from one part of an organ or body to another. The process may occur naturally as a result of a congenital defect or as a result of a surgical procedure as in the artificial s. of cerebrospinal fluid from the brain to the external jugular vein to relieve symptoms of hydrocephalus.

shut-in personality a withdrawn, isolated, asocial type of individual, common among persons who become schizophrenic. This type is also described as schizoid.

shuttle box a multicompartment box used for avoidance-conditioning research. Performance of animals in the s.b. varies with different types of CNS lesions; e.g., ablation of one side of the neocortex or a particular sensory area may affect acquisition or retention of conditioned responses. See SHUTTLE-RESPONSE METHOD.

shuttle-response method avoidance conditioning in which the animal must shuttle from one compartment of a cage or box to another to avoid a shock. The compartments are separated by a swinging door, hurdle, or some other obvious dividing line. See SHUTTLE BOX.

shyness disorder a disorder characterized by avoidance of other people, or excessive discomfort, embarrassment, and inhibition in the presence of others. See AVOIDANT DISORDER OF CHILDHOOD OR ADOLESCENCE.

-sial-; -sialo- a combining form relating to saliva.

Siamese twins a term applied to any anomaly of monozygotic twins whose bodies fail to separate completely during embryonic life. The result is a teratomorph at birth of two conjoined bodies that may be separated by surgery, or variations of one body with two heads or four legs, or two individuals with shared vital organs, or some other combination. The term is derived from a famous set of S.t., Eng and Chang (1811–74), who were born in Thailand (Siam) and exhibited in sideshows. Their livers and hepatic vessels communicated, and they shared one umbilicus; yet they led a relatively normal life, married two sisters, and had more than 20 children between them. (Many of their descendants, all entirely normal, live in North Carolina to this day.)

sibilant a fricative produced by forcing the air through an opening between the tongue and the roof of the mouth, e.g., /s/, /z/, or /sh/.

sibling one of two or more children born of the same two parents. In strict usage, the term applies only to full brothers and sisters and excludes children born simultaneously, e.g., twins.

sibling rivalry competition among siblings for the attention, approval, or affection of one or both parents, or for other recognition or rewards, as in sports or school grades.

sibship method a technique used in genetics, particularly in determining inherited psychiatric factors, in which the incidence of a mental disorder among blood relatives is compared with the distribution of the disorder in the general population. S.m. studies have found a higher incidence of schizophrenia in twins and close family members than in the general population.

sick headache = MIGRAINE.

sickle-cell anemia a severe chronic form of anemia marked by joint pain, fever, weakness, thrombosis, and infarctions. It is caused by the presence of crescent-shaped red blood cells that are distorted and fragile. The condition—which afflicts mainly individuals of African descent—is due to inheritance of a genetic trait that produces hemoglobin S (Hb S), in which there is an error in the arrangement of amino acids in the hemoglobin molecule so that valine occurs in the position normally occupied by glutamic acid. Also see BLOOD DISORDER; HEMOGLOBINOPATHIES.

sick role the protective role provided a person who is physically or mentally ill or injured as a matter of common social custom.

s.i.d. an abbreviation used in prescriptions, meaning "once a day" (Latin *semel in die* /dē′ā/).

side effects additional, and usually undesirable, reactions that may occur following administration of a drug. S.e. can occur (a) as a result of an interaction between drugs with opposing effects, because of an additive or synergistic effect of drugs with the same or similar effects, (b) as an allergic reaction or extreme sensitivity of a patient due to genetic or other factors, or (c), in some cases, as an emotional effect.

-sider-; -sidero- a combining form relating (a) to iron (from Greek *sideros*, "iron"), (b) to the stars or destiny (from Latin *sidus*, "star, constellation, destiny").

siderodromophobia a morbid fear of railroads or of traveling by train (from Greek *sideros*, "iron," and *dromos*, "course, running").

siderophobia a morbid fear of the stars or any evil that might come down from them (from Latin *sidus*, "star, constellation, destiny"). Also see URANOPHOBIA.

Sidman avoidance schedule an avoidance-conditioning technique in which a subject learns to avoid an adverse effect without an external signal, e.g., by pressing a lever repeatedly to delay a shock indefinitely. Also called **free operant avoidance**.

SIDS: See CRIB DEATH.

SIECUS /sē′kəs/ *S*ex *I*nformation and *E*ducation *C*ouncil of the *U*nited *S*tates, a nonprofit health organization (New York City). Its aim is "to establish man's sexuality as a health entity; to identify the special characteristics that distinguish it from . . . human reproduction"; and to give aid "toward responsible use of the sexual faculty and toward assimilation of sex into . . . individual life patterns as a creative and recreative force."

sig. an abbreviation used in prescriptions, meaning "write on label" (Latin *signa*).

sighting line a visual axis that extends along a line from a point of fixation to the point of clearest vision on the retina.

sight method a reading technique in which a student is taught to recognize entire words rather than parts of words that represent sounds. Compare PHONICS.

sight words in reading, words that are recognized instantly without additional analysis.

sigma /sig′mə/ 18th letter of the Greek alphabet (Σ, σ, ς).

sigmation = INTERDENTAL SIGMATISM.

sigmatism = LISPING.

sign an objective, observable indication of a disorder or disease. Also see SOFT S.

signal a stimulus pattern leading to a response; also, a sign communicated from one individual or electromagnetic device to another.

signal anxiety in psychoanalysis, a reaction in which anxiety is a sign or anticipation of impending threat, either from internal or external sources. It serves the purpose of warning the individual to mobilize his resources in order to deal with danger through fight, flight, or surrender.

signal-detection task an experimental task consisting of several trials in which the subject attempts to detect weak auditory signals embedded in noise backgrounds. See DETECTION THEORY.

signal-detection theory = DETECTION THEORY.

signaling system a stimulus pattern that serves to arouse a response. In explaining the functioning of the nervous system, Pavlov distinguished between the first signaling system, or sensory conditioning system, which enables the organism to adapt to changes by "tying" the original unconditioned reflex to environment signals (a deer, e.g., learns to react by fleeing when he scents a predatory animal); and a second signaling system involving language, which makes it possible for the individual to think before acting and to generalize from experience. Also see FIRST S.S.; SECOND S.S.

sign Gestalt Tolman's term for a cognitive process consisting of a learned relationship between an environmental cue and a subject's expectations.

significance in statistics, a measure of the probability that a result is due to chance. Statistical s. at the one-percent or .01 level means that there is one chance in 100 that a result is due to chance, but does not necessarily imply importance or meaningfulness of the result. Also see TEST OF S.

significant others a term coined by H. S. Sullivan for individuals such as parents and teachers who have a profound influence on our emotional security and interpersonal relations.

sign language communication with and among the deaf by means of hand or body movements representing ideas, actions, or objects. See FINGER SPELLING.

sign-significance relation expectancy of a given phenomenon.

sign stimulus = RELEASER.

sign system a term used by Schilder to characterize psychotherapy since it depends upon language as the major tool for exploring and understanding the hidden causes of a patient's problems, and gaining access to his inner personality.

sign test a statistical test in which cases are classified into two groups (e.g., present versus absent, or above versus below mean), and this classification is tested for deviation from a chance distribution.

silence deliberate muteness on the part of a patient in analysis, in contrast to mutism, which may be due to organic or psychological causes. S. of this kind may indicate that the patient's emotional responses are temporarily blocked by internal conflicts and acute anxiety. S. may also be a form of unconscious resistance to the therapy, or hostility (negative transference) to the therapist. See MUTISM; RESISTANCE.

Silver, Henry K. American pediatrician, 1918—. See SILVER-RUSSELL SYNDROME.

silver-cord syndrome a parental relationship in which the father is absent or passive and the mother is domineering. The family pattern is believed to increase susceptibility of the offspring to development of schizophrenia. See SCHIZOPHRENOGENIC MOTHER.

silver-fork deformity an orthopedic disorder of the wrist, involving the distal end of the radius bone of the lower arm which displaces the wrist backward. The disorder, sometimes identified as a **Colles' fracture**, may result from a sports injury or workplace accident.

silver nitrate AgNO₃—a topical antiinfective medication applied to the eyes of newborn infants to prevent **ophthalmia neonatorum**, an acute form of conjunctivitis. The disease is contracted during birth from the vaginal discharge of a mother infected with gonorrhea.

Silver-Russell syndrome a congenital disorder characterized by short stature, hemihypertrophy, and elevated urinary gonadotropin hormones without precocious sexual maturity. Motor development often is delayed because of muscle weakness. Physical features include **pseudohydrocephalus**, a condition of normal head circumference but a small face, giving the appearance of an enlarged head. Various studies have found a higher-than-average incidence of mental retardation among the patients. Also called **Silver's syndrome; Russell's dwarf**.

silver stain a tissue dye used in histological studies of neurons. The s.s. contains a silver salt that marks the location of neurons as black lines against white or transparent neighboring tissues, which will not absorb the silver salt. The technique is similar to that of making photographs with films and papers impregnated with silver salts.

similarities: See DISCRIMINATION.

similarities test a test in which the subject must either state the likenesses between items or arrange items in categories according to their similarities.

similarity paradox = SKAGGS-ROBINSON HYPOTHESIS.

Simmonds, Morris German physician, 1855–1925. See SIMMONDS' DISEASE; HYPOPHYSEAL CACHEXIA.

Simmonds' disease a pituitary-gland disorder caused by necrosis of adenohypophysis tissue. Failure of the anterior portion of the pituitary, which may be partial or complete, causes secondary failure of the gonads, adrenal cortex, and thyroid gland which depend upon the hormonal stimulation of the pituitary. Anorexia, atrophy of sexual features, absence of libido, hypotension, bradycardia, and hypoglycemia are symptoms of the disorder.

Simon, Théodore /simôN'/ French psychologist, 1873–1961. See BINET TEST (there: **Binet-Simon test**); STANFORD-BINET INTELLIGENCE SCALE. Also see BINET.

simple depression = MILD DEPRESSION.

simple mastectomy: See MASTECTOMY.

simple phobia an anxiety disorder characterized by a persistent, irrational fear of specific objects such as knives, or specific animals (e.g., dogs, snakes, insects, mice), or specific situations (e.g., heights, closed spaces), together with a compelling desire to avoid these sources of distress, and a recognition that the fear is excessive or unreasonable. See PHOBIA. (DSM-III)

simple schizophrenia one of the four major types of schizophrenia described by Kraepelin and Bleuler, and characterized primarily by gradual withdrawal from social contact, lack of initiative, and emotional apathy.

simple structure a set of criteria for adequacy of a rotated factor-analytic solution. These criteria call for each factor to show a pattern of high loadings on some variables, and near-zero loadings on others, with each factor showing a different pattern. This arrangement makes each factor as clear-cut as possible. These criteria were developed by Thurstone.

simple tone: See PURE TONE.

simple type: See AGGRESSIVE TYPES.

simulated environment = SIMULATION.

simulated family a teaching technique in which hypothetical family situations are enacted by clinicians or other professional persons. The method is also used in family therapy, with one or more members of the family participating along with others who play the roles of other family members.

simulation an experimental method used to investigate the psychological mechanisms and processes of individuals in real social environments by "simulating" those environments in a realistic way, usually through role-playing by subjects informed about the purposes of the research. Simulated encounters provide the opportunity to explore psychosocial determinants of behavior in environments and institutions to which investigators can not gain access easily, e.g., prisons. Also called **simulated environment**.

simulator a training device, e.g., a Link trainer, that resembles the actual equipment to be used.

simulator-real model: See REAL-SIMULATOR MODEL.

simultanagnosia an impairment in the ability to perceive or integrate visual stimuli appearing simultaneously, possibly due to a lesion in the anterior portion of the left occipital lobe. An example is ability to name the objects represented in a picture but not the action that is taking place.

simultaneous conditioning a classical-conditioning technique in which the conditioned stimulus and the unconditioned stimulus are presented together or in which the conditioned stimulus is presented a second or two before the unconditioned stimulus and continues until the unconditioned stimulus is presented.

simultaneous contrast: See COLOR CONTRAST; CONTRAST EFFECT.

simultaneous fertilization the fertilization of more than one ovum at approximately the same time by the spermatozoa of one or more males. Also see SUPERFECUNDATION.

sin: See DELUSION OF SIN AND GUILT.

sine /sē'nā/ or /sīn'ə/ a term used in prescriptions, meaning "without" (Latin).

Sinemet a trademark for a drug combination of **levadopa** and **carbidopa**, used in the treatment of Parkinson's disease.

sine wave a theoretical shape of a sound wave or electromagnetic wave as plotted on a graph with rectangular coordinates. The plot shows a curve that gradually increases to a maximum point then falls to a minimum point over the time span of one cycle. A pure s.w. may not be observed in clinical research because of modifying influences on recordings.

single blind an experimental condition in which the subject or patient, but not the experimenter or physician, is unaware of the experimental treatment, manipulation, or drug administered. Also see DOUBLE BLIND.

single-case experimental design in behavior therapy, a method of investigating treatment techniques and their effects by focusing on changes in the behavior of individual clients, as contrasted with group research and average change among many clients. The individual serves as his own control. This approach usually involves a number of observations obtained at different times. Also called **single-subject design; intrasubject replication design**.

single-episode depression: See MAJOR DEPRESSION.

single-gene defect: See GENETIC DEFECT.

single-major-locus model a mode of inheritance in which only two alleles are believed to be involved in manifestation of the trait in question, that is, the normal allele and abnormal allele responsible for the trait. Abbrev.: **SML**.

single-room occupancy a term referring to the splitting of a large, frequently dilapidated building into one-room units occupied by persons who often include the mentally ill, addicts, physically disabled, and eccentric individuals who are reduced to living solitary, dehumanized lives with no ties to the community and its activities. Abbrev.: **SRO**.

single-subject design = SINGLE-CASE EXPERIMENTAL DESIGN.

sing-song theory: See ORIGIN-OF-LANGUAGE THEORIES.

-sinistr-; -sinistro- a combining form relating to the left side (from Latin *sinister*, "left, on the left").

sinistrality a tendency or preference to be left-handed or to use the left side of the body in motor activities. Also see LEFT-HANDEDNESS.

sinning-fear = ENOSIOPHOBIA; PECCATOPHOBIA.

sissa = CITTOSIS.

sissy behavior: See TOMBOYISM.

-sito- a combining form relating to food (from Greek *sitos*, "wheat, corn, meal").

sitophobia a morbid fear of food. Also called **sitiophobia; cibophobia**. Also see PHAGOPHOBIA.

sitting-fear = THAASSOPHOBIA. Also see KATHISOPHOBIA.

situated identities the theory that one takes on different social roles in different social settings; that is, one's appropriate role or behavior pattern shifts according to the situation. Also see EXTRAINDIVIDUAL BEHAVIOR.

situational analysis a method of studying behavior in a natural setting, as opposed to a laboratory.

situational attribution the ascription of external or circumstantial causes to one's own or another's behavior. Also called **environmental attribution**. See ATTRIBUTION THEORY. Compare DISPOSITIONAL ATTRIBUTION.

situational conditions in educational psychology, all the relevant external variables within the classroom setting that influence students' learning and achievement, e.g., physical environment, social relationships, goals, organization of material, teaching methods, time factors, methods of testing, consequences of performance, and type of reinforcement.

situational crisis = ACCIDENTAL CRISIS.

situational determinants the environmental conditions that exist before and after a behavioral activity and which serve as the basis of behavior assessment.

situational homosexuality homosexual activity that develops from a more or less transient situation or environment. S.h. may occur in a prison, school, or military setting where individuals are segregated according to their sex. Also see PSEUDOHOMOSEXUALITY; FAUTE DE MIEUX; OCCASIONAL INVERSION.

situationalism the concept that the environment and situational factors are of primary importance as determinants of behavior. Also called **situationism**.

situational orgasmic dysfunction the inability of a woman to experience orgasm with a particular sex partner or in a particular situation.

situational psychosis a severe but temporary disturbance involving such symptoms as delusions and hallucinations, resulting from a traumatic situation such as imprisonment. Also called **reactive psychosis**.

situational reaction a disturbance precipitated by severe, disrupting conditions of life as opposed to unconscious conflicts or other internal sources of maladjustment. See TRANSIENT SITUATIONAL DISTURBANCE.

situational restraint a form of restraint that depends upon environmental arrangements (screens on windows, immovable furniture) so that the risk of dangerous or destructive acts by patients will be minimized, as opposed to physical restraint of the individual.

situational sampling the observation of an individual in significant real situations as part of the study of his behavior.

situational-stress test a situation test with stress as an integral component. See SITUATION TEST.

situational test = SITUATION TEST.

situational therapy = ENVIRONMENTAL THERAPY.

situation ethics: See MORAL RELATIVISM.

situationism = SITUATIONALISM.

situation neurosis a neurosis that is induced by a situation, usually a highly stressful situation such as rape or combat, as opposed to a character neurosis with roots in a childhood personality disturbance.

situation set a state of readiness for a situation, e.g., preparation for an expected thunderstorm.

situation test a test that places a subject in a natural setting or in an experimental setting that approximates a natural one to test either the ability to solve a problem that requires adaptive behavior under stressful conditions or to test reactions to what is believed to be a stressful experience. E.g., a course of desensitization therapy aimed at reducing phobic reactions might begin with a s.t. in which the individual encounters the phobic object. The subject's reactions are then assessed and considered in relation to individual needs for a specific therapy program. Also called **situational test**.

Six-Hour Retarded Child a child mistakenly judged to be retarded or a slow learner in school (for about six hours a day) while functioning well outside in a complex social world without any signs of retardation. This mistake—which often leads to a lifelong programing for failure—is made by middle-class teachers and psychologists who fail to realize that the child simply may not have middle-class habits such as sitting still and following instructions. See IQ.

Sixteen D scale an IQ scale based on a multiple of the standard deviation of the mean score on other tests at age 16. Also spelled **16-D scale**.

Sixteen Personality Factor Questionnaire a comprehensive personality inventory developed by Cattell and his associates for ages 16 and over, yielding 16 scores on various traits: aloof versus warm, submissive versus dominant, glum versus enthusiastic, emotional versus calm, reserved versus outgoing, humble versus assertive, shy versus venturesome, trusting versus suspicious.

sixth cranial nerve = ABDUCENS NERVE.

size-age confusion the tendency to assume that children who are larger than normal for their age also will be more mature.

size constancy the awareness that objects do not change size when the retinal image changes as they move closer or farther away. S.c. has been demonstrated in infants as young as two months, and also in fish, ducklings, kitttens, and monkeys. Also see PERCEPTUAL CONSTANCY.

size discrimination the ability to distinguish differences in the sizes of objects. The ability depends, in the absence of visual clues, on tactile sensation, which can be affected by lesions in either hemisphere but mainly by lesions in the right hemisphere. Micropsia and macropsia may be caused by temporal-lobe epilepsy.

size perception: See RETINAL SIZE.

size-weight illusion the tendency to equate weight with size; the tendency to perceive an object of larger dimensions as having greater weight than an equally heavy but smaller object.

Sjögren, Torsten Swedish physician, 1896—. See SJÖGREN-LARSSON SYNDROME; MARINESCO-SJÖGREN SYNDROME; ASCORBIC ACID.

Sjögren-Larsson syndrome an autosomal-recessive condition of scaly skin, spasticity, and mental retardation. Sweat glands are sparse or deficient. The scaliness varies in specific cases among populations from different regions of the world.

Skaggs, Ernest Burton American psychologist, fl. 1923, 1947. See SKAGGS-ROBINSON HYPOTHESIS.

Skaggs-Robinson hypothesis the hypothesis that in learning identical materials, one set enhances the retention of the other, but as the materials become dissimilar, one interferes with the retention of the other—however, when the materials are completely dissimilar, retention increases again, but not to the level achieved when the materials were identical. Also called **similarity paradox**.

skeletal muscles the muscles that provide the force to move a part of the skeleton. S.m. are attached to the bones by tendons and usually span a joint so that one end of the muscle is attached through a tendon to one bone and the other end of the s.m. to another bone. S.m. occur in reciprocal pairs so that a bone can be moved in opposite directions. Also called **voluntary muscles**.

skeletal-system deformity any structural or functional defect that interferes with normal actions of the bones, the muscles, and the nerves supplying the muscles. The term usually is applied to the spinal column and the limbs, and may include disorders such as osteoporosis, achondroplasia, Marfan's syndrome, torticollis, acromegaly, clubfoot, clawhand, and scoliosis.

skelic index the ratio between length of the legs and length of the trunk. The s.i. is used in anthropometry.

Skene, Alexander Johnston Chalmers Scottish-born American gynecologist, 1838–1900. See SKENE'S GLANDS.

Skene's glands small mucous glands that open into the female urethra near the orifice. They are regarded as homologous to the prostate gland of the male.

skewness a measure of the deviation from normality of a distribution of scores, in which cases pile up at one extreme of the distribution and are reduced at the other extreme. Adjective: **skewed**.

-skia- a combining form relating to shadow (Greek *skia*).

skiascope an instrument for measuring the refractive condition of the eye. Also called **sciascope**.

skid row a deteriorated area comprising shoddy bars, shabby hotels, and cheap luncheonettes frequented by alcoholics and vagrants.

skill an acquired high-order ability to perform complex motor acts smoothly and precisely.

skilled-nursing facility a nursing home or similar extended-care facility that provides continuous nursing service on a 24-hour basis. The nursing care may be administered by registered nurses, licensed practical nurses, and nursing aides as directed by a licensed physician. A s.-n.f. emphasizes medical nursing care with restorative therapy, physical therapy, occupational therapy, and other special services. Abbrev.: **SNF**.

skimming a rapid, somewhat superficial, reading of material to get the general idea of the content.

skin the external covering of the body, consisting of an outer layer (epidermis) and a deeper layer (dermis) resting on a layer of subcutaneous tissue.

skin cancer any malignant tumor involving the skin cells. Most kinds of s.c. are **melanomas**, formed from pigment-producing melanocytes, **squamous-cell carcinomas** that originate on the surface and ulcerate inward, and **basal cell papillomas** that begin beneath the surface of the skin and erupt over the surface. Contrary to popular belief, skin cancers can metastasize and spread to other body areas; e.g., melanomas can evolve from moles and migrate to produce lung cancer.

skin-disease fear = DERMATOSIOPHOBIA.

skin disorders in psychiatry, skin conditions exacerbated by or resulting from internal conflicts and emotional situations, e.g., hives, urticaria, eczema, pruritus, and neurodermatitis. Attempts have been made to explain these conditions in terms of such concepts as self-punishment (e.g., scratching oneself), expressions of hostility, acute stress, threatening situations, sexual conflicts (e.g., itching in the genital region), or marital irritations (ring-finger dermatitis). For a dramatic illustration, see STIGMATA.

skin eroticism sexual pleasure derived from stroking, rubbing, or licking the skin, especially during the forepleasure stage of sexual excitement. Painful stimulation of the skin is basic in masochism. According to Freud, the skin is the erotogenic zone par excellence (1905).

skin-injury fear = DERMATOPHOBIA.

Skinner, Burrhus Frederic American psychologist, 1904—. S. is known chiefly for studies of operant conditioning and its application to language, learning, educational methods, psychotherapy, and cultural analysis. See SKINNER BOX; BEHAVIOR ANALYSIS; DESCRIPTIVE BEHAVIORISM; DRL; EXPERIMENTAL ANALYSIS OF BEHAVIOR; MAND FUNCTION; OPERANT CONDITIONING; RADICAL BEHAVIORISM; RESPONDENT CONDITIONING; SHAPING; TEACHING MACHINE.

Skinner box a box with a bar or lever at one end in which a laboratory animal can be placed for operant-conditioning experiments. The animal must learn to operate the bar or lever in order to receive rewards or avoid punishment. The laboratory device was introduced by B. F. Skinner in the 1950s and has been modified in many ways for specific types of experiments although the basic principle of the apparatus is unchanged.

skin-popping a street-slang term for injection of narcotics into the skin, as opposed to mainlining, or injecting into a vein.

skin receptors nerve endings in the skin that respond to pain, pressure, temperature, or other stimuli.

skin-sensory spots areas of the skin that contain nerve endings for stimuli such as heat, cold, pain, and touch. Some areas of the skin have a greater concentration of s.-s.s. than others. E.g., the fingertips are likely to have more s.-s.s. per square centimeter than the skin of the back.

skin stimulation a cutaneous sensation experienced as pain, pressure, cold, warmth, tickle, or itch through nerve receptors in the skin.

Skoptsy a religious sect (from Russian *skopets*, "eunuch") whose members practice a castration ritual based on their interpretation of a passage in the Book of Saint Matthew (19:12) regarding eunuchs. In their first degree of castration, called the small seal, the scrotum and testicles are removed. The second stage, or grand seal, requires removal also of the penis. Women members of the sect, which originated in Russia, also participate in ceremonies that include removal of the breasts or genital excisions.

skull-lifting headache: See LEAD-CAP HEADACHE.

skull trephining: See TREPHINATION.

skyscraper fear: See BATOPHOBIA.

slashers: See CUTTING.

Slavson, Samuel Richard Russian-born American psychotherapist, 1890—. See ACTIVITY GROUP THERAPY; ACTIVITY-INTERVIEW GROUP PSYCHOTHERAPY; ANALYTIC GROUP PSYCHOTHERAPY; COLLECTIVE EXPERIENCE; DIRECTIVE GROUP PSYCHOTHERAPY; IDENTIFICATION TRANSFERENCE; INTERVIEW GROUP THERAPY; LIBIDO-BINDING ACTIVITY; MULTIPOLARITY; NEUTRALITY; NEUTRALIZER; PLAYGROUP PSYCHOTHERAPY; SUPPORTIVE EGO.

SLE: See LUPUS ERYTHEMATOSUS.

sleep a state of the organism characterized by partial or total suspension of consciousness, muscular relaxation and inactivity, reduced metabolism, and relative insensitivity to stimulation. See ACTIVATED S.; CONTINUOUS-S. THERAPY; DELTA-WAVE S.; DESYNCHRONIZED S.; DREAM STATE; HYPOSOMNIA; MONOPHASIC S. RHYTHM; NEUROTIC-S. ATTACKS; NREM S.; ORTHODOX S.; PARADOXICAL S.; PARASOMNIA; POLYPHASIC S. RHYTHM; SYNCHRONIZED S.; TEMPLE S.; TWILIGHT S.

sleep apnea: See APNEA.

sleep center a nucleus in the hypothalamus which, when stimulated, induces sleep.

sleep characteristics the conditions of mental and somatic rest that include reduced levels of certain physiological activities, increased thresholds of many reflexes and responses to stimulation, and amnesia for events occurring during the loss of consciousness associated with sleep. The s.c. help distinguish normal sleep from a loss of consciousness due to injury, disease, or drugs.

sleep deprivation deliberate prevention of sleep, usually for experimental purposes, but also used as a form of punishment or a means of exacting a "confession" from a prisoner. Studies show that the loss of one night's sleep does not have a substantial effect on physical or mental functioning, and subjects kept awake for 30 to 60 hours show little impairment in performing novel or challenging tasks, but cannot tolerate boring tasks such as keeping watch. After this, speech begins to be slurred and performance on psychological tests becomes increasingly poor. Many of the symptoms of psychosis, such as disorientation, detachment from reality, perceptual distortion, and paranoid reactions, appear after six or seven days without sleep.

sleep disorders disordered sleep or disorders occurring during sleep, including INSOMNIA, HYPERSOMNIA, NARCOLEPSY, NIGHTMARE, SLEEP-TERROR DISORDER, NOCTURNAL ENURESIS, NOCTURNAL MYOCLONUS, PHASE SHIFT, APNEA, SLEEP-WALKING DISORDER, and EKBOM'S SYNDROME. See these entries.

sleep drive the basic physiological urge to sleep, which appears to be governed, at least in part, by sleep and waking centers in the hypothalamus, and by deactivation of the reticular activating system. The s.d. does not vary materially from the general average of eight hours per night, since one rarely finds a person in good health who requires less than six hours or more than nine hours. The deepest and most restorative sleep occurs in the first four hours, and periods of light sleep, during which we usually dream, occur approximately every 90 minutes, mostly in the last four hours.

sleep drunkenness a state of being half-awake and half-asleep, with normal orientation absent while the mind is under the influence of nightmarish thoughts. Some individuals become dangerously violent during this state and may inflict injury on persons nearby. The condition was formerly called **somnolentia**.

sleep epilepsy an obsolete term for narcolepsy.

sleeper effect the observation that a persuasive communication reaches its maximum effect after a delay.

sleep fear = HYPNOPHOBIA.

sleepiness: See SOMNOLENCE.

sleeping sickness: See HYPERSOMNIA.

sleep inversion a tendency to sleep or somnolence by day and to remain awake at night when not required by one's work schedule. S.i. is frequently observed in patients with schizophrenia or organic brain damage.

sleeplessness: See INSOMNIA.

sleep paralysis = NOCTURNAL HEMIPLEGIA.

sleep patterns habitual, individual patterns of sleep such as two four-hour periods, daytime napping, various forms of insomnia (initial, intermittent, matutinal), or excessive sleep as a means of evading reality or regressing to an infantile state.

sleep research ongoing research on such questions as sleep stages, REM versus NREM sleep, phasic activity, the reticular activating system, EEG-wave patterns, sleep deprivation, dream deprivation, dream interpretation, circadian rhythms, and sleep disorders.

sleep rhythm = SLEEP-WAKE CYCLE.

sleep spindles an EEG pattern that is observed during the first few minutes of sleep when the relatively slow alpha-wave pattern changes suddenly to bursts of waves with a frequency of about 15 spikes per second. The bursts of rapid EEG waves are the spindles, indicating a state of light sleep.

sleep stages the five-step progression that, according to EEG recordings, occurs in a normal night's sleep. Stage zero, characterized by a waking alpha rhythm (ten cycles per second), is followed by stage-1 sleep, marked by drowsiness and irregular low-voltage waves of four to six cycles per second with rolling eyeball movements; stage 2 is characterized by sleep spindles at 12 to 14 cycles per second and high-voltage slow-wave complexes; in stages 3 and 4, waves of one to two cycles per second predominate. These stages comprise orthodox sleep (or NREM, slow-wave, or synchronized sleep), and are interspersed with periods of paradoxical sleep (or REM, desynchronized, or activated sleep) accompanied by a low-voltage EEG with waves of four to ten cycles per second and frequent bursts of conjugate rapid eye movements associated with dreaming.

sleep state: See DREAM STATE; W-STATE.

sleep talking verbalization during sleep, either in the form of mumbling or an approximation of waking speech. S.t. usually but not always occurs during NREM sleep, and the sleeper is sometimes responsive to questions or commands. It is not considered pathological in most cases, and occurs at one time or another in the majority of persons.

sleep-terror disorder a sleep disorder characterized by repeated episodes of abrupt awakening from NREM, delta-wave sleep with signs of extreme panic and intense anxiety, such as screaming, profuse perspiration, a frightened expression, dilated pupils, and rapid breathing and heartbeat. Efforts to comfort the individual are unavailing until the agitation and confusion subside, and only fragmentary dream images of threatening nature can be recalled. Also called **pavor nocturnus; night terror**. Also see NIGHT-MARE. (DSM-III)

sleep treatment the use of prolonged sleep as a psychiatric modality, usually in cases of agitated depression, manic excitement, and acute anxiety neurosis. S.t. has a long history, dating back to the Egyptians and, later, the Greeks who prescribed "temple sleep" for both mental and physical disorders. In the 1920s, Jacob Klaesi used barbiturates and other drugs to keep schizophrenic patients asleep for eight to ten days, calling the technique **prolonged narcosis**. The technique, which is rarely used today, was often called continuous-sleep therapy. Also see TEMPLE SLEEP.

sleep-wake cycle the natural process of brain-controlled bodily rhythms that results in alternate periods of sleep and wakefulness. The patterns vary with animal species; rabbits, rats, and other rodents tend to follow polyphasic sleep-wake cycles, with six or more short periods of sleep each 24-hour period. Humans, as well as canaries and snakes, tend to have monophasic sleep-wake cycles, with one long period of sleep and one long period of wakefulness each day. The s.-w.c. may be disrupted by such factors as flights across time zones, switching to daylight saving time and back, changing from a day to a swing or night shift and back, drug use, and space flight. Periods of stress or extreme boredom, as well as manic and depressive episodes, also disrupt the cycle. Also called **sleep-wakefulness cycle; sleep rhythm**. See MONOPHASIC SLEEP RHYTHM; POLYPHASIC SLEEP RHYTHM.

sleepwalking disorder a disorder occurring repeatedly during NREM, delta-wave sleep: The individual sits up, picks at the blanket, then gets up and walks about or opens doors, eats, etc., for up to a half hour. If challenged, the **sleepwalker** will stare blankly and unresponsively, and can be awakened only with great difficulty. The episode will not be remembered the next morning. Also called **somnambulism; noctambulation**. See NREM SLEEP; DELTA WAVES. Also see MONOIDEIC SOMNAMBULISM. (DSM-III)

slice-of-life commercials: See NONOVERT APPEALS.

slip of the pen = LAPSUS CALAMI.

slip of the tongue = LAPSUS LINGUAE.

slippage: See COGNITIVE S.

slipped disk a condition in which one of the cartilage disks separating two adjacent vertebrae slips out of its normal position. The displaced disk may press on the spinal cord or a nerve root, causing severe pain. The s.d. usually is corrected by surgery unless it returns to its normal position by other therapies, such as prolonged bed rest. Also see RADICULOPATHIES.

slipped epiphysis the displacement of the cartilage head of the femur, or thigh bone, from its normal position near the hip socket. The disorder may occur in growing children, and the onset usually is marked by a sudden pain and limp. The s.e. can be manipulated back into its normal position in some cases or corrected with KNOLLS PINS. See this entry.

slogans phrases developed as attention-getting advertising devices that are associated with product images. S. also help the consumer recall the name of a product brand, as in "good to the last drop" for Maxwell House Coffee, or "99 and 44/100 percent pure" for Ivory Soap. S. may be revised periodically as a result of continuing studies of consumer psychology. E.g., Coca-Cola in 1982 introduced "Coke is it," as a successor to "it's the real thing," "I'd like to buy the world a Coke," and others, including "thirst knows no season" in 1923 and "delicious and refreshing" in 1904.

slow learner the child of somewhat lower-than-average intelligence, usually measured at 80 to 95 on IQ tests. Slow learners are estimated at 15 to 17 percent of the average school population. They do not show marked variations from physical, social, and emotional norms and are usually placed in regular classes. The term is often imprecisely applied to the educable mentally retarded as well as children of normal capacity whose intellectual progress is nonetheless slow. Also see MENTAL RETARDATION.

slow virus a virus that may be present in the body for many years before producing clinical signs or symptoms. A s.v. theory is employed to explain the development of several degenerative brain diseases such as kuru and Creutzfeldt-Jakob disease, which develop long after exposure to known sources of infection.

slow waves = DELTA WAVES.

slow-wave sleep a stage of deep sleep that is characterized by slow, synchronous EEG waves. It is controlled by serotonin-rich cells in the brainstem; increased levels of serotonin stimulate s.-w.s. while abnormally low levels of the substance result in insomnia. S.-w.s. has a restorative function that helps eliminate feelings of fatigue. See DELTA-WAVE SLEEP.

S-M: See SADOMASOCHISTIC RELATIONSHIP.

small-for-dates a phrase indicating that a baby is underweight for his GESTATIONAL AGE. See this entry.

small-object fear = MICROPHOBIA.

small-penis complex an emotional concern by some males that they possess a penis too small to give a female partner adequate sexual satisfaction. The s.-p.c. often is given impetus by the visual distortion that results when the male looks downward toward his genitals, a perspective that can make an average penis appear smaller than average.

small-sample theory a concept that population or other data can be extrapolated from a small number of cases if certain mathematical techniques are used.

smegma a thick, cheesy residue of secretions of Tyson's glands, or the glandulae preputiales, of the corona glandis of the penis and the inner surface of the prepuce. These sebaceous secretions sometimes accumulate under the foreskin of the penis or in the area of the clitoris.

smell the olfactory sensation that enables an organism to detect particles of substances in inhaled air; also, the odors themselves. Molecules of odorous chemicals are carried by air currents to olfactory receptors where they are dissolved in mucus and analyzed in a manner similar to the way that taste buds evaluate flavors. See OLFACTION; S. MECHANISM; ODOR.

smell mechanism the sense of smell originating in olfactory receptors which extend numerous cilia into the mucosal layer in the roof of the nasal cavity. The cilia, along with villi of supporting tissue cells, form a feltlike layer if hairlike projections. Ions of molecules of substances carried to the olfactory mucosa by air currents stimulate the receptors which carry impulses in axonal bundles through tiny holes in the bony layer separating the base of the skull from the nasal cavity. On the top surface of the perforated bony layer, the cribiform plate, rests the olfactory bulb which receives the impulses and sends them on to the telencephalon through the olfactory nerve. Also see INFRARED-THEORY OF SMELL; STERIC THEORY OF ODOR; RAMAN SHIFT.

smell prism = ODOR PRISM.

Smets, G. Belgian psychologist, fl. 1973. See SMETS-PATTERN RESPONSES.

Smets-pattern responses responses by test subjects to Smets patterns, or checkerboard patterns in which the checkered elements have been rearranged. The various patterns contain from 64 to 900 elements, or grains. The subjects are asked to judge the patterns for beauty, visual discomfort, or other factors.

Smirnov, Nikolai Vasilevich Russian mathematician, 1900—. See KOLMOGOROV-SMIRNOV TEST.

Smith, David W. American pediatrician, 1921—. See SMITH-LEMLI-OPITZ SYNDROME.

Smith-Lemli-Opitz syndrome an autosomal-recessive disorder marked by microcephaly, broad, short nose, syndactyly, polydactyly, and mental retardation. Nearly all male S.-L.-O.s. patients have hypospadias or other genital anomalies while females have no obvious abnormalities of the external genitalia, a factor that led early investigators to believe erroneously that the syndrome affected only males.

SML = SINGLE-MAJOR-LOCUS MODEL.

smoking the act of drawing the smoke of burning tobacco or other substances, such as marijuana, into the mouth or lungs. The motives for s. cigarettes, cigars, or pipes range widely: relaxation of tension; having something to do with the hands; a means of curbing appetite; the sociable thing to do; and, according to some psychoanalysts, erotic pleasure derived from oral stimulation. Also, in view of statistics on lung cancer and other serious disorders, heavy smoking may reflect a self-destructive impulse. See TOBACCO DEPENDENCE; TOBACCO WITHDRAWAL.

smooth curve a curve with little if any deviation in direction.

smoothed curve a curve that has been adjusted to eliminate erratic or sudden changes in slope, so that its fundamental shape and direction will be evident.

smooth muscles muscles that are short-fibered and under control of the autonomic nervous system. They function primarily as involuntary muscles, and are able to remain in a contracted state for long periods of time or maintain a pattern of rhythmic contractions indefinitely without fatigue. Smooth-muscle tissues are found in the digestive organs and the muscles of the eyes. Unlike skeletal muscles, they do not require exercise. Also called **involuntary muscles**.

smooth-pursuit eye movements normal eye movements that present a disordered pattern in 70 to 80 percent of schizophrenic patients and 45 to 50 percent of their first-degree relatives, but only in six percent of normal subjects. The schizophrenic patterns are believed to be due to dysfunction in the area of the reticular activating system.

smothering-fear = PNIGEROPHOBIA.

snake phobia = OPHIDIOPHOBIA.

snake symbol in psychoanalysis, the penis. The s.s. is frequently found in dreams and in primitive rites and art productions in which it probably represents life. Also see OPHIDIOPHILIA; OPHIDIOPHOBIA.

SNE = SUBACUTE NECROTIZING ENCEPHALOMYELOPATHY.

Snellen, Hermann Dutch ophthalmologist, 1834–1908. See SNELLEN CHART.

Snellen chart a device for testing visual acuity, consisting of printed letters ranging in size from very small to very large and read by the subject at a given distance. Also called **Snellen test**.

SNF = SKILLED-NURSING FACILITY.

sniffing of chemicals: See VOLATILE-CHEMICAL INHALATION.

sniff sign a term used to identify a type of breathing experienced by persons with tracheal tumors who inhale with small, sharp, sniffing breaths. The s.s. is an example of an organic disorder that often is mistaken as a symptom of a psychiatric condition.

snow = COCAINE.

snow blindness a visual distortion caused by exposure to extreme intensities of white light, marked by photophobia, an illusion that all objects are red, or a temporary loss of vision.

snow fear = CHIONOPHOBIA.

SOAP /sōp/ an acronym for the four aspects of the progress notes on a problem-oriented record (POR): S for subjective report, O for objective findings, A for assessment of the patient's response, and P for plan, or statement of what is to be done about the problem.

sobbing: See CRYING.

sociability the need or tendency to seek out companions, friends, and social relationships. See AFFILIATION.

sociability rating an evaluation of an individual's degree of sociability based on the amount of time devoted to social activities.

sociable type: See SOCIAL TYPE.

social action a group action that is directed to achieve social benefits for the community or a segment of the population.

social-action program a planned and organized effort to change some phase of society, such as enactment of gun-control legislation or initiating improvements in mental hospitals.

social activities events that bring individuals together in a pleasurable environment, e.g., dancing, singing, games, or cocktail parties. S.a. are frequently a part of the rehabilitation process for mentally or physically disabled persons because of their need to experience contacts with other individuals of their community in order to gain self-confidence, self-acceptance, and self-esteem.

social adaptation an adequate adjustment to the demands, restrictions, and mores of a particular society, including the ability to live and work with others in a reasonably harmonious manner, and to carry on social interactions and relationships that are satisfying to oneself as well as others. Also called **social adjustment**.

social-adequacy index = SAI.

social adjustment = SOCIAL ADAPTATION.

social age: See VINELAND SOCIAL MATURITY SCALE.

social agency an organization, private or governmental, that supervises or provides personal services, especially in the fields of health, welfare, and rehabilitation. The general objective of a s.a. is to improve the quality of life of its clients.

social aggregate all the individuals inhabiting a designated geographical area.

social anchoring the inability to make up one's mind without relying on group trends or on an interpretation of group attitudes.

social animal: See SOCIAL INSTINCT.

social animism a concept of the world that is fashioned to fit the emotions of the individual, as observed in the schizophrenia patient who believes, if he feels inferior, that everyone views him as an inferior person.

social anorexia a loss of appetite associated with starvation or malnutrition, as in cases of indigent individuals who are undernourished.

social anthropology: See ANTHROPOLOGY.

social anxiety feelings of apprehensiveness about one's social status, social role, and social behavior. According to Davis and Havighurst, s.a. is a prime characteristic of middle-class adolescents.

social assimilation the process by which two or more cultures or cultural groups become fused, although one is likely to remain dominant.

social atom the smallest social structure in the community, which may be represented by the interactions of one individual with others to whom he is attracted or by whom he is repelled.

social attitude an attitude toward social responsibilities, as opposed to private matters; an attitude toward other people, e.g., friendly or hostile; also, an opinion shared by many people.

social behavior behavior that is under the control of or influenced by society or a social group; also, behavior of a group or organization.

social being an organism that, in the interests of survival and propagation, lives with other species members in a social setting where regular patterns are established for nurturance of the young, food-gathering or cultivation, and mutual aid. See SOCIAL INSTINCT.

social bond the link that unites members of a social group such as a club or gang. A s.b. is usually established by such factors as similar interests, aims, or feelings.

social-breakdown syndrome a symptom pattern observed primarily in chronic institutionalized mental patients, but also in long-term prisoners. It consists of such reactions as withdrawal, loss of interest and initiative, submissiveness and passivity, and progressive social and vocational incompetence—all of which were at one time attributed to mental illness itself, but are now believed to be due to lack of stimulation, overcrowded conditions, unchanging routine, and disinterest on the part of the staff. Also called **chronicity; institutionalism; institutional neurosis; social-disability syndrome**.

social case work a type of social work that is concerned with the personal needs, social relationships, and environmental pressures of individual clients. Also called **case work**.

social change the process of altering the general character of a society, as in the Industrial Revolution of the 19th century, and the introduction of nuclear technology and freer sexual expression in the 20th. Rapid s.c. increases stress and creates many psychological problems. See FUTURE SHOCK.

social class a large group or division of society that shares a common level of education, occupation, and income as well as many common values and, in some cases, similar religious and social patterns. Child-rearing practices, physical setting, social environment, educational opportunities, emotional adjustment, and occupational opportunities may all be affected by s.c.

social climate the character of the milieu in which individuals and groups live, that is, prevailing customs, mores, and social attitudes that influence their behavior and adjustment.

social climbing the attempt to improve one's social standing through acceptance in a higher class.

The term implies an attempt to cater to or hobnob with selected members of the higher class.

social code a general term for laws and other social rules and standards accepted by a specific community or society.

social cohesion the tendency of individuals with similar interests to integrate into a meaningful group. S.c. is one of the most effective forces in group therapy.

social-comparison theory the idea that people partially or primarily assess their accomplishments, abilities, talents, values, and attitudes in relation to those of others, that is, through a process of comparison.

social competence the ability to handle a variety of social situations effectively; skill in interpersonal relations.

social compliance a term coined by H. Hartmann for the influence of the social structure upon the individual's personality development and characteristic modes of adaptation. He believed that an analytic study of interactions with the environment would be a major contribution to sociology.

social consciousness an awareness of the needs of others and the fact that our experiences are shared by others.

social contact in psychiatry and rehabilitation, any personal communication or relationship between a patient and other individuals, particularly persons who are not members of the immediate family or health-care team. The s.c. often is a means of preventing or overcoming the tendency of some patients to withdraw from reality.

social context the specific circumstances or general environment that serve as a backdrop for social status or interpersonal behavior.

social control the power of the institutions, organizations, and laws of society to influence or regulate the behavior of individuals and groups; the impact of religion, the economic system, education, the communications industry, and other social forces on individual or group behavior. Widespread conformity increases the power of social institutions to shape behavior. S.c. may be positive. However, in the mental-health and legal communities, there is growing concern over the administration of psychotropics and certain aversive-conditioning procedures to patients in mental-health facilities and individuals in prisons with behavior control in mind. See BEHAVIOR CONTROL.

social decrement: See SOCIAL INCREMENT.

social density the number of individuals per given unit of space. The term applies not only to the amount of space for each person but also to the number of interpersonal interactions likely to occur. Also see SPATIAL DENSITY.

social deprivation lack of adequate opportunity for social experience, frequently due to parental overprotection or an isolated environment.

social-desirability bias in surveys and interviews, the widespred tendency for respondents to shift their answers to personal questions in the direction of majority opinion or social consensus. The s.-d.b. necessitates control measures. See RESPONSE SET.

social determinism: See CULTURAL DETERMINISM.

social development the gradual acquisition of attitudes, relationships, and behavior that enable the individual to function as a member of society.

social diagnosis a term used in psychiatric social work to identify the environmental conditions related to a patient's disorder.

social disability syndrome = SOCIAL-BREAKDOWN SYNDROME.

social disintegration the disruption and fragmentation of a social group or community, with legal and institutional breakdowns and individual demoralization and emotional disturbances.

social distance the relative degree of association and acceptance between members of different social groups such as racial, religious, or national groups. See PROXEMICS.

social-distance scale a rating scale on which the subject indicates the degree of intimacy he would accept in association with a specific individual or with a member of a specific social group. See BOGARDUS S.-D.S.

social drive the drive to establish social relationships and to be gregarious.

social dyad two interacting persons or groups in which varied social relationships take place, e.g., (a) rivalry between two brothers or two teams, (b) symbiosis between mother and infant, (c) positive or negative transference between therapist and patient, or (d) harmony or hostility between business partners.

social dynamics a branch of social psychology that focuses on the processes and effects of social and cultural changes.

social ecology the study of organisms, human or animal, in relation to their social environment.

social engineer an individual engaged in social-policy planning and in organizing community-action programs dealing with such problems as crime, drug abuse, and urban decay.

social-exchange theory the theory that behavior is primarily motivated by reciprocity and expectation of reward; the idea that social interaction is based on the exchange of various emotional, social, and material benefits. S.-e.t. derives from the stimulus-response orientation.

social facilitation the term given to the finding that a person's ability to quickly and correctly carry out a task is improved when others are present. However, some social psychologists maintain that this effect only applies to uncomplicated tasks or tasks previously mastered through practice. Also see SOCIAL INCREMENT.

social factors in rehabilitation psychology, social influences such as the attitudes of members of the community toward a disability and the resultant effect on the patient's self-image and morale. Such factors can, e.g., play a major role in the efforts to rehabilitate a patient who has suffered facial disfigurement and is concerned about sexual attractiveness, about rejection by employers or fellow workers, or about being the object of curiosity or pity.

social feedback a direct report of the effect of one's behavior or verbal communications on other people in the form, e.g., of laughter after telling a joke, or a warm handclasp after telling someone you like him.

social fission the division of a social group into smaller groups owing to internal dissension or environmental conditions that endanger the survival of the group as originally constituted.

social fixity = SOCIAL IMMOBILITY.

social flexibility = SOCIAL MOBILITY.

social gerontology the study of old age from the viewpoint of society, including the contributions of the elderly to the community, health problems of the aged, provision of appropriate medical care, and residences and communities for retirees.

social group a cluster of two or more persons with a common interest or a common goal.

social habit a common form of social behavior that is deeply ingrained and often appears to have an automatic quality, e.g., saying "Thank you."

social hunger a desire to be accepted by a group. It is a primary incentive for improvement in a therapy group.

social immobility a feature of rigid class systems such that a person's or a group's movement from one social class to another is impossible or only possible in very rare cases, e.g., the traditional Hindu caste system. Also called **social fixity**. Compare SOCIAL MOBILITY.

social-impact assessment the evaluation of the social effect of a proposed construction project while it is in the planning stage. The s.-i.a. is based on studies of project effects on land values, traffic flow, displacement of jobs and homes, ecological balance, air pollution, and related factors, as well as predicted benefits to the environment and people who would utilize the proposed new facility.

social imperception the inability to perform social activities commensurate with chronological age and intelligence because of neurological dysfunction and poor impulse control.

social increment for any behavioral variable, such as manners or speech, an increase or improvement when the subject is with others as compared to being alone. A **social decrement** is a decline in performance that occurs when the subject is in the presence of others. Also see SOCIAL FACILITATION.

social indicators variables by which the quality of life of a society can be assessed. Many s.i. have been suggested by different authorities—among them, poverty, unemployment, mental health, general health, air pollution, public safety, per capita income, cost of housing, leisure and re-creation, crime rate, nutrition, life expectancy, labor conditions, and status of the elderly.

social-inquiry model a teaching model that emphasizes the role of social interaction and is concerned with methods of resolving social issues through a process of logical reasoning and academic inquiry.

social instinct the basic tendency for individuals to congregate, affiliate, and engage in group activities. In psychoanalysis, the s.i. is a basic craving for social contact, which first manifests itself in love for the parents and gradually spreads to encompass brothers, sisters, friends, and in some cases humankind in general. In Adlerian psychology, the s.i. is an innate drive for cooperation, which leads normal individuals to incorporate social interest and the common good into their efforts to achieve self-realization. (Aristotle had defined the human being as the *zoon politikon*, the "social animal.") See GRE-GARIOUSNESS; HERD INSTINCT.

social integration the process by which an individual is assimilated into a group; also, the process of bringing together different groups to form a unified society.

social intelligence the degree of ease and effectiveness displayed by a person in social relationships.

social interaction any process that involves reciprocal stimulation and response between two or more people, ranging from the first encounters between mother and infant to the complex interactions of adult life. S.i. studies cover major areas, including the development of cooperation and competition, the influence of status and social roles, and the dynamics of group behavior, leadership, and conformity.

social interest in Adler's individual psychology, the key concept of communal feeling (German *Gemeinschaftsgefühl*) based on the idea that man lives in a social context, is an integral part of his family, community, humanity, and the cosmos itself, and has a natural aptitude for acquiring the skills and understanding necessary to solve social problems and to take socially affirmative action—an aptitude, however, that needs to be trained and developed if we are to be mentally healthy and socially useful.

social intervention in evaluation research, social-action programs designed to produce an increased level of some type of social goods or services. The effects of the intervention may be compared with levels before the intervention occurred or with levels of change in alternative existing programs.

social introversion a behavioral trait manifested by shy, inhibited, and withdrawn attitudes.

social island = ISOLATE.

social-isolation syndrome in animal experiments, a syndrome produced in rhesus monkeys by raising them in total isolation, and consisting of severely abnormal behavior of an apparently autistic nature such as rocking, huddling, self-clasping, self-mouthing, retreat into a corner, as well as impaired sexual behavior. It has been found that this syndrome can be reversed by administration of chlorpromazine and interaction with younger, normal monkeys who serve as "monkey psychiatrists."

sociality willingness to cooperate with and adapt to the demands of a group gregariousness; sociability.

socialization of individuals in consumer psychology, the process whereby individuals become aware of alternative life-styles and behaviors. The process enables the individual to learn the value-system behavior pattern, and what is considered normal for the social environment in which he will be a member.

socialization process acquisition of roles, behavior, and attitudes expected of the individual in society. According to Bowlby (1969), the s.p. starts as soon as the child (a) orients toward people, tracks them with the eyes, and smiles, (b) makes differential responses to the mother, (c) approaches, climbs on, clings to the mother, and (d) at the age of four begins to manipulate others through gestures, crying, and requests, and starts to establish reciprocal relationships with others. In psychiatry, socialization is equivalent to sublimation, the process in which instinctual energies are converted into higher, socially acceptable forms of behavior. See SUBLIMATION.

socialize to work, play, or mingle well with other members of a group; also, to encourage social behavior.

socialized, aggressive reaction: See CONDUCT DIS-ORDER, SOCIALIZED, AGGRESSIVE.

socialized drive a primary drive that has been modified to make it conform to acceptable social behavior, e.g., eating without gorging.

socialized, nonaggressive reaction: See CONDUCT DISORDER, SOCIALIZED, NONAGGRESSIVE.

socialized speech: See EGOCENTRIC SPEECH.

socializing activity an activity that helps a patient interact with other members of a group, such as movement therapy or participating in a party.

social-learning theory an approach to behavior therapy in which behavior is assumed to be developed and regulated (a) by external stimulus events, such as the influence of other individuals, (b) by external reinforcement, such as praise, blame, and rewards, and, most importantly, (c) by the effects of cognitive processes, such as thinking and judgment, on the individual's behavior and on the environment that influences him or her. The term also applies to the general view that learning is largely or wholly due to social influences, as in imitating or emulating others.

social maladjustment the inability to develop relationships that satisfy affiliative needs; the lack of social finesse or tact; also, a breakdown in the process of maintaining constructive social relationships.

social masochism a term used by Theodore Reik

to identify the attitude of giving up, as when a patient becomes submissive and passive in order to tolerate defeat and misfortune.

social maturity the development of social standards and behavior that are the norm for adults or the particular age of the individual.

social mind the hypothetical concept of a group mind that cannot be explained in terms of the traits of the individual members of the group. See GROUP MIND.

social-mindedness a term used by the psychoanalyst O. Sperling for a form of altruism which is directed toward the search for the causes and solutions of social problems. Also called **social-mindfulness**. See ALTRUISM.

social mobility social flexibility; the capacity of a society or social group to allow for changes in social status and social roles, and to permit or encourage free interactions among its members. S.m. is also the tendency to move upward or downward in social status. See UPWARD MOBILITY; DOWNWARD MOBILITY; VERTICAL GROUP; HORIZONTAL GROUP. Compare SOCIAL IMMOBILITY.

social mores customs and codes of behavior established by a social group that are not necessarily supported by legal sanction, but which may be as binding as laws.

social motive any motive acquired as a result of experience in interaction with others; a learned motive in contrast to a physiological motive. A. s.m. may be universal as in the need for affiliation, or it may be culture-specific as in the achievement drive. **Personal-s.m.** is a somewhat broader term that embraces the individual variations within cultures.

social movement a collective effort of individuals and groups to resolve a major social problem or in some way to alter the existing social structure.

social needs: See NEED-HIERARCHY THEORY.

social-network therapy a form of psychotherapy in which various persons who maintain significant relationships with the patient in different aspects of life (relatives, friends, fellow workers) are assembled in small or larger group sessions. Also see NETWORK THERAPY.

social norms the standards of correct or acceptable behavior as defined and required in a specific group; the combined attitudes and concepts approved by the group and used by the group member to interpret and explain the environment. S.n. set forth the feelings, attitudes, thoughts, and behavior expected of the group member. Also called **group norms**.

social object any person, group, or animal with whom an individual establishes a social relationship in actuality or fantasy. Imaginary companions and inanimate objects (e.g., dolls, teddy bears) may fall into this category.

social organism a term sometimes applied to a social group or society when emphasizing its dynamic or "living" qualities, e.g., the complexity of social structure, processes, and interrelationship of subsystems.

social organization a system that links individual humans into groups through kinship, age, sex, religion, matrimony, area of residence, or common interests. The s.o. usually implements the system by rules of behavior.

social pathology the study of patterns of social organization, attitudes, and behaviors that tend to influence the mental health of individuals.

social perception an awareness of social objects or events, or awareness of the personality traits of others as expressed in their behavior.

social phenomenon any process, event, or accomplishment that results from the interaction of two or more individuals.

social phobia an anxiety disorder characterized by a persistent, irrational fear of, and a compelling desire to avoid, situations in which the individual is exposed to scrutiny by others (speaking, eating or writing in public, or using a public lavatory), together with a distressing fear of behaving in a humilating or embarrassing manner. (DSM-III)

social pressure any unofficial or implicit social process that has the effect of encouraging or inducing conformity.

social psychiatry a broad area of psychiatric research and practice covering the relation between mental disorder and the social environment. The social viewpoint is an outgrowth of three major forces: (a) recognition of sociological, anthropological, ecological, and epidemiological factors in the etiology of mental illness, (b) the social emphasis of Horney, Sullivan, Fromm, and others, and (c) development of the public-health approach, and the field of community psychiatry. S.p. focuses on such subject matter as cross-cultural concepts of normality, social patterns of drug abuse and sexual behavior, social attitudes toward illness, community mental-health centers, and other forms of social treatment and prevention. Also called **sociocultural psychiatry**. See COMMUNITY PSYCHIATRY; CROSS-CULTURAL PSYCHIATRY.

social psychology a branch of psychology that deals with the psychological processes of individuals in groups, the interactions of groups, and factors that affect social life, such as status, role, and class.

social quotient: See VINELAND SOCIAL MATURITY SCALE.

social reality the shared attitudes and opinions held by members of a group or society; the network of information, interpretations, and commonly held social beliefs that influence the individual.

social recovery a term used by H. S. Sullivan for restoration of a normal or near-normal mental state through social therapy and improvement in social skills. See SOCIAL THERAPY.

social-reform programs in evaluation research, intervention programs developed and instituted to counter deleterious aspects of social systems—programs whose primary objective is to reduce the effects of malfunctions in the social system. Also called **countermeasure-intervention programs**.

social rehabilitation the achievement of a higher level of social functioning among mentally or physically disabled individuals through social and recreational activities and participation in clubs and other organizations of their own.

social resistance in environment psychology, group opposition to environmental changes that may clash with traditional use of areas, buildings, or facilities. E.g., a demand for personal privacy may be expressed as s.r. to open planning in homes, offices, or public buildings.

social-responsibility norm the social standard or ideal that one should assist those in need of assistance.

social role the functional position and the part played by the individual in a group situation, such as the role of squadron leader, teacher, or vice-president of an organization. Positions of this kind are termed **role categories**, and the attitudes and behavior associated with each category are termed **role expectations** or **role behaviors**.

social rules and standards: See SOCIAL CODE.

social sanction a method of social control that enforces a group's standards by authorizing punishment for violation of the group's rules.

social scale a system of assigning individuals to various social classes or categories.

social self the aspects of the self that are important to or influenced by social relations; our characteristic behavior in social situations; also, the role or façade that an individual may exhibit in contact with other people, as contrasted with the real self.

social services services arranged by trained professionals, usually social workers, including visiting-nurse service, homemaking assistance, mental-health counseling, housing for the physically disabled and mentally retarded, and government benefits.

social-sexual relationships: See NORMALIZATION PRINCIPLE.

social situation the effect of a configuration of social factors on the behavior of an individual or his reaction to a particular situation. A s.s. may vary according to the set of social factors influencing an individual at a particular time, and his reactions usually reveal information about his self-image.

social-skills training a form of therapy for individuals who need to overcome social inhibition or ineffectiveness. The techniques of behavior rehearsal, cognitive rehearsal, and assertiveness training are applied to essentially normal and functioning persons as well as certain psychiatric patients who may be taught to substitute direct verbal expression for violence, withdrawal, or other maladaptive patterns. Abbrev.: **SST**.

social status the position or rank of an individual in a social group or class in relation to other members.

social stimulus any nonphysical stimulus that elicits a social response; also, an individual or group that elicits a response.

social stratification the existence of separate socioeconomic levels in a society. See SOCIAL CLASS.

social-stress theory the concept that endocrine and other physical effects increase among individual members of a group as the size of the group increases beyond an optimal number. The increased social competition, according to the theory, leads to adrenal and other glandular stresses and, in turn, to physiological and behavioral deficits. Some investigators state that social stress moderates population density because it tends to diminish the birth rate.

social structure the distinctive organization of a group in terms of internal relationships, objectives, and stratification of members.

Social Studies Reading Test: See ACT ASSESSMENT.

social technology the use of the principles and methodology of the social sciences (e.g., economics, sociology, psychology) to develop practical strategies for confronting and resolving conflicts and problems of society.

social therapy therapeutic and rehabilitative approaches focused on improved social functioning of psychiatric patients through such means as milieu therapy, recreational therapy, occupational therapy, patient government, work therapy, remotivation, and the therapeutic community.

social-therapy club: See MENTAL-PATIENT ORGANIZATION.

social transmission the transfer from one generation to the next of customs, language, or other aspects of the cultural heritage of a group.

social trap a conflict situation that cannot be resolved without negative consequences or one that is embedded in the nature of a society and its relationships, e.g., a government policy that benefits one group and inevitably harms another, or an established societal pattern that is recognizably irrational and destructive but cannot be abandoned.

social type a person whose goals and values are primarily socially determined. The term is also used as the equivalent of E. Spranger's social or **sociable type**, who is friendly, compassionate, considerate, and congenial.

social withdrawal retreat from society and interpersonal relationships, usually accompanied by an attitude of indifference, detachment, and aloofness. S.w. is a common expression of schizophrenic autism. See AUTISM; WITHDRAWAL REACTION; WITHDRAWAL.

social-work aide a nonprofessional social worker who performs limited social-work duties, such as interviewing patients and providing practical services to patients and families under the supervision of professional social workers.

social worker a person trained in an accredited college or graduate school to help individuals and families deal with personal and practical problems, including problems related to mental or physical disorder, poverty, living arrangements, social life, marital relationships, child care, occupational stress, and unemployment. Social workers are major members of treatment and rehabilitation teams in clinics, social agencies, mental-health centers, mental hospitals, and general hospitals. See PSYCHIATRIC SOCIAL WORK; MEDICAL S.W.; COMMUNITY S.W.; FAMILY SOCIAL WORK.

social zone in social psychology, the area of physical distance between persons engaged in business interactions or relationships of a relatively formal nature, e.g., that of attorney and client. The s.z. is defined as the area from 1¼ to 3½ m (4 to 11½ ft.). See PROXEMICS.

societal-reaction theory = LABELING THEORY.

society a large group of individuals of a species, particularly humans, whose members are more or less formally organized and mutually interdependent; also, a social organization within a s. as a whole.

sociobiology the systematic study of the biological basis for social behavior, a field pioneered by E.O. Wilson. An example is his theory that populations tend to maintain an optimal level of density (neither overpopulation nor underpopulation) by such controls as aggression, stress, fertility, emigration, predation, and disease. According to Wilson, such controls operate through the Darwinian principle of natural selection. S. has also been termed **Darwinian psychology.**

sociocenter = STAR.

sociocentrism the tendency to identify with one's own social group to the extent that its group norms and prescriptions form a relatively inflexible standard against which other people are judged. S. usually refers to smaller social groups whereas ethnocentrism refers to larger ethnic, religious, racial, or national groups.

sociocognitive biases in evaluation research, the realization that evaluators may be susceptible to subtle biases in judgment. These biases differ from values in that the biases are inaccurate judgments that result from shortcomings in cognitive processing. S.b. appear to be universals that intrude regardless of values or ethics.

sociocultural factors in psychiatry and clinical psychology, environmental conditions that play a part in normal behavior but also in the etiology of mental disorder, mental retardation, or social pathology. Examples of s.f. of a negative nature are slum conditions, poverty, occupational pressures, lack of good medical care, inadequate educational opportunities, and in some cases disruptive ethnic or religious beliefs such as demonomania. See CULTURE-SPECIFIC SYNDROMES.

sociocultural psychiatry = SOCIAL PSYCHIATRY.

sociocusis the loss of hearing acuity due to all of the hazards of living in our modern society including disease, noise exposure, and aging.

sociodrama a technique for human relations and social skills that utilizes dramatization and role-playing.

socioeconomic factors: See SOCIOECONOMIC STATUS.

socioeconomic status the position, or level, of an individual or group on the socioeconomic scale, which is determined by a combination or interaction of social and economic factors such as income, amount and kind of education, type of occupation (e.g., blue-collar, white-collar), place of residence, and in some areas ethnic, nationality, or religious background.

socioempathy in social or interpersonal interactions, the awareness or intuitive recognition of the roles or status of others in relation to oneself.

sociofugal space a physical environment designed to discourage interpersonal interaction, e.g., the design of church pews. See PROXEMICS. Compare SOCIOPETAL SPACE.

sociogenesis the process by which an individual's ideas or development are affected or influenced by social experience.

sociogenetics the study of the origin and development of societies.

sociogenic characterizing an idea, attitude, or other mental process that is based on sociocultural influences.

sociogram a diagram depicting the interactions and interrelationships between members of a group, such as a class, gang, team, or work group. J. L. Moreno employed four types of sociograms in psychodrama: **intuitive s.**, based on relationships noted by the therapist in the first session; **observer's s.**, consisting of the cotherapist's impressions; **objective s.**, based on a sociometric test; and **perceptual s.**, in which each member indicates which other members appear to accept or reject him. See SOCIOMETRY.

sociolinguistics the study of language in society, applying techniques and findings from linguistics and various social sciences. S. is mainly concerned with the individual's language in the context of his community or culture.

sociological factors social conditions that affect human behavior. These conditions determine, in part at least, the types and incidence of mental disorder. Examples are socioeconomic and educational level, urban decay, the customs and mores of particular groups such as the Tennessee hill people, the Welsh coal miners, or the Russian Skoptsy sect.

sociological measures: See PRIMARY PREVENTION.

sociology the scientific study of the formation, structure, and functioning of organizations, groups, societies, and institutions. See CLINICAL S.

sociometric analysis = SOCIOMETRY.

sociometric cleavage the absence of sociometric

choices between two or more subgroups, indicating that they are socially separate or at odds. See SOCIOMETRY.

sociometric clique on a sociometric test, a group of individuals who nominate each other by the same criterion while infrequently selecting persons outside the group. See SOCIOMETRY.

sociometric distance the degree of closeness or acceptance between individuals or groups as measured on a social-distance scale. See SOCIAL DISTANCE; SOCIAL-DISTANCE SCALE; PROXEMICS.

sociometry a field originated by J. L. Moreno in which the interpersonal structure and dynamics of groups are determined and plotted by asking each member to choose one or more individuals with whom he would like to work, eat, study, or share an apartment. This method (**nominating technique**) reveals significant information, such as which members are considered most popular ("stars"), which tend to be rejected or asocial ("isolates"), and which are the best leaders. It also brings to light the existence of cliques, pairs, triangles, and other patterns of group structure. Also called **sociometric analysis; sociometrics**. See SOCIOGRAM.

socionomics the study of nonsocial influences on social groups, that is, the ways in which physical environment modifies society, e.g., the effects of different terrains and climactic conditions on economic and social organization.

sociopath an obsolete term for an individual with an ANTISOCIAL-PERSONALITY DISORDER. See this entry. Also see NEUROTIC S.; PRIMARY S.

sociopathic behavior an older term for socially pathological behavior such as stealing, rape, child molestation, embezzlement, prostitution, burglary, murder, drug abuse, and sexual sadism. See DYSSOCIAL BEHAVIOR.

sociopathic personality: See ANTISOCIAL-PERSONALITY DISORDER.

sociopathic-personality disturbance a DSM-I category characterized primarily by failure to adapt to prevailing ethical and social standards, and lack of social responsibility. The term comprised ANTISOCIAL REACTION, DYSSOCIAL REACTION, SEXUAL DEVIANCY, and ADDICTION. See these entries.

sociopetal space a physical environment designed to encourage interpersonal interaction, e.g., a restaurant. See PROXEMICS. Compare SOCIOFUGAL SPACE.

sociotaxis in social psychiatry, any social stimulus that impinges on the individual, such as stimulation from social groups that are part of the social network, or field of relationships.

sociotherapy a supportive approach based on modification of the patient's environment, and improvement in the patient's interpersonal adjustment. The approach includes establishment of a therapeutic community, and such procedures as working with parents, foster-home placement, family counseling, vocational retraining, and assistance in readjusting to community life following hospitalization.

socius the individual as a member of society. He or she is the primary social unit.

Socrates /sok′rətēz/ Greek philosopher, ca. 470–399 B.C. See DIALECTICAL METHOD; EXISTENTIALISM.

sodium-Amytal interview a diagnostic or therapeutic interview conducted with a patient who has been injected intravenously with sodium Amytal, or amobarbital, a short-acting hypnotic and sedative drug which relaxes the patient and facilitates the expression of repressed feelings and memories. Also called **Amytal interview**. See NARCOTHERAPY.

sodium glutamate a chemical compound used in the treatment of ammonia poisoning and certain types of encephalopathies. Intravenous injection of s.g. allows it to combine with the ammonia to form glutamine, which the body can dispose of through excretion or absorption. Ammonia poisoning, resulting from liver and kidney deficiencies, can cause coma, brain damage, and death if untreated.

sodium pentothal: See PENTOTHAL SODIUM.

sodium pump the process whereby adenosine triphosphate pumps out of a nerve cell the sodium ions that crossed the cell membrane from the outside during the previous nerve-impulse transmission. By restoring the balance of sodium ions outside the cell and potassium ions inside the cell, the neuron is primed to fire again.

sodium regulation the maintenance of sodium ions in the blood plasma where the element functions as the primary cation. An adrenal-cortical hormone, aldosterone, is released when extracellular levels of sodium fall below a minimum level. The hormone enhances reabsorption of sodium that otherwise might be excreted in the urine. A severe sodium deficiency can be fatal, while an excess of sodium in the blood may result in hypertension.

sodomy anal intercourse between human beings; also, sexual intercourse of any kind between a human being and an animal. (The term is derived from the corrrupt town of Sodom described in Genesis 18–19.) Also see ANAL INTERCOURSE; ZOOERASTY.

soft determinism: See DETERMINISM.

soft palate the fibromuscular tissue that is attached to the posterior portion of the hard palate. It separates the oral cavity from the pharynx and, when elevated, closes off the nasopharynx to produce normal speech sounds. Also called **velum palatinum**.

soft signs diagnostic clues that suggest a possible but hard-to-demonstrate organic basis for a mental disorder. S.s. may be involved in cases of mild mental retardation, minimal brain dysfunction, learning difficulties, and presenile dementias associated with idiosyncratic behavior. Perceptual deficit, mixed laterality, short attention span, and borderline EEG records are examples of s.s.

Sohval-Soffer syndrome a rare, presumably

hereditary, disease characterized by mental retardation and testicular deficiency. The few patients studied were psychotic and had subnormal intelligence. Penis and testes are small, and facial and pubic hair is sparse. Other physical traits of patients include skeletal anomalies and diabetes mellitus.

sol. an abbreviation used in prescriptions, meaning "solution" (Latin *solutio*).

solanacea the nightshade family of trees, shrubs, and herbs. The family includes the white potato and other plants of economic importance as well as sources of belladonna, stramonium, and other drugs.

soldier's heart = DA COSTA'S SYNDROME.

solipsism the philosophical viewpoint that there can be no proof that anything exists outside my mind because, after all, everything else is dependent upon my perception of it (from Latin *solus ipse*, "I alone").

solitude fear = AUTOPHOBIA.

Solomon, Richard American psychologist, 1918—. See OPPONENTS-PROCESS THEORY OF ACQUIRED MOTIVATION.

solvent inhalation the practice of inhaling fumes of industrial solvents and aerosol sprays that usually contain hydrocarbons capable of producing intoxication. The fumes may contain alcohol, ether, chloroform, or trichloroethylene. The substances generally produce a state of euphoria followed by CNS depression. Tolerance to the solvents develops, followed by tissue damage to the brain, liver, and kidneys.

-som-; -somat- a combining form relating to the body.

soma the body as a whole (Greek, "body"); all organic tissue; the body as distinguished from the mind; also, body cells with the diploid set of chromosomes as distinguished from the haploid gamete cells produced by the gonads. Adjective: **somatic.**

The word s., with different etymology, is also an alternative term for FLY AGARIC. See this entry.

somaesthesia = SOMESTHESIA.

somatic: See SOMA.

somatic areas = SOMATIC SENSORY AREAS.

somatic cell = BODY CELL.

somatic compliance the tendency to express psychological disturbances through bodily functions. The reasons one organ rather than another becomes the locus for psychogenic symptoms (e.g., why a conversion neurotic becomes hysterically blind rather than paralyzed) are often conjectural. One theory is that the organ is constitutionally predisposed to breakdown; another, that it has been weakened by illness; still another, that it symbolizes or otherwise represents the individual's unconscious impulses or conflicts. See SYMPTOM CHOICE.

somatic concern anxious preoccupation with bodily complaints and bodily processes such as digestion and elimination. See HYPOCHONDRIASIS.

somatic delusion the false belief that individual bodily organs, or the body as a whole, are disturbed or disordered, e.g., that the stomach or heart is missing, or that the legs are two yards long. Such reactions are most frequently observed in paranoid schizophrenia. Also called **somatopsychic delusion.**

somatic disorders organic disorders, as distinguished from functional or psychogenic disorders. The term refers also to behavior disorders resulting from organic factors such as hereditary conditions, infections, or drugs such as heroin or alcohol.

somatic hallucination the false perception of a physical occurrence, such as electric currents or a cancerous growth, within the body. The symptom is frequently observed in paranoid schizophrenia.

somatic nervous system the part of the nervous system that involves sensory and motor neurons innervating the skeletal muscles and related skin receptors.

somatic obsession the preoccupation of a person with his body or a part of the body. The patient often has a monosymptomatic neurosis and may spend much time comparing his physical features with those of other people he encounters.

somatic receptors the sensory organs located in the skin including the deeper kinesthetic sense organs. Kinds of s.r. include free nerve endings, Merkel's cells, Meissner corpuscles, Krause end bulbs, Golgi tendon organs, and hair-follicle-basket nerve endings.

somatic senses the senses of pressure (or touch), pain, heat, coldness, and movement (kinesthetic sense), mediated by receptors in the skin, visceral organs, muscles, tendons, and joints.

somatic sensory areas the two main areas of the cortex mapped with evoked potentials to locate projection points associated with the various somatic senses. The s.s.a. vary somewhat with different species; in humans one is located in the region of the postcentral gyrus and the other is on the lateral surface of the cortex near the temporal auditory area. Also called **somatosensory cortex; somatic areas.**

somatic therapy in psychiatry, the treatment of mental disorders by organic methods such as electroshock therapy, psychotropic drugs, or megavitamins.

somatic weakness the vulnerability of an organ or organ system to the effects of psychological stress. The organ usually becomes the focus of a psychophysiological disorder. S.w. is believed to be a congenital susceptibility because of evidence in infants who may, e.g., develop colic when their routine is changed. In later life, the individual may develop peptic ulcers or another digestive disorder as a result of psychological stress.

somatization the organic expression of neurotic disturbance. The term was used by W. Stekel for what is now called conversion. Some investigators apply the term **s. reaction** not merely to the bodily symptoms that occur in almost every neurosis but regard it as a separate category that includes such psychophysiologic disorders as psychogenic asthma and peptic ulcers. See ORGAN NEUROSIS; PSYCHOLOGICAL FACTORS AFFECTING PHYSICAL CONDITION.

somatization disorder a somatoform disorder involving a history of multiple physical symptoms (at least 14 for women and 12 for men) of several year's duration, for which medical attention has been sought, but which are apparently not due to any physical disorder or injury. The complaints are often presented in a dramatic, vague, or exaggerated way, and are usually accompanied by an anxious and depressed mood. Among them are feelings of sickliness, difficulty in swallowing or walking, blurred vision, abdominal pain, nausea, diarrhea, painful or irregular menstruation, sexual indifference, painful intercourse, pain in back or joints, shortness of breath, palpitations, and chest pain. (DSM-III)

somatization reaction: See SOMATIZATION.

somatoform disorders /sōm'-/ a group of disorders marked by physical symptoms suggesting specific disorders for which there are no demonstrable organic findings or known physiological mechanisms, and for which there is positive evidence or a strong presumption that they are linked to psychological factors. See SOMATIZATION DISORDER; CONVERSION DISORDER; PSYCHOGENIC PAIN DISORDER; HYPOCHONDRIASIS; ATYPICAL SOMATOFORM DISORDER. (DSM-III)

somatogenesis the origin of behavioral or personality traits or disorders in organic factors, such as anatomical or physiological changes; also, the transformation of germ-cell material into body cells. Also see ORGANOGENESIS.

somatognosia the awareness that one's own body is a functioning entity. An abnormal perception of the body or body parts as unusually large is called **macrosomatognosia**; a perception of the body or its parts as abnormally small is known as **microsomatognosia**. The abnormal perceptions may be due to neurological lesions, epilepsy, schizophrenia, migraine, or the use of certain drugs that distort perception.

somatopathic drinking = BETA ALCOHOLISM.

somatoplasm the tissue cells of the body as distinguished from the gametes, or germ cells. Also see GERM PLASM.

somatopsychic delusion = SOMATIC DELUSION.

somatopsychic disorders psychological disturbances resulting from organic factors, as in the effects of opiates on behavior, or the postencephalitic syndrome consisting of impulsivity and overactivity, resulting from epidemic encephalitis.

somatopsychosis a psychosis in which the patient's delusions involve his body or body parts.

somatosensory cortex = SOMATIC SENSORY AREAS.

somatosensory systems the sensory nerve systems that transmit impulses to and from the skin, muscles, joints, and certain parts of the viscera. The receptors in all those areas are similar in appearance and function, and their fibers follow the same general pathways through the central nervous system.

somatostatin a substance that inhibits the release of the growth hormone, somatotrophin, by the anterior lobe of the pituitary gland. S. is found in the hypothalamus, the pancreas, the stomach, and the duodenum portion of the intestine. It is used therapeutically in the control of acromegaly. Because the growth hormone is associated with carbohydrate metabolism, s. activity also inhibits secretion of insulin and glucagon. Also called **somatotrophin-release-inhibiting factor (SRIF)**.

somatotonic temperament: See MESOMORPH.

somatotopagnosia = AUTOTOPAGNOSIA.

somatotopic organization the distribution of motor areas of the cortex relating to specific activities of skeletal muscles. The hemispheres can be mapped to locate s.o. areas by electrical stimulation of a point in the cortex that results in the movement of a particular skeletal muscle in the face, trunk, or a limb. See SOMATIC SENSORY AREAS.

somatotrophin a growth hormone secreted by the pituitary gland.

somatotrophin-release-inhibiting factor: See SOMATOSTATIN.

somatotype the body build or physique of a person as it relates to his temperament or behavioral characteristics. Numerous categories of somatotypes have been proposed by various investigators since ancient times.

somatotypology the classification of individuals according to somatotypes, or body builds, usually correlated with personality characteristics.

somber-bright dimension in psychological esthetics, a system of classifying artistic styles on the basis of emotional effects. Experimental evidence shows that intense brightness, high saturation, and hues that correspond to long wavelengths of light tend to excite a subject.

somesthesia the body or somatic senses: kinesthetic, tactile, and organic or internal sensitivity. Also called **somesthesis; somaesthesia**. Adjective: **somesthetic**.

somesthetic area a region of the parietal lobe in which sensory impulses from somatic receptors are received. Studies indicate that the body surface is projected in the postcentral gyrus area in the same relationship as the dermatomes represented by the nerve fibers.

somesthetic disorders dysfunctions involving the somatic senses, such as visual-spatial or body-image disturbances, difficulty in maintaining postural awareness, or lack of sensitivity to pain, touch, or temperature. S.d. usually are related to brain damage in the parietal lobe, e.g., from gunshot wounds. A form of temporal-lobe epilepsy is also marked by body-image distortions.

somesthetic stimulation stimulation of kinesthetic, tactile, or visceral receptors, which constitute our bodily senses.

somnambulism = SLEEPWALKING DISORDER.

somnambulistic state a state of mind in which walking or talking or other complex acts occur during sleep (somnambulism). The term refers also to a hypnotic phase in which the subject, in a deep trance, may appear to be awake and in control of his actions but is actually under the control of the hypnotist.

somnifacients agents that are capable of inducing sleep. The term is sometimes applied to sedative-hypnotic drugs, and is essentially synonymous with SOPORIFICS. See this entry.

somniferous /-nif'-/ sleep-inducing; soporific.

somnium dream: See INSOMNIUM DREAM.

somnolence pathological sleepiness or drowsiness, sometimes prolonged for days. The condition may be due to narcotic drugs, overmedication with sedatives, conversion disorder, or epidemic encephalitis. Also see TWILIGHT SLEEP.

somnolentia: See SLEEP DRUNKENNES.

sonant in phonetics, a **voiced sound** produced by means of vocal-cord vibrations, e.g., /b/, /v/, or /z/, as opposed to a voiceless sound; in phonology, a **semivowel**, that is, a speech sound that can have features of both a vowel and a consonant, e.g., /r/ as in "read," /w/ as in "well," or /y/ as in "yellow."

sone a unit of the ratio scale of loudness that is approximately 40 decibels above the mean threshold at 1,000 cycles per second.

sonic boom a severe noise stressor caused by aircraft or projectiles traveling at supersonic speeds. The nose of the craft compresses air ahead of it, and the rear end produces a cone of reduced pressure behind it. The result is two successive shock waves, a fraction of a second apart, experienced by people on the ground as a startling loud noise that resembles the shock wave of an earthquake or thunderclap, great enough to rattle windows and vibrate walls. Because of the psychological stress of a s.b., supersonic-aircraft flights usually are routed away from populated areas.

sonoencephalogram an alternative term for echoencephalogram. Abbrev.: **SEG.** See ECHOENCEPHALOGRAPH.

sonogram: See BIOMEDICAL ENGINEERING; ULTRASOUND TECHNIQUE. Also see SONOENCEPHALOGRAM.

sonometer an instrument for auditory experiments and demonstrations made by stretching one or more strings over a resonating box.

soothability; soothing: See PACIFICATION.

sophism a plausible but subtly fallacious argument that is usually intended to deceive.

soporifics agents that are capable of producing sleep, particularly a deep sleep (Latin *sopor*). Also called **sopoforics.** See SEDATIVE-HYPNOTICS; SOMNIFACIENTS.

S-O-R: See DYNAMIC PSYCHOLOGY.

SORC /sôrk/ an acronym for the four types of variables employed in behavioral assessment: *s*ituational determinants, *o*rganismic variables, overt *r*esponses, and reinforcement *c*ontingencies.

sorcery drugs a group of plant alkaloids that includes belladonna, opium, mandrake, aconite, and hemlock. The substances have been chewed, smoked, or brewed into potions since primitive times for therapeutic and intoxicating purposes. Medicinal herbs were usually grown and administered by witches or sorcerers until physicians discovered the value of s.d.

sororate marriage to a deceased wife's sister. Marriage to a deceased wife's brother is termed **levirate**. These situations are sometimes encountered in family therapy.

sorting test a technique for assessing the ability to conceptualize. The subject, usually a child, is asked to arrange an assortment of common objects by categories. The method used in this task reflects the level of cognitive development; e.g., a very young child may group random objects together for entirely subjective reasons while an older child will categorize objects on the basis of functional relationships. Also see CLASS INCLUSION.

sotalol a potent beta-adrenergic blocking agent derived from the stimulant isoproterenol. The hydrochloride form of s. is employed in the control of heart arrhythmias. Although a close chemical relative of propranolol, s. does not have the anesthetic effect on cell membranes that can occur with propranolol.

soteria the possessions or other objects, including collections, that are acquired for a feeling of security. The term is distinguished from accumulation, which refers to the continued possession of unclassified, useless, or meaningless objects. Also see HOARDING CHARACTER.

soul a metaphysical entity that is hypothesized to have a permanent existence beyond mortal life. In his *De Anima*, Aristotle anticipated modern psychology by describing the soul, or mind, as the activity of the body. As synonym for mind, however, the term is now obsolete. Also see CREATIVE SELF.

soul image in Jungian psychology, the deeply unconscious portion of the psyche that is composed of the animus (male) and anima (female) archetypes.

soul kiss = FRENCH KISS.

sound vibrations of molecules in the air, particularly those in the frequency range that can be detected by the human ear. Some s. vibrations are outside the auditory spectrum of human adults but can be heard by human infants and by certain animals. S. waves can be converted from air vibrations to fluid vibrations, as occurs in the cochlea, or to electromagnetic vibrations, as in radio broadcasting.

sound cage a device for measuring sound localization.

sound direction; sound distance: See AUDITORY SPACE PERCEPTION.

sound fear = PHONOPHOBIA.

sound frequency: See FREQUENCY OF SOUND.

sounding out = PHONICS.

sound intensity the strength of the particle vibration, or the rate of sound-energy transmission through a medium. It is related to the square of the amplitude and the square of the frequency of a sound wave.

sound localization the ability to determine the direction of the source of a sound. S.l. is experienced more or less unconsciously by intensity, phase differences, and differences in the time of arrival of the sound waves at the right and left ears.

sound perimetry a method of measuring the ability of a subject to localize sounds in space.

sound-pressure level the common reference level (.0002 dyne per square centimeter) used in specifying sound intensity in decibels, e.g., "30 db (SPL)." Abbrev.: SPL.

sound shadow an area in which sound is blocked by a nontransmitting object, such as the head.

sound spectrogram an image of a pattern made by sounds. The image shows not only the pattern of the frequencies or wavelengths but the effects of various modulating influences such as the resonant cavities formed during speech by changes in the muscles of the tongue, lips, cheeks, and nasopharynx.

sound spectrum an analysis of complex tones into their component frequencies and intensities. Also called **acoustic spectrum; tonal spectrum.**

sound wave a periodic pressure fluctuation in a plastic medium, such as air or water, that may be perceived as a sound by a human if the frequency is between 20 and 20,000 cycles per second.

source language the language of the learner of a foreign language or of an artificial (e.g., computer) language system; also, the language from which a translation is made. Compare TARGET LANGUAGE.

sourness fear = ACEROPHOBIA.

source traits a term applied by R. B. Cattell to 12 personality traits determined by factor analysis, which underlie and determine our surface traits. Examples are cyclothymia (emotionally expressive and changeable) and schizothymia (reserved, anxious, laconic). Also see SURFACE TRAITS; PERSONALITY SPHERE.

sour-grapes mechanism a form of rationalization in which the individual expresses disdain for something he does not or cannot have ("She would have been fat before 30"). Also see SWEET-LEMON MECHANISM.

sp. an abbreviation used in prescriptions, meaning "spirit" (Latin *spiritus*).

spaced practice a learning procedure in which practice periods are separated by long, regular time intervals or rest periods. Distributed practice is similar. Also called **spaced learning; spaced repetition.** Compare MASSED PRACTICE.

space error an error in judging the position of a stimulus due to its spatial relationship to the observer.

space factor an ability, identified by factor analysis, which accounts for individual differences in the capacity to perceive spatial relations.

space orientation the ability to locate or adjust one's position in space.

space perception an awareness derived from sensory inputs of the spatial properties of objects in the environment, including their shape, dimension, and distances.

Space, Quantity, Time: See BOEHM TEST OF BASIC CONCEPTS.

Spalding, D. A. English naturalist, fl. 19th century. See IMPRINTING.

Spanish fly an insect, Cantharis vesicatoria, that is used as a source of the skin irritant cantharidin, employed primarily in the treatment of warts. Also called **Russian fly.** Also see CANTHARIDES.

span of apprehension; span of attention = ATTENTION SPAN.

spasm a sudden involuntary muscle contraction, which may vary in severity from a twitch to a convulsion. A s. that is continuous or sustained is called a **tonic s.**; one that alternates between contraction and relaxation is known as a **clonic s.** A s. also may be identified with a body part, e.g., **vasospasm** when a blood vessel is involved, **bronchial s.** when the bronchi are involved. A common form of clonic s. is the disorder usually known as **hiccups.** Adjective: **spastic.** Also see HABIT S.; BRISSAUD'S DISEASE; TONIC.

spasmoarthria a term literally meaning a joint spasm but applied occasionally to spasms involving the muscles and cartilaginous rings of the throat, affecting speech. The condition occurs in spastic paralysis.

spasmodic ergotism: See ERGOTISM.

spasmodic flatfoot: See FLATFOOT.

spasmodic torticollis = WRYNECK SYNDROME.

spasmophemia a disturbance in the rhythm of speech; a blocking or hesitation in speech production, more frequently called STUTTERING. See this entry.

spastic: See SPASM.

spastic colitis: See COLITIS.

spastic diplegia = LITTLE'S DISEASE.

spastic dysphonia a functional voice disorder characterized by intermittent laryngeal spasms which interfere with normal speech. S.d. is not uncommon to public speakers.

spastic hemiparesis a condition of partial paralysis on one side of the body complicated by muscle spasms of the limbs on the affected side. The dystonic muscle contractions may be quite painful. Treatment may include biofeedback training and cryothalectomy, in addition to traditional procedures of medications and braces.

spasticity a motoneuron disorder marked by rigidity and clonus, which in turn is due to involuntary resistance to stretching of a muscle by increased tension. The condition involves deep tendon reflexes and results in a jerking action of the limbs.

spastic paralysis a type of paralysis marked by increased muscle tension, with a flexed limb that may show spasmodic movements. The cause usually is a motoneuron lesion, and the condition frequently occurs in cerebral palsy.

spastic paraplegia a form of paraplegia in which the lower part of the body is paralyzed and there is increased irritability and spasmodic contraction of the muscles of the legs. Also called **tetanoid paraplegia**.

spastic speech a type of difficult, labored speech associated with spastic paralysis.

spatial ability the ability of an individual to orient, or perceive his body, in space, or to detect spatial relationships. A deficit in s.a. may be observed in persons with brain injuries who are unable to perform effectively in map-reading tests and jigsaw puzzles or who have difficulties in recognizing shapes tactually.

spatial apractagnosia = APRACTAGNOSIA.

spatial conformance: See BEHAVIORAL FACILITATION; CONFORMANCE.

spatial density the amount of space per individual in a given area. The term is sometimes used in relation to experiments on the effects of crowding in which a same-size group is observed interacting in different-size areas. Also see SOCIAL DENSITY.

spatial disorders disorders of space perception, usually associated with parietal-lobe lesions and including impaired memory for locations, route-finding difficulties, constructional apraxia, and poor judgment of the localization of stimuli. The patient may underestimate the distance of far objects and overestimate the distance of near objects, or may be unable to align objects according to instructions.

spatial relationships the three-dimensional relationship of objects in space, such as their distance apart and their position relative to each other. Abbr.: **S.** Also called **spatial relations**. Also see PRIMARY ABILITIES; DEPTH PERCEPTION.

spatial-reversal learning a form of conditioning in which goals and rewards are reversed during the training. E.g., an animal first learns it will receive a reward if it goes to a white object and ignores another that is black; then the problem is reversed so that black becomes the proper goal and white must be ignored.

spatial summation a neural mechanism present in the spinal-motor system in which a neuron is fired by the sum of several synaptic inputs being discharged simultaneously. S.s. firings occur at points where the discharge of a single synapse would not be sufficient to produce the energy needed to activate the neuron.

spatial threshold the point of stimulus separation, that is, the smallest distance on the skin, at which two stimuli are perceived as two stimuli rather than a single stimulus. Also called **two-point threshold**. Also see TWO-POINT DISCRIMINATION.

spatial vision the perception of patterns and details in images observed through the visual sense. The term is used to distinguish the sensations from visual acuity, movement vision, or other categories of visual perception and discrimination.

Spatz, Hugo /shpäts/ German neuropathologist, fl. 1922. See HALLERVORDEN-SPATZ DISEASE.

spaying the surgical removal of the ovaries of a female mammal as a sterilization procedure.

speaking-fear = LALOPHOBIA.

speaking in tongues: See GLOSSOLALIA.

Spearman, Charles Edward English psychologist, 1863–1945. S. made many lasting contributions to statistical methods and psychological testing, including the distinction between general intelligence and special abilities, the rank-difference coefficient of correlation, and techniques of factor analysis. See SPEARMAN-BROWN PROPHECY FORMULA; RANK-ORDER CORRELATION (also called **Spearman's rho; Spearman rank-order correlation**); GENERAL FACTOR; SPECIFIC FACTOR; SPECIFIC ABILITY.

Spearman-Brown prophecy formula a statistical equation used to correct a reliability coefficient for the length of the test.

special aptitude = SPECIFIC ABILITY.

special child a term that is roughly equivalent to exceptional child, except that the emphasis is usually more on children with special problems, who need special education and training, e.g., slow learners, the retarded, the physically disabled, and the emotionally handicapped. Also see EXCEPTIONAL CHILD; ATYPICAL CHILD; SPECIAL EDUCATION; SPECIAL CLASSES.

special classes educational programs designed specifically for students with particular intellectual, behavioral, or physical disabilities, e.g., blindness, deafness, or speech impairment. The s.c. also may serve as training facilities for teachers who plan to specialize in teaching disabled students and are required to work in s.c. as part of their graduate-level university education. Also see SPECIAL EDUCATION; SPECIAL CHILD.

special education education provided to children with learning disabilities such as perceptual deficit, minimal brain dysfunction, blindness, deafness, and neurological disorders, or to children with intellectual ability so far above or below the norm that they require special curricula or special classes. See SPECIAL CHILD; SPECIAL CLASSES.

special factor a specialized ability which, according to Spearman, comes into play in particular kinds of cognitive tasks. Special factors, such as mathematical ability, are contrasted with the general intelligence factor, or g, which underlies every cognitive performance. Compare GENERAL FACTOR.

special schools facilities that provide education for disadvantaged or disabled children who are not prepared to cope with the intellectual and social skills demanded of children in regular schools.

special-symptom reaction a DSM-I category of personality disorders comprising such conditions as stuttering, nail-biting, enuresis, tics, and compulsive gambling.

special vulnerability a particularly low tolerance for certain kinds of stress.

species-specific behavior behavior that is common to all members of a particular species, appears to be unlearned, and is manifested by all species members in essentially the same way. This term is often preferred to use of the word instinct.

specific ability a special ability or aptitude that does not correlate with other abilities, as opposed to general ability, which correlates at least moderately with other abilities (Spearman). Also called **special aptitude**.

specific aptitude: see APTITUDE.

specific-attitudes theory the viewpoint that certain psychosomatic disorders are associated with particular attitudes. An example is an association between the feeling of being mistreated and the occurrence of hives. A similar concept is the SPECIFIC-REACTION THEORY. See this entry.

specific developmental disorders a group of childhood disorders involving specific areas of functioning, but not due to any other disorder such as infantile autism or mental retardation. See DEVELOPMENTAL READING DISORDER; DEVELOPMENTAL ARITHMETIC DISORDER; DEVELOPMENTAL LANGUAGE DISORDER; DEVELOPMENTAL ARTICULATION DISORDER; MIXED SPECIFIC DEVELOPMENTAL DISORDER; ATYPICAL SPECIFIC DEVELOPMENTAL DISORDER. (DSM-III)

specific dynamic pattern according to Franz Alexander, the specific nuclear conflict or dynamic configuration of a particular psychosomatic disorder.

specific-energy doctrine a concept advanced originally in the 1830s by Johannes Peter Müller, who held that the quality of a sensory experience is determined by the type of receptor. Although the s.-e.d. has been challenged by some investigators from time to time, it is still generally agreed that the sense of pain originates with pain receptors, hearing with receptors in the inner ear, and so on. Also called **nerve-energy doctrine**.

specific excitant the special kind of stimulus that is required to fire an impulse in a particular receptor. A sensory receptor may be sensitive only to the specific stimulus for which it was designed by nature; e.g., a s.e. for the retinal cells would be light, rather than sound or temperature.

specific hunger an urge to eat that is directed toward foods required by the animal in order to maintain constant weight, adequate energy, and normal health. An animal may, e.g., have a s.h. for protein and by self-selection seek protein-rich foods even though more palatable or attractive but protein-deficient foods are available. Also see SELF-SELECTION OF DIET.

specific inhibition an ego function inhibition, expressed, e.g., as anorexia or impotence. A s.i. is regarded as a renunciation of the functon which if exercised would result in severe anxiety.

specificity a quality of being unique, of a particular kind, or limited to one phenomenon, e.g., a stimulus that elicits a specific response, or a psychosomatic symptom localized in a particular organ such as the stomach.

specific learning disability a learning disorder such as reading or arithmetic difficulty that cannot be associated with a physical or mental defect such as mental retardation, epilepsy, or cerebral palsy, and is possibly due to developmental lag.

specific phobias: See PHOBIA.

specific-reaction theory a concept that an innate tendency of the autonomic nervous system to react in a particular way to a stressful situation accounts for psychosomatic symptoms. A similar concept is the SPECIFIC-ATTITUDES THEORY. See this entry.

specific thalamic projection system the direct sensory pathways via the thalamus for visual, auditory, and somesthetic impulses.

specific transfer the ability to apply skills and knowledge acquired in one field to problems in the same field. Also see GENERAL TRANSFER.

specimen record in observational studies, a written, chronological account of a subject's behavior during a given observational session. A s.r. should be as complete a description as possible, ideally excluding no behavioral details.

spectator role a term introduced by Masters and Johnson to identify a behavior pattern in which one's natural sexual responses are blocked by observing oneself closely and worrying about how well or poorly one is performing, rather than participating freely.

spectator therapy the tendency of group-therapy members to benefit from observing the therapy of other patients with similar problems. Imitating others is often a constructive way of experimenting with new behavior.

spectral absorption the ability of chemicals to absorb light of specific wavelengths, as determined by passing lights of nearly pure wavelengths through solutions of the chemicals and measuring the amount of light absorbed. In visual s.a. the principle is applied by measuring the degree to which wavelengths of light decompose retinal pigment molecules.

spectral color one of the colors of the spectrum produced when white light is refracted by a prism.

spectral sensitivity the relative degree of spectral absorption by retinal pigments at various wavelengths of light. The s.s. is recorded as a curve plotted on a graph of rectangular coordinates.

spectrometer a device that measures the wavelengths of colors in a spectrum.

spectrophobia = EISOPTROPHOBIA.

spectrophotometry a technique of photometric analysis in which a complete light spectrum is produced and the desired wavelength is isolated for use in analyzing chemicals in a body substance such as blood. It is based on a principle that physiological substances such as carotene, uric-acid, and hemoglobin components absorb light of precise wavelengths, thereby revealing their presence.

spectroscope an instrument designed to make the spectrum visible for study.

spectrum the series of visible colors produced when white light, e.g., sunlight, is refracted through a prism; also, the radiant energy that can be projected after refraction.

speculation conjectural thinking that is not supported by scientifically determined evidence.

speech communication through conventional vocal and oral symbols.

speech-and-hearing centers: See COMMUNITY S.-A.-H.C.

speech areas areas of the cerebral cortex that are associated with voice communication. Speech-association areas generally are located in the left hemisphere. Maps of the s.a. have been quite well plotted by studying left-hemisphere lesions that are found in patients with specific speech defects, e.g., Broca's area in the third convolution of the frontal lobe, and the "naming area" of the temporal lobe where lesions block ability to name objects.

speech audiometry the measurement of hearing in terms of the reception of spoken words presented at controlled levels of intensity.

speech block a temporary inability or a delay in producing the proper speech sounds, as in stuttering.

speech conservation a term coined by the military during World War II referring to preventive speech therapy given to newly deafened persons in order to keep their speech and voice disturbance to a minimum.

speech correction the "professional field which deals with the elimination and alleviation of speech defects or with the development and improvement of speaking intelligibility; sometimes distinguished from speech improvement." (L. E. Travis, *Handbook of Speech Pathology and Audiology*, 1971) Also see SPEECH PATHOLOGY.

speech derailment a type of paraphasia, or perverted speech, seen primarily in schizophrenia, and characterized by disconnected and apparently meaningless sounds which are usually whispered or screeched.

speech development: See ORIGIN-OF-LANGUAGE THEORIES.

speech disorders any disorder arising from defective speech apparatus (spasticity, cleft-palate speech), faulty functioning of the speech mechanism (stuttering, tachyphemia), or psychiatric symptoms that seriously interfere with communication (echolalia, verbigeration, word salad, mutism).

speech disturbance any language or communication disorder, such as mutism or stuttering, that is not due to impaired speech muscles or organs of articulation. For details, see COMMUNICATION DISORDER; LANGUAGE DISORDER; SPEECH DISORDERS.

speech functions the variety of purposes for which speech is used: to communicate ideas, maintain social relationships, or express feeling and emotion. The style of speech, choice of words, and use of linguistic expressions such as clichés and metaphors are reflections of the individual's personality and level of development. Speech may also be used for attack, for exhibitionistic display, for settling differences, for calming the disturbed or overwrought. And speech disorders such as verbigeration, circumstantiality, and paralogia, may be symptoms of mental or emotional disturbance. See SPEECH DISORDERS.

speech impairment any difficulty in communicating by voice due to organic or nonorganic causes. Types of **nonorganic s.i.** include neurotic-telegraphic speech, aphonia, and elective mutism. Types of **organic s.i.** include global aphasia, Broca's aphasia, conduction aphasia, and anomic aphasia.

speech lateralization the role of hemispheric asymmetry in the control of verbal communication. For most individuals, speech centers are located in the left hemisphere, which is relatively dominant for the speech function. Also see LANGUAGE LOCALIZATION; WADE DOMINANCE TEST.

speech origin: See ORIGIN-OF-LANGUAGE THEORIES.

speech pathology the "study and treatment of all aspects of functional and organic speech defects and disorders; often the same as speech correction." (L. E. Travis, *Handbook of Speech Pathology and Audiology*, 1971) Also see SPEECH CORRECTION.

speech-reading = LIP-READING.

speech-reception threshold the measurement of a person's threshold for speech for individual frequencies to determine the level at which he can repeat simple words, or understand simple connected speech. Abbrev.: **SRT.**

speech rehabilitation the training to restore a lost or disabled speech function. Also called **speech reeducation.**

speech theories: See ORIGIN-OF-LANGUAGE THEORIES.

speech therapy the application of remedies, treatment, and counseling for the improvement of speech functions.

speed a street term for amphetamine compounds, in particular for methamphetamine (or methamphetamine chloride), which is sold under the trademark Methedrine. See AMPHETAMINES; METHEDRINE.

speedball a popular name for a drug of abuse that is composed of heroin and a powerful stimulant, e.g., cocaine or amphetamine.

speed test a type of test intended to calculate the number of problems or tasks a subject can solve or perform under time pressure; any test in which the testee must operate within specified time restraints; or a test in which the subject's speed contributes to his score. Also called **timed test.** Compare POWER TEST.

sperm a general term for the male gamete (sex

cell), or for the semen containing male gametes (spermatozoa).

sperm analysis a part of the evaluation of male fertility based on the sperm count per milliliter of ejaculate and the degree of spermatozoa motility. The average male ejaculate after three days of continence is at least three milliliters of semen with approximately 100,000,000 spermatozoa per milliliter of which at least 60 percent show adequate motility for movement from the vagina to the Fallopian tubes. See SPERMATO-ZOON.

spermatic duct = DUCTUS DEFERENS.

spermatid a primitive form of spermatozoa that begins to develop in the male testis at the start of puberty. The s. develops from a secondary spermatocyte after the individual's pituitary begins secreting interstitial-cell-stimulating hormone. After puberty, production continues at a rather constant rate.

spermatocyte an intermediate stage in the development of spermatozoa from spermatogonia in the male testis. Each spermatogonium divides by mitosis into two cells, one of which becomes a primary s. Each primary s. divides into two secondary spermatocytes, each of which divides again into two spermatids.

spermatogenesis the process of production of spermatozoa in the seminiferous tubules of the male testis. S. is continuous in humans after the onset of puberty and seasonal in some other animal species.

spermatogonia cells in the seminiferous tubules of the male testis that are the first stage of spermatogenesis. As puberty approaches in the human male, each **spermatogonium** divides by mitosis into two cells, one of which develops into a primary spermatocyte. The other daughter cell remains a spermatogonium which can divide again repeatedly to produce a continuous supply of spermatocytes.

spermatophobia a morbid fear of sperm.

spermatorrhea the involuntary discharge of semen, in the absence of orgasm.

spermatorrhea ring an infibulation device for men promoted in the late 19th century as a method of preventing unlawful intercourse. The s.r. consisted of a small belt or ring lined with teeth or spikes that made painful contact with the penile shaft during erection. Also see INFIBULATION.

spermatozoon /-zō'ən/ the male gamete or sex cell. The human s., containing 23 chromosomes, is about 60 microns in length and consists of an oval head about five microns in length, a middle piece packed with mitochondria immediately below the head, and a long tail, a filament approximately 50 microns in length. The mitochondria provide the energy for propelling the s. after ejaculation. Enzymes in the acrosome of the head of the s. enable the male gamete to dissolve the protective barriers on the surface of the female ovum. Sperm counts in men who have fathered children have ranged from 5,000,000

spermatozoa per milliliter to 500,000,000 per milliliter. Plural: **spermatozoa**. Also see SPERM ANALYSIS.

spermaturia the presence of semen in the urine. Also called **semenuria**.

spermicide any natural or synthetic agent that kills spermatozoa. Some contraceptive jells and foams contain a s.

Sperry, Roger Wolcott American neurobiologist, 1913—. See CHIMERIC STIMULATION.

spherical aberration the failure of light rays to converge at the same focal point because of the curvature of a lens. Rays at the outer surface are bent more than those refracted at the inner surface.

sphincter control the ability to control the muscles that open and close the openings of the body, particularly the anal and urinary sphincters. This ability is an important stage in physical development and, according to psychoanalysis, in psychosexual development as well, since the capacity to accede to the wishes of others with respect to elimination, and to renounce immediate gratification, constitute an essential step in the development of the personality. See ANAL CHARACTER; TOILET TRAINING. Also see DEFECATION REFLEX.

sphincter cunni = bulbospongiosus muscle.

sphincter morality in psychoanalysis, the child's obedience to parental demands in toilet training, which Ferenczi considered the precursor of the superego. S.m. is also used for personality characteristics such as obstinacy, extreme orderliness, and parsimony, which are believed to result from overly strict toilet training. See ANAL CHARACTER; TOILET TRAINING.

sphingolipid a fatty substance that occurs in high concentrations in the brain and other nerve tissues. An excess of s. is associated with Tay-Sachs, Gaucher's, and Niemann-Pick diseases, and other disorders marked by mental-retardation symptoms.

sphingolipidoses a group of diseases characterized by abnormal metabolism of sphingomyelins and other long-chain fatty molecules. Examples include gangliosidosis, Gaucher's disease, and Niemann-Pick disease. The cerebral s. include the amaurotic familial idiocy diseases: Tay-Sachs, Spielmeyer-Vogt, Kuf's, and Bielschowsky-Jansky diseases.

sphingomyelin a fatty substance that contains phosphoric acid, choline, and a long-chain complex alcohol. It occurs naturally in tissues of the central nervous system and is present in certain food items, e.g., egg yolk.

sphingomyelin lipidosis: See NIEMANN-PICK DISEASE.

-sphygmo- a combining form relating to the pulse (from Greek *sphygmos*, "pulse").

sphygmograph an instrument for measuring the strength and rapidity of the pulse.

sphygmomanometer an instrument for measuring blood pressure in the arteries. The term is derived from the Greek work *sphygmos*, "pulse," and *manometer*, an instrument for the measurement of gases and fluids. A s. actually measures the amount of pressure required to stop the pulse sounds of blood flowing through the artery.

spider cells: See STELLATE CELLS.

spider fantasy spider images or stories that occur in dreams, phobias, and folklore. These fantasies are so prevalent that psychoanalysts believe this insect has special significance. They suggest, e.g., that spiders may represent, ambivalently, either a good or a bad omen, or that their web may represent pubic hair; also, since some females of some species kill the male after copulation, spiders may represent being killed by the mother during incestuous intercourse.

spider phobia = ARACHNEOPHOBIA.

Spielmeyer, Walter /shpēl′mī·ər/ German physician, 1879—. See SPIELMEYER-VOGT DISEASE; CEREBROMACULAR DEGENERATION (there: **Batten-Spielmeyer-Vogt disease**); SPHINGOLIPIDOSES.

Spielmeyer-Vogt disease a form of juvenile amaurotic familial idiocy that is inherited as an autosomal-recessive chromosomal abnormality. The onset of symptoms usually is between the ages of five and six years when progressive blindness begins with degeneration of rods, cones, and ganglia of the visual system. It is followed by cerebral lesions, mental deterioration, and death before the age of 20 years. Also called **Vogt-Spielmeyer disease**.

spike-and-dome discharges a pattern of brain waves that provides a diagnostic clue to petit mal epilepsy. It consists of a sharp spike followed by a low-amplitude slow wave that occurs at a frequency of three per second and indicates a thalamic lesion.

spike potential the change in electrical potential produced by the transmission of a nerve impulse. It is marked by a rapid swing of perhaps 100 millivolts from a negative charge through a positive charge and back to a resting potential stage, all within 1/1,000 of a second.

spike-wave activity the pattern produced by the electrical discharge of a neuron when amplified and projected onto the screen of an oscilloscope. The wave form appears as a sharp high peak, followed by a short dip below the horizontal line, then a return to the predischarge level. The size of the wave spike usually indicates the intensity of the discharge.

spina bifida /spɪ′nə bī′fədə/ or /spē′nä bif′idä/ a developmental defect, also known as open or split spine, resulting from a failure of the vertebral canal to close normally around the spinal cord. In **s.b. occulta** the problem is minimal since the spinal cord is essentially normal despite the fact that some of the vertebrae are defective. In s.b. with myelomeningocele (**s.b. manifesta** or **s.b. cystica**) part of the spinal cord protrudes from the body surface. In extreme cases, this may lead to weakness or paralysis of the muscles of the legs or feet, club foot, dislocated hips, in-

adequate control of bladder or bowel, susceptibility to infection, and, in 80 percent of cases, hydrocephalus, which usually leads to brain damage. Some of the symptoms may be avoided or modified if the protruding cord is surgically buried below the skin surface soon after birth. See HYDROCEPHALUS; MYELOMENINGOCELE. Also see RACHISCHISIS.

spinal animal a laboratory animal whose spinal cord has been separated from the brain so that nerve processes of the body are spinal only.

spinal canal a small tube that runs through the center of the spinal cord and carries cerebrospinal fluid.

spinal conditioning a theory suggesting that conditioned reflexes might be established through circuits in the spinal cord that lack interconnections to CNS structures above the cord. The experiments have failed to demonstrate discriminative-learning functions in the spinal circuits.

spinal cord the part of the central nervous system that extends from the lower end of the medulla, at the base of the brain, down to the lumbar area of the vertebral column. The s.c. is enclosed in a spinal canal formed by openings in the vertebrae of the spinal column.

spinal-cord disease any pathologic condition caused by infection, injury, or congenital defect that involves the spinal cord. Examples of s.-c.d. include Brown-Sequard's and Bernard-Horner syndromes, spinal meningitis, amyotrophic lateral sclerosis, Oppenheim's disease, multiple sclerosis, syringomyelia, acute transvere myelitis, and hereditary ataxias.

spinal-cord injury any wounding, maiming, or similar damage to the spinal cord due to sudden or progressive external forces. Kinds of s.-c.i. include contusion, hemorrhage, laceration, transection, spinal shock, or compression. See RADICULOPATHIES; SLIPPED DISK; FORAMINOTOMY; LAMINECTOMY.

spinal curvature any deviation from the normal cervical, thoracic, lumbar, and sacral curves of the spinal column. S.c. may be due to muscle spasm, or diseases of the ligaments or joints, in the absence of an orthopedic disorder. Kinds of s.c. include SCOLIOSIS, KYPHOSIS, and LORDOSIS See these entries.

spinal fusion a surgical procedure in which two or more adjacent vertebrae are fused into a single segment of spinal column. The procedure may be performed in the treatment of a spinal-cord-compression disorder. See FORAMINOTOMY; LAMINECTOMY.

spinal ganglia clumps of sensory-neuron-cell bodies that form the dorsal roots of the spinal cord.

spinal gate according to the gate-control theory of pain, a mechanism in cells of the substantia gelatinosa that transmits the net effect of both excitatory and inhibitory signals to the brain. In addition, the mechanism modifies the pain signals themselves in accordance with messages from higher centers which reflect previous experience and the influence of emotional factors and personality on pain perception. The theory also suggests that pain may be relieved by interrupting excitatory fibers or stimulating inhibitory pain fibers. Also called **gating mechanism**. See GATING.

spinal meningitis an acute inflammation of the meningeal membranes surrounding the spinal cord, usually caused by a bacterial infection.

spinal nerves the 31 pairs of nerves that originate in the spinal cord and extend into the body's dermatomes (skin areas) through openings between the vertebrae of the spinal column. The s.n. include eight cervical, 12 **thoracic**, five **lumbar**, five **sacral**, and one **coccygeal** nerve. Also see CERVICAL NERVES.

spinal pia mater: See PIA MATER.

spinal poliomyelitis: See POLIOMYELITIS.

spinal reflexes a set of reflexes that are involved in functions such as posture or locomotion. They are sometimes classed as segmental s.r., if the circuit involves only one segment of the spine, or intersegmental s.r., if the impulses must travel through more than one spinal segment. Reflexes that require brain activity are suprasegmental s.r.

spinal root the junction of the spinal nerve and the spinal cord; the sensory roots on the dorsal side of the cord and motor roots on the ventral side.

spinal shock a failure of motor nerves following injury to the spinal cord because of inability of impulses from the brain to maintain excitability of neurons and interneurons below the site of the injury. The period of recovery is longer for humans and other higher animals than for lower vertebrates, such as amphibia, with less complex nervous systems.

spinal stenosis a narrowing of the spinal canal of the vertebral column. The condition is one of the types of orthopedic pathology observed in dwarfism.

spinal tonus a continuous degree of spinal-cord contractility maintained after connections to the brain have been severed.

spinal transection a lesion that cuts across the spinal cord. **Complete s.t.**, caused by disease or injury, results in paraplegia and paralysis of the body area below the site of the lesion. Some reflex functions may be retained, such as penile erection in paraplegic men by stimulation of the genital area.

spinal trigeminal nucleus the nucleus of the descending or spinal branch of the fifth cranial, or trigeminal, nerve with extensions into the spinal cord. It sometimes is described as part of the medulla and a continuation of the substantia gelatinosa of Rolando in the spinal cord.

spinal tumor any abnormal tissue growth that may arise from the layers of the spinal cord, the nerve roots, or the vertebrae. A s.t. also may develop as a secondary cancer from cells that have metastasized from the lung, breast, prostate, kidney, or other organs. About two-thirds of primary spinal tumors are meningiomas or neurofibromas. The symptoms usually are pain and paresthesia resulting from spinal-cord compression. Spinal tumors are treated by surgery or radiation.

spindle waves electroencephalogram patterns associated with light sleep and characterized by delta-wave forms that occur at a frequency of about 14 per second.

spindling in EEG bursts of EEG activity that follow positive reinforcement during conditioning. The postreinforcement synchronization involves cholinergic neurons in the cortex and can be controlled by cholinergic blockers and cholinesterase inhibitors. The effect indicates a state of attention or excitement.

Spinnbarkeit/shpin′bärkīt/literally, "spinnability" (German), a term referring to the threadlike, viscous character of cervical mucus crystal that forms when a sample of mucus taken at the time of ovulation is allowed to dry on a microscope glass slide. The mucus forms a fern pattern as it crystallizes. See FERNING.

spinocerebellar tract a major nerve tract that carries impulses from the muscles and other proprioceptors through the spinal cord to the cerebellum.

spinothalamic tract one of the ascending pathways for somatic sensory impulses that travel through the spinal cord to the thalamus. The s.t. contains two groups of fibers: one, the **central s.t.**, carries pressure sensations; the second, the lateral s.t., carries pain and temperature information. See LATERAL S.T.

-spir-; -spiro- a combining form relating to (a) respiration, (b) a spiral formation.

spiral ganglion the site of the cell bodies for the hair cells of the auditory nerve. The s.g. is in the inner wall of the cochlea, near the organ of Corti.

spiral organ = ORGAN OF CORTI.

spiritism: See SPIRITUALISM.

spiritual factors in psychiatry and psychology, moral and religious influences on behavior; transcendental forces and values.

spiritualism the metaphysical belief that the universe is basically nonmaterial, or incorporeal; also, the belief that it is possible to communicate with the deceased through mediums. The latter is sometimes called **spiritism**.

Spirocheta pallida: See SYPHILIS.

spirograph an instrument for measuring and recording the rate and amount of breathing.

spirometer an instrument used for measuring the air capacity in the lungs. It provides information regarding the amount of inhaled and exhaled air during speech production.

Spitz, René A. Austrian-born American psychologist, 1887–1974. See EMOTIONAL RESPONSE; HOSPITALISM.

SPL = SOUND-PRESSURE LEVEL.

-splanch-; -splanchno- a combining form relating to the viscera (Greek *splanchnon*).

splanchnic a term that refers to the abdominal organs, or viscera, and is employed in the definitions of various body types in which the abdomen is a prominent feature, e.g., normosplanchnic, microsplanchnic, megalosplanchnic.

spleen a large, flat organ located under the ribs on the left side of the upper abdomen. Before birth and when there is bone-marrow failure after birth, the s. produces red blood cells. It also stores and cleans red blood cells and helps clean the blood of worn-out blood cells and waste products, releasing stored blood in emergencies. **Splenectomy**, or surgical removal of the s., may be performed in the treatment of certain diseases, and in conjunction with kidney transplants.

-splen-; -spleno- a combining form relating to the spleen (Latin *splen*).

splenectomy: See SPLEEN.

splenium a blunt enlargement at the posterior end of the corpus callosum where it overlaps a portion of the third ventricle.

splinter skill a skill that is not an integral part of the systematic sequential development in a child, e.g., learning how to write before physiological readiness for this skill.

splints the rigid or flexible devices used mainly to immobilize fractures and dislocated joints. The purpose of s. is to provide a means of isolating the fracture or joint from wear and tear while natural healing takes place. S. may be applied internally in certain orthopedic procedures, e.g., rebuilding a hip joint for an older patient, as well as externally.

split brain the phenomenon of the two cerebral hemispheres functioning independently. The s.b. effect is produced experimentally on laboratory animals and occurs in humans as a result of injury or disease resulting in damage to the corpus callosum connecting the two hemispheres. In the classic pioneering Déjérine case, a s.b. patient could write and copy words but could not remember or understand what he had written since the visual images could not reach the speech center. Normally, however, visual and other inputs can be received and stored as memory traces in both hemispheres through interhemispheric transfer of information—but not in an individual with a s.b. Also called **divided brain**. See CEREBRAL DOMINANCE; LATERALITY; FUNCTIONAL PLASTICITY.

split-brain technique a method of studying the process of bilateral transfer in the brain by separating the hemispheres at the corpus callosum, with or without severing also the optic chiasma.

split-half reliability a measure of the internal consistency of a test, obtained by correlating responses on half the test with responses on the other half. Also see ODD-EVEN RELIABILITY.

split personality a popular term for multiple personality. It is sometimes confused with schizophrenia (which literally means a splitting of the mind but does not involve the formation of a second personality).

splitting headache: See LEAD-CAP HEADACHE.

spoiled-child reaction a behavior pattern marked by a lack of self-care, independence, and responsibility, attributed to parental overindulgence and oversolicitude.

-spondyl-; -spondylo- a combining form relating to the vertebrae or the spine.

spondylitis an inflammation of any part of the spinal column.

spondyloepiphysial dysplasia congenita a type of dwarfism characterized by a short trunk, round face, protruding abdomen, and broad chest with extreme lordosis. The patient also is likely to show a leg deformity such as bowleg or knock-knee.

spongioblast an embryonic ectodermal cell that develops along the neural tube and evolves into neuroglial tissue.

spongy degeneration of the CNS in infancy = CANAVAN'S DISEASE.

spontaneity test a type of sociometric test, devised by Moreno, in which the subject is encouraged to improvise freely in typical life situations with members of the group who have been judged to be emotionally related, positively or negatively, to the subject. The object is to elicit insight into interpersonal relationships not revealed by the standard sociometric test, which deals only with attraction and repulsion.

spontaneity training a more or less formal personality training program in which the patient learns to act naturally and spontaneously in real-life situations by practicing such behavior in graduated sessions (Moreno). Also called **spontaneity therapy.**

spontaneous abortion an interruption of pregnancy with loss of the fetus as a result of natural causes. A common cause of s.a. is an imbalance of hormones required to support the pregnancy. Emotional disturbances also may be causative factors. More than ten percent of all human pregnancies are terminated by s.a. Also see MISCARRIAGE.

spontaneous behavior behavior that is not the result of an external stimulus.

spontaneous discharge the firing of neural impulses or spike potentials without direct influence of an external stimulus.

spontaneous movement movement occurring in the absence of any particular stimulus. Spontaneous neuron firing is common in auditory, visual, and neuromuscular fibers, as a result of metabolic activity or hypersecretion of synaptic transmitter chemicals, e.g., acetylcholine.

spontaneous neural activity the apparent automatic firing of neurons, or firing in the absence of observable stimuli. The effect has been attributed to an excessive buildup of neurotransmitter chemical at the synapses.

spontaneous recovery the reappearance of a

conditioned response after it has been experimentally extinguished. The response strength is usually very weak.

spontaneous regression a phenomenon of hypnosis in which a subject suddenly relives an event from an earlier age, e.g., childhood, and may even exhibit appropriate behavior for that age.

spontaneous remission recovery or partial recovery independent of formal treatment.

spontaneous thought an alternative term for daydreaming.

spoonerism a form of jumbled speech, or cluttering, in which initial sounds are transposed. The condition is named after the English clergyman W. A. Spooner (1844–1930), who habitually made such mistakes as referring to "our queer old dean" when he meant "our dear old queen."

s population = STIMULUS POPULATION.

sport in genetics, an organism that has undergone mutation and is distinctly different from its parents.

Spranger, Edward /shpräng'ər/ German philosopher, 1882–1963. S. developed a holistic view of personality, and a typology based on six cultural values: theoretical, economic, political, esthetic, social, and religious. See ALLPORT-VERNON-LINDZEY STUDY OF VALUES; PERSONALISTIC PSYCHOLOGY; PERSONALITY TYPES; SOCIAL TYPE.

spread of effect a generalization that satisfaction or dissatisfaction associated with a response will spread to other aspects of the situation.

spurious correlation any correlation that may be coincidental or only partly the result of factors attributed to it, e.g., the increase in lung cancer may show a s.c. to the use of television.

spurt a sudden sharp increase in the rate of a process, e.g., a growth s. around the time of puberty. Also see INITIAL S.; END S.

Spurzheim, Johann Caspar /shpoŏrts'hīm/ German philosopher and anatomist, 1776–1832. S. was a pupil of Franz Joseph Gall, the founder of phrenology. He is credited with coining this word. See PHRENOLOGY; CRANIOLOGY.

squamous-cell carcinoma: See CARCINOMA; SKIN CANCER.

square sum: See SUM OF SQUARES.

squeeze technique a technique devised by J. H. Semans for overcoming premature ejaculation. The partner squeezes the head of the penis until the urge to ejaculate and some of the erection disappear. By repeating this maneuver, the male becomes conditioned to last longer before ejaculation.

squiggle game a technique devised by D. W. Winnicott, in which a child patient and the therapist take turns in drawing lines that gradually evolve into a significant object. The drawing elicits comments or stories from the child and paves the way toward dealing with anxiety-laden situations.

squint: See STRABISMUS; CROSS-EYE.

S-R an abbreviation of *s*timulus-*r*esponse. Also see DYNAMIC PSYCHOLOGY.

S-R psychologists psychologists whose work emphasizes the role of the *s*timulus-*r*esponse effect in learning and other forms of conditioning. Also called **associationists.**

SRA Mechanical Aptitude Test a test that measures mechanical aptitude in three ways: by identification of different tools; by fitting pieces together as a test of space relations; and by solving problems in shop arithmetic involving the use of tables and diagrams.

SRIF: See SOMATOSTATIN.

SRO = SINGLE-ROOM OCCUPANCY.

Srole, Leo American social scientist, 1908—. See MIDTOWN MANHATTAN STUDY.

SRT = SPEECH-RECEPTION THRESHOLD.

ss an abbreviation used in prescriptions, meaning "half" (Latin *semi* or *semis*).

SSPE = SUBACUTE SCLEROSING PANENCEPHALITIS.

SST = SOCIAL-SKILLS TRAINING.

S-state: See DREAM STATE; W-STATE.

stabilimeter an instrument for measuring postural stability and body sway when the subject is standing erect and blindfolded and asked to remain immobile.

stability the absence of variation or motion, as applied to genetics (invariance in characteristics), personality (few mood changes), or body position (absence of body sway).

stability coefficient: See COEFFICIENT OF STABILITY.

stability-lability a dimension of sensitivity to stimuli due to individual variations in autonomic nervous systems. Thus, a labile individual would be expected to react to a wider range of stimuli than a stable person.

stabilized image an image on the retina that does not fade away during visual-system studies. The image may be stabilized (a) by a bright flash that in effect burns the image onto the retina for a few seconds or, as has been found to be more effective, (b) by attaching a contact lens on which the image has been imprinted.

stage a natural division in a changing process, usually characterized by biological or other qualities.

stage fright an anxiety reaction associated with speaking or performing before an audience or being otherwise subjected to public scrutiny. The individual becomes tense and apprehensive, perspires profusely, and may stutter, forget lines, or run away. Some psychoanalysts explain the reaction in terms of a defense against exhibitionist tendencies and the unconscious fear of castration which these tendencies produce. See SOCIAL PHOBIA.

stage of exhaustion = EXHAUSTION STAGE.

stage of resistance in H. Selye's general adaptation syndrome, the second major phase of the body's response to an extended period of stress in which the organism combats or defends itself against the stressor. Adaptation is manifested, in part, by the increased secretions of the adrenal glands. Also called **resistance stage**. See GENERAL ADAPTATION SYNDROME. Also see ALARM REACTION; EXHAUSTION STAGE.

stagnation: See GENERATIVITY VERSUS SELF-ABSORPTION.

stains chemical dyes that are applied to microscopic sections of tissues to render them more easily visible. The choice of s. is determined by the type of tissue and the study objective. A stain that dyes an unmyelinated nerve may not be as effective in staining a myelinated fiber.

staircase illusion the line drawing of a staircase in which the stairs may appear to ascend or descend depending on the point of fixation.

stair phobia = CLIMACOPHOBIA.

stalking behavior: See PREDATION.

stammering = STUTTERING.

standard a criterion model against which performances are judged or evaluated; also, a fixed unit such as the nautical mile.

standard deviation a measure of the dispersion of a set of scores, indicating how narrowly or broadly they are distributed around the mean, and symbolized by s (**sample s.d.**) or σ (**population s.d.**). One s.d. above and below the mean includes about 68 percent of the cases, two standard deviations include about 95 percent of the cases, and three standard deviations include about 99 percent of the cases. S.d. is also the square root of the variance. Symbol: $\sigma = \sqrt{x^2/N}$.

standard difference the difference between two means divided by the standard error of that difference.

standard error the standard deviation of a sampling distribution. Every statistic varies from sample to sample, and the s.e. indicates how much spread a particular statistic will show around its central value.

standard error of estimate a measure of the degree to which a regression line fits a set of data; the error in estimating one variable from another.

standard error of the mean the standard deviation of a sampling distribution of means, showing how much successive samples of means vary. A large s.e.o.t.m. indicates that there is much variation in successive samples of the mean. Symbol: $\sigma_{\bar{x}} = \sigma/\sqrt{n}$.

standardization a method of establishing norms or standards and uniform procedures for a test by administering it to a large group of representative individuals.

standardization group a sample to whom a test is administered to ascertain the average level of performance and the relative frequency of different degrees of deviation above and below the average for the purpose of establishing reliable norms and scoring standards for the population that the s.g. represents. Also called **standardization sample**.

standardized in statistics, compared with the responses of a known group, and therefore having known characteristics.

standardized interview schedule a type of structured interview with preestablished questions and procedures designed to enhance the technique's predictive value, provide criteria for objective scoring, and eliminate interviewer bias and other sources of variability.

standardized measuring device a test or instrument that has been administered to a large and representative sample of the population for which it is to provide reliable norms of achievement or aptitude in a designated area or areas.

standardized test a test whose validity and reliability have been established by thorough empirical tryouts and analysis and which has clearly defined time limits and instructions for administration and scoring.

standard ratio: See STANDARD DIFFERENCE.

standard scores a set of scores with a mean of 0 and a standard deviation of 1. Raw scores may be standardized or transformed to s.s. Also called **z scores**. Symbol: $z = (X - \bar{X})/s$.

standard stimulus a stimulus that is used as the basis of comparison for other stimuli applied in a psychological experiment, e.g., in comparing loud sounds to a sound of a given intensity.

Stanford Achievement Test a test designed to measure progress in word meaning, paragraph meaning, and grammatical usage.

Stanford-Binet Intelligence Scale an individual test designed primarily for school children, but with a range of age two to adult. The present S.-B.I.S. is a revision, by L. M. Terman and M. Merrill, of the first intelligence test created by A. Binet and T. Simon in 1905. It consists of scale items for each half year or year, with heavy emphasis on verbal ability (information, vocabulary, memory span, use of words), and yields an MA (mental age) which, when divided by the CA (chronological age), can be translated into an overall IQ without separate scores for special abilities. See IQ. Abbrev.: **S-B**.

Stanford-Binet Scale the 1916 revision of the original scale developed in 1905 by Binet and Simon, to fit American conditions. The scale was again revised in 1937 and 1960. See STANFORD-BINET INTELLIGENCE SCALE.

Stanford Diagnostic Arithmetic Test; Stanford Diagnostic Reading Tests: See DIAGNOSTIC EDUCATIONAL TESTS.

Stanford Hypnotic Susceptibility Scale a standardized 12-item scale used to measure hypnotizability by means of the subject's response to such suggestions as swaying backward, closing the eyes, lowering an outstretched arm, and fingerlock for mild hypnosis, and such responses as hallucinating a fly and posthypnotic amnesia for deeper hypnosis.

stapedectomy a surgical procedure used to restore hearing in individuals with otosclerosis: The stapes bone is removed and replaced with a prosthetic ossicle. See OSSICLES.

stapedes: See STAPES.

stapedius a muscle that controls the movement of the stapes in the middle ear. It is innervated by the facial nerve. The s. has a modulating control on the stapes, reducing vibrations caused by very intense noises which might otherwise damage delicate inner-ear structures.

stapes a stirrup-shaped ossicle that is the innermost of the three bones of the middle ear. The flat side of the s. is attached to the oval window on the side of the cochlea, allowing vibrations received from the tympanic membrane, or ear drum, to be relayed by the chain of ossicles to the oval window which converts sound vibrations to changes in fluid pressure. Plurals: **stapes; stapedes**.

star on a sociometric test designed to reveal relationship patterns within a group, the group member most frequently designated as the person with whom other members would wish to work or spend time in some way. Also called **sociocenter**. Compare ISOLATE.

star cells: See STELLATE CELLS.

star fear = SIDEROPHOBIA.

startle reaction a rapid, pervasive reflex response to a sudden, unexpected stimulus such as a pistol shot, or a face looming up in the darkness. The reaction involves closing of the eyes, widening of the mouth, increased heartbeat and respiration, flexion of the trunk and extremities, and increased alertness. This pattern is so uniform from individual to individual that many psychologists consider it an inborn, primitive self-preservation mechanism. It occurs in normal persons as well as in acute anxiety disorders. Also called **startle response**.

starvation reactions physical and psychological effects of chronic undernourishment, which is experienced by perhaps well over one-quarter of the world's population. Common physical effects include general weakness or asthenia, hunger pangs, sluggishness, and susceptibility to disease. Common psychological effects are slowing down of thought processes, difficulty in concentration, apathy, irritability, reduced sexual desire, and loss of pride in appearance. Psychotic reactions seldom occur except when starvation is accompanied by infection or extreme stress.

stasibasiphobia a morbid fear of standing upright and walking. Also called **stasobasophobia**.

stasiphobia a morbid fear of standing or getting up, sometimes resulting in a psychogenic inability to do so. See ASTASIA-ABASIA. Also called **stasophobia**.

stasis a state of inactivity and stagnation in an organism, a person, or a society; a sterile equilibrium in which change and growth do not occur.

-stasis a combining form relating to stagnation or to the stoppage of the flow of a liquid.

stasobasophobia = STASIBASIPHOBIA.

stasophobia = STASIPHOBIA.

stat. an abbreviation used mainly in prescriptions, meaning "immediately" (Latin *statim*).

state-dependent learning learning that occurs in association with a particular biological or psychological state. S.-d.l. will not transfer to or cannot be retrieved in states unrelated to the state in which learning originally occurred. E.g., an animal trained to run a maze while under the influence of a certain drug may not run it successfully without the drug. Also called **dissociated learning**.

state-dependent memory a condition in which memory for a past event is improved when the person can be in the same mental state as when the event occurred. Thus, a person who is sad may have difficulty in recalling details of a happy event.

states of arousal the states experienced by infants in fairly even alternation, e.g., regular, periodic, and irregular sleep, crying, waking activity, and alert inactivity.

static response a postural reflex that orients the body against a force, such as gravity. Also called **static reflex**.

static sense = SENSE OF EQUILIBRIUM.

statistic: See STATISTICS.

statistical control the use of statistical methods to reduce the effect of factors that could not be eliminated or controlled during an experiment.

statistical error any error of sampling, measurement, or treatment that interferes with drawing a valid conclusion from experimental results.

statistical inference: See INFERENTIAL STATISTICS.

statistical paradigm in abnormal psychology, a set of conditions by which a substantial deviation from the average is considered abnormal.

statistical psychology a branch of psychology that uses statistical models and methods to derive explanations for phenomena.

statistical regression: See REGRESSION TOWARD THE MEAN.

statistical significance: See SIGNIFICANCE.

statistics a branch of mathematics that uses data descriptively or inferentially to find or support answers for scientific and other quantifiable questions. A **statistic** is a numerical datum; or a mathematical summary or description of a body of data; also, an estimate of a parameter, obtained by sampling. Also see DESCRIPTIVE S.; INFERENTIAL S.; NONPARAMETRIC S.; DISTRIBUTION-FREE S.; PSYCHOLOGICAL S. (Example: page 710)

statoacoustic nerve the eighth cranial nerve, which also is the auditory nerve. It is a sensory nerve with tracts that innervate both the sense of hearing and the sense of balance. It has two roots, the vestibular branch originating in the vestibule and the semicircular canals, and the cochlear branch originating in the cochlea. The s.n. transmits impulses from the inner ear to the medulla and pons, with fibers that continue into

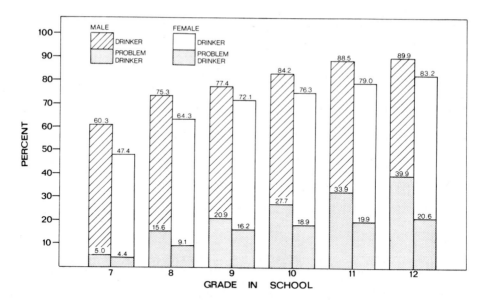

STATISTICS. Example: Percentages of students who admittedly were drinkers or
problem drinkers (Califano, 1979, and Donovan & Jessor, 1978).

the cerebrum and cerebellum. The s.n. is referred to as "cranial nerve VIII." Also called
vestibulocochlear nerve; auditory nerve; acoustic nerve.

statoconia = OTOLITHS.

statocyst a basic device found mainly in lower
animals that functions as a receptor for the sense
of balance. The s. is a sac containing small solid
particles, called otoliths, which shift with the
force of gravity when the animal moves its head.
The movements of the otoliths (literally, ear
stones) indicate to the animal which countermovements are needed to maintain balance.
Also see GEOTAXIS.

statokinetic responses postural reflexes and other
muscular reactions that enable a person to maintain balance and orientation while walking, running, or jumping.

statue of Condillac a hypothetical model proposed by Condillac to explain the gradual acquisition of human senses, using an imaginary
statue that first develops an olfactory apparatus,
and then the other senses, one by one.

status the state or position of an individual or
group, e.g., one's standing in a social group;
also, a persistent condition, as in status epilepticus.

status comparison the comparison by an individual of his own abilities and shortcomings with
the same or similar qualities in others.

status disraphicus a hereditary disorder marked
by a number of developmental anomalies which
result from faulty development of the spine or
spinal cord during the embryonic stage. It is believed to be the basis for such neurological diseases as syringomyelia and hereditary ataxia.

status epilepticus a continuous series of grand mal
seizures, sometimes resulting in death.

status grouping a grouping of individuals according to their social standing.

status need the need to attain a high degree of social recognition, prestige, or power.

status role the function fulfilled by an individual
who, through membership in a group, lends status to the group as a whole because of reputation, special abilities, or achievements. E.g., an
internationally recognized professor fulfills a s.r.
in his or her university.

statutory rape a legal term applied in cases in
which a girl consents to sexual intercourse
although she is not qualified because of her age
to give lawful consent. Most state laws make no
provision for the age of the male, who may
actually be younger than the girl. Thus a boy of
15 can be charged with s.r. of a 16-year-old girl
even though the girl seduced the boy. Also see
RAPE.

Stauder's lethal catatonia = CATATONIC CEREBRAL
PARALYSIS.

stealing: See KLEPTOMANIA.

stealing-fear = KLEPTOPHOBIA.

-steat-; -steato- a combining form relating to fat or
fatty tissue.

steatopygia the presence of large quantities of fat
in the buttocks. In some cultures s. is considered
a prerequisite for female beauty. As the condition is commonly observed among the Hottentots of southern Africa, it is also called **Hottentot
bustle.**

Steele, John C. Canadian physician, fl. 1951,
1968. See STEELE-RICHARDSON-OLSZEWSKI SYN
DROME.

Steele-Richardson-Olszewski syndrome a form of ocular-muscle paralysis in the sixth decade marked by a fixed downward gaze and limited upward gaze. Lateral gaze is not affected. The condition may be accompanied by rigidity of the neck and trunk and a mild form of dementia. Pathology often shows demyelination in various regions of the brainstem, basal ganglia, and cerebellum. Also called **supranuclear palsy**.

Stegreiftheater = THEATER OF SPONTANEITY.

Steinert, Hans Gustav Wilhelm /shtī′nərt/ German physician, 1875—. See CURSCHMANN-BATTEN-STEINER SYNDROME; MYOTONIC DYSTROPHY (also called **Steinert's disease**).

Stekel, Wilhelm /shtā′kəl/ Austrian psychiatrist, 1868–1940. S. was an early associate of Freud and developed a shortened form of psychoanalysis in which the therapist plays an active role (in collaboration with the patient) in interpreting dreams, exposing inner conflicts, and directing the discussion of resistances and repressions. See ACTIVE ANALYTIC PSYCHOTHERAPY; FALSE ASSOCIATION; FINAL TENDENCY; INTEREGO; KATA-GOGIC TENDENCY; MASK; PARAPATHY; PROPHETIC DREAMS; SOMATIZATION; SUBJECT-ILL; TELEPATHIC DREAM.

stellate cells any of a number of the larger pyramidal cells below the plexiform layer of the cortex. Generally, the s.c. are named for their shape, such as **star cells, bushy cells**, or **spider cells**. At the bottom of the outer pyramidal layer, most of the cells are s.c.

-steno- a combining form meaning narrow.

stenosis the abnormal narrowing of a body conduit or passageway. E.g., an **aortic s.** is a narrowing of the blood vessel leading from the left ventricle, thereby restricting blood flow from the heart to the general body circulation; a **pyloric s.** restricts the flow of stomach contents into the small intestine; and a spinal s. is a narrowing of the opening in the spinal column that restricts the space needed for the spinal cord. Also see SPINAL S.

stenosis of aqueduct of Sylvius a hereditary or familial disorder marked by massive head enlargement at birth and hydrocephalus. One study found 37 males in five families affected by the disorder, indicating the cause is transmitted as an X-linked recessive gene. In some cases, the disorder develops insidiously after adulthood rather than as a congenital condition.

step-down test a test used in studies of the amount of time required for a memory trace to become permanently established in the cortex. The test involves giving an animal an electroconvulsive shock after it steps down from an elevated platform and in some trials also giving the animal a foot shock at various intervals before the electroconvulsive shock, which tends to wipe out a recent memory trace.

step interval = CLASS INTERVAL.

steppage gait: See FOOT DROP.

stepping reflex a reflex movement elicited during the first two weeks of life by holding the infant

with his feet touching a surface, and moving him gently forward.

stereognosis the ability to recognize an object by touch (from Greek *stereos*, "hard, solid," and *gnosis*, "knowledge").

stereopsis = DEPTH PERCEPTION.

stereopsyche a term used by Storch to identify certain motor activities of schizophrenic patients, such as catatonic postures and a fetal position. The movements and postures appear to be isolated from the rest of the psychic structure of the patient. They are believed to be a manifestation of the primitive part of the mind performing primitive types of motility.

stereoscope a device that presents two slightly disparate pictures of the same scene, one to each eye, the separate retinal images fusing to produce a binocular, three-dimensional image. The device is used for vision-testing and -training.

stereoscopic vision = DEPTH PERCEPTION.

stereotactic tractotomy a form of psychosurgery in which radioactive yttrium seeds are implanted below the head of the caudate nucleus for the relief of symptoms of anxiety, severe depression, and obsessional states. Also called **seed psychosurgery**.

stereotaxic instrument a device designed to permit experimental work on the brains of animals without damaging neighboring tissues. The s.i. holds the animal's head in a position which, when coordinated with information from the coordinates of brain atlases, allows an electrode to be inserted into a precise area or structure of the brain.

stereotaxy /ster′-/ the precise positioning of a point in three-dimensional areas, e.g., the exact location of a nerve center in the brain. S. is employed in the positioning of an electrode in the brain for diagnostic, experimental, or therapeutic purposes. It is also of increasing importance in intrauterine treatment and surgery. Also called **stereotaxic technique**.

stereotype /ster′ē-ōtīp/ a biased, oversimplified, and inflexible, frequently erroneous conception usually of an ethnic or social group, e.g., "all teen-agers take drugs and play loud music." The s. ignores the unique, individual qualities of persons belonging to the stereotyped group, and may reflect many different motives, such as scapegoating, ignorance, fear, or economic considerations. Also see RACISM; PREJUDICE.

stereotype accuracy the ability to determine accurately in what way a person's traits correspond to a stereotype associated with his age group, ethnic group, professional group, or some other group. Compare DIFFERENTIAL ACCURACY.

stereotyped behavior = STEREOTYPY.

stereotyped-movement disorders (DSM-III): See TRANSIENT-TIC DISORDER; CHRONIC MOTOR-TIC DISORDER; TOURETTE'S DISORDER; ATYPICAL TIC DISORDER; ATYPICAL STEREOTYPED-MOVEMENT DISORDER. Also see STEREOTYPY.

stereotypy /-ot′ipē/ persistent pathological repetition of the same words, phrases, or movements. It is a common symptom in autistic children and in patients with obsessive-compulsive disorder or catatonic schizophrenia. The condition is frequently interpreted as an unconscious effort to allay anxiety and gain a feeling of security. Also called **stereotyped behavior**.

steric theory of odor the concept that certain odors are perceived because they are produced by chemical molecules of certain shapes. The molecules that fit a receptor in a lock-and-key manner cause the neural membrane to become depolarized or hyperpolarized, an effect which in turn signals the cue that identifies the odor. Also see SMELL MECHANISM.

sterility a condition of being infertile, or incapable of contributing to the production of living organisms. The term may be applied to an individual incapable of reproducing his own species or, in another sense, to a person or object rendered incapable of supporting microbial life because of treatment with chemicals, radiation, or heat. Also see INFERTILITY; FECUNDITY.

sterilization the process of rendering a person incapable of sexual reproduction. S. may be performed surgically by vasectomy or castration in the male or by excision of the Fallopian tubes, ovaries, or uterus in the female. S. also may result from injury or from exposure to radiation, heat, or chemicals.

Stern, Wilhelm /shtern/ German psychologist, 1871–1938. See AUSSAGE TEST; PERSONALISTIC PSYCHOLOGY; PHENOMOTIVE.

sternocleidomastoid a muscle originating in the sternum and clavicle and passing obliquely across the neck to the mastoid process behind the ear. When the s. muscle contracts, it rotates the head and draws it toward the shoulder on the same side. Contraction of both s. muscles bows the head.

Stern's disease a form of presenile psychosis associated with thalamic degeneration.

steroids complex organic molecules which have in common four interconnected hydrocarbon rings, three with six carbon atoms and one with five. The molecules are the basic form of male and female sex hormones, adrenal-cortical hormones, and other natural substances such as vitamin D and cholesterol.

stertorous breathing: See GRAND MAL.

-steth-; -stetho- a combining form relating to the chest.

Stevens, Albert Mason American pediatrician 1884–1945. See STEVENS-JOHNSON SYNDROME.

Stevens, Stanley Smith American psychophysicist, 1906–73. See STEVENS' LAW; STEVENS' POWER LAW.

Stevens-Johnson syndrome a condition sometimes associated with infections or reaction to drugs such as tranquilizers and barbiturates and marked by acute inflammation of the skin and mucous membranes particularly in the anogenital region, also by prostration, headache, fever,

joint pain, and conjunctivitis. Also called **erythema multiforme major; ectodermosis erosiva pluriorificialis; Baader's dermatostomatitis; Fiessinger-Rendu syndrome; Klauder's syndrome; Neumann's aphthosis**.

Stevens' law a psychophysical relationship stating that the psychological magnitude of a sensation is proportional to a power of the stimulus producing it. Symbol: $\psi = ks^n$, in which ψ is the sensation, k is a constant of proportionality, s is the stimulus magnitude, and n is a function of the particular stimulus. Also see FECHNER'S LAW; WEBER'S LAW.

Stevenson, Robert Louis Scottish novelist and poet, 1850–94. See BEHAVIOR METAMORPHOSIS.

Stevens' power law a logarithmic relationship between the impulse frequency of a visual stimulus and its intensity. It is expressed as $S = I^b$, where b is an empirical constant that is approximately 0.33 for the human eye.

Stewart, Douglas Hunt American surgeon, 1860–1933. See STEWART-MOREL SYNDROME.

Stewart, Dugald Scottish philosopher, 1753–1828. See FACULTY PSYCHOLOGY.

Stewart-Morel syndrome a disorder characterized by hypertrophy of the frontal bone of the skull, obesity, headache, nervous-system disturbances, and a tendency toward mental retardation. Also called **Morel's syndrome**.

-sthen- a combining form relating to strength or force (from Greek *sthenos*, "strength").

sthenic type a constitutional type characterized by strength and vigor and roughly equivalent to Kretschmer's athletic type.

stiff-man syndrome a voluntary-muscle disorder characterized by severe intermittent painful spasms of the muscles of the trunk, shoulders, and upper arms and legs. The onset of symptoms is sudden but the condition spreads gradually through the other skeletal muscles. The s.-m. s. occurs in cases of hyperthyroidism and certain other diseases.

stigma a personal trait that clearly distinguishes the individual from others and which constitutes or is believed to constitute a physical, psychological, or social disadvantage, e.g., a physical deformity, mental retardation, a known history of criminal conduct or psychiatric illness, and differences of race, religion, or sexual preference. The term signifies social disapproval that may have economic, social, and psychological consequences, e.g., discrimination and social isolation, as well as negative effects on the individual's self-image and expectations. Plurals: **stigmas; stigmata**.

For another meaning of the term, primarily in the plural, see STIGMATA.

stigmata /stig'mətə/ or /stigmä'tə/ spontaneous development of sores or wounds (Greek, "marks") on the head, hands, feet, and side corresponding to the location of wounds suffered by Christ during the crucifixion. S. are believed to have appeared for the first time on the body of Saint

Francis of Assisi, but since that time, about 300 cases have been reported, chiefly among deeply religious women. Many psychiatrists regard s. as a hysterical, or conversion, reaction, pointing out that the wounds most frequently bleed spontaneously on days that commemorate Christ's life or death, such as Good Friday, when religious suggestibility and masochistic identification with the sufferings of Christ are at their height. Some psychiatrists, however, regard the hand wounds as punishment for forbidden masturbatory impulses. Singular: **stigma**. Adjective: **stigmatized**. Also called **stigmatization**. Also see SKIN DISORDERS.

For another meaning of the term, primarily in the singular, see STIGMA.

stigmata of degeneracy a term applied by Cesare Lombroso to certain physical characteristics which, in his view, indicated a hereditary tendency to criminal behavior. Among them were small, pointed ears, a low forehead, and close-set eyes. See DEGENERACY THEORY; PHYSIOGNOMY.

Stiller, Berthold Hungarian physician, 1837–1922. See STILLER'S SIGN.

Stiller's sign a floating tenth rib, which is associated with a tendency to neurasthenia. Also called **costal stigma: Stiller's rib**.

Stilling, Benedikt /shtil'ing/ German anatomist, 1810–79. See CLARKE'S COLUMN (also called **Stilling's nucleus**).

Stilling, Jakob /shtil'ing/ German ophthalmologist, 1842–1915. See **Stilling Test**.

Stilling Test a test consisting of a chart containing dots of various hues, saturations, and intensities developed for the detection of color weakness. Some of the dots form numbers that are visible to the normal eye but not to the color-blind or color-weak eye.

stilted speech formal, affected, or pompous speech, characteristic of a self-conscious, arrogant, or rigid personality; also, a speech disturbance observed in some schizophrenic patients.

stimulants agents that excite functional activity in an organism or in a part of an organism. S. may be classified according to the body system or function excited, e.g., cardiac, CNS, genital, and by the type of drug or other agent producing the stimulation, such as amphetamine, methylxanthine, convulsants, analeptics. Analeptic drugs generally are s. that excite the central nervous system.

stimulating occupation an occupational-therapy activity that has an arousing and stimulating effect on slow or depressed patients, e.g., dancing or music therapy.

stimulation effects physiologic changes produced when a stimulus alters the electrical potential of a neuron by producing an irritating effect on the cell membrane which in turn disrupts the ionic balance on either side of the membrane. The potential change travels along the nerve fiber to a terminus or synapse, which can pass the impulse along to a neighboring fiber. *In vitro* (test-

tube) experiments find increased temperature, increased oxygen consumption, and other metabolic effects when neurons are exposed to electrical stimulation.

stimulation method an approach to the treatment of speech disorders in which the emphasis is placed on the development of auditory concepts; the learning of speech sounds by listening to them.

stimulator a device used to excite or stimulate a receptor. An early type of s. was an induction coil wired to a vibrator that would convert direct-current electricity into pulsations. An important part of today's s. is a device for controlling the rate of change in the electric current since a steady current flow has little stimulus effect.

stimulus in general, any event or situation, internal or external, that elicits a response from the organism (Latin, "goad"); or, more specifically, any change in the physical-energy level that activates a sense organ, or receptor. The activity of the sense organ is termed the proximal stimulus, and the physical energy that excites it is termed the distal stimulus. Human receptors are limited to a relatively small range of energy changes (in hearing, 20 to 20,000 cycles per second), and are also limited to only six types of stimuli: photic (eyes), acoustic (ears), chemical (nose, tongue), thermal (skin), mechanical (pressure, touch), and destruction of tissue (pain). Electrical energy has the unique ability of exciting all sense channels. See CONDITIONED S.; UNCONDITIONED S.; SUBLIMINAL STIMULATION.

stimulus attitude an expectant set in which the subject is ready to respond to a particular stimulus.

stimulus barrier in psychoanalytic theory, the early pre-ego process in which the infant protects himself from unbearable overstimulation. It is based on an innate ability to perceive and differentiate painful states of increasing tension and pleasurable states of decreasing tension. Later on, the s.b. serves as a shield against the flood of excitations that occurs in traumatic situations, and helps to keep us from becoming disorganized and confused.

stimulus-bound pertaining to a perception that is more or less dependent upon the qualities of the stimulation; also, characterizing an individual whose behavior tends to be inflexible and determined primarily by the stimulus situation.

stimulus continuum a series of stimuli related to each other along a specific dimension, e.g., a series of tones in the diatonic scale, or an unbroken series of shades of blue.

stimulus differentiation a process whereby an organism learns to discriminate between two stimuli capable of eliciting the same reponse. S.d. is also a Gestalt term for distinguishing different parts or patterns in a visual field.

stimulus discrimination the ability to distinguish different stimuli, e.g., to distinguish a circle from an ellipse.

stimulus equivalence the condition in which two

or more related stimuli elicit the same response or allied responses. The term is related to stimulus generalization, the chief difference being that equivalence implies less similarity between the stimuli whereas generalization denotes stimuli that are very similar.

stimulus error according to E.B. Titchener's introspective method, the error involved in responding to a stimulus in terms of its meaning (e.g., "chair") instead of its properties as a stimulus (size, shape, etc.).

stimulus generalization the tendency for a conditioned response to be evoked by stimuli that are similar to the conditioned stimulus. E.g., if a dog is conditioned to bark when a particular bell is sounded, he tends to make the same response to a wide range of bells; and a child who nearly drowns in the bathtub may develop a fear of wading and swimming. In experiments, alternate stimuli are employed to determine the extent of s.g., by noting which stimuli produce the same response. Also see RESPONSE-GENERALIZATION PRINCIPLE.

stimulus hunger a need to receive new and varied stimulation from the environment. The satisfaction of this need is believed to be essential to normal functioning. See SENSORY DEPRIVATION.

stimulus object any object or person that elicits a response from an organism.

stimulus overload the condition in which the environment presents too many stimuli to be comfortably processed, resulting in stress and behavior designed to restore equilibrium. According to S. Milgram, the "unfriendliness" of urbanites may represent a necessary strategy for screening out environment stimuli in the effort to maintain psychological balance. See HOMEOSTATIC MODEL.

stimulus pattern the grouping of stimuli into an organized configuration, as in a painting or sonata.

stimulus population a finite or measurable number of independent events in the environment, of which only one sample is effective at a given time. Abbrev.: **s population**.

stimulus-processing function: See DUAL-AROUSAL MODEL.

stimulus-response theory a concept introduced in 1898 by E. L. Thorndike, and later supported by Pavlov and others, which holds that learning is primarily a trial-and-error process in which connections, or "S-R" bonds, are established between stimuli and responses.

stimulus set in reaction-time experiments, the expectancy or readiness associated with concentration on the stimulus rather than the response.

stimulus situation all the components of an occurrence or experience that, taken as a whole, comprise a stimulus to which an organism responds. The term is used to accentuate the complexity of behavior-arousing events. That is, a stimulus is perceived as a unitary pattern but is composed of many elements. An example is a concert, another is a championship bout.

stimulus tension the tension induced by a stimulus. According to Freud, pain increases the s.t. and pleasure lowers it.

stimulus value the strength of a given stimulus as measured in standard units, e.g., a shock of 40 volts; also, the effectiveness of any stimulus in eliciting a response or series of responses.

stimulus variable the stimulus as one of a group of variables; the independent variable in a psychological experiment.

stimulus word a word presented to a subject to elicit a response. Many tests and procedures employ the oral presentation of stimulus words, e.g., learning experiments or projective techniques such as the word-association test.

stinginess miserliness; extreme lack of generosity. In psychoanalysis, this trait is believed to stem from the anal-retention stage of psychosexual development. See ANAL CHARACTER; ANAL-RETENTIVE STAGE.

stirpiculture: See GROUP MARRIAGE.

STM = SHORT-TERM MEMORY.

stochastic referring to a system of events whose occurrence probability changes constantly, although the probability of a predictable occurrence increases with the number of events. A s. model is opposed to a strictly deterministic one. Also see PROBABILISM.

Stockholm syndrome the bond that sometimes develops between captor and captive, in particular between terrorist and hostage. The term stems from the case of a woman held hostage at a bank in Stockholm, Sweden, who became so emotionally attached to one of the robbers that she broke her engagement to another man and remained faithful to her former captor during his prison term. (Another recent example is Patty Hearst.) Unconscious identification with the aggressor is also one of the symptoms of the persecution syndrome. See IDENTIFICATION WITH THE AGGRESSOR; PERSECUTION SYNDROME.

stocking anesthesia: See GLOVE ANESTHESIA.

Stokes, William Irish physician, 1804–78. See CHEYNE-STOKES BREATHING.

stoma an opening from an area within an organism to a free surface outside. The term often is used as a combining form (-stomy) and linked to a name suggesting the internal source of the s., e.g., colostomy when the s. is an opening through the abdominal wall leading to the colon. Plurals: **stomata; stomas**.

-stoma-; -stomat-; -stomato- a combining form relating to the mouth (Greek *stoma*).

stomach activity activity marked by gastrointestinal effects of intense emotion, such as inhibition of muscular contractions, and flow of gastric juices, which are under the control of the autonomic nervous system.

stomach loading the effect of a distended stomach on appetite. In animal experiments, expanding a balloon in the subject's stomach or filling the stomach with water or an inert substance decreases the amount of food eaten. The distention of the stomach walls triggers nerve impulses to the hypothalamus, which results in inhibition of the urge to eat.

stomach reactor a person who reacts to stress through symptoms of gastrointestinal distress. e.g., colitis or peptic ulcers.

stomas; stomata: See STOMA.

-stomy; -ostomy a combining form relating to an opening, especially a surgical opening. Also see -STOMA-; OSTOMY.

stop = PLOSIVE.

storm-and-stress period a period of emotional turmoil. The term is derived from the German words *Sturm und Drang* (literally, "storm and urge, or pressure"), which was the title of a 1776 drama by Friedrich Maximilian von Klinger, set in America at the time of the Revolution, and which became the name of the period of German literary romanticism in the late 18th century. A century later, G. Stanley Hall used s.-a.-s.p. to characterize adolescence, which be believed to correspond to the turbulent transition from savagery to civilization. Also called **Sturm und Drang period**.

stormy personality a term applied by S. Arieti to individuals whose lives are punctuated by an unending series of crises and abrupt changes in occupation and relationships.

story fear = MYTHOPHOBIA.

story-recall test a test which requires the subject to recall details of a story that is told or read to him.

STP: See PSYCHEDELICS; PHENYLETHYLAMINE DERIVATIVES; AMPHETAMINES.

strabismus any abnormal alignment of the eyes; squint. Also called **heterotropia**. See CROSS-EYE; GRIEG'S DISEASE; BRAID'S S.; DOUBLE VISION.

strain a term used to indicate excessive tension in a muscle or nerve unit, usually due to an activity overload, or in psychological adjustment, usually due to an emotional overload.

straining at the leash: See METAPHORIC LANGUAGE.

straitjacket = CAMISOLE.

strange-hand sign a tactile perceptual disorder characterized by an inability of the subject to recognize his own left hand. The person may be able to write with his left hand but does not believe the writing is his own. Or when clasping his two hands, he may be unable to acknowledge without visual clues that the left hand is his own. The disorder is due to a corpus callosum defect. Also called **la main étrangère** /lämen′äträNzher′/.

strangeness fear = NEOPHOBIA.

stranger anxiety; stranger fear: See SEPARATION ANXIETY; FEAR OF STRANGERS; XENOPHOBIA.

strangulated affect in psychoanalysis, an inhibition or retention of the normal discharge of emotion, which leads to a substitute discharge in the form of physical symptoms. This theory was advanced by Freud and Breuer in 1893 to explain the dynamics of conversion hysteria, but the concept of s.a. was later supplanted by the concept of REPRESSION. See this entry.

stratification a horizontal layering or organization. The term is usually applied to such divisions of a social group or society as a whole.

stratified sample a sample drawn in such a way as to include or exclude representation of a particular group. If an experimenter wishes to insure representation of all ages, he might stratify by, or include, children, adolescents, and adults, and sample equal numbers within each of these classifications.

Stratton, George Malcolm American psychologist, 1865–1957. See STRATTON'S EXPERIMENT.

Stratton's experiment a visual and tactual-motor study technique in which a subject wears special eye glasses that turn the visual field through an angle of 180 degrees so that retinal images are inverted.

Strauss, Alfred A. American (?) psychologist, fl. 1940, 1947. See STRAUSS' SYNDROME.

Strauss' syndrome a term used to describe the behavioral characteristics of brain-injured children based upon clinical studies by Alfred Strauss and Laura Lehtinen (1947). See LEARNING DISABILITIES; MINIMAL BRAIN DYSFUNCTION.

stream of action the continuous activities of an organism, as opposed to the stream-of-consciousness concept applied by William James to thought processes.

stream of consciousness a term introduced in 1890 by William James, who described consciousness as a continuous, dynamic flow of ideas and images rather than a static series of discrete components. The term differentiates between the functionalist and structuralist approaches. Also called **stream of thought**.

street fear = AGYIOPHOBIA.

street hustlers: See MALE HOMOSEXUAL PROSTITUTION.

Streiff, Enrico Bernard /shtrīf/ Italian-born Swiss ophthalmologist, 1908—. See HALLERMANN-STREIFF SYNDROME.

stren a term used by W. G. Hollister to denote an experience that *stren*gthens the individual's personality by producing greater maturity, sensitivity, self-confidence, or depth. Strens are contrasted with traumas, but may be initially viewed as traumatic events.

strephosymbolia the term used by Orton (1937) to define reading difficulties as a failure to establish the left-hemisphere dominance, the speech area of the brain, because the child tends to reverse letters in reading or writing (as "gril" for "girl"). Also called **twisted symbols**.

stress a state of physical or psychological strain which imposes demands for adjustment upon the indivdual. S. may be internal or environmental, brief or persistent. If excessive or prolonged, it may overtax the individual's resources and lead to a breakdown of organized functioning, or decompensation. Types of situation that produce s. include frustrations, deprivations, conflicts, and pressures, all of which may arise from internal or external sources. The term is also used to denote emphasis put on a word or thought in speaking or writing. (The concept of s. was introduced to psychology by Hans Selye, around 1940.) Also see s. THEORY; SELYE.

stress-decompensation model a concept of the development of abnormal behavior as a result of stress that leads to decompensation, or to the gradual but progressive deterioration of normal behavior.

stress immunity a highly developed capacity to tolerate emotional strain; failure to react to stressful situations or events.

stress-inoculation training a type of cognitive-behavioral therapy designed to help patients cope by altering their attitudes toward the stressors and themselves.

stress interview an interview in which the individual is subjected to conditions of emotional strain, as in questioning him under a glaring light or conducting a merciless cross-examination. A s.i. is sometimes used to test an individual's ability to withstand pressure.

stressor any event or force that results in physical or emotional stress.

stress reaction faulty, maladaptive, or pathological behavior resulting from conditions of pressure or strain. Examples are extreme feelings of tension or panic, disorganized speech patterns, and accidents incurred under the influence of alcohol, drugs, or emotional stress. Reactions to stress may also be "task-oriented," which involves an objective appraisal of the situation with an eye toward choosing the most constructive, rational way of handling it.

stress situation any condition that puts an extra burden on the organism's capacity to adapt. Examples are extreme hunger, an overcompetitive environment, combat conditions, bankruptcy, marital conflicts, and a new and taxing job.

stress test a test conducted in a natural "real-world" setting designed to ascertain the subject's capacity to perform a relatively complex task under purposefully stressful conditions. The term is also applied to a medical test in which the subject runs on a treadmill while his cardiac, respiratory, or other processes are being measured.

stress theory the theory that certain stimuli perceived as noxious or threatening cause reactions that have adverse emotional, behavioral, and physiological reactions. See STRESS; GENERAL ADAPTATION SYNDROME; SELYE.

stress tolerance the capacity to withstand pressures and strains; the ability to function effectively under conditions of stress. See STRESS; STRESS SITUATION.

stretch reflexes spinal reflexes that involve increased tension or contraction in extensor muscles which support the body against the pull of gravity. Also called **myotatic reflexes**. Also see EXTENSOR THRUST.

striate cortex an area of the occipital lobes of the cortex where the visual functions are centered. The entering fibers are so concentrated in this region that they form a white band, the stripe of Gennari, and suggest the name striate (from Latin *stria*, "furrow, channel").

striated muscle a term generally applied to the tissue of skeletal, or voluntary, muscles. It is striated ("striped") in appearance under a microscope because of the alternation of muscle fibers that permit the muscle to shorten and thicken during contraction. An exception is cardiac-muscle tissue which is striated but involuntary.

stria terminalis a tract of fibers running between the amygdala and hypothalamus. The fibers carry impulses from the amygdaloid nuclei to the septal, hypothalamic, and thalamic areas. Experimental stimulation of the s.t. may evoke escape or other forms of defense behavior in animals.

striatum the portion of the developing forebrain that becomes the basal ganglia. The s. tissues are forced back over the thalamus during the forebrain growth, leaving the cell bodies as basal ganglia nuclei.

stridor a shrill, high-pitched sound (Latin).

stridor dentium = BRUXISM.

string phobia = LINONOPHOBIA.

striped muscle: See STRIATED MUSCLE.

stripe of Gennari a collection of optic-nerve fibers in the striate cortex. The bundle forms a white band that is visible to the naked eye.

strip key a test-scoring key in the form of a long strip of paper that aligns with the test answers.

striving for superiority the basic concept of individual psychology, which holds that human beings are motivated by an innate, sovereign drive for self-realization. This drive is defined as the urge for completion and perfection rather than for superiority in the sense of social status or domination over others. See INDIVIDUAL PSYCHOLOGY.

stroboscopic illusion the apparent motion of a series of separate stimuli occurring in close consecutive order, as in motion pictures; also, making a moving object such as a rotating fan appear motionless, or move in reverse, by illuminating it with a series of intermittent light flashes. Also called **stroboscopic effect**.

Strohl, André French physician, 1887—. See GUILLAIN-BARRÉ SYNDROME (also called **Guillain-Barré-Strohl syndrome**).

stroke a sudden and severe attack, especially a cerebrovascular accident (CVA) which may be due to a hemorrhage of a blood vessel in the brain or an embolism or thrombus blocking an artery in the brain (**apoplexy**). Either type of s. can deprive brain tissue of oxygen and nutrients, thereby causing a loss of normal function. See CEREBROVASCULAR ACCIDENT. Also see ARTERIOSCLEROTIC BRAIN DISORDER; CEREBRAL INFARCT.

Strong, Edward Kellogg, Jr. American psychologist, 1884–1963. See STRONG-CAMPBELL INTEREST INVENTORY; INTEREST TESTS.

Strong-Campbell Interest Inventory the 1974 revision of the **Strong Vocational Interest Blank**, based upon the concept that persons engaged in one occupation are characterized by common interests that differentiate them from persons in other occupations. The test therefore presents an inventory of 325 items which the subject marks Like, Indifferent, or Dislike. The items include occupations, school subjects, amusements, activities, contact with various kinds of people, self-descriptive statements, and preference between such items as dealing with things versus dealing with people. The test provides 124 occupational scales and six general occupational themes. Abbrev.: **SCII**.

Stroop, J. R. American (?) psychologist, fl. 1935. See STROOP TEST.

Stroop Test a three-part test in which (a) color names are read as fast as possible, (b) the colors of rows of dots are rapidly named, and, most important, (c) cards are presented on which color names are printed over the wrong colors to test the ability of the subject to name the color in spite of the conflict. The degree to which the person is subject to interference by the printed words is a measure of his cognitive control.

structural analysis a term sometimes applied to the recognition of words through the analysis of such word units as prefixes, suffixes, and root words.

structural approach = STRUCTURAL MODEL.

structural family therapy a general type of family therapy which provides a built-in method for the rational solution of problems, based on the theory that these problems are the result of a poorly structured life. To modify this structure, the entire relationship system of the family and the part each person plays in that system must be modified. Also called **structured family therapy**. Compare EXPERIENTIAL PSYCHOTHERAPY.

structural hypothesis in psychoanalysis, the view that the total personality is divided into three divisions, or functions: the id, which represents instinctual drives; the ego, which controls id drives and mediates between them and external reality; and the superego, which comprises moral precepts and ideals. Freud proposed this hypothesis in 1923 to replace the "topographic" division of the mind into three regions: the unconscious, preconscious, and conscious, which was advanced in 1913.

structuralism the dominant school of psychology in Germany and the United States between 1890 and 1920, led by Wilhelm Wundt and E. B. Titchener. The school based its approach on the introspective analysis of the structural, or morphological, components of consciousness, namely sensations, images, and affective or emotional states. It sought to describe these irreducible mental contents in terms of the *what* (quality, intensity, clearness, duration), the *how* (interrelationships), and the *why* (investigation of physiological correlates on the principle that mental and physiological events run a parallel course). Also called **structural psychology**. See TITCHEN-

ER; WUNDT. Also see ATOMISM; REDUCTIONISM. Compare GESTALT PSYCHOLOGY; FUNCTIONALISM; BEHAVIORISM.

structural matrix: See STRUCTURED INTERACTIONAL GROUP PSYCHOTHERAPY.

structural model in psychoanalysis, the topographic organization of the psyche developed by Freud in 1923. In the s.m., the total personality is divided into three components: the id, ego, and superego (literally, from German, the I, it, and upper-I), in contrast to the earlier division into conscious, preconscious, and unconscious. Also called **structural approach**. For details, see PSYCHIC APPARATUS; ID; EGO; SUPEREGO.

structural psychology = STRUCTURALISM.

structural scoliosis: See SCOLIOSIS.

structural therapy a system of treatment for autistic children who are provided a structured environment that emphasizes physical and verbal stimulation in a gamelike setting. The purpose is to increase the amount and variety of stimuli received by the patients, thereby helping them to relate to their environment in a more realistic manner.

structured autobiography: See AUTOBIOGRAPHY.

structured exercises a technique used in personal-change groups, in which the members engage in leader-arranged exercises, including games and experiments, such as (a) staging a fantasy fight between one's weak and strong self, (b) describing the most joyous moment of one's life in words and then actions, or (c) shrinking oneself in imagination in order to take a trip to the most troublesome part of one's body.

structured family therapy = STRUCTURAL FAMILY THERAPY.

structured group a therapy group in which members are selected on the basis of their potential for effecting therapeutic changes in each other.

structured interactional group psychotherapy a form of group therapy in which the therapist provides a "structural matrix" for the group's interactions, particularly by selecting a different member of the group to be the focus of the interaction in each session. This technique was developed by Harold Kaplan and Benjamin Sadock.

structured interview an interview based on a predetermined set of questions or topics. Structured interviews are used in market research to determine consumer reactions to ads or products, or the reasons for purchasing a particular product or service. This type of interview is also used in personnel departments. Also see PATTERNED INTERVIEW.

structured stimulus a complex, organized stimulus with interrelated parts, e.g., the pictures in the Rosenzweig Picture-Frustration Study.

structure word = FUNCTION WORD.

structuring a counselor's explanations of the specific procedures and conditions of the counseling process, including the anticipated results of treatment, time restrictions, fees, and the function and responsibilities of both client and counselor.

Strümpell, Adolph von /shtrim′pəl/ German neurologist, 1853–1925. See ANKYLOSING SPONDYLITIS (there: **Marie-Strümpell disease**).

strychnine $C_{21}H_{22}N_2O_2$—an alkaloid derived from Strychnos nux vomica and other species of strychnos plants. It stimulates the entire central nervous system, and has been used as a stomachic despite its intensely bitter taste. It also has been used in the treatment of heart disease, as an antidote for overdoses of depressant drugs, and as a lacing agent for drugs of abuse. No marked tolerance develops for s., and increased susceptibility to poisoning is likely from repeated use. Also see NUX VOMICA.

student's disease a term applied to students or other individuals who believe they have the symptoms of a disease or mental disorder that they have been studying, or which they have read or heard about.

study a research project that is less formal than a controlled experiment that involves independent and dependent variables.

study of values: See ALLPORT-VERNON-LINDZEY S.O.V.

study skill any method used to facilitate the process of studying, such as outlining, taking notes, underlining, or silent recitation.

stupor a mental state in which the individual is totally or almost totally unresponsive and immobile. In organic cases, such as toxic states, brain disease, and epilepsy, s. involves complete suspension of conscious thought processes and unawareness of the surroundings. In functional conditions, such as catatonic and depressive stupors, the patient is mute and motionless, but there is no loss of consciousness or sensation; mental activity may be intense, and the patient may be well aware of his surroundings.

stuporous depression: See DEPRESSIVE STUPOR.

stuporous mania = MANIC STUPOR.

Sturge, William Allen English physician, 1850–1919. See STURGE-WEBER SYNDROME; AMENTIA; PORT-WINE STAIN.

Sturge-Weber syndrome a congenital disorder marked by a facial port-wine stain, birthmark, glaucoma, and focal-motor seizures. The skin pigmentation may be on one or both sides of the face or extend into the scalp area. About half the patients are mentally retarded. Other symptoms may include contralateral hemiplegia and intracranial calcification. Also called **encephalofacial angiomatosis**.

Sturm und Drang period = STORM-AND-STRESS PERIOD.

stuttering frequent repetition or prolongation of sounds, syllables, or words, with hesitations and pauses that disrupt speech. The disorder occurs in about one percent of all children. Mild cases usually recover spontaneously; chronic stutterers experience exacerbations in situations where communication is required. Also called

stammering. Also see PRIMARY S.; SECONDARY S.; DYSPHEMIA; PSELLISM. (DSM-III)

stuttering gait a gait characterized by hesitancy in taking steps, a walking pattern observed in certain schizophrenic or hysterical patients. In some cases it is organic in origin. Also called **gait stuttering**.

stygiophobia a morbid fear of hell. Also called **hadephobia**.

style of life: See LIFE-STYLE.

stylistic ratings a system of evaluating works of art in terms of technical attributes, as opposed to reactions or moods of subjects who view the art. S.r. may be based on such factors as importance of shapes, lines, composition, surface textures, and reproduction of objects or people portrayed. Stylistic dimensions may include classicism, subjectivism, and expressionism.

stylus maze a maze that is "run" by moving a stylus through the various pathways. The test may be performed visually or tactually. The performance of an individual may indicate his ability to handle spatial tasks. Lesions in the right hemisphere seem to affect performance. Also see MAZE.

subacute necrotizing encephalomyelopathy a rare hereditary disorder of thiamine metabolism, characterized by ataxia, nystagmus, mental retardation, seizures, peripheral neuropathy, difficulty in swallowing, and inhibition of growth. The symptoms usually appear before one year of age, and death follows within a year unless massive doses of thiamine are administered. Abbrev.: SNE.

subacute sclerosing panencephalitis a rare progressive disease of children and young adults with onset five to seven years after infection with measles. Symptoms include awkwardness, stumbling, mental deterioration, and memory loss followed by convulsions and myoclonus, and, in the final stage, stupor, coma, and increased spasticity, with death occurring one to three years after onset. Abbrev.: SSPE. Also called **sclerosing encephalitis**.

subarachnoid hemorrhage bleeding in the brain area that sometimes is the result of a ruptured congenital aneurysm. Headache and loss of consciousness usually result as escaping blood distends the basal cisterns, causing compression or spasm of the blood vessels of the thalamus and upper brainstem.

subarachnoid space a space beneath the delicate arachnoid membrane surrounding the brain and spinal cord. It is occupied by cerebrospinal fluid, which drains into the superior sagittal sinus through villi that protrude through the arachnoid membrane.

subcallosal gyrus a portion of the medial limbic system behind the cingulate gyrus but with functions reciprocal to those of the cingulate gyrus. E.g., the s.g. has functions inhibitory to motoneuron activity, whereas the cingulate gyrus enhances the motoneuron functions.

subception a reaction to an emotion-provoking stimulus that is not clearly enough perceived to be reportable, although its effects may be observed indirectly by a galvanic skin response or a longer-than-expected reaction time.

subclavian steal syndrome a form of impaired blood circulation to the brain due to a stenosis or occlusion of the subclavian artery in the shoulder area. Because of the shunting of blood flow at this point in the circulation, the blood that normally would flow to the brain is in effect stolen.

subcoma insulin treatment treatment of severe anxiety and tension states by intramuscular injection of small doses of insulin that induce drowsiness and hypoglycemia but not coma. Also called **subshock insulin treatment; ambulatory insulin treatment** (since the patient may walk about during the treatment period).

subcommissural organ a group of cells on the dorsal wall of the third ventricle, near the aqueduct of Sylvius. They are secretory cells believed to be associated with the body's water-sodium balance. Lesions in the area are followed by reduced fluid intake.

subconscious the area of the mind beneath the level of consciousness, comprising the preconscious and unconscious. The term is used more popularly than technically today, and as an adjective more than a noun, referring to memories or other events of which we are not now aware, or only dimly aware, but which can be brought to consciousness.

subconscious personality the personality in a multiple-personality individual that is not dominant at the time. When a s.p. becomes dominant, the previously dominant personality becomes the s.p.

subcortical relating to a nervous-system structure or process that is below the level of the cortex, e.g., spinal reflexes.

subcortical arteriosclerotic encephalopathy = BINSWANGER'S DISEASE.

subcortical centers any of the CNS nuclei located at levels below the cerebral cortex, including such structures as the thalamus, hypothalamus, and basal ganglia. Within each structure may be several special s.c., such as nuclei of the hypothalamus that regulate sleep, water balance, protein metabolism, and sexual activity. Sensory relay nuclei within the thalamus link skin, muscle, and other body tissues with the cortex.

subcortical dementia a disorder marked by excessive slowness in making intellectual responses. The cause is an abnormality of the subcortical structure resulting in a malfunction of the activating mechanisms. The diagnosis is based in part on the length of time considered to be normal for responding to a question.

subcortical learning a type of learning that occurs under certain conditions during cortical-spreading depression which is produced by a temporary lesion, e.g., induced by an injection of potassium chloride into the cortex. The technique may be used to study interhemispheric transfer when one hemisphere is affected by the temporary chemical lesion.

subculture a group that maintains a characteristic set of religious, social, ethnic, or other customs that serve to distinguish it from the larger culture in which the members live. Subcultural groups usually share with the larger society a common language as well as certain basic values and behavioral traits, but they retain their separate group identity.

subcutaneous injection injection of a drug beneath the skin. S.i. may be applied at points in the body, e.g., the upper arm or thigh, where there is an adequate layer of subcutaneous tissue. While s.i. is used mainly to inject fluids, medications also may be administered subcutaneously in the form of slowly absorbed pellets. Also called **hypodermic injection**. Also see ADMINISTRATION.

subcutaneous sensibility the sensitivity of nerve receptors beneath the skin, e.g., Pacinian-corpuscle sensitivity.

subdelirious state the precursor of a full delirium, marked by restlessness, headache, irritability, hypersensitivity to sound and visual stimuli, and emotional lability. A subacute delirious state may also appear independently or after an episode of delirium and persist for months. In these cases the typical symptoms are clouding of consciousness, perplexity, and incoherent thinking. Also called **subdelirium**.

subdural hematoma a type of brain bruise that involves bleeding between the dura mater membrane and the brain surface. Since the lost blood cannot escape through the skull, it causes pressure that distorts brain structures. The bleeding may occur over a period of days or weeks following a seemingly minor injury, producing symptoms of confusion, memory loss, or other neurologic deficits that may be mistaken as signs of senile dementia in an older person.

subdural hemorrhage bleeding beneath the dura mater, the outer layer of the meningeal membranes. S.h. may occur as a result of injury, stroke, or brain tumor. The specific symptoms may vary according to the brain area affected by the bleeding. A s.h. usually occurs in the parietal region and may result from a fall. See SUBDURAL HEMATOMA.

subfecundity a below-average ability to reproduce an adequate number of offspring. See FECUNDITY.

subictal epilepsy a form of epilepsy that is marked by muscle twitchings or uncoordinated involuntary movements, depression, anxiety, or hysterical behavior. The condition is difficult to diagnose because no convulsions occur and EEG findings are negative. However, the patient responds to antiepileptic drugs.

subitizing /sōōb'-/ perceiving at a glance how many

objects are presented, without estimating or counting (from Latin *subito*, "at once"). The limit appears to be seven, for humans and trained birds as well.

subject the individual—human or other organism —used in an experiment. The s. may be further identified as an experimental s. or control s. The term applies also to a person whose experiences are being reported or evaluated.

subject-ill a term applied to the use by a patient of his own body to symbolize his emotions in a kind of organic language. Stekel distinguishes between the s.-i. patient and the **object-ill** patient, who expresses his emotions through symbolization of objects outside his body. See SOMATIZATON DISORDER.

subjection the state of being under the control of another individual or an organization.

subjective characterizing a perception, construct, or internal state that is intrinsically inaccessible to the experience or observation of other persons.

subjective attributes perceptual qualities that are uniquely dependent on the person, or subject, who experiences them, e.g., a particular taste or color.

subjective colors the pastel colors perceived when viewing interleaved black and white disks rotating on a color wheel.

subjective error in experimental psychology, any error caused by prejudice, bias, or unsystematic procedures; an error attributable to individual variations in perception and interpretation of experience.

subjective examination a test, usually of the essay type, whose scoring depends upon the interpretation of the examiner.

subjective orientation the type of moral reasoning typical of childen over age ten and characterized by the ability to take an individual's motives into account when judging an act. Younger children do not usually consider motives; they focus only on the physical consequences of an act. Compare OBJECTIVE ORIENTATION.

subjective-outcome value a term sometimes used by social-learning theorists to refer to the fact that behavior is influenced by the personal or subjective value placed by an individual on a specific act or outcome.

subjective psychology a psychological approach that focuses on introspective or phenomenological data.

subjective-quality point: See POINT OF SUBJECTIVE QUALITY.

subjective scoring: See OBJECTIVE SCORING.

subjective sensation a sensation, e.g., an illusion, that is produced without external stimulation.

subjective test a test that is scored according to personal judgment or nonobjective, unsystematic standards, e.g. certain long-essay examinations.

subjective tone = OTOGENIC TONE.

subjectivism a tendency to be influenced in perception and thinking by the conviction that personal experience is the basis of reality and should be evaluated in terms of one's own feelings, needs, and frame of reference.

subjectivism factor possible bias contributed to data because of the intrusion of the conscious or unconscious viewpoint of the subject. S.f. also may be applied to expressionism or surrealism types of paintings in which the illustration is influenced by the artist's personal psychology.

subjectivity a mental state that focuses on the individual and his personal feelings and thoughts, and his own interpretation and evaluation of events or ideas in the light of personal experience.

subject variable a variable of individual differences in an experiment, e.g., the subject's sex or occupation. The s.v. is neither manipulated by the experimenter, as an independent variable would be, nor is it usually changed in the experiment, as a dependent variable would be.

sublimation in pychoanalysis, the unconscious process of channeling unacceptable sexual or aggressive drives into acceptable expression. A guilt-laden heterosexual drive may be transformed into romantic poetry or other artistic creation; an exhibitionistic impulse may gain a new outlet in choreography; a voyeuristic urge may lead to scientific research; and a dangerously aggressive drive may be expressed with impunity on the football field. The outlets may not only protect us from the anxiety which the original drive would produce, but also bring us new satisfactions, such as recognition from other people.

subliminal consciousness a level of consciousness in which a stimulus may affect behavior even though one is not aware of it.

subliminal learning learned material or habits that cannot be directly recalled because they were acquired without awareness, that is, subliminally.

subliminal perception the perception of stimuli below the level of awareness, or perception of stimuli that are too weak (or too rapid) to affect the individual on a conscious level. Questions have been raised as to (a) whether response to subliminal stimuli actually occurs, and (b) whether it is possible for subliminal commands or advertising messages to influence behavior. However, studies indicate that subliminal commands do not significantly affect behavior.

subliminal stimulation stimulation that is below the threshold intensity required to produce a spike potential. The threshold is the critical level at which a stimulus of sufficient strength will carry the potential from a graded to a suddenly explosive spike discharge. See SUBLIMINAL PERCEPTION.

submissiveness: See COMPLIANCE.

subnormal inferior, or below the normal level by a given standard.

subnormal period of neuron a period of time, measured in milliseconds, when neuron excitability is below normal. It follows a refractory period or a supernormal period of excitability.

suboccipital puncture an alternative procedure to lumbar puncture for obtaining access to the CNS subarachnoid space for diagnostic or therapeutic purposes. S.p. also is a procedure used for determining spinal arachnoid block. In s.p., a needle is inserted into the cisterna magna through an area near the base of the skull. Also called **cistern puncture**.

subshock insulin treatment = SUBCOMA INSULIN TREATMENT.

subshock therapy shock treatment, e.g., ECT, administered at a mild level.

subsidiation the relationship of means to an end, e.g., the achievement of a series of subgoals that are necessary to reach an ultimate objective.

substance abuse a term applied to a pattern of pathological use of alcohol or drugs (that is, need for daily use, inability to cut down) with impairment in social and occupational functioning (e.g., failure to meet family obligations, erratic or criminal behavior, missing work or school), and a minimal duration of disturbance of at least one month. Also called **drug abuse**. (DSM-III)

substance dependence a substance-use disorder (generally more severe than substance abuse) involving physiological dependence as manifested in (a) tolerance (that is, markedly increased amounts of the substance are required to reach the desired effect, or a markedly diminished effect occurs with regular use of the same dose) and (b) withdrawal (that is, a set of specific symptoms, such as restlessness, anxiety, and insomnia, occurs when the use of a particular substance is suspended or reduced). (DSM-III)

Substance P: See ENKEPHALIN.

substance-use disorders a diagnostic category that comprises pathological behavioral changes associated with more or less regular use of substances that affect the central nervous system. The substances include, among others, alcohol, barbiturates, opioids, cocaine, amphetamines, cannabis, and hallucinogens; the behavioral changes include inability to control or stop taking these substances, withdrawal symptoms if use is suspended, and impaired social and occupational functioning. (DSM-III)

substance withdrawal the cessation or sharp reduction of intake of a substance that was previously used regularly to induce a state of intoxication. See ALCOHOL WITHDRAWAL; AMPHETAMINE OR SIMILARLY ACTING SYMPATHOMIMETIC WITHDRAWAL; BARBITURATE OR SIMILARLY ACTING SEDATIVE OR HYPNOTIC WITHDRAWAL; OPIOID WITHDRAWAL; TOBACCO WITHDRAWAL; WITHDRAWAL.

substantia gelatinosa a gelatinous-appearing mass of extensively interconnected small neurons at the tip of the dorsal horn of the spinal cord.

They communicate with collaterals of branches of peripheral fibers of the extralemniscal system. The s.g. cells appear to affect only neighboring cells in the dorsal horn. S.g. neurons extend into the medulla where they form the spinal nucleus of the trigeminal nerve.

substantia nigra a part (Latin, "black substance") of the extrapyramidal motor system composed of gray matter and lying between the tegmentum of the midbrain and the crus cerebri.

substituted phenyl alkylamines = PHENYLETHYLAMINE DERIVATIVES.

substitute formation = SYMPTOM FORMATION.

substitution the replacement of blocked or unattainable goals with alternative satisfactions, as in resorting to adoption when one cannot have a child of one's own, or raiding the refrigerator after a disappointment in love. Also, s. denotes replacing unacceptable drives with socially approved pursuits; e.g., a compulsive drive to keep the house spotlessly clean may be a substitute for the "unclean" impulse to be promiscuous.

substitution test any test in which the subject substitutes one set of symbols for another, e.g., a code test in which symbols or letters are substituted for numbers.

substrate a chemical compound whose reaction is catalyzed by an enzyme. The enzyme locks with the s. in a manner similar to the fitting together of two pieces of a jigsaw puzzle. While locked in place, the enzyme places specific stress upon the s. to break its chemical bonds and reorganize the molecules in it. When the process is over and they break away, the enzyme is unchanged but the s. has been changed into different molecules called reaction products. The released enzyme then repeats the process with another s. of the same composition as before.

subtest a separate division of a test or test battery.

subthalamic nuclei a part of the thalamus that receives fibers from the globus pallidus and peduncle as a part of the descending pathway from the corpus striatum. It is an oval mass in a transition zone between the dorsal thalamus and the tegmentum, and functions as part of the extrapyramidal system.

subthalamus a transitional zone of tissue between the thalamus and the mesencephalic tegmentum. It contains portions of the red nucleus and the substantia nigra, as well as groups of fibers known as fields of Forel.

subthreshold potential a type of graded potential resulting from a stimulus that is not of sufficient intensity to produce a spike potential. Because of its below-threshold intensity, the impulse does not travel beyond the immediate region of its own fiber. Also see LOCAL POTENTIAL.

subtotal hysterectomy: See HYSTERECTOMY.

subtraction method a technique for determining reaction time involving a choice, e.g., subtracting sensory time and motor time from total time to calculate the time used to decide on a response.

subtractive mixture: See COLOR MIXTURE.

subvocal speech faint movements of the lips, tongue, and larynx. These movements resemble speech movements but are inaudible.

success: See S. NEUROSIS; FAILURE THROUGH S.

successive-approximations method = METHOD OF SUCCESSIVE APPROXIMATIONS.

successive contrast: See COLOR CONTRAST; CONTRAST EFFECT.

successive induction the succession of movements of limbs or other body parts in a pattern of antagonistic reflex actions. In walking, e.g., s.i. requires alternate flexion and extension of muscles of the lower limbs.

successive-intervals method a variation of the equal-appearing intervals method in which intervals are defined verbally or by the use of samples.

successive-practice method a technique for assessing transfer of learning by measuring the saving in time or trials when B is learned after A has been learned, in comparison with a control group that learns B without learning A.

successive reproduction a method used to study the way in which information in long-term memory is altered by reconstruction. In this technique, subjects are asked to reproduce or recall the same material at successive time intervals, and the variations in their reproductions are recorded. Also see RECONSTRUCTION.

success neurosis in psychoanalysis, neurotic illness in individuals who have accumulated wealth. This type of neurosis is believed to be due to the arousal of unconscious guilt feelings and castration fears stemming from early rivalry with the father. The guilt feelings lead to such neurotic symptoms as masochistic tendencies and a need to suffer. Also see POLYCRATES COMPLEX.

succinic acid: See GABA SHUNT.

succinimides a group of chemically related drugs that are effective in the treatment of petit mal epilepsy. S. were discovered in a search for an antidote for drug-induced convulsions. S. produce a sedative effect, and may cause behavioral changes. Kinds of s. include **ethosuximide**—$C_7H_{11}NO_2$, **methsuximide**—$C_{12}H_{13}NO_2$, and **phensuximide**—$C_{11}H_{11}NO_2$.

succinylcholine a skeletal-muscle-relaxant drug used intravenously in anesthesia and before electroconvulsive treatment.

succorance need H. A. Murray's term for the need for protection, aid, and support.

succubus a medieval term for a demon or evil spirit in female form who is believed to have intercourse with a sleeping man (from Latin *succubare*, "to lie under").

sucker: See BARNUM EFFECT.

sucking reflex a basic reflex in which the infant grasps the nipple with its lips and draws milk into its mouth by suction. Among lower animals, the s.r. is used by leeches and biting insects to draw blood from a host. In psychoanalysis, **sucking** is considered the earliest autoerotic gratification and a prime activity of the oral stage of psychosexual development. See THUMB-SUCKING.

suckling: See ETERNAL S.

-sud- a combining form relating to sweat (from Latin *sudor*, "sweat, moisture").

sudanophilic leukoencephalopathy = ADRENO-LEUKODYSTROPHY.

sudden-infant-death syndrome = CRIB DEATH.

sudden insight: See AHA EXPERIENCE; DISCONTINUITY HYPOTHESIS.

sudoriferous glands the glands that secrete sweat.

suffering the experience of pain or acute distress, either psychological or physical. Psychologically speaking, suffering may be proportionate to the situation, such as loss of a loved one or a physical trauma, or it may be grossly exaggerated to satisfy a need for sympathy, attention, or control over others. It may also be self-induced, as in self-mutilation and martyrdom. See MASOCHISM; SADISM; SEXUAL MASOCHISM; SEXUAL SADISM. Also see PAIN; UNPLEASURE.

suffering-hero daydream: See DAYDREAM.

suffocation fear a common conversion symptom associated with acute anxiety that interferes with respiration. In psychoanalysis, this fear is explained in terms of anxiety aroused by respiratory changes occurring during sexual excitement. Also see PNIGOPHOBIA.

sugar self-selection a food-preference effect observed in rats that have been allowed to choose between sugar and a protein such as casein. Normally, an animal will select the food that is required by the body. But rats will develop a fondness for sugar and continue to choose sugar rather than protein even when the body needs the protein. Also see BLOOD SUGAR.

suggestibility a state in which the ideas, beliefs, or attitudes of others are uncritically adopted. Examples can be found in individuals with hysterical personalities or persons under hypnosis.

suggestible stage: See DISASTER SYNDROME.

suggestion the process of inducing uncritical acceptance of an idea or course of action. S. is usually expressed in words, as in hypnotic commands, "pep talks," or testimonials, but it may also be pictorial, as in ads for beauty creams. For different types of s., see AUTOSUGGESTION; PROPAGANDA; S. THERAPY; PRESTIGE S.

suggestion therapy a type of psychotherapy in which distressing symptoms are alleviated through direct suggestion and reassurance. The technique, sometimes coupled with a hypnotic trance, has been found to be effective in relieving the effects of stress and the more superficial conversion symptoms. It may be accompanied by an explanation of the meaning and the purpose of the symptoms, but no attempt is made to modify the patient's basic personality.

suicidal crisis an emergency situation in which suicide is threatened or attempted. Among the factors that most frequently precipitate such a situation are (a) severe depression, including involutional psychosis and the depressive phase of bipolar disorder, (b) schizophrenic disorders, and, less frequently, (c) alcoholism, ill health, marital conflict, loss of a loved one, and business failure.

suicidal ideation thoughts of suicide, or preoccupation with suicide. S.i. is frequently associated with depression (especially the simple and claiming types), bipolar disorder (especially the depressive phase), pathological grief reaction, aging (especially when accompanied by isolation or rejection), terminal illness, or alcoholism (especially involving self-loathing). S.i., though always of great concern to the clinician, leads to suicidal attempts in only a small minority of cases, and various studies indicate a ratio of about eight or nine attempted suicides to one successful suicide in England and the United States.

suicide the act of killing oneself. In psychiatry, s. threats and gestures are always taken seriously, since they may be forerunners of actual s. Also, half-hearted attempts may be desperate cries for help, and may succeed by accident. The motives and conditions for s. vary widely. It may be a symptom of deep depression or schizophrenic withdrawal; a turning of hostility inward to the self; an attempt to make others feel guilty; a reaction to personal guilt; a means of obtaining release from unbearable pain, failure, grief, or fear of old age; or, in occasional cases, an act of revenge or spite; also, in exceptional cases, an expression of adventurousness or playfulness or an assertion of intellectual freedom. Also see ALTRUISTIC S.; ANOMIC S.; COLLECTIVE S.; EGOISTIC S.; PARASUICIDE; PSYCHIC S.; PSYCHOSOMATIC S.

S. has been an age-old theme in literature (Hamlet's "To be, or not to be: that is the question") and in philosophy, in particular in existentialism (Albert Camus' "There is but one truly serious philosophical problem, and that is suicide").

suicide attempt: See SUICIDAL IDEATION; SUICIDE.

suicide-prevention center an emergency, or crisis-intervention, facility dealing primarily with individuals with suicidal thoughts, or who make suicidal threats or attempts. Such centers are usually manned by social workers with mental-health preparation and trained to deal with such emergencies in person or over a telephone hot-line.

suicidology a multiprofessional discipline devoted to the study of suicidal phenomena and their prevention. Major groups involved are (a) scientists (epidemiologists, sociologists, statisticians, demographers, and social psychologists), (b) clinicians (psychiatrists, clinical psychologists, psychiatric social workers, trained volunteers, and clergymen), and (c) educators (health educators and school and college personnel).

suigenderism the nonsexual relationship between children of the same gender, as during the period of childhood when boys prefer to play with boys and girls prefer to be with girls. The situation is natural until the period when sexual feelings develop.

suk-yeong = KORO.

sulcus = FISSURE.

sulcus principalis a groove in the contours of the cerebral-cortex frontal lobe. It is an area of the brain associated with the sense of hearing.

sulfonamides a group of drugs derived from the sulfur-based compound sulfanilamide and used as antibiotics because of their ability to inhibit the proliferation of disease organisms while the body's immune system fights the infection. Side effects include depression, headache, dizziness, and listlessness and other neurologic symptoms resembling alcoholism.

sulfone a chemical unit of sulfur and oxygen that is a component of some drugs used as antibacterial agents, e.g., dapsone, the leprosy medication. S. drugs also have been employed in the treatment of malarial and rickettsial infections. Also see DAPSONE.

Sullivan, Harry Stack American psychiatrist, 1892–1949. S. is chiefly recognized for his systematic approach to human development, personality, and psychotherapy—all in terms of interpersonal relations. The individual's development is primarily portrayed as a process of socialization in which the values of the culture are gradually absorbed. Personality is defined as a "relatively enduring pattern of recurrent interpersonal situations," especially involving our relations with "significant others." Mental illness is attributed to misperceptions of the self or others ("parataxic distortions"), which produce loss of security and self-esteem. Therapy is directed toward correcting faulty "security operations," or defenses, which the patient has adopted as a reaction to these distortions. Adjective: **Sullivanian.** See AS-IF PERFORMANCE; BAD-ME; COLLABORATION; CONSENSUAL VALIDATION; DEPTH PSYCHOLOGY; DYNAMISM; EMOTIONAL SECURITY; GOOD-ME; INTERPERSONAL PSYCHIATRY; INTERPERSONAL RELATIONS; INTERPERSONAL THEORY; ISOPHILIA; LONG-TERM PSYCHOTHERAPY; LUST DYNAMISM; MALEVOLENT TRANSFORMATION; MOTHERING ONE; NEO-FREUDIAN; NOT-ME; OBSESSIONALISM; PARATAXIC DISTORTION; PARATAXIC MODE; PARTIAL ADJUSTMENT; PARTICIPANT-OBSERVER; PERSONIFICATION; PERSONIFIED SELF; PROTOTAXIC MODE; PSYCHIATRIC INTERVIEW; RECONSTRUCTIVE PSYCHOTHERAPY; SECURITY OPERATIONS; SELECTIVE INATTENTION; SELF-DYNAMISM; SELF-SYSTEM; SIGNIFICANT OTHERS; SOCIAL PSYCHIATRY; SOCIAL RECOVERY; SYNTAXIC MODE; SYNTAXIC THOUGHT; UNCANNY EMOTIONS.

sulthiame: See CARBONIC ANHYDRASE INHIBITORS.

summa libido = ACME.

summating potential a type of electrical potential detected in the cochlea that builds up slowly and persists beyond the instant of stimulation.

summation the increased intensity experienced in a sensation when two stimuli are presented to a receptor in rapid succession (temporal s.) or to adjacent areas (spatial s.). See TEMPORAL S.; SPA-TIAL S.

summation effect: See BINOCULAR CELLS.

summation tone a tone that is the sum of the frequencies of two tones differing by more than 50 cycles per second when sounded simultaneously.

summative evaluation the appraisal of a student's achievement at the conclusion of an educational program. Also called **terminal assessment**.

In evaluation research, s.e. means attempts to assess the overall effectiveness of a program after it is in operation (whereas the purpose of formative evaluation is generally to help in the development of the program). S.e. reports are directed primarily toward those who set policy at various levels. Sometimes called ex post facto evaluation. Also see FORMATIVE EVALUATION; EX POST FACTO RESEARCH.

sum of squares the total of the squared differences between each score and the mean.

Sunday neurosis the aggravation of neurotic symptoms on Sunday or during weekends and holidays. Psychoanalysts, such as Ferenczi, suggest that repressed impulses may come to the surface on nonworking days, and that in some cases weekend events such as family outings that once aroused guilty fantasies (such as the primal scene) are revived. If the patient is in analysis, a S.n. may also be due to separation from the analyst. Also called **weekend neurosis**. Also see HOLIDAY SYNDROME.

sundowner a term used to characterize an elderly individual whose intellectual and emotional adjustments are relatively satisfactory during the day, but who becomes confused and agitated at night. This condition, termed **deliriant confusion**, is believed to be due to cerebral hypoxia resulting from cerebrovascular inadequacy accentuated by hypnotic medication.

sunlight fear = HELIOPHOBIA.

sunrise fear = EOSOPHOBIA.

Sunset procedures federal legislation requiring (a) that all federal programs be reauthorized every ten years according to an established schedule and that reauthorization be preceded by standardized committee reviews, (b) that inventories of federal programs be established and maintained, and (c) that Congressional committees select a few programs for in-depth reexamination. **Sunset bills** are laws proposed to the legislature recommending standards and guidelines for formalized procedures of evaluating programs that are funded by federal and/or state governments; and the term **Sunset acts** is applied to legislation established by federal and state governments that requires assessment of federally or state-funded programs by evaluation researchers.

supercold surgery: See CRYOGENIC METHODS.

superego in psychoanalysis, the ethical component of the personality, which represents society's standards and determines our own standards of right and wrong (our conscience) as well as our aims and aspirations (our ego ideal). Our con-

scious self, or ego, which controls our impulses and directs our actions, operates by the rules and principles of the s., which basically stem from parental demands and prohibitions. We adopt, or "introject," them because we need our parents' love and fear their disapproval. The formation of the s. occurs on an unconscious level. The process begins in the first five years of life but continues throughout childhood and adolescence and into adulthood, largely through identification with admired models of behavior. Also see DOUBLE S.; GROUP S.; HETERONOMOUS S.; PARASITIC S.; PRESUPEREGO PHASE; PRIMITIVE S.; REWARD BY THE S.

superego anxiety a type of anxiety caused by unconscious superego activity that produces feelings of guilt and demands for atonement.

superego lacunae superego defects in psychopathic persons that are believed to be acquired from parents with similar defects, indicating that antisocial behavior may represent an acting-out of the unconscious impulses of the parents.

superego resistance a type of resistance to the psychoanalytic process created by the superego, which generates a sense of guilt that gives rise to the need for punishment in the form of persistent symptoms. S.r. is observed in obsessionals and cases of masochistic behavior. An often synonymously used term is NEGATIVE THERAPEUTIC REACTION. See this entry.

superego sadism in psychoanalysis, the aggressive, rigid, punitive aspect of conscience, with energy derived from the destructive forces of the id, and its intensity and strength dependent upon the violent and sadistic fantasies of the child's primordial strivings.

superfecundation the fertilization of an ovum immediately after another ovum has been fertilized; also, the nearly simultaneous fertilization of two separate ova by the spermatozoa of different males. Also see SIMULTANEOUS FERTILIZATION.

superfemale a term sometimes applied to a female born with more than the normal XX complement of female chromosomes. In some rare cases of sex-chromosome aberrations, females have been found with as many as five X chromosomes. Women born with three or more X chromosomes occur at a frequency slightly greater than one per thousand. However, the additional X chromosomes often are associated with mental retardation, sterility, and, despite the term s., underdeveloped female sexual characteristics. Also see SUPERSEX.

superfetation the development and fertilization of an ovum when the mother already is pregnant. See SUPERFECUNDATION.

superficial burns: See BURN INJURIES.

superior brachium: See BRACHIUM.

superior colliculus one of a pair of rounded prominences near the cerebral peduncle and immediately beneath the pineal gland. The s.c. receives fibers from the optic tract through the superior brachium. The four adjoining colliculi, two superior and two inferior, form the corpora quadrigemina.

superior function the function among Jung's four basic psychological types that dominates the other three, which become **inferior functions**.

superior intelligence an arbitrary category of general intelligence attained by only 15 percent of the population. It includes individuals with an IQ of 120 or more on both the Wechsler and Stanford-Binet scales.

superiority feelings an attitude characterized by an exaggerated idea of one's physical or mental abilities, or both, in comparison with the abilities of others. S.f. are often a defense against inferiority feelings.

For a different meaning of superiority, see STRIVING FOR SUPERIORITY.

superior longitudinal fasciculus a bundle of nerve fibers that runs from front to back, extending from the frontal lobe to the occipital lobe, with fibers that also communicate with the temporal lobe.

superior oblique: See EYE MOVEMENTS.

superior olivary complex a collection of nuclei appearing as small masses of gray matter in the pons. The cells receive terminals and collaterals from the cochlear nuclei on the same and opposite sides through the trapezoid body, a concentration of transverse nerve fibers in the pons.

superior olive a structure in the medulla that receives fibers from auditory nerves of both ears. It consists of two or three small masses of gray matter in the tegmentum of the pons.

superior rectus: See EYE MOVEMENTS.

superior sagittal sinus a part of the system of veins that drain blood from the cerebral tissues. The s.s.s. runs approximately across the top of the cerebral cortex, draining venous blood from an area above the eye to the transverse sinus which empties into the internal jugular vein.

superjoint: See PHENCYCLIDINE.

supermale a term sometimes applied to men born with more than the usual complement of male chromosomes. Early study findings suggested that men with XYY chromosome sets were large and aggressive because of the extra male chromosome. However, the first cases were discovered in prison inmates, and further study showed that normal, average men in the general population also may have an extra male chromosome. Also see SUPERSEX.

supernormal period a brief time span, of between 15 and 100 milliseconds, that may occur immediately after the refractory period of a neuron-firing cycle. During the s.p., excitability is greater than normal. A cause may be the overshooting of the resting potential.

superordinate goal an objective that is meaningful for a number of persons or groups but can only be attained if they work as a team. In studies on aggression, the hostility of rival groups was significantly lessened by the experimenter's introduction of a s.g.

supersex a popular term applied to individuals who have inherited an excess of either male or female sex chromosomes. A person with an excess of female chromosomes, e.g., a 47,XXX complement, would be considered a superfemale, and one with a 47,XYY complement of chromosomes would be a supermale. A s. person may be sterile or fertile, depending upon other factors than the number of sex chromosomes in their gametes. Also see SUPERFEMALE; SUPERMALE.

supersonic transport: See SONIC BOOM.

superstition a belief or practice based on the operation of supernatural or magical forces, such as charms, omens, prayers, or exorcism. Also, s. may denote any unscientific belief accepted without question. See ANIMISM; MAGICAL THINKING; SUPERSTITIOUS CONTROL; FAITH HEALING.

superstitious control the illusion that one can influence outcomes through various practices designed to protect oneself or alter the environment, e.g., a rain dance, incantation, or other kind of prayer. Certain writers maintain that s.c. serves a positive psychological function in averting the development of LEARNED HELPLESSNESS. See this entry. Also see MAGICAL THINKING; FAITH HEALING.

supervalent characterizing an idea that takes on excessive intensity and cannot be eliminated by the individual's efforts, either because "it itself reaches with its roots down into the unconscious, repressed material, or because another unconscious thought lies concealed beneath it" (Fred, 1905). An example is extreme jealousy stemming from a source that is now concealed in the unconscious.

supervision clinical guidance and direction of a trainee in the field of psychotherapy or psychoanalysis, provided by an experienced therapist.

supination the act of assuming a **supine** position, or of turning the palm forward or upward by lateral rotation of the forelimb.

supplementary motor area one of the regions of the cortex in which motor tracts have somatotopic organization, with neurons distributed in a pattern that more or less resembles the general design of the body. Cells relating to eye function, e.g., occur near motoneurons associated with face muscles, and so on.

supportive ego a term introduced by S. R. Slavson to describe a member of an activity-therapy group who helps a fellow member work out his intrapsychic difficulties.

supportiveness in counseling, an attitude or response of acceptance, encouragement, or reassurance displayed by the counselor. See REASSURANCE. Also see SUPPORTIVE PSYCHOTHERAPY.

supportive personnel health professionals who function in special areas of diagnosis, therapy, and rehabilitation in support of activities of the medical-surgical personnel. S.p. may, e.g., include occupational, recreational, and physical therapists.

supportive psychotherapy a form of "surface therapy" directed to reinforcing existing defenses, and relieving emotional distress and symptoms without probing into the sources of conflicts or attempting to alter basic personality structure. Specific methods used include reassurance, reeducation, advice, persuasion, hypnotic suggestion, ventilation, environmental manipulation, pastoral counseling, art therapy, dance therapy, music therapy, occupational therapy, recreational therapy, bibliotherapy, remotivation, and encouragement of desirable behavior. Such measures may be used as adjuncts to depth therapy, and are frequently applied to patients with relatively minor or limited problems, as well as hospitalized patients, as a means of maintaining morale and preventing deterioration.

supportive services functions of the sheltered workshop that are in support of the needs of the client, e.g., employment counseling, psychologic or psychiatric service, medical supervision, and physical-tolerance review to determine the ability of the patient to cope with job demands outside the sheltered-workshop environment.

suppos. an abbreviation used in prescriptions, meaning "suppository" (Latin *suppositorium*).

suppression a conscious effort to put disturbing thoughts and experiences out of mind, or to control and inhibit the expression of unacceptable impulses and feelings. Though salutary when used in moderation, it should be recognized that "out of consciousness isn't out of mind," and that rigidly suppressed drives may seek drastic expression or give rise to distressing symptoms. Also see REPRESSION.

suppressive therapy a form of psychotherapy directed to the reinforcement of the patient's defense mechanisms and the suppression rather than expression of distressing experiences and feelings. Compare EXPRESSIVE THERAPY.

suppressor area an area of the cortex which, when stimulated, inhibits cortical activity of other areas.

supraliminal above the difference threshold or absolute threshold. **S. difference** refers to a difference between stimuli that are above the difference threshold.

supramarginal gyrus: See POSTERIOR PARIETAL LOBE.

supranuclear palsy = STEELE-RICHARDSON-OLSZEWSKI SYNDROME.

suprarenalectomy = ADRENALECTOMY.

suprarenal gland = ADRENAL GLAND.

suprasegmental reflexes reflexes that require some control by brain areas as well as the spinal cord and the various neuromuscular connections of the limbs and trunk. Segmental and intersegmental reactions are a part of the s.r. with coordination by the brain.

surd a **voiceless sound** produced without vibration of the vocal cords, e.g., /p/, /t/, or /f/.

-surd- a combining form meaning deaf or silent (Latin *surdus*).

surdimutism an alternative term for deaf-mutism.

surdity an alternative term for deafness.

surface color a color that is perceived as localized on the surface, as opposed to a color that permeates an object.

surface structure the linear relationship between the words of a sentence, that is, the relationship that is merely formal or grammatically consistent. The s.s. may or may not contain real meaning, and may not reveal the underlying grammatical DEEP STRUCTURE. See this entry.

surface therapy psychotherapy carried out on a conscious level and directed toward relieving the patient's symptoms and emotional stress through such measures as reassurance, suggestion, reinforcement of present defenses, and direct attempts to modify attitudes and behavior patterns. Compare DEPTH THERAPY.

surface traits a group of 35 characteristics which R. B. Cattell found to be highly correlated in the same individual. E.g., warmth versus aloofness correlates highly with responsiveness versus unresponsiveness, affectionate versus cold, and even-tempered versus sensitive. Also see SOURCE TRAITS; PERSONALITY SPHERE.

surfactin the liquid that coats the air sacs of the lungs, and which, by reducing surface tension, enables them to transmit oxygen from the air to the blood. See HYALINE-MEMBRANE DISEASE.

surgency Cattell's term for a personality trait marked by cheerfulness, responsiveness, and sociability, but at a level below that of extraversion or mania.

surplus meaning a connotation or implication that goes well beyond the observable. Explanatory concepts that refer to vague or undetectable internal processes are said to contain s.m.

surprisal a term used in information theory meaning the surprise value of a message. The greater the s., the more information the message relates; e.g., "Man gives birth to twins" would have more s. than "Woman gives birth to twins."

surprisingness the measure of the degree to which one's expectations are disconfirmed. The term is used in psychological esthetics and in environmental psychology.

surrogate a person or object that substitutes for the role of an individual who has a significant position in a family or group. The s. may substitute for a parent, child, or mate who is absent from the scene. Young animals may use soft-cloth material as a s. mother, and young humans may use stuffed toys as s. companions. See MOTHER S. Also see S. PARTNER.

surrogate father = FATHER SURROGATE.

surrogate mother = MOTHER SURROGATE.

surrogate partner in sex therapy, a professional substitute trained to help the patient overcome inhibitions and resistances so that satisfactory intercourse can be achieved.

sursumvergence the deviation or turning upward of one eye in relation to the other.

survey research a research method utilizing written questionnaires or personal interviews to discover the attitudes and beliefs of a given population, as in a public-opinion poll. Many variables must be controlled including experimenter bias, sampling procedures, interview format, and question-wording. Also called **survey method**.

survey tests tests designed to yield accurate information about a large group of individuals.

survival guilt feelings of guilt for having survived when others did not, as in the concentration-camp syndrome. Such feelings may be accentuated by real or fancied actions that are interpreted as endangering the lives of others, or merely the vague unspecified conviction of having done something wrong though that was not the case. In other situations, s.g. may take the form of feeling that "I should have done something" to avert the tragedy or, as with children, "Maybe my mom died because I did something bad." See CONCENTRATION-CAMP SYNDROME; SURVIVOR SYNDROME; PERSECUTION SYNDROME.

survival of the fittest: See NATURAL SELECTION.

survival value the capacity of an attitude or physical quality to contribute to the survival of an individual or population.

survivor syndrome a constellation of symptoms observed in survivors of a disaster such as a flood, earthquake, or hurricane. Among the symptoms found by Lifton (1976) and others are indelible images of death, continuing anxiety, guilt over having lived while others died, numbing, depression, withdrawal, loss of interest and enjoyment in activities, and increased smoking and drinking. See SURVIVAL GUILT; CONCENTRATION-CAMP SYNDROME.

susceptibility rhythms cyclical variations in sensitivity to infections or allergic responses.

suspiciousness an attitude of mistrust toward the motives or sincerity of others. Extreme, pervasive s. is a common characteristic of the paranoid personality.

sustenacular cells cells that provide structural support for other cells or tissues. Examples include s.c. that surround the olfactory neurons and the Sertoli cells which house the spermatids in the testes.

sustenacular fibers = MÜLLER'S FIBERS.

susto a culture-specific syndrome (Spanish, "fright") occurring among children throughout Central and South America. In a typical case the child becomes highly irritable, easily frightened, cries constantly, resists being left alone, and loses his appetite. The natives believe the illness is due to the fact that the child's soul has fled his body, but observers have found that the condition usually follows a traumatic experience such as encountering a snake or other frightening animal. S. is sometimes called **espanto**, meaning "terror" or "ghost."

swallow-belch method a technique of speaking without a larynx by swallowing air, then belching while the lips, teeth, and tongue are manipulated to form word sounds as the air is expelled. See LARYNGECTOMY.

swallowing the process of moving food, liquid, or medications from the oral cavity to the stomach through a complex series of muscle contractions and relaxations. The muscles of the cheeks, tongue, and roof of the mouth first contract to form a chute, after which the tongue presses upward and backward against the hard palate. As the substance to be swallowed passes toward the back of the mouth, the soft palate is raised to close the opening to the nasal area of the pharynx. At the same time, the epiglottis is lowered over the opening to the trachea to prevent ingestion of food or fluid into the respiratory system and the larynx moves upward to form a seal against the lower side of the epiglottis. As the substance swallowed enters the esophagus, it is moved along by contractions of two layers of muscles, one composed of longitudinal muscles fibers and the other of circular muscle fibers. By alternate contractions of the separate muscle-fiber layers, the food or fluid is advanced toward the stomach. The esophageal contractions enable the s. process to function regardless of body position.

sway-back: See LORDOSIS.

sweet-lemon mechanism a form of rationalization in which a disappointment is justified by giving reasons for being satisfied with the status quo. E.g., a woman who has been rejected by a new acquaintance will find that her present boyfriend has sterling qualities she had overlooked. Also see SOUR-GRAPES MECHANISM.

sweet taste a gustatory sensation associated with a sugary effect on the taste buds. It sometimes is described as the opposite of sour or bitter, although very small concentrations of table salt, sodium chloride, may produce a sweet taste on the tongues of some individuals. Sweet-sensitive taste buds are concentrated at the tip of the tongue.

swimming reflex a reflex of the healthy newborn infant consisting of "paddlelike" motions of the limbs when the baby is placed in water. See REFLEX.

Swindle, Percy Ford American physiologist, 1889–1916. See SWINDLE'S GHOST.

Swindle's ghost a prolonged positive afterimage.

swinging a popular term for uninhibited sexual expression, including such activities as wife-swapping, "one-night stands," group sex, homosexual encounters, and experimentation with such deviations as sadism and masochism.

switch process behavioral phenomena observed during the spontaneous transition from depression to mania and mania to depression in cases of bipolar disorder. **Switches** into mania are usually preceded by a moderate depression followed by a brief, relatively normal period, but with reduction in total sleep and REM sleep. The switch into depression goes through the following stages: transition from mania to hypomania, then to a short period characterized by a labile mood and activity, and finally to psychomotor retardation.

Sydenham, Thomas English physician, 1624–89. See CHOREA (there: **Sydenham's chorea**).

syllabic synthesis a term for the process of forming bizarre new words or neologisms from parts of other words, as occurs in dreams and in the language of certain schizophrenic patients.

syllogism a form of reasoning in which a major and a minor premise yield a conclusion, which is true only if the two premises are true.

Sylvius, Franciscus Dutch physician, 1614–72. See AQUEDUCT OF SYLVIUS; FISSURE OF SYLVIUS (also called **Sylvian fissure**); STENOSIS OF AQUEDUCT OF SYLVIUS; INTERIOR COLLICULI; ISLAND OF REIL; LATERAL SULCUS; MIDDLE CEREBRAL ARTERY; SUBCOMMISSURAL ORGAN; THIRD VENTRICLE.

sym = SYMPTOM.

-sym-; -syn- a combining form relating to a union or fusion.

symbiosis literally, living together. In psychiatry, s. is a relationship between two disturbed people characterized by excessive dependence and mutual exploitation for neurotic needs. The term is also used to denote the stage in infantile development when the infant's dependence is total and he is neither biologically nor psychologically separated from the mother; this is a normal phase promoting further development, but failure to progress beyond this stage may lead to severe pathology. Also called **symbiotic relationship**. See SYMBIOTIC PSYCHOSIS.

symbiotic infantile psychosis; symbiotic infantile psychotic syndrome = SYMBIOTIC PSYCHOSIS.

symbiotic marriage a marriage of two individuals who are dependent upon each other for the gratification of certain psychological needs. Both partners may have neurotic or otherwise unusual needs that could not be satisfied easily outside the marriage. Also see SYNERGIC MARRIAGE.

symbiotic psychosis a major mental illness occurring between the ages of two and five. The condition was first described by M.S. Mahler, and is characterized by complete emotional dependence on the mother, inability to tolerate separation from her, reactions of anger and panic if any separation is threatened, and developmental lag. Aso called **symbiotic infantile psychotic syndrome; symbiotic infantile psychosis**.

symbiotic relatedness a close, parasitic attachment of one individual for another, involving the satisfaction of neurotic needs. As used by E. Fromm, the term refers to the condition in which an individual does not achieve psychological autonomy and develops a style of relating based on merging with the other partner and characterized by abnormal dependence and sadistic or masochistic trends. The original relationship between mother and child may provide the pattern for later symbiotic relationships.

symbiotic relationship = SYMBIOSIS.

symbol any object, figure, or image that represents something else. A s. may appear as a musical notation, letter, word, pictograph, or activity. In psychoanalysis, a s. may appear as a disguised representation of a repressed idea, impulse, or wish. See PHALLIC S.

symbolic action a simple or complex action that is unconscious and automatic but expresses an underlying meaning, e.g., pulling one's ear lobe. Also see SYMPTOMATIC ACT.

symbolic displacement transferring a response, usually emotional, from its original stimulus to one that represents it. E.g., a man who harbors homicidal impulses might develop a morbid fear of knives or guns.

symbolic loss in psychoanalysis, an unconscious ego interpretation of a rejection as a complete loss that is equivalent to a death in the family.

symbolic masturbation the handling of body parts that are symbolic substitutes for the penis or clitoris, e.g., the nose, ear lobe, mouth, or fingertips. S.m. also may be expressed in the twisting or pulling of garments or hair strands.

symbolic mode Bruner's third stage of cognitive development, following the enactive and iconic periods. Symbolic representation enables the young child to depict and convey ideas through the use of words, sounds, and play. He can, e.g., imagine he is a fire engine, and make siren noises while pushing a block that represents a speeding engine. See ENACTIVE MODE; ICONIC MODE.

symbolic parricide: See SACRIFICE.

symbolic play: See MAKE-BELIEVE.

symbolic process a cognitive activity involving the use of symbols, such as words or formulae, as in thinking, remembering a theory, or problem-solving. Also called **symbolic thinking**.

symbolic realization fulfillment of a blocked desire or goal through a substitute that represents it. E.g., a person who has not been able to rebel against an authoritarian father, may rebel against all symbols of authority such as the laws or customs of the society in which he lives.

symbolic stage = PREOPERATIONAL STAGE.

symbolic synthesis a form of abstract reasoning involved in problems of logic and mathematics. S.s. may require spatial concepts in placing numbers in the proper sequence in order to obtain the correct answer. Persons with certain left-hemisphere lesions may experience difficulty in such tasks because of confusion about the spatial relationship of numbers.

symbolic thinking = SYMBOLIC PROCESS.

symbolism in psychoanalysis, the substitution of a representation, or symbol, for a repressed impulse or threatening object in order to avoid censorship by the superego, e.g., dreaming of a steeple instead of a male organ. Jung maintained that mythological and religious symbols throw special light on the racial unconscious. See THRESHOLD S.; PHALLIC SYMBOL.

symbolization in psychiatry, an unconscious mental process in which images, objects, or gestures come to represent repressed thoughts, feelings, or impulses. Through this mechanism, emotionally charged material may frequently obtain expression without arousing excessive anxiety. A mute patient, e.g., always communicated with her husband in red ink, which symbolized both the fact that he had taken her money and left her "in the red" and the rage she felt toward him ("seeing red"). S. is found in many mental disorders, such as phobic reactions, obsessive-compulsive rituals, the body language of conversion hysterics, and the gestures and grimaces of schizophrenics.

symbolophobia a morbid fear of symbolism, especially of other people's seeing something symbolic in one's words or actions.

symbol-substitution test = CODE TEST.

symmetrical distribution a distribution in which the values above the mean are a mirror image of those below the mean.

symmetry balance and harmony in the proportions of objects or works of art, an esthetically pleasing quality; also, in a narrower sense, the mirrorlike correspondence of parts on opposite sides of a center.

Symonds, Percival Mallon American psychologist, 1893–1960. See SYMONDS PICTURE-STUDY TEST.

Symonds Picture-Study Test a projective test for adolescents, consisting of 20 pictures of interpersonal situations. The subject tells a story about each of the pictures, and the psychologist analyzes these productions in terms of their dynamics.

sympathectomy a surgical procedure in which the sympathetic division of the autonomic nervous system is partially excised or severed to eliminate its influence, to study its effects in experimental animals, or to alleviate intractable pain.

sympathetic division a part of the autonomic nervous system that consists of preganglionic and postganglionic fibers from the spinal cord, innervating organs from the eye to the reproductive organs. The vagus nerve is an example of a fiber of the s.d.

sympathetic dyspraxia an apraxia affecting the left limbs in patients who are afflicted with a right hemiplegia and aphasia due to lesions in Broca's area.

sympathetic ganglion any of the nerve clusters of the sympathetic division of the autonomic nervous system that form a beadlike chain on either side of the spinal cord.

sympathetic nervous system a part of the autonomic nervous system with fibers from the thoracolumbar portion innervating the heart and smooth muscles and glands throughout the body, from the eyes to the urogenital organs. Typical sympathetic changes take place during heavy exertion or emergency situations, e.g., the pupils widen to facilitate vision, the arteries constrict to supply more blood to the muscles and the brain, adrenaline is secreted to raise the blood-sugar level and increase metabolism, the skin perspires to eliminate waste products, and stomach and intestinal activities cease so that energy can be directed elsewhere. In a word, the s.n.s. mobilizes the entire organism to meet the situation.

sympathicotonia a syndrome involving increased sympathetic-nervous-system tonus, with a marked tendency to vascular spasms and hypertension, and hyperfunctioning of the adrenal glands with hypersensitivity to epinephrine.

sympathin a neurohormonal nerve-impulse mediator secreted at sympathetic-nerve synapses. The term usually is applied only when the mediator cannot be identified as epinephrine or norepinephrine. One form, I, has an inhibitory effect; another, E, has an excitatory effect.

sympathism the tendency to seek emotional support by arousing sympathy; the habit of eliciting the concern and assistance of others by dwelling on one's misfortunes and bad breaks, which are usually ascribed to an unkind fate or the faults of others. It is more commonly called **sympathy-seeking**.

sympathomimetics agents that mimic the activities of the sympathetic nervous system. Amphetamines are s. as they can cause the release of norepinephrine from sympathetic-nervous-system fiber terminals and stimulate body tissues innervated by sympathetic fibers.

sympathy compassion for an individual or group experiencing distress; concern and consideration for others based on a capacity to share their feelings. Most children, by four years of age, perceive the misfortunes of others and respond in a variety of ways, such as by comforting, helping, punishing the cause of the distress, telling an adult, and asking the cause of the trouble. Also see EMPATHY.

sympathy-seeking: See SYMPATHISM.

sympatric species species that occupy the same habitat or overlapping habitats. Species that do not occur together or occupy the same habitat are **allopatric**.

symptom in psychiatry and general medicine, any deviation from normal functioning which is considered indicative of physical or mental disorder. In general, a s. is any event that is indicative of another event; e.g., a series of strikes is symptomatic of economic unrest. Abbrev.: **sym**. For s. in the medical meaning, also see SIGN.

symptomatic act in psychoanalysis, an action that appears to be meaningless but which, if analyzed, reveals a hidden motivation, e.g., playing with one's watch chain, or constantly adjusting one's necktie. These are sometimes called symbolic actions, since they may represent repressed impulses such as an urge to masturbate. See PARAPRAXIS; SYMBOLIC ACTION.

symptomatic alcoholism = ALPHA ALCOHOLISM.

symptomatic autoscopy: See AUTOSCOPIC SYNDROME.

symptomatic epilepsy a type of epilepsy in which a seizure represents a symptom of a CNS disorder, e.g., carbon-monoxide poisoning, meningitis, cerebral hemorrhage, or a congenital brain defect.

symptomatic psychosis a severe mental disorder associated with impairment of brain-tissue function. See ORGANIC BRAIN SYNDROMES; ORGANIC MENTAL DISORDERS.

symptomatic schizophrenia a term applied by E. A. Rodin to a recurrent episodic psychotic reaction characterized by clouded sensorium, partial memory loss, and schizophrenic behavior. Some investigators, however, find these episodes closer to either centrencephalic or temporal-lobe epilepsy than to schizophrenia. See ONEIROPHRENIA.

symptomatic treatment treatment directed toward the relief of distressing symptoms as opposed to treatment focused on underlying causes and conditions and the reconstruction of the patient's personality. The leading exponent of this approach is the English psychologist H. J. Eysenck. Major techniques used in symptom removal are behavior therapy, hypnotherapy, suggestion therapy, and narcotherapy.

symptom choice the unconscious "selection" of one symptom or symptom pattern rather than another as an expression of underlying pathology. It is often difficult or impossible to explain why a given patient develops a compulsion rather than a phobia, or becomes hysterically blind rather than paralyzed, but among the explanations frequently given are constitutional predisposition, parental behavior patterns, fixation at an early psychosexual stage, and specific traumatic experiences. Also called **choice of a neurosis**. See SOMATIC COMPLIANCE. Also see LOCALIZATION OF SYMPTOMS.

symptom cluster a group of related symptoms that usually occur together, as in a syndrome.

symptom complex = SYNDROME.

symptom formation in psychoanalysis, the process of developing a somatic or behavioral substitute for an unconscious impulse or conflict that provokes anxiety. Examples are conversion symptoms such as glove anesthesia, or phobias such as fearful avoidance of crowds. Also called **substitute formation**.

symptom localization: See LOCALIZATION OF SYMPTOMS.

symptom neurosis a psychoneurotic disorder with a specific pattern of symptoms (such as obsessive-compulsive, phobic, dissociative, anxiety), as opposed to individual neurotic traits and tendencies such as meticulousness, apprehensiveness, or irrational fears that may or may not develop into one or another neurotic reaction type. See NEUROTIC PERSONALITY.

symptom specificity the group of symptoms involving an organ that is the focus of a psychosomatic disorder. E.g., a person whose psychosomatic problem is the heart is likely to have an unusually large variety of complaints expressed as cardiovascular symptoms, rather than complaints about other possible organs or disorders.

symptom substitution the development of a symptom to replace one that has cleared up as a result of treatment. It is often observed in hysteric patients, and frequently occurs if the unconscious impulses and conflicts responsible for their formation are not dealt with. S.s. is often used as an argument against therapies aimed at symptom removal alone, as in behavior therapy, suggestion, and some forms of hypnotherapy.

-syn-; -sym- a combining form relating to a union or fusion.

synapse an area between two adjacent neurons where a nerve impulse is transmitted across the intervening space. Synapses in vertebrates usually are **axodendritic synapses**, between the axon of one neuron and the dendrites of the other, or **axosomatic synapses**, as between the axon of one neuron and the body of another. **Axodendrosomatic synapses**, between an axon and the dendrites and body of a neighboring neuron, are found in motor-nerve tracts. Also called **synaptic junction**. Verb: **to s**. See AXOAXONAL S.

synaptic cleft the space between the synaptic knob of a neuron and the membrane of a neighboring dendrite. The s.c. may actually be no larger than 1/50 of a micron in width. Also called **synaptic gap**.

synaptic junction = SYNAPSE.

synaptic knobs the terminal portion of an axon from which a nerve impulse is transmitted to a neighboring neuron's dendrites or cell membrane. S.k. are about one micron in diameter, and there may be several on a single axon. The normal direction of travel of a nerve impulse is from one dendritic zone toward the s.k. of the same neuron. Also called **end buttons; terminal boutons; boutons terminaux** /bo͞otôN′terminō′/; **terminal bulbs**.

synaptic resistance a condition that inhibits the transmission of a nerve impulse across a synapse, usually due to lack of electrical energy needed to cross the gap rather than a true opposition to the impulse.

synaptic vesicles small granules in the cytoplasm of synaptic knobs. The s.v. are believed to be the sources of the transmitter substance released by the synaptic knobs when a nerve impulse arrives at the terminus of an axon.

synchronism the occurrence of several developmental disorders at about the same time of embryonic or fetal life, as in Down's syndrome. The term s. is also used by Jung to describe events that occur at the same time but independently of each other despite what appears to be a causal relationship, as in purported examples of telepathy or clairvoyance.

synchronization a pattern of brain waves that appears to be coordinated with mental or physical activity. Alpha-wave s. may be observed during periods of relaxed mental states in one hemisphere during split-brain verbal and spatial tasks while theta-wave synchronization can be recorded during slow-wave sleep, in which the EEG rhythm may be coordinated with the heartbeat.

synchronized sleep the type of sleep associated primarily with stage 4, or deep-sleep states, when EEG recordings show slow synchronous waves. The waves appear to follow a rhythm of cell activity; brain-cell metabolism is at a minimum level; and the brain is in a resting state.

synchrony a term used in dance therapy to denote moving together in harmony, which tends to bring people closer together. Other forms of s. are self-s., or movement in relation to one's own speech; and **interactional s.**, in which the movement of a listener is synchronous with the speech and movements of the speaker.

syncope /singk′əpē/ a transient fainting spell (Greek, "cutting short") resulting from cerebral anemia, that is, sudden reduction in the blood supply to the brain. **Syncopal** attacks may be experienced by patients with cerebral arteriosclerosis, cardiovascular disorders coupled with emotional stress, and hysterical, or conversion, tendencies.

syncratic decisions: See ROLE SPECIALIZATION.

syncretic thought a term applied by Piaget to the first or prelogical, stage of thinking in the child's life, characterized by egocentric and frequently animistic thought processes; e.g., a simple block may be called a car, or a broomstick may be ridden as a horse. At this stage, connections are likely to be purely accidental; e.g., if the sun shines brightly on the child's birthday, he may think it shines *because* it is his birthday. See PHYSIOGNOMIC THINKING; SYNCRETISM. Compare PRIMARY PROCESS.

syncretism the integration of elements from two or more systems, theories, or concepts into a new system, theory, or concept. The system may represent cultures, beliefs, or doctrines that may appear incompatible or inconsistent. The terms s. or syncretic thought are also used by Piaget to refer to representational thinking typical of children in the preoperational or symbolic stage. (The term s. is derived from the Greek word *synkretismos*, meaning a confederation like that of Cretan cities against a common enemy, from *syn-* and *Kret*, "Cretan.")

syndrome a constellation of symptoms and signs which together constitute a recognizable illness, physical or mental. The term is frequently used as a synonym for disease. Also called **symptom complex**. See METHODOLOGICAL NOTES, 3.3 (d).

syndrome of approximate answers = GANSER SYNDROME.

syndrome of extra-small acrocentric chromosome = CAT'S-EYE SYNDROME.

syndrome of missing fifth-digit nails a congenital condition apparently affecting only unrelated females and marked by the absence of fifth fingernails and toenails, short distal phalanges, and lax joints. All patients studied have been microcephalic and mentally retarded with IQs estimated at less than 30.

syndrome of obstinate progression a term applied by Bailey and Davis (1942) to the effect of surgery performed on the brainstems of cats: Apparently the balance between excitation and inhibition was so severely disrupted that the cats walked forward persistently until they finally became exhausted and died.

synectics model an educational approach that emphasizes creative problem-solving and the development of teaching methods that enhance student creativity, e.g., encouraging metaphorical thinking.

synergic: See SYNERGY.

synergic autonomy a psychological balance of dependence on others and independence, with the ability to function effectively in either manner under appropriate conditions. S.a. is regarded by some psychiatrists as evidence of psychological well-being.

synergic marriage a marriage that is enhanced by the contributions the partners can make in satisfying each other's psychological needs in a positive manner. Also see SYMBIOTIC MARRIAGE.

synergism the concept that ideas and reactions are the product of combinations of factors working together and reinforcing each other.

synergistic: See SYNERGY.

synergistic muscles muscles that work together to produce a specific action, such as flexion or extension of a limb. S.m. are classed according to homonymous reflex action, in which stimulation of a muscle causes contraction of that muscle, and heteronymous reflex action, in which stimulation begins in one muscle but causes another member of the synergistic-muscle group to contract.

synergy a coordination of forces or efforts to achieve a goal, e.g., a group of muscles working together to move a limb. Adjectives: **synergic; synergistic**.

synesthesia literally, feeling together; a condition in which stimulation of one sensory modality also arouses sensations in another; e.g., sounds (and sometimes tastes and odors) may be experienced as colors while they are being heard, and specific sounds, such as different musical notes, may yield specific colors. A small proportion of the general population reports such experiences, but they are especially vivid in persons under the influence of hallucinogenic drugs, and are occasionally experienced during epileptic seizures. Also called **crossed perception; secondary sensation**. Also see CHROMESTHESIA.

synkinesia an involuntary movement that accompanies a voluntary action. S. is often a sign of neurologic damage, as in movement in paralyzed muscles when other muscles are contracted. Also called **synkinesis**.

synonym-antonym test a type of test in which the

subject is given word pairs to be identified as equal or opposite in meaning.

synoptic a term describing a brief sketch, or **synopsis**; also, referring to a form of synesthesia in which sounds are perceived as colors.

synorchidism a congenital fusion of the testes in the abdominal cavity. Also called **synorchism**.

syntactical aphasia a form of aphasia characterized by grammatical errors, particularly in the combinations or sequences of words in sentences.

syntality the characteristic of consistent behavior in a social group which makes its performances predictable (Cattell).

syntax the rules for the combination of words into grammatical sentences; the way words are combined in this manner.

syntaxic mode a term used by H. S. Sullivan for the highest stage in experiencing the world, characterized by consensual validation, the development of rational or "syntaxic" thought, and the expression of ideas in a commonly accepted language. Also see SYNTAXIC THOUGHT.

syntaxic thought H. S. Sullivan's term for the highest level of cognition, which includes logical, goal-directed, reality-oriented thinking. See SYNTAXIC MODE.

synthesis in psychiatry and psychology, the integration of personality factors such as attitudes, impulses, and traits into a totality. This process requires a perception of one's personality as a whole (as emphasized by Gestaltists); reconciliation of conflicting values and tendencies, and the achievement of a new balance among all aspects and levels of the psyche, both conscious and unconscious (as emphasized by Jung). See PSYCHOSYNTHESIS.

synthetic approach a perceptual method in which the observer tends to make judgments based on an integrated whole, as opposed to analysis of the parts. Experimental evidence indicates that individual personality factors are associated with synthetic and analytic perceivers.

synthetic narcotics any of the numerous compounds created in the laboratory in a search for drugs that provide the pain relief of morphine without the undesirable side effects, e.g., addiction or depressed respiration. One of the s.n., **Bentley's compound**, was found to be up to 10,000 times as potent as morphine in analgesic effects but was also much more potent in adverse effects and could not be used therapeutically. One of the first practical s.n. was **meperidine hydrochloride (pethidine)**—$C_{15}H_{22}ClNO_2$—developed in 1930, but also found later to be addictive. One of the most commonly used s.n. today, **methadone hydrochloride**—$C_{21}H_{28}ClNO$—was developed by German chemists during World War II and introduced in other countries in 1946. Other s.n. include **alphaprodine**—$C_{16}H_{23}NO_2$, **anilerdine**—$C_{22}H_{28}N_2O_2$, **dextromoramide**—$C_{25}H_{32}N_2O_2$, **dextropropoxyphene**—$C_{22}H_{29}NO_2$, **dipipanone**—$C_{24}H_{31}NO$, LEVOR-

PHANOL (see this entry), **pentazocine**—$C_{19}H_{27}NO$, **phenadoxone hydrochloride**—$C_{24}H_{30}ClNO_2$, PHENAZOCINE (see this entry), **piminodine**—$C_{23}H_{30}N_2O_2$, and **propoxyphene**—$C_{22}H_{29}NO_2$. See OPIOIDS; OPIUM ALKALOIDS.

synthetic speech sounds that resemble speech but are made by machine.

synthetic trainer a device used to train individuals under conditions that closely resemble actual operating situations.

synthetism a form of abstract painting developed in the 1880s mainly by Paul Gauguin and characterized by brilliant colors separated by black lines. The art form was explained as an expression of ideas, moods, and emotions synthesized into an abstract illustration. Also called **cloisonnism**.

syntone: See HYSTEROSYNTONIC.

syntropy literally, turning together; a term used by Adolf Meyer to characterize healthy, hormonious, mutually beneficial relationships and associations.

syphilis a contagious venereal disease caused by an infection of the spirochete organism Treponema pallidum (Spirocheta pallida). S. is usually, but not always, transmitted by sexual contact and through a break or cut in the skin or mucous membrane. S. also can be transmitted by an infected pregnant woman to an unborn child. Untreated, s. is progressively destructive of body tissues, particularly those of the heart and nervous system. The term s. comes from the thus infected hero of a 16th-century play by Girolamo Fracastoro, a shepherd named Syphilus (literally translating from the Greek as "lover of swine"). A synonymously used term is LUES. See this entry. Also see GENERAL PARESIS; BAYLE'S DISEASE; CONGENITAL S.; CEREBRAL S.; WASSERMANN TEST; MENINGEAL S.; INTRACRANIAL GUMMA.

syphiloma: See INTRACRANIAL GUMMA.

syphilophobia a morbid fear of syphilis.

syr. an abbreviation used in prescriptions, meaning "syrup" (Latin *syrupus*).

-syring-; -syringo- a combining form relating to a long cavity, as in the spinal cord.

syringomyelia a disease marked by the destruction of CNS tissue because of fluid-filled cavities in the spinal cord. One of the effects is a loss of temperature sensations in dermatomes innervated by tracts that communicate with the diseased part of the spinal cord. Also see STATUS DYSRAPHICUS.

system a set of elements that are organized to work together to perform a function; a method of classification or procedure; or a set of facts and concepts that serve as the framework of a service or program.

systematically biased sampling a sampling procedure that is not representative of the major traits of a population and which errs in a consistent manner, e.g., drawing a sample from the dean's list of the senior class when the entire senior class is the population under study.

systematic approach Freud's original division of the psyche (1913) into three regions or "systems": the system unconscious (Ucs), made up of unconscious impulses clustering around specific drives or instincts, such as hunger, thirst, and sex, as well as repressed childhood memories associated with them; the system conscious (Cs), which enables the individual to adapt to society, distinguish between inner and outer reality, delay gratification, and anticipate the future; and the system preconscious (Pcs), which stands between the Cs and Ucs systems and is made up of logical, realistic ideas intermingled with irrational images and fantasies. Also called **descriptive approach; qualitative approach; topographic model.** See PRECONSCIOUS; CONSCIOUS; UNCONSCIOUS; PSYCHIC APPARATUS. Compare DYNAMIC APPROACH.

systematic desensitization a form of behavior therapy, developed by J. Wolpe and others, in which (a) the patient is trained in deep muscle relaxation, (b) various anxiety-provoking situations related to a basic problem, such as fear of death or a specific phobia, are listed in order from weakest to strongest, and (c) each of these situations is presented in imagination or in reality, beginning with the weakest, while the patient practices muscle relaxation. Since the muscle relaxation is incompatible with the anxiety, this process gradually desensitizes the patient to the anxiety-provoking situations. See RECIPROCAL INHIBITION.

systematic distortion the process by which memory traces show gradual, progressive changes with time in a more or less orderly pattern. Also see LEVELING-SHARPENING.

systematic error an error in data or conclusions that is regular and repeatable due to improper collection or statistical treatment of the data.

systematic observations the gathering of data according to an objective, systematic method that will yield reliable information about some aspect of behavior. S.o. often constitutes the initial stage of a study, preceding the formation of hypotheses.

systematic rational restructuring a system of psychotherapy in which the patient is encouraged to imagine anxiety-provoking situations while discussing them with himself in a realistic manner that reduces his anxieties.

systematic reinforcement a broad term denoting some form of consciously planned reinforcement. The term is nonspecific as to particular schedules of reinforcement.

systematics = BIOLOGICAL TAXONOMY.

systematic sampling a type of probability sampling in which all population members can be accounted for and listed. The sample is systematically selected without bias, e.g., by alphabetically listing all members and then selecting every seventh name.

systematized delusion a false, irrational belief that is highly developed, superficially coherent and convincing, and resistant to change. Systematized delusions are characteristically found in paranoid states and stand in sharpest contrast to the transient, fragmentary delusions that occur in delirium. Most delusions fall between these two extremes.

system conscious: See SYSTEMATIC APPROACH.

systemic concerning a condition that involves an entire organ system or the body's total organ systems rather than individual areas or parts.

systemic lupus erythematosus: See LUPUS ERYTHEMATOSUS.

systemic mucopolysaccharidosis: See MAROTEAUX-LAMY SYNDROME.

systemic routes of administration: See ADMINISTRATION.

systemic sense the part of the nervous system that receives signals from receptors in the body's internal organs. Also called **interoceptive sense**.

system model of evaluation in evaluation research, a method of assessing organizational effectiveness in terms of a working model of a social unit that is capable of achieving a goal. It is concerned with assessing the allocation of resources by the organization to reach an optimum level of operation, rather than with assessing the effectiveness of the organization in achieving public goals.

system preconscious: See SYSTEMATIC APPROACH.

systems theory: See GENERAL-SYSTEMS THEORY.

system unconscious: See SYSTEMATIC APPROACH.

systolic blood pressure the pressure of the blood against the arterial walls produced by the contraction of the heart muscles, as the blood is forced into the aorta and the pulmonary artery (from Greek *systole*, "contraction"). See BLOOD PRESSURE.

Szasz, Thomas Stephen /säs/ Hungarian-born American psychiatrist, 1920—. See ANTIPSYCHIATRY; ASCRIPTIVE RESPONSIBILITY.

Szondi, Lipot /sōn'dē/ Hungarian-born Swiss psychiatrist, 1893—. See SZONDI TEST; FAMILIAL UNCONSCIOUS; FATE ANALYSIS; GENOTROPISM.

Szondi test an unsubstantiated projective test introduced by Lipot Szondi in 1947, consisting of 48 photographs of psychiatric patients divided into six sets of the following eight types: sadistic, homosexual, epileptic, hysteric, catatonic, paranoiac, depressive, and manic. One set is presented at a time, and the subject is instructed to select the two pictures he likes best and the two he dislikes most. According to Szondi, these choices are determined by recessive hereditary factors and therefore reveal the subject's true personality. See FATE ANALYSIS.

T

TA = TRANSACTIONAL ANALYSIS.

tabel. an abbreviation used in prescriptions, meaning "lozenge" (Latin *tabella*).

tabes dorsalis: See LOCOMOTOR ATAXIA.

tabetic curve a pattern produced in Lange's colloidal gold-reaction test by the precipitation of samples of cerebrospinal fluid from patients suffering from tabes or meningovascular syphilis. Also called **luetic curve**.

tabetic psychosis a psychotic state that occasionally occurs in cases of tabes dorsalis, due to syphilitic endarteritis of the small cortical vessels.

taboo an object, person, word, or act that is at once sacred, dangerous, uncanny, and surrounded by religious prohibitions; something that inspires "holy dread" (Freud, 1913). (The term is Polynesian.) Also spelled **tabu**. Also see INCEST T.; VIRGINITY T.

tabula rasa concept the view, advanced by John Locke, that at birth the mind is a blank tablet devoid of ideas, and that all knowledge is subsequently derived from sensory experience. See EMPIRICISM.

tachisme /täshism'/ a form of painting in which fortuitous abstract patterns are sought by unconventional techniques, e.g., allowing paint to splash, dribble, trickle, or be slapped more or less randomly onto the canvas (from French *tache*, "blot, stain"). Also called **action painting**.

tachistoscope an instrument that exposes visual material on a screen for very brief intervals. Words, numbers, pictures, and symbols can be rapidly presented in the right or left visual field. The t. has experimental, diagnostic, and other practical uses; e.g., it is sometimes used in training individuals in speed-reading and remedial-reading programs. Also called **T-scope**.

-tachy- a combining form meaning fast (Greek *tachys*).

tachyathetosis = EKBOM'S SYNDROME.

tachycardia pathologically rapid heartbeat, often associated with drugs or anxiety. See ARRHYTHMIA.

tachylalia; tachylogia = LOGORRHEA.

tachyphagia a term used to describe a morbid form of rapid eating observed in regressed schiz-

ophrenia patients. The patient may place any object, food or inedible substances, in his mouth and swallow it.

tachyphemia speech characterized by persistent volubility and rapidity. It is a condition which may interfere with educational and emotional growth if left untreated. The term is essentially equivalent to LOGORRHEA. See this entry. Also see PRESSURE OF SPEECH.

tachyphrasia: See LOGORRHEA.

tachyphylaxis an acute tolerance for a substance as indicated by progressively decreasing response to repeated administration. In a case of t., the blood pressure of a patient might continue to rise despite repeated injections of a drug that normally would lower the blood pressure.

-tact- a combining form relating to touch (Latin *tactus*). Adjectives: **tactile; tactual**.

tactic: See TAXIS.

tactile: See -TACT-.

tactile agnosia = ASTEREOGNOSIS.

tactile amnesia a loss of the ability to judge the shape of objects by touch, due to brain injury or disease. It is a form of ASTEREOGNOSIS. See this entry.

tactile circle an area of the skin where two tactile stimuli presented simultaneously are perceived as one.

tactile hallucination a false perception involving the sense of touch. The patient may feel he is being slowly electrocuted by a distant apparatus, or masturbated by an unknown hand, or bitten by an army of fleas. Also called **haptic hallucination; tactual hallucination**.

tactile perception the ability to perceive sensations from nerve receptors that react to touch stimuli. Touch stimuli generally involve contact with the skin or mucous membranes. Other cutaneous sensations, e.g., itch and tickle, are due to mild stimulation of pain receptors. Cold and warmth also are cutaneous sensory qualities.

tactile-perceptual disorder a condition due to brain damage resulting in difficulty in discrimination of sensations that involve touch receptors. Patients with this disorder may be unable to determine the shape, size, texture, or other physical aspects of an object merely by touching it.

tactile sense = TOUCH SENSE.

tactile stimulation activation of a sensory receptor by a touch stimulus.

tactual: See -TACT-.

tactual hallucination = TACTILE HALLUCINATION.

tactual shape discrimination the ability to determine shapes of objects by touch alone. A subject may be required to tell the difference between a cylinder and another object when he is unable to see the objects.

tactual size discrimination the ability to judge the comparative size of two objects that cannot be seen and may be evaluated through the sense of touch. It is used as a test for the possible presence of a cortical lesion that would interfere with this ability.

Tadoma method a technique of communicating with patients who are both deaf and blind. The deaf-blind person places his fingers on the cheek and his thumb on the mouth of the person speaking and translates the vibrations and muscle movements into words. The name is derived from Tad and Oma, two young students of Sophia Alcorn, who originated the technique in the 1930s.

taeniophobia a morbid fear of tapeworms.

tagging: See RADIOACTIVE TRACERS.

tag question the type of question posed as a declarative sentence with the query tacked on at the end, e.g., "We have ice cream, don't we?" During the fourth year, most children develop the ability to ask a t.q. correctly.

Takayasu, Michishige Japanese physician, 1872 —. See TAKAYASU'S DISEASE.

Takayasu's disease a circulatory disorder involving arteries that carry blood from the aortic arch above the heart toward the brain. Obliteration of the innominate, left subclavian, and left carotid arteries results in a loss of pulses in the arms and neck, intermittent claudication of the arms, and fainting spells due to cerebral ischemia. The disease seems to affect mainly young females.

Talbot, William Henry Fox English pioneer photographer, physicist, and mathematician, 1800–77. See TALBOT-PLATEAU LAW.

Talbot-Plateau law the principle that if a light flickers so rapidly that it is perceived as continuous, its brightness will be reduced by the ratio between the period when the light actually reaches the surface and the whole period.

talent a high level of inborn ability in a special area, e.g., music, which can be enhanced by training or practice to a greater level of proficiency. See GENIUS.

tales /tä′läs/ a term used in prescriptions, meaning "such, like this" (Latin).

talion retaliation; especially, retaliation in kind, according to the early biblical injunction, "an eye for an eye, a tooth for a tooth." The **t. prin-**ciple, or **t. law**, plays an important part in psychoanalysis, since it includes the general idea of retribution for defying the superego, and the specific fear, or **t. dread**, that all injury, accidental or intentional, will be punished in kind. E.g., a voyeur may be afflicted with a visual disturbance (like the legendary, 11th-century Peeping Tom); a boy who harbors incestuous thoughts toward his mother may fear castration by the father; and an unconscious wish for the death of another person may precipitate a hysterical attack in which the patient feels he himself is dying. See PEEPING TOM.

talipes = CLUBFOOT.

talipes equinus = PES EQUINUS.

talis a term used in prescriptions, meaning "such, like this" (Latin).

talking books phonograph recordings or tape recordings of persons reading novels or other published works, produced mainly for the benefit of the blind and paralyzed. Copies of the t.b. are circulated by mail to the homes of these individuals who are provided with special turntable devices or cassette players. Many actors and actresses and others with professional speaking experience contribute their time to reading the books into recording microphones.

talking cure a superficial and usually derogatory characterization of psychoanalysis based on the idea that the technique involves only the verbal expression of feelings and experiences. See VERBALIZATION.

The term t.c. was first applied by Josef Breuer's landmark patient "Anna O." to his largely successful attempts to rid her of a variety of hysterical symptoms, including paralyzed limbs and impaired sight and hearing, through a combination of hypnosis and the "cathartic method." This case was an important precursor of psychoanalysis; it was cited by Breuer and Freud in their celebrated *Studies in Hysteria* (1895). Anna O. was in reality Bertha Pappenheim (1859–1936), a pioneer social worker, writer, and feminist.

talking-fear = LALOPHOBIA.

talking it out a popular term for freely ventilating one's conscious problems and immediate feelings. Anxious, upset individuals may gain temporary relief through verbally unburdening themselves and "letting off steam," but in genuine therapy the patient gives voice to what is innermost in his mind, not what is uppermost.

talking typewriter a typewriter designed for use by blind individuals. When the key for a letter or number is pressed, an electronic device emits the sound of the symbol.

tall tales: See PATHOLOGICAL LYING; PSEUDOLOGIA FANTASTICA.

tambour a membrane, usually flexible, that is used on certain recording devices: It is sensitive to pressure changes and moves a stylus to produce a written record.

taming: See NEUTRALIZATION.

tandem reinforcement an intermittent-reinforcement schedule in which a single reinforcement is contingent upon successful completion of two units of behavior.

tangential thinking a thought disturbance in which the patient constantly interrupts himself and digresses to irrelevant topics. In extreme form it is a manifestation of loosening of associations, a symptom most frequently found in schizophrenia. Also called **tangentiality**.

tangent screen a black screen, which may be a sheet of black felt material, used for testing or plotting the area an individual can see while looking straight ahead as the tester moves a light or small white object about the periphery of the subject's field of view. The subject reports whether or not the light or object can be seen, and the point on the t.s. is marked.

Tangier disease: See LIPID-METABOLISM DISORDERS.

tantrum = TEMPER T.

tanyphonia an abnormally thin, weak, and metallic voice caused by excessive tension in the vocal apparatus. Also called **thin voice**.

tapetum a light-reflecting layer in the retina of some animals. Kinds of t. include **t. lucidum** in elasmobranches (rays, sharks), **t. fibrosum** in ungulates (hoofed animals), and **t. cellulosum**, in carnivores and lower primates.

tapeworm fear = TAENIOPHOBIA.

taphephobia a morbid fear of being buried alive.

taphophilia a morbid attraction for cemeteries. See NECROMANIA; NECROPHILIA.

Tapia, Antonio García Spanish otolaryngologist, 1875–1950. See TAPIA'S SYNDROME.

Tapia's syndrome a unilateral paralysis of the larynx, tongue, and other throat and mouth structures, often accompanied by atrophy of the tongue. The disorder is due to a lesion involving the vagus and hypoglossal nerves.

tapping test: See DOTTING TEST.

tarantism the name given by the Italian physician Giorgio Baglivi to the compulsive dancing of the late Middle Ages in which an entire populace attempted to rid itself of overexcitement and convulsions which they believed were due to being bitten by the spider Lycosa tarantula. The lively tunes to which the people danced, known as the tarantella, are still popular. Also called **tarantulism**. See CHOREOMANIA; MASS HYSTERIA.

taraxein a protein substance obtained from blood samples of schizophrenia patients. Investigators have claimed that the substance produces symptoms of schizophrenia when injected into normal persons. Analysis of t. indicates it contains a copper compound. See ANTIBRAIN ANTIBODY.

Tarchanoff, Ivan Romanovich Russian physiologist, 1846–1908. See TARCHANOFF PHENOMENON.

Tarchanoff phenomenon an electrodermal effect in which the body produces a very weak electric current on the skin surface, probably due to emotional strain.

tardive dyskinesia a form of oral-facial dyskinesia that may be induced in older patients and those with brain injuries by the administration of large doses of phenothiazines and related agents over a long period of time. The symptoms include oral and facial grimaces, tongue movements, and torticollis that do not disappear when the medication is discontinued and which resist other therapies. Also see BLM.

target behavior behavior selected for modification by behavior therapy.

target language the foreign language that is being taught, or the artificial (e.g., computer) language system that is being acquired; also, the language into which a translation is made. Compare SOURCE LANGUAGE.

target patient the group member who becomes the focus of attention and discussion in STRUCTURED INTERACTIONAL GROUP PSYCHOTHERAPY. See this entry.

target response the designated response, response sequence, or behavior that constitutes the goal of shaping. The t.r. is the desired result of the shaping process. See SHAPING.

target stimulus in a test or experimental procedure, a specific stimulus to which subjects must attend, e.g., in tests of hearing, a specific tone that one must identify.

Tartar type a term that refers to patients with Down's syndrome, or Mongolian idiocy, whose facial features have been likened to those of Mongols or Tartars.

Tartini, Giuseppe /tärtē′nē/ Italian violinist, 1692–1770. See DIFFERENCE TONE (also called **Tartini's tone**).

Tarui's disease a rare form of muscular dystrophy characterized by an abnormal accumulation of glycogen in the skeletal muscles. The condition is due to an absence of the enzyme phosphofructokinase in the muscle tissue. Like similar glycogen-storage disorders, e.g., McArdle's and Pompe's diseases, T.d. is inherited as an autosomal-recessive trait.

task analysis an analysis or breakdown of a subject into component tasks to identify the different skills the student must possess in order to master the subject. The term is also used to refer to the detailed breakdown of a job into its component skills, required knowledge, and specific operations. Also see TASK INVENTORY.

task inventory in industrial psychology, a list of the specific tasks required by a job or position, such as jet-engine mechanic or hospital attendant. Also called **job inventory**. Also see TASK ANALYSIS.

task-oriented approach = TASK-ORIENTED REACTION.

task-oriented group a group of persons primarily devoted to solving a problem, creating or producing a product, or other goal-directed behavior.

task-oriented reaction a realistic manner of coping with stressors as opposed to dependence on an ego-defensive approach. Also called **task-oriented approach.**

taste the sensation produced by stimulation of the taste buds in the mouth. The t. sense depends upon molecules of food substances entering pores or other openings in and around t. buds where they react chemically with receptors to trigger nerve impulses. The t. experienced is influenced by the type of receptor and the concentration of flavor substance. Also see GUSTATION; SWEET T.; SALT T.

taste bud a sensory receptor containing gustatory cells, located primarily on the tongue but ocasionally present in other areas of the mouth in different species. The catfish has 100,000 taste buds over its whole body, while a chicken has only 24 taste buds. A human adult has approximately 10,000.

taste fear = GEUMAPHOBIA.

taste solitary tract a neural pathway that receives impulses from a receptor that is differentially sensitive to only one kind of taste stimuli.

taste tetrahedron a graphic representation in the shape of a tetrahedron showing the relationships of the four basic tastes: sweet, sour, salty, bitter.

TAT = THEMATIC APPERCEPTION TEST.

ta-ta theory: See ORIGIN-OF-LANGUAGE THEORIES.

tau /tou/ or /tô/ 19th letter of the Greek alphabet (T, τ).

tautophone a projective device consisting of a recording of random indistinct vocal sounds which the subject is asked to interpret.

taxes movements of motile organisms in response to a stimulus. T. can be a negative response, marked by movement away from the stimulus, or positive, in which case the organism moves toward the stimulus. T. differ somewhat from tropism, which tends to be an involuntary reaction to a natural force such as light or gravity. Kinds of t. include phototaxis, in which movement is toward a light source; geotaxis, marked by a movement toward the earth; and **chemotaxis**, in which an animal directs its orientation by chemicals in the environment. **Tropotaxis** indicates a direct path orientation toward a source, such as a food smell, and **klinotaxis**, a movement interrupted by pauses to evaluate stimuli sources. Singular: **taxis.** Adjectives: **tactic; taxic.** See TROPISM; PHOTOTAXIS; GEOTAXIS.

taxonomy a system of classifying items, e.g., biological specimens, according to their natural relationships. See BIOLOGICAL T.

Tay, Warren English physician, 1843–1927. See TAY-SACHS DISEASE; AMAUROTIC IDIOCY; AUTOSOMAL ABERRATIONS; BATTEN'S DISEASE; BIRTH DEFECT; CEREBROMACULAR DEGENERATION; CNS ABNORMALITY; DOLLINGER-BIELSCHOWSKY SYNDROME; GANGLIOSIDOSIS; HEXOSAMINIDASE A; INBORN ERROR OF METABOLISM; SPHINGOLIPID; SPHINGOLIPIDOSES.

Taybi, Hooshang Iranian-born American radiologist, 1919—. See RUBINSTEIN-TAYBI SYNDROME.

Taylor, Frederick Winslow American inventor and efficiency engineer, 1865–1915. See TAYLORISM.

Taylorism the first important scientific management system in industrial psychology, developed by F. W. Taylor starting in 1899. He sought to increase worker efficiency and productivity through time-motion studies and wage incentives. Also called **Taylor system.**

Taylor Manifest Anxiety Scale a system of measuring anxiety based on responses to a series of 50 questions selected from the MMPI.

Tay-Sachs disease an autosomal-recessive disorder affecting primarily Ashkenazi Jews, of central and eastern European origin. The disease appears due to a deficiency of hexosaminidase A enzyme. Abnormally high levels of gangliosides and sialic acid are found in all tissues. Motor-nerve development is normal until the sixth month of infancy, followed by a loss of acquired skills. Startle reactions to sound are exaggerated. Vision deteriorates in the second year so that the eyes no longer follow a light. The brain becomes progressively larger due to edema and gliosis of the white matter. Children who survive beyond the age of two tend to be bedridden and fail to respond to stimulation. Abbrev.: TSD. Also called **familial amaurotic idiocy; G_{M2} gangliosidosis.**

TB = TUBERCULOSIS.

TC = THERAPEUTIC COMMUNITY.

TCA = TRICYCLIC ANTIDEPRESSANTS.

T-data information that has been obtained through *t*ests (Cattell).

t distribution a probability curve used for testing hypotheses about differences between means. As the sample size (degrees of freedom) increases, the t d. approximates the normal distribution more and more closely.

tea the leaves of the plant Thea sinensis ("Chinese tea"), indigenous to central Asia but also grown commercially in Africa, South America, and the Black Sea region of the U.S.S.R.; also, an infusion made from the dried and treated leaves, consumed world-wide as a stimulating beverage. The active ingredients are caffeine, from two to six percent, and a related substance, theophylline. T. originated as a medicinal herb in China as early as 2737 B.C. and became a popular caffeine beverage about 780 A.D. in China, and in Europe in the 17th century.

teaching games classroom instruction in the form of games designed to engage students' active interest as they work on specific skills, e.g., vocabulary or mathematics games. T.g. provide incentives to students in the form of rewards or the pleasure of winning.

teaching machine an instrument, simple or elaborate, which (a) automatically presents programed material to the learner, (b) provides an opportunity to check understanding at each step through problems or questions, and (c) provides feedback as to whether the response is right or wrong. The modern-day prototype of the t.m. is associated with B. F. Skinner who advocates more use of programed instruction, of which the t.m. is an example. Although possibly useful in teaching some fundamental, delimited, structured tasks, teaching machines have not found wide acceptance and may not be highly effective in teaching complex tasks, concepts, or behavior that involve complicated skills. See PROGRAMED INSTRUCTION; BRANCHING PROGRAM.

teaching model: See DEVELOPMENTAL T.M.

teaching style those personal attributes that define a teacher's classroom methods and behavior. Some qualities associated with teacher effectiveness are mastery of subject matter, pedagogical thinking, organizational ability, enthusiasm, warmth, calmness, and the establishment of rapport with students.

team approach a multidisciplinary approach to diagnosis and therapy combining the services of psychiatrists, clinical psychologists, psychiatric social workers, and other specialized personnel such as movement, occupational, and recreational therapists.

teamwork working together toward a common goal or on a common project. At six a child may participate in easily organized games involving several children; in first grade, a class is divided into small groups, but by the fourth grade it is capable of acting as a whole on a project, especially if one or two children take the lead. From there on, teams and clubs with complex rules develop rapidly.

tears: See CRYING; BOGORAD'S SYNDROME.

technological illiteracy: See COMPUTER ILLITERACY.

tectal nuclei nerve cells located in the superior and inferior colliculi of the corpora quadrigemina. They receive fibers from the upper neurons of the extralemniscal system, inherited from the afferent-nerve system of primitive ancestors.

tectorial membrane a membrane that covers the organ of Corti in the cochlea. It contains a gelatinous substance in which the hair cells of the auditory organ are embedded. Also called **Corti's membrane; tectorium**.

tectum the part of the midbrain that literally is the "roof" (Latin), to distinguish the structure from the "floor" of the midbrain. The t. contains the superior colliculi sensory centers for visual impulses and the inferior colliculi sensory centers for auditory impulses.

tegmentum a part of the cerebral peduncle above the substantia nigra and a structure associated with sensory and motor tracts passing through the midbrain. Adjective: **tegmental**.

-tel-; -tele-; -telo- a combining form relating to (a) distance, (b) an end (from Greek *tele*, "far off, at a distance").

tele /tel′ə/ J. L. Moreno's term for a feeling projected toward others, sometimes further identified as **positive t.** for attraction or **negative t.** for repulsion. T. is used as the unit of measurement in sociometry.

telebinocular a type of stereoscope used in visual tests.

telecanthus-hypospadias syndrome a hereditary disorder marked by widely spaced eyes, a high nose bridge, and a urethral opening on the ventral side of the penis. Some of the patients also are mentally retarded, with IQs in the 40s and 50s. The condition is believed to be transmitted as a dominant trait.

teleceptor a receptor for distant stimuli, e.g., the eye or ear.

telegnosis in parapsychology, a term for alleged knowledge of distant events without direct communication, as a form of clairvoyance.

telegrammatism the reduction of a spoken message to words conveying basic meaning, analogous to a telegram message.

telegrapher's cramp a painful spasm in the fingers making it impossible to operate a telegraphic key. See OCCUPATIONAL NEUROSIS.

telegraphic speech a descriptive term for the speech of very young children in the "duos-stage," that is, roughly between the ages of 18 and 30 months when most speech is in the form of two-word expressions known as duos. Such speech is telegraphic in that it utilizes only the most germane and prominent features of language while by-passing articles, prepositions, and other ancillary words. Also see DUOS.

telekinesis = PSYCHOKINESIS.

telencephalic sleep = NREM SLEEP.

telencephalon = CEREBRUM.

teleological: See TELEOLOGY.

teleologic hallucination a hallucination in which the patient receives advice as to the course he should follow.

teleologic regression: See PROGRESSIVE T.R.

teleology the doctrine that the existence of everything in nature can be explained in terms of purpose. In psychology and psychiatry, t. is the concept that mental processes are purposive, that is, directed toward a goal. The view that behavior is to be explained in terms of ends and purposes is frequently contrasted with explanations in terms of causes, such as instincts and childhood experiences. Adler's emphasis on goals and ideals chosen by the individual to fulfill himself ("fictional finalism") is **teleological**, as is Jung's emphasis on moral and religious values and on the development of individual aims and purposes. Also see HORMIC PSYCHOLOGY.

teleonomy the study of behavior patterns that appear to be a function of a concealed purpose. A human child or a pet dog may behave in an antisocial manner that actually is a **teleonomic** approach to obtaining a display of attention or affection from the parent or pet owner.

telepathic dream according to W. Stekel, a dream that is allegedly stimulated or influenced by the dream of another person sleeping in the same room.

telepathy the alleged direct communication from mind to mind, in the absence of any known

means of transmission. It is a form of EX-
TRASENSORY PERCEPTION. See this entry.

telephone scatologia a form of psychosexual disorder in which an individual obtains sexual
pleasure by making obscene telephone calls.

telephone support service a service provided by
mental-health clinics, community mental-health
centers, and drug-treatment centers in which a
trained individual gives emotional support and
practical guidance over the telephone to individuals undergoing emergencies.

telephone theory the concept of auditory-nerve
transmission that proposes a rate of impulse frequencies that is the same as those of the sound
waves perceived, as in the principle of the telephone wire. Because a nerve fiber would be unable to transmit sounds above 1,000 cycles per
second, the t.t. has been modified to propose
that nerve fibers fire in groups to carry higher
sound-frequency impulses; this is called the volley theory. The term t.t. is essentially equivalent
to FREQUENCY THEORY. See this entry. Also see
HEARING THEORIES; VOLLEY THEORY.

teleplasm in parapsychology, a term for a hypothetical substance that emanates from a psychic
medium in the form of a human being and is presumably capable of telekinetic activities.

telesthesia in parapsychology, a term for the
alleged ability to perceive objects or events
beyond the normal range of human perception.

teletactor a device that amplifies and transmits
sounds to the skin, for use in teaching speech to
the deaf.

telodendria the terminal fibrils of an axon, with
further branchings of the synaptic knobs. T.
usually wind through dendrites and other structures of neighboring neurons, making synaptic
associations with them.

temperament an individual's constitutional pattern of reactions, including such characteristics
as general energy level, emotional make-up, and
intensity and tempo of response. Though such a
pattern is believed to have an inherent basis, and
is manifested early in life, it may be modified in
some degree by life experiences: A placid person may become more vigorous, and a volatile
person may learn to control his emotions.

temperature drive a form of behavior observed in
both cold-blooded and warm-blooded animals
and characterized by activities designed to
achieve an optimum temperature in their environment. Fish and rats, e.g., can learn to press
a bar that adjusts the temperature of the water
or air around them; humans adjust thermostats
or change their clothing. (The anterior part of
the hypothalamus contains a center for temperature regulation, which appears to produce circulatory changes throughout the body.)

temperature effects stress effects, both psychological and physical, to wide variations from
optimal environmental temperatures. The
effects on comfort are also dependent upon such
influences as humidity, wind, and personal acclimatization. See COLD EFFECTS; HEAT EFFECTS.

temperature eroticism in psychoanalytic theory,
the erotic pleasure of feeling warm, which is believed to stem from the oral stage of psychosexual development when the child was cuddled by
the mother. In later stages the sensation of heat
is a normal accompaniment of sexual excitation,
and may also be experienced when an individual
desires or fantasies sexual activity.

temperature sense a part of the somatosensory
system with receptors at various depths in the
skin and other body surfaces that may be exposed to the environment, such as the tongue.
Temperatures generally above 33°C (91°F) on
the skin produce a sensation of warmth while
those below cause a feeling of coolness. The impulses generated are carried by slow A fibers to
the thalamus.

temperature spots areas of the skin that contain
temperature-sensitive receptors.

temper tantrum a violent outburst of anger commonly occurring between the ages of two and
four and involving such behavior as screaming,
kicking, biting, hitting, and head-banging. The
episodes are usually out of proportion to immediate provocation and are regarded as an
expression of accumulated tensions and frustrations. Also called **tantrum**. See OPPOSITIONAL
DISORDER.

temple sleep a forerunner of modern sleep treatment in which Egyptian, Babylonian, and Greek
citizens with various disorders slept on a temple
floor in order to learn through dreams what
treatments would be most effective. In the cult
of Aesculapius, sleep was apparently induced by
drugs, potions, hypnosis, or ventriloquism. The
dreams were interpreted by a priest or oracle. In
some cases, it was claimed, Aesculapius himself
would appear in a dream to heal the patient out-
right. See THEURGIC APPROACH. Also see SLEEP
TREATMENT.

-tempor- a combining form relating to (a) the tem-
ple, (b) the temporal lobe of the brain (from
Latin *tempus*, "temple of the head"), (c) time
(Latin *tempus*). Adjective: **temporal**.

temporal arteritis: See ARTERITIS.

temporal conditioning a learning procedure similar to that of trace conditioning except that an
unconditioned stimulus is offered at regular intervals but in the absence of an accompanying
conditioned stimulus. The alpha-wave-blocking
effect is approximately the same, for both
procedures.

temporal-frequency discrimination = PATTERN
DISCRIMINATION.

temporal hallucinations = TEMPORAL-LOBE ILLU-
SIONS.

temporal lobe an area of the cerebral hemisphere
immediately behind the lateral fissure, on the
lower outside surface of the hemisphere, containing the auditory projection and auditory association areas, and an area for visual processing.
Lesions of the t.l. result in visual deficits and
memory loss. The degree of memory loss depends in part on the size and location of the

lesion. Lost learning skills can be restored in most cases. See BRAIN.

temporal lobectomy the surgical excision of a temporal lobe or a portion of the lobe. T.l. may be performed in the treatment of temporal-lobe epilepsy, the location and size of the lesion determining which tissues and related functions may be affected. Verbal deficits may be observed after **left t.l.** and performance deficits after **right t.l.**, but in many cases functional disturbances existed before the surgery.

temporal-lobe epilepsy = PSYCHOMOTOR EPILEPSY.

temporal-lobe illusions distorted perceptions associated with temporal-lobe epilepsy seizures. T.-l.i. often include distortions of the sizes or shapes of objects, recurring dreamlike thoughts, sensations of déjà vu or jamais vu, or feeling of g forces as if rapidly accelerating or decelerating in an airplane or elevator, an effect linked to labyrinthine involvement in the seizure. Hallucinations such as the sensation of the head separating from the body or the sound of threatening voices may also be experienced. Also called **temporal-lobe hallucinations; temporal hallucinations**.

temporal-lobe syndrome a complex of personality traits associated with temporal-lobe epilepsy in some patients. The traits include a profound sense of righteousness, preoccupation with details, compulsive writing or drawing, religiosity, and changes in sexual attitudes.

temporal maze a maze in which the subject must choose among alternative pathways that follow a particular sequence without being given external cues. The subject must therefore use memory and reasoning alone, as in turning right twice, then left twice (RRLL) at the same choice point in a T-maze.

temporal-perceptual disorder a condition observed in some patients with lesions in the left hemisphere who have difficulty in temporal perception of visual and auditory stimuli. E.g., patients with t.-l.d. may be unable to identify the sequences of vowels repeated at measured time intervals.

temporal summation an effect sometimes produced as a motoneuron response to two successive impulses, neither of which is of sufficient intensity to cause the response. The partial depolarization of the first firing continues for a few milliseconds and is able, with the additive effect of the second, to produce the energy to complete the neuronal discharge.

temporary commitment involuntary emergency hospitalization of a mental patient for a limited period of observation or treatment. See COMMITMENT.

temporary threshold shift a temporary condition in which the normal level of hearing is altered or disrupted. E.g., after relatively prolonged exposure to very loud noise, the absolute threshold may shift so that minimal sound intensities one could normally detect are temporarily inaudible; a similar shift can occur in vision. Abbrev.: **TTS**.

temporizers in child psychology, a descriptive term for parents who have not worked out a consistent pattern of parental and authoritative behavior. Drifting from one situation to the next, they seem unsure how to resolve conflicts with their children. They are not consistently authoritarian nor do they consistently emphasize reason and cooperation (Lafore, 1945). Also see APPEASERS; COOPERATORS; DICTATORS.

temporomandibular joint: See TMJ SYNDROME.

tendency wit a type of wit that has some deep meaning or that serves some purpose, as opposed to abstract or harmless wit. According to Freud, t.w. is a means of gratifying a craving which may be crude or hostile.

tendentious apperception a tendency to perceive what one wishes to perceive in an event or object, e.g., Adler's tendency to interpret human experience in terms of the drive for superiority.

tender-minded a term used by William James to denote a personality trait characterized by intellectualism, idealism, optimism, dogmatism, religiosity, and monism. Compare TOUGH-MINDED.

tendon a band of tough fibrous tissue that links a muscle to a bone.

tendon reflexes reflexes that involve the muscle-spindle feedback circuit so that when a tendon to an extensor muscle is tapped, the muscle is suddenly stretched. This results in impulses being fired from the spindle receptors to the spinal cord, followed by a reaction in which the muscle contracts suddenly. The t.r. can be demonstrated with the knee-jerk reflex action.

tendon sensation the kinesthetic sensation produced by stimulation of receptors in a tendon, e.g., by stretching it.

Tensilon = EDROPHONIUM.

tension a feeling of physical and psychological strain accompanied by discomfort, uneasiness, and pressure to seek relief through talk or action; also, strain resulting from contraction or stretching of a muscle or tendon. Also see PSYCHIC T.

tension headache a persistent headache produced by acute or prolonged emotional tension, and usually accompanied by insomnia, irritability, and painful contraction of the neck muscles.

tension reduction alleviation of feelings of tension through such means as relaxation therapy, tranquilizing drugs, muscle relaxants, hypnotic suggestion, periods of meditation, verbal catharsis, movement therapy, or sex therapy.

tensor tympani one of the two muscles involved in movements of the middle-ear ossicles. The t.t. reacts automatically to help disengage the ossicles briefly when very loud noises are received as air vibrations at the eardrum. The subject hears a distorted sound but the t.t-reflex action protects the inner ear structures from damage.

tenth cranial nerve = VAGUS NERVE.

tentorium cerebelli a fold of dura mater that separates the surface of the cerebellum from the basal surfaces of the occipital and temporal lobes of the cerebral cortex. The t.c. is attached at the midline to the falx cerebri which separates the two cerebral hemispheres except in areas through which vital tissues communicate.

teonanactl a Mexican mushroom that is the source of the psychedelic drugs psilocybin and psilocin. The botanical name of the plant is Psilocybe mexicana. Also called **magic mushroom; God's flesh**.

-terat-; -terato- a combining form relating to a deformed being or a congenital abnormality (from Greek *teras*, "monster, sign, marvel").

teratogenic literally, monster-producing; inducing developmental abnormalities in the fetus. A **teratogen** is an agent or process that causes such abnormal developments, a process called **teratogenesis**; a **teratomorph** is a fetus or offspring with developmental abnormalities; the study of such developments and their causes is called **teratology**.

teratogenic X-ray the ionizing radiation of machines or chemicals used in radiology for diagnosis or therapy and which may damage the reproductive cells of the testes and ovaries. The gonads are particularly sensitive to the energy effects of radioactivity, which can alter molecular structures in tissues. The effects may include mutations of genes and resulting birth defects.

teratological defects structural or functional abnormalities in an individual caused by hereditary factors or an environmental influence such as exposure to drugs or X-rays during the mother's pregnancy. Down's syndrome is among t.d. associated with abnormal genetic factors. The thalidomide syndrome, marked by deformed arms and legs, is an example of t.d. caused by a drug used during pregnancy.

teratology; teratomorph: See TERATOGENIC.

teratophobia a morbid fear of monsters; also, the fear of bearing and giving birth to a monstrously deformed child.

term the gestational age of 266 days from conception, usually marking the end of pregnancy. Also see GESTATION PERIOD.

Terman, Lewis Madison American psychologist, 1877–1956. Terman's career was primarily devoted to the development and application of psychological tests. He was responsible for validation and revision of the Binet scales for use in America, resulting in the Stanford-Binet Intelligence Scale; construction of the Army Alpha and Beta Tests administered during World War I; development of the Stanford Achievement Test; and questionnaires designed to reveal *Psychological Factors in Marital Happiness* (1938); as well as a series of studies of gifted children and eminent adults. See TERMAN-MCNEMAR TEST OF MENTAL ABILITY; MASCULINITY-FEMININITY TESTS (there: **Terman-Miles Attitude-Interest Analysis Test**); ARMY TESTS; GENIUS; STANFORD-BINET INTELLIGENCE SCALE.

Terman-McNemar Test of Mental Ability a group-intelligence scale designed for grades 7 through 12, and consisting of seven types of verbal tests: synonyms, classification, logical selection, information, analogies, opposites, and best answer.

terminal assessment = SUMMATIVE EVALUATION.

terminal boutons; terminal bulbs = SYNAPTIC KNOBS.

terminal care service for the terminally ill, most recently provided by hospices, which are usually free-standing units or associated with a hospital, nursing home, or extended-care facility. The emphasis is on palliative care, pain control, supportive psychological services, and involvement in family and social activities, to enable these patients to live out their lives in comfort, peace, and dignity.

terminal insomnia a form of insomnia in which the individual habitually awakens very early, feels unrefreshed, and cannot go back to sleep. The condition is common in the elderly, in patients with cerebral arteriosclerosis, and in persons suffering from chronic anxiety, depression, and severe daytime fatigue, as well as in recently widowed and divorced women. Also called **matutinal insomnia**.

terminal reinforcement a reward delivered at a goal or after the organism performs the correct response or response sequence.

terminal stimulus the maximum stimulus to which an organism can respond.

terminal threshold the maximum stimulus intensity that will produce a sensation.

territorial aggression the act of defending or enlarging one's territory by fighting or threatening intruders. T.a. is characteristic of rats, chimpanzees, wolves, and other animals, but also observed in children laying claim to a sandbox, and street gangs defending their turf.

territorial dominance the tendency of territorial animals to protect their areas as well as their ability to drive out stronger trespassers. By extension, the term refers to the observation that people tend to dominate interpersonal interactions to a greater extent when in their own homes or offices. See TERRITORIALITY.

territoriality a form of behavior observed in animals from arthropods to mammals and characterized by the acquisition of an area in which individuals, pairs, or family groups confine their activities and guard against intrusion from other members of the same or other species. The male cichlid fish fails to develop nuptial color markings unless it can establish and defend its territory. If the dominant male is removed, the next in rank develops the coloring. By extension, t. refers to characteristic human attitudes toward and use of dwellings or other essential spaces. Human aggression is considered by some theorists to be related to human t. Also see PROXEMICS; GROUP TERRITORIAL BEHAVIOR.

terror dream: See SLEEP-TERROR DISORDER.

tertiary circular reaction according to Piaget, an infant's action, usually emerging near the beginning of the second year, that creatively alters former schemes to fit the requirements of new situations. The t.c.r. differs from earlier behavior in that the child can, for the first time, develop new schemes to achieve a desired goal. This is sensorimotor stage 5. See SCHEMES. Also see PRIMARY CIRCULAR REACTION; COORDINATION OF SECONDARY SCHEMES; SECONDARY CIRCULAR REACTION.

tertiary cortical zone: See CORTICAL ZONES.

tertiary cortex a region of the cytoarchitecture of the cerebral cortex in which zones of overlapping parietal, temporal, and occipital sensory activities are located. The cells are mainly from the upper layers of the cortex and are involved in integration of auditory, somatosensory, and visual impulses.

tertiary gains a term sometimes used to describe benefits obtained by someone other than the patient as a result of the patient's illness or injury. See PRIMARY GAINS; SECONDARY GAINS.

tertiary prevention in psychiatry, application of rehabilitative measures designed to prevent relapse and to forestall or reduce handicaps arising out of mental disorder, such as difficulty in finding and adjusting to work, and problems relative to participating in family, social, and community life. Also see PREVENTIVE PSYCHIATRY.

tertiary-process thinking a term applied by S. Arieti to innovative, imaginative, creative thought processes that transcend both primary- and secondary-process thinking. See CREATIVE THINKING; DIVERGENT THINKING; PRIMARY PROCESS; SECONDARY PROCESS.

test a standardized set of questions or other criteria designed to assess knowledge, skills, interests, or other characteristics of a subject; also, a set of operations designed to assess the validity of a hypothesis. See PSYCHOLOGICAL T. Also see the Appendix for TESTS.

testability the ability of a scientific proposition to withstand challenges to the data, design, or other aspects of the premise on which it is based.

test administration the process of administering tests under conditions that put individuals at ease and enable them to give a fair accounting of themselves, that is, by giving tests in a quiet, well-lighted room, by providing a comfortable chair and table, by strict adherence to instructions for administration, and by reassurance as to confidentiality.

test age the score obtained on a test that is standardized in age units or age equivalents.

testamentary capacity /-men'-/ the legal ability to make a will; in forensic psychiatry, the mental competence to make a will.

test anxiety: See PERFORMANCE ANXIETY.

test battery a group or series of related tests administered at one time, with scores recorded separately or combined to yield a single score. Also called **battery of tests**.

testes: See TESTIS.

test for contrasts = SCHEFFÉ TEST.

testicle the male gonad or reproductive gland. The term is commonly used to describe the testis and its surrounding structures, including the scrotum. See TESTIS.

testicular atrophy the loss of size or function of a testis as a result of infarction of the blood supply, injury, infection by syphilis, mumps, or filariasis, or of surgical repair of an inguinal hernia. **Pressure t.a.** may result from failure of a testis to descend normally from the abdominal cavity during sexual development.

testicular-feminization syndrome a form a pseudohermaphroditism in which an individual who is genetically a male acquires external genitalia and secondary sexual characteristics of a female but also has male testes. The internal female reproductive organs, the uterus and Fallopian tubes, are absent.

testing: See PSYCHOLOGICAL T.

testis one of the male gonads, or reproductive glands, normally located in the scrotum. Plural: **testes**. Also called **orchis**. See TESTICLE. Also see ARRESTED T.; ECTOPIC T.; HYPERMOBILE TESTES.

testitis an inflammation of the testis. Also called **orchitis**.

test of hypothesis: See DIRECTIONAL T.O.H.; NONDIRECTIONAL T.O.H.

test of significance a measure of the probability that a result can be attributed to chance. Some tests of significance consist of a measure divided by its expected variability.

testophobia a popular term for a fear of taking tests or of being tested. T. may account for test results that do not accurately reflect the normal standard of physical or mental performance by a subject. E.g., blood pressure frequently shows a much higher reading when tested by an examining physician than it would be during a typical day at home or at work. Also see PERFORMANCE ANXIETY.

testosterone a male sex hormone and one of the most active of the androgens produced by the testes. It stimulates the development of male reproductive organs, including the prostate, and secondary features such as the beard and bone and muscle growth. Women normally secrete small amounts of t., but above-normal levels in women can result in traits of masculinity. The main function of the Y sex chromosome is the production of enzymes that build t. molecules.

test power: See POWER OF A TEST.

test profile a chart or similar graphic representation depicting a subject's relative standing on a series of tests.

test-retest coefficient; test-retest method = COEFFICIENT OF STABILITY.

test-retest reliability the degree of correlation between scores of the same subjects on an identical test administered two separate times. The resulting test-retest coefficient is the value that expresses the correlation and helps to indicate the test's reliability. A coefficient of .70 to .90 is an acceptable indication of reliability. Also see COEFFICIENT OF STABILITY.

test score a numerical value assigned as a measure of performance on a test.

test selection the choice of a test or set of tests that can be the most useful in providing accurate diagnostic or other psychological information. T.s. is made on the basis of medical or psychological history, interviews, or other pretest knowledge of the individual or group to be tested.

test-study-test method an approach to the teaching of spelling that utilizes a pretest to determine the words a child knows, followed by study of the words that are failed, then by a retest.

test sophistication past familiarity with a particular test or type of test, which might affect the present score. Also see TEST-WISE.

test-wise a descriptive term applied to an individual who has taken a number of tests, and who is presumably less naive about tests and more adept at taking them than a person who is relatively new to the testing process. Also see TEST SOPHISTICATION.

tetanoid paraplegia = SPASTIC PARAPLEGIA.

tetanus an acute infectious disease marked by skeletal-muscle spasms and convulsions. The infection is caused by a sporulating bacillus, Clostridium tetani. The disease agent enters the body through a wound and produces a toxin, **tetanospasmin**, which is carried by the bloodstream or peripheral motor nerves to the central nervous system and blocks synaptic membranes. Also called **lockjaw**.

tetanus dorsalis = OPISTHOTONOS.

tetanus posticus = OPISTHOTONIC MOVEMENTS.

tetanus anticus = EMPROSTHOTONOS.

tetany: See HYPOPARATHYROIDISM; CALCIUM-DEFICIENCY DISORDERS.

tetany type = T TYPE.

-tetart- a combining form meaning fourth (Greek *tetartos*).

tetartanopia a form of color blindness marked by difficulty in discriminating among yellow and blue shades. The person has a normal luminosity function. But yellow and blue processes have confused or possibly merged connections. T. is one of the rare forms of color blindness.

-tetra- a combining form meaning four (Greek *tetra-*).

tetrabenazine a drug that is used as a tranquilizer in some subjects. It produces a sedative effect similar to that of reserpine, depleting brain stores of norepinephrine and serotonin.

tetrachoric correlation a correlation estimated from a 2×2 table, but nevertheless assuming that both variables are continuous and not merely dichotomous.

tetrachromatism the theory that normal color vision is based upon perception of four primary colors: red, green, blue, yellow.

tetrahydrocannabinols: See PSYCHEDELICS.

tetralogy of Fallot a congenital heart disorder that includes four structural defects: pulmonary stenosis; an opening between the left and right ventricles; a malpositioned aorta that receives blood from both the left and right ventricles; and an enlarged right ventricle. Also see CARDIAC DISORDERS.

tetraparesis = QUADRIPARESIS.

tetraphocomelia a congenital disorder in which all limbs are missing. X-ray pictures or autopsy examination generally show that arm or leg bones are entirely absent or very small. See ROBERT'S SYNDROME.

tetraplegia = QUADRIPLEGIA.

texture gradient: See GRADIENT OF TEXTURE.

T function = REDUNDANCY.

TGA = TRANSIENT GLOBAL AMNESIA.

T-group *t*raining group; the type of experiential group concerned with fostering the development of leadership skills, communication skills, and attitude change. T-groups grew out of K. Lewin's work in the area of small-group dynamics. Though sometimes used synonymously with encounter group, the emphasis is less on personal growth and more on practical interpersonal skills, e.g., as stressed in management training. Also called **training group**.

thaassophobia /thā·asō-/ a morbid fear of sitting, of being seated. Also see KATHISOPHOBIA.

thalamic lesion a loss of structure or function of a part of the thalamus resulting in such effects as avoidance-learning deficits. Animals that have experienced a t.l. take much longer to learn to avoid an electric shock, although they learn eventually. Effects vary somewhat with the part of the thalamus affected.

thalamic nucleus: See LATERAL T.N.

thalamic pacemaker groups of nuclei in the thalamus that trigger waves of electrical activity in the cerebral cortex. Several nuclei have been found to initiate cortical discharges, including the intralaminar, midline, reticular, and ventralis anterior nuclei.

thalamic theory of Cannon: See CANNON'S THEORY.

thalamotomy = THALECTOMY.

thalamus /thal'-/ a two-lobed gray-matter structure situated at the bottom of the cerebral hemispheres that serves as a relay point for nerve impulses traveling between the spinal cord and brainstem and the cerebral cortex. The t. is structured so that specific areas of the body surface and cerebral cortex are related to specific parts of the t. It is considered to be a part of the forebrain. Also see POSTERIOR T.; EXTRINSIC T.

thalassemia a category of anemias, all inherited, each of which is caused by a deficiency in the synthesis of hemoglobin molecules. Each type of t. is classified according to the hemoglobin chain involved (e.g., alpha, beta, delta), the kind of hemoglobin, and whether the disorder is inherited as a heterozygous or homozygous trait. E.g., Cooley's anemia is a homozygous beta-t. involving hemoglobin A. (The term t. is derived from the Greek words *thalassa*, "sea," and *haima*, "blood," because the disorder was first observed in the blood of persons living around the Mediterranean Sea.) Also see COOLEY'S ANEMIA.

thalassophobia a morbid fear of the sea.

thalectomy a psychosurgical procedure in which lesions are made in the thalamus by electrocoagulation. Also called **thalamotomy; grantham lobotomy.**

thalidomide $C_{13}H_{10}N_2O_4$—a tranquilizing drug used during pregnancy, especially in Europe in 1960–61, until it was discovered to be a human teratogen. The drug produced undeveloped arms and legs, but it also had neurologic effects which included deafness, sixth- and seventh-cranial-nerve palsies, microcephaly, meningoencephalocele, and a greater-than-average incidence of mental retardation. (T. is still used in treating leprosy, though not when pregnancy is possible.) Also see PIPERIDINEDIONES.

-thanat-; -thanato- a combining form relating to death (Greek *thanatos*).

thanatology the study of death and dying, including psychological preparation for death, attitudes toward dying, and techniques of counseling and psychotherapy appropriate for the dying individual and his or her family.

thanatomania an obsolete term for an uncontrollable impulse to commit suicide.

thanatophobia a morbid fear of death or dying. Also called **death phobia.** Also see NECROPHOBIA.

Thanatos in psychoanalysis, the death instinct, which is directed toward destruction of life and a return to the inorganic state (Greek, "death"). The aggressive drive in all its forms—violence, hostility, sadism, etc.—is regarded as an expression of T. See DEATH INSTINCT; DESTRUDO; MORTIDO.

THC: See CANNABIS ORGANIC MENTAL DISORDERS.

Theater of Spontaneity an experimental theater established by J. L. Moreno in Vienna in 1921, in which the process of playing unrehearsed, improvised parts proved to be not only effective training for actors, but frequently had a salutary effect on their interpersonal relationships. This technique evolved into the psychotherapeutic approach which Moreno named psychodrama and brought to America in 1925. The T.o.S. is also called by its original German name, **Stegreiftheater** /shtäg'rĭf-/ (from *aus dem Stegreif*, "extempore"). See PSYCHODRAMA.

thebaine $C_{19}H_{21}NO_3$—an opium alkaloid that has an action resembling that of strychnine. About one-third of one percent of natural opium is t., compared with ten percent for morphine. T. is similar in structure to morphine, but it lacks the analgesic effect of morphine. However, t. molecules can be converted to other drugs that are much more potent than morphine, e.g., etorphine and cyprenorphine. (T. was named for Thebes, the city of ancient Egypt.)

theft: See KLEPTOMANIA.

thema H. A. Murray's term for the unit of interplay between an individual and the environment in which a need and a press interact to yield satisfaction.

Thematic Apperception Test a projective technique developed by H. A. Murray and his associates, in which subjects reveal their attitudes, feelings, conflicts, and personality characteristics by making up stories about a series of relatively ambiguous pictures. The examiner assures the subject that there are no right or wrong answers, and that the stories should have a beginning, middle, and ending. At the end, the stories are discussed for diagnostic purposes. Abbrev.: **TAT.**

thematic paralogia a speech characteristic marked by the incessant, distorted dwelling of the mind on a single theme or subject.

thematic paraphrasia incoherent speech that wanders from the theme or subject.

theme interference a cognitive conflict in the preconscious mind of the patient that is emotionally charged and related to an actual life experience or fantasies of the patient without being adequately resolved. The therapist must identify the themes and reduce or eliminate them because they interfere with the therapy.

theobromine $C_7H_8N_4O_2$—a methylated xanthine that occurs naturally in the seeds of Theobroma cacao, the cocoa plant. T. is structurally similar to caffeine in coffee and theophylline in tea but has less pharmacologic potency than the other xanthines in CNS stimulation, diuresis, skeletal-muscle stimulation, or cardiac effects. Also see METHYLXANTHINES.

theophobia a morbid fear of gods or God.

theophylline: See METHYLXANTHINES.

theorem a scientific proposition or premise that can be proved in a series of logical steps; or a statement that is generally accepted as true.

theories of color vision: See COLOR THEORIES.

theory a body of interrelated principles that explain or predict; a hypothesis that has been largely verified by facts; also, in popular usage, a guess, conjecture, or supposition.

theory of aging: See CYBERNETIC T.O.A.; EVERSION T.O.A.

theory of situated identities: See SITUATED IDENTITIES.

therapeutic abortion an abortion that is induced legally by a qualified physician for medical or other reasons. A t.a. may be performed because of results of an amniocentesis test showing the presence of a genetic abnormality associated with a congenital defect such as mental retardation.

therapeutic agent any instrumentality used to advance the treatment process, such as a drug, the therapist, a therapeutic group, electroshock, occupational therapy, or a therapeutic community.

therapeutic atmosphere an aura of acceptance, empathic understanding, and "unconditional positive regard" (C. Rogers) in which the patient feels free to verbalize his feelings and emotions, and make constructive changes in his attitudes and reactions.

therapeutic communication any comment or observation by the therapist that increases the patient's awareness or self-understanding.

therapeutic community a term applied by the English psychiatrist Maxwell Jones (1953) to a mental hospital that utilizes milieu therapy. In this approach the entire environment and every detail of institutional life are organized into a continuous all-embracing program aimed at promoting recovery and preventing institutional disability. Such a program includes not only the standard treatment processes but also the interactions between the patient and all members of the staff; the development of constructive social relationships among the patients; the esthetic character of the architecture, grounds, and furnishings; participation in patient government and community meetings; and all types of supportive therapy, recreational, occupational, industrial, and educational. Abbrev.: **TC**. See MILIEU THERAPY; SOCIAL-BREAKDOWN SYNDROME.

therapeutic crisis a turning point in the treatment process, usually due to sudden insight, acting out, or a significant revelation on the part of the patient. The crisis may have positive or negative implications, and may lead to a change for the better or the worse, depending on how it is handled.

therapeutic group a group of patients who meet under the leadership of a therapist for the express purpose of working together toward improvement in the mental and emotional health of the members.

therapeutic group analysis = GROUP-ANALYTIC PSYCHOTHERAPY.

therapeutic impasse a situation in which progress in the treatment process has ceased, and failure is imminent. This situation occurs when further insight is not forthcoming, or when the process is blocked by extreme resistance or severe transference and countertransference conflicts.

therapeutic matrix in marital therapy, the specific combination of therapist and patients that is used in the sessions, e.g., a different therapist for each spouse in collaborative therapy, or seeing the couple together in conjoint therapy.

therapeutic recreation a rehabilitation program that involves disabled persons in community recreation activities, such as the arts, theater, music, sports, and hobby and craft projects. T.r. is designed to provide patients with opportunities to interact with other individuals in the community, thereby gaining experience and confidence in independent living.

therapeutic relaxation: See RELAXATION THERAPY.

therapeutic role the functions of the therapist or other therapeutic agent in treating disorders or alleviating a distressing condition. See THERAPEUTIC AGENT.

therapeutic window the range of plasma (not dosage) levels of a drug within which optimal therapeutic effects occur. With psychotropic drugs the range may be different for different patients depending on such factors as age, sex, constitutional characteristics, and concurrent medications.

therapist an individual who has been trained to treat mental or physical disorders or diseases in a professional manner. Also see PSYCHOTHERAPIST.

therapist obligations: See CONTRACT.

therapy a system of treatment designed to cure a pathological condition or relieve the symptoms of the condition (from Greek *therapeia*, "service, attendance, waiting on"). See PSYCHOTHERAPY. Also see the Appendix for THERAPIES.

therblig a unit of movement used by F. B. Gilbreth in describing and recording industrial operations in standard terms ("Gilbreth" spelled backward).

there-and-then approach a term applied to a historical approach to therapy focusing on the roots of the patient's difficulties in past experience. Compare HERE-AND-NOW APPROACH.

-therm-; -thermo- a combining form relating to heat (Greek *therme*).

thermal discrimination the ability to detect changes in temperatures. Although some animals, e.g., snakes, are able to locate prey by differences of a fraction of a degree between the environment and body heat, efforts to locate cortical centers of t.d. have failed.

thermalgesia a state in which a warm stimulus produces pain.

thermal sensitivity: See TEMPERATURE SENSE; VASCULAR THEORY OF T.S.

thermic fever = HEAT STROKE.

thermistor a device used to measure temperatures according to their effects on the electrical resistance of semiconducting materials. Tiny thermistors can be implanted in neurons to measure such data as the energy of metabolic activity during nervous-system functions.

thermoanesthesia a loss of the ability to distinguish between heat and cold by touch; the absence of heat sense. Also called **thermanesthesia**.

thermode a device made of copper through which water can be circulated at a controlled temperature. A t. can be implanted in an organ of an animal in order to determine the effects of temperature changes on surrounding tissues. Much information about thermal receptors has been obtained in this manner.

thermography a diagnostic technique using thermally sensitive liquid crystals to detect temperature changes over the body. Chronic pain secondary to reflex-sympathetic dystrophy is frequently present, though undiagnosed, and produces a characteristic hypothermia. (Thus, t. functions on the basis that diseased tissues, such as tumors, produce more heat than surrounding tissues and the heat can be measured in terms of infrared radiation; a breast cancer, e.g., could appear on a **thermograph** as an area of relatively intense infrared activity.) This new imaging technique correlates well with clinical and surgical findings and is an attempt to document objectively the subjective complaint of pain.

thermohypesthesia = HYPOTHERMESTHESIA.

thermophobia a morbid fear of heat. Also called **heat phobia**.

thermoreceptor a part of the nervous system that has the function of monitoring and maintaining the temperature of the body core and its vital organs. It is believed to be separate from the temperature-sensitivity network of receptors and fibers located in the skin. In some animals, the t. is presumed to be located in areas of the hypothalamus that have a blood temperature approximating that of the heart and that are sensitive to cooling effects.

thermoregulation behavioral characteristics associated with voluntary adjustments of an organism to less-than-optimum temperatures in the environment. T. behavior may be involved in moving closer to or farther away from hot or cold areas of a room. T. does not include autonomic reactions such as shivering in cold or sweating or panting in hot environments.

thermotropism the tendency of an organism to orient itself toward or away from heat or cold.

thesis a proposition that is formally offered for proof or disproof; also, a systematic treatise required for an advanced academic degree.

theta /thēt′ə/ or /thāt′ə/ eighth letter of the Greek alphabet (Θ, θ).

theta waves sine-wave patterns, recorded with electroencephalography equipment, that are regular, occurring at a rate of four to seven cycles per second. T.w. are observed in paradoxical sleep of animals, light (stage-2) sleep in humans, and in the drowsiness state of newborn infants.

theurgic approach an ancient Egyptian system of magic based on a belief in divine intervention in human affairs, and in beneficent dieties who may come to the aid of the mentally or physically ill. The term theurgic is derived from the Greek word for magic (*theourgia*, literally, "divine work"). See TEMPLE SLEEP.

they-group = OUT-GROUP.

thiamine the B_1 component of the B-vitamin complex present in various foods and also normally present in blood plasma and cerebrospinal fluid. Deficiency of t. results in neurological symptoms, as in beriberi and alcoholic peripheral neuropathy. Also spelled **thiamin**.

thiamine deficiency a disorder caused by a lack of vitamin B_1 and marked by anorexia, neuritis, and, in severe cases, beriberi, which can result in damage to the heart and central nervous system. A type of cardiomyopathy, or cardiovascular beriberi, is associated with alcoholism. Also see WERNICKE'S DISEASE.

thiazides a group of synthetic chemicals developed in the 1950s and widely used as diuretics in the treatment of hypertension. T. compounds cause the excretion of approximately equal amounts of sodium and chloride with an accompanying volume of water lowering blood pressure. Also called **benzothiadiazides**.

thinking cognitive behavior in which images or ideas that represent objects and events are ex-perienced or manipulated; symbolic or implicit mental processes. These processes include imagining, remembering, problem-solving, daydreaming, free association, concept formation, and creative thought. See ABSTRACT T.; ALLUSIVE T.; ANIMISTIC T.; ARCHAIC THOUGHT; ARTIFICIAL INTELLIGENCE; ASSOCIATIVE T.; ASYNDETIC T.; AUDIBLE THOUGHT; AUTISTIC T.; CATEGORICAL THOUGHT; CONCRETE T.; CONSTRAINT OF THOUGHT; CONTENT-THOUGHT DISORDER; CONVERGENT T.; CREATIVE T.; CRITICAL T.; DICHOTOMOUS T.; DIRECTED T.; DIVERGENT T.; FORMAL-THOUGHT DISORDER; FRAGMENTATION OF T.; GROUPTHINK; IMAGELESS THOUGHT; JANUSIAN T.; MAGICAL T.; MOTOR THEORY OF THOUGHT; OMNIPOTENCE OF THOUGHT; PALEOLOGIC T.; PARALOGIA; PHYSIOGNOMIC T.; PRECAUSAL T.; PRECONSCIOUS T.; PREDICATE T.; PRELOGICAL T.; PRIMARY-PROCESS T.; PRIMARY THOUGHT DISORDER; PRODUCTIVE T.; REALISTIC T.; SECONDARY PROCESS; SPONTANEOUS THOUGHT; STREAM OF CONSCIOUSNESS; SYMBOLIC PROCESS; SYNCRETIC THOUGHT; SYNTAXIC THOUGHT; TANGENTIAL T.; TERTIARY-PROCESS T.; TREND OF THOUGHT; UNEMOTIONAL THOUGHT; VERBAL THOUGHT; WISHFUL T.

thinking aside a form of asyndesis observed in schizophrenics whose thinking patterns drift into insignificant side associations so that speech and thought appear incoherent and lacking in unity of ideas.

thinking-fear = PHRONEMOPHOBIA; PSYCHOPHOBIA.

thinking horse: See CLEVER HANS.

thinking, opinion, belief: See THOBBING.

thinking through a profound thought process in which the individual attempts to understand and achieve insight into his own reactions.

thinking type one of Jung's rational functional psychological types, exemplified by the individual whose life is ruled by reasoning and reflection.

thin voice = TANYPHONIA.

thiopental one of the ultrashort-acting barbiturates. It is used primarily as an anesthetic that can be administered intravenously to produce almost immediate loss of consciousness. T. also may be used as an antidote in the treatment of patients experiencing overdoses of stimulants or toxic substances that produce convulsions.

thiopental sodium: See PENTOTHAL SODIUM; BARBITURATES.

thioproperazine: See PHENOTHIAZINES.

thioridazine $C_{21}H_{26}N_2S_2$—a phenothiazine compound used as an antianxiety drug or tranquilizer in the treatment of hyperactive children as well as agitated, aggressive, and acutely or chronically psychotic adults. See PHENOTHIAZINES.

thiothixene; thiothixene hydrochloride: See THIOXANTHINES.

thiouracil an antithyroid substance derived from a compound of urea and sulfur. It is employed in the treatment of hyperthyroidism because t. suppresses thyroid-hormone synthesis.

thioxanthines a group of drugs that resemble the phenothiazine neuroleptics both in pharmacologic activity and molecular structure. T. are used mainly in the treatment of schizophrenias. The prototype drug of the group is **chlorprothix-ene**—$C_{18}H_{18}ClNS$—which is analogous to chlorpromazine. Other t. include **thiothixene**—$C_{23}H_{29}N_3O_2S_2$—and **thiothixene hydrochloride** —$C_{23}H_{29}N_3O_2S_2.2HCl.2H_2O$.

third cranial nerve = OCULOMOTOR NERVE.

third dimension: See DEPTH PERCEPTION.

third ear: See LISTENING WITH THE T.E.; SENSORY-AWARENESS GROUPS.

third eye: See PINEAL BODY.

third-force therapy a relatively new trend in psychotherapy contrasting with both the psychoanalytic and behavior-therapy approaches, and comprising various humanistic, existential, and experiential therapies. In general t.-f. t. revolves around direct experience; the here-and-now; concrete, immediate personality change; responsibility for oneself; group interactions; trust in natural processes and spontaneous feeling rather than reason; emphasis on personal growth rather than cure or adjustment; and self-exploration and self-discovery. Also called **humanistic therapy**. For examples of t.-f.t., see CLIENT-CENTERED PSYCHOTHERAPY; TRANSACTIONAL ANALYSIS; RATIONAL PSYCHOTHERAPY; IMAGERY THERAPY; GESTALT THERAPY; PRIMAL THERAPY; BIOENERGETICS; EXISTENTIAL PSYCHOTHERAPY; EXPERIENTIAL PSYCHOTHERAPY; REALITY THERAPY.

third nervous system a term applied by Trigant Burrow to neural processes involved in communication through the use of symbols. He believed that misuse of these processes is responsible for behavior disorders.

third sex an infrequently used term for homosexuals.

third-variable problem an effect posed by a third factor confounding a correlational research effort involving two other variables.

third ventricle a cerebrospinal fluid-filled cavity of the brain, appearing as a cleft between the two thalami of the hemispheres. It communicates with the lateral ventricles at the anterior end and with the fourth ventricle through the aqueduct of Sylvius.

thirst a sensation caused by a need for increased fluid intake in order to maintain an optimum balance of water and electrolytes in the body tissues. As fluid is lost from the body through urine and feces, through water vapor exhaled from the lungs, and as perspiration, sensory cells associated with the lateral hypothalamus register the condition as a dryness in the mouth and throat and a craving for fluids. Neural factors also include changes in the chemical composition of blood as the fluid component is reduced, resulting in a chemical stimulus to the thirst receptors, and a cholinergic mechanism for drinking. In animal experimentation, stimulation of the lateral hypothalamus with crystals of carbachol, a cholinergic drug, e.g., is followed by a greatly increased urge to drink water. Also see HEMORRHAGE AND T.; LOCAL THEORY OF T.; ELECTROLYTE IMBALANCE; WATER REGULATION.

thobbing a type of thinking that is distorted by emotions, prejudice, or bias. The term is derived from *th*inking, *o*pinion, *b*elief.

Thomas, André /tōmä'/ French physician, 1867—. See DÉJÉRINE-THOMAS SYNDROME.

Thomas Aquinas, Saint /əkwī'nəs/ Italian theologian, ca. 1225–74. T. tried to make faith and intellect compatible, and founded a philosophical system now called Thomism. He held—more than six centuries before Freud—that "Any idea that is hurtful to the mind does harm in just the proportion that it is repressed. The reason is that the mind is more intent on a repressed idea than it is if the idea is brought to the surface and allowed to escape."

Thomsen, Asmus Julius Thomas Danish physician, 1815–96. See THOMSEN'S DISEASE; MYOTONIC DISORDERS.

Thomsen's disease a rare inherited form of muscular dystrophy in which the patient has extreme difficulty in relaxing a muscle that has undergone forceful contraction. The condition includes ocular symptoms, such as difficulty in opening the eyes rapidly and in turning them from one side to the other. The disorder usually begins in childhood, and while the muscles may become hypertrophied and stiff, they do not develop the progressive weakness of other forms of myotonia. Also called **myotonia congenita; ataxia muscularis**.

Thomson, Matthew Sidney English dermatologist, 1894–1969. See ROTHMUND-THOMSON SYNDROME.

-thorac-; -thoraco- a combining form relating to the *thorax* or chest (Greek). Adjective: **thoracic**.

thoracic nerves: See SPINAL NERVES.

thoracolumbar system the portion of the spinal cord that extends along the 12 thoracic and three lumbar sections of the spine, including roots of the autonomic nervous system's sympathetic fibers. Fibers of the t.s. innervate structures of the head, such as the eye and salivary glands, well beyond the usual range of nerves from the thoracic region of the spinal cord.

Thorazine a trademark for the hydrochloride form of chlorpromazine, a sedative, antiemetic, and tranquilizer.

Thorndike, Edward Lee American psychologist and lexicographer, 1874–1949. A pioneer in his field, T. carried out the first laboratory studies of animal learning; developed the concept of trial and error and the theory of "connectionism" (associative bonds); devised the laws of exercise and effect; compiled a junior dictionary based on frequency of word use; published treatises on military and applied psychology; and through these and other contributions earned the honorary title of Dean of American Psychology. See THORNDIKE'S HANDWRITING SCALE; THORNDIKE'S TRIAL-AND-ERROR LEARNING; ASSOCIATIVE SHIFTING; CAVD TEST; CONNECTIONISM; DRIVE-REDUCTION THEORY; LAW OF READINESS; LEARNING THEORY; PRINCIPLE OF BELONGINGNESS; PUZZLE BOX; SATISFIER; STIMULUS-RESPONSE THEORY;

TRANSFER OF TRAINING. Also see CATTELL, JAMES MCKEEN; JAMES.

Thorndike's Handwriting Scale a graded series of handwriting samples with which the subject's handwriting can be compared.

Thorndike's trial-and-error learning the theory that learning involves an S-R process in which neural connections are established when a response to a stimulus results in satisfaction or pleasure.

thought: See THINKING.

thought-broadcasting the feeling that one's thoughts are being disseminated throughout the environment for all to hear. The symptom occurs in schizophrenia.

thought deprivation = BLOCKING.

thought derailment a disorder characterized by disorganized, disconnected thought processes, most commonly observed in schizophrenic disorders. Also called **thought disorganization**. The term is essentially equivalent to COGNITIVE SLIPPAGE and COGNITIVE DERAILMENT. See these entries.

thought disorder any disturbance in the thinking processes that affects communication, language, or thought content, including such disorders as blocking, poverty of ideas, loosening of associations, verbigeration, circumstantiality, neologisms, paralogia, concrete thinking, incoherence, word salad, and delusions. T.d. is considered the single most important mark of schizophrenia. Also called **thought disturbance**. See CONTENT-T.D.; FORMAL-T.D.

thought disorganization = THOUGHT DERAILMENT.

thought disturbance = THOUGHT DISORDER.

thought-echoing = ÉCHO DES PENSÉES.

thought fear = PHRONEMOPHOBIA; PSYCHOPHOBIA.

thought obstruction = BLOCKING.

thought pressure the feeling that thoughts are irresistibly forced into one's mind. T.p. is a characteristic symptom of paranoid schizophrenia, in which the ideas are ascribed to outside sources. It is also observed in the manic phase of bipolar disorder, but in this case the patient insists that the pressure arises from within his own mind. Also called **pressure of ideas**.

thought-process disorder: See THOUGHT DISORDER.

thought processes a general term for any type of thinking or symbolic process involved in such activities as judgments, imagination, problem-solving, and drawing inferences.

thought-stopping a type of behavior therapy in which the therapist shouts "Stop!" to interrupt a trend toward undesirable thoughts, and the patient learns to apply this technique to himself or herself.

thought transference a form of alleged mental telepathy in which the mental activities of one person are thought to be transmitted without physical means to the mind of another person.

threat any real or imagined danger to an individual or group, or an indication of an impending disas-

ter. The term is also used to suggest a degree of coercion.

threctia Cattell's term for a personality trait consisting of timidity, susceptibility to threat, and withdrawal.

three-component theory = TRICHROMATIC THEORY.

three-cornered therapy = MULTIPLE THERAPY.

three-day schizophrenia a brief psychotic episode involving schizophrenialike symptoms such as agitation, incoherence, hallucinations, and poorly organized delusions. The condition is precipitated by extreme external stress, as in situations involving earthquakes, fires, flood, or combat.

three-dimensionality: See DEPTH PERCEPTION.

3,4-dimethoxyphenethylamine: See PINK SPOT.

3-methoxy-4-hydroxyphenylethylene glycol one of the metabolites of norepinephrine and epinephrine. The process involves the action of the enzyme catechol-O-methyltransferase on either of the neurotransmitters, followed by the action of a second enzyme, monoamine oxidase. About seven percent of epinephrine in the body is metabolized to 3-m.-4-h.g. Abbrev.: **MHPG**. See HIAA; UNIPOLAR DEPRESSION.

Three Mile Island: See NUCLEAR NEUROSIS.

threshold the magnitude of a stimulus that will lead to its detection 50 percent of the time; also, a usually very narrow transitional level below which a certain action or response is unlikely to occur without additional intensity of stimulus or similar influencing factors. E.g., an auditory t. is the slightest perceptible sound—a stimulus of less than t. intensity will be unable to trigger a neuron spike potential; a renal t. is the concentration of a substance in the blood required before the excess is excreted. Also called **limen**.

threshold symbolism a term used by Silberer (1911) to denote a dream image that symbolizes the desire to wake up. Images of this kind are believed to occur during the hypnagogic state between sleep and waking. See HYPNAGOGIC HALLUCINATION.

-thrix- a combining form relating to hair or hairlike formations.

-thromb-; -thrombo- a combining form relating to a blood clot (thrombus).

thromboangiitis obliterans = BUERGER'S DISEASE.

thrombosis the presence or formation of a blood clot, a thrombus, in a blood vessel, including the heart as well as arteries and veins. It is likely to develop where the flow of blood is impeded by disease, injury, a foreign substance, or simply by physical inactivity. A t. in the brain tissues can cause a stroke or cerebrovascular accident. Adjective: **thrombotic**. Also see CORONARY T.; THROMBUS.

thrombotic microangiopathy: See MICROANGIOPATHY.

thrombus a blood clot that forms in the heart or blood vessels. A t. that blocks a blood vessel in the heart is termed a coronary thrombosis while the blockage of a blood vessel in the brain by a t.

is a cerebral thrombosis. In a vein, the condition is a venous thrombosis. Also see THROMBOSIS.

thumb opposition the ability to coordinate the thumb and index finger in pincerlike movements. T.o. begins to develop around the third or fourth month, although it is not fully achieved until the second half of the first year, as eye-hand coordination grows more skillful.

thumb-sucking a common though not universal phenomenon among infants and young children, formerly classified as a habit disturbance if it persists beyond three or four years. The common explanation is in terms of a basic sucking impulse from which the child derives pleasure as well as comfort and relaxation. Psychoanalysts regard it as a form of neurotic gratification derived from the oral stage of psychosexual development.

Thurstone, Louis Leon American psychologist, 1887–1955. See THURSTONE ATTITUDE SCALES; INTEREST TESTS (there: **Thurstone Interest Schedule**); GENERAL FACTOR; LIKERT SCALE; PRIMARY ABILITIES; SIMPLE STRUCTURE.

Thurstone Attitude Scales a series of statements, each selected according to the method of equal-appearing intervals, and assigned a scale value on the basis of the judgment of at least 100 raters, on such subjects as capital punishment, communism, the church, and censorship. Also see LIKERT SCALE.

thwart to prevent a subject from achieving a goal or completing an S-R sequence.

-thym-; -thymo- a combining form relating (a) to the mind (from Greek *thymos*, "soul, mind"), (b) to the thymus gland (from Greek *thymos*, "warty excrescence, thymus gland").

thymectomy a surgical procedure in which the thymus, a ductless gland beneath the breastbone, is removed. The thymus normally produces a type of lymphocyte essential to the immune reaction. Excision of the thymus or its failure reduces the ability of the body to resist infection or reject tissue transplants. However, an enlarged or malfunctioning thymus may be a cause of myasthenia gravis or autoimmune diseases, e.g., rheumatoid arthritis.

thymeretics = MONOAMINE OXIDASE INHIBITORS.

thymergasia one of the "ergasias" established by Adolf Meyer as terms to describe forms of human behavior. T., derived from the Greek words for "mind" and "work," was applied to the category of manic-depressive disorders.

-thymia a combining form relating to a condition of the mind. See -THYM-.

thymogenic drinking = ALPHA ALCOHOLISM.

thymoleptics agents that have a mood-changing effect, particularly drugs that can relieve the symptoms of severe depression without also acting as CNS stimulants. The term may be applied to the tricyclic antidepressants or lithium carbonate.

thymopathic a term introduced by Bleuler to describe an abnormal disruption of mood that he believed was evidence of a genetic susceptibility to manic-depressive psychosis.

thymus a ductless, glandlike body in the lower neck region that reaches a maximum size at puberty, then undergoes involution. It is associated with the body's immune-response system. Also see THYMECTOMY.

-thyro- a combining form relating to the thyroid gland.

thyroidectomy the surgical removal of the thyroid gland or a portion of the gland. Total t. usually is performed only when the thyroid gland is cancerous. But more than half of the thyroid gland may be excised to control hyperthyroidism. A complication of both hyperthyroidism and t. is a thyroid crisis in which pulse, respiration, body temperature, and other vital functions rage out of control.

thyroid gland the largest of the human body's endocrine glands, appearing as a shieldlike structure on the front and sides of the throat, just below the thyroid cartilage. It produces the hormones thyroxine and triiodothyronine, which stimulate a number of organs and systems involved in skeletal growth and sexual development, and calcitonin, which controls calcium and phosphate levels in the blood.

thyroid-stimulating hormone = THYROTROPIC HORMONE.

thyrotoxic myopathy an acquired myopathy marked by proximal limb weakness with no clinical signs of inflammation or rash. Evidence of hyperthyroidism and hypermetabolism may or may not be present; those signs are lacking in apathetic hyperthyroidism. The symptoms subside when normal thyroid function is restored.

thyrotoxicosis a toxic condition caused by an excess of thyroid hormone which may be produced by an overactive thyroid gland or administered therapeutically. **Endogenous t.** may be familial and can involve an autoimmune reaction in which the patient's antibodies stimulate rather than destroy thyroid-hormone cells. T. is characterized by nervousness, tremor, palpitation, weakness, heat sensitivity with sweating, and increased appetite with weight loss. Ocular effects include the exophthalmos condition associated with goiter, lid lag, and an apparent fixed stare. T. frequently is associated with hyperplasia of the thyroid gland, excessive thyroid-hormone secretion, and increased metabolic-rate symptoms of Graves' disease, or the development of thyroid nodules, or Plummer's disease, which occurs in older persons. See GRAVES' DISEASE; EXOPHTHALMIC GOITER. Also see APATHETIC HYPERTHYROIDISM; THYROTOXIC MYOPATHY.

thyrotropic hormone the hormone thyrotropin, produced by the anterior pituitary gland to control the growth and function of the thyroid gland. T.h. has no therapeutic value but is used in the differential diagnosis of thyroid-gland disorders. When t.h. is injected into a patient, followed by a dose of radioactive iodine, the rate of uptake of the iodine indicates, e.g., whether the patient has myxedema or hypopituitarism. Also called **thyroid-stimulating hormone (TSH)**.

thyroxine a hormone of the thyroid gland that catalyzes a number of metabolic activities and influences growth and development. Vitamin requirements, defense against infection, and metabolism of fats, carbohydrates, and proteins depend upon t. levels in the body.

thyroxine-hormone-deficient dwarf: See DWARF-ISM.

TIA: See CEREBRAL ISCHEMIA.

tic a repeated, involuntary contraction of a small group of muscles, as in continually clearing the throat, shrugging the shoulders, or grimacing. These automatisms may be either psychogenic (tension-reducing behavior or reactions to repressed experiences) or neurogenic (after-effects of encephalitis). See TOURETTE'S DISORDER.

tic convulsif with coprolalia; tic de Guinon = TOURETTE'S DISORDER.

tic douloureux /tik'dŏolŏorœ'/ a form of facial neuralgia involving the trigeminal nerve, characterized by paroxysms of excruciating pain (French, "painful tic").

tickle experience a sensation produced by impulses from skin receptors that are adjacent and stimulated lightly in rapid succession. It is assumed that the involved receptors also are those for itch and pain and the method of stimulation accounts for the different sensation. Also see HYPERGARGALESTHESIA.

t.i.d. an abbreviation used in prescriptions, meaning "three times a day" (Latin *ter in die* /dē'ā/).

tight-rope test a test of the ability of rats to maintain balance while climbing a sloping wire in order to obtain food. The t.-r.t. has been employed in experiments to determine if the learning process is accompanied by changes in RNA composition of neurons, such as in the nuclei of vestibular neurons.

tigroid bodies particles observed in the protoplasm of neurons, including their dendrites. They consist of granular cytoplasmic reticulum and ribosomes, and can be identified by the way in which they absorb certain histological stains. Also called **chromophil substance; Nissl granules; Nissl bodies.**

timbre a tonal quality, as determined by the complexity of the sound waves that impinge on auditory receptors. We rarely encounter pure tones; most tones are "colored" since they result from composite sound waves. T. accounts for the different sound qualities of the same note played by different musical instruments, since the fundamental tone is accompanied by different harmonics and overtones generated by the instruments' individual structure.

time agnosia an inability to perceive the passage of time, usually due to a disorder involving the temporal area of the brain. Causes may include a stroke or alcoholic coma, as well as a head injury; soldiers have experienced t.a. after a combat trauma. The patient is unable to estimate short time intervals, and long periods of time appear much shorter than they actually are. The patient, however, is aware of the fact of time.

time and rhythm disorders speech and language problems related to the timing of sounds and syllables, including repetitions and prolongations and stuttering. The disorders often are functional, and complicated by guilt feelings of the afflicted person. The condition may be treated with a combination of psychotherapy and speech therapy, using such techniques as cancellation (interrupted stuttering), voluntary stuttering, or rewarding or reinforcing fluent speech efforts.

time consciousness: See HURRY SICKNESS.

time disorientation loss of the ability to keep track of time or the passage of time. The inability to say what day or hour it is is a common psychiatric symptom. See DISORIENTATION.

time distortion a type of perceptual distortion, sometimes experienced in altered states of consciousness, in which time appears to pass either with great rapidity or with extreme slowness. Perception of past and future may also be transformed.

timed test = SPEED TEST.

time error a tendency to misjudge items that are dependent upon their relative position in time; e.g., the first of two identical tones sounded consecutively tends to be judged as louder.

time-extended therapy a form of group psychotherapy in which prolonged sessions replace or alternate with the usual 90-minute sessions. The experience is usually highly emotional and revealing since "there's no place to hide" and, due to fatigue, the participants do not have the energy to play defensive games. The overall value of six-hour or weekend sessions is yet to be demonstrated, but as I. D. Yalom points out in *The Theory and Practice of Group Psychotherapy* (1975), "such experiences as commitment, responsibility, intimacy, and trust cannot be compressed without grotesquely distorting their nature." See MARATHON GROUP; ACCELERATED INTERACTION.

time fear = CHRONOPHOBIA.

time-motion study analysis of industrial operations into their component movements, noting the time required for each, for the purpose of increasing productivity, setting pay rates, reducing fatigue, and preventing accidents. See THERBLIG; EQUIPMENT DESIGN.

time out from reinforcement a behavior-therapy technique in which undesirable behavior is weakened by moving the patient into a nonreinforcing area.

time-out procedures in operant conditioning, a time interval during which a behavior does not occur. A time-out procedure may be used to eliminate stimulus effects of earlier behaviors or as a marker in a series of events.

time perception awareness of the passage of time, including the ability to estimate time intervals, to tell time accurately by clocks or approximately by the position of the sun, as well as the ability to judge time duration by circadian rhythms, and to recognize that time appears to pass more rapidly when we are engaged in an absorbing activity than when we are bored or waiting for a train. In t.p. testing, subjects are required to perform an act, such as pushing a lever, at regular intervals of a fixed number of seconds. Studies have found a close correlation between t.p. performance and alertness as measured by a high percentage of alpha waves on EEG recordings. Also see TIME SENSE.

time samples in testing or research procedures, those samples in which cases are drawn or observed in a sequence of relatively brief, specific time frames, e.g., the observation of covert smoking in high-school stairwells between 2 P.M. and 3 P.M. over a period of one month.

time score a score based on the amount of time used to complete a particular task, sequence, or series of problems, e.g., the number of minutes a three-year-old child requires to solve a simple puzzle.

time sense the direct experience of the passage of time; also, the ability to judge an interval of time. Time perception is highly variable, but, in general, time passes more slowly when we are bored or inactive than when we are active and interested. Drugs and hypnosis can be used to speed up or slow down the passage of time. Intervals of up to five or six seconds are judged most accurately; biological rhythms and standard events such as school and college classes enhance our judgment of longer intervals. Also see PSYCHOLOGICAL TIME; TIME PERCEPTION.

time series a statistical series ordered sequentially in time, e.g., a learning curve, accident rates over a number of years, or monthly rates of admission to mental hospitals.

timidity the tendency to experience anxiety when meeting new persons or situations; shyness and avoidance of other people; inability to assert oneself.

Tinbergen, Nikolaas Dutch experimental zoologist, 1907—. See HIERARCHICAL THEORY OF INSTINCT.

tinct. an abbreviation used in prescriptions, meaning "tincture" (Latin *tinctura*).

tinnitus noises in one or both ears, including ringing, buzzing, or clicking sounds due to acute ear ailments, such as Ménière's disease, disturbances in the receptor mechanism, drug side effects (especially tricyclics), and epileptic aura. Occasionally t. is due to psychogenic factors (conversion symptom).

tip foot = PES EQUINUS.

tip-of-the-tongue phenomenon the experience of attempting to retrieve from memory a specific fact, often a name or word, that eludes one but seems to hover tantalizingly on the rim of consciousness. The tip-of-the-tongue feeling illus-

trates a preconscious process in that the given fact is ordinarily accessible and is only temporarily unavailable to consciousness. Abbrev.: TOT.

tiqueur /tikœr'/ a person afflicted with a tic (French).

tissue an organic structure composed of identical or similar cells with the same or similar function.

tissue damage a measure of the intensity of a pain experience, or in some cases the anticipation of a pain experience. Studies show that blows resulting in cuts, pin pricks, or other painful experiences are accompanied by the release of histamine or other substances known to be pain-receptor excitants. Similar effects are observed in hypnotized subjects who are told they are experiencing severe pain although no painful stimulus is applied. Also see PAIN.

tissue need the requirements of cells of an organism for oxygen, water, and appropriate nutrients, as well as a suitable environment for growth.

tissue rejection the natural resistance of the body tissues to transplants or grafts of cells or organs from the body of a genetically different individual. See ORGAN TRANSPLANTS; IMMUNITY FACTORS.

Titchener, Edward Bradford English-born American psychologist, 1867–1927. T. studied under Wundt, and in 1895 became a professor of psychology at Cornell University. Still under the influence of Wundt's theories, he became the chief exponent of structuralism in America, emphasizing the use of introspection to uncover the elements of experience (sensations, images, feelings). He also developed experimental techniques that were more fully accepted than his atomistic approach. See ATTENSITY; CONTEXT THEORY OF MEANING; IMAGELESS THOUGHT; STIMULUS ERROR; STRUCTURALISM.

titration a technique employed in the determination of an optimum dose of a drug needed to produce a desired effect in a particular individual. The dosage may be gradually increased until a noticeable improvement is observed in a patient or adjusted downward from a level that is obviously excessive because of overdose or other adverse effects. Many people self-titrate optimum levels of caffeine or alcoholic beverages in this manner.

TL = TOLERANCE LEVEL.

TM = TRANSCENDENTAL MEDITATION.

TMA: See COMBINED TRANSCORTICAL APHASIA.

T-maze a simple type of maze shaped like the letter T and consisting of one choice point and two paths, one of which is incorrect while the other leads to the goal box. Frequently, more complicated structures are designed by joining several T-m. components. See MAZE.

TMJ syndrome a degenerative disease of the *tem-poromandibular joint*, at the point of articulation of the upper and lower jaws. The condition, which may be due to nervous tension, arthritis, or a tumor, often is marked by headaches, deafness, tinnitus, or pain in the ear. TMJ s. frequently is associated with bruxism and may respond to biofeedback training.

T-mycoplasma a category of microorganisms responsible for a type of genital-tract disease known as ureaplasma urealyticum. **Mycoplasmas** are themselves the smallest known free-living organisms. (The T stands for "*t*iny" mycoplasma colonies.)

tobacco the dried leaf of the plant Nicotiana tabacum and other Nicotiana species, which is smoked, chewed, and sniffed for its stimulant effects. The main active ingredient is nicotine, which stimulates the autonomic ganglia in the same manner as acetylcholine. T. was used by the native tribes of North and South America when the first European explorers arrived and was quickly transplanted to gardens and plantations throughout the world. T. has no therapeutic value but is of interest because of its universal use by individuals who smoke or chew the dried, processed leaves. In addition to nicotine, the t. leaves contain volatile oils that give t. its characteristic odor and flavor. Also see NICOTINE.

tobacco dependence a disorder characterized by continuous use of tobacco for at least one month (usually cigarette-smoking, but may be pipe- or cigar-smoking, snuff use, or tobacco-chewing), and one or more of the following: unsuccessful attempts to stop or significantly reduce tobacco use; tobacco withdrawal during these attempts; and continued use despite a serious physical disorder (bronchitis, emphysema, cardiovascular disease, cancer) which the user knows to be aggravated by tobacco use. (DSM-III)

tobacco withdrawal a symptom pattern developing within 24 hours of abrupt termination or reduction in tobacco use, and consisting of four or more of the following: craving for tobacco, irritability, anxiety, difficulty in concentrating, restlessness, headache, drowsiness, or gastrointestinal disturbances. (DSM-III)

-toco- a combining form relating to childbirth or labor (from Greek *tokos*, "childbirth").

toe drop a loss of muscular control of the toes. T.d. is a sign of the onset of Charcot-Marie-Tooth (C-M-T) disease; the peripheral nerves gradually cease transmitting impulses to the tips of the fingers and toes, causing a loss of muscle tone, after which the disorder spreads toward the body core. T.d. progresses to foot drop, resulting in a slapping gait.

togetherness need the infant's need for psychic union with the mother; also, the general need for close attachments to other persons.

toilet training the process of teaching a child to control the emptying of the bowel or urinary bladder by learned inhibition of natural reflexes; and to excrete in the "proper" place and manner. Although defecation and urination involve autonomic-nervous-system functions, t.t. conditions the individual to override the reflex action with voluntary nerve control. The t.t. period of a child's life is particularly sensitive because of its

influence on mental health in later years. See DEFECATION REFLEX; MICTURITION REFLEXES.

token economy a behavior-therapy program usually conducted in a hospital or classroom setting, in which desired behavior is reinforced by offering tokens that can be exchanged for special foods, television time, passes, or other rewards. See BEHAVIOR MODIFICATION; OPERANT CONDITIONING.

token reward any object that has no value in itself but can be exchanged for a true reward or reinforcer.

tolerance a condition resulting from persistent use of a drug, and characterized by a markedly diminished effect with regular use of the same dose, or a need to increase markedly the dose to achieve the same desired effect. T. is one of the two prime indications of physiological dependence on a drug, the other being withdrawal. Also called **drug t**. See SUBSTANCE DEPENDENCE.

tolerance level the hearing level at which speech becomes uncomfortably loud. It also represents the level of maximum amplification the person can tolerate in a hearing aid. Abbrev.: **TL**.

Tolman, Edward Chase American psychologist, 1886–1959. T. developed a neobehaviorist approach which held that behavior is purposive and goal-directed, and that we learn sequences and solutions by establishing meaningful connections between stimuli and by developing "expectations," which may or may not be confirmed. See TOLMAN'S PURPOSIVE BEHAVIORISM; CAUSAL TEXTURE; CONFIRMATION; EXPECTANCY THEORY; INTERVENING VARIABLE; LEARNING THEORY; MEANS-END CAPACITY; MEANS-END RELATIONSHIP; MEANS-ENDS READINESS; PLACE LEARNING; RESPONSE LEARNING; REWARD EXPECTANCY; SIGN GESTALT.

Tolman's purposive behaviorism a combination of Gestalt concepts with behaviorism applied primarily to the study of animal learning. In maze-running, the animal creates a cognitive map out of sign Gestalts which consist of environmental cues and subjective expectations. Other influential factors are place-learning (starting from the same place), reward expectancy, and latent learning (incidental learning, without reward). The total process involves a combination of variables: physiological drive, environmental stimuli, heredity, previous training, and maturity or age.

toloa a species of Datura, closely related to the jimson weed of eastern North America. T. is an herb used by the Algonquin, the Zuñi, and other Native American nations in rituals that included an adolescent search for identity. T. also is the Yaqui's herb described by Carlos Castenada as having powers to permit humans to fly like birds. Also called **wysocean**.

Toluene: See GLUE-SNIFFING.

toluidine blue: See NISSL METHODS.

toluol: See PSYCHEDELICS.

-tom-; -tomo-; -tomy; -otomy a combining form relating to sections or surgical operations (from

Greek *tome*, "a cutting, a section," and *tomos*, "a cutting, a piece cut off").

tomboyism the tendency of girls to adopt behavior associated with boys in our society. By present cultural standards, such behavior is more acceptable than "sissy" behavior in the boy. Ordinarily t. diminishes as the girl grows older, and does not lead to transsexualism. However, girls with adrenogenital syndrome and a high androgen level may remain masculine in their interests and behavior. Also, over half of female homosexuals have been found to be tomboyish in childhood. Also see ROLE CONFUSION.

Tomkins, Silvan S. American psychologist, 1911 —. See TOMKINS-HORN PICTURE ARRANGEMENT TEST.

Tomkins-Horn Picture Arrangement Test a projective test in which the subject arranges sets of three sketches of the same interpersonal scene in the sequence "which makes the best sense," after which he writes a sentence that tells the story depicted. Scoring is both qualitative and quantitative, and there are norms for normal and abnormal subjects.

tomography a system of radiological examination using a series of X-rays, each of which shows a section of the body or an organ that is adjacent to the next section. Special X-ray equipment is used to produce consecutive pictures of adjacent sections or slices of the body tissues. See COMPUTERIZED AXIAL T.

tomomania a compulsive urge to be operated on. Also see MUNCHAUSEN SYNDROME.

-tomy: See -TOM-.

-ton-; -tono- a combining form relating (a) to a sound or tone, (b) to tension or pressure (both meanings from Greek *tonos*, "a stretching, straining").

tonal attribute a measurable characteristic of a tone, e.g., pitch, volume, timbre, and loudness.

tonal bell a bell-shaped model used to demonstrate the relationships of the various tonal attributes.

tonal chroma = TONALITY.

tonal fusion the blending of two or more tones into a single tonal experience.

tonal gap a range of pitches to which a person may be partially or totally insensitive (**island deafness**), although able to perceive tones on either side of the gap.

tonal island a region of normal pitch acuity surrounded by tonal gaps (**island deafness**).

tonality a pitch attribute by which a tone sounds more closely related to its octave than to the adjacent tone on the scale; also, the sum of the relationships between the tones of a musical scale. Also called **tonal chroma**.

tonal patterns the sequence of tones or musical notes that forms a tune. Tonal-pattern discrimination requires a cortical mechanism for storing tonal information. Lesions in the temporal lobe can result in tonal-pattern deficits, particularly when there is a long time span between two notes in a usual sequence.

tonal pencil a graphic representation of the relationship between pitch and volume.

tonal scale the normal range of sound frequencies perceived by a young adult, that is, from 20 to 20,000 cycles per second.

tonal spectrum = SOUND SPECTRUM.

tonal volume the extensity or space-filling quality of a tone. E.g., an organ has greater t.v. than a flute.

tone a sound caused by a periodic vibration or sound wave in an elastic medium; also, a unit of measure of the musical interval; and the characteristic timbre of an instrument or voice.

tone deafness = ASONIA.

tone variator a device that can produce pure tones of variable pitch.

tongue kiss = FRENCH KISS.

tongue thrust a reflexive extension of the tongue, especially during the feeding process, a symptom occurring in some cases of cerebral palsy and other musculoskeletal disorders.

tongue tie: See ANKYLOGLOSSIA.

tonic a condition of continuous muscle tension that can occur either as a normal or abnormal bodily activity. A t. phase of facial muscles prevents the lower jaw from falling open, a normal function. In a grand mal epileptic attack, muscles controlling respiration may become t. so that breathing is suspended temporarily. Also see TONUS; SPASM.

tonic activation a form of arousal mediated by the reticular activating system, and identified as tonic because of its persistent effect. Also see PHASIC ACTIVATION.

tonic conduction = ELECTROTONIC CONDUCTION.

tonic contraction the contraction of groups of muscles whose fibers maintain muscular tonus.

tonic epilepsy a type of epilepsy in which tonic, but not clonic, muscle contractions occur.

tonic immobility an alternative term for DEATH-FEIGNING. See this entry.

tonicity the normal state of tension of a muscle or other organ. The term is sometimes used for a degree of mental tension, which is, e.g., very high in a manic episode.

tonic pupil of Adie a unilateral eye defect in which the pupil responds poorly to light and very slowly to convergence.

tonic reflex a complex set of reflexes that may involve muscle groups throughout the body as muscle tonus is increased in preparation for an activity. An example is the general head- and body-postural changes observed when a boxer or a football player prepares to meet an opponent in bodily contact.

tonic spasm: See SPASM.

tonitophobia: See ASTRAPHOBIA.

tonometer a device that can produce a tone of a given pitch or can measure the pitch of other tones.

For a different meaning of t., see TONOMETRY.

tonometry a method of measuring **intraocular pressure (IOP)** in the diagnosis of glaucoma and ocular hypertension. T. usually is performed with a Schiotz indentation tonometer or a Goldmann applanation tonometer. The Schiotz device is placed on the anesthetized cornea and measures intraocular pressure in terms of resistance of the surface of the eye to a scale of weights on the instrument. The Goldmann instrument measures pressure as the patient rests his chin on a head support while the applanator is adjusted by slowly moving the tip toward the eye until the ophthalmologist sees two overlapping semicircles and a dial reading that indicates the intraocular pressure. T. also can be performed with a device that blows a puff of air against the eyeball and automatically measures the amount of indentation in terms of intraocular pressure.

tonotopic organization the arrangement of centers and pathways of neural sensations in the cochlea and auditory areas of the cortex with respect to different sound frequencies. The orderly relationship of responsiveness to different frequencies can be projected as a cochlear map in the cortical auditory areas I and II.

tonus a continuous slight stretching or tension in muscles when they are not active. E.g., the jaw muscles exhibit t. when not used for eating or talking. T. serves to keep the muscles ready for action. Also see TONIC.

tool design in industrial psychology, design of instruments and tools in terms of such human factors as efficiency and avoidance of muscle fatigue or injury. See EQUIPMENT DESIGN.

tool subjects academic subjects, e.g., reading or arithmetic, that are regarded as basic tools for gaining advanced knowledge.

tool-using behavior in comparative psychology, the ability of animals to use objects as tools. Man is not the only tool-using animal, as previously thought: A finch may use a cactus spine to probe for insects; an antlion may hurl grains of sand at prey to make them fall into a pit; and chimpanzees frequently use sticks to push into ant nests and use leaves as sponges for drinking or cleaning themselves. And, in a laboratory situation, chimpanzees have been known to pile up five boxes to reach hanging food. The use of tools requires a capacity to generalize relationships between the presence, e.g., of a stick lying randomly in the environment, and its usefulness in extending the animal's reach. While chimpanzees may use tools to hunt food, baboons, e.g., seem to lack the ability.

toot = COCAINE.

Tooth, Howard Henry English physician, 1856–1925. See CHARCOT-MARIE-TOOTH DISEASE; BRAIN ATROPHY; PROGRESSIVE SPINAL-MUSCULAR ATROPHY; TOE DROP.

tooth fear = ODONTOPHOBIA.

-top-; -topo- a combining form relating to place, location, or position (from Greek *topos*, "place").

topalgia a pain that is localized in one spot or small area. T. often is a symptom of hysteria or neurasthenia, particularly in cases in which the pain seems to occur in unlikely segments of nerve or circulatory patterns.

topdog the descriptive term with which F. Perls refers to those internal moral standards or rules of conduct that produce anxiety and conflict in the individual when they are not fulfilled or carried out. See GESTALT THERAPY. Also see UNDERDOG.

topectomy a psychosurgical procedure in which selected areas of the frontal cortex are excised in cases of refractory mental illness (schizophrenia, obsessive-compulsive disorder) that have not responded to electroconvulsive or other types of treatment.

topical application the administration of an agent by applying it to the surface of the skin or similar covering tissue such as a mucous membrane. The drug is absorbed through the surface and produces its effects on lower layers of cells. Certain substances, e.g., dimethyl sulfoxide, have greater capacity than others for penetrating skin surfaces and may be used as carriers for therapeutic drugs. Also see ADMINISTRATION.

topical flight = FLIGHT OF IDEAS.

topographagnosia a disturbance of topographical orientation due to parietal damage in either hemisphere. The patient gets lost in the streets, cannot find his way about the ward, and cannot draw or locate significant features on a map.

topographical disorientation a disorder of spatial visualization due to cortical lesions. T.d. is exemplified by difficulty or inability to recall the arrangement of rooms in a house or the furniture in a room of a house in which the subject lives. A t.d. patient also may be unable to recall or describe the location of landmarks or other objects in his or her neighborhood.

topographical organization the arrangement of structures in an organism, as in the orderly relationship between distribution of neural receptors in an area of the body and a similar distribution of neurons representing the same functions in cortical cells. Auditory and visual receptors occur twice in the cortex in patterns representing their positions in respective sense organs.

topographical psychology the process of mapping the mind, or locating the various mental processes in different regions of the mind. E.g., Jung located the archetypes in the deeper regions of the unconscious, and Freud divided the mind into three strata, or layers—conscious, preconscious, and unconscious. Also called **mental topography**.

topographic hypothesis Freud's original view of the psyche, in which mental functioning was divided into three systems, conscious, preconscious, and unconscious. See SYSTEMATIC APPROACH.

topographic model = SYSTEMATIC APPROACH.

topological psychology K. Lewin's system of psychology in which phenomena are described and classified in terms of the formal relationships, or valences, that obtain in an individual's life space. The result is a geometric map, or topology, of needs, purposes, and goals. Also see VECTOR ANALYSIS; TOPOLOGY.

topology in general, the study of geometric forms and their transformations in space. Piaget found that most children three or four years of age could identify common objects (key, comb, pencil) by haptic perception (exploring through touch alone), but only about one in five could identify simple geometric shapes without using sight. Also, K. Lewin used topological concepts in describing behavior in the LIFE SPACE. See this entry. Also see TOPOLOGICAL PSYCHOLOGY.

topophobia a morbid fear of a particular place or of the place where one happens to be. The term is also used synonymously with AGYIOPHOBIA. See this entry.

torpillage a form of aversion therapy in which a strong electric current is applied to a person in a state of hysteria. The practice, sometimes used in war-time conditions, produces a painful shock that is more aversive than the situation the person tries unconsciously to escape. Also called **torpedoing**.

torpor a condition of total inactivity that may occur in a case of severely disordered consciousness. Only a very strong stimulus can arouse a patient from the stupefaction of t.

Torrance, Ellis Paul American psychologist, 1915 —. See TORRANCE TESTS OF CREATIVE THINKING.

Torrance Tests of Creative Thinking three batteries of test items (thinking creatively with words, with pictures, with sounds and words) applicable from kindergarten to graduate school. Typical "activities," as they are called, are listing possible consequences of the action in an intriguing picture, citing ways of improving a toy, incorporating a curved line in drawing an unusual picture, and writing down whatever is suggested by a series of sounds played on a record. The object is to test for three characteristics identified by Guilford: fluency, flexibility, and originality. See CREATIVITY TEST; ARP TESTS.

torsion dystonia; torsion spasm = DYSTONIA MUSCULORUM DEFORMANS.

torticollis a continuous or spasmodic contraction of the neck muscles, resulting in rotation of the chin and twisting of the head to one side. The condition may be neurological and may respond to drug treatment or biofeedback training. However, it may also be psychogenic, and the turning of the head may, e.g., symbolize avoidance of a feared or guilt-laden sight. T. is sometimes classed as a tic. The term is essentially equivalent to WRYNECK SYNDROME. See this entry.

Torula = CRYPTOCOCCUS.

TOT = TIP-OF-THE-TONGUE PHENOMENON.

Total Battery Composite: See BRUININKS-OSERETSKY TEST OF MOTOR PROFICIENCY.

total color blindness = ACHROMATISM.

total hysterectomy: See HYSTERECTOMY.

totalism a term applied by E. Erikson to an or-

ganization of the self-concept that has rigid, arbitrary boundaries.

totality of possible events: See LIFE SPACE.

total lipodystrophy a form of lipodystrophy that often is congenital, although it may be acquired. It is characterized by an absence of adipose tissue in the subcutaneous tissues, perirenal area, epicardium, and mesentery. Also see PARTIAL LIPODYSTROPHY.

total-push therapy a supportive approach originated by Myerson (1939) primarily for the treatment of chronic institutionalized schizophrenics. To maintain their morale and prevent deterioration, he sought to surround them with a highly stimulating environment and engage them in constant activities such as daily walks, sports, massages, bowling, and, as they improved, music, dance, crafts, and occupational therapy. He also advocated greater attention to attractive clothing and a neat appearance. This approach had considerable effect on the improvement of institutional conditions. See MILIEU THERAPY; THERAPEUTIC COMMUNITY.

totem in anthropology, a revered animal, plant, natural force, or inanimate object that is conceived as the tribal ancestor, symbol, protector, and tutelary spirit of the clan in preliterate society. It is usually associated with tribal prohibitions against destroying the plant or animal or having sexual relations with a member of the same totem, which Freud interpreted in terms of prevention of incest (*Totem and Taboo*, 1913). Also see TOTEMISM.

totemism the practice of using nonhuman objects, such as animals, plants, or inanimate objects, to represent individuals or groups as a refuge for the soul. In several non-Western cultures, the person or group believes the totem symbol offers protection for those who adhere to certain rules of the tribe or clan whose members are forbidden to harm the totem animal, plant, or object. Also see TOTEM.

touch the sensation produced by contact of an object with the surface of the skin. Sensitivity to touch varies in different parts of the body; the lips and fingers are far more sensitive than the trunk or back.

touch fibers nerve fibers that are receptors for mechanical stimuli, such as stroking or light contact.

touching an association disorder of schizophrenics who are unable to recognize an object unless they can touch it, a disturbance similar to naming. The term applies also to the practice of sensitivity-group members who use physical contact with others as a means of breaking down barriers in interpersonal communication.

touch sense the ability to perceive a stimulus applied in the form of cutaneous stroking or light contact with a hair or similar object. Also called **tactile sense; cutaneous sense**. Also see HAPTIC PERCEPTION.

touch spot any of the small areas of the skin that are particularly sensitive to light contact.

tough-minded William James' term for a personality type which he described as empirical, materialistic, skeptical, and fatalistic. Compare TENDER-MINDED.

Tourette: See GILLES DE LA T.

Tourette's disorder a stereotyped-movement disorder characterized by repeated, involuntary rapid movements of various muscle groups, and involving vocal tics such as grunts, yelps, barks, sniffs, and in most cases an irresistible urge to utter obscenities. It is a lifelong disorder of unknown origin, which usually starts with eye spasms before age 13. It was first described by the French physician Georges Gilles de la Tourette in 1885, and is considered by many to be a schizophrenic condition. Also called **Gilles de la Tourette's syndrome; tic convulsif with coprolalia; multiple tics with coprolalia; maladie des tics; tic de Guinon; Guinon's disease**. See GILLES DE LA TOURETTE. (DSM-III)

Towne, Edward Bancroft American physician, 1883–1957. See ROENTGENOGRAM (there: **Towne projection roentgenogram**).

-tox-; -toxi-; -toxo-; -toxic- a combining form relating to poison or poisoning (from Greek *toxikon*, "arrow poison"). Adjective: **toxic**. Noun: **toxin**.

toxemia an illness characterized by toxins, or poisons, in the blood. The poisons may be caused by an infectious disease or by exposure to ingested or environmental substances. Also see BLOOD-POISONING.

toxemia of pregnancy a syndrome of edema, hypertension, and proteinuria that may develop in the last trimester of a pregnancy. The onset also may be delayed until the first days after childbirth. T.o.p. complicated by convulsions and coma may be identified as **eclampsia** while the syndrome without the complications is called **preeclampsia**. It occurs most often with first pregnancies, regardless of age. Also see ECLAMPTIC SYMPTOMS.

toxic: See -TOX-.

toxic delirium delirium resulting from infectious diseases (such as pneumonia, scarlet fever, malaria, uremia, rheumatic fever) in their acute or convalescent stage. See DELIRIUM.

toxic diffuse goiter = GRAVES' DISEASE.

toxic disorders brain syndromes due to acute or chronic intoxication, including mercury, manganese, lead, bromide, alcohol, and barbiturate poisoning.

toxic-infectious psychosis a severe mental disorder occurring during or after an infectious disease or poisoning by an exogenous toxin. Major symptoms are delirium, stupor, epileptiform attacks, hallucinosis, confusion, and incoherence. See TOXIC DELIRIUM; TOXIC DISORDERS.

toxicity the capacity of a substance to produce toxic, or poisonous, effects in an organism. The t. of a substance, whether a drug or industrial or household chemical, generally is related to the size of the dose per body weight of the individual, expressed in terms of milligrams of chemical per kilogram of body weight. T. also may be expressed in terms of the minimum dose needed to affect a laboratory animal or 50 percent of the animal population. Also see BEHAVIORAL T.

toxicomania a morbid desire to consume poisons, or a severe dependency on drugs.

toxicophobia = TOXIPHOBIA.

toxic psychosis an acute or chronic brain disorder resulting from ingestion of poisons or drugs, infectious diseases, or exhaustion. The most common manifestation is delirium: restlessness, apprehensiveness, and frightening images, often followed by clouding of consciousness, disorientation, and in some cases hallucinations, delusions, and coma. If the toxic condition is only temporary and the personality is well-integrated, the delirium clears up rapidly; if it does not, a lasting psychosis may result. Examples of toxic conditions are diphtheria, typhoid fever, ingestion of barbiturates or amphetamines, carbon-monoxide inhalation, and postoperative disturbances.

toxin: See -TOX-.

toxiphobia a morbid fear of being poisoned or of poison. Also called **toxicophobia; iophobia**.

toxoplasmosis a disease caused by the infection of a warm-blooded animal by a protozoan parasite, Toxoplasma gondii, which invades the tissue cells and multiplies. T. parasites also reproduce in the intestinal cells of cats, the disease being spread by cat feces. When acquired by a pregnant woman, t. can be transmitted to the fetus, causing hydrocephalus, blindness, mental retardation, and other nervous-system disorders. Also see CONGENITAL T.

TPR an abbreviation of *t*emperature, *p*ulse, and *r*espiration.

tr. an abbreviation used in prescriptions, meaning "tincture" (Latin *tinctura*).

trace conditioning a learning procedure in which a conditioned stimulus and an unconditioned stimulus are separated by a constant interval. The effectiveness of the method can be measured in terms of alpha-wave blocking to a previously neutral stimulus.

trace-decay theory = DECAY THEORY.

tracers: See RADIOACTIVE T.

-trache-; -tracheo- a combining form relating to the windpipe (**trachea**).

tracheostomy the surgical creation of an opening through the neck to the trachea with insertion of a tube. A t. may be performed in order to remove secretions from the respiratory tract or to enhance the ability of the patient to breathe normally. Special care must be taken by the t. patient to maintain the integrity of the opening, which could become blocked by a pillow while sleeping or a means of drowning while taking a bath or swimming.

tracheotomy a surgical incision in the trachea, made to form an opening to facilitate breathing or to begin a TRACHEOSTOMY. See this entry.

trachoma an infection of the eye, involving mainly

the conjunctiva and cornea, caused by the bacterial strain Chlamydia trachomatis. T. begins with pain, tearing, and photophobia and, untreated, progresses to blindness. T. is common in Asia and Africa where 400,000,000 persons have been infected and 20,000,000 blinded; in some parts of Africa, entire populations are infected with t. The same bacterium is responsible for a form of nongonococcal urethritis. Also called **Egyptian ophthalmia**. See OPHTHALMIA.

trachyphonia an abnormal hoarseness of the voice.

tracing: See RADIOACTIVE TRACERS.

tract a bundle or group of nerve fibers. The term usually is applied to groups of fibers within the central nervous system, or in the brain or spinal cord. A bundle of nerve fibers outside the central nervous system often is identified as a nerve.

trademark any word, symbol, or device that is used by a manufacturer or merchant to identify his products. Examples include Coca-Cola, Pepsi-Cola, and Polaroid. The t. may be a pattern of display that is associated with a particular product or a unique package or container. Trademarks are an important part of a product image, especially after they have been established for a number of years in association with acceptable and reliable products.

While a t. identifies goods or services, a **trade name** identifies the company that makes or sells them. According to the United States Trademark Association, the term trade name should therefore not be used (as it is still used, e.g., in several drug reference sources) to refer to a product; its use should be restricted to its manufacturer or purveyor, e.g., E. I. Du Pont de Nemours. However, under certain conditions t. and trade name can be identical, e.g., Christian Dior or Jordache. See PROPRIETARY DRUG. Also see METHODOLOGICAL NOTES, 7.3.1.

trade test a test designed to measure competence in a trade such as electrician or draughtsman, based on either information questions or job-skill items usually of the work-sample variety.

tradition a set of social customs or other ethnic or family practices handed down from generation to generation (from Latin *traditio*, "handing down").

traditionalist: See ETHICAL HIGHBROW.

traditional marriage a formal relationship of husband and wife joined in wedlock for the primary purpose of establishing a family. Although prenuptial customs vary in different cultures, a t.m. generally follows a period of courtship approved by families of both the bride and groom, public announcement of wedding plans, and a religious wedding ceremony. In some cultures, a t.m. requires that the bride and groom be forbidden to meet before the wedding ceremony.

traditional psychotherapies: See PSYCHOTHERAPY.

tradition-directed the term used by D. Riesman and applied to those persons whose values,
goals, and behavior are largely determined by their traditional cultural heritage, that is, by the social norms transmitted by their parents. Compare INNER-DIRECTED; OTHER-DIRECTED.

Trail-Making Test: See CEREBRAL-DYSFUNCTION TESTS.

trainability the capacity of an individual to benefit from training in a particular skill.

trainable a term applied to the mentally retarded, usually in the moderate category (IQ 35 to 49), who cannot profit from academic education even in special classes, but who are capable of achieving a degree of self-care and social adjustment at home, and vocational usefulness in a closely supervised setting such as a sheltered workshop. See MENTAL RETARDATION.

trainer in psychiatry, a professional leader or facilitator of a sensitivity-training group, or T-group. The term is also applied to teachers or supervisors of individuals learning to practice psychotherapy.

train fear = SIDERODROMOPHOBIA.

training systematic instruction and practice by which an individual acquires competence in a vocational or recreational skill or activity.

training aids the use of devices that simulate or resemble equipment used on the job to train personnel, especially when the actual equipment may be impractical due to cost or possible injury.

training analysis = DIDACTIC ANALYSIS.

training evaluation: See EVALUATION OF TRAINING.

training group = T-GROUP.

training school a rehabilitation facility for mentally retarded children utilizing interdisciplinary teams of therapists in a homelike setting. The children are given medical and psychological care while being carefully evaluated and trained in vocational areas in which they show the greatest promise of success. The t.s. also provides full social and recreational experiences.

training transfer: See TRANSFER OF TRAINING.

trait an enduring personality characteristic that determines the individual's behavior; in genetics, an attribute resulting from a hereditary predisposition, e.g., hair color or facial features.

trait organization the way in which an individual's personal traits are related and comprise a unique, integrated whole.

trait profile a diagram which charts test scores that represent individual traits. These scores or ratings are arranged on a common scale to depict the pattern of traits visually. Also called **psychograph**.

trait-rating an observation technique in which a given behavioral trait or feature is observed, rated, and recorded, e.g., a character trait such as industriousness in a school child.

trait theory: See ALLPORT'S PERSONALITY-T. T; CATTELL'S FACTORIAL THEORY OF PERSONALITY.

trait variability the scattering or dispersion of various trait measures shown by the individual.

trance a sleeplike state characterized by markedly diminished consciousness and responsiveness to stimuli. T. is also a hypnotic state, which may vary from a **light t.**, characterized by inability to open the eyes, limb catalepsy or rigidity, and hand anesthesia, to a **medium t.**, in which there is partial amnesia, posthypnotic amnesia, and suggestion, to **deep t.**, characterized by inability to open the eyes without affecting the trance, complete somnambulism, positive and negative posthypnotic hallucinations, and hyperesthesias.

trance logic a descriptive term for the tendency of hypnotized subjects to engage simultaneously in logically contradictory or paradoxical trains of thought. It has been suggested that t.l. may be viewed as evidence for the parallel-processing theory in that there appears to be simultaneous registration of information at different levels of awareness. That is, incoming information appears to be processed by separate systems, some information being recorded consciously while other information does not reach consciousness.

trance state a hypnotic state of dissociation and diminished response to external stimuli, induced by hypnosis, occurring in catalepsy, or found in groups undergoing religious excitement, as in revivalist meetings. See TRANCE.

tranquilizer a drug that is used to relieve tension or combat psychotic symptoms without significant sedation. A t. that reduces agitation is a minor t., e.g., meprobamate or diazepam, and may be identified as an anxiolytic. A t. used as an antipsychotic agent or neuroleptic is a major t., e.g., chlorpromazine. Anxiolytics tend to depress the limbic and reticular activating systems, although specific drugs may have other effects such as relaxing skeletal muscles or inhibiting reflexes. Neuroleptics generally cause gross behavioral changes such as reducing motor activity, decreasing emotionality, and producing an indifference to external stimuli. Neuroleptics are administered primarily to psychotic patients rather than neurotics. Also see ATARACTICS.

tranquilizer chair a heavy wooden chair in which patients of Benjamin Rush, the first American psychiatrist, were strapped at the chest, abdomen, ankles, and knees, with their head inserted in a wooden box. He preferred this method of restraint to the straitjacket for "maniacal" patients because it reduced the flow of blood to the head and did not interfere with bloodletting, one of the standard treatments of the time. See RUSH.

tranquilosedatives = ATARACTICS.

transaction any interaction between the individual and the social or physical environment, especially during encounters between two or more persons. In some psychotherapies, such as R. R. Grinker's and Eric Berne's approaches, t. is the interplay between the therapist and the patient, and ultimately between the patient and other individuals in his or her environment.

transactional analysis a form of dynamic group or individual psychotherapy originated by Eric Berne, which focuses on characteristic interactions which reveal internal "ego states," and the "games people play" in social situations. Specifically, the approach involves (a) a study of the three primary ego states (parent, child, adult) and determination of which one is dominant in the transaction in question, (b) identification of the tricks and expedients, or games, habitually utilized in the patient's transactions (called by popular names such as "payoff," "con," and "Ain't it awful?"), and (c) analysis of the total "script," or unconscious plan, of the patient's life, in order to uncover the sources of his emotional problems. Abbrev.: **TA**. See BERNE; EGO STATE.

transactional evaluation in evaluation research, an attempt to apply systems-theory principles to the area of program innovation. It is designed to minimize the disruption of the reallocation process occurring when changes are introduced in an organization and thereby minimize personal threat and defensiveness felt by the system participants.

transactional theory of perception a generalization that fundamental perceptions are learned reactions based on interactions with the environment. These reactions generate expectancies to which new experiences tend to conform.

transaxial: See COMPUTERIZED AXIAL TOMOGRAPHY.

transcendence need according to E. Fromm, the need to create so as to rise above passivity and attain a sense of meaning and purpose in an impermanent and seemingly random or accidental universe. Both creativity and destructiveness are considered by Fromm to be manifestations of the t.n.

transcendental meditation a technique for achieving a transcendental state of consciousness, introduced in the United States in 1959 by the Maharishi Mahesh Yogi, but based upon the Bhagavad-Gita and other ancient Hindu writings. In essence, the modernized version of the original discipline consists of a series of six steps which culminate in sitting with one's eyes closed for two 20-minute periods a day, while repeating a mantra. Repetition of the mantra serves to block distracting thoughts and to induce a state of relaxation in which images and ideas can arise from deeper levels of the mind and from the cosmic source of all thought and being. The result is said to be not only a greater sense of well-being, but more harmonious interpersonal relations and the achievement of a state of "absolute bliss." Abbrev.: **TM**. Also see MYSTIC UNION; MANTRA.

transcendental state a level of consciousness believed to reach beyond waking, sleeping, and hypnotic states, characterized physically by lowered metabolism and reduced adrenergic functions, and psychologically by alleviation of tension, anxiety, and frustration, and a high level of tranquillity. Claims to achieve a t.s. have frequently been made by individuals under the influence of hallucinogens and by religious devotees who seek to be "in tune with the infinite" through prayer and meditation.

transcervical uterine aspiration the removal by suction of fluid or other materials from the uterus by a device inserted via the vagina and cervix.

transcortical aphasia a type of aphasia due to a lesion that may be extensive without damaging the Broca or Wernicke areas. Those areas, however, may become isolated from the rest of the brain, and as a result the patient will be able to repeat spoken words even though he may have difficulty in producing or understanding speech.

transcortical motor aphasia: See COMBINED TRANSCORTICAL APHASIA.

transcortical pathways a concept associated with Pavlov experiments of the 1920s indicating the presence in the neocortex of direct links between sensory and motor areas. Pavlov argued that conditioning was not possible in decorticated animals, but other researchers demonstrated that conditioning was difficult but possible in the absence of t.p.

transcortical sensory aphasia: See COMBINED TRANSCORTICAL APHASIA.

transcultural psychiatry = CROSS-CULTURAL PSYCHIATRY.

transducing the neurological process of converting information within the brain from one sensory modality to another, such as auditory-to-visual-to-motor.

transection the severing or cutting across a nerve tract, fiber, axon, or the spinal cord.

transfer by generalization the transfer from one situation to another of general principles rather than behavior patterns. Also called **transfer of principles.**

transference /-fur'-/ in psychoanalysis, the projection or displacement upon the analyst of unconscious feelings and wishes originally directed toward important individuals, such as parents, in the patient's childhood. This process, which is at the core of psychoanalysis, brings repressed material to the surface where it can be reexperienced, studied, and "worked through." In the course of this process, the sources of neurotic difficulties are frequently discovered, and their harmful effects alleviated. See NEGATIVE T.; POSITIVE T.; ANALYSIS OF T.; COUNTERTRANSFERENCE; INSTITUTIONAL T.; IDENTIFICATION T.; DISTORTION BY T.; DUAL-T. THERAPY; LIBIDINAL T.

transference cure = FLIGHT INTO HEALTH.

transference improvement alleviation of neurotic symptoms through a transference relationship involving the therapist who is perceived unconsciously as the reincarnation of the parents.

transference-love in psychoanalysis, feelings of affection and attachment transferred from the original love objects, such as parents, to the analyst. This type of love is an artifact of the analysis, not the "real thing," since it is a reenactment of infantile feelings and is not related to the character or even sex of the analyst as a person. Ses POSITIVE TRANSFERENCE.

transference neurosis in psychoanalysis, neurotic reactions released by the transference process, due to the fact that the patient's early conflicts and traumas are revived and relived. These reactions are an artificial illness which replaces the original neurosis and helps the patient become aware that his attitudes and behavior are actually repetitions of infantile drives. The t.n. must be resolved if the patient is to free himself from the harmful effects of past experiences, and adopt more appropriate attitudes and responses.

transference remission = FLIGHT INTO HEALTH.

transference resistance in psychoanalysis, a form of resistance to the disclosure of unconscious material, in which the patient maintains silence or attempts to act out feelings of love or hate transferred from past relationships to the analyst. See RESISTANCE; NEGATIVE TRANSFERENCE; POSITIVE TRANSFERENCE; ANALYSIS OF TRANSFERENCE.

transfer of learning a theory associated with 1960s experiments with RNA molecules as possible units of stored information or engrams. T.o.l. presumes that RNA molecules from a trained animal can be ingested by or injected into a naive animal which will then have the memory trace of the trained animal. Experiments have involved the feeding of minced trained flatworms to naive flatworms and injecting naive rats with RNA extracted from the brains of trained rats.

transfer of principles = TRANSFER BY GENERALIZATION.

transfer of training the influence of prior learning on new learning, either to enhance it (positive transfer) or to hamper it (negative transfer). Solving a new problem is usually easier if we can apply previously-learned principles or components. The general principles of mathematics, e.g., transfer to computer programing, but a knowledge of Spanish may have both positive and negative effects in learning Italian. At one time, a study of mathematics, Greek, and Latin was believed to enhance learning ability in all subjects—until Thorndike and Woodworth showed that no single high-school subject trained the intellect better than any other. See FACULTY PSYCHOLOGY; FORMAL DISCIPLINE; POSITIVE TRANSFER; NEGATIVE TRANSFER.

transfer RNA a ribonucleic-acid molecule that has the ability to transfer specific amino acids to protein molecules during the synthesis of proteins. Each amino acid has a corresponding t.RNA molecule.

transformation in psychoanalysis, the change in feelings or impulses as a means of disguising them to gain admittance to consciousness.

transformational grammar grammar that describes a language by laying down procedures for transforming one grammatical pattern into another, e.g., changing sentence types and adding or deleting elements or modifying their order. The most advanced t.g. is Noam Chomsky's **transformational-generative grammar**.

transformation of affect the transformation of a feeling, or affect, into its opposite in dreams. E.g., a feeling of love may be obscured in the dream as a feeling of hatred.

transfusion the introduction of whole natural blood, blood components, or synthetic blood substitutes into the circulation of a patient. A t. is performed to restore depleted blood supplies in a person who has experienced hemorrhage, shock from burns or surgery, or similar trauma, and also in the treatment of certain kinds of anemias and other blood diseases.

transfusional hemosiderosis an abnormal increase in iron levels in the body tissues as a result of a blood transfusion. Except in certain diseases, e.g., Cooley's anemia, t.h. is not a serious problem.

transgenderism a form of psychosexual dysfunction marked by a confusion of sex roles. T. usually is associated with a failure by one or both parents to establish strong gender model roles with which the person could identify adequately for proper gender identification. Also see ROLE CONFUSION.

transience in psychiatry, a feeling of impermanence combined with an anticipation of loss. The idea that everything is transitory may, according to Freud (1916), interfere with enjoyment and preclude the establishment of deep or lasting relationships. The normal individual, on the other hand, focuses primarily on the here and now and is not frightened by the idea of eventual loss of love objects.

transient ego ideal a concept suggested by the psychoanalyst S. Lorand (1962) to denote the function of the analyst in serving as a temporary object of love and acceptance during the transference process. This constitutes an important step toward satisfying the patient's needs and correcting the original ego ideal, especially when the parent has been cold or severe during the patient's childhood. See EGO IDEAL.

transient group: See NATURAL GROUP.

transient global amnesia a sudden, temporary loss of memory ability apparently due to a transient cranial ischemia (inadequate blood flow). Other functions may continue normally during the memory disruption. Abbrev.: **TGA**.

transient ischemic attack: See CEREBRAL ISCHEMIA.

transient situational disturbance an acute, temporary reaction to an overwhelmingly stressful situation, experienced by an individual who does not have an underlying personality disorder. The disturbance may occur at any period of life, and is due, e.g., to separation from the mother in infancy, rejection or frightening experiences during childhood, parental conflict or natural catastrophe in adulthood, or menopause and forced retirement in later life. Such disturbances

are termed "transient situational personality disorder" in DSM-I, "t.s.d." in DSM-II, and ADJUSTMENT DISORDER in DSM-III. See this entry.

transient situational personality disorder a DSM-I category replacing the older term traumatic neurosis. Acute reactions such as insomnia, loss of appetite, tremors, stuttering, anxiety attacks, irritability, and tics are experienced by basically stable individuals in response to situations of overwhelming stress; and "in the presence of good adaptive capacity recession of symptoms generally occurs when the situational stress diminishes" (DSM-I). Subcategories include GROSS STRESS REACTION, ADULT SITUATIONAL REACTION, ADJUSTMENT REACTION OF INFANCY, ADJUSTMENT REACTION OF CHILDHOOD, ADJUSTMENT REACTION OF ADOLESCENCE, and ADJUSTMENT REACTION OF LATER LIFE. See these entries.

transient-tic disorder a stereotyped-movement disorder involving repeated involuntary purposeless movements, such as an eye blink or twitches of the face or limbs. Transient tics appear in childhood or adolescence, are aggravated by stress, subside during sleep or absorbing activities, and ordinarily last no more than a year. (DSM-III)

transient tremor: See TREMOR.

transitional cortex the portion of the cortex that lies between the primitive cortex, or archipallium, and the neocortex, which is believed to represent the newest phase of animal-brain development in terms of evolution.

transitional employment workshop a sheltered workshop, or similar rehabilitation facility, that is specifically designed to advance a disabled person toward the open job market. The transitional period may be extended as needed for patients unable to cope with a rapid change from sheltered workshop to competitive employment situations.

transitional object an object selectively acquired by an infant because of its anxiety-reducing value, e.g., a "security blanket" that helps induce sleep. Some authors differentiate between a **primary t.o.** acquired during the first year of life and a **secondary t.o.** adopted around the age of two. Also see SYMBIOSIS; INDIVIDUATION.

transitional probability the likelihood of one event's being followed by a second event.

transitional program a rehabilitation project in which a disabled patient lives with his family on the hospital grounds for several days before being transferred to home-care treatment. During the transitional period, the patient and family members occupy a cottage where nurses, dietitians, psychotherapists, and other hospital-staff members instruct the family members in the methods of medical care and rehabilitation required for the patient's disability.

transitivism the illusory transfer of symptoms or other characteristics to other people, e.g., a schizophrenic patient's belief that other persons are also experiencing his hallucinations, are also being persecuted, or are also lacking a stomach or another internal organ.

transitivity a concept in which a relationship between two entities is transferred to a third; e.g., A includes B and B includes C, therefore A includes C. Also, the term t. is sometimes applied to a schizophrenic process which is more commonly called TRANSITIVISM. See this entry.

translocation: See AUTOSOMAL ABERRATIONS.

transmission the sending or dispatching of objects, words, symbols, or neural impulses; the spreading of a disease; passing hereditary traits on from one generation to the next; or handing down customs and mores from generation to generation. Also see HORIZONTAL T.

transmitter an instrument or device that encodes and sends a message or impulse to a receiver or aids in its transmission, e.g., a synaptic t.

transmitter substance a chemical released by a nerve impulse as it arrives at a synapse of a neuron. The chemical is presumably produced by the synaptic vesicles and is discharged across the synaptic cleft to render the postsynaptic membrane more permeable.

transmuted scores a set of scores or values that have been converted from one scale to another.

transorbital lobotomy a psychosurgical procedure in which a leukotome (a narrow rotating blade) is introduced through the socket above the eyes and carefully swung through a 30-degree angle to sever connections between the frontal lobe and the thalamus. The technique is preferred by some neurosurgeons since undesirable side effects such as incontinence and apathy are less frequent than in classical prefrontal lobotomy.

transpersonal psychology an area in humanistic psychology concerned with the exploration of "higher" states of consciousness and transcendental experiences. "Transpersonal" refers to the concern with ends that transcend personal identity and individual, immediate desires.

transplacental transmission: See HORIZONTAL TRANSMISSION.

transplantation the removal of something from one place to another, as in the t. of a body organ or skin graft; also, the removal of a person from a permanent home to a transient residence or nursing home, a situation that may result in emotional disturbances such as anxiety, depression, and other effects. The mental distress of t. of a person sometimes is called **t. shock.** Also see ORGAN TRANSPLANTS.

transplantation reactions immune reactions in which donor tissue, such as an organ, is rejected by antibodies of the recipient. T.r. are comparable to a severe reaction by the body tissues to the foreign protein of an infectious organism. T.r. may be less severe when the donor and recipient are genetically identical or similar. Chemicals that suppress the immune reaction may be administered to control t.r. Also see ORGAN TRANSPLANTS; ANTIBODY.

transplantation shock: See TRANSPLANTATION.

transposition an interchange of positions of two or more elements in a system; in a learning situation, a reaction of the subject to a relationship of the elements rather than the elements per se; in music, the change from one key to another.

transposition of affect the transfer of the affective component of an unconscious idea to an unrelated idea or object, as frequently occurs in obsessive-compulsive disorder. Also called **displacement of affect.**

transsexualism a psychosexual disorder consisting of a persistent sense of discomfort and inappropriateness relating to one's anatomic sex, with a persistent wish to be rid of one's genitals and live as a member of the other sex. In DSM-III, the diagnosis is made only if the condition has been continuous for at least two years, is not due to another mental disorder, such as schizophrenia, and is not associated with physical intersex or genetic abnormality. Some **transsexuals** dress in clothes of the other sex (cross dressing), and some seek to change their sex through surgical or hormonal means. Also see AMBISEXUALITY; VAGINAL ENVY. (DSM-III)

transsynaptic filament a filament that extends between the membranes of an axon and a neighboring dendrite. It is believed the structure, observable only with an electron microscope, is involved in an exchange of materials during the growth period when axons and dendrites are moving toward each other as part of the development of an organism's nervous system.

transverse colostomy: See COLOSTOMY.

transverse flatfoot: See FLATFOOT.

transverse myelitis a type of CNS inflammation that involves an entire cross section of the spinal cord at one level. The long-range effects may include progressive degeneration of the nervous system to an eventual state of quadriplegia. Also called **transverse myelopathy.**

transvestism a psychosexual disorder consisting of persistent cross dressing by a heterosexual male (initially at least to achieve sexual excitement) and intense frustration if the cross dressing is interfered with. Though these males are basically heterosexual, their sexual experience with women is limited, and occasional homosexual acts may occur. The cross dressing usually begins in childhood or adolescence, sometimes secretly, and in some cases may have been inflicted as "petticoat punishment." Also see CROSS DRESSING. (DSM-III)

T. is also occasionally found in women, but then, according to P. Friedman (1959), it has more of a "make-believe character" and often stems from bravado and defiance rather than from a genuine transvestite impulse.

transvestitism the pathological impulse to wear the clothes and accessories of the opposite sex; cross dressing. The term is essentially equivalent to TRANSVESTISM. See this entry for details.

Transylvania effect a term sometimes applied to abnormal behavior that is correlated with the phases of the moon. (The term is derived from a novel by Bram Stoker, *Dracula*, a wild tale of vampires and werewolves affected by phases of the moon in Transylvania, a region in Romania.) Also see MOON-PHASE STUDIES.

tranylcypromine; tranylcypromine sulfate: See MONOAMINE OXIDASE INHIBITORS.

trapezius muscle a triangular muscle that covers much of the back of the body, its base extending from the back of the skull to the level of the 12th thoracic vertebra. The t.m. is composed of numerous muscle fibers that converge at the apex of the triangle at the collar bone. Portions of the t.m. working independently can draw the head to one side, turn the face, raise or lower the shoulder blade, or help move the arm.

trapezoid body a bundle of transverse nerve fibers in the pons with origins in the cochlear nucleus.

t ratio the ratio used to determine whether differences between two items are larger than could be expected by chance. In this case the statistical study usually involves fewer than 30 subjects.

trauma an injury (Greek, "wound"), either physical or psychological. In psychiatry, physical traumas include blows to the head, brain insults such as hemorrhages and cerebrovascular accidents, or injuries to other parts of the body such as burns or amputated limbs. Psychological traumas include emotional shocks that have a more or less permanent effect on the personality, such as rejection, divorce, combat experiences, civilian catastrophes, and racial or religious discrimination. These are often referred to as **traumatic experiences.** Plurals: **traumas; traumata.**

traumatic anxiety a state of apprehensiveness or an anxiety attack precipitated by a physical or psychological trauma such as a natural catastrophe, combat experience, business loss, or marital failure.

traumatic delirium an acute delirium following a head or brain injury. In some patients the delirium may become chronic, with symptoms of confabulation, disorientation, and memory deficit.

traumatic encephalopathy a diffuse brain disease caused by an injury to the brain. Among various symptoms are headaches, dizziness, poor concentration, personality changes, drowsiness, and insomnia.

traumatic event a physical or psychic injury that is the immediate cause of an emotional or mental disorder, e.g., of a traumatic neurosis or psychosis.

traumatic experience: See TRAUMA.

traumatic hemorrhage the type of brain hemorrhage that results from a severe head injury, such as a skull fracture. The bleeding usually involves a meningeal-artery rupture, with rapid and extensive loss of blood requiring emergency treatment. An example of a t.h. is EXTRADURAL HEMORRHAGE. See this entry.

traumatic neurasthenia a type of neurasthenia

that follows a physical injury experienced in an accident. The neurasthenia may have been an underlying neurosis that was aggravated by the trauma.

traumatic neurosis an emotional disorder precipitated by an acutely disturbing situation or experience, and characterized by such symptoms as preoccupation with the trauma, at least partial amnesia for the event, reduced efficiency, nightmares, irritability, and autonomic dysfunction. In DSM-I, the term was replaced by "transient situational personality disorder," and in DSM-III, by POSTTRAUMATIC STRESS DISORDER. See this entry. Also see COMBAT FATIGUE; PSYCHORRHEXIS.

traumatic pseudocatatonia a state of catatonia that is the result of an injury.

traumatophilic diathesis an alternative term for accident proneness, or predisposition to accidents. See VICTIM RECIDIVISM.

traumatophobia a morbid fear of sustaining an injury.

traveling wave a wave of pressure that follows a course, affecting objects in its path which may in turn continue the effect in different physical media. E.g., a sound wave of pressure is converted in the middle ear to a mechanical vibration which in turn is translated into a fluid pressure wave in the cochlea and finally into nerve impulses that are tuned to the sound wave's frequency.

travel phobia = HODOPHOBIA.

Treacher Collins: See COLLINS.

Treacher Collins' syndrome an autosomal-dominant hereditary disorder characterized by facial anomalies including a small retracted chin, small eyes with iris colobomas, and deformed external ears. Many of the patients have conductive-hearing loss and some are mentally retarded. Also called **mandibulofacial dysostosis; Franceschetti-Zwahlen-Klein syndrome.**

treatment the administration of appropriate measures, e.g., drugs or psychotherapy, designed to relieve a pathological condition; also, the manner in which experimental procedures are applied and the resulting data evaluated.

treatment-evaluation strategies in behavior therapy, the determination of the effects of a particular treatment through application of different procedures, such as the TREATMENT-PACKAGE STRATEGY and the DISMANTLING-TREATMENT STRATEGY. See these entries.

treatment-package strategy in behavior therapy, application of several therapeutic components, such as modeling, guided practice, and positive reinforcement, as a means of determining if treatment alters the problem for which it is designed.

tremograph an instrument for measuring body tremors.

tremophobia a morbid fear of trembling.

tremor any trembling of the body or a part of the body, e.g., the hands, due to organic or psychologic causes. **Psychologic tremors** may be mild, due to tension, or violent and uncontrolled in severe disturbances. Toxic effects of drugs or heavy metals may produce a **transient t.** A **coarse t.** involves a large muscle group in slow movements while a **fibrillary t.** is caused by a small bundle of muscle fibers which, when moving rapidly, produce a **fine t.** Some tremors occur only during voluntary movements, e.g., the **volitional t.** associated with multiple sclerosis. **Hunt's t.** is a trembling during voluntary movements that is caused by lesions of the cerebellum. A parkinsonism t. involves cerebral motor neurons. A senile t. is one that is associated with aging. Also see INTENTION T.

trend analysis the analysis of a set of variable measurements, taken at different intervals, to determine if there is evidence of a trend.

trend of thought in psychiatry, a tendency to think in terms of a particular pattern of ideas with an affective tone, especially when it is associated with a pathological condition, e.g., a delusional system, or an autistic fantasy.

trephination a surgical procedure in which a disk of bone is removed, usually from the skull, with a circular instrument (a **trephine**) with a sawlike edge. **Skull trephining** is believed to be one of the oldest types of surgery, based on evidence found in skulls of prehistoric humans with round holes that apparently had healed. Also called **trepanation**.

Treponema pallidum: See SYPHILIS.

treppe /trep′ə/ the graduated sequence of increasingly stronger muscle contractions that occur when a corresponding sequence of identical stimuli is applied to a rested muscle (from German *Treppe*, "stairs"). It may be explained as a warm-up effect.

triad a set of three persons involved in a dynamic relationship, especially a father, mother, and child, or the therapist and a couple being seen in marriage therapy.

triadic therapy = CONJOINT THERAPY.

triage situations /trē·äzh′/ in psychiatry, catastrophic situations such as earthquakes and bombings, in which it is necessary to select and sort out psychiatric casualties and route them to the most appropriate treatment services available.

In evaluation research, triage is a method of allocating scarce resources among social programs such that only programs that are in need and are most likely to benefit from the resources are considered. It is usually a method of resource allocation that makes more help available to those that are likely to become self-sufficient.

trial in tests or experiments, one practice session or performance of a given task, e.g., one run through a maze.

trial analysis in psychoanalysis, a provisional period of one or two weeks during which the analyst diagnoses the patient, determines if he is an appropriate case, and acquaints him with the analytic approach. Most analysts of today do not set aside a special period for these purposes,

since they are incorporated in the general procedure.

trial and error: See VICARIOUS T.A.E.

trial identification a term used by R. Fliess (1942) for a process in which the analyst puts himself in the patient's shoes, so that he can obtain "an inside knowledge that is almost firsthand." See EMPATHY.

trial lesson a diagnostic technique that provides information about a child's learning style and the teaching approaches most effective for him.

trial marriage = EXPERIMENTAL MARRIAGE.

triamterene a diuretic that sometimes is combined with thiazide drugs to enhance their hypotensive activity. T. is related chemically to folic acid and other vitamins but has no important pharmacologic action except on the kidneys. T. increases the excretion rate of sodium and, to a lesser extent, of the chloride ion.

triangular therapy = CONJOINT THERAPY.

tribade /trib′-/ a woman, usually one with a large clitoris, who plays the male role in Lesbian practices (from Greek *tribein*, "to rub," referring to the rubbing of female genitalia against each other).

tribadism /trib′-/ a seldom used term for Lesbianism. Adjective: **tribadic** /-bad′ik/.

triceps reflex the extension of the forearm by tapping the triceps tendon at the elbow when the forearm is partly flexed.

triceptor theory the theory that the retina contains three types of receptors, one for each of the primary colors of trichromatism.

-trich-; -tricho- a combining form relating to hair or hairlike formations (from Greek *trichos*, "hair").

trichinosis an infection caused by a parasitic roundworm, Trichinella spiralis, which enters the body through the ingestion of improperly prepared pork products. Larvae of the parasite are released from muscle cysts of the meat by the digestive juices of the host and migrate to various organs. A target tissue in humans is the eyelid, which develops edema from the infection, followed by photosensitivity and retinal hemorrhage. T. infections may result also from eating the meat of bears and certain marine animals. The disease rarely occurs in countries such as France where hogs are fed root vegetables.

trichomegaly-retinal degeneration syndrome a rare disorder marked by abnormally short stature, long eyebrows and eyelashes, and poor vision due to retinal pigmentary degeneration. Some of the patients show slow psychomotor development and may have IQs of less than 70; in others, normal intelligence has been reported.

trichomoniasis a sexually transmitted disease caused by the protozoan Trichomonas vaginalis. T. may be symptomless in men, although it can be a cause of epididymitis or prostatic disorders; but the disease organism usually causes severe genital itching and edema in women with eventual cervical erosion and possible cervical cancer if the infection is repeated or untreated.

trichopathophobia = TRICHOPHOBIA.

trichophagy /trikof'-/ a term applied to persistently biting and eating one's hair.

trichophobia a morbid fear of hair. Also called **trichopathophobia**.

trichorrhexis nodosa with mental retardation a congenital disorder marked by stubby, brittle hair, thin tooth enamel, defective nails, and severe mental retardation. The patients studied have been microcephalic. X-rays have revealed a small cranial vault.

trichorrhexomania the compulsion to break off one's hair with the fingernails.

trichotillomania = HAIR-PULLING.

trichromat: See TRICHROMATISM.

trichromatic theory one of several concepts of the physiological basis of color vision, based on evidence that normal color perception depends upon retinal pigments that are sensitive to three primary wavelengths, blue, green, and red. Some investigators have argued that the retina also may have special sensitivity to yellow or violet, or both. Also called **three-component theory**.

trichromatism normal color vision; the capacity to distinguish the three primary color systems of light-dark, red-green, and blue-yellow. A **trichromat** is one who possesses normal color vision. Also called **trichromatopsia**. For the major forms of color blindness, see ANOMALOUS T.; DICHROMATISM; ACHROMATISM.

triclofos sodium: See CHLORAL DERIVATIVES.

tricyclic antidepressants a group of drugs developed in the 1950s and found to be effective in treating depression. T.a. function by preventing the passage of norepinephrine through the presynaptic membrane. T.a. are identified by their molecular structure which consists of three conjoined benzene rings with varied radicals attached to the middle ring. The prototype drug of the group is **imipramine hydrochloride**—$C_{19}H_{25}ClN_2$, which is used mainly in the treatment of psychotic, or endogenous, depression. Other t.a. are **amitriptyline**—$C_{20}H_{23}N$, **amitriptyline hydrochloride**—$C_{20}H_{23}N.HCl$, **desipramine hydrochloride**—$C_{18}H_{23}ClN_2$, **doxepin hydrochloride**—$C_{19}H_{22}ClNO$, **nortriptyline**—$C_{19}H_{21}N$, **nortriptyline hydrochloride**—$C_{19}H_{21}N.HCl$, **protriptyline hydrochloride**—$C_{19}H_{22}ClN$. A tricyclic drug that has hydantoinlike effects although it is related chemically to imipramine, **carbamazepine**—$C_{15}H_{22}N_2O$, is employed sometimes as an antiepileptic. T.a. are occasionally called thymoleptics. Abbrev.: TCA. See ANTIEPILEPTICS; HYDANTOINS; THYMOLEPTICS.

tridimensional theory of feeling Wundt's viewpoint that feeling has three dimensions: pleasantness-unpleasantness, tension-relaxation, and excitement-depression.

triethylene tetramine a substance sometimes used in the treatment of hepatolenticular degeneration, or Wilson's disease, a condition caused by excessive amounts of copper in the body tissues. T.t. was developed as an alternative medication for Wilson's-disease patients who develop tolerance with prolonged use of penicillamine, a previously developed treatment for this disease.

triflupromazine: See ALIPHATIC PHENOTHIAZINES.

trigeminal nerve the fifth and largest cranial nerve, which carries both sensory and motor fibers. The motor fibers are primarily involved with the muscles used in chewing, tongue movements, and swallowing. The sensory fibers innervate the same areas, including the teeth and most of the tongue in addition to the jaws. Some t.n. fibers innervate the cornea, face, scalp, and the dura mater membrane of the brain. The t.n. is referred to as "cranial nerve V."

trigeminal neuralgia: See TIC DOULOUREUX.

trigeminal nucleus either of two nuclei associated with the three main roots of the trigeminal nerve. One, the spinal t.n., extends downward in the medulla to the upper region of the spinal cord and receives fibers from pain and temperature receptors. The other, the main sensory t.n., receives large myelinated fibers from pressure receptors in the skin and relays impulses upward to the thalamus. Also see SPINAL T.N.

trigram a three-letter nonsense syllable used for experimental purposes.

trigraph: See DIGRAPH.

trihexyphenidyl hydrochloride: See ANTICHOLINERGICS.

triiodothyronine an iodine-containing amino acid that is one of the active principles of the thyroid gland. It has been found to be very similar to but much more potent than thyroxine, once believed to be the primary thyroid hormone.

trimester a period of approximately three months, as in referring to the first or third t. of pregnancy.

trimethadione: See OXAZOLIDINEDIONES.

trimipramine $C_{20}H_{26}N_2$—a tricyclic antidepressant drug. It is related structurally and pharmacologically to the other imipramine types of tricyclic antidepressants.

triolist a person who, in a three-way sexual relationship, enjoys both a heterosexual relationship with a partner and observing the partner in homosexual activities with a third person. The heterosexual relationship may be maintained with either or both of the homosexual partners.

triorchid a male having three testes.

triple alternation: See ALTERNATION METHOD.

triple insanity = FOLIE À TROIS.

triple-X condition a sex-chromosomal aberration characterized by the inheritance of three rather than the normal two X chromosomes which determine that an individual is a female. At one time considered to be a factor in mental retardation because the condition was found initially in mental hospital patients, the t.-X c. now is known to occur also in normal females who give birth to normal children.

triploid karyotype a chromosome combination in a cell nucleus that consists of three copies instead of the normal diploid (or two copies) for a tissue cell, or haploid (or one copy) for a germinal cell or gamete. An example would be an XXX sex-chromosome combination.

trisexuality in psychoanalysis, the representation in dreams of three aspects of sexuality—man, woman, and child—at the same time. The concept of the patient's desire to play the three roles symbolically and simultaneously is regarded as a manifestation of a tripartition of the mind.

triskaidekaphobia a morbid fear of the number 13; a superstitious attitude toward situations or events involving the number 13, such as 13 dinner guests, Friday the 13th, or a house, hotel room, or floor with that number. (T. sufferers could try to find solace in contemplation of the one-dollar bill: There are 13 stars over the eagle, 13 arrows in his claw, 13 stripes on his shield, and 13 leaves on his olive branch; the pyramid has 13 steps, and the legends "Annuit coeptis" and "E pluribus unum" each have 13 letters.)

trisomy /trī′sōmē/ a condition in which there are three instead of the usual two chromosomes in each cell nucleus. T. is the cause of several disorders.

trisomy 17-18 a congenital disorder marked by small-for-full-term offspring, with various facial anomalies, a prominent occiput, overlapping of the index finger over the third finger, and visual abnormalities. Severe mental retardation accompanies the defect which is due to nondisjunction of one of the chromosomes in the 17-18 group. Also called **Edward's syndrome**; **E trisomy**.

trisomy 13-15 = CHROMOSOME-13 TRISOMY.

trisomy 21 a condition associated with 85 percent of Down's-syndrome cases, characterized by the presence of three No. 21 chromosomes in the body cells rather than the normal pair. The extra chromosome may be contributed by either the father or the mother. Also called **21 trisomy; chromosome-21 trisomy; 47,XX+21**. This condition is often treated as synonymous with DOWN'S DISEASE. See this entry.

tristimulus value a hue as defined in terms of the percentage of the trichromatic primaries—red, green, and blue—needed to match it.

tritanopia a form of color blindness in which the subject has some loss of luminosity in the blue portion of the visual spectrum, apparently as a result of a blue-pigment deficiency. The condition differs from tetartanopia which is marked by a confusion of yellow and blue without loss of blue luminosity.

trochlear nerve the fourth cranial nerve containing the motor components of the superior oblique muscle of the eyeball. The t.n. is referred to as "cranial nerve IV." Also called **pathetic nerve**.

-trop-: See -TROPIC-.

Tropenkoller /trō′pənkôlər/ a culture-specific syndrome occurring among young males in Africa (German, "tropic rage"). Victims of the disorder, as well as victims of a similar disorder called **misala**, start quarrels and rapidly work themselves up to a frenzy of speech and wild gesticulation without apparent purpose or cause. The attack lasts from a few minutes to a few hours, after which the victim collapses in exhaustion.

-troph-; -tropho-; -trophy a combining form relating to nourishment or development (from Greek *trophe*, "food, nourishment"). Also see -TROPIC-.

Trömner, Ernst L. O. /trem′nər/ German neurologist, 1868—. Also spelled **Troemmer**. See HOFFMANN'S SIGN (also called **Trömner's sign**).

trophic function the activities associated with the ingestion of food substances and metabolism of the nutrient components. The term may also be applied to the perikaryon (cytoplasm) portion of a neuron to distinguish that function from the activity of impulse reception and transmission.

trophotropic process a term introduced in the 1930s by W. R. Hess to identify the CNS functions associated with arousal. T.p. was an outgrowth of the theory proposed earlier by Walter Cannon to explain the sympathetic and parasympathetic networks. Compare ERGOTROPIC PROCESS.

trophotropics drugs or other substances that may affect the brain so as to produce a condition of apathy.

-tropic-; -trop-; -tropy a combining form denoting a turning toward, influencing, or having an affinity for (from Greek *trope*, "turning"). This combining form is sometimes used instead of -trophic-; this use is wrong, but has become established as an alternative in certain expressions. See -TROPH-.

tropism a form of behavior observed in both plants and animals in which there is movement away from or toward a stimulus which often exists as a natural force, such as sunlight or gravity. The flower of a plant, e.g., may turn gradually to face the sun as it moves across the sky (heliotropism) while its roots follow magnetic lines of force and the pull of gravity. Also see NEGATIVE T.; POSITIVE T.; TAXES; GEOTROPISM; HELIOTROPISM; THERMOTROPISM; RHEOTROPISM.

tropotaxis: See TAXES.

Trotter, Wilfred Batten Lewis English surgeon, 1872–1939. See HERD INSTINCT.

truancy absence from school without permission. Persistent t. is described in DSM-III as a chronic violation of important rules, within the diagnostic category CONDUCT DISORDER, SOCIALIZED, NONAGGRESSIVE. See this entry.

true anxiety: See INSTINCTUAL ANXIETY.

true-false test: See SELECTIVE-ANSWER TEST.

true microcephaly = PURE MICROCEPHALY.

true self the total of an individual's potentialities that could be developed under ideal social and cultural conditions. The term is used in the context of Fromm's approach to neurosis as a reaction to cultural pressures and repressed potentialities. The realization of the t.s. is a major goal of therapy.

true symbolism symbolism that meets the following standards suggested by Ernest Jones, Rank, and Sachs: representation of unconscious material; constant or limited meaning; an evolutionary basis with regard to individual and race; nondependence on individual factors only; phylogenetic parallels with the symbolism found in myths, cults, and religions; and a linguistic link between the symbol and the symbolized idea.

truncated distribution a distribution of cases that lacks one or both extreme ends of the distribution of values, usually through a failure to obtain the appropriate cases.

trust: See BASIC T.; INTERPERSONAL T.

trust versus mistrust the first in the series of Erikson's eight stages of man. It covers the first year of life and corresponds roughly to Freud's oral stage. During this stage, the individual's attitudes toward trust or mistrust of other people and himself is influenced by the kind of care he receives. See ERIKSON'S EIGHT STAGES OF MAN. Also see BASIC TRUST; BASIC MISTRUST.

truth serum a common term for narcotic-type drugs such as Pentothal Sodium, ultrashort-acting barbiturates injected intravenously in subjects to help elicit information that has been consciously or unconsciously repressed. The term is derived from the reported use of narcotic drugs by police to extract confessions from criminals. T.s. has been used in war time to help identify amnesia victims found wandering in combat areas.

tryptamine derivatives a group of drugs that bear a chemical relationship to serotonin (5-hydroxytryptamine) and include a number of agents with psychedelic effects similar to those of LSD. The prototype of the series is **dimethyltryptamine (DMT)**—$C_{12}H_{16}N_2$—which occurs naturally in a variety of plants in many areas of the world. Other t.d. include **diethyltryptamine** —$C_{14}H_{20}N_2$, BUFOTENINE (see this entry), **psilocin**—$C_{12}H_{16}N_2O$, **psilocybin**—$C_{12}H_{17}N_2O_4P$. Psilocybin is essentially the same as psilocin, differing only by the addition of a phosphate radical which is rapidly metabolized in the body so that psilocybin is converted to psilocin. T.d. also may be classified as substituted indole alkamines. See PSYCHEDELICS.

tryptamines: See PSYCHEDELICS; TRYPTAMINE DERIVATIVES.

tryptophan one of the essential amino acids of the human diet and a precursor of the vasoconstricting drug serotonin. T. also is a precursor of the B vitamin niacin, which is needed to prevent the neurologic and other effects of pellagra.

TSA: See COMBINED TRANSCORTICAL APHASIA.

T-scope = TACHISTOSCOPE.

T scores a set of scores with mean equal to 50 and standard deviation equal to 10.

TSD = TAY-SACHS DISEASE.

TSH = THYROTROPIC HORMONE.

t test a statistical test giving the probability that two means have been drawn from the same population; also, a statistic divided by its standard error. Symbol: $t = (\bar{X}_1 - \bar{X}_2)/\sigma_{(\bar{x}_1 - \bar{x}_2)}$.

t test for independent groups a t test comparing two separate groups, each measured once, e.g., comparing hypnotizability of college students and high-school students. Also see T TEST FOR MATCHED GROUPS.

t test for matched groups a t test for the difference between two means obtained on a single group of subjects, or for the difference between two means in which the scores are significantly correlated. Also see T TEST FOR INDEPENDENT GROUPS.

TTS = TEMPORARY THRESHOLD SHIFT.

T type a type of eidetic imagery that persists after adolescence and is associated with *t*etany on the basis of blood mineral tests of the patients. In the T t. the imagery resembles the afterimage rather than the memory image (**B type**). Also called **tetany type**.

tubal ligation a surgical procedure leading to female sterilization by severing and closing the Fallopian-tube passageway between the ovaries and the uterus. T.l. does not affect sex drive, ability for coitus, or menstrual cycles, and in many cases the tubes can be reconnected if the woman desires to have more children.

tubal pregnancy = FALLOPIAN-TUBE PREGNANCY.

tubectomy the excision or tying of one or both of the Fallopian tubes.

tuberculomania an unfounded obsession that one has developed tuberculosis. Also called **phthisiomania**.

tuberculophobia = PHTHISIOPHOBIA.

tuberculosis an infectious inflammatory disease caused by the bacillus Mycobacterium tuberculosis. T. usually involves the lungs, mainly because the common route of infection is by inhaling infected droplets, although it also can be transmitted by infected urine or milk. By metastasis, t. can spread to the bones, kidneys, bladder, genitalia, adrenal glands, skin, and central nervous system. Abbrev.: **TB** (from *t*ubercle *b*acillus). Also see TUBERCULOUS MENINGITIS.

tuberculous meningitis a complication of tuberculosis in which an area of infection in the membrane lining the cerebral ventricles ruptures into the subarachnoid space. The invasion of the meninges may follow involvement of the blood vessels as a focus of tuberculosis. The symptoms resemble bacterial meningitis and may cause mental retardation, convulsions, or a form of hydrocephalus.

tuberous sclerosis a congenital disorder, transmitted as an autosomal-dominant trait, characterized by adenoma sebaceum, mental retardation, and seizures. Other anomalies may include brain tumors, visual disorders, and multiple large white macules that are present on the skin at birth. Many patients have average intelligence, but the IQ tends to decline as they grow older. Also called **epiloia; Bourneville's disease**.

tubocurarine an alkaloid drug obtained from the stems of Chondodendron and used to produce muscle relaxation during surgery. It raises the threshold for acetylcholine at the junctions of nerves and muscles by occupying the receptor sites. T. also blocks nerve transmission at ganglia.

tufted cell one of the special types of cells of the sense of smell. The tufted cells are found in a layer adjacent to the glomeruli of the olfactory bulb. Axons of the tufted cells pass through the anterior commissure to the olfactory bulb on the other side of the head while the dendrites join thousands of afferent fibers and the dendrites of the mitral cells in the olfactory glomeruli.

tuitional analysis = DIDACTIC ANALYSIS.

Tuke, Daniel Hack British psychiatrist, 1827–95. See MOON-PHASE STUDIES; DOUBLE INSANITY.

Tuke, William English philanthropist, 1732–1822. After visiting an asylum in which a fellow Quaker had mysteriously died, this coffee and tea merchant devoted 30 years of his life to improving the care of the mentally ill. Appalled by current conditions, he and the Society of Friends founded the York Retreat, and instituted a policy of nonrestraint, activities, and "personalized attention" that inaugurated a new era of humane treatment. However, this era did not come to full fruition until about 1850. See MORAL TREATMENT.

tulipmania: See MASS HYSTERIA.

tumescence a **tumefaction**, or condition of swelling or being swollen. The term sometimes is applied to the swelling of the cavernosum bodies of the penis or clitoris as a result of sexual stimulation or a similar **tumefacient**. Adjective: **tumescent**. Compare DETUMESCENCE.

tumor: See NEOPLASM.

tunica dartos a thin layer of smooth-muscle fibers around the base of the scrotum and extending along the undersurface of the penis. The fibers also form a septum of the scrotum. The action of the t.d. is one of slow contractions or relaxations that raise or lower the testes.

tuning fork a fork-shaped device with two tines, made of specially tempered steel, that emits a specific pure tone when struck.

tunnel vision a restriction in the field of vision that produces the effect of perceiving the world through a long tunnel or tube. Peripheral vision may be entirely lost. T.v. occurs in uncontrolled glaucoma and retinitis pigmentosa, and may also be a hysterical (conversion) symptom.

turbinator one of the raised, conchlike structures within the nasal cavity that deflect currents of inhaled air. The t. provides a blood-warmed surface that helps raise the temperature of inhaled air before it continues into the pharynx and lungs. It also directs an increased flow of air over olfactory receptors when an individual sniffs an aroma.

turf: See TERRITORIAL AGGRESSION.

Turner, Henry Hubert American endocrinologist, 1892–1970. See TURNER'S SYNDROME; MOSAICISM.

Turner's syndrome a chromosomal disorder marked by the absence of all or a part of one of the two X chromosomes in a female karyotype. The effects include sexual infantilism, webbing of the neck, short stature, and an IQ that is slightly below normal. Nerve deafness and space-perception abnormalities also may be present. The karyotype in most cases is 45,X, resulting in infertility, but the syndrome may occur in females who are fertile because of a 46,XX karyotype, or in 46,XY males. Also called **XO syndrome; gonadal dysgenesis; 45,X**.

turning inward: See ENTROPY.

turnover in industrial psychology, the tendency to change jobs voluntarily. T. records are frequently used to measure job tenure (how long workers remain on the job) as well as job satisfaction or dissatisfaction.

twelfth cranial nerve = HYPOGLOSSAL NERVE.

twenty-minute hour a term used by Castelnuovo-Tedesco for brief, supportive psychotherapy administered by a general physician. Suggestion, exhortation, advice, environmental manipulation, and prescription of drugs are among the techniques used in this type of therapy.

21 trisomy = TRISOMY 21.

twilight attacks a type of psychomotor seizure characterized by sudden changes in consciousness accompanied by meaningless speech and automatic movements.

twilight sleep a state of somnolence, or prolonged drowsiness, observed in cases of sleep drunkenness and sometimes maintained by hypnotic drugs for therapeutic purposes. In the latter case, interviews may be conducted during this state. The term t.s. applies also to a form of anesthesia induced during labor that permits the woman to remain sufficiently alert during pains to assist delivery-room personnel but at the same time keeps her drowsy enough to sleep between pains. This t.s. usually is produced by administration of a combination of a barbiturate drug and scopolamine. A possible complication is that the anesthetic tends to depress respiration for the infant. Also see SLEEP DRUNKENNESS; SLEEP TREATMENT; SOMNOLENCE.

twilight state a clouded state of consciousness in which the individual is temporarily unaware of his surroundings, experiences fleeting auditory or visual hallucinations, and responds to them by performing irrational acts such as undressing in public, running away, or committing violence. The disturbance occurs primarily in psychomotor epilepsy, dissociative reactions, and alcoholic intoxication. On regaining normal consciousness, the patient usually reports that he felt he was dreaming, but has little or no recollection of his behavior. Also see DREAM STATE; POSTEPILEPTIC T.S.

twilight vision = SCOTOPIC VISION.

twinning the simultaneous production of two or more embryos within a single uterus; or the production of two symmetrical objects from a single object by division.

twin studies research on twins with the *general* purpose of throwing light on the question of heredity versus environment with respect to intelligence, personality, and mental disorder, and for such *specific* purposes as (a) comparing the physical, mental, and social characteristics of identical and fraternal twins, (b) comparing twins of both types who have been reared together or reared apart, and (c) comparing twins with regard to such questions as prematurity, language use, gestures, mutual dependence, various forms of maladjustment, and severe illnesses such as bipolar disorder and schizophrenia. The twin-study procedure was originated by Francis Galton. Also called **twin-study method**. See KALLMANN; CONCORDANCE; DIZYGOTIC TWINS; MONOZYGOTIC TWINS; CO-TWIN CONTROL. Also see SIAMESE TWINS; SIBLING.

twisted symbols = STREPHOSYMBOLIA.

two-dimensional leader-behavior space = MANAGERIAL GRID.

two-factor design a factorial design in which two independent variables are manipulated.

two-factor theory a concept of avoidance learning proposed by O. H. Mowrer in which fear is attached to a neutral stimulus by pairing it with an adverse UCS, after which the subject learns to avoid the fear of the conditioned stimulus and thereby escapes the UCS.

two-neuron arc a type of polysynaptic nerve circuit in which an impulse must pass through an interneuron before firing a motoneuron. Each synapse adds about 8/10 of a millisecond to the travel time of a nerve impulse, thus responses that pass through multiple neurons and synapses usually require more time compared with more direct routing of impulses.

two-point discrimination the ability to sense the contact of a touch stimulus at two different points on the hand at the same time. The t.-p.d. test is employed in studies of the effects of parietal lesions of the brain, particularly in patients who have suffered missile wounds in the head. Also see SPATIAL THRESHOLD.

two-point threshold = SPATIAL THRESHOLD.

two-sided message a consumer-pychology technique in which an attempt is made to change the attitude of a subject by presenting both favorable and unfavorable arguments, rather than one side of an issue. Studies indicate the t.-s.m. has a greater effect on persons with higher education and those who believe that a source that presents both sides has greater credibility.

two-stage-memory theory a concept that information acquired by learning processes is stored first in an immediate-memory mechanism from which items are transferred into a permanent memory. The transfer priority may be based on the frequency of repetition in the immediate memory, as in the example of one's ability to store in the permanent memory telephone numbers that are repeated in the immediate memory.

two-tailed probability: See ONE-TAILED TEST; TWO-TAILED TEST.

two-tailed test a statistical test of an experimental hypothesis that does not specify the expected direction of an effect or a relationship; twice the probability of a one-tailed test. A **two-tailed probability** of .10 corresponds to a **one-tailed probability** of .05.

2,3,-benzopyrrole = INDOLE.

two-way analysis of variance a statistical test analyzing the joint and separate influences of two independent variables on a dependent variable.

two-way table a scatter diagram showing the distribution of two variables.

two-word stage of language development: See DUOS; TELEGRAPHIC SPEECH.

tybamate $C_{13}H_{26}N_2O_4$—a short-acting anxiolytic with pharmacologic effects similar to those of meprobamate. Because of its short metabolic half-life and its lack of risk of physical dependence, t. often is the drug of choice in treatment of certain anxiety and tension states associated with psychoneurotic disorders. Although t. is a butylcarbamic-acid derivative, its chemical formula is similar in structure to those of the propanediols.

tympanic cavity = MIDDLE EAR.

tympanic membrane a diaphragm that separates the external ear from the middle ear and serves as a device for transferring the pressure waves of sounds to a mechanical device in the form of the bony ossicles. Also called **eardrum**.

tympanic reflex a reaction of the muscles of the middle-ear ossicles to very loud sounds. The stapedius muscle and to a lesser extent the tensor tympani attenuate the sound intensity by deflecting the ossicles. Studies show the t.r. can reduce sound intensities transmitted through the middle ear by the equivalent of as much as 20 decibels.

tympanometry the measurement of mobility, or changes in pressure of the external and middle ear. Negative pressure would be an index of congestion and possible transitory hearing loss.

tympanoplasty a reconstructive surgical procedure on the eardrum or the middle ear to improve hearing. The extent of preoperative conductive-hearing loss is determined by audiometric testing.

tympanum /tim'-/ an alternative term for (a) the middle ear, or tympanic cavity, and (b) the eardrum, or tympanic membrane.

Type A behavior a life-style pattern associated with increased risk of coronary heart disease and marked by a tendency to clench teeth and fists, rapid body movements, impatience, and **polyphasic activity** such as shaving or eating while reading a newspaper or making business telephone calls. Some research also indicates an obsession with numbers. See TYPE A PERSONALITY.

Type A personality a personality pattern outlined by California physicians Meyer Friedman and Ray H. Rosenman in the 1970s to identify a person whose life-style predisposes him or her to coronary heart disease. The Type A individual is highly competitive in recreational activities as well as in work, suppresses fatigue, and shows hostility when efforts to meet deadlines are frustrated.

Type B behavior a behavior pattern that is free of aggression and hostility, marked by an absence of time urgency and lack of a compulsive need to display or discuss one's accomplishments and achievements. See TYPE B PERSONALITY.

Type B chronic bronchitis: See BLUE BLOATER.

Type B personality a personality pattern outlined by California physicians Meyer Friedman and Ray H. Rosenman to distinguish the patient from the Type A personality. The Type B individual can relax without feeling guilty, work without being easily frustrated, and participate in sports or other recreational activities without feeling a need to prove his superiority or abilities.

type fallacy the view that individuals can be classified as distinct types, although evidence shows that human characteristics form a continuum.

Type V glycogen-storage disease = MCARDLE'S DISEASE.

Type I conditioning = PAVLOVIAN CONDITIONING.

Type I error the rejection of the null hypothesis when it is in fact true. An experimenter makes this error when he believes he has detected an effect or a relationship, although neither is present in reality.

Type R conditioning = INSTRUMENTAL CONDITIONING.

Type S conditioning = PAVLOVIAN CONDITIONING.

Type III glycogenosis = CORI'S DISEASE.

type-token ratio an index of the ratio between repetition and variety of words used by an individual in verbal communication. The t.-t.r. is used in psychotherapy to evaluate a patient. The greater the variety of words compared with the repetition of words the higher the index.

Type II conditioning = INSTRUMENTAL CONDITIONING.

Type II error the acceptance of the null hypothesis when it is false. An experimenter makes this error when he concludes that a particular effect or relationship is not present, whereas in fact it is. Also called **beta error**.

Type II hyperlipoproteinemia: See XANTHOMATOSIS.

typewriter for the blind: See TALKING TYPEWRITER.

typhoid fever a bacterial infection caused by Salmonella typhi, which is harbored in human excrement and transmitted through contaminated foods and beverages, e.g., shellfish collected near a sewage outlet. About five percent of recovered patients become carriers and are thereafter able to transmit the disease to others. Symptoms mainly are sore throat, vomiting, bronchitis, or nephritis. A neural effect is **meningismus psychosis**.

typhomania = HYPERMANIA.

typology in psychiatry, a classification of individuals into types according to specific criteria. The first known t. was Hippocrates' humoral theory. See CONSTITUTIONAL TYPE; HUMORAL THEORY; PERSONALITY TYPES.

tyramine a sympathomimetic substance found in a variety of sources, including ripe cheese, ergot, mistletoe, wines, and decaying animal tissue. T. resembles epinephrine, producing increased blood pressure and heart action. Foods containing t. react with MAO inhibitor drugs which prevent normal metabolism of the t., resulting in a greatly aggravated effect on blood pressure. As a consequence, the patient may suffer a hypertensive crisis.

tyrosinase-negative albinism; tyrosinase-positive albinism: See ALBINISM.

tyrosine a nonessential amino acid present in most proteins and a precursor of the adrenergic stimulators dopamine, norepinephrine, and epinephrine, which differ structurally only in the radicals at one position of the molecule. T. is in turn derived from the essential amino acid phenylalanine.

Tyson, Edward English anatomist, 1649–1708. See TYSON'S GLANDS; SMEGMA.

Tyson's glands sebaceous glands located on the corona glandis of the penis and the inner surface of the prepuce. Also called **preputial glands; glandulae preputiales**. Also see SMEGMA.

U

UCR = UNCONDITIONED RESPONSE.

Ucs: See SYSTEMATIC APPROACH.

UCS = UNCONDITIONED STIMULUS.

U fibers nerve pathways that run through pyramidal-cell white matter from one cortical neuron to another. The U f. are believed to be the fastest route of impulses in cortical transmission, as the alternative pathway is composed of very fine fibers that are associated with slow transmission rates.

UFOs /yōō′ef′ōs′/ or /yōō′fōs/ unidentified flying objects; in Jung's view, "a living myth... a product of the unconscious archetype... involuntary, automatic projections based on instinct... whose simple, round form portrays the archetype of the self... and is therefore best suited to compensate the split-mindedness of our age." ("*Should* it be that an unknown physical phenomenon is the outward cause of the myth, this would detract nothing from the myth...") (*Civilization in Transition*) See MYTHOLOGICAL THEMES; MANDALA.

ulcer an erosion of a tissue surface, such as the mucosal lining of the digestive tract. **Peptic ulcers**, which affect the stomach and duodenum, are associated with increased secretion of hydrochloric acid and **pepsin**, a digestive enzyme, during periods of emotional stress. Other causative factors of peptic u. may include the patient's blood group and the use of certain medications such as aspirin. Also see GASTRODUODENAL ULCERATION.

ulcerative colitis: See COLITIS.

ulcer personality a personality pattern that appears to be associated with proneness to the formation of peptic ulcers. According to Franz Alexander, ulcer patients tend to be tense, hard-driving, and aggressive on the surface but passive and dependent underneath. B. Mittelmann and H. G. Wolff denied that they are always hard-driving, but agreed that they have strong dependency longings which, if frustrated, lead to gastric disturbances.

-ule-; -ulo- a combining form relating to (a) scars and scar tissue, (b) the gums.

Ullrich, Otto /ōōl′rish/ German pediatrician, 1894 –1957. See BONNEVIE-ULLRICH SYNDROME; NIELSEN'S DISEASE.

ultradian rhythm a periodic change in physiological and psychological processes that is believed to have a cycle shorter than one day. Also see INFRADIAN RHYTHM.

ultrashort-acting barbiturates barbiturates that are rapidly absorbed from the stomach and usually produce an immediate effect on the subject. U.-a.b. apparently are absorbed more rapidly because they have a weaker level of acidity, a factor which also enhances rapid absorption from the small intestine. Fast-acting barbiturates are almost completely metabolized while long-acting barbiturates may be excreted in virtually unchanged form.

ultrasonic irradiation in psychiatry, a substitute for prefrontal lobotomy in which sound waves of a frequency of approximately 1,000,000 cycles per second are directed through trephine openings in the skull, as opposed to surgical excision of prefrontal tissue. The risk is said to be minimized, the damage less severe, and the results at least as positive.

ultrasound technique the use of devices, e.g., **sonogram**, that generate sound frequencies beyond the range of human hearing for diagnostic and therapeutic procedures. By analyzing echoes of the sound waves reflected from tissue surfaces of varying densities, images of internal organs and structures can be recorded. Heat generated by ultrasound waves can also be utilized to destroy areas of diseased tissue, e.g, nervous-system lesions.

ultraviolet absorption absorption of ultraviolet wavelengths of light by substances. U.a. activity by olfactory receptors is necessary for the perception of odors, according to one theory.

ululation the incoherent wailing of a psychotic or hysterical individual (from Latin *ululare*, "to cry out, yell").

umbilical cord a cordlike structure containing two arteries and a vein in a cylindrical membrane that connects the fetus to the placenta during pregnancy.

umbilicus the navel. Also called **omphalus**.

Umwelt /ōōm′velt/ in the existential philosophy of Martin Heidegger, the first and nearest world of the body and its attributes (German, "surrounding world"). Also see EIGENWELT; MITWELT.

unanticipated crisis = ACCIDENTAL CRISIS.

unbiased estimate an estimate formulated on the basis of a representative sample. See U.E. OF VARIANCE.

unbiased estimate of variance a variance estimate that has been corrected for the fact that extremely high or low scores are unlikely to occur in a small sample, leading to an underestimate of the variance. The correction is made by using N–1 in place of N in the denominator, thereby slightly increasing the estimate: $s^2 = \Sigma(X-\bar{X})^2/(N-1)$.

uncanny emotions a term used by Sullivan for the sense of weirdness and unreality that sometimes accompanies dreams, nightmares, states of intoxication, and schizophrenic reactions. These feelings are believed to hark back to anxiety-provoking experiences in childhood, which now threaten to invade consciousness and therefore inspire dread, horror, and a feeling of unfamiliarity. See NOT-ME.

uncertainty-arousal factor in psychological esthetics, a scale of visual-pattern response that may reflect autonomic reactions by a subject to a work of art, as opposed to cortical arousal. The factor contains simple-complex, clear-indefinite, and disorderly-orderly components, which are said to reflect subjective uncertainty.

uncertainty factor a term used in psychological esthetics to describe subject responses to a work of art that include high positive ratings on simple-complex and clear-indefinite scales and high negative ratings on a disorderly-orderly scale.

uncertainty level in psychological esthetics, the interval between the upper and lower levels of differences in judgments.

uncinate fasciculus a bundle of nerve fibers that connects the anterior and inferior portions of the frontal lobe, appearing as a compact bundle as the fasciculus bends around the lateral sulcus while spreading into a fan shape at either end.

uncivilized: See PRIMITIVE.

unconcernedness: See BOHEMIAN U.

unconditional positive regard a term used by C. Rogers for an attitude of concern, acceptance, and warmth on the part of the therapist, which he considered most conducive to self-awareness and personality growth on the part of the client. Rogers applies the term also to the mother's spontaneous love and affection given without conditions, a universal need in infancy and a prerequisite for healthy development. The mother's u.p.r. is internalized by the child and contributes to the development of an enduring sense of self-worth. U.p.r. does not imply license; Rogers maintains that disapproval of specific types of behavior can be expressed without withdrawing love or inducing feelings of unworthiness. Compare CONDITIONAL POSITIVE REGARD.

unconditioned reflex an innate, unlearned, reflexive response to a stimulus, as in salivation at the sight or smell of food. See UNCONDITIONED RESPONSE.

unconditioned response the unlearned response to an unconditioned stimulus; any original response that occurs naturally and in the absence of conditioning, e.g., in Pavlov's experiment, the dog's salivation. The u.r. serves as the basis for establishment of the conditioned response, and it is frequently reflexive in nature. Abbrev.: **UCR; UR**. Compare CONDITIONED RESPONSE.

unconditioned stimulus a stimulus that elicits an unconditioned response, as in withdrawal from a hot radiator, contraction of the pupil to light, or salivation when food is in the mouth. Abbrev.: **UCS; US**. Also see CONDITIONED STIMULUS.

unconscious a term meaning, as an adjective, an absence of awareness, as in a coma or sleep, or in phrases like "u. prejudice." As a noun, particularly in psychoanalytic theory, it refers to the division or region of the psyche that contains memories, emotional conflicts, wishes, and repressed impulses that are not directly accessible to awareness, but which have dynamic effects on thought and behavior. Dreams, fantasies, slips of the tongue, and neurotic symptoms are all manifestations of u. processes. See COLLECTIVE U.; FAMILIAL U.; PERSONAL U.; RACIAL U. Also see SYSTEMATIC APPROACH.

unconscious cerebration thinking that occurs in the absence of awareness. See INCUBATION.

unconscious factors influences operating beneath the level of consciousness, such as repressed experiences, latent impulses, defense mechanisms, buried feelings, memories, and, in Jung, the contents of the racial or collective unconscious.

unconscious fantasies = PRIMAL FANTASIES.

unconscious guilt a sense of guilt or, as Freud preferred to say, an unconscious need for punishment, produced by hidden impulses that conflict with the precepts of the superego.

unconscious homosexuality: See LATENT HOMOSEXUALITY.

unconscious impulses: See UNCONSCIOUS MOTIVATION.

unconscious memory in psychoanalysis, a memory that has been forced from the conscious into the unconscious level of the mind. See REPRESSION.

unconscious motivation wishes, impulses, aims, and drives of which we are not aware. Examples of behavior produced by u.m. are purposive accidents, slips of the tongue, and dreams that express unfulfilled wishes.

unconscious process a psychic process that takes place in the unconscious, e.g. repression or symbolization.

unconscious resistance: See RESISTANCE.

unconventional virus one of the slow viruses, disease agents that are viruslike and may remain dormant in the body for a number of years before producing signs or symptoms of disease. Disorders associated with u.v. include kuru and

Creutzfeldt-Jakob disease. Compare CONVEN-
TIONAL VIRUS.

uncorrelated axes: See ORTHOGONAL.

uncovering techniques techniques directed toward breaking through the patient's repressions
to bring latent conflicts and traumatic experiences to the surface where they can be studied.
Such techniques include sodium-Amytal interviews, hypnotherapy, and free association.

uncriticalness a nonjudgmental attitude on the
part of the therapist, which is considered essential in C. Rogers' nondirective approach as well
as other forms of psychotherapy, since criticism
tends to inhibit the patient's efforts to recognize
and revise his own self-defeating patterns.

uncus a part (Latin, "hook") of the rhinencephalon
near, but separated from, the temporal pole of
the cerebral cortex. It is associated with neural
pathways of the olfactory-organ connections to
the brain.

underachiever a person, usually a student, who
achieves far below his demonstrated capacity,
especially if aptitude or general-intelligence
scores exceed achievement scores by 30 percent.
Underachievement may be specific to an area of
study or it may be general. It is far more prevalent among boys than girls and is quite common
in bright and even gifted children. It is also
prevalent among average students and the educable mentally retarded. Also see ACADEMIC-
UNDERACHIEVEMENT DISORDER. Compare OVER-
ACHIEVER.

underage: See OVERAGE.

underarousal a physiological response to a stimulus that is inadequate to initiate an expected
action.

undercontrolled pertaining to a type of childhood
behavior that is marked by a lack of sufficient
self-control expected for a person of a particular
age and in a particular setting. Kinds of u.
behavior include hyperactivity and conduct
disorders.

underdog the descriptive term with which F. Perls
refers to the rationalizations and self-justifi-
cations employed by an individual to allay the
sense of guilt or shame arising from an inability
to meet the demands of internal moral standards
or other rules of conduct. See GESTALT THERAPY.
Also see TOPDOG.

undermanning the condition in which the number
of persons available for a program or function
falls below the MAINTENANCE MINIMUM. See this
entry. Compare OVERMANNING.

underpayment in industrial psychology, a form of
inequity that leads to job dissatisfaction, lack of
motivation, and in some cases lowered productivity.

undersocialized characterizing an individual
who has not developed adequate social feelings
and social relationships, and who tends to be
egocentric and unconcerned about others. See
CONDUCT DISORDER, UNDERSOCIALIZED, AGGRES-
SIVE; CONDUCT DISORDER, UNDERSOCIALIZED,
NONAGGRESSIVE.

undersocialized, aggressive reaction: See CON-
DUCT DISORDER, UNDERSOCIALIZED, AGGRESSIVE.

undersocialized, nonaggressive reaction: See
CONDUCT DISORDER, UNDERSOCIALIZED, NON-
AGGRESSIVE.

understanding the process of insight or comprehension of information acquired from unrelated
or related observations and organized through a
flexible framework of personal knowledge. In
counseling and psychotherapy, u. may refer to
the process of discerning the network of relationships existing between a client's behavior
and his environment, history, aptitudes, motivation, ideas, feelings, relationships, and modes
of expression.

understimulation theory the theory that severe
anxiety and other psychological disturbances can
be caused by insufficient stimulation. The theory
is based on studies of sensory-deprivation
effects. The u.t. has been used to explain vandalism and other crimes that occur in urban settings where young people lack exposure to a
great variety of environmental stimuli. See DI-
VERSIVE EXPLORATION.

undescended testicle = ARRESTED TESTIS.

undifferentiated schizophrenia a term applied to
schizoprenic cases that exhibit a wide variety of
symptoms cutting across the four major types
(simple, catatonic, paranoid, hebephrenic or
disorganized). Two types have been distinguished in some classifications: In the acute undifferentiated type, the symptoms manifest
themselves suddenly, but unrelated to external
stress. In the chronic undifferentiated type, they
develop insidiously and there is no acute attack;
the patient grows apathetic and "settles down"
with the disorder despite poor adjustment. See
SCHIZOPHRENIC DISORDER, UNDIFFERENTIATED
TYPE.

undinism an alternative terms for UROLAGNIA and
UROPHILIA. See these entries.

undoing in psychoanalysis, an unconscious defense
mechanism in which attempts are made to counteract guilty impulses or behavior through acts
of atonement and expiation. A healthy individual tries to make amends by apologizing,
making restitution, or bestowing gifts. An obsessive-compulsive individual, on the other hand,
seeks to rid himself of guilt by magical or symbolic means, such as washing his hands every few
minutes, repeatedly saying the same prayer, or
counting to one hundred all day long. A catatonic schizophrenic may go to the further extreme
of seeking to undo the sins of mankind by holding his arms in a gesture of blessing for days or
weeks on end. Also see SACRIFICE.

undulant fever: See BRUCELLOSIS.

unemotional thought a term employed by S.
Rado for the highest evolutionary level of integration, at which action and self-control are
based on reason, logic, science, and common
sense.

ung. an abbreviation used in prescriptions, meaning "ointment" (Latin *unguentum*).

ungual fibromas small tumors that develop along the nail beds. The wartlike growths are composed of connective tissue and may be a diagnostic sign of tuberous sclerosis.

unidentified flying objects = UFOS.

unidimensional containing a single dimension, or composed of a pure factor. Compare MULTIDIMENSIONAL.

uniform-density factor: See LAW OF COMMON FATE.

uniformism a concept applied to total adherence to the standards and behavior of one's peer group.

unilateral lesion a lesion that involves an area of one hemisphere, left or right, with effects that may vary according to the dominance of the hemisphere and the function affected. The u.l. effect generally is on the contralateral side.

unilateral neglect a visual-spatial disorder associated with lesions of the parietal lobe. It is characterized by a tendency of the patient to neglect or ignore the extrapersonal space on the side of the body opposite the location of the lesion. A patient with a right-side lesion may show inattention for space on the left side, an effect that can influence reading or drawing performance.

unilateral sensorimotor cortex lesion any interruption of function caused by destruction of normal tissue in the sensorimotor area of a single hemisphere of the brain. A u.s.c.l. may affect certain tactual functions such as roughness discrimination without altering the ability of a subject to make size judgments through the sense of touch.

unimodal describing a frequency distribution having a single mode, that is, one peak; describing anything that has only one dimension.

unio mystica = MYSTIC UNION.

uniovular twins = DIZYGOTIC TWINS.

uniparous = PRIMIPAROUS.

unipolar depression a form of manic-depressive illness in which there are recurrent episodes of depression without episodes of mania. The term also may be applied to depression patients whose first-degree relatives have not exhibited symptoms of mania.

unipolar manic-depressive psychosis a manic-depressive illness characterized by one type of episode, usually recurrent depression.

unipolar neuron a nerve cell in which the cell body is connected to an axon but there is no dendrite. The term may be misleading since a u.n. has a dendritic zone at the end opposite from the synaptic terminals, as does a normal bipolar cell. However, the cell body, or perikaryon, of a u.n. is outside the fibrous process rather than inside as is the case with other types of neurons.

unipolar psychosis a severe affective disorder characterized by recurrent depressive episodes or, far more rarely, recurrent manic episodes. See BIPOLAR DISORDER, DEPRESSED; BIPOLAR DISORDER, MANIC; BIPOLAR DISORDER, MIXED.

unique trait a personality trait that is observed in only one individual or one member of a population, or seldom found in the same form.

unisex a life-style marked by an interchange of sex roles in clothing choices, work assignments, and other environmental factors, such as gifts of dolls or other traditional "female" toys to boys and "male" gifts to girls.

unitary consciousness: See CROWD BEHAVIOR.

unit character an inherited characteristic that is transmitted to an offspring in its entirety.

United Nations Declaration on the Rights of Mentally Retarded Persons: See RIGHTS OF THE MENTALLY RETARDED.

United States Employment Service Basic Occupational Literacy Test: See USES BASIC OCCUPATIONAL LITERACY TEST.

unitization of services the administrative division of a large hospital into several autonomous units, usually on the basis of function (psychiatry, obstetrics, etc.), but sometimes on the basis of geographical areas from which it draws its patients.

unity and fusion in altered states of consciousness, an affective state in which the normal differentiation between self and environment may seem to recede or disappear while the individual experiences a sense of merging, fusing, or uniting with persons, objects, nature, or the universe. Also see MYSTIC UNION.

univariate characterized by a single variable.

universality: See MOB PSYCHOLOGY.

universal phobias a term applied by Freud to "common phobias," which consist of an exaggerated, intensified fear of situations and objects which everyone detests or fears to some extent, such as night, death, illness, solitude, snakes, and dangers in general.

universal psychological motives: See PSYCHOLOGICAL MOTIVE.

universal symbol in psychoanalysis, an object or idea that has the same significance for all humans, regardless of their culture, e.g., dreams of pointed objects symbolizing the penis.

unlearning: See DECONDITIONING.

Unlust: See UNPLEASURE.

unobtrusive measures measures that can be obtained without the subject's awareness, or without disturbing or alerting the subject, whose behavior is thus assumed to be unaffected by the investigative process. Compare REACTIVE MEASURES.

unpleasantness an affect or feeling characterized by disagreeableness, dislike, and aversion.

unpleasure in psychoanalysis, a term used to describe the psychic pain, tension, and "ego suffering" that is consciously felt when instinctual needs and wishes (such as hunger and sex) are blocked by the ego and denied gratification. (The term is a translation of the German word *Unlust*, meaning literally "listlessness.") See EGO.

unproductive mania = MANIC STUPOR.

unreality: See DEPERSONALIZATION.

unselective observation: See NATURALISTIC OBSERVATION.

unsocialized disturbance of conduct a childhood behavioral disorder marked by disobedience, hostility, and aggressiveness.

unspaced practice a learning method in which no intervals or rest periods are allowed between trials.

unspecified mental retardation a diagnostic category comprising individuals of any age who are presumed to be retarded, but who are too impaired or uncooperative to be evaluated by standard intelligence tests. (DSM-III)

unspecified substance dependence a substance-use disorder in which the individual is dependent on a substance that is not yet known. (DSM-III)

unstructured characterizing an object or stimulus that does not have a definite pattern, such as materials used in projective techniques (ink blots, ambiguous pictures).

unstructured autobiography: See AUTOBIOGRAPHY.

upper respiratory infection: See COMMON COLD.

uppers a colloquial term for STIMULANTS. See this entry.

uprooting neurosis a term applied by Hans Strauss (1957) to neurotic reactions precipitated by immigrating to a strange land with residence among people who speak a different language and have a different life style. Also see MIGRATION ADAPTATION.

upsilon /yōŏp′silon/ or /up′-/ 20th letter of the Greek alphabet (Υ, υ).

upward mobility the movement of a person or group from one social class to a higher social class. U.m. tends to be a feature of certain relatively relaxed class systems operating within expanding economies. Also see SOCIAL MOBILITY. Compare DOWNWARD MOBILITY.

UR = UNCONDITIONED RESPONSE.

UR = UTILIZATION REVIEW.

-uran-; -urano- a combining form relating (a) to the palate, (b) to the sky (from Greek *ouranos*, "sky, roof of the mouth").

uraniscolalia a speech difficulty due to a CLEFT PALATE. See this entry.

uranism homosexuality, usually in the male. The term, now obsolete, was coined by K. H. Ulrichs in 1862, derived from Aphrodite Urania, the source of heavenly love between males according to Greek mythology.

uranophobia a morbid fear of heaven or the sky. Also see SIDEROPHOBIA.

uranoschisis = CLEFT PALATE.

Urbach, Erich American dermatologist, 1893–1946. See URBACH-WIETHE DISEASE.

Urbach-Wiethe disease an inherited lipid-protein-storage disease marked by lipid-protein deposits in cutaneous and mucous tissues, calcification of brain tissues, photosensitivity, alopecia-type loss of hair, short stature, and mental disturbances including epileptic seizures, memory loss, and rage attacks. Also called **Rössle-Urbach-Wiethe lipoproteinosis.**

Urban, Frank M. American (?) psychophysicist, fl. 1927. See MÜLLER-URBAN WEIGHTS.

urbanization the trend toward living in cities, which are defined by the United States Bureau of the Census as all central cities with populations of 50,000 or more. Some studies in sociocultural psychiatry have shown that overall rates of psychiatric disorder are higher in urban than in rural areas and are disproportionately concentrated in the lowest social class, especially in the case of schizophrenia and personality disorders with their antisocial subtypes. These findings, however, are contradicted by other studies that indicate better overall mental health among urban dwellers than among the rural population. There are also studies that indicate that the effect on mental health of migration to the city varies with the degree of discrimination and acceptance in the new setting.

Urban's weights = MÜLLER-URBAN WEIGHTS.

Ur-defenses /ŏŏr′-/ a term applied by J. Masserman to three fundamental beliefs that help to protect us from anxiety: the delusion of invulnerability and immortality; the delusion of the omnipotent servant in the form of an abstract being or principle; and the conviction of man's ultimate goodness and kindness (from German *Ur-*, "primeval").

ureaplasma urealyticum one of the infectious mycoplasma strains associated with NONGONOCOCCAL URETHRITIS. See this entry. Also see T-MYCOPLASMA.

uremia the accumulation in the blood of waste products ordinarily excreted in the urine. U. is a complication of several forms of kidney disease resulting in a failure of the functioning units of the organ to filter out the urine products. If uncorrected at an early stage, u. may be fatal. Also see AZOTEMIA; KIDNEY DISEASE.

-ureter-; -uretero- a combining form relating to the ureters, the pair of tubes that conduct urine from the kidneys to the bladder.

ureterostomy an artificial opening in the body surface to permit the excretion of urine. In most cases, the u. is created in the perineum, or pelvic floor; an alternative procedure involves joining the ureters to the digestive tract at the colon. A u. is performed in the treatment of cancer or a dysfunction of the kidneys or bladder. It also may be performed when spinal-cord damage causes incontinence.

urethra a membrane-lined tube or canal that carries urine from the bladder to an external opening of the body. In the male, the u. is contained in the corpus spongiosum column of the penis and extends over a distance of about 20 centimeters (8 inches). In the female, the u. is less than four centimeters in length and runs almost directly to an opening above the vaginal orifice.

urethral anxiety a type of anxiety and tension

associated with urination, particularly when urinating in a public place.

urethral character in psychoanalysis, a personality type characterized by a long-term history of bed-wetting and a pattern of traits acquired as a reaction formation to the shame and humiliation associated with enuresis, namely, excessive ambition, lack of perseverance, and boastfulness.

urethral complex a concept introduced by H. A. Murray to describe a psychological state between the Freudian oral and anal stages of development. The u.c. personality is manifested by an overly ambitious, strongly narcissistic adult with an obsession for immortality. Also called **Icarus complex**.

urethral eroticism in psychoanalysis, sexual pleasure derived from urination. Fixation at the urethral stage may lead to fantasies or wishes concerning urinating on others or being urinated on. See UROLAGNIA.

urethral phase a stage of psychological development that represents a transition from the anal to the phallic stage with some characteristics of both stages. It involves conflicts about urethral control, resolution of which leads to pride, self-competence, and gender identity.

urethritis an inflammation of the urethra. The causative agent may be a sexually transmitted disease, e.g., gonorrhea, or a nonspecific organism. See GONORRHEA; NONGONOCOCCAL U.

URI: See COMMON COLD.

-uria; -urin-; -uro- a combining form relating to urine or the urinary system.

urinary-tract infection an infection, usually bacterial, that affects the genitourinary (GU) system from the kidneys to the urethra. GU infections are a common type of bacterial invasion and are ten times as likely to affect females as males. A u.-t.i. usually enters the GU tract of small children through the circulatory or lymphatic system, but in older children and adults the infection generally spreads upward from the urethra through the bladder. A u.-t.i. can be a serious complication in a case of spinal-cord injury. Until World War II, a u.-t.i. was a leading cause of death among persons suffering a spinal-cord injury.

urination: See MICTURITION REFLEXES.

urning an obsolete term for a male homosexual who plays the female role in contacts with other males. **Urninde** is the corresponding term for a female homosexual playing the passive role with other females. For the derivation of these terms from Aphrodite Urania, see URANISM.

-uro-: See -URIA-.

urolagnia a morbid preoccupation with urine and urination; the tendency to derive pleasure or sexual excitement from watching others urinate, from being urinated on during sexual intercourse, or from drinking one's own urine. Also see URETHRAL EROTICISM.

urophilia a psychosexual disorder marked by a pathologic interest in urine. Also see UROLAGNIA; URETHRAL EROTICISM.

urticaria = HIVES.

US = UNCONDITIONED STIMULUS.

use law: See LAW OF FREQUENCY.

USES Basic Occupational Literacy Test a test provided by the United States Employment Service for assessing the literacy skills of educationally deficient adults, and evaluated in terms of occupational literacy requirements. The test covers vocabulary, reading comprehension, arithmetic computation, and arithmetic reasoning. Abbrev.: **BOLT**.

ut dict. an abbreviation used in prescriptions, meaning "as directed" (Latin *ut dictum*).

-uter-; -utero- a combining form relating to the womb (uterus).

uteromania an obsolete term for NYMPHOMANIA. See this entry.

uteroplacental insufficiency an inability of the placenta to sustain the life of a fetus because of hormonal, circulatory, or other types of dysfunction that interfere with normal exchange of metabolic products between the uterus and the placenta.

uterus the hollow muscular organ in female mammals in which the offspring develops from a fertilized ovum until birth. Also called **womb**. Also see WANDERING U.; -HYSTER-.

utilization review periodic review by a specially appointed committee of the quality of services rendered in a hospital, as well as the use of its facilities. Abbrev.: **UR**.

utricle the larger of the two membranous sacs in the labyrinth of the inner ear. It communicates with the semicircular canals associated with the sense of balance and also receives the utricular filaments of the acoustic nerve.

uveal tract: See EYE STRUCTURE.

uvula a fleshy appendage that hangs from the soft palate as the palatine u. Other uvulas are located in the urinary bladder and the cerebellum. Plurals: **uvulas; uvulae**.

uxoricide the murder of a wife by her husband (from Latin *uxor*, "wife," and *-cide*, from *caedere*, "to kill").

V

V = VERBAL ABILITY. Also see PRIMARY ABILITIES.

vaccination the introduction into the body of a suspension of killed or attenuated bacteria, viruses, or rickettsiae to produce an immunity. The immunity results from the body's production of antibodies which will resist the invasion of live organisms of the same specific species and strain in future contacts with the disease agents.

vaccinophobia a morbid fear of being vaccinated.

vacuum activity a distorted or incomplete response that may be observed when motivational energy accumulates in a neural center but an appropriate releasing stimulus does not occur. The motivational energy forces its way past the inhibitory blocking system to cause the v.a.

vagabond neurosis = DROMOMANIA.

vagal lobes bulges of new tissue that appear on the medulla of some species, e.g., fish, representing the solitary tracts and nuclei of the sense-of-taste system. The relative size of the v.l. is related to the importance of the sense of taste in the species and the number of taste buds. In fish, which may have 100,000 taste buds over the entire body, the v.l. can be extremely large.

vagina a sheathlike structure (Latin, "sheath") in a mammalian female that leads from the uterus to the external genital-canal orifice.

vagina dentata in psychoanalysis, the fantasy, usually unconscious, that the vagina is a mouth "with teeth" (Latin *dentata*) that can castrate the male partner. In females the fantasy is believed to stem from intense penis envy and a desire to castrate the partner as an act of revenge. In males it is believed to stem from castration anxiety.

vaginal administration: See ADMINISTRATION.

vaginal barrel an alternative term for vagina.

vaginal canal the portion of the vagina that extends from the orifice to a point just behind its attachment to the cervix. The walls of the canal, formed by a muscular coat with an internal mucous lining, contain a layer of erectile tissue.

vaginal envy a psychological characteristic of males who desire the ability to become pregnant and bear children. V.e. may be expressed by male transsexuals and transvestites in Western cultures and has been observed in rituals and ceremonies of societies that regard menstruation and childbirth as sacred functions. Also see WOMB ENVY; FEMININITY COMPLEX.

vaginal father in psychoanalysis, a male who dreams or fantasizes that he has a vagina. This wish is believed to arise from strong identification with the mother and is associated with feminine, nonaggressive behavior, an intense rivalry with women, and the performance of wifely duties in marriage.

vaginal hypoesthesia relative frigidity, in which sensitivity is limited to the clitoral area.

vaginal orgasm a peak of genital excitation experienced through the vagina and usually marked by vasocongestion and contraction of the vaginal tissues during the plateau phase of the female sexual response.

vaginalplasty: See PLASTIC SURGERY.

vaginal plethysmograph: See PLETHYSMOGRAPH.

vaginismus a painful vaginal spasm that occurs during or immediately preceding sexual intercourse, causing intercourse to be painful or impossible. No physical cause can be ascertained in most cases, and psychological factors can often be found. Also called **vaginism**. See FUNCTIONAL V.; PSYCHIC V.

vaginitis an inflammation of the vagina, often characterized by the appearance of a whitish, nonbloody discharge from the vagina. The cause may be postmenopausal use of estrogens, gonorrhea, Trichomonas, Candida infections, or a nonmalignant cervical disorder.

vagus nerve the tenth cranial nerve, a mixed nerve with both sensory and motor fibers. The sensory fibers innervate the external ear, vocal organs, and thoracic and abdominal viscera. The motor nerves innervate the tongue, vocal organs, and thoracic and abdominal viscera. The v.n. is referred to as "cranial nerve X." Also called **pneumogastric nerve**.

Vagusstoff /-shtôf'/ the original name (from German *Stoff*, "matter") of a substance released by the terminal fibers of the vagus nerve when it is stimulated. The substance has now been identified as the neurotransmitter acetylcholine.

Vaihinger, Hans /fī'ingər/ German philosopher, 1852–1933. See AS-IF HYPOTHESIS; AS-IF PERSONALITY.

VAKT /vakt/ or /vē'ā'kā'tē'/ a multisensory

teaching method involving the *v*isual, *a*uditory, *k*inesthetic, and *t*actile modalities. Also called **Fernald method**.

valence a quality of objects that affects their attractiveness to organisms. An object that attracts has positive v., while one that repels has negative v.

valgus a deformity in which the body part is bent outward, or away from the midline. E.g., talipes valgus denotes the eversion or turning outward of the affected foot.

valid in statistics and tests, accurately measuring what is intended to be measured. A test is v. if it selects, predicts, or assesses correctly. See VALIDITY.

validation the process of determining the accuracy of an instrument or device in measuring what it is designed to measure; also, the accuracy of the data or other information produced by its use.

validity the characteristic of being founded on truth, accuracy, fact, or law; the ability of a test to measure what it purports to measure. See VALID; FACE V.; CONSTRUCT V.; EMPIRICAL V.; EXTERNAL V.; INTERNAL V. Also see CRITERION V.; CONCURRENT V.; ETIOLOGICAL V.

validity criterion an independent and external measure of what a test is presumed to measure.

Valium: See BENZODIAZEPINES.

value a goal or standard that is considered especially worthy by an individual or society. In psychoanalysis, the moral values of society are incorporated into the superego through identification with the parents. The term may also denote: the degree of excellence assigned to an object or activity; the mathematical magnitude, or quantity, of an object; or the market price of an item or service.

value judgment an assessment of persons, objects, or events in terms of their value or worth rather than of their objective characteristics; also, a **qualitative judgment**, in contradistinction to a **quantitative judgment**.

value system the moral, social, esthetic, economic, and religious concepts accepted either explicitly or implicity by an individual or a particular society.

valve replacement a surgical procedure in which one or more of the heart valves is replaced with an artificial device, usually made of plastic, metal, or rubber, or a combination of materials. A v.r. also may be performed by transplanting a human heart valve from the body of a donor.

vampirism a belief in blood-sucking creatures. In literature, v. is often portrayed in a manner suggesting sexual pleasure associated with sucking blood from a person of the opposite sex, a representation of the "love bite." V. also is interpreted by some psychiatrists as oral sadism, oedipal strivings, fear of castration, or aggressive hostile feelings.

van Bogaert, Ludo /fän bō′gärt/ Belgian neurologist, fl. 1923, 1952. See CEREBROTENDINOUS XANTHOMATOSIS (also called **van Bogaert's disease**); XANTHOMATOSIS.

van Buchem, Francis Steven Peter Dutch internist, 1897—. See VAN BUCHEM'S SYNDROME.

van Buchem's syndrome an autosomal disorder marked by thickening and osteosclerosis of bones of the face, skull, and trunk, resulting in facial paralysis and loss of hearing and vision. The symptoms usually begin around the age of puberty.

van Creveld: See CREVELD.

vandalism willful defacement or destruction of property ("acting like a Vandal"). A persistent pattern of v. is a common symptom of CONDUCT DISORDER, UNDERSOCIALIZED, AGGRESSIVE. See this entry. Also see SEXUAL V.

variability the ability of an individual, situation, or species to change; in statistics, the degree to which scores differ from each other or from their central tendency.

variable an element in an experiment or test that varies, that is, takes on different values, while other conditions remain constant.

variable chorea of Brissaud a condition described by E. Brissaud in 1899, characterized by highly variable choreiform movements that come and go, increase and decrease, and appear to be quick at one time and slow at another. Some authorities believe it is a form of Tourette's disease.

variable error = RANDOM ERROR.

variable-interval reinforcement schedule in operant conditioning, a type of interval reinforcement in which the reinforcement or reward is presented after varying periods of time. Reinforcement is not contingent on the number of correct responses emitted during the intervals. See INTERVAL REINFORCEMENT. Compare FIXED-INTERVAL REINFORCEMENT SCHEDULE.

variable-ratio reinforcement schedule in operant conditioning, an intermittent reinforcement schedule in which a response is reinforced after a variable number of responses, determined by a random series of values having a certain mean and lying within a certain range. Compare FIXED-RATIO REINFORCEMENT SCHEDULE.

variable stimulus any one of a set of experimental stimuli that vary from a constant stimulus; also, the independent variable.

variance the variation in a set of scores; also, the square of the standard deviation. Symbol: s^2 or σ^2

varicella; varicella-zoster virus: See CHICKEN POX.

varimax a criterion for rotation in factor analysis.

varus a deformity in which the body part is turned inward, or toward the midline. E.g., genu varum, or bowleg, is marked by a deviation of the legs toward the midline so that the knees are farther apart than normally and the patient walks with the feet turned inward.

-vas-; -vaso- a combining form relating to a vessel (Latin *vas*), especially (a) a blood vessel, (b) the vas deferens.

vascular accident an alternative term for CEREBROVASCULAR ACCIDENT or STROKE. See these entries.

vascular insufficiency a failure of the cardiovascular system to deliver adequate blood flow to body tissues. The v.i. may involve large regions of the body or a particular organ or area of an organ. Atherosclerosis can narrow arteries supplying the leg muscles, causing intermittent claudication (limping), the arteries to the heart, resulting in angina pectoris, or arteries to the brain, causing symptoms of stroke.

vascular surgery the repair or replacement of damaged or diseased blood vessels. E.g., an artery that is blocked by atherosclerotic disease may be replaced or by-passed by a length of blood vein removed from another part of the patient's body or by a piece of plastic tubing. In some instances, a blood vessel may be opened so that an obstructing substance can be removed, or the blood vessel may be cleaned by a reaming technique.

vascular theory of thermal sensitivity the theory that temperature sensations are related to the constriction or dilation of blood vessels.

vas deferens = DUCTUS DEFERENS.

vasectomy a surgical procedure leading to male sterilization by severing and blocking the vas deferens which carries spermatozoa from the testes to the urethra. A v. usually involves an incision through the scrotum and cutting the vas deferens, or removing a section of the tube on either side, then tying the openings. Because of stored spermatozoa beyond the incision, sterilization of the male is not effective immediately.

vasoconstriction the constriction or narrowing of a blood vessel. V. is controlled by the fibers of the sympathetic nervous system or by agents such as amphetamine or epinephrine. Also see ERGOT DERIVATIVES.

vasoconstrictors drugs or other agents, e.g., the hormone vasopressin, that cause constriction of the blood vessels so that the caliber of the vessel is reduced. The vasomotor nerves of the sympathetic system also serve as v.

vasodilation the dilation of blood vessels. The term commonly is applied to the size of the bore of the arterioles.

vasomotor a nerve, drug, or other agent that can affect the caliber of a blood vessel.

vasopressin = ANTIDIURETIC HORMONE.

vasospasm: See SPASM.

Vasoxyl a trademark for methoxamine hydrochloride, a sympathetic amine administered as a vasopressor drug because of its action on the adrenergic nerves. See METHOXAMINE.

Vater, Abraham /fä′tər/ German anatomist and botanist, 1684–1751. See PACINIAN CORPUSCLES (also called **Vater's corpuscles**).

VD = VENEREAL DISEASE.

Vecchi, V. /vek′ē/ Italian physician, fl. 1956. See ZANOLI-VECCHI SYNDROME.

vector a force of a specific magnitude acting in a specific direction (Latin, "bearer, carrier"), rep-resented by a line of specific length with an arrow indicating the point of application of the force. In field theory, the term denotes a method of indicating forces involved in "psychological locomotion" within an individual's life space. In statistics, a v. is the representation of a score or a variable as a line with a specific length and direction.

vector analysis a mathematics term applied by K. Lewin to a technique for studying an individual's relationships within his "life space," and for depicting the forces, or vectors, that act upon him at any given moment. The vectors, such as conflicting goals, are represented diagrammatically by lines of different length and direction. Also called **vector psychology**. See VALENCE; VECTOR; FIELD THEORY; TOPOLOGICAL PSYCHOLOGY.

vegetative pertaining to basic physiological functions such as those involved in growth, respiration, sleep, digestion, elimination, and homeostasis, and governed primarily by the autonomic nervous system. Many of these functions, such as respiration and digestion, become disturbed when the individual faces extreme stress, and many of the characteristic symptoms of depression, such as decreased appetite, insomnia, and diminished sexual response, are vegetative in nature.

vegetative level = VEGETATIVE STATE.

vegetative nervous system an obsolescent term for the autonomic nervous system based on the fact that it controls the internal functions of the organism but not movement, sensation, or thought.

vegetative neurosis = VISCERAL NEUROSIS.

vegetative retreat a tendency to regress to infantile behavior marked by visceral reactions when facing a dangerous reality situation. Examples include adults who express a need for help by developing diarrhea or turning to thumb-sucking instead of taking an appropriate action.

vegetative state a passive, "dilapidated," state of deterioration in which the patient is immobile, out of contact with the environment, and unresponsive to questioning, and ultimately has to be fed and toileted. The condition occurs primarily in chronic schizophrenics and patients with advanced senile brain disease or cerebral arteriosclerosis. Also called **vegetative level**.

vegetotherapy = ORGONE THERAPY.

vehicle fear = AMAXOPHOBIA.

velar: See GUTTURAL.

velum a veil of white matter, such as the superior and inferior medullary **vela** that form a part of the cerebellar-medullary roof over the fourth ventricle. See SOFT PALATE.

velum palatinum = SOFT PALATE.

-vene-; -veno- a combining form relating to veins (from Latin *vena*, "vein, artery").

venereal disease any infectious disease that is transmitted through heterosexual or homosexual contact. The term is connected with Venus, the Roman goddess of love, although venereal diseases may also be transmitted by person-to-person or indirect contacts that do not involve lovemaking. There are approximately 20 known kinds of v.d., including syphilis, gonorrhea, herpes simplex Type 2, and granuloma inguinale. Abbrev.: **VD**. Also called **sexually transmissible disease**.

venereal-disease phobia = CYPRIPHOBIA.

venesection = BLOOD-LETTING.

Venezuelan equine encephalitis: See EQUINE ENCEPHALITIS.

Venn, John English logician and man of letters, 1834–1923. See VENN DIAGRAMS.

Venn diagrams charts of partially overlapping circles that indicate logical relations between sets or proposition terms, and operations on sets or proposition terms. The relations or operations are expressed by exclusion, inclusion, or intersection of the circles and by different kinds of shading for empty areas, areas that are not empty, and areas that may be either. V. d. were developed by the English 19th-century logician John Venn, based on the similar work of the Swiss mathematician Leonhard Euler in the preceding century (**Euler diagrams**).

venous thrombosis: See THROMBUS.

ventilation a free expression of feelings or emotions, especially in a therapy session.

-ventr-; -ventro- a combining form relating to the abdomen (Latin *venter*).

ventral pertaining to the abdomen, belly, or anterior surface or side of an organism. Compare DORSAL.

ventral tegmental area of Tsai an area below the medial lemniscus. The v.t.a.o.T. appears to be one of the structures in the rat brain that is a source of rewarding effects when wired with microelectrodes for self-stimulation.

ventral white commissure = WHITE COMMISSURE.

ventricle any small cavity in the body, including the brain which has several ventricles that serve as reservoir of cerebrospinal fluid. They include the two lateral ventricles, the third v., and the fourth v., which communicate with each other and with the spinal cord and subarachnoid spaces.

ventricle puncture a surgical procedure in which an opening from the outside is made to the lateral ventricle areas of the brain. The procedure may be performed in order to reduce intracranial pressure, to inject medications such as antibiotics directly into the brain, to obtain cerebrospinal fluid, or as part of the technique of making X-ray pictures of the brain that requires injecting air into the spaces normally filled with fluid.

ventricular system a network of ventricles and passageways to the spinal cord and subarachnoid spaces of the brain through which the cerebrospinal fluid circulates as a possible source of nutrients for CNS tissues.

ventriculoatrial shunt a surgically created passage for draining cerebrospinal fluid from the ventricles of the brain to the external jugular

vein, as in the treatment of hydrocephalus. The shunt carries the fluid through a catheter to the venous system which empties into the right atrium of the heart.

ventromedial nucleus an area of the hypothalamus that is associated with the inhibition of eating after certain nutritional requirements of the body have been met. If the v.n. suffers loss of structure or function, a condition of hyperphagia, or overeating, results. Also called **satiety center**.

veratrine: See HELLEBORE.

verbal ability the demonstrated capacity to communicate effectively by speech. Brain areas necessary for normal speech appear to be distributed over a broad region of the cerebral cortex and can be mapped by electrical stimulation. However, stimulation of a specific area will produce only phonemes or vocalizations; complete words apparently require simultaneous stimulation of combinations of speech areas. Abbr.: **V**. Also see PRIMARY ABILITIES.

verbal alexia a form of agnosia in which individual letters may be recognized but not whole words or combinations of letters, such as APA.

verbal amnesia a loss of the ability to remember words due to neurological disorder or disease. See NEUROLOGICAL AMNESIA.

verbal aphasia = EXPRESSIVE APHASIA.

verbal automatism: See AUTOMATISM.

verbal generalization a statement of a universal principle or general judgment.

verbal intelligence the ability to use words and symbols effectively in communication and problem-solving.

verbalization the expression of thoughts, feelings, and fantasies in words. In psychoanalysis, which has been popularly described as "the talking cure," the patient is encouraged to freely associate in words rather than to act out or rely on gestures. V. is a major procedure in other forms of psychotherapy as well, such as the nondirective approach. It may also take extreme, pathological form, as in circumstantiality or the pressured speech of the manic patient.

verbal leakage a term sometimes applied to slips of the tongue and dreams that reveal information about a patient's motives and behavior that he has attempted to conceal. Body language that tries to conceal information is described by some psychologists as **nonverbal leakage** (Freud: "If his lips are silent, he chatters with his fingertips").

verbal learning the process of learning to respond verbally to verbal stimuli, which may include symbols, nonsense syllables, lists, or words, and the solution of complex problems stated in words.

verbal masochism a psychosexual disorder in which an individual enjoys hearing words that are humiliating and insulting, and derives sexual excitement from the abuse. According to Theodore Reik, the sexual excitement may depend upon the choice and emphasis of words or sentences used.

verbal memory the capacity to remember something written or spoken that was previously learned, e.g., a poem. Also see MOTOR MEMORY; VISUAL MEMORY.

verbal paraphasia inclusion of inappropriate words and phrases in one's speech, a condition associated with lesions in the auditory speech areas of the cortex. See PARAPHASIA.

verbal proposition Piaget's term for a construct or abstraction that represents a given fact or phenomenon, e.g., an algebraic formula or a concept in sociology. The capacity to manipulate verbal propositions in reasoning signals the adolescent's arrival at the stage of FORMAL OPERATIONS. See this entry.

verbal suggestion a term introduced by Ernest Jones to describe the method of influencing, or molding, a patient's mind by hypnotic suggestion. See IDEOPLASTY.

verbal summator a projective method in which an instrument produces low-intensity vowel sounds that the subject is asked to translate into words.

verbal test any test or scale in which performance depends upon the ability to deal with words; also, any test that measures verbal ability.

verbal thought according to Vigotsky, a reasoning process that requires language and thus represents the merging of language and thought, e.g., in political discourse or in the field of history (H. Gardner, *Developmental Psychology*, 1978). Also see INNER LANGUAGE; PURE MEANING.

verbatim recall = ROTE RECALL.

verbigeration = CATAPHASIA. Also see HALLUCINATORY V.

verbochromia a condition in which a person experiences color sensations at the sound of certain words. V. is regarded as a form of synesthesia. (Rimbaud, in his celebrated poem "Voyelles," 1871, said "A" is black, "E" is white, "I" is red, "U" is green, and "O" is blue.)

verbomania = LOGORRHEA.

verbone H. A. Murray's term for a verbal-action pattern.

vergence a turning movement of the eyes. If they turn inward, the movement is convergence; if outward, divergence.

verification the use of objective empirical data to test or support the truth of a statement, conclusion, or hypothesis.

vermis the median lobe of the cerebellum that lies between the two hemispheres. Also called **v. cerebelli**.

vernix the fatty substance that covers and lubricates the skin of the fetus for passage through the birth canal.

Vernon, Philip Ewart English psychologist, 1905—. See ALLPORT-VERNON-LINDZEY STUDY OF VALUES.

verrucose dysplasia any abnormal development of adult tissue cells that acquire a rough, wart-

like appearance. V.d. usually involves the epidermis, but the abnormal cells also may develop on tissue surfaces in other body areas; e.g., verruca of the endocardium is associated with several types of heart-muscle inflammation.

Verstehen /fershtā′ən/ in evaluation research, a precondition to research involving understanding of language, cultural-symbol systems, and behavior, usually by participant observation; an understanding of mental constructs, as well as behavior, in the studies of programs and cultures; or vicarious understanding and empathy in evaluation (German, "understanding").

vertebral artery a branch of the left or right subclavian artery which in turn arises from the aorta, beginning at a point deep in the neck area and running upward through the foramina, or openings, of the neck vertebrae. The v.a. enters the skull near the top of the vertebral column. After passing through the foramen magnum, it joins the v.a. from the other side of the body to become the basilar artery, forming a part of the collateral circulation of the brain.

vertebrobasilar system the blood-supply system to the brain areas provided by the combined basilar and vertebral artery networks, which are joined in the arterial circle. Their branches provide blood flow to the spinal cord, brainstem including medulla, pons, and midbrain, posterior diencephalon, and temporal and occipital lobes of the cerebrum.

vertex potential a potential recorded by electrodes placed at the vertex of the skull. The v.p. seems to be evoked by a variety of stimuli but is closely associated with attention. In some studies, it has been found to be the only evoked potential related to changes in attention.

vertical axis a direction that is perpendicular to the horizon, or head-to-foot in an animal body; also, the ORDINATE. See this entry.

vertical group a group composed of individuals who come from different social classes. Vertical mobility refers to progress or displacement from one class to another. Also see SOCIAL MOBILITY. Compare HORIZONTAL GROUP.

vertical job enlargement: See JOB ENLARGEMENT.

vertical mobility movement from class to class in a social system. See VERTICAL GROUP.

vertical transmission: See HORIZONTAL TRANSMISSION.

vertigo dizziness and head spinning due to organic disorder (such as Ménière's disease or brain tumor), psychological stress (conflicts, tensions, anxieties), or activities that disturb the labyrinthine mechanism in the inner ear (as in a roller-coaster ride or flying in a small airplane).

vesania an obsolete term for insanity, or mental disorders, especially those not known to be organic in origin, such as mania, melancholia, and paranoia. The term was introduced by B. de Sauvages in 1763.

vesicle a fluid-filled saclike structure. E.g., synaptic vesicles contain transmitter fluid.

-vesico- a combining form relating to the urinary bladder (Latin *vesica*).

vestibular adaptation an effect of repeated suppression of the vestibular function observed in individuals whose daily activities require frequent or repeated turning of the head. Examples are found in ballet dancers and figure skaters. The v.a. effect may be permanent as evidenced by an absence of nystagmus during standard tests of balance sensitivity.

vestibular glands two small roundish glands situated on either side of the vaginal orifice. For the function of the greater v.g., see BARTHOLIN'S GLANDS.

vestibular hallucination a visual or cutaneous sensation that is due to an irritation or disorder of the vestibular apparatus. The v.h. may occur as a result of alcoholism or during passive rotation of the patient, appearing as the image of a person or several persons.

vestibular membrane = REISSNER'S MEMBRANE.

vestibular nerve a part of the eighth cranial nerve that carries cochlear nerve fibers associated with the sense of balance or orientation in space. It consists of a group of fibers that serve as pathways for impulses transmitted from the vestibular receptors in the cochlea to the cortex through the ascending limb of the medial longitudinal fasciculus. Most of the ascending fibers terminate in the oculomotor nuclei, although some probably communicate with neurons in the thalamus.

vestibular nuclei the cell bodies of the neurons associated with the sense of balance that are located in the posterior part of the fourth ventricle. Fibers of the v.n. may join the eighth cranial nerve, the statoacoustic nerve, that enters the brainstem below the pons.

vestibular receptors nerve cells associated with the sense of balance located in the cristae of the semicircular canals and the maculae of the utricle and saccule of the cochlea. They occur in two similar forms, a hair cell enclosed in a chalicelike nerve ending and a cylindrical hair cell that synapses at its base with a nerve ending.

vestibular sense = SENSE OF EQUILIBRIUM.

vestibular system a network of receptors and nerve fibers that comprise the sense of balance. It consists of sensory hair cells in compartments of the cochlea that detect movements of the head, with implied movements of the body, through the shifting of fluid, granules, or other substances (depending upon the species) due to the force of gravity. Impulses generated by the hair cells are transmitted automatically to the cerebellum, spinal cord, and other structures, such as the vagus nerve. The response to stimulation of the vestibular receptors may require complex reflex actions intended to compensate for a loss of balance. The complete v.s. may, under appropriate conditions, involve the ocular system, as evidenced by signs of nystagmus, and the digestive tract, as demonstrated by symptoms of motion sickness.

vestibule a cleft between the labia minora and behind the clitoris, containing the vaginal and urethral orifices and the vestibular glands. Also called **v. of the vagina**.

vestibule school a vocational term for the short-term intensive course provided to new workers in a building or area separate from the area of production.

vestibulocochlear nerve = STATOACOUSTIC NERVE.

vestibulospinal system one of the suprasegmental routes of reflex action, involving one or more segments of the spinal cord and connections of the sensory and motor nerves in brain areas. The v.s. has a facilitating effect on stretch reflexes. A lesion that decerebrates will affect the v.s. and result in a form of muscular rigidity.

VI an abbreviation of *v*ariable *i*nterval.

vibration a periodic motion of an object, e.g., a tuning fork, with a frequency that is usually measured in cycles per second.

vibrational theory one of several explanations for the phenonemon of odor discrimination, based on a concept that variations in the structure and movement of molecules of aroma particles enable olfactory receptors to distinguish between substances. Other theories relate to infrared, ultraviolet, or Raman-shift optical properties of odor particles.

vibration experience a sensation produced by contact with a pulsating, or rapidly vibrating, object that stimulates somatic receptors in the skin. The vibration sense can be measured with a mechanical vibrator that can be adjusted for threshold frequencies of the effect.

vibration receptors nerve endings that respond to various ranges of vibration frequencies. The v.r. have been identified through histological studies as Pacinian corpuscles. They have been located at depths ranging from the skin surface to as deep as the periosteal membrane covering the bone. Some v.r. seem most sensitive to vibrations between 100 and 600 cycles per second while others react only to those below 100 cycles per second.

vibration sense: See VIBRATION EXPERIENCE.

vibrator a cylinder, usually manufactured with a plastic outer casing, containing a small electric motor that produces a vibrating action. A typical v. is about six inches in length, but may range in length from three to ten inches. Smaller models are often inserted in the rectum and larger models in the vagina for sexual arousal. The motor may be powered by batteries or by household electric current. Also see DILDO.

vibratory sensitivity responsiveness to contact with a vibrating stimulus.

vicarious describing the substitution of one object or function for another, as in obtaining substitutive satisfaction by viewing the experiences of others in television programs.

vicarious function a theory intended to explain the ability of humans and other animals to recover from effects of brain damage, based on the assumption and some evidence that many functions are not well localized in the brain, and that many brain areas can assume a function previously performed by a brain area that has been damaged. Also see LOCALIZATION.

vicarious learning learning that is wholly a result of indirect experience and observation, as contrasted with learning based on direct experience and practice.

vicarious living a life-style in which one's behavior is identified with some hero or ideal, thereby avoiding a need for self-fulfillment by developing one's own personality.

vicarious trial and error mental trial and error; the mental testing out of several possible responses before making a decision or committing oneself to overt action, as in playing checkers.

vicious circle a situation in which a person's problems become increasingly difficult because of a tendency to solve them through unhealthy defensive reactions which in turn merely complicate the earlier problems.

victim psychology: See VICTIM RECIDIVISM.

victim recidivism /-sid'-/ the tendency of a victim of rape or other type of crime to be involved repeatedly in the same type of situation. According to some surveys, at least 25 percent of these victims had previous experiences of the same general kind. The reasons are only a matter of conjecture: masochistic tendencies, defiant or thoughtless behavior (walking alone at night), living in a risky environment, a timid manner that may attract a mugger, or possibly accident proneness. See ACCIDENT-PRONE PERSONALITY; TRAUMATOPHILIC DIATHESIS.

vidarabine = ARA-A.

videotape methods in psychiatry and clinical psychology, the use of videotape recordings of patient behavior or group-therapy sessions for therapeutic, research, or teaching purposes. Among the areas of application are dance therapy, speech therapy, family therapy, group therapy, behavior therapy, mental-retardation programs, psychiatric-nursing instruction, and psychodrama.

Vienna Psychoanalytic Society: See WEDNESDAY EVENING SOCIETY.

Viennese School a term applied to a group of practitioners of psychoanalysis who followed the theories of Freud. Also called **Vienna School; Wiener Schule**. Also see WEDNESDAY EVENING SOCIETY.

Vierordt, Karl /fēr'ôrt/ German physiologist, 1818–84. See VIERORDT'S LAW.

Vierordt's law the principle that the two-point threshold for a stimulus is lower in mobile body parts than in those less mobile.

vigilambulism a form of unconsciousness which resembles somnambulism but occurs in the waking state. The patient's behavior is one of automatism.

vigilance the alerting function of the nervous system. In conditioning experiments, v. is repre-

sented by a sudden sharp spike of alertness or arousal following a positive or negative conditioned stimulus. The spike of alertness is sometimes identified as a stimulus-v. spike.

For use of the term in a different context, see GENERALIZED-ANXIETY DISORDER.

Vigotsky, Lev Semionovich Russian psychologist, 1896–1934. Also spelled **Vygotsky**. See VIGOTSKY TEST; CONCEPT-FORMATION TESTS; EGOCENTRIC SPEECH; INNER LANGUAGE; PURE MEANING; VERBAL THOUGHT.

Vigotsky Test an instrument devised to study the process of thinking and concept formation and to detect thought disturbances and impaired ability to think abstractly. The test activity consists of sorting and classifying blocks of different sizes, shapes, and colors, each with a nonsense syllable printed on the underside. The subject devises and verbalizes hypotheses as he attempts to find the correct categories which require grouping according to combinations of characteristics that are not readily apparent, such as green-flat-circular. See HANFMANN-KASANIN CONCEPT FORMATION TEST.

vinbarbital sodium: See BARBITURATES.

Vincent curve a group-learning curve used to compare the performances of individuals who require different lengths of time or numbers of trials to achieve a specified learning level.

Vineland Social Maturity Scale a test developed by E. A. Doll (1936) to assess the development of individuals, including possible mental deficiency, from infancy to 30 years of age. Persons acquainted with the subject rate him or her in terms of self-help, locomotion, communication, self-direction, socialization, and occupation. The resulting scores yield a social age which, when divided by the chronological age, yields a social quotient.

Viola, Giacinto Italian physician, 1870–1943. See MICROSPLANCHNIC TYPE; NORMOSPLANCHNIC TYPE.

violence the expression of hostility and rage through physical force directed against persons or property. V. is aggression in its most extreme and unacceptable form, and most investigators believe it has no therapeutic justification, since there are more constructive and humane ways of expressing anger. It may, however, be socially justified in defensive wars or in combatting terrorism.

violinist's cramp a symptom of occupational neurosis in which the musician experiences a psychogenic spasm of the arm or hand muscles and is unable to play his instrument. See OCCUPATIONAL NEUROSIS.

Vira-a = ARA-A.

viraginity the tendency of a woman to act like a man and to possess masculine qualities, including sexuality (from Latin *virago*, "female warrior, manlike heroic maiden," from *vir*, "adult male").

viral cerebral infection: See CEREBRAL INFECTION.

viral meningitis: See MENINGITIS.

virginal anxiety anxiety associated with a first heterosexual encounter.

virginal tribute = JUS PRIMÆ NOCTIS.

virgin fear = PARTHENOPHOBIA.

virginity the state of a girl or woman who has not participated in sexual intercourse. Traditionally, a woman was assumed to possess v. if the hymen was not ruptured, but a ruptured hymen is no longer regarded as prima facie evidence of loss of v. V. was regarded as a sign of magical qualities in several cultures, e.g., by the ancient Romans who assigned virgins to guard sacred objects and to deal with the gods. Also see HYMEN; DEFLORATION; WEDDING NIGHT.

virginity taboo a social prohibition against defloration of the woman (elimination of the hymen) before marriage. This taboo appears to be a means of keeping women in social bondage, restricting their sexual activity, and insuring that they have not been impregnated.

virilism the presence in a female of sexual characteristics that are peculiar to men, such as absence of breasts and menstruation. The condition is due to overactivity of the adrenal cortex, with excessive secretion of androgen, which can be corrected in some cases. Also called **masculinization**.

virility the composite features of normal primary male sexual characteristics (from Latin *vir*, "adult male"). Also see MASCULINITY.

Virola a genus of South American trees used in Colombia, Brazil, and Venezuela as a source of hallucinogenic snuffs. The trees are cut down so that the bark can be removed and boiled to extract a red resin that is dried, ground, and mixed with wood ash. An effect of the snuff is microscopia and an "ability to talk with the little people."

virus: See CONVENTIONAL V.; UNCONVENTIONAL V.; SLOW V.

virus infections diseases caused by viral invasion of tissue cells, in which a cell becomes a host for the production of materials that can be utilized in manufacturing additional viruses. A virus may live in a body cell for years without causing damage by intracellular parasitism, and the condition would not be considered an infection in the absence of cell injury.

Visatoner an electronic device that enables a blind person to read printed material. Moving the V. over a line of print results in a series of tones that can be translated after extensive training by the user into patterns of letters of the alphabet. Also see OPTACON.

viscera the organs in any great body cavity, particularly the abdominal and thoracic cavities. Singular: **viscus**. Also see SPLANCHNIC.

visceral drive a motive that is derived from a physiological need.

visceral epilepsy a type of epilepsy in which the symptoms are expressed through a visceral organ disturbance, e.g., in the gastrointestinal organs. The association is believed to involve lesions in brain areas from which visceral sensations arise.

visceral learning = LEARNED AUTONOMIC CONTROL.

visceral neurosis a neurosis in which chronic internal conflicts and repressed emotions produce disturbances in the internal organs resulting in such symptoms as duodenal ulcer and essential hypertension. Also called **vegetative neurosis**.

visceral sensations = ORGANIC SENSATIONS.

visceral sense the sense or sensation associated with functions of the viscera.

visceroceptor a nerve-receptor organ in one of the visceral organs. Also called **visceroreceptor**.

viscerogenic needs a term applied by H. A. Murray to primary, physiological needs that arise from organic processes and lead to physical gratification. Among them are the need for air, water, food, sex, urination, and defecation. Also see PHYSIOLOGICAL NEEDS.

visceroreceptor = VISCEROCEPTOR.

viscerotonic temperament: See ENDOMORPH.

viscosity of libido in psychoanalysis, the fluidity of the libido, which moves slowly through phase after phase from infancy to maturity, and can remain fixed at, or return to, an earlier phase at slight provocation.

viscus: See VISCERA.

visibility coefficient a numerical designation of the visibility of a wavelength of radiant energy relative to a standard maximum visibility of a wavelength of 554 millimicrons.

visibility curve a graphic representation of the relative visibility, or brilliance, of various wavelengths of radiant energy.

visible speech a representation of vocal sound produced by converting sound waves into visible light patterns that can be photographed.

vision the sense of sight in which the eye is the receptor and the stimulus is radiant energy in wavelengths ranging from approximately 400 to 760 millimicrons; or that which is seen; also, a visual hallucination. Also see VISUAL SYSTEM; VISUAL PERCEPTION.

visiting nurse a nursing-school graduate who provides usual nursing services to patients in their homes. The responsibilities may include carrying out of physicians' orders, bedside care, health education, and supervising or coordinating activities with home health aides, or special therapists, e.g., physical therapists. A v.n. usually is employed by a local voluntary agency, such as a v.n. association.

visual accommodation = ACCOMMODATION.

visual acuity the degree of clarity, or sharpness, of visual perception. V.a. may be measured in one or more of several ways, such as the ability to detect very small gaps between two parts of a figure, called the **minimum separable method**, or the ability to discern a fine dark line on a light background or a fine light line on a dark background. Also see ACUITY GRATING.

visual adaptation the ability of the retina to adjust

to either continued stimulation or a lack of stimulation.

visual agnosia an inability to recognize visual stimuli, such as objects. The condition is observed in humans with brain lesions. A similar effect has been noted in experimental animals, who must touch objects in order to identify them. Also called **object blindness**.

visual agraphia an impaired ability to write due to failure to recognize letters, numbers, or words. The condition results from lesions in the occipitoparietal areas.

visual allachesthesia a symptom of a parietal lobe lesion manifested as a transposition of visual images to an opposite point in space.

visual amnesia a loss of the ability to recognize familiar objects, printed words, or handwriting by sight, due to neurological disease or injury. See APHASIA.

visual aphasia = ALEXIA.

visual aura a type of sensory seizure in which flashes of light precede a grand mal seizure. The aura also may occur without the seizure. The focus usually is in the temporooccipital area.

visual axis a straight line that extends from the external fixation point through the nodal point of the eye to the fovea.

visual cliff an experimental apparatus for testing depth perception in human and animal infants. The v.c. is a structure topped by heavy glass. One half of the surface below the glass is a short drop (the shallow side) while the other half is a drop of several feet (the deep side). The infant subject is placed on a board in the middle of the structure and must crawl to one of the two sides to get off. Most children and animal subjects refuse to crawl over to the "deep side," indicating the presence of depth perception at a very early age.

visual closure the ability to identify a familiar object from an incomplete visual presentation.

visual cortex the region of the cerebral cortex in which retinal images are projected by impulses carried from the eyes by the optic nerves. It is located in the Brodmann Areas 17, 18, and 19 of the occipital lobe of the cortex, a site sometimes identified as the **calcarine cortex** because it is located beneath the calcarine sulcus.

visual cycle the system of metabolic phases of visual pigments, particularly rhodopsin which during periods of vision goes through simultaneous and continuous cycles of breaking down into opsin and retinene and being reformed from the same substances. An equilibrium between the processes depends upon the intensity of the light stimulus, which energizes the breakdown of rhodopsin, and upon the oxidation energy for the reverse action.

visual discrimination the ability to distinguish shapes, patterns, hidden figures, or other images from similar objects that differ in subtle ways. Some species suffer a loss of this function after brain lesions and bump into objects that normally would be avoided.

visual-distortion test a test of a subject's psychological reaction to the visual distortion produced by wearing a pair of glasses with lenses of +6.00 or −6.00 diopters for several minutes. The distortion is assumed to cause a temporary breakdown of the synthetic and integrative functions of the ego, and is therefore a measure of ego strength.

visual field the total amount of the external world that is visible to the immobile eye at a given time; also, the subjective three-dimensional space in which objects, distances, and movements are perceived.

visual-field defect any of a number of types of partial or total blindness due to an interruption in the flow of visual impulses between the retina and the visual cortex. The interruption may be caused by a lesion before, after, or in the optic chiasm, in all or a part of the optic-radiation fibers, and involving tracts of one or both eyes. Each possible lesion produces a different v.-f.d.

visual fixation the orientation of the eyes so that images fall on the foveas, in the central part of the retinas.

visual hallucination false perception of visual images in the absence of external stimulation, such as seeing visions of angels, large animals, or insects crawling on the walls or on the individual's skin. It is most common in delirium tremens (alcohol-withdrawal delirium), paranoid schizophrenia, and ingestion of hallucinogenic drugs. For examples, see FORMICATION; LILLIPUTIAN HALLUCINATION.

visual impairment the partial or complete loss or absence of vision, due to disease, injury, or congenital defect. V.i. also may result from degenerative disorders, such as cataracts, glaucoma, refractive errors, and certain cases of astigmatism.

visual induction the effect on the perception of one area of a visual field of stimulation of a different area. E.g., a small yellow square may cause surrounding gray areas to appear blue.

visualization the ability to create a visual image in one's mind. In consumer psychology, the term refers to a motivation-research technique that utilizes imaginary or fictitious situations or conditions in order to induce consumers to reveal the true reasons for their choice of products. E.g., instead of being asked why he likes or dislikes a product, the consumer may be asked to characterize the type of individual who would buy the product.

visualization technique a hypnotic method in which the subject is asked to imagine that he is sitting comfortably and calmly at home, and then use all his senses in perceiving the scene, e.g., by noticing the color of the walls, the curtains blowing in the windows, the smells coming from the kitchen, the texture of the armchair under his fingers, and the relaxing support of the chair itself. The more fully the subject concentrates on these familiar features, the more deeply relaxed he or she becomes. Any number of other visualization techniques can then be used to promote hypnotic relaxation, e.g., sailing through the sky like a balloon, or lying on a beach in the warm sun. The technique can be used by itself or as a means of enhancing other suggestion procedures.

visual learning training or conditioning that depends upon visual cues. The brain center for v.l. is believed to be in the inferotemporal area where experiments indicate cortical cells are highly active in analyzing visual inputs. However, lesions in the center reduce but do not eliminate performance of this function, indicating that other cortical areas also are involved.

visual memory the capacity to remember in the form of visual images what has previously been seen. Also see MOTOR MEMORY; VERBAL MEMORY.

visual memory span: See MEMORY SPAN.

visual-motor coordination the ability to synchronize visual information with the movements of different parts of the body, as in learning to play volleyball.

visual organization a Gestalt term for a visual field that appears to be organized and meaningful.

visual perception the visual observation and recognition of objects. The process is initiated by light reflected from the objects onto nerve receptors in the retina that transduce the nerve impulses and project them onto cortical cells, which in turn transmute them into images. Recognition is achieved by relating the viewed object to similar images stored in the memory.

visual phosphene a visual sensation produced by a stimulus other than visual light. A v.p. may occur with the eyes closed, and the stimulus may be pressure on the eyeball or an electrical current. The sensation appears as a flicker, and in the case of the electrical stimulation the response varies with the frequency of alternating current.

visual-placing reflex the act of animals in placing their legs so as to reach a surface they can see. Animals that have undergone surgical decortication may lose their normally automatic response and fail to stretch their legs toward a visible surface.

visual projection the act of attributing a spatial object location to a visually perceived object.

visual purple: See RHODOPSIN.

visual pursuit = OCULAR PURSUIT.

visual-righting reflexes the reflexes that automatically orient the head to the visual fixation point of the moment.

visual search a type of test sometimes employed in diagnosis of visual-perception disorders. The subject is asked to seek a number or other item from a random display distributed over areas of both the left and right visual fields. Results are based on the relative amount of time required to find the items on the left and right sides of a midline.

visual-search perceptual disorder a disorder exemplified by difficulty in locating a specific number from a random array on a board as a result of a lesion in one of the hemispheres. Normal subjects perform better when the number sought is to the left of the midline. Patients with left-hemisphere damage also do better when the number is on the left of the midline, while those with right-hemisphere damage perform better in the search when the number is to the right of the midline.

visual sequential memory the ability to recall a sequence of visual stimuli such as letters, words, or pictures.

visual space the three-dimensional perspective of the visual field.

visual-spatial ability the ability to comprehend and conceptualize visual representations and spatial relationships in learning and in the performance of such tasks as reading maps, navigating mazes, conceptualizing objects in space from different perspectives, and various geometric operations. Beginning in adolescence, males, on the average, show a definite superiority in v.-s.a. while females, on the average, display superiority in verbal ability. See FROSTIG DEVELOPMENTAL TEST OF VISUAL PERCEPTION.

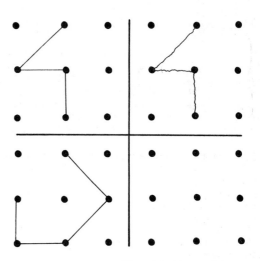

VISUAL-SPATIAL ABILITY. The task in this example is to reproduce the design on the left (from Frostig Developmental Test of Visual Perception).

visual stimulation the stimulation by light of a frequency and intensity that will trigger a response by receptor cells in the retina. The stimulus is measured in **photons**, units of radiant energy that are capable of altering the composition of visual pigments in the retinal cells.

visual system the network of receptors and nerve cells and fibers that enable an organism to perceive the external environment through the medium of electromagnetic energy with wavelengths between 4/10 and 7/10 of a micron. The receptor is the eye, which protects the receptor cells in the retinal membrane which is technically an extension of the brain. In most species a lens mechanism helps focus the electromagnetic waves reflected from an object onto the receptors. The v.s. also includes nerve cells and fibers in the retina, between the retina and the visual cortex, and within the visual cortex where images from the eyes are projected and analyzed. A feature of the v.s. is the optic chiasm that routes part of the fibers from the retina of the left eye to the visual cortex on the right side of the brain, and vice versa. Also see EYE STRUCTURE.

visual tracking = OCULAR PURSUIT.

visual type an individual who tends to think in visual terms and whose imagery is predominantly visual.

visuoconstruction defect a disorder associated with a parietal-lobe dysfunction. It is characterized by difficulty in assembling the various parts of an object into a complete structure. See CONSTRUCTIONAL APRAXIA.

visuomotor theory a model of the development of the motor system and its interaction with learning. The theory focuses on the dependence of each successive state of development upon an earlier level (Getman, 1965).

visuospatial agnosia a disorder of spatial orientation, which may be tested by such techniques as having the subject point to objects or other stimuli located in different parts of his visual fields.

vital capacity the capacity of the lungs to hold air, measured by the greatest volume of air that can be expressed after maximum inspiration.

vitalism the theory that the functions of living organisms are determined, at least in part, by an inorganic force or principle. The biologist Hans Driesch was the chief exponent of this view, holding that life processes are autonomous and purposive, and that potentialities for growth and development are realized through the operation of an agent to which he applied Aristotle's term **entelechy** /entel'əkē/ (Greek *entelecheia*, "full reality"). The philosopher Henri Bergson termed this creative, vital force the **élan vital** /āläN'vētäl'/.

vital spirits: See HYDRAULIC MODEL.

vital statistics data, usually compiled by a government agency or insurance firm, on the rates of birth, death, and disease in a population.

vitamin an organic substance generally found in food sources and essential in minute quantities for normal growth and health maintenance. A v. may function as a coenzyme, aiding in the various metabolic steps of utilization of carbohydrates, fats, and proteins. The term was coined in 1913 by the Polish biochemist Casimir Funk, the discoverer of vitamins, from the Latin word *vita*, "life," and the German word *Amin*, because vitamins were originally thought to be amines.

vitamin A in vision the influence of vitamin A on normal vision. The nutrient vitamin A is a component of the visual pigments rhodopsin and porphyropsin. Rhodopsin is formed from opsin and retinene which in turn is formed from vitamin A and opsin. Porphyropsin is similar to rhodopsin except that it contains a form of vitamin A with a double carbon bond and is sometimes designated vitamin A_2 to distinguish it from the A_1 in rhodopsin. A vitamin-A deficiency results in night blindness and other visual disorders. Also see VISUAL CYCLE.

vitamin-A toxicity: See HYPERVITAMINOSES.

vitamin B_5 = NICOTINIC ACID.

vitamin B_6: See GLUMATIC ACID; GLYCINE.

vitamin deficiency lack of a vitamin needed for normal body-system functions. A deficiency of the vitamin niacin may result in severe disorders including pellagra and a form of dementia. A thiamine deficiency is associated with alcoholism symptoms and beriberi. Several B vitamins, including thiamine and niacin, are important for normal metabolism of neurons. Others, such as A and D, may affect mental functions indirectly through a debilitating effect that makes it difficult to perform learning tasks. Also see THIAMINE DEFICIENCY; RIBOFLAVIN.

vitamin-D toxicity: See HYPERVITAMINOSES.

vitrectomy a surgical procedure in which vitreous humor between the lens and retina of the eye is removed. The procedure is performed when the vitreous humor has become clouded or discolored by disease or injury; it is then replaced with a clear fluid.

vitreous hemorrhage a visual complication of diabetes mellitus marked by bleeding within the eyeball due to the rupture of capillaries of the retina. Also see DIABETIC RETINOPATHY; MICROANGIOPATHY.

vitreous humor: See HUMOR; EYE STRUCTURE.

Vitus, Saint Christian child martyr, fl. third century. See CHOREA (there: **Saint Vitus' dance**).

Vives, Juan Luis /vē'ves/ Spanish humanist, 1492–1540. This Renaissance educator was one of the first to hold that individual emotional experience rather than abstract reason plays the primary role in human life, and that we should attempt to understand the emotions of the mentally ill and treat them with compassion.

vocabulary growth linguistic development as measured by the increase in the child's vocabulary. Studies indicate that the recognition vocabulary increases from about 20 words at 15 months to 270 at two years, 900 at three, 1,500 at four, 2,000 at five. By the end of elementary school, the child recognizes up to 20,000 words; by the end of high school, a few students recognize up to 80,000; and by the end of four-year college, some students recognize 250,000 or more. However, the writing vocabulary is seldom more than 15 to 20 percent of the total, and the speech vocabulary is even smaller. Girls progress more rapidly than boys in this and all other features of language development. (While "unabridged" dictionaries list hundreds of thousands of words, the educated adult rarely uses over 12,000 in writing, and in ordinary speech 2,000 words are enough to express 99% of what we have to say. The Old Testament has only 6,000 different words; and Shakespeare's vocabulary, which is considered huge, is "limited" to 20,000.) Also see ACTIVE VOCABULARY; PASSIVE VOCABULARY.

vocabulary test a test designed to determine the number and level of words that a subject can use (active vocabulary) or understand (passive vocabulary).

vocabulary word = CONTENT WORD.

vocal cords a set of ligaments in the larynx that produce sounds by vibrating when respiratory air passes through them.

vocal-image voice the audible speech patterns that have been electronically transformed into visual patterns which can be read by the deaf.

vocalization use of the voice in uttering sounds without words, as in babbling, screaming, barking, and singing arpeggios or scales in music practice.

vocal register the tonal or pitch range of an individual's voice.

vocational adjustment the degree to which an individual makes use of his abilities in obtaining the kind of work or career best suited to his desires and talents. The term emphasizes the relations between personal aptitudes, interests, and achievement whereas occupational adjustment focuses on the relationship between the individual and objective work conditions. See OCCUPATIONAL ADJUSTMENT. Also see VOCATIONAL CHOICE.

vocational appraisal the prediction by a vocational counselor of a client's potential for success and fulfillment in a particular occupation. A v.a. is based on the counselor's understanding of occupational opportunities considered in relation to the client's personality, intelligence, abilities, and interests as revealed in interviews and tests.

vocational-aptitude test a test designed to assess the ability, interest, personality, and other factors deemed essential for success in a particular occupation.

vocational choice a process that may begin in adolescence or before with an examination of individual interests, strengths, and limitations in light of their meaning within a given vocational context. A mature v.c. involves sufficient self-understanding to correctly match up personal interests and resources to the perceived requirements and conditions that obtain in a specific vocation or profession. Also see VOCATIONAL ADJUSTMENT.

vocational counseling the process of counseling an individual on job selection, where and how to seek employment, adjustment to the job, and human relations or other personal problems affecting job satisfaction and job performance.

vocational education a training program designed

to help an individual meet the necessary qualifications for a particular job or profession.

vocational evaluation = WORK EVALUATION.

vocational guidance the process of helping an individual choose an appropriate vocation through such means as (a) depth interviews, (b) administration of aptitude, interest, and personality tests, and (c) discussion of the nature and requirements of specific types of work in which the individual expresses an interest.

vocational maladjustment a broad term referring to inadequate job performance or a lack of personal satisfaction with or fulfillment in a job or profession. V.m. may result if an individual's ability level is not matched to his job or if a variety of social or psychological factors inhibit harmonious functioning on the job, e.g., insufficient compensation or benefits, or friction with superiors or fellow workers.

vocational rehabilitation the process of developing or restoring the productivity of mentally or physically handicapped persons through vocational guidance, testing, training, and adjustment to the work situation. A v.r. program involves development of skills that have been lost or neglected, and helping the individual find employment either in the business or industrial world or in a sheltered workshop. An effective program enables the disabled person to become a contributing member of society and promotes psychological adjustment by enhancing self-esteem and morale.

vocational selection the process of selecting the most likely candidates from a group of applicants for a job in terms of probability for success.

vocational services vocational testing, guidance, counseling, training, and assistance in finding employment, as provided by a school, hospital, clinic, or rehabilitation center.

vocational training an organized program of instruction designed to equip individuals with the requisite skills for placement in specific jobs or trades. Also see VOCATIONAL REHABILITATION.

vodun = VOODOO.

Vogt, Oskar /fōkt/ German neurologist, 1870–1959. See SPIELMEYER-VOGT DISEASE; CEREBRO-MACULAR DEGENERATION (there: **Batten-Spielmeyer-Vogt disease**); SPHINGOLIPIDOSES.

voice disorders phonatory voice deviations affecting pitch, loudness, and quality of voice.

voiced sound: See SONANT.

voiced stop: See PLOSIVE.

voiceless sound = SURD.

voiceless stop: See PLOSIVE.

voice quality: See PARALINGUISTIC FEATURES.

voice-stress analyzer an instrument that records alterations in the voice that are undetectable to the human ear and that occur automatically when an individual is under stress. The v.-s.a. is employed in lie detection.

voice therapist a specialist knowledgeable in the areas of physiology and pathology of voice production and concerned with diagnosis and re-mediation of voice disorders. The specialist is often part of a team which includes an otolaryn-gologist, internist, neuropsychiatrist, psychol-ogist, and audiologist.

void-fear = KENOPHOBIA.

volatile-chemical inhalation the act of sniffing of volatile chemicals for their intoxicating effects. Substances involved in v.-c.i. include paint thin-ners, methyl alcohol, spray-can freons, lacquer thinners, plastic-glue solvents, gasoline, and kerosene. The fumes are absorbed directly into the bloodstream through the lungs and are, therefore, capable of producing immediate euphoria. Also see INHALATION OF DRUGS.

volatile-solvent dependence tolerance for chemi-cals whose fumes produce an intoxicating effect. Most volatile solvents are fat soluble and are re-tained in the body tissues for a long period of time instead of being rapidly metabolized. V.-s.d. often occurs as a form of cross addiction with alcohol and barbiturate abuse. Workers ex-posed to industrial solvents frequently develop dependence.

volition will, or the act of willing; the process of choosing a course of action voluntarily or with-out direct external influence. Also see DERAIL-MENT OF V.

volitional tremor: See TREMOR.

volley theory a variation of the alternation-of-response theory in which individual fibers re-spond to one stimulus of a burst of stimuli while others in the group respond to the second, third, or Nth stimulus. The result is that successive vol-leys of impulses are fired to match the inputs of stimuli; yet, no single fiber is required to re-spond to each of the individual stimuli in the group. Also called **volley principle**. Also see TELEPHONE THEORY; HEARING THEORIES.

volubility in psychiatry, excessive, uncontrollable talkativeness. See LOGORRHEA.

voluntarism the philosophical view that volition is the fundamental mental process and voluntary actions can change the course of events.

voluntary admission in psychiatry, admission of a patient to a mental hospital or unit at his own request. Also called **voluntary commitment; voluntary hospitalization**.

voluntary agencies and organizations nonprofit groups supported in whole or in part by public contributions and devoted to the amelioration of public-health or social-welfare problems. The term voluntary usually is applied to distinguish the groups from government agencies. E.g., the American Heart Association, March of Dimes, and United Cerebral Palsy Associations are v.a.a.o. The American Red Cross is a combined voluntary-government agency.

voluntary ataxia an effect of damage to the nerve tracts carrying kinesthetic impulses to the brain and marked by a lack of control over movement of the limbs. Because of ineffective restraint on the movements, through absence of feedback signals, the patient tends to make overextended

actions such as reaching far beyond an object he is attempting to grasp.

voluntary commitment = VOLUNTARY ADMISSION.

voluntary control the regulation of activities such as movements, impulses, or affects by conscious intention.

voluntary dehydration: See DEHYDRATION.

voluntary hospitalization = VOLUNTARY ADMIS-SION.

voluntary movement movement by choice or in-tention, in contrast to automatic movements such as reflexes.

voluntary muscle = SKELETAL MUSCLES.

voluntary nervous system = CENTRAL NERVOUS SYSTEM.

voluntary processes processes marked by inten-tion and volition, that is, activities that are con-sciously desired, chosen, planned, regulated, and under cortical control, in contrast to reflex actions or involuntary behavior. Also see VOLUNTARY RESPONSE.

voluntary response a deliberately chosen reaction to a stimulus that may require a complex suprasegmental coordination of excitatory and inhibitory impulses with feedback signals from the visual and other systems. A v.r. could occur in a situation as simple as walking or as difficult as playing in a doubles tennis match. Also see VOLUNTARY PROCESSES.

volunteer in the health field, an individual who contributes his services without compensation to a hospital, social agency, rehabilitation center, or nursing home. Today many volunteers re-ceive special orientation and training under the guidance of a qualified v. director. Among their duties are teaching crafts, feeding incapacitated patients, assisting the librarian, and providing clerical assistance.

volunteer bias error resulting from differences be-tween volunteers and nonvolunteers in attitudes or personality. Volunteers may have stronger motivation, may want more excitement, may be seeking self-understanding, etc., and these attri-butes may in part account for their responses in an experiment.

vomiting ejecting the contents of the stomach through the mouth. In psychiatry, this process, especially when repeated, is frequently inter-preted in psychogenic terms as a symbolic expression of anger, hatred, or rejection of a situation that arouses internal conflict, such as a forced marriage or an unwanted pregnancy. V. also signifies expulsion of dangerous wishes in-volving the mouth, e.g., fellatio. Also see NERV-OUS V.

vomiting-fear = EMETOPHOBIA.

von Domarus principle an explanation of schiz-ophrenic thinking developed by Eilhard von Domarus in 1946, based on the concept that the schizophrenic perceives two things as identical merely because they have identical predicates or properties. This principle appears to be denied in the paranoid delusion in which individuals are perceived as impostors (Cotard's syndrome).

von Economo: See ECONOMO.

von Gierke: See GIERKE.

von Gierke's syndrome a disorder characterized by an accumulation of glycogen in the liver and kidney cells. The condition is due to an enzyme deficiency. Symptoms, which may be present at birth or develop soon afterward, include enlarged liver, kidney lesions, ketosis, and convulsions. Because of frequent occurrence of v.G.s among siblings and offspring of consanguineous marriages, it is assumed to be an inherited disorder. Also called **glucogenosis**.

von Helmholtz: See HELMHOLTZ.

von Recklinghausen, Friedrich Daniel /-housən/ German pathologist, 1833–1910. See VON RECKLINGHAUSEN'S DISEASE.

von Recklinghausen's disease an autosomal-dominant disorder in which the common anomalies are café-au-lait skin-pigmentation areas and peripheral-nervous-system tumors. The tumors, or **neurofibromas**, may be firm subcutaneous nodules or soft cutaneous lumps that invaginate (form a pocket) when pressed. Visual, hearing, and other neurologic anomalies may occur, and about one-fourth of the patients are mentally retarded. Also called **neurofibromatosis** and, more popularly, **Elephant Man's disease** (so named after a 19th-century victim of the disease, John Merrick, who was known as the Elephant Man).

von Restorff, Hedwig German psychologist, fl. 1933, 1935. See VON RESTORFF EFFECT.

von Restorff effect a memory-process theory introduced in 1933 by H. von Restorff. It states that in a series of learning experiences or items of information, the items that contrast categorically with most of the others in the series will be retained better than items that are categorically similar.

voodoo a polytheistic religion, practiced chiefly in the West Indies, in which the tradition of African cults and magic is intermingled with rites derived from Catholicism. Also called **voodooism; vodun**. Adjective: **voodooistic**. Also see V. DEATH; FAITH HEALING.

voodoo death a culture-specific syndrome observed in natural societies in most parts of the world, in particular, Africa, New Zealand, Australia, the Islands of the Pacific, and the Caribbean, especially Haiti. In a typical case, a medicine man discovers that a healthy individual has transgressed a taboo, draws a magic bone from his robe and points it at the culprit while uttering an incantation. The culprit withdraws to a dark corner of his hut, refuses to talk or eat, and within 24 to 48 hours withers away and dies. The physiologist W. Cannon has pointed out that the victim is literally "frightened to death," and has compared the phenomenon to "wound shock," which produces a vasomotor paralysis. Other explanations include heart arrhythmias, adrenaline shock, vagal-nerve overstimulation, anorexia, poisoning, and increased susceptibility to serious disease due to "giving up." Also see CURSING MAGIC; MAGICAL THINKING; PSYCHIC SUICIDE.

Vorbeireden /fôrbī'rādən/ a German word meaning to talk (or a talking) past the point or beside the point, used in psychiatry to characterize the tendency of patients with Ganser syndrome to give nonsensical or approximate answers to questions. See GANSER SYNDROME.

voyeurism a psychosexual disorder in which the preferred or exclusive method of achieving sexual excitement consists of observing unsuspecting people who are nude or in the act of disrobing or engaging in sexual activity. Though the **voyeur** seeks no sexual activity with the person he observes, orgasm is usually produced through masturbation during the act of "peeping" or in retrospect. Also called **inspectionalism**. Also see PEEPING TOM. (DSM-III)

voyeuse a female voyeur.

VR an abbreviation of *v*ariable *r*atio.

vulnerable-child syndrome the symptoms observed in the behavior of a child who has recovered from a serious illness but is overly protected by his parents as if he were still in danger of his life.

-vulv-; -vulvo- a combining form relating to the vulva.

vulva the external genital features of the female, including the mons pubis, the labia majora, the labia minora, the clitoris, the vestibule of the vagina, the bulb of the vestibule, and the greater vestibular or Bartholin's glands. Also called **pudendum; cunnus**.

vulvectomy the surgical excision of the external female genitalia. V. is performed as a form of treatment for cancer of the vulva and, in some cultures, for esthetic reasons.

Vygotsky: See VIGOTSKY.

W

w = WILL FACTOR.

W = COEFFICIENT OF CONCORDANCE.

Waardenburg, Petrus Johannes Dutch ophthalmologist, 1886—. See WAARDENBURG'S SYNDROME; FISCH-RENWICK SYNDROME (there: **Klein-Waardenburg syndrome**).

Waardenburg's syndrome a familial or hereditary disorder marked by a white or gray forelock of hair, abnormal pigmentation of the iris, nerve deafness due to malfunction of the auditory nerves, and lateral displacement of the eyelids giving a false appearance that the eyes are widely separated. Mental retardation may occur, but deafness can be a factor in testing for intelligence.

Wada, Juhn Atsushi Japanese-born Canadian neurologist, 1924—. See WADA DOMINANCE TEST.

Wada dominance test a test of speech lateralization in which a dose of sodium Amytal is injected into the carotid artery on the left or right side to anesthetize the hemisphere on the injected side. Evidence of dysphasia is produced if the side injected is dominant for language for that patient. Both sides are tested on different days. Speech representation generally is in the left hemisphere for right-handed persons, with many exceptions. Also called **Wada technique**.

Wadsworth, Guy Woodbridge, Jr. American psychologist, 1901—. See HUMM-WADSWORTH TEMPERAMENT SCALE.

WAIS = WECHSLER ADULT INTELLIGENCE SCALE.

wakefulness a condition of awareness of one's surroundings coupled with an ability to communicate with others or to understand what is being communicated by others. W. also can be a relaxed state that is characterized by EEG alpha waves that border on signs of drowsiness. See SLEEP CHARACTERISTICS; INSOMNIA.

waking center an area of the posterior hypothalamus that includes fibers of the reticular activating system, and which may extend through the system to the brainstem. Laboratory animals subjected to lesions of the posterior hypothalamus and humans suffering tumors or inflammations in that structure develop abnormal tendencies to sleep. A similar effect also results from lesions in the reticular activating system.

waking hypnosis a state of hypnosis induced without reference to sleep by having the subject fix his attention on an object and close his eyes tightly. Wells (1924) found that the waking method has a distinct advantage over the sleeping method; it is easier to learn, easier to apply, appears less occult, and a higher percentage of subjects can be hypnotized.

waking state = W-STATE.

Waldenström, Jan Gosta Swedish physician, 1906—. See LEGG-CALVÉ-PERTHE DISEASE (also called **Waldenström's syndrome**).

Walker, Arthur Earl American neurologist and surgeon, 1907—. See DANDY-WALKER SYNDROME; DYSMORPHOGENESIS OF BRAIN, JOINTS, AND PALATE.

walk-in clinic a clinic in which diagnostic or therapeutic service is available without an appointment.

Wallenberg, Adolf /väl'ənberk/ German physician, 1862–1949. See WALLENBERG'S SYNDROME.

Wallenberg's syndrome a circulatory disorder of the brainstem caused by restricted blood flow in the inferior cerebellar artery. The interruption of arterial circulation results in ipsilateral loss of pain and temperature sensations of the face, soft palate, pharnyx, and larynx as well as contralateral hypoesthesia of the trunk and extremities. Similar effects are observed in the Bernard-Horner syndrome and Opalski's syndrome.

Waller, August Volney English physiologist, 1816–70. See WALLERIAN DEGENERATION.

Wallerian degeneration the deterioration of the myelin sheath and axis cylinder from the point of injury of a peripheral sensory or motor nerve toward the periphery, regenerating if the neurilemma is left intact.

walleye: See GRIEG'S DISEASE; EXOTROPIA; DIVERGENCE.

Wallis, Wilson Allen American statistician and economist, 1912—. See KRUSKAL-WALLIS TEST.

Walpole, Horace English writer, 1717–97. See SERENDIPITY.

wandering attention an attention disturbance in which a patient appears fully alert but is distracted by almost any external stimulus. The condition may result from focal or widespread CNS disease such as subfrontal tumors occurring higher in the neuraxis than in drifting attention. A similar disorder may occur in severely depressed or acutely schizophrenic patients. Also see DRIFTING ATTENTION.

wandering-impulse a strong desire to leave home and travel or change surroundings. Also see DROMOMANIA.

wandering uterus a uterus that is not fixed in the same position at all times. The uterus normally changes positions according to the posture of the woman. However, anterior, lateral, or posterior displacement of the uterus can produce signs or symptoms of infertility, menstrual aberrations, or aches and pains anywhere from the diaphragm to the pelvic floor. In Hippocrates' theory, hysteria (now termed conversion disorder) was attributed to a uterus (Greek *hystera*) that had wandered to different parts of the body in search of a child. Also see -HYSTER-.

wanderlust a love to wander, or roam (from German *Wanderlust*). Some psychiatrists associate w. with an oedipal conflict manifested by a morbid urge to wander incessantly in an effort to reestablish a relationship with one or both parents as the individual experienced it or wished to experience it as a child.

Ward Atmosphere Scale: See ENVIRONMENTAL ASSESSMENT.

warehousing a popular term for the practice of confining mental patients to large institutions for long-term, and in many cases lifetime, custodial care.

warfarin an anticoagulant drug that may have teratogenic effects when used by pregnant women. Infants born to some mothers using w. have been found to suffer seizures, severe mental retardation, or blindness or other visual disorders. W. has been used as a human heart-disease medication and as a rodent poison.

war footing: See FIGHT-FLIGHT REACTION.

warm-blooded animals = HOMOIOTHERMS.

warming-up period an initial period in learning and motor activities in which responses are slow and inexact, followed by a gradual increase in speed and accuracy with practice.

warm spot any of the skin areas that are particularly sensitive to warm stimuli.

warmth a feeling or sensation experienced when a stimulus warmer than the skin—normally a temperature greater than 33°C (91°F)—is applied to the skin. Slightly warmer temperatures may be required to produce the w. sensation internally.

war neurosis a traumatic neurosis precipitated by war-time experiences, including not only catastrophic events like bombings but long exposure to combat conditions, and internal conflicts over killing or the expression of fear. Symptoms include persistent anxiety and tension, nightmares, irritability, exhaustion, depression, and in some cases phobias and conversion symptoms such as paralysis or bent back (camptocormia). See COMBAT FATIGUE; COMBAT REACTIONS; SHELL SHOCK.

Wassermann, August Paul von /väs′ərmän/ German bacteriologist, 1866–1925. See WASSERMANN TEST; JUVENILE TABES.

Wassermann test one of several types of blood tests for the detection of syphilis. Variations of the W.t. include **Eagle, Hinton,** and **Kahn serological tests.** The blood tests are only about 90 percent accurate as blood changes caused by malaria and certain forms of arthritis may indicate falsely the presence of the syphilis spirochete in the blood sample.

wastebasket diagnosis = NEGATIVE DIAGNOSIS.

watch test a crude test of auditory acuity based on determining the distance from which the subject can hear a watch ticking.

water phobia a morbid fear of water. The term is equivalent to one of the meanings of HYDROPHOBIA. See this entry. Also see AQUAPHOBIA.

water on the brain = CEREBRAL EDEMA.

water regulation a complex mechanism for maintaining optimum fluid balance in the body cells and extracellular liquids. W.r. involves secretion of an antidiuretic hormone to increase reabsorption of water from urine-producing structures in the kidneys, and transfer of water from one type of tissue to another. In some species, body fat can be oxidized to produce water as a metabolic byproduct. Also see THIRST.

Waters, Charles Alexander American radiologist, 1888–1961. See ROENTGENOGRAM (there: **Waters view roentgenogram**).

water-seeking behavior behavior observed in animals that have been deprived of water. Animals usually follow visual and olfactory clues toward possible water sources. An untrained animal, e.g., may be attracted by a reflecting surface that shows movement until it discovers that the visual cue does not lead to water. It then seeks other areas or objects that project the sight and smell of wetness.

watershed infarction an interruption of the normal blood flow to an area between two of the major arteries of the brain. Although the cerebral cortex is well supplied by arteries with collateral branches, there are areas near the junction of the parietal and occipital lobes and between the parietal and temporal lobes that are watershed areas.

Waters view roentgenogram: See ROENTGENOGRAM.

Watson, John Broadus American psychologist, 1878–1958. W. was the founder of behaviorism, which ruled out the then current emphasis on introspection, instincts, and consciousness, in favor of an objective study of observable, measurable behavior, molded after the methods of natural science. In applying this approach, major emphasis was placed on learned behavior, stimulus-response connections, and conditioning. See BEHAVIORISM.

wave forms: See BRAIN WAVES.

wave-interference patterns the principle of holographic photography in which a three dimensional image can be projected in space by light waves that converge from different angles at the site of the image. The principle has been proposed as an explanation for the ability of the mind to store spatial information and reconstruct the image of the original by recall processes.

wavelength thresholds the minimum and maximum light or sound wavelengths that can be perceived. In the visual system, w.t. vary somewhat with intensity but are generally around a minimum of 380 and a maximum of 760 millimicrons. Rod and cone functions also may be limiting factors, while species differences account for w.t. beyond human limits. W.t. also vary in the auditory system for different species and intensities of sound.

waxy flexibility = CATALEPSY.

WAY technique = WHO ARE YOU?

weak ego an ego, or conscious self, that is domineered by urges of the moment and cannot control the individual's emotions and actions. In psychoanalytic terms, a w.e. is an ego that is subject to unconscious impulses and which may disintegrate under strain, developing mental symptoms or character defects.

weakness fear = ASTHENOPHOBIA.

Weber, Ernst Heinrich /vā'bər/ German physiologist, 1795–1878. Recognized as the founder of psychophysics, W. did basic research on the skin and muscle senses, and discovered that we perceive relative rather than absolute changes in the intensity of stimuli. See WEBER'S LAW; DIFFERENCE THRESHOLD; FULLER-CATTELL LAW; MATHEMATICAL MODEL; PSYCHOPHYSICAL LAW. Also see MÜLLER, GEORG ELIAS.

Weber, Frederick Parkes English physician, 1863(?)–1962. See STURGE-WEBER SYNDROME; AMENTIA; PORT-WINE STAIN.

Weber's law the principle that the ratio of the stimulus change that is just noticeable to the level of the stimulus equals a constant, or $\triangle I/I = C$. The more intense the stimulus, the greater the change that must be made in it to be noticed. Also see FECHNER'S LAW; STEVENS' LAW.

Wechsler, David Rumanian-born American psychologist, 1896–1981. See WECHSLER ADULT INTELLIGENCE SCALE; WECHSLER BELLEVUE SCALE; WECHSLER INTELLIGENCE SCALE FOR CHILDREN; WECHSLER PRESCHOOL AND PRIMARY SCALE OF INTELLIGENCE; CULTURE-FAIR TESTS; DETERIORATION INDEX; INDIVIDUAL TEST; INFANT AND PRESCHOOL TESTS; INTELLIGENCE TEST; MISSING-PARTS TEST; PICTURE-ARRANGEMENT TEST; SUPERIOR INTELLIGENCE.

Wechsler Adult Intelligence Scale a modification of the Wechsler-Bellevue Scale containing the same six verbal subtests (Information, Comprehension, Arithmetic, Similarities, Digit Span, Vocabulary), and the same five performance subtests (Digit Symbol, Picture Completion, Block Design, Picture Arrangement, Object Assembly), with many of the individual items changed. The test yields a Verbal IQ, a Performance IQ, and a Full Scale IQ with a mean of 100 and a standard deviation of 15. In scoring the

test, the examiner notes strengths and weaknesses, the amount of scatter among the scores, and any significant discrepancy between the verbal and performance portions. The test was standardized on subjects ages 16 to 64. On the WAIS-R (revised 1981) a number of items have been updated and others involve both sexes and different races. Abbrev.: **WAIS**. See CULTURE-FAIR TESTS; IQ.

Wechsler-Bellevue Scale an individual intelligence scale for adults and older children developed by David Wechsler in 1939, and consisting of six verbal and five performance subtests which yield separate verbal and performance IQs as well as an overall IQ. The test has been replaced by the Wechsler Adult Intelligence Scale.

Wechsler Intelligence Scale for Children an intelligence test developed and standardized for children ages five years (zero months) to 15 years 11 months. The subtests are the same as those on the WAIS except for the alternate test (Mazes), and like the WAIS they measure verbal, numerical, social, and visual-motor capabilities, yielding a Verbal IQ, a Performance IQ, and a Full Scale IQ with a mean of 100 and a standard deviation of 15. Abbrev.: **WISC**.

Wechsler Preschool and Primary Scale of Intelligence an intelligence test for children ages four years to six years six months that includes five verbal subtests (Information, Vocabulary, Arithmetic, Similarities, Comprehension) and an alternate test (Sentences), and five performance subtests (Animal House, Picture Completion, Mazes, Geometrical Design, Block Design). These tests yield Verbal, Performance, and Full Scale IQs with a mean of 100 and a standard deviation of 15. Abbrev.: **WPPSI**.

wedding night the traditional time for the beginning of sexual adjustment between the bride and groom. The w.n. and honeymoon period immediately following marriage can be distressful for the man and woman, particularly if they have entered into marriage in the belief that the principal purpose of the union is to provide sexual satisfaction. If both husband and wife are virgins, they may be unduly concerned about differences in sexual desire, the pain or pleasure of the first sexual experience, or whether the vagina or penis may be too large or too small to afford proper sexual satisfaction. Cultural influences regarding the w.n. vary considerably, from the Victorian concept that a true lady might submit to her husband's sexual desires but would never enjoy it or take an active part, to the custom of permitting coitus by the couple before marriage, to prove their fertility, with the w.n. scheduled only after the woman has become pregnant. Also see DEFLORATION; VIRGINITY.

Wednesday Evening Society an informal group of Freud's disciples who met with him for instruction in psychoanalysis beginning in 1902. The Society evolved into the larger **Vienna**

Psychoanalytic Society in 1910. Also see VIEN-
NESE SCHOOL.

weekend hospital a form of partial hospitalization
in which psychiatric patients function in the
community during the week but spend the
weekend in the hospital.

weekend neurosis = SUNDAY NEUROSIS.

weekend parents parents who tend to devote only
their weekends to personal contact with their
children because both husband and wife work
full-time outside the home. The children of w.p.
as a result acquire life-style and behavioral influences from babysitters, day-care-center personnel, schools, and media, particularly television.
In 1982, more than 50 percent of married
women in America worked outside the home.

weeping = CRYING.

we-group = IN-GROUP.

Weigert, Carl /vī'gərt/ German histologist and
pathologist, 1845–1904. See WEIGERT STAIN.

Weigert stain a tissue dye used in the study of
myelinated axons. W.s. contains a substance,
hematoxylin, that does not stain the neuron but
rather the surrounding cells so that the neuron
appears as a clear area against a dark background on a microscope slide. Also see HEMA-
TOXYLIN STAIN.

weight a coefficient or multiplier indicating the relative importance of a statistic. The term is used
as noun or verb. (Thus **weighting** is the process
of assigning test-score values according to their
relative importance in determining the total
score.)

weight discrimination the ability to distinguish
weight differences of identical or similar objects.
The w.d. ability is believed to be controlled by
neurons in the postcentral gyrus of the parietal
lobe. Induced lesions of the postcentral gyrus in
monkeys result in w.d. impairment.

weighting: See WEIGHT; ITEM W.

weight regulation a process of body-energy
homeostasis that is under control of a center in
the hypothalamus. The w.r. mechanism seeks an
optimum balance between food intake and energy expenditure by the organism after a certain
body weight is achieved. Experimental evidence
indicates that obese animals usually reduce food
intake after reaching a certain weight level and
eat only enough to maintain the much-higher-
than-average weight.

Weight Watchers: See SELF-HELP GROUPS.

Weigl, Egon Rumanian-born psychologist, fl.
1929, 1968. See WEIGL-GOLDSTEIN-SCHEERER
TEST; CONCEPT-FORMATION TESTS.

Weigl-Goldstein-Scheerer Test a concept-
formation test requiring the subject to sort
geometric figures according to shape and color,
and to shift from one category to another. At the
same time, and subject is asked to verbalize
what he is doing in order to distinguish concrete
from abstract behavior. The test has been used
in studying brain injury.

Weill, Georges French ophthalmologist, 1866–

1952. See ADIE'S SYNDROME (also called **Weill**'s
syndrome).

Weinberg, Wilhelm /vīn'berk/ German physician,
1862—. See HARDY-WEINBERG LAW.

Weiss, Edoardo Austrian-American psychoanalyst, 1889–1970. See DESTRUDO; EGO NUCLEI;
EGO PSYCHOTHERAPY; EGO STATE.

Weiss, Nathan /vīs/ Austrian physician, 1851–83.
See CHVOSTEK'S TREMOR (also called **Weiss' sign**).

Welander, Lisa Swedish neurologist, 1909—. See
PROGRESSIVE SPINAL-MUSCULAR ATROPHY (there:
Wohlfart-Kugelberg-Welander disease).

Wells, Herbert George English novelist and science writer, 1866–1946. See MASS HYSTERIA.

Wells, William D. American psychologist, fl.
1975, 1982. See ETHICAL HIGHBROW.

Weltanschauung /velt'änshou·ŏong/ the total
body of an individual's philosophic beliefs and
observations about human life, society, and the
world at large (German, "world view").

Weltschmerz /velt'shmerts/ a sentimental melan-
choly and pessimism over the state of the world,
accompanied by a romantic acceptance of this
sadness as a natural aspect of human life (German, literally, "world pain").

Wepman Test of Auditory Discrimination an
individual test for assessing auditory deficits, in
which words that are alike or that vary by only
one phoneme are pronounced by the examiner,
and the subject must determine whether they
are the same or different.

Werdnig, Guido Austrian neurologist, 1844–
1919. See PROGRESSIVE SPINAL-MUSCULAR ATRO-
PHY (there: **Werdnig-Hoffmann disease**).

werewolf a person who supposedly has been
changed into a wolf, or is capable of changing
himself into a wolf. See LYCANTHROPY; MASS HYS-
TERIA; TRANSYLVANIA EFFECT.

Wermer, Paul American physician, fl. 1954, 1974.
See WERMER'S SYNDROME.

Wermer's syndrome a form of the Zollinger-
Ellison syndrome in which the peptic-ulcer-
pancreatic-tumor combination is complicated by
other endocrine-gland disorders. W.s. involves
tumors of the pituitary gland, adrenal cortex,
thyroid, and parathyroid glands, as well as the
pancreatic tumors and peptic ulcers.

Werner, Heinz German-born American psychologist, 1890–1964. See FORMAL PARALLEL-
ISM; PHYSIOGNOMIC PERCEPTION.

Werner, Otto German physician, 1879—. See
WERNER'S DISEASE.

Werner's disease a rare hereditary disorder affecting both sexes and characterized by signs of premature aging that may appear before the age of
20. The patients usually are of short stature. The
symptoms include graying and loss of hair, skin
atrophy, hypofunction of the endocrine glands,
accumulation of calcium deposits in the tissues,
and a form of arthritis. Also called **progeria
adultorum; Werner's syndrome**. Also see
PROGERIA.

Wernicke, Carl /ver'nikə/ German neurologist,

1848–1905. Wernicke's studies of brain pathology extended our knowledge of aphasia, established the dominance of one hemisphere of the brain, and gave us new information on brain damage associated with alcoholism. See WERNICKE'S APHASIA; WERNICKE'S AREA; WERNICKE'S CRAMP; WERNICKE'S DISEASE; WERNICKE'S ENCEPHALOPATHY; WERNICKE-KORSAKOFF SYNDROME; WERNICKE-MANN HEMIPLEGIA; PRESBYOPHRENIA (also called **Wernicke's dementia**); ACULALIA; ALCOHOL-AMNESTIC DISORDER; AUDITORY AMNESIA; AUTOPSYCHIC DELUSION; CONFABULATION; DEMENTIA; HYSTERICAL PSEUDODEMENTIA; NEUROLOGICAL IMPAIRMENT; SEMANTIC JARGON; THIAMINE DEFICIENCY; TRANSCORTICAL APHASIA.

Wernicke-Korsakoff syndrome an episode of Wernicke's encephalopathy followed by alcohol-amnestic disorder, or Korsakoff's disease. Both conditions are believed to be due to thiamine deficiency, but differences in the localization of the lesions produce different clinical pictures. For details, see ALCOHOL-AMNESTIC DISORDER; AMNESIC-CONFABULATORY SYNDROME; WERNICKE'S DISEASE.

Wernicke-Mann hemiplegia partial hemiplegia of the extremities with posture and gait abnormalities. The condition is caused by lesions of the central nervous system.

Wernicke's aphasia a loss of the ability to comprehend sounds or speech, and in particular to understand or repeat spoken language (word deafness) and to name objects or qualities (anomia). The condition is due to brain damage. The patient's auditory sensory organs beyond the brain may be normal. Other disorders of communication may be associated with the condition, including alexia, acalculia, or agraphia. Also called **Bastian's aphasia**; **cortical sensory aphasia**. See APHASIA; AUDITORY AMNESIA.

Wernicke's area a region in the posterior temporal gyrus containing nerve tissue associated with the interpretation of sounds. The area is named for Carl Wernicke who first reported, in 1874, a lack of comprehension of speech in patients who had suffered a brain lesion in that part of the brain.

Wernicke's cramp a muscle cramp that is due to psychogenic factors, such as fear or anxiety. Also called **cramp neurosis**. Also see OCCUPATIONAL NEUROSIS.

Wernicke's dementia = PRESBYOPHRENIA.

Wernicke's disease a symptom triad of ocular palsy, ataxia, and polyneuropathy associated with a thiamine, or vitamin-B$_1$, deficiency. The patient also may exhibit signs of mental confusion and aphonia. Cerebral blood flow is usually reduced significantly. The condition is observed in chronic alcoholism. Also called **cerebral beriberi**. See WERNICKE'S ENCEPHALOPATHY.

Wernicke's encephalopathy a brain disorder caused by a deficiency of vitamins, particularly thiamine and niacin, first described by the German neurologist Carl Wernicke in 1881. The principal symptoms are clouding of consciousness, ophthalmoplegia (paralysis of the eye muscles), failure of pupils to respond to light changes (Argyll-Robertson pupil), and ataxia. The disorder is most frequently seen in chronic alcoholics, but is also found in cases of pernicious anemia, gastric cancer, and vitamin-starved prisoners of war. If thiamine is not administered, W.e. may advance to Korsakoff's psychosis, in which memory loss and confabulation are major symptoms. See ALCOHOL-AMNESTIC DISORDER.

Wertheimer, Max /vert′hīmər/ German-born American psychologist, 1880–1943. After a broad education in philosophy and psychology, W. served as professor at Frankfurt, Germany, between 1909 and 1933, then accepted a post at the New School in New York. In opposition to the atomistic approach of structuralism, he founded the Gestalt movement, which holds that many of our perceptions and experiences comprise unique wholes that cannot be reduced to individual sensations, because the relationships between sensations are as important as the sensations themselves. With the assistance of his associates, Köhler and Koffka, he applied the Gestalt approach not only to an understanding of perception, but to the process of creative thinking and the solution of problems through insight. See GESTALT PSYCHOLOGY; LAW OF COMMON FATE. Also see KOFFKA; KÖHLER.

West, W. J. English physician, fl. 1840. See WEST'S SYNDROME.

western equine encephalitis: See EQUINE ENCEPHALITIS.

Western perspective: See PRIMITIVE.

Westphal, Alexander Karl Otto /vest′fäl/ German neurologist, 1863–1941. See WESTPHAL-LEYDEN SYNDROME.

Westphal, Karl Friedrich Otto /vest′fäl/ German neurologist, 1833–90. See WESTPHAL'S SIGN; EDINGER-WESTPHAL NUCLEUS.

Westphal-Leyden syndrome a neurologic disorder marked by slow scanning speech, ataxia with slow jerky action, faulty memory, excitability, and dementia. The onset may be marked by dizziness, vomiting, and coma. The cause of the disease is unknown. Also called **Leyden's ataxia**; **Westphal's ataxia**.

Westphal's sign the absence of the knee-jerk reflex as a sign of tabes dorsalis, or degeneration of the dorsal columns of the spinal cord and sensory-nerve trunks. The effect is observed in advanced cases of syphilis. Also called **Westphal's phenomenon**.

West's syndrome a progressive neurologic disorder affecting infants and marked by convulsions and mental retardation. The convulsions usually involve the neck, trunk, and limbs, causing a flexing of the arms and nodding of the head, as in a bowing movement. Also called **salaam convulsions; infantile spasms; eclampsia nutans**.

wet brain = CEREBRAL EDEMA.

wet dream a popular expression for nocturnal

emission, or ejaculation, occurring during an erotic dream. See NOCTURNAL EMISSION.

wet packs: See HYDROTHERAPY.

Wever, Ernest Glen American psychologist, 1902 —. See WEVER-BRAY EFFECT; HEARING THEORIES.

Wever-Bray effect the electrical activity generated in the cochlea as a response to external stimuli. It is not identical with the electrical nerve impulse carried by the auditory nerve, but seems to be due to conversion of sound energy to the electrical energy of the nerve impulse. Also called **aural microphonics**.

Weyer, Johann Dutch physician, fl. 1530. W. is sometimes regarded as the founder of modern psychiatry. Living at a time when witchcraft was rampant and abnormal behavior was blamed on the devil, W. insisted that witches were not possessed but were sick people who should be treated rather than punished. He also recommended that superstitions and dogma be replaced by naturalistic observation of mental life, and set an example by describing schizophrenic delusions and hallucinations in great detail, and by attributing the epidemics of mental illness of his time to mass suggestion. The reaction of the theologians was to accuse him of sorcery and place his name on the *Index Expurgatorius*. See WITCHCRAFT.

WF = WORD FLUENCY. Also see PRIMARY ABILITIES.

W factor = WILL FACTOR.

wheel: See COMMUNICATION NETWORKS.

wheelchair sports a type of recreational and rehabilitative activity in which disabled persons confined to wheelchairs participate in competitive individual and team sports. W.s. include basketball, bowling, archery, table tennis, and many standard track and field events, e.g., shot-put, discus, javelin, sprints, and relays. W.s. programs originated among World War II veterans in California, and at the Stoke Mandeville Hospital in England, and involve 10,000 disabled persons in 50 countries.

whiplash effect common name for a cervical syndrome that is associated with painful injury to soft tissues of the neck. The w.e. results from a sudden change of motion of the body, as when the patient is a passenger in a car involved in an accident; the momentum of forward movement may carry the head forward while the rest of the body is halted. Or, in a parked car struck by a moving vehicle, the head may be snapped back suddenly.

whipping in psychiatry, a common form of sexual sadism and masochism. Krafft-Ebing's accounts of both children and adults who derived sexual excitement from watching others being whipped, being whipped themselves, or from fantasies of whipping or being whipped, are considered classic. See FLAGELLATION.

Whipple, George Hoyt American pathologist, 1878—. See LIPODYSTROPHY (there: **Whipple's disease**).

whisper aphonia oral communication without complete vocal-cord function, a physiological laryngeal sound phenomenon.

whisper test a crude test of auditory acuity in which the examiner whispers test words from a distance of 20 feet while the subject, with one ear plugged, responds without watching the examiner.

whistling-face syndrome a congenital disorder characterized by flat facial bones that contribute to a stiff, masklike face. The patients also have a high arched palate, small tongue, small mouth, and thin protruding lips that create the appearance of a person who is whistling. The condition occurs in first children born prematurely. Also called **Freeman-Sheldon syndrome**.

White, Samuel American psychiatrist, 1777–1845. W. was one of the original 13 founders of the Association of Medical Superintendents of American Institutions for the Insane, which later evolved into the American Psychiatric Association.

White, Sheldon American psychologist, 1928—. See FIVE-TO-SEVEN SHIFT.

White, William Alanson American psychiatrist, 1870–1937. As lifetime superintendent of the Government Hospital for the Insane in Washington (now St. Elizabeth's), W. transformed it from a custodial institution to a center for active, holistic treatment, research, and psychiatric training—a veritable "scientific community." W. also taught at Washington medical school; played a leading role in forensic psychiatry, and in disseminating the psychoanalytic approach; served as president of the American Psychiatric Association, the American Psychoanalytic Association, and the American Psychopathological Association; and wrote 17 influential books on psychiatry, diseases of the nervous system, psychopathology, and mental hygiene. Also see BLUE-COLLAR THERAPY.

white commissure a bundle of myelinated fibers that crosses from one side of the spinal cord to the other, linking the ascending and descending columns of white-matter fibers on either side. It is located between the ventral gray commissure and the ventral median fissure of the spinal cord. Also called **ventral w.c.**

white lies: See LYING.

white matter the portion of the nervous system that is composed of nerve fibers that are enclosed in myelin sheaths which contribute a white coloration to otherwise grayish structures. The sheaths cover only the fibers, however, so the cell bodies of the myelinated nerves are gray.

whiteness constancy a perception of white surfaces as having the same brightness even when lighting changes are made. Also see PERCEPTUAL CONSTANCY; BRIGHTNESS CONSTANCY.

white noise a sound pattern composed of pure tones, harmonics, and discordants presented as background noise. W.n. is used as background noise to modulate the effects of intrusive or distracting sounds in the environment, e.g., sounds that normally disturb sleep or concentration. W.n. frequently is employed as background sound for speech-intelligibility tests.

white-out syndrome a psychosis occurring in arctic explorers and mountaineers exposed to the same white environment for long periods of time. Also see SENSORY DEPRIVATION.

white rami communicantes the myelinated fibers of the preganglionic branches of the sympathetic-nervous-system ganglia. They are located along the thoracic and upper lumbar segments of the sympathetic tract and function as input fibers from the spinal nerves.

whitiko = WINDIGO.

Whitney, Donald Ransom American mathematical statistician, 1915—. See MANN-WHITNEY U TEST.

WHO the common abbreviation of World Health Organization.

Who Are You? a projective test in which the subject is asked to write three short answers to the question "Who are you?" The answers are analyzed for the information they reveal about the subject's identity or self-concept. Also called **WAY technique; Who Am I?**

whole method of learning a learning technique in which the total material is repeated until it is memorized, as opposed to learning the material in parts. Compare PART METHOD OF LEARNING.

whooping cough a highly contagious bacterial infection that affects the respiratory tract from the nasopharynx to the bronchioles. W.c. is characterized clinically by spasmodic coughing that commonly ends in a prolonged high-pitched whooping inspiration. Complications can include brain hemorrhage, convulsions, anoxia, and damage to vision and hearing abilities. Also called **pertussis.**

Whorf, Benjamin Lee American anthropological linguist and chemical engineer, 1897–1941. See WHORF'S HYPOTHESIS.

Whorf's hypothesis a generalization that differences in language and linguistic habits produce differences in perception and thought, so that variations in languages are derivable from diverse world-views and cultures. Also called **Sapir-Whorf hypothesis.**

Wide Range Achievement Test an individual achievement test used primarily for remedial and vocational as well as general educational purposes, measuring the subject's level of skill in reading, spelling, and computation, with an adjustable range from kindergarten to college.

widowhood crisis a period, often lasting at least a year because of anniversaries and fresh memories, in which a widow must adjust to the loss of her husband and readjust her life accordingly. Typically, she goes through the stages of grief delineated by E. Kübler-Ross: denial, anger, negotiation with God, depression, acceptance. Group therapy and the experimental Widow-to-Widow Program have been found particularly effective in helping to meet this crisis. Also see GRIEF; MOURNING.

Widow-to-Widow Program: See WIDOWHOOD CRISIS; DEATH NEUROSIS.

Wiener, Norbert American mathematician, 1894–1964. See CYBERNETICS.

Wiener Schule = VIENNESE SCHOOL.

Wiesengrund Adorno: See ADORNO.

Wiethe, Camille /vē′tə/ Austrian otologist, 1888–1949. See URBACH-WIETHE DISEASE.

wife-beating: See BATTERED WIVES.

wife-swapping a form of group sex in which two or more married couples by mutual agreement exchange spouses for the purpose of sexual intercourse. The practice of w.-s. also may include watching the husband or wife participate in sexual intercourse with another's spouse. Also called **partner-swapping.** Also see SWINGING.

Wiggly Block Test a manual-dexterity test in which nine wavy blocks are reassembled into a single rectangular block from which they have been cut.

wihtigo; wihtiko = WINDIGO.

Wilcoxon, Frank Irish-born American chemist and statistician, 1892—. See WILCOXON TEST.

Wilcoxon test a nonparametric test of statistical significance in which two matched sets of observations are ranked and the difference between the ranks is tested for significance.

wild boy of Aveyron a supposed feral child, unsocialized and nonliterate, found living in the woods near Aveyron around 1800 and studied by a French physician, Jean Itard. It has been suggested that the boy actually was a subnormal child abandoned in the woods by his parents. Itard's attempts to teach the boy inspired his pupil, Edouard Seguin, to develop materials and methods for training the retarded. Also see WOLF CHILDREN; FERAL CHILDREN; SEGUIN.

Wilder, Joseph American neuropsychiatrist, 1895—. See LAW OF INITIAL VALUES (also called **Wilder's law of initial values).**

Wildervanck, L. S. /vil′dərfängk/ Dutch physician, fl. 1960. See WILDERVANCK'S SYNDROME.

Wildervanck's syndrome a hereditary disorder associated with Klippel-Feil syndrome and characterized by deaf-mutism and abducens paralysis. Cranial asymmetry also may occur. See KLIPPEL-FEIL SYNDROME.

wild psychoanalysis a term used by Freud (1910) for procedures that depart from the technical process of psychoanalysis, e.g., offering direct advice to a patient, or making dynamic interpretations before the patient is ready for them.

will: See FREE W.; FREEDOM OF W.; DYSBULIA; VOLITION.

will disturbances the deficiency or lack of will power identified by Bleuler as a basic symptom of schizophrenia. The patient may appear lazy and lacking in objectives and motivation. Another form of w.d. observed in schizophrenics is characterized by a high degree of activity that is bizarre, trivial, inappropriate, or purposeless.

Wille zur Macht: See WILL TO POWER.

will factor in factor analysis, the factor correlated with persistence, purpose, striving, and effort. Abbrev.: **w**. Also called **W factor**.

Willi, Heinrich Swiss pediatrician, fl. 1956. See PRADER-LABHART-WILLI SYNDROME.

Willis, Thomas English physician, 1621–75. See ARTERIAL CIRCLE (also called **circle of Willis**).

Willowbrook Consent Judgment a landmark agreement between agencies, parents, friends of the court (plaintiffs), and the Division of Mental Retardation of the New York State Department of Mental Hygiene (defendant) detailing the rights of the retarded (1972) regarding such questions as the resident-living environment, program, evaluation of program, personnel, education, recreation, food and nutrition service, dental services, psychological services, physical-therapy services, speech and audiology, medical and nursing services, safety procedures, treatment and medication, building maintenance, emergencies, records, and community placement.

will therapy a form of psychotherapy developed by Otto Rank, who held that neuroses can be avoided or overcome by asserting one's will (or "counterwill"), and by achieving independence. According to his theory, life is a long struggle to separate oneself from the mother psychologically, just as one separates oneself physically during birth. Also called **Rankian therapy**. See BIRTH TRAUMA; LIFE FEAR; RANK.

will to live = WILL TO SURVIVE.

will to meaning the term introduced by V. Frankl to denote the need to find a suitable meaning and purpose for one's life. The w.t.m. is the basis and fundamental motivation of logotherapy, developed by Frankl as a technique for addressing problems related to the contemporary experience of meaninglessness. See LOGOTHERAPY; EXISTENTIAL VACUUM.

will to power a term used by Adler for the determination to strive for superiority and domination, which he believed to be particularly strong in males who feel a need to escape the feelings of insecurity and inferiority which they associate with femininity. The term was borrowed from Nietzsche (German *Wille zur Macht*). See MASCULINE PROTEST.

will to survive the determination to live in spite of an adverse situation such as a severe illness, disabling disorder, or extreme conditions such as lack of food and water, or entrapment in a mine shaft. There is considerable evidence, mostly anecdotal, that a strong w.t.s. can in some cases enhance the chances for recovery, or at least prolong the life of the individual, and can enable many persons to endure deprivation, incarceration, and both physical and mental punishment. Also called **will to live**.

Wilm, Marx German surgeon, 1867–1918. See WILM'S TUMOR.

Wilm's tumor a type of congenital kidney tumor that may lie dormant for several years before producing symptoms. First signs may be an abdominal mass, fever, bloody urine, pain, nausea, and vomiting. W.t. is the second most common type of childhood tumor and usually is treated with chemotherapy, surgery, and radiation, with a 50-percent chance of extending survival by five years.

Wilson, E. O. American social scientist, 1929—. See SOCIOBIOLOGY.

Wilson, Samuel Alexander Kinnier English neurologist, ca. 1877–1937. See HEPATOLENTICULAR DEGENERATION (also called **Wilson's disease**); BRAIN DAMAGE; TRIETHYLENE TETRAMINE.

wind-chill index a system of determining the combined effect of air temperature and wind speed on human body temperature. At an air temperature of 32°F (0°C), the wind-chill factor when the wind speed is five miles an hour is 29°F (–1.7°C). As the wind speed increases to 35 miles an hour, at the same air temperature, the wind-chill factor is –1°F (–18.3°C). A wind-chill factor of –40°F (–40°C), produced by a 30-mile-an-hour wind at 0°F (–17.8°C), will freeze human skin in less than one minute.

wind effects in environmental psychology, the influence of winds on feelings and comfort. A light wind can have a refreshing effect, particularly on a hot or humid day; a strong, howling wind can cause feelings of fear and anxiety, which may be aggravated by news reports of tornadoes and hurricanes. W.e. generally are associated with AIR-PRESSURE EFFECTS. See this entry. Also see BEAUFORT WIND SCALE.

wind fear = ANEMOPHOBIA.

windigo a severe culture-specific syndrome occurring primarily in Cree Eskimos and Canadian Ojibwas. Initial symptoms are usually anorexia, nausea, and vomiting accompanied by the brooding fear of a supernatural man-eating witch, or w., made of ice. If the phobia is not dispelled by a medicine man, the patient may feel that he himself has been transformed into a w., and proceed to kill and eat one or more members of his household. Also called **whitiko; wihtigo; wihtiko; witigo**.

windmill illusion an illusion of motion of rotating objects such as windmills and automobile wheels, in which they appear to reverse direction intermittently.

window: See THERAPEUTIC W.

wind-swept deformity a term applied to the appearance of some cases of pseudoachondroplasia dwarfism in which there is a bowing of the lower legs. The left knee may turn outward and the right knee inward, or vice versa.

wind tunnel a structure designed as a corridor through which air can be blown at controlled velocities and patterns of turbulence to test the performance of aircraft or other objects or materials in a simulated outdoor environment. A w.t. also may be utilized in environmental-psychology experiments to study effects of wind or changing air pressures on the performance or behavior of humans. See AIR-PRESSURE EFFECTS.

Winiwarter, Felix von /vin'ēvärtər/ Austrian surgeon, 1852–1931. See BUERGER'S DISEASE (also called **Winiwarter-Buerger syndrome**).

winning back: See DEPROGRAMING.

wiring in evaluation research, "a situation in which the federal system issues a request for proposals and receives bids, however[,] a pre-existing special relationship virtually assures the contract to a specific bidder; transmitting advance knowledge of a program only to a favored bidder." (M. R. Meyers, *The Evaluation Enterprise*, 1981)

WISC = WECHSLER INTELLIGENCE SCALE FOR CHILDREN.

wish a term denoting ordinarily a desire or longing, but more broadly used in psychoanalysis to denote any urge, striving, tendency, or impulse that operates on a conscious or unconscious level.

wish-fulfillment in general, the gratification or realization of one's desires; in psychoanalysis, the drive to free oneself from the tension created by instinctual needs such as sex and hostility.

wishful thinking thought processes governed by inner wishes and desires rather than by logic or reality; believing what we want to believe.

wit a mental function consisting of the ability to make amusing, incisive comments that throw light on a subject or person. In psychoanalysis, wit means a verbal retort, jibe, or pun that suddenly and strikingly releases a repressed or hidden feeling or attitude. Also see EXAGGERATION IN WIT; TENDENCY WIT.

witchcraft sorcery practiced by a woman reputed to possess supernatural powers derived from a compact with the devil. Witch-hunting received its greatest impetus in 1487 when two German theologians and inquisitors, Heinrich Krämer and Johann Sprenger, published a manual entitled the *Malleus Maleficarum* ("the witches' hammer"), with the approval of the church. This work not only argued for the existence of witches, but insisted that they could be identified by pigment spots or anesthetic areas on their bodies left by the "devil's claw." It also gave detailed instructions for trying them. Witches were blamed for all types of natural catastrophes and all types of abnormal and criminal behavior. As a result, thousands were tortured and burned at the stake, until the beginning of the 19th century. See DEMONOLOGY; INCUBUS; SUCCUBUS; WEYER. Also see CURSING MAGIC; SORCERY DRUGS; HEX DOCTORS.

witch doctor = SHAMAN.

witches' sabbath a ceremony observed by some groups during the Middle Ages in defiance of the church and including the drinking of wine spiked with henbane or belladonna. The concoction reportedly produced frenzied sexual arousal accompanied by vivid hallucinations. If the participants were caught, they were usually tortured into confessions, then burned alive.

withdrawal an organic mental disorder following cessation or reduction in intake of a substance such as alcohol, an opioid, amphetamines, tobacco, or sedatives that have previously been used regularly to induce intoxication. W. symptoms vary in intensity depending upon the substance, but they usually include some degree of anxiety, restlessness, insomnia, impaired attention, and irritability. See ALCOHOL W.; ALCOHOL-W. DELIRIUM; AMPHETAMINE OR SIMILARLY ACTING SYMPATHOMIMETIC W.; BARBITURATE OR SIMILARLY ACTING SEDATIVE OR HYPNOTIC W.; OPIOID W.; TOBACCO W.; INFANTILE NARCOTIC W.; SUBSTANCE W. Also see SOCIAL W.; APATHETIC W.; W. REACTION. (DSM-III)

withdrawal-destructiveness according to E. Fromm, a style of relating based on withdrawal and isolation from others, destructive behavior directed toward others, or a combination of the two trends. Fromm held that the motivation for w.-d. styles lies in the need to establish emotional distance due to the fear of dependency.

withdrawal reaction a defensive reaction consisting of retreat from social contact and involvement, or from threatening situations. In its extreme form, withdrawal is characterized by retreat from reality as a whole. Pathological withdrawal occurs primarily in schizophrenia and depression. The term withdrawal also applies to physical retraction of a hand or foot from a painful stimulus. See ADJUSTMENT DISORDER WITH WITHDRAWAL; SOCIAL WITHDRAWAL; WITHDRAWAL.

withdrawal reflex a response that may be stimulated by any unexpected threat to the well-being of the individual. It is characterized by sudden movement away from the potentially damaging stimulus as a natural survival procedure. It requires rapid coordination of neuromuscular units and thus may not involve impulse circuits above the primitive brain areas.

within-groups variance a variation in scores occurring among the subjects in an experiment and not resulting from an experimental treatment. Also see BETWEEN-GROUPS VARIANCE.

witigo = WINDIGO.

witness: See EXPERT W.

Wittmaack, Theodor /vit'mäk/ German physician, fl. 1861. See EKBOM'S SYNDROME (also called **Wittmaack-Ekbom syndrome**).

wit work a Freudian term used to describe the psychic processes involved in producing witticisms.

Witzelsucht /vit'səlzo͞okht/ a German word meaning literally "compulsive wisecracking"; in psychiatry, a type of joking mania, a symptom occurring in lesions in the frontal association areas, often resulting from tumors or cerebral arteriosclerosis. The patient's facetiousness is probably defensive in nature and is manifested in a jocular manner and a euphoric attitude. It is often accompanied by childish behavior and indifference to the seriousness of the situation.

Wiveleslie: See ABNEY SIR WILLIAM DE W.

wobbly knee a condition in which lowered muscle tonus causes a laxness of the knee. It is often a sign of cerebellar disorder.

Wohlfart, Gunnar Swedish neurologist, 1910–61. See PROGRESSIVE SPINAL-MUSCULAR ATROPHY (there: **Wohlfart-Kugelberg-Welander disease**).

Wohlwill, Joachim Friedrich German-Portuguese physician, 1881—. See ANDRADE'S SYNDROME (also called **Wohlwill-Corino Andrade syndrome**).

Wolberg, Lewis Robert Russian-born American psychiatrist, 1905—. See PSYCHOTHERAPY.

wolf children a term applied, particularly, to two girls who were apparently raised by wolves in India, and who adopted all their major life patterns, such as bolting their food, howling in the night, and running on all fours. When captured, they were approximately 18 months and eight years old, but the younger girl died within a year. The older girl lived till about age 17 and, though never fully civilized, learned to walk on two feet in a half-crouch, ate without devouring her food, acquired a 50-word vocabulary, and learned to wear clothes and run errands. Also see WILD BOY OF AVEYRON; FERAL CHILDREN.

Wolf Man a landmark case reported by Freud in 1918, involving a conversion symptom (constipation), a phobia (for wolves and other animals), a religious obsession (piety alternating with blasphemous thoughts), and an appetite disturbance (anorexia), all of which proved to be reactions to early experiences. The case helped to confirm Freud's theory of infantile sexuality.

Wolman, Moshe Polish-born Israeli pathologist, 1914—. See WOLMAN'S DISEASE; XANTHOMATOSIS.

Wolman's disease a genetic metabolic disorder characterized by a deficiency of an acid-lipase enzyme needed to break down lipid molecules. Adrenal glands become enlarged and calcified. Psychomotor development in affected infants appears delayed, and mental retardation may be present but difficult to document due to overriding effects of vomiting, diarrhea, and other signs of acute illness. Also called **primary familial xanthomatosis.**

womb = UTERUS.

womb envy a psychological characteristic of a transsexual or transvestite male whose gender identity is female. Also see VAGINAL ENVY.

womb fantasy the fantasy of returning to the womb or existing in the womb, usually expressed in symbolic form, e.g., living under water, or being alone in a cavern.

women's liberation movement a trend among women, or certain groups of women, to free themselves (a) from the sexual double standard, (b) from being relegated to inferior positions in business, (c) from receiving lower pay than men for the same work, (d) from the total responsibility for child-rearing and homemaking, (e) from the dominance of the male not only in the home and in business but in the arts and sciences as well, and (f) from the traditional stereotype of women as fragile, passive, dependent individuals who are governed by emotion rather than reason. Also see CLITORIDECTOMY; CONSCIOUSNESS-RAISING; DOUBLE STANDARD; FEMINISM; FEMININITY; GENDER ROLE; HOUSEWIFE SYNDROME; JUS PRIMAE NOCTIS; PIBLOKTO; RADICAL THERAPY; RAPE COUNSELING; RAPE-TRAUMA SYNDROME; RAP GROUP; SEX DISCRIMINATION; SEXISM; SEX ROLES; SEX-TYPING; TOMBOYISM; UNISEX; WORKING MOTHERS.

women's roles the functions of women in society, which have recently been expanded to include increasingly active participation in business, industry, the armed forces, courts, police departments, and every other major function of local and national government, in addition to their traditional roles in homemaking, child-rearing, and volunteer service.

women with penis a childhood concept that every female possesses or once possessed a penis. The discovery by small boys that girls lack a penis reinforces their concern about castration.

Woodworth, Robert Sessions American psychologist, 1869–1962. W. studied with James at Harvard and Cattell at Columbia, later serving as professor at Columbia, experimentalist, educational psychologist, and textbook writer (*Psychology*, 1921; *Contemporary Schools of Psychology*, with M. R. Sheehan). He developed a basic personality inventory during World War I, to be used as a screening device for neurosis, and formulated the dynamic approach in psychology based on the importance of motivation. See WOODWORTH-MATHEWS PERSONAL DATA SHEET; DRIVE; RACE DIFFERENCES; TRANSFER OF TRAINING. Also see JAMES; CATTELL, JAMES MCKEEN.

Woodworth-Mathews Personal Data Sheet a personality inventory containing 116 yes-no items designed to be used in educational institutions as a screening device for neurosis.

Wooldridge, Dean Everett American scientist, 1913—. See MECHANICAL-MAN CONCEPT.

woolly mammoth a term introduced by Paul Wachtel to describe repressed conflicts encapsulated in the unconscious for many years, like prehistoric mammoths that were frozen alive and preserved for millennia.

word approximation a schizophrenic speech disturbance in which conventional words are used in unconventional or inappropriate ways (as in metonymy), or new but understandable words are constructed out of ordinary words, e.g., "easify" for "simplify."

word-association test a projective test in which the subject responds to a stimulus word with the first word that comes to mind. The technique was invented by Francis Galton in 1879 for use in exploring individual differences, and Kraepelin was the first to apply it to the study of abnormality. Jung compiled a list of 100 words designed to uncover complexes, and Kent and Rosanoff (1910) and Rapaport and colleagues (1946) also compiled lists to be used for clinical purposes.

word blindness = ALEXIA. Also see AGNOSIC ALEXIA.

word-building test a test in which the subject constructs as many words as possible out of a given group of letters.

word configuration the overall visual pattern projected by a written word; the general visual effect of a word as produced by the combination of shapes or particular typeface or script.

word count a study of the rate of occurrence or the prevalence of specific words in a designated sample of spoken or written speech, e.g., in 50 children's books for third- and fourth-graders or in a particular Presidential address.

word deafness = AUDITORY APHASIA.

word dumbness = EXPRESSIVE APHASIA.

word fluency the ability to list words rapidly in certain designated categories, such as words that begin with a particular letter of the alphabet. The ability is associated with a part of the brain anterior to the Broca area of the dominant frontal lobe. Persons with lesions in that part of the brain are likely to suffer w.f. deficits in verbal tests and tasks. Abbr.: **WF**. Also see PRIMARY ABILITIES.

word-frequency study: See WORD COUNT.

word hash = WORD SALAD.

word realism = NOMINAL REALISM.

word-recognition skills a cluster of word-recognition strategies used in reading, such as use of sight words, context clues, phonics, and structural analysis.

word salad incoherent, unintelligible speech associated with advanced schizophrenic states, seemingly a hodgepodge of both real words and neologisms. Although usually incomprehensible, w.s. is not necessarily meaningless; but uncovering the meaning requires a patient process of association and interpretation. The term is essentially equivalent to NEOLOGISTIC JARGON. See this entry. W.s. is also called **jargon aphasia; paraphrasia; word hash**.

work addiction a compulsive dependence on work as the only means of maintaining self-esteem and self-worth.

workaholic a popular term for an individual who has a craving for working night and day even when it is not necessary.

work decrement a decline in the size or rate of output of a task per unit of time; also, in experimentation, a decline in the magnitude of responses as a function of frequency of the response.

work ethic an emphasis, and frequently overemphasis, on the value of work as a goal in life and as a justification for one's existence. Also see ACHIEVEMENT ETHIC.

work evaluation assessment of an individual worker's job performance in terms of such factors as productivity, number and kind of errors, safe operation of machines, special skills and abilities, ability to learn new methods, and potential for progress to a higher level. Also called **vocational evaluation**.

work-for-pay unit an in-patient or aftercare work facility constituting a component of a comprehensive rehabilitation program for mental patients. Such units offer prevocational screening and evaluation, vocational training, ego-strength assessment, and simple-to-complex industrial operations performed under supervision. See SHELTERED WORKSHOP.

work hours in industrial psychology, the effects of the total number of hours worked per week, as well as overtime work, moonlighting, shift work, and a flexible work schedule, upon such factors as productivity, injuries, absenteeism, and worker satisfaction.

working conditions in industrial psychology, the conditions under which employees carry out their job, including such variables as illumination, atmospheric conditions, noise, work schedule, shift work, and rest periods.

working mean an assumed mean, usually an arbitrary value near the middle of a series. Also called **assumed mean**.

working mothers mothers of small and school-aged children who work outside the home. The growing number of w. m. has exposed them to added stresses, and has frequently created role conflicts and role strain which lead to an identity crisis. These are counterbalanced in varying degrees by feelings of self-fulfillment, economic advantages, availability of day-care facilities, and a more cooperative role for the father in the home.

working over a term used by Freud to describe the psychic processes involved in reorganizing, adjusting, and otherwise modifying excitations to prevent the harmful effects of discharging outward undesirable responses.

working through in psychoanalysis, the process in which the patient gradually overcomes his resistances to the disclosure of unconscious material and is repeatedly brought face to face with the repressed feelings, threatening impulses, and internal conflicts that are at the root of his difficulties. The purpose of this process is to increase the patient's insight and to help him master his conflicts and assimilate new and constructive attitudes and reactions into his personality.

working vocabulary = ACTIVE VOCABULARY.

work inhibition: See ADJUSTMENT DISORDER WITH WORK OR ACADEMIC INHIBITION.

work-limit test a test in which all subjects perform the same task but scores are based on the time required for the performance.

work motivation: See EXISTENCE, RELATEDNESS, AND GROWTH THEORY.

work phobia = PONOPHOBIA.

work rehabilitation center a facility, such as a sheltered workshop, in which efforts are made to habilitate or rehabilitate the physically or mentally disabled through a paid work program geared to their abilities and interests.

work-sample test a job-specific test in which the individual either (a) performs specific operations in a controlled testing situation, using actual or simulated equipment (e.g., driving a loaded fork-lift truck around a standard course), or (b) takes a written test on the knowledge required for a particular job, such as operating a tool-grinding machine.

work-space design the design of fixed work stations for effective, comfortable, and safe performance of tasks. Examples are placement of materials, tools, machines, and controls within easy reach, and a comfortable, adjustable seat adapted to the particular job.

work-study program any of a variety of educational programs combining classroom study with job experience for the purpose of providing students with financial assistance or practical training.

work therapy the use of paid work activities, e.g., weaving, packaging, assembly, or ceramics, as a therapeutic agent for persons with mental or physical disorders. Productive work keeps them from lapsing into inertia, focuses their attention outside themselves, provides healthy physical activity, develops their skills, and helps to maintain their sense of self-esteem.

world-destruction phantasies: See SCHIZOPHRENIC SURRENDER.

World Test: See BOLGAR-FISCHER W.T.

wormwood the common name of Artemisia absinthium, the source of absinthe, which is prepared from the dried leaves and flowering tops of the plant. See ABSINTHE.

worry a state of mental distress or agitation due to concern for an impending or anticipated event, threat, or danger.

WPPSI = WECHSLER PRESCHOOL AND PRIMARY SCALE OF INTELLIGENCE.

writer's block inhibited creativity in a professional writer, due to unconscious factors. Psychoanalysts cite such factors as fear of success or revival of rivalry with the father, along with oedipal anxieties associated with it. The block may result in WRITER'S CRAMP. See this entry.

writer's cramp a painful spasm of the muscles involved in writing or typing, usually considered a conversion or hysterical symptom due to unconscious conflicts. The patient may be able to use the same muscles in other activities such as shuffling cards. Also called **mogigraphia**. See COMPENSATION NEUROSIS; OCCUPATIONAL NEUROSIS.

writing-fear = GRAPHOPHOBIA.

wryneck syndrome intermittent or continuous spasms of the neck muscles, causing a turning and tipping of the head. The direction of head movement depends upon which of the several neck muscles are involved. The condition is commonly associated with psychologic disorders, and usually responds to psychiatric treatment in lieu of surgical correction of the neck nerves and muscles. Also called **spasmodic torticollis**. Also see TORTICOLLIS.

W-state the *w*aking state, as contrasted with the S-state (sleep state) and D-state (dream state).

Wundt, Wilhelm Max /voont/ German psychologist and physiologist, 1832–1920. W. became the founder of experimental psychology when he established the first official psychological laboratory in Leipzig, in which introspective and psychophysical methods were applied to a wide range of subjects, including reaction time, word associations, attention, judgment, and emotions. A man of encyclopedic mentality, he not only published monumental works on the history and foundations of psychology, but on logic, ethics, and the psychological interpretation of the data of history and anthropology. See WUNDT CURVE; ACT PSYCHOLOGY; STRUCTURALISM; TRIDIMENSIONAL THEORY OF FEELING. Also see BRENTANO; CATTELL, JAMES MCKEEN; TITCHENER.

Wundt curve an illusion described in 1898 by Wilhelm Wundt who found that straight lines that appeared to be curved when viewed through a prism appeared to curve in the opposite direction when the prism was removed.

Würzburg School a school of psychology developed by Oswald Külpe and his associates in Würzburg, Germany, largely as a reaction to the structuralist approach of Wundt and Titchener. Instead of reducing experience to its basic elements (sensations, images, feelings), the W.S. focused on intangible mental activities such as judgments, meanings, determining tendencies (or sets), all of which were termed conscious attitudes (German *Bewusstseinslage*, "state of consciousness"). See AUFGABE; DETERMINING TENDENCY; IMAGELESS THOUGHT; SET; KÜLPE.

Wyatt v. Stickney decision: See FORCED TREATMENT.

Wyburn-Mason, Roger English physician, fl. 1943, 1972. See WYBURN-MASON'S SYNDROME.

Wyburn-Mason's syndrome a brain disease caused by an arteriovenous aneurysm on one or both sides of the midbrain. The condition may be accompanied by ocular anomalies and cutaneous nevi (moles). Symptoms include speech disorders, headache, facial paralysis, and hydrocephalus. Mental retardation is a common complication. Also called **cerebroretinal arteriovenous aneurysm**.

wysocean = TOLOA.

X

-xanth-; -xantho- a combining form meaning yellow (Greek *xanthos*).

xanthines a group of stimulants related chemically to the xanthine bodies in urine and animal tissues. See CAFFEINE EFFECTS; METHYLXANTHINES.

xanthocyanopsia a form of color blindness in which red and green are not perceived and objects are seen in shades of yellow or blue.

xanthomatosis any of several disorders marked by an accumulation of excess lipids, such as cholesterol, in the body due to a metabolic disturbance. The lipids lead to the formation of foam cells in skin lesions and other symptoms. Types of x. include bulbi x., marked by fatty degeneration of the cornea; Wolman's disease; cerebrotendinous x., or van Bōgaert's disease, characterized by ataxia, dementia, and cataracts; hypercholesterolemic x., or Type II hyperlipoproteinemia, associated with accelerated atherosclerosis and premature heart attacks; and normal cholesterolemic x., or Hand-Christian-Schüller syndrome. A related form of x. results in cutaneous lesions and other effects in some cases of diabetes. Also see HAND-CHRISTIAN-SCHÜLLER SYNDROME; CEREBROTENDINOUS X.; WOLMAN'S DISEASE.

xanthopsia yellow-sightedness, or an excessive visual sensitivity to yellow.

X axis: See ABSCISSA.

X chromosome the female sex chromosome, which controls sex differentiation. A normal female complement of sex chromosomes consists of a pair of X chromosomes, even though one of the X chromosomes is inactivated in a tissue cell. Also see FRAGILE X C.

-xen-; -xeno- /-zen-/ a combining form meaning different, strange, alien (from Greek *xenos*, "stranger, guest").

xenoglossophilia a tendency to use strange or foreign words, particularly in a pretentious manner.

xenophobia a pathological fear of strangers. X. also refers to hostile attitudes or aggressive behavior toward people of other nationalities or minority groups. Also see FEAR OF STRANGERS.

-xer-; -xero- /-zērŏ-/ a combining form relating to a dry condition or process (from Greek *xeros*, "dry").

xeroderma pigmentosum an autosomal-recessive syndrome characterized mainly by hypersensitivity to sunlight and by skin cancer. The patients usually are freckled, suffer from photophobia, and have delayed or deficient sexual maturation. Microcephaly, spasticity, and mental retardation occur in many cases.

xerodermic idiocy a syndrome acquired as an autosomal-recessive trait marked by microcephaly and mental retardation combined with dwarfism and XERODERMA PIGMENTOSUM. See this entry.

xi /zī/ or /sī/ 14th letter of the Greek alphabet (Ξ, ξ)

X-linked abnormalities sex-chromosomal aberrations that result in disorders such as gonadal dysgenesis (defective development) in a female who fails to inherit a complete XX set of chromosomes. In some cases, one normal and one abnormal X chromosome will form a ring. The incidence of X-l.a. is reduced, according to the Lyon hypothesis, because one of the X chromosomes in a female is genetically inactivated.

X-linked anophthalmia a hereditary disorder marked by microcephalic skull and the clinical absence of eyeballs. All patients examined have had subnormal intelligence and slow psychomotor development during childhood.

XO syndrome = TURNER'S SYNDROME.

X-O Test one of the first tests of attitudes and interests, on which the subject crosses out or circles certain preferences. The test was designed by S. L. Pressey.

X-ray a short-wavelength electromagnetic emission produced by passing a high-voltage current through a vacuum tube. Because the radiation can produce images of objects on photographic film or can cause certain chemicals to fluoresce, the X-ray is used in medical diagnosis to visualize internal body-tissue structures. The energy of the rays also is utilized therapeutically to destroy malignant cells. X-ray emissions also are produced by the sun and radioactive isotopes. Also called **Roentgen ray**. Also see DIAGNOSTIC X-RAY TECHNOLOGIST; ROENTGENOGRAM.

XXXX syndrome /fôreks'/ a chromosomal disorder in which the individual acquires four X chromosomes, or double the number that identifies a human as female. There is no specific phenotype for this condition although 48,XXXX females are likely to have minor physical anomalies and be mentally retarded. IQs of tested patients have ranged from 30 to 80. The mature patients have menses and can bear children. Also called **48,XXXX**.

XXXXX syndrome /fīveks´/ a rare chromosomal disorder in which a female child acquires five X chromosomes instead of the normal pair. All five-X-chromosome patients studied have been mentally retarded, and some had ocular disturbances or other anomalies such as patent ductus arteriosus, microcephaly, or abnormalities of the limbs. Also called **49,XXXXX**.

XXXXY syndrome /fôr´ekswī´/ a rare chromosomal disorder in which a male offspring inherits three extra X chromosomes and a variety of anomalies including abnormally small genitalia, a short broad neck, and muscular hypotonia. Most patients are mentally retarded, with IQs of less than 60. One child appeared normal until his second year when mental retardation developed. Also called **49,XXXXY**.

XXXY syndrome /trip´əlekswī´/ a relatively rare chromosomal disorder in which an offspring inherits the full complement of both male and female sex chromosomes. The patients have a normal penis but small testes and prostate, and about half develop enlarged breasts. IQs of those tested ranged from 20 to 76, although most cases have been found by screening patients in mental institutions and may not represent the frequency for the general population. Also called **48,XXXY**.

XXY syndrome = KLINEFELTER'S SYNDROME.

XXYY syndrome /dubəleks´dubəlwī´/ a chromosomal abnormality in which a male offspring is born with a double complement of the normal XY chromosome pair. Skeletal deformities, genital anomalies, and mental retardation are common effects. More than half the patients tested had IQs below 70, and some exhibited bizarre behavior. Enlarged breasts and eunuchoid abdominal and hip fat also are among the physical traits. Also called **48,XXYY**.

XYY syndrome /eks´dubəlwī´/ a chromosomal anomaly discovered in 1961 and associated with males who were aggressive or violent in institutions for criminals. It was originally assumed that the extra Y chromosome predisposes males to such behavior, but the theory was modified as XYY anomalies were later found among normal males. Also called **47,XYY**.

Y

yagé = CAAPI.

yakee = EPENA.

yantra a visual pattern on which attention is focused during meditation.

Yates, Frank English statistician, 1902—. See YATES CORRECTION.

Yates correction a statistical adjustment in computing chi-square from small samples, in which the differences between observed and expected frequencies are decreased by 0.5. Also called **correction for continuity**.

yaupon: See CASSINA LEAVES.

YAVIS /yāvis/ an abbreviation of *y*oung, *a*daptable, *v*erbal, *i*ntelligent, and *s*uccessful—referring to the group for whom psychoanalysis is said to work best.

Y axis: See ORDINATE.

Y chromosome the male sex chromosome, which controls sex differentiation. It normaly occurs in tissue cells as part of a pair of sex chromosomes, the other member being the female X chromosome.

yellow-blue response a graded potential reaction that is correlated with the spectral sensitivity of the retinal receptors. The response at the blue end of the spectrum is negative, or hyperpolarized, while the response at the yellow end is positive, or depolarized. Thus, blue may have an inhibitory and yellow an excitatory influence on retinal receptors and ganglia in producing color vision.

Yellow Dye No. 5; Yellow Dye No. 6: See RED DYE NO. 3.

yellow-sightedness = XANTHOPSIA.

yellow spot: See RETINAL MACULA.

yerba maté = PARAGUAY TEA.

Yerkes, Robert Mearns /yur'kis/ American psychobiologist, 1876–1956. Y. is chiefly noted for his illuminating experiments carried out at the Yale Laboratories of Primate Biology, later renamed the Yerkes Laboratories in his honor. There he broadened our knowledge of animal behavior by showing, e.g., that chimpanzees are capable of imitating humans and each other, and can stack boxes to reach for food (and transfer this learning to other problems). He also proved that lower animals can solve simple multiple-choice problems, and that mouse-killing in kittens is not instinctual, but learned. Experiments of this kind earned him recognition as America's leading comparative psychologist. See YERKES-DODSON LAW.

Yerkes-Dodson law the rule that task performance is an inverted U-shaped function of arousal. E.g., performance is enhanced by moderate arousal conditions and is reduced at low and very high levels of arousal.

Yin and Yang in Chinese philosophy, two forces or principles whose interactions determine the fate of individuals as well as the universe: The Yin is seen as negative, passive, and feminine, complementary to the Yang, which is seen as positive, active, and masculine.

ylophobia = HYLOPHOBIA.

yoga a school of Hindu philosophy which seeks to achieve union with the Supreme Being or supreme principle through a prescribed mental discipline and physical exercises. Y. exercises are frequently used as a means of releasing tension and achieving a state of contemplation, self-control, and mental relaxation. (The term is a Sanskrit word meaning "union" or—derived from the same word—"yoke".)

yo-he-ho theory: See ORIGIN-OF-LANGUAGE THEORIES.

yohimbine an alkaloid stimulant derived from the bark of the African tree Corynanthe yohimbi, with limited action as a blocker of alpha-adrenergic receptors. Y. has been valued locally as a reputed aphrodisiac. It is related in chemical structure to the Rauwolfia alkaloids and LSD through an indole group; but y. has little value as a therapeutic tool. Y. effects reportedly are similar to those of cocaine.

yoked control in operant conditioning, an experimental procedure designed to insure that both a control and an experimental animal receive the same stimuli at the same time, but in which only one animal may respond. E.g., the experimental animal may be able to postpone electric shocks by pressing a lever, while the control animal receives as many shocks but cannot postpone them.

yopo a beverage made from the bark of a South American plant, Paullinia yopo. Y. is similar to guarana paste but contains about half as much caffeine, or about two and one-half percent. It is consumed mainly by Native Americans of Colombia as a stimulant and to reduce feelings of hunger.

Young, Thomas English physician and physicist, 1773–1829. See YOUNG-HELMHOLTZ THEORY OF COLOR VISION; COLOR THEORIES.

young adulthood the period in which the young man or woman who has passed through adolescence reaches the height of physical and mental vigor, has attained basic independence from his or her family, and is ready to achieve an intimate, meaningful relationship with a member of the opposite sex. During this period, two major choices, choice of an occupation and choice of a marriage partner, take place—both of which are tests of adaptability and maturity.

Young-Helmholtz theory of color vision a concept developed by physicians Thomas Young and Hermann von Helmholtz to explain color vision in terms of retinal cones sensitive to three different wavelengths of light: red, green, and blue. Other colors are perceived by stimulation of two of the three kinds of cones; e.g., yellow is produced by simultaneous stimulation of red and green cones. Light that stimulates all three cones equally is perceived as white. Partial or total absence of certain cones accounts for color blindness, according to the theory.

youpon: See CASSINI LEAVES.

youth culture a society that places a high premium on youth, youth values, and perpetuation of youth, and usually tends to derogate the values and needs of the mature and the elderly. Also see COUNTERCULTURE.

youth period the stage of life between childhood and maturity, or adulthood.

Youtz, Richard P. American psychologist, 1910—. See DERMO-OPTICAL PERCEPTION.

Z

Z a statistic used to transform correlation coefficients, often for the purpose of averaging them.

Zange, Johannes /tsäng'ə/ German otorhinolaryngologist, 1880–1969. See ZANGE-KINDLER SYNDROME.

Zange-Kindler syndrome a neurological disorder caused by inflammations, tumors, or other lesions that block cerebrospinal-fluid circulation in the cisterna magna. Also called **cisternal-block syndrome**.

Zanoli, Raffaele /tsänō'lē/ Italian physician, 1897–1971. See ZANOLI-VECCHI SYNDROME.

Zanoli-Vecchi syndrome a condition that may follow spinal surgery, due to hemorrhage with blood draining into the cerebral ventricles. Symptoms include loss of consciousness, apnea, and convulsions, which usually begin within two or three hours after surgery.

Zappert, Julius Czech-born physician, 1867–1942. See ZAPPERT'S SYNDROME.

Zappert's syndrome a disorder that occurs suddenly in some children following a viral infection. It is characterized by slurred speech, ataxia, nystagmus, and intention tremor. Also called **acute cerebellar ataxia; acute cerebral tremor; hypertonic-dyskinetic syndrome**.

Zeigarnik, Bluma Russian psychologist, 1900—. See ZEIGARNIK EFFECT.

Zeigarnik effect the tendency for interrupted, uncompleted tasks to be better remembered than completed tasks if the tasks are performed under nonstressful conditions. Under conditions of stress, the Z.e. may be reversed. Also called **Zeigarnik phenomenon**.

Zeitgeist /tsīt'gīst/ the spirit of the times (German, literally, "time spirit"). The term is applied to the cultural flavor that appears to pervade the ideas, attitudes, and feelings of a particular society in a specific historical period. It may also be used in relation to the theory of history that stresses the role of economics, technology, and social influences in contrast to the great-man theory of leadership. The term was first used in English by the 19th-century poet and literary critic Matthew Arnold.

zelophobia a morbid fear of jealousy or having reason to be jealous.

Zen Buddhism a Japanese form of Buddhism in which spiritual unity and illumination, or **satori**, are achieved through direct, intuitive experience as contrasted with the scientific, intellectual approach. One method of preparing the way for such insight is to devote oneself to the solution of an insoluble problem such as "What is the sound of one hand clapping?" See BUDDHISM.

Zen therapy a form of psychotherapy which, like existentialism, is concerned with the unique meaning of the patient's life rather than improvement of his adjustment or removal of his symptoms. The goal is sought through contemplation of his own existence, and grappling with the nature of humankind. This process helps the patient release inner tension and, if it is fully effective, leads to a climactic experience of oneness with the universe and the feeling that one's entire life has been transformed. See EXISTENTIALISM; MYSTIC UNION; ZEN BUDDHISM.

zeppia a term applied by Cattell to a factor trait described as a flexible superego.

zero-base budgeting an approach to budgeting in which each item proposed is evaluated on its own current merits, regardless of its merits in any previous budget. This method helps to identify unnecessary allocations of resources, investments, and personnel.

zero-order correlation a correlation between two variables without partialing out, or allowing for the influence of, other related variables. A z.-o.c. may have any value between 1 and –1, since this term does not mean "nearly zero."

zero population growth a condition in which the number of births and deaths is balanced and there is no increase or decrease in population, or very little change. In the United States, the effect of this trend has been to raise the mean age from 28 to 40, to reduce the proportion of those under 15 years of age from 30 to 20 percent, and to increase the proportion of those over 65 from ten to 20 percent. Psychological and social effects of this generally older population are extensive: a shifting of values, beliefs, and behavioral traits away from those associated with youth, and toward those characteristic of mid- and later life; an altering of the tempo of life, the rate of social change, and the types of recreation desired; and a retarding of the process of job advancement for the young, while retaining the elderly in industry as long as possible.

zeta /zēt′ə/ or /zāt′ə/ sixth letter of the Greek alphabet (Z, ς).

Zieve, Leslie American physician, 1915—. See ZIEVE'S SYNDROME.

Zieve's syndrome a condition of hyperlipemia, jaundice, and hemolytic anemia, with fatty infiltration of the liver due to the consumption of excessive amounts of alcoholic beverages.

Zilboorg, Gregory Russian-born American psychiatrist, 1890–1959. Z. is noted for his studies of ambulatory schizophrenia, criminology, and the history of psychiatry.

Zimmerman, Wayne S. American psychologist, 1916—. See GUILFORD-ZIMMERMAN TEMPERAMENT SURVEY; INTEREST TESTS (there: **Guilford-Zimmerman Interest Inventory**); MASCULINITY-FEMININITY TESTS.

Z lines: See MUSCLE FIBER.

zoanthropy = LYCANTHROPY.

Zollinger, Robert Milton American surgeon, 1903—. See ZOLLINGER-ELLISON SYNDROME; WERMER'S SYNDROME.

Zollinger-Ellison syndrome a form of peptic-ulcer disease associated with a tumor of the non-insulin-producing cells of the pancreas. The ulcers may appear anywhere from the lower esophagus to the jejunum of the small intestine. The tumors produce enormous amounts of **gastrin**, a substance that stimulates a flow of gastric acid that in turn causes the ulcers. A serious symptom is diarrhea, which in a case of Z.-E. s. may result in fatal complications.

Zöllner, Johann Karl Friedrich /tsel′nər/ German astrophysicist, 1834–82. See ZÖLLNER ILLUSION.

Zöllner illusion a visual illusion in which parallel lines appear to diverge when one of the lines is intersected by short diagonal lines slanting in one direction, and the other by lines slanting in the other direction.

zombie: See PHENCYCLIDINE.

-zoo- /-zō·ə-/ a combining form relating to animals (from Greek *zoon*, "animal, living being").

zooerasty /zō·ə·ēras′tē/ sexual excitement or gratification through intercourse or other sexual contact with an animal, such as masturbation, fellatio, rubbing, or anal or genital penetration (from Greek *zoon*, "animal," and *erastes*, "lover"). Also called **zooerastia; bestiality**. In

DSM-III, the corresponding term is ZOOPHILIA. See this entry. Also see SODOMY.

zoolagnia a sexual attraction to animals. See ZOOPHILIA; ZOOERASTY.

zoomorphism the attribution of animal traits to humans, deities, or inanimate objects; also, the use of animal psychology or physiology to explain human behavior. Compare ANTHROPOMORPHISM.

zoon politikon: See SOCIAL INSTINCT.

zoophilia a psychosexual disorder in which animals are repeatedly preferred or exclusively used to achieve sexual excitement. The animal, usually a household pet or farm animal, is either used as the object of intercourse or is trained to lick or rub the human partner. Also see ZOOERASTY. (DSM-III)

zoophobia a morbid fear of animals in general. See ANIMAL PHOBIA.

zoopsia /zō·op′-/ the visual hallucinations in which the patient sees insects or other animals, as in cases of delirium tremens.

zoosadism sadistic satisfaction obtained from torturing an animal, with or without direct sexual contact with the victim.

z scores: See STANDARD SCORES.

Zurich School a group of psychoanalysts who were followers of Jung, as opposed to the Viennese School of Freud's followers.

Zwahlen, P. /tsvä′lən/ Swiss physician, fl. 1944. See TREACHER COLLINS' SYNDROME (also called **Franceschetti-Zwahlen-Klein syndrome**).

zygomaticus the set of muscles innervated by the facial nerve (the seventh cranial nerve) which activate the movement of the upper lip outward, upward, and backward.

zygosis the union of two gametes.

zygosity specific inheritance; zygotic characteristics. See TWIN STUDIES.

zygote /zī′gōt/ or /zig′ōt/ a fertilized egg, or ovum, with a diploid set of chromosomes, half contributed by the mother and half by the father (from Greek *zygotos*, "yoked"). By repeated mitosis, or cell division, the z. can evolve from a single cell into an adult member of the species with hereditary traits of the genetic lines of both parents. The term also has been applied to a thus developing organism in the first two weeks after conception. Adjective: **zygotic**.

-zym-; -zymo- /-zīm-/ a combining form relating to (a) fermentation, (b) an enzyme (from Greek *zyme*, "leaven, ferment").

DSM-III CLASSIFICATION

This table groups the official DSM-III terms of this Dictionary in the order and context in which they are grouped in the DSM-III Classification (*DSM-III*, pages 15–19).

The numbers in parentheses are the official DSM-III codes, which are also codes of the *International Classification of Diseases*, 9th Edition. See the entry DSM-III in this Dictionary.

A few of the terms below are followed by only one digit after the decimal point. This indicates flexibility for further diagnostic specification, such as "chronic," "with depression," or "unspecified." For details, consult the *DSM-III*.

All terms of this table, other than the headings, appear as entries in this Dictionary. When a heading (capital letters or italics type) is also a Dictionary entry, the term is repeated (in light roman type).

There are 238 entry terms on this table. The corresponding definitions are followed by the reference "(DSM-III)." This reference is also given after the definitions of another 22 Dictionary terms that are DSM-III-related though they are not verbatim among the terms of the table.

DISORDERS USUALLY FIRST EVIDENT IN INFANCY, CHILDHOOD, OR ADOLESCENCE

Mental Retardation
mental retardation
mild mental retardation (317.0)
moderate mental retardation (318.0)
severe mental retardation (318.1)
profound mental retardation (318.2)
unspecified mental retardation (319.0)

Attention-Deficit Disorders
attention-deficit disorder with hyperactivity (314.01)
attention-deficit disorder without hyperactivity (314.00)
attention-deficit disorder, residual type (314.80)

Conduct Disorders
conduct disorder, undersocialized, aggressive (312.00)
conduct disorder, undersocialized, nonaggressive (312.10)
conduct disorder, socialized, aggressive (312.23)
conduct disorder, socialized, nonaggressive (312.21)
atypical conduct disorder (312.90)

Anxiety Disorders of Childhood or Adolescence
anxiety disorders of childhood or adolescence
separation-anxiety disorder (309.21)

avoidant disorder of childhood or adolescence (313.21)
overanxious disorder (313.00)

Other Disorders of Infancy, Childhood, or Adolescence
reactive-attachment disorder of infancy (313.89)
schizoid disorder of childhood or adolescence (313.22)
elective mutism (313.23)
oppositional disorder (313.81)
identity disorder (313.82)

Eating Disorders
anorexia nervosa (307.10)
bulimia (307.51)
pica (307.52)
rumination disorder of infancy (307.53)
atypical eating disorder (307.50)

Stereotyped-Movement Disorders
transient-tic disorder (307.21)
chronic motor-tic disorder (307.22)
Tourette's disorder (307.23)
atypical tic disorder (307.20)
atypical stereotyped-movement disorder (307.30)

Other Disorders with Physical Manifestations
stuttering (307.00)
functional enuresis (307.60)
functional encopresis (307.70)
sleepwalking disorder (307.46)
sleep-terror disorder (307.46)

Pervasive Developmental Disorders
pervasive developmental disorders
infantile autism (299.0)
childhood-onset pervasive developmental disorder (299.9)
atypical pervasive developmental disorder (299.8)

Specific Developmental Disorders
specific developmental disorders
developmental reading disorder (315.00)
developmental arithmetic disorder (315.10)
developmental language disorder (315.31)
developmental articulation disorder (315.39)
mixed specific developmental disorder (315.50)
atypical specific developmental disorder (315.90)

ORGANIC MENTAL DISORDERS

organic mental disorders

Dementias Arising in the Senium and Presenium
primary degenerative dementia, senile onset
primary degenerative dementia, senile onset, with delirium (290.30)

primary degenerative dementia, senile onset, with delusions (290.20)
primary degenerative dementia, senile onset, with depression (290.21)
primary degenerative dementia, senile onset, uncomplicated (290.00)
primary degenerative dementia, presenile onset (290.1)
multiinfarct dementia (290.4)

Substance-Induced Organic Mental Disorders
alcohol intoxication (303.00)
alcohol idiosyncratic intoxication (291.40)
alcohol withdrawal (291.80)
alcohol-withdrawal delirium (291.00)
alcohol hallucinosis (291.30)
alcohol-amnestic disorder (291.10)
dementia associated with alcoholism (291.2)

barbiturate or similarly acting sedative or hypnotic intoxication (305.40)
barbiturate or similarly acting sedative or hypnotic withdrawal (292.00)
barbiturate or similarly acting sedative or hypnotic withdrawal delirium (292.00)
barbiturate or similarly acting sedative or hypnotic amnestic disorder (292.83)

opioid intoxication (305.50)
opioid withdrawal (292.00)

cocaine intoxication (305.60)

amphetamine or similarly acting sympathomimetic intoxication (305.70)
amphetamine or similarly acting sympathomimetic delirium (292.81)
amphetamine or similarly acting sympathomimetic delusional disorder (292.11)
amphetamine or similarly acting sympathomimetic withdrawal (292.00)

phencyclidine (PCP) or similarly acting arylcyclohexylamine intoxication (305.90)
phencyclidine (PCP) or similarly acting arylcyclohexylamine delirium (292.81)
phencyclidine (PCP) or similarly acting arylcyclohexylamine mixed organic mental disorder (292.90)

hallucinogen hallucinosis (305.30)
hallucinogen-delusional disorder (292.11)
hallucinogen-affective disorder (292.84)

cannabis intoxication (305.20)
cannabis-delusional disorder (292.11)

tobacco withdrawal (292.00)

caffeine intoxication (305.90)

The DSM-III Classification also lists Other or Unspecified Substance intoxication (305.90), withdrawal (292.00), delirium (292.81), dementia (292.82), amnestic disorder (292.83), delusional disorder (292.11), hallucinosis (292.12), affective disorder (292.84), personality disorder (292.89), and atypical or mixed organic mental disorder (292.90). For these categories, the corresponding

entries in this Dictionary are INTOXICATION, WITHDRAWAL, etc.

Organic Brain Syndromes
organic brain syndromes
delirium (293.00)
dementia (294.10)
amnestic syndrome (294.00)
organic-delusional syndrome (293.81)
organic hallucinosis (293.82)
organic-affective syndrome (293.83)
organic personality syndrome (310.10)
atypical or mixed organic brain syndrome (294.80)

SUBSTANCE-USE DISORDERS

substance-use disorders
alcohol abuse (305.0)
alcohol dependence (alcoholism) (303.9)
barbiturate or similarly acting sedative or hypnotic abuse (305.4)
barbiturate or similarly acting sedative or hypnotic dependence (304.1)
opioid abuse (305.5)
opioid dependence (304.0)
cocaine abuse (305.6)
amphetamine or similarly acting sympathomimetic abuse (305.7)
amphetamine or similarly acting sympathomimetic dependence (304.4)
phencyclidine (PCP) or similarly acting arylcyclohexylamine abuse (305.9)
hallucinogen abuse (305.3)
cannabis abuse (305.2)
cannabis dependence (304.3)
tobacco dependence (305.1)
other, mixed, or unspecified substance abuse (305.9)
other specified substance dependence (304.6)
unspecified substance dependence (304.9)
dependence on combination of opioid and other nonalcoholic substance (304.7)
dependence on combination of substances, excluding opioids and alcohol (304.8)

SCHIZOPHRENIC DISORDERS

schizophrenic disorders
schizophrenic disorder, disorganized type (295.1)
schizophrenic disorder, catatonic type (295.2)
schizophrenic disorder, paranoid type (295.3)
schizophrenic disorder, undifferentiated type (295.9)
schizophrenic disorder, residual type (295.6)

PARANOID DISORDERS

paranoid disorders
paranoia (297.10)
shared paranoid disorder (297.30)
acute paranoid disorder (298.30)
atypical paranoid disorder (297.90)

PSYCHOTIC DISORDERS NOT ELSEWHERE CLASSIFIED

schizophreniform disorder (295.40)
brief reactive psychosis (298.80)

schizoaffective disorder (295.70)
atypical psychosis (298.90)

NEUROTIC DISORDERS

(Included in affective, anxiety, somatoform, dissociative, and psychosexual disorders, below. And see the entry NEUROTIC DISORDER.)

AFFECTIVE DISORDERS

affective disorders

Major Affective Disorders
bipolar disorder, mixed (296.6)
bipolar disorder, manic (296.4)
bipolar disorder, depressed (296.5)

major depression, single episode (296.2)
major depression, recurrent (296.3)

Other Specific Affective Disorders
cyclothymic disorder (301.13)
dysthymic disorder (depressive neurosis) (300.40)

Atypical Affective Disorders
atypical affective disorders
atypical bipolar disorder (296.70)
atypical depression (296.82)

ANXIETY DISORDERS

anxiety disorders

phobic disorders (phobic neuroses)
agoraphobia with panic attacks (300.21)
agoraphobia without panic attacks (300.22)
social phobia (300.23)
simple phobia (300.29)

anxiety states (anxiety neuroses)
panic disorder (300.01)
generalized-anxiety disorder (300.02)
obsessive-compulsive disorder (obsessive-
   compulsive neurosis) (300.30)

posttraumatic stress disorder
acute posttraumatic stress disorder (308.30)
chronic posttraumatic stress disorder (309.81)
atypical anxiety disorder (300.00)

SOMATOFORM DISORDERS

somatoform disorders
somatization disorder (300.81)
conversion disorder (hysterical neurosis, conversion
   type) (300.11)
psychogenic pain disorder (307.80)
hypochondriasis (hypochondriacal neurosis)
   (300.70)
atypical somatoform disorder (300.70)

DISSOCIATIVE DISORDERS (HYSTERICAL NEUROSES, DISSOCIATIVE TYPE)

dissociative disorders
psychogenic amnesia (300.12)
psychogenic fugue (300.13)
multiple personality (300.14)
depersonalization disorder (depersonalization
   neurosis) (300.60)
atypical dissociative disorder (300.15)

PSYCHOSEXUAL DISORDERS

psychosexual disorders

Gender-Identity Disorders
gender-identity disorders
transsexualism (302.5)
gender-identity disorder of childhood (302.60)
atypical gender-identity disorder (302.85)

Paraphilias
paraphilias
fetishism (302.81)
transvestism (302.30)
zoophilia (302.10)
pedophilia (302.20)
exhibitionism (302.40)
voyeurism (302.82)
sexual masochism (302.83)
sexual sadism (302.84)
atypical paraphilia (302.90)

Psychosexual Dysfunctions
psychosexual dysfunctions
inhibited sexual desire (302.71)
inhibited sexual excitement (302.72)
inhibited female orgasm (302.73)
inhibited male orgasm (302.74)
premature ejaculation (302.75)
functional dyspareunia (302.76)
functional vaginismus (306.51)
atypical psychosexual dysfunction (302.70)

Other Psychosexual Disorders
ego-dystonic homosexuality (302.00)
psychosexual disorders not elsewhere classified
   (302.89)

FACTITIOUS DISORDERS

factitious disorders
factitious disorder with psychological symptoms
   (300.16)
chronic factitious disorder with physical symptoms
   (301.51)
atypical factitious disorder with physical symptoms
   (300.19)

DISORDERS OF IMPULSE CONTROL NOT ELSEWHERE CLASSIFIED

disorders of impulse control not elsewhere classified
pathological gambling (312.31)
kleptomania (312.32)
pyromania (312.33)
intermittent explosive disorder (312.34)
isolated explosive disorder (312.35)
atypical impulse-control disorder (312.39)

ADJUSTMENT DISORDERS

adjustment disorder
adjustment disorder with depressed mood (309.00)
adjustment disorder with anxious mood (309.24)
adjustment disorder with mixed emotional features
   (309.28)
adjustment disorder with disturbance of conduct
   (309.30)
adjustment disorder with mixed disturbance of
   emotions and conduct (309.40)

adjustment disorder with work or academic inhibition (309.23)
adjustment disorder with withdrawal (309.83)
adjustment disorder with atypical features (309.90)

PSYCHOLOGICAL FACTORS AFFECTING PHYSICAL CONDITION

psychological factors affecting physical condition (316.00)

PERSONALITY DISORDERS

personality disorders
paranoid-personality disorder (301.00)
schizoid-personality disorder (301.20)
schizotypal-personality disorder (301.22)
histrionic-personality disorder (301.50)

narcissistic-personality disorder (301.81)
antisocial-personality disorder (301.70)
borderline personality disorder (301.83)
avoidant personality disorder (301.82)
dependent-personality disorder (301.60)
compulsive-personality disorder (301.40)
passive-aggressive-personality disorder (301.84)
atypical, mixed, or other personality disorder (301.89)

The DSM-III Classification also lists Conditions Not Attributable to Mental Disorder That Are a Focus of Attention or Treatment (e.g., MALINGERING and BORDERLINE INTELLECTUAL FUNCTIONING — included throughout this Dictionary) and Additional Codes. Details are given on page 19 of the *DSM-III*.

APPENDIX B

488 TEST ENTRIES

This Appendix is a compilation of 488 entries that denote primarily psychological and neurological tests. Not listed are the numerous test entries of this Dictionary in such areas as statistics, market research, and medicine other than neurology.

An asterisk means that the entry referred to does not appear in this Appendix.

ability test
absurdities test
accuracy test
ACE test
achievement battery
achievement tests
ACT Assessment (also called **American College Testing Program**)
Adaptive Behavior Scale
adaptive testing
adjective check list
adjustment inventory
adrenaline-Mecholyl test
aiming test
Akerfeldt test
Allport A-S Reaction Study
Allport-Vernon-Lindzey Study of Values
Alpha verbal test: See ARMY TESTS
alternate binaural loudness-balance test
alternate-response test
alternate-uses test
altitude test
American College Testing Program = ACT ASSESSMENT
American Home Scale

amniocentesis
analogies test
anchor test
antonym test
anxiety scales
aptitude tests
Army General Classification Test
Army tests
ARP tests
articulation test
art test
association test
attitude scale
Attitude Scale Toward Disabled Persons
attitude survey
Auditory Apperception Test
Aussage test
Bárány test
Barron-Welsh Art Scale
Bayley Scales of Infant Development
behavior check list
Bem Sex-Role Inventory
Bender-Gestalt test
Benton Visual Retention Test
Bernreuter Personal Adjustment Inventory
best-answer test (also called **best-reason test**)
Beta test: See ARMY TESTS
Binet Test
binomial test
Black Intelligence Test of Cultural Homogeneity (abbrev.: **BITCH test**)
block-design test
Boehm Test of Basic Concepts
Bolgar-Fischer World Test
BOLT = USES BASIC OCCUPATIONAL

LITERACY TEST
bone-conduction testing
Brainerd Occupational Preference Inventory: See INTEREST TESTS
brand-use survey
Brief Psychiatric Rating Scale (abbrev.: **BPRS**)
Briggs-Myer Type Indicator = MYER-BRIGGS TYPE INDICATOR
Broadbent test
Bryngelson-Glaspey test
Caine-Levine Social Competence Scale
California Achievement Tests
California Infant Scale for Motor Development
California Psychological Inventory
California Tests of Mental Maturity
California Tests of Personality
cancellation test
card-sorting test
Category Test: See CEREBRAL-DYSFUNCTION TESTS
Cattell inventories
cause-and-effect test
CAVD Test
cerebral-dysfunction tests
Children's Apperception Test
Children's Personality Questionnaire: See CATTELL INVENTORIES
CIRCUS
classification test
Classroom Environment Scale: See ENVIRONMENTAL ASSESSMENT*
classroom test
clerical-aptitude tests
cochleopalpebral-reflex test
code test (also called **coding test; sym-**

bol-substitution test)
coin test
college admission tests
color sorting test: See HOLMGREN TEST
Columbia Mental Maturity Scale
Comfortable Interpersonal Distance
  Scale: See INTERPERSONAL DIS-
  TANCE*
Compass Diagnostic Test of Arithmetic: See DIAGNOSTIC EDUCATIONAL
  TESTS
completion, arithmetic, vocabulary,
  direction-following: See CAVD TEST
completion test
comprehension test
Comrey Personality Scales
concept-formation tests
Concept Mastery Test
Conflict Resolution Inventory
Cornell Medical Index
Cornell Word Form
Crawford Small Parts Dexterity Test
creativity test
criteria-referenced testing
cross-cultural testing
Culture-Fair Intelligence Test: See
  CROSS-CULTURAL TESTING
culture-fair tests
culture-free tests
cumulative scale (also called Guttman
  scale; scalogram)
cumulative tests
DAH test; DAP test: See MACHOVER
  DRAW-A-PERSON TEST
DAT: See MULTIPLE-APTITUDE TEST
delayed-alternation test
delayed-matching test
design-judgment test: See GRAVES
  DESIGN JUDGMENT TEST
developmental scale
Developmental Test of Visual Perception: See FROSTIG D.T.O.V.P.
dexamethasone suppression test
diagnostic educational tests
diagnostic test
Differential Aptitude Test: See MULTI-
  PLE-APTITUDE TEST
difficulty scale
digit-span test
directions test
disarranged-sentence test
distribution-free tests
Doerfler-Stewart test
dotting test
double-simultaneous stimulation
Downey's Will-Temperament Tests
Draw-a-House Test; Draw-a-Person
  Test: See MACHOVER DRAW-A-
  PERSON TEST
DTVP = FROSTIG DEVELOPMENTAL
  TEST OF VISUAL PERCEPTION
Duncan multiple-range test
Durham rule. (also called Durham
  test)
Durrell Analysis of Reading Difficul-
  ty: See DIAGNOSTIC EDUCATIONAL
  TESTS
Early School Personality Question-
  naire: See CATTELL INVENTORIES
educational tests: See DIAGNOSTIC E.T.
Edwards Personal Preference
  Schedule
EGY test = KENT SERIES OF EMERGEN-

CY SKILLS
Elgin check list
Elithorn maze
Embedded Figures Test
empirical test
English Usage Test: See ACT ASSESS-
  MENT
essay test: See OBJECTIVE EXAMINA-
  TION*
Examining for Aphasia
Eysenck Personality Inventory
fables test
face-hand test
feasibility test
Fels Parent Behavior Rating Scales
ferric-chloride test
figure-drawing test
finger-nose test
Fink-Green-Bender test: DOUBLE-
  SIMULTANEOUS TACTILE SENSATION*
Fölling test
forced-response test (also called
  forced-choice test; objective test)
Forer Vocational Survey: See IN-
  TEREST TESTS
formboard test
Fournier tests
free-association test
free recall
free-response test
Frostig Developmental Test of Visual
  Perception (abbrev.: DTVP)
Frostig Movement Skills Test Battery
Gates-MacGinitie Reading Tests
Geist Picture Interest Inventory: See
  INTEREST TESTS
General Anxiety Scale for Children:
  See ANXIETY SCALES
General Aptitude Test Battery
Gesell Development Scales
Gmelin test (also called Rosenbach-
  G.t.)
Goldstein-Scheerer tests
go-no-go test
good-and-evil test
Goodenough Draw-a-Man Test
Goodenough-Harris Drawing Test
Gordon Occupational Check List: See
  INTEREST TESTS
Gough Femininity Scale: See MASCU-
  LINITY-FEMININITY TESTS
Gough Adjective Check List: See
  ADJECTIVE CHECK LIST
Graduate Record Examination
graphometry
Graves Design Judgment Test
Gray Oral Reading Tests
Griffiths Mental Development Scale
group test
guess-who technique
Guilford-Zimmerman Interest Inven-
  tory: See INTEREST TESTS
Guilford-Zimmerman Temperament
  Survey
Guttman scale = CUMULATIVE SCALE
Halstead Impairment Index
Halstead-Reitan Neuropsychological
  Battery: See CEREBRAL-
  DYSFUNCTION TESTS
Hampton Court maze
Hanfmann-Kasanin Concept Forma-
  tion Test
Harris Tests of Lateral Dominance

heel-to-knee test
Heidbreder test
Hejna test
hidden-clue test
hidden-figures test
High School Personality Question-
  naire: See CATTELL INVENTORIES
Hiskey-Nebraska Test of Learning
  Aptitude
Holland Vocational Preference Inven-
  tory: See INTEREST TESTS
Holmes' phenomenon = REBOUND
  PHENOMENON
Holmgren test
Home Index: See AMERICAN HOME
  SCALE
Hoover's sign
Hopkins symptoms check list
  (abbrev.: HSCL)
House-Tree-Person Technique
  (abbrev.: HTP)
HSCL = HOPKINS SYMPTOMS CHECK LIST
HTP = HOUSE-TREE-PERSON TECH-
  NIQUE
Humm-Wadsworth Temperament
  Scale
Hunt-Minnesota Test for Organic
  Brain Damage
identification test
Illinois Test of Psycholinguistic Abili-
  ties
impairment index
in-basket test
incomplete-pictures test
incomplete-sentence test = SENTENCE-
  COMPLETION TEST
Index of Adjustment and Values
individual test
induction test
infant and preschool test
Infant Behavior Record: See BAYLEY
  SCALES OF INFANT DEVELOPMENT
infant test
informal test
Information Test
ink-blot test: See RORSCHACH TEST
Inpatient Multidimensional Psychiat-
  ric Scale: See ANXIOUS INTROPUNI-
  TIVENESS*
intelligence test (also called intelli-
  gence scale)
interest tests
inventory test
Iowa Silent Reading Test: See
  DIAGNOSTIC EDUCATIONAL TESTS
Iowa Stuttering Scale
Iowa Tests of Basic Skills
IQ
Ishihara test
Janet's test
job-specific test
Jung association test
Kahn Test of Symbol Arrangement
Kent-Rosanoff Test
Kent Series of Emergency Skills (also
  called EGY test)
Knox Cube Test
Kohnstamm test
Kohs Block Design Test
Kolmogorov-Smirnov test
Kuder Preference Record
Kuhlmann-Anderson Tests
Lange's colloidal gold reaction (also

called **Lange's test**)
Least-Preferred Coworker Test
Leiter International Performance Test
Levy Draw-and-Tell-a-Story Technique
Lichtheim's test
Likert scale (also called **Likert procedure**)
Lincoln-Oseretsky Motor Development Scale
literacy test
locomotor maze
Lorr Scale = MULTIDIMENSIONAL SCALE FOR RATING PSYCHIATRIC PATIENTS
Luria-Nebraska Neuropsychological Battery: See CEREBRAL-DYSFUNCTION TESTS
Luria technique
Machover Draw-a-Person Test (abbrev.: **DAP test**)
MacQuarrie Test for Mechanical Ability
Maddox rod test
Make a Picture Story (abbrev.: **MAPS**)
Manifest Anxiety Scale: See ANXIETY SCALES
manikin test
Mann-Whitney U test
man-to-man rating scale
map-reading test
MAPS = MAKE A PICTURE STORY
masculinity-femininity tests
matching test
Mathematics Usage Test: See ACT ASSESSMENT
Maudsley Personality Inventory
maze
McCarthy Scales of Children's Abilities
mechanical-aptitude tests
Meier Art Judgment Test
Memory-for-Designs Test
Mental Scale: See BAYLEY SCALES OF INFANT DEVELOPMENT
Mental Status Examination Report (abbrev.: **MSER**)
mental test
Merrill-Palmer Scale
methacholine infusion test
Metropolitan Achievement Tests
Miller Analogies Test
Minnesota Clerical Aptitude Test
Minnesota Mechanical Assembly Test
Minnesota Multiphasic Personality Inventory (abbrev.: **MMPI**)
Minnesota Paper Formboard Test
Minnesota Rate of Manipulation Test
Minnesota Spatial Relations Test
Minnesota Vocational Interest Inventory: See INTEREST TESTS
missing-parts test
MMPI = MINNESOTA MULTIPHASIC PERSONALITY INVENTORY
Mooney Problem Check List
mosaic test
Motor Scale: See BAYLEY SCALES OF INFANT DEVELOPMENT
motor tests
MSER = MENTAL STATUS EXAMINATION REPORT

Multidimensional Scale for Rating Psychiatric Patients (abbrev.: **MSRPP**; also called **Lorr Scale**)
multiple-aptitude test
multiple-choice test
Myer-Briggs Type Indicator (also called BRIGGS-MYER TYPE INDICATOR)
myokinetic-psychodiagnosis test
Nalline test
National Reference Scale: See ANCHOR TEST
Natural Science Reading Test: See ACT ASSESSMENT
Nelson-Denny Reading Test: See DIAGNOSTIC EDUCATIONAL TESTS
nonlanguage test (also called **nonverbal test; performance test**)
norm-referenced testing
number-completion test
object-assembly test
objective test = FORCED-RESPONSE TEST
object-reversal test
occupational test
omnibus test
opposites test
oral test
Otis Quick Scoring Mental Ability Test
Otis Self-Administering Test of Intelligence
Paper-and-pencil test
paragraph-meaning test
Peabody Picture Vocabulary Test
performance test = NONLANGUAGE TEST
Periodic Evaluation Record: See MENTAL STATUS EXAMINATION REPORT
Personal Experience and Attitude Questionnaire
personal-history questionnaire
personality inventory
personality test
personnel tests
Phillips Scale
photometrazol test
picture-anomalies test
picture-arrangement test
picture-completion test
picture-frustration study: See ROSENZWEIG P.-F.S.
picture-interpretation test
picture world test
Pigem's question
Pintner-Paterson Scale of Performance Tests
placement test
point-localization test
point scale
Porteus maze
power test
Present State Examination (abbrev.: **PSE**)
pressure-threshold test
Primary Abilities Test: See PRIMARY ABILITIES*
probing technique
problem box
problem check list
professional-aptitude tests
prognostic test
Progressive Matrices: See CROSS-CULTURAL TESTING

projective test
proverb test
PSE = PRESENT STATE EXAMINATION
psychological test
psychomotor tests
psychopenetration test
Quick Test
reaction-time test
readiness test
rebound phenomenon (also called **Holmes' phenomenon**)
recurring-figures test
referenced recognition test
remote-association test
REP Test = ROLE CONSTRUCT REPERTORY TEST
right-and-wrong test
Rinné test
Role Construct Repertory Test (abbrev.: **REP Test**)
Rorschach test
Rosenbach-Gmelin test = GMELIN TEST
Rosenberg Draw-a-Person Technique
Rosenzweig Picture-Frustration Study
Ross-Jones test
rotary-pursuit test
roughness discrimination
SAI (social-adequacy index)
sales-aptitude tests
Sarason Test Anxiety Scale: See ANXIETY SCALES
SAT = SCHOLASTIC APTITUDE TEST
S-B = STANFORD-BINET INTELLIGENCE SCALE
scalogram = CUMULATIVE SCALE
SCAT = SCHOOL AND COLLEGE ABILITY TEST
scholastic achievement test
Scholastic Aptitude Test (abbrev.: **SAT**)
School and College Ability Test (abbrev.: **SCAT**)
SCII = STRONG-CAMPBELL INTEREST INVENTORY
Seashore Measures of Musical Talent
selective-answer test
self-administered test (also called **self-administering test**)
self-concept tests
self-inventory
self-marking test
self-rating scale
self-report inventory
semantic differential
sensory tests
sentence-completion test (also called **incomplete-sentence test**)
sentence-repetition test
short-answer test
similarities test
situation test
Sixteen D Scale
Sixteen Personality Factor Questionnaire
Smets-pattern responses
Snellen chart (also called **Snellen test**)
social-adequacy index = SAI
Social Studies Reading Test: See ACT ASSESSMENT
sorting test
speech-reception threshold

(abbrev.: **SRT**)
speed test (also called **timed test**)
spontaneity test
SRA Mechanical Aptitude Test
SRT = SPEECH-RECEPTION THRESHOLD
standardized test
Stanford Achievement Test
Stanford-Binet Intelligence Scale
(abbrev.: **S-B**)
Stanford-Binet Scale
Stanford Diagnostic Arithmetic Test;
Stanford Diagnostic Reading Tests:
See DIAGNOSTIC EDUCATIONAL TESTS
Stanford Hypnotic Susceptibility
Scale
step-down test
Stilling Test
story-recall test
stress test
Strong-Campbell Interest Inventory
(abbrev.: **SCII**)
stylus maze
subjective examination
subjective test
substitution test
subtest
survey tests
symbol-substitution test = CODE TEST
Symonds Picture-Study Test
synonym-antonym test
Szondi test
tapping test: See DOTTING TEST
TAT = THEMATIC APPERCEPTION TEST
Taylor Manifest Anxiety Scale

temporal maze
Terman-McNemar Test of Mental
Ability
Terman-Miles Attitude-Interest
Analysis Test: See MASCULINITY-
FEMININITY TESTS
test-study-test method
Thematic Apperception Test
(abbrev.: **TAT**)
Thurstone Attitude Scales
Thurstone Interest Schedule: See IN-
TEREST TESTS
tight-rope test
timed test = SPEED TEST
T-maze
Tomkins-Horn Picture Arrangement
Test
Torrance Tests of Creative Think-
ing
trade test
Trail-Making Test: See CEREBRAL-
DYSFUNCTION TESTS
true-false test: See SELECTIVE-
ANSWER TEST
USES Basic Occupational Literacy
Test (abbrev.: **BOLT**)
verbal test
Vigotsky Test
Vineland Social Maturity Scale
visual-distortion test
vocabulary test
vocational-aptitude test
Wada dominance test
WAIS = WECHSLER ADULT

INTELLIGENCE SCALE
Ward Atmosphere Scale: See EN-
VIRONMENT ASSESSMENT*
watch test
WAY technique = WHO ARE YOU?
Wechsler Adult Intelligence Scale
(abbrev.: **WAIS**)
Wechsler-Bellevue Scale
Wechsler Intelligence Scale for Chil-
dren (abbrev.: **WISC**)
Wechsler Preschool and Primary
Scale of Intelligence (abbrev.:
WPPSI)
Weigl-Goldstein-Scheerer Test
Wepman Test of Auditory Discrim-
ination
whisper test
Who Are You? (also called **WAY**
technique; Who Am I?)
Wide Range Achievement Test
Wiggly Block Test
Wilcoxon test
WISC = WECHSLER INTELLIGENCE
SCALE FOR CHILDREN
Woodworth-Mathews Personal Data
Sheet
word-association test
word-building test
work-limit test
work-sample test
WPPSI = WECHSLER PRESCHOOL
AND PRIMARY SCALE OF
INTELLIGENCE
X-O Test

APPENDIX C

216 THERAPY ENTRIES

This Appendix is a compilation of 216 therapy entries with headwords that include the term "therapy." Not listed are the numerous therapies defined in this Dictionary under headwords that end in "analysis," "conditioning," "counseling," "modification," "technique," "treatment," or similar terms, and under one-word designations such as **autocatharsis** or **rolfing**.

An asterisk means that the entry referred to does not appear in this Appendix.

aboriginal therapies
active analytic psychotherapy
active therapy
activity-group therapy
activity-interview group psychother-
apy
activity-play therapy
activity therapy
adjuvant therapy
adolescent psychotherapy
ambulatory psychotherapy
anaclitic therapy
analytic group psychotherapy

antiandrogen therapy
art therapy
assertion-structured therapy
atropine-coma therapy
attitude therapy
aversive therapy (also called **aversion**
therapy)
behavior therapy (also called **be-**
havioral psychotherapy)
benzodiazepines pharmacotherapy
bibliotherapy
biological therapy
blue-collar therapy
body therapies
brief group therapy
brief psychotherapy = SHORT-TERM
THERAPY
brief-stimulus therapy
carbamates pharmacotherapy
carbon-dioxide therapy
cerebral electrotherapy
character-analytic vegetotherapy
chemotherapy = DRUG THERAPY
chromotherapy: See PHOTOBIOLOGY*
clay-modeling therapy
client-centered psychotherapy
cognitive therapy

collaborative therapy
combined therapy
computerized therapy
concurrent therapy
conditioned-reflex therapy
conditioning therapy
conjoint therapy (also called **conjoint**
marital therapy; triadic therapy;
triangular therapy)
continuous-sleep therapy
controlled-drinking therapy
convulsive therapy
cooperative therapy = MULTIPLE
THERAPY
corticoid therapy
corticosteroid therapy
cotherapy = MULTIPLE THERAPY
counselor-centered therapy: See
DIRECTIVE COUNSELING*
couples therapy = MARRIAGE THERAPY
crisis-intervention group psycho-
therapy
crisis therapy
dance therapy
delay therapy
depth therapy
deterrent therapy

didactic group therapy
directive group psychotherapy
directive-play therapy
directive therapy: See DIRECTIVE COUNSELING*
drama therapy: See PSYCHODRAMA*
drug therapy (also called chemotherapy)
dual-leadership therapy = MULTIPLE THERAPY
dual-sex therapy
dual-transference therapy
dyadic therapy = INDIVIDUAL THERAPY
dynamic psychotherapy
educational therapy: See EDUCATIONAL THERAPIST*
ego psychotherapy
electro-sleep therapy
electrotherapy
emergency psychotherapy
emotive therapy
environmental therapy (also called situational therapy)
existential-humanistic therapy (also called humanistic-existential therapy)
existential psychotherapy
experiential psychotherapy
expressive therapy
extended-family therapy
family therapy
focal psychotherapy
food therapy
Gestalt therapy
goal-limited adjustment therapy: See SECTOR THERAPY
goal-limited therapy
graphic-arts therapy
group-analytic psychotherapy (also called therapeutic group analysis)
group psychotherapy
humanistic-existential therapy = EXISTENTIAL-HUMANISTIC THERAPY
humanistic therapy = THIRD-FORCE THERAPY
hydrotherapy
hypnodelic therapy
hypnotherapy
imagery therapy
implosive therapy
indirect method of therapy
individual therapy (also called dyadic therapy)
industrial therapy
inhalation therapy = RESPIRATORY THERAPY
insight therapy
inspirational group therapy
instigation therapy
insulin-coma therapy (also called insulin-shock therapy)
interpersonal therapy
interpretive therapy (also called interpretative psychiatry)
interview group psychotherapy
interview therapy
leaderless-group therapy

lithium therapy
logotherapy
long-term psychotherapy
LSD psychotherapy
ludotherapy = PLAY THERAPY
major-role therapy
marriage therapy (also called marital therapy; couples therapy)
medical psychotherapy
megadoses pharmacotherapy
megavitamin therapy: See ORTHOMOLECULAR PSYCHIATRY*
Metrazol therapy: See METRAZOL SHOCK TREATMENT*
milieu therapy
minimum-change therapy
Morita therapy
movement therapy
multimodal behavior therapy
multiple family therapy
multiple therapy (also called cooperative therapy; cotherapy; dual-leadership therapy; role-divided therapy; three-cornered therapy)
music therapy
narcotherapy
network therapy
nondirective play therapy
nude-group therapy
objective psychotherapy
occupational therapy
organic therapies
organotherapy
orgone therapy (also called vegetotherapy)
paraverbal therapy
persuasion therapy
pharmacotherapy
physical therapy (also called physiotherapy)
plastic-arts therapy
play-group psychotherapy
play therapy (also called ludotherapy)
polyvitamin therapy
primal therapy (also called primal-scream therapy)
projection therapy
projective psychotherapy
psychedelic therapy
psychoanalytic group psychotherapy
psycholytic therapy
psychopharmacotherapy
psychosocial therapy
psychotherapy
psychotherapy by reciprocal inhibition
puppetry therapy
quadrangular therapy
radical therapy
radioactive-iodine therapy
radiotherapy
Rankian therapy = WILL THERAPY
rational psychotherapy (also called rational-emotive therapy)

recreational therapy
reeducative therapy: See REEDUCATION*
reality therapy
reconditioning therapy
reconstructive psychotherapy
regressive electroshock therapy
relationship therapy
relaxation therapy
release therapy
religious therapy
remedial therapy
replacement therapy
replication therapy
repressive-inspirational group psychotherapy
respiratory therapy (also called inhalation therapy)
restitutive therapies
restoration therapy
retroactive therapy
rhythmic sensory-bombardment therapy
Rogerian therapy: See CLIENT-CENTERED PSYCHOTHERAPY
role-divided therapy = MULTIPLE THERAPY
sector therapy
semantic therapy
sensate-focus-oriented therapy
sex therapy
shame-aversion therapy
shock therapy: See SHOCK TREATMENT*
short-term therapy (also called brief psychotherapy)
situational therapy = ENVIRONMENTAL THERAPY
social-network therapy
social therapy
sociotherapy
somatic therapy
spectator therapy
speech therapy
structural family therapy
structural therapy
structured interactional group psychotherapy
subshock therapy
suggestion therapy
supportive psychotherapy
suppressive therapy
surface therapy
therapy
third-force therapy (also called humanistic therapy)
three-cornered therapy = MULTIPLE THERAPY
time-extended therapy
total-push therapy
triadic therapy; triangular therapy = CONJOINT THERAPY
vegetotherapy = ORGONE THERAPY
will therapy (also called Rankian therapy)
work therapy
Zen therapy

177 RELATED FIELDS

This Appendix is merely a sampling of the many entry headwords that delineate the extent to which psychology and psychiatry interact with other fields of endeavor, as treated in this Dictionary.

See the INVENTORY OF ARTICLE ENTRIES for the number of entries that this Dictionary lists for many of these fields (e.g., **behavioral medicine**, 70 entries; **sexology** 320 entries; **linguistics**, 130 entries).

acoustics
adoptive studies
advertising research
advocacy research
alchemy
anthropology
anthropometry
audiology
audiometry
behavioral endocrinology
behavioral medicine
behavioral neurochemistry
behavioral sciences
behavior genetics
bioengineering
biogenetics
biomechanics
biomedical engineering
biometry
bionomics
biophysics
biotechnology
brain research
clinical psychopharmacology
clinical sociology
cognitive science
communication engineering
communications theory
communicology
community mental health
constitutional medicine
consumer education
consumerism
consumer research (market research)
content analysis
control-devices research
cosmology
counseling services
craniology
criminology
cytotechnology
demography
demonology
developmental psycholinguistics
ecological studies
ecology
ecopharmacology
educational counseling
electrophysiology
environmental esthetics
epidemiology

esthetics
ethics
ethnography (ethnology)
ethnopsychopharmacology
eugenics
euthenics
evaluation research
existential phenomenology
experimental analysis of behavior
experimental esthetics
factor analysis
feminism
genealogy
general semantics
general-systems theory
genetic engineering
genetics
genetic technology
geriatric psychopharmacology
geriatrics
grammar
graphology
health insurance
holistic medicine
human engineering
hypnosis
immunology
information theory
kinesiology
lexicology (and lexicography)
linguistics
logopedics
mathematical biology
mental hygiene
microsocial engineering
micropsychophysiology
mind control
motivation research
mythology
neuroanatomy
neurochemistry
neuroendocrinology
neuroethology
neurology
neurometrics
neuropathology
neuropharmacology
neurophysiology
neuroscience
operant conditioning
operations research
outcome research
paralinguistics: See PARALINGUISTIC FEATURES
parapsychology
parent-effectiveness training
pathophysiology
pediatric psychopharmacology
penology
pharmacogenetics
philosophy
phonetics
phonology

photobiology
photochemistry
phrenology
phylobiology
physical education
physical medicine
physical therapy (physiatrics)
physiology
physiopathology
plastic surgery
political genetics
proxemics
pseudosciences
psychiatric epidemiology
psychoacoustics
psychoanalytic anthropology
psychobiology
psychochemistry
psychodietetics
psychoendocrinology
psychohistory
psycholinguistics
psychological esthetics
psychological statistics
psychometry
psychopathology
psychopharmacology
psychophysics
psychophysiology
psychopolitics
psychosomatic medicine
psychosurgery
public-opinion poll
rehabilitation
rehabilitation medicine
rights of patients
self-help groups
semantics
semasiology (historical semantics)
semiotic movement (semiotics)
sexology
social ecology
social gerontology
social pathology
social services
social technology
sociobiology
sociogenetics
sociolinguistics
sociology
sociometry
socionomics
speech pathology
spiritualism
statistics
suicidology
thanatology
time-motion study
topology
transcendental meditation
twin studies
wheelchair sports
women's liberation movement